Your
Health
Today

This book is dedicated to our families

To my children, Ryan and Josh, and my daughters-in-law, Shannon and Jamie, who continuously reinforce that family is one of nature's most precious gifts—M.T.

To my husband, Paul, and my daughters, Lila and Sydda, who fill my life with laughter and balance—S.M.

To my wife, Jane, and my children—Daniel and Rebecca; daughter-in-law, Courtney; son-in-law, Chris; and their children, Isaac, Darby, Emily, and Cyrus—the people to whom I feel closest and who provide daily inspiration—D.R.

Your Health Today

Choices in a Changing Society

Second Edition

Michael L. Teague
University of Iowa

Sara L. C. Mackenzie
University of Washington

David M. Rosenthal
Lower East Side Harm Reduction Center

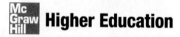

Higher Education

Published by McGraw-Hill, a business unit of The McGraw-Hill Companies, Inc., 1221 Avenue of the Americas, New York, NY 10020. Copyright © 2009 and 2007 by The McGraw-Hill Companies, Inc. All rights reserved. No part of this publication may be reproduced or distributed in any form or by any means, or stored in a database or retrieval system, without the prior written consent of The McGraw-Hill Companies, Inc., including, but not limited to, any network or other electronic storage or transmission, or broadcast for distance learning.
Some ancillaries, including electronic and print components, may not be available to customers outside the United States.

This book is printed on acid-free paper.

1 2 3 4 5 6 7 8 9 0 DOW/DOW 0 9 8

ISBN: 978-0-07-722858-3
MHID: 0-07-722858-8

Editor-in-Chief: Michael Ryan
Publisher: William R. Glass
Executive editor: Christopher Johnson
Marketing manager: William Minick
Director of development: Kathleen Engelberg
Developmental editors: Carlotta Seely,
    Kathleen Engelberg, Sarah Hill
Development editor for technology: Julia D. Akpan
Text permissions coordinator: Marty Moga
Production editor: Leslie LaDow

Manuscript editor: Amy Marks
Art editor: Robin Mouat
Designers: Jeanne Schreiber and Amanda Kavanagh
Photo research coordinator: Alexandra Ambrose
Photo researcher: Jennifer Blankenship
Production supervisor: Randy Hurst
Media project manager: Ron Nelms
Composition: 10/12 Times by Argosy
Printing: 45# Pub Matte Plus by R.R. Donnelley

The credits for this book begin on page C-1, a continuation of the copyright page.

Library of Congress Cataloging-in-Publication Data

Teague, Michael L., 1946–
    Your health today: choices in a changing society / Michael l. Teague, Sara L.C.
Mackenzie, David M. Rosenthal—2nd ed.
        p. cm.
    Includes bibliographical references and index
    ISBN-13 978-0-07-722858-3
    ISBN-10 0-07-722858-8
        1. Health education. 2. Health promotion. I. Mackenzie, Sara L.C. II.
        Rosenthal, David M. III. Title.

RA440.T43 2009
362.I–dc22

                                    2008939105

The Internet addresses listed in the text were accurate at the time of publication. The inclusion of a Web site does not indicate an endorsement by the authors or McGraw-Hill, and McGraw-Hill does not guarantee the accuracy of the information presented at these sites.

Brief Contents

Contents

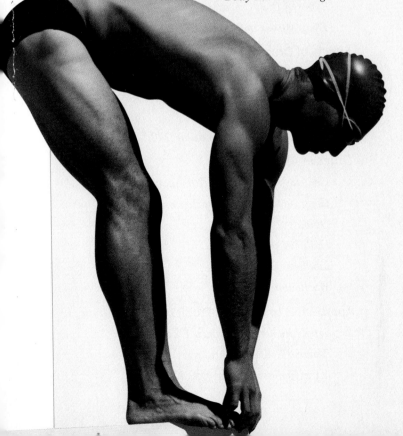

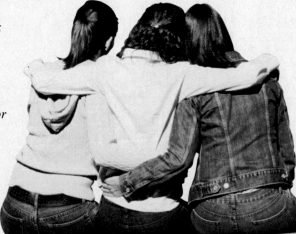

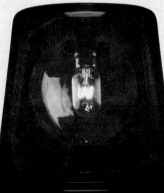

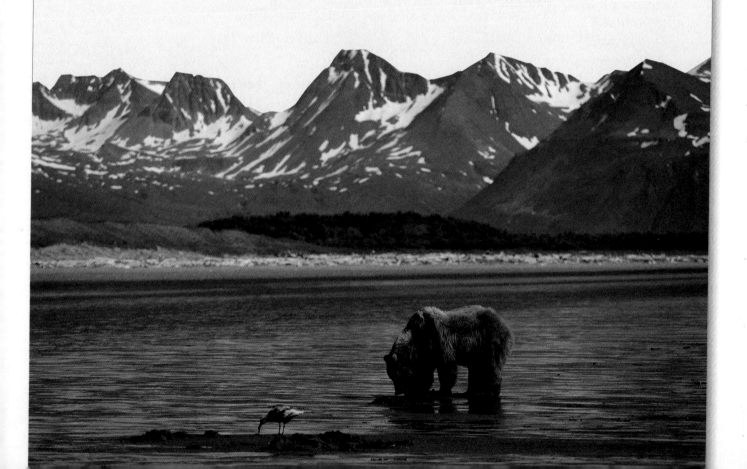

Special Features

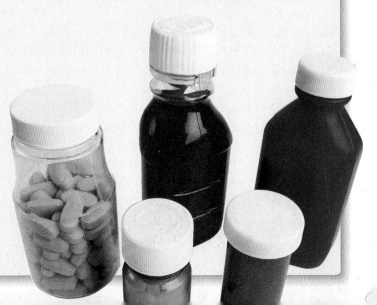

Highlight on Health

Consumer Clipboard

You Make the Call

Add It Up!

Preface

Your Health Today is the product of a collaboration among a health educator teaching at a large Midwestern university (Michael Teague), a family physician working at a large university in the Northwest (Sara Mackenzie), and a family therapist working in New York City (David Rosenthal). Each of us interacts with students in a different way, yet we all share an intense interest in student health and a commitment to student well-being. When we first began talking about this text, we found we also shared a belief that more could be done to engage students in their own health care and health-related decisions. Further, we believed that students could benefit from an expanded view of the factors that influence their health today—and of ways they can influence the health of their campuses and communities. We endorse the vision of *Healthy People 2010*—"Healthy People in Healthy Communities"—and we wanted to embed that vision in our book.

The Story Behind *Your Health Today* —Not "Just Another Health Book"

Most college personal health books focus almost exclusively on health-related lifestyle behaviors. We agree that encouraging students to take responsibility for their behaviors is a critically important goal, and we cover this aspect of health fully in our text. But if students walk away from their personal health course thinking that their health depends only on their personal choices, they are missing some important parts of the picture. Our text presents a more comprehensive view, taking into account the complex factors that play a role in our health today.

BEHAVIOR CHOICE: WHY OUR SUBTITLE IS "CHOICES IN A CHANGING SOCIETY"

Three broad threads are woven into the story of personal health throughout this text. One is lifestyle behavior choice and change. As is well known, almost half of all premature deaths in the United States are caused in part by lifestyle-related behaviors. Thus, we wanted to raise awareness among students about how their daily choices contribute to their health today—whether they are overweight or lean, out of shape or fit, depressed or engaged with life—and to their health later in life.

We provide the information students need to make healthy choices, and we support students in changing unhealthy behaviors with full coverage of behavior change strategies and skills. We also encourage students to look at the promotion of unhealthy choices in our society, as well as the uneven distribution of health resources, especially for minority populations—the societal context of choice. Thus, our subtitle—"Choices in a Changing Society."

GENETIC ENDOWMENT AND FAMILY HEALTH HISTORY: THE MISSING LINK

The second thread woven into *Your Health Today* is the role of genetic makeup in individual health and well-being. With rapidly advancing knowledge and technology in the field of genetics, students have the opportunity to understand their health in a new way. All too often, the influence of genetic inheritance on a person's health and well-being is overlooked. In including this information, we explain that a person's genes represent a blueprint for health and wellness, not a final outcome, and that genetics and behavior choice interact in a dynamic way. Our hope is that students will investigate their own family health histories and take a proactive approach in any areas in which they may be at increased risk.

We address genetic issues not just at the individual and family level but also at the group and population level. College populations today reflect the growing diversity of American society at large. Both family health history and racial, ethnic, and cultural factors contribute to students' health status and that of any children they may choose to have. We explain the prevalence of certain genetic conditions in particular racial and ethnic groups, and we describe current screening, testing, and treatment options. Our intent is to make sure students are informed about both the risks and the opportunities associated with their many layers of identity.

SOCIAL DETERMINANTS OF HEALTH: WHY PERSONAL HEALTH IS "NOT JUST PERSONAL"

The third thread woven in our text is the influence of broader factors in the social environment, such as a person's socioeconomic status, community resources, and access to health care. These social determinants of health, along with environmental conditions like air quality and climate, are receiving increasing attention today as critical factors in the opportunities any individual or group has for a healthy life. We want students to understand that, as important as behavior choice and genetic makeup are in personal health, they are not the whole story. It also matters whether the corner store sells fresh produce or liquor, whether neighborhood streets have bike lanes or are dominated by highway overpasses, and whether there's a nearby clinic that offers prenatal care and HPV vaccinations.

We challenge students to grapple with the complexities of personal health in the context of social, economic, and political conditions in a rapidly changing and multicultural society. We also encourage students to participate in their communities and to contribute to the creation of healthy environments, whether by advocating for smoke-free environments, joining in "safe spring break" campaigns, or getting involved in the "greening" of their campus. To us, this is the true meaning of "healthy people in healthy communities."

What Else Is *Your Health Today* About?

Of course, there's more to our text that this broad framework. We have many more specific goals, and we've developed a variety of features to address them.

THE SCOOP ON HEALTH: CURRENT, RELIABLE INFORMATION

To make wise health choices, students need the basics—accurate, up-to-date information on topics and issues relevant to their lives. The second edition of *Your Health Today* has been thoroughly updated throughout, with topics of special interest addressed in "Highlight on Health" boxes in every chapter. Some current topics covered are overweight and obesity, diabetes and metabolic syndrome, prescription drug abuse, the latest American College of Sports Medicine and American Heart Association physical activity guidelines, and climate change and the actions students can take to reduce their ecological footprints.

BEHAVIOR CHANGE: WHAT IT TAKES

Changing an entrenched health behavior is difficult, whether it's quitting smoking, reducing stress, achieving a healthy weight, improving sleep habits, communicating more effectively, or choosing a heart-healthy diet. We discuss behavior change in Chapter 1 and offer strategies, skills, tips, and behavior change plans throughout the text and in "Challenges & Choices" boxes in every chapter.

HEALTH LITERACY: DECONSTRUCTING MEDIA MESSAGES

Preparing students to be informed consumers of health information, health care services, and health-related messages in the media is a key function of a college personal health course. We discuss the basics of health literacy in Chapter 1 and address a wide range of consumer issues in "Consumer Clipboard" boxes in every chapter. A few topics: Choosing sunscreen, tap water versus bottled water, understanding media messages about body size and shape, buying running shoes, reducing antibiotic resistance, and preventing identity theft.

CURRENT ISSUES: WEIGHING THE PROS AND CONS

Life in the 21st century presents us with complex and difficult issues, including those that arise when technological advances outpace our ethics and values. By discussing controversies throughout the text and in the "You Make the Call" feature at the end of every chapter, we encourage students to consider issues in depth and develop their critical thinking skills. Issues include egg and sperm donation, embryonic stem cell research, gene therapy, the right to die, violence in the media, college vaccination requirements, public smoking restrictions, and many more.

EMBRACING DIVERSITY AND CONFRONTING DISPARITIES

As our society becomes more diverse, national attention focuses on disparities in health status across different segments of the population, including racial and ethnic groups, younger and older adults, males and females, and residents of urban versus rural settings. We consider diversity-related health issues as well as health disparities both in the text narrative and in "Who's at Risk" boxes in every chapter, new to the second edition.

TAKING HEALTH TO THE NEXT LEVEL: THE COMMUNITY AND PUBLIC HEALTH PERSPECTIVES

In line with our emphasis on the social determinants of health, we explore the role of community, society, social structures, and government at all levels in personal and public health. This perspective is included in the text and highlighted in "Public Health in Action" boxes in every chapter, new to the second edition.

BEYOND THE USUAL CONTENT: SPECIAL TOPICS THAT STUDENTS WANT TO KNOW ABOUT

We believe that certain important topics have been generally overlooked in the personal health course, and we have included coverage of the following:

- **Spirituality** Spiritual wellness is increasingly recognized as a vital part of overall wellness. In Chapter 4,

Spirituality, we discuss the many ways that humans fulfill their longing for meaning and purpose, and we offer a variety of suggestions for building a spiritual life.

- **Sleep** Sleep is such a vital part of wellness that we often simply take it for granted—until it eludes us. In Chapter 6, Sleep, we explain why adequate, high-quality sleep is critical to good health, how sleep deprivation—so common among college students—affects performance and well-being, and how to establish good sleep habits.

- **Body Image** Although national attention is currently focused on overweight and obesity, eating disorders and body image issues remain a challenge for many women and men in our society, especially adolescents and young adults. Chapter 10, Body Image, includes discussion of cultural and media messages about beauty, signs and symptoms of eating and exercise disorders, and awareness and prevention of body image problems.

- **Family Health History** As noted earlier, a person's genetic endowment, especially as evidenced through family health history, is an important component of health. In Chapter 2, Your Family Health History, we discuss the role of genes in health, personality, and behavior, the relationship between ethnicity and certain genetic disorders, the circumstances in which genetic counseling and testing are appropriate, and the social and ethical implications of genetic research.

THE TEACHING CHALLENGE: GETTING STUDENTS ENGAGED

We know students lead busy lives filled with entertaining distractions. We've designed this book to engage them and help them make the best use of their time:

- Every topic suggests questions we've all wondered about. In this text we've sought to tap into that curiosity by opening every chapter with a few short questions labeled "Ever Wonder...?"—

  - Ever wonder if sexual orientation could be genetic?

  - Ever wonder if sleeping in on weekends makes up for the sleep you lost during the week?

  - Ever wonder what your chances of getting pregnant are if you are sexually active and don't use any form of contraception?

  - Ever wonder if there's any risk in getting a tattoo or piercing?

- Similarly, every group of related topics suggests broader questions for reflection, and we've posed some of these on Part-opening pages under the heading "Think It Over"—

  - Are you working to prevent stress, or are you reacting to it?

  - Where does physical fitness fall in your list of priorities?

  - What does being sexually responsible mean to you?

  - If all drugs were legal, would the drug problem be solved?

- For every chapter, we've focused more on the student population and the relevance of these topics to students' lives. For example, we discuss campaigns to reduce the stigma of mental illness on campus, improvements in campus communication systems since the shootings at Virginia Tech, college efforts to curb binge drinking and provide interventions for at-risk drinkers, the top infectious diseases on campus, and efforts by schools and universities to be environmentally responsible.

- Students want to know how they measure up, and the "Add It Up!" feature gives them a chance to assess themselves in relation to each chapter topic—

  - Are You at Risk for Drug Dependence?

  - Do You Worry Too Much About Your Appearance?

  - What Is Your Risk for Coronary Heart Disease?

  - Are You an Aggressive Driver?

  - Is Your Lifestyle Environmentally Friendly?

- In our visual culture, people respond to bright, attention-grabbing images. Our book team has come up with a bold, visually exciting design to engage students and help them learn, and we've doubled or tripled the number of illustrations and photos in each chapter.

  - We've also streamlined the narrative text in each chapter, chunking and bulleting information for better learning and retention and easier review. Key terms are called out in bold type and defined in the margins next to the text where they occur.

  - To further support learning, we've ended each chapter with a concise summary called "In Review." Students can also access detailed chapter summaries and review questions on the Online Learning Center, the Web site that accompanies the book.

- When it comes to researching topics for assignments, students turn to the Internet. We include a short selection of highly reliable Web sites at the end of each chapter under the heading "Web Resources"—sites like the Centers for Disease Control (CDC), the National Mental Health Association, Planned Parenthood, and Alcoholics Anonymous.

DIGITAL SOLUTIONS FOR A DIGITAL AGE

We also know that students learn differently today and are used to getting information via current technology. This text is accompanied by *Connect Personal Health,* a Web-based assignment and assessment platform with benefits for both students and instructors. *Connect Personal Health* is described in more detail in the Teaching Tools section of the Preface. Students can also access a wide range of electronic study aids on the Online Learning Center.

YOU *CAN* TELL A BOOK BY ITS COVER

The covers of most health books depict vibrant-looking young people engaged in healthy activities. Although we heartily endorse such activities, we wanted our cover to convey more about the message of our book—"Choices in a Changing Society." In keeping with the cover of the first edition of *Your Health Today,* our cover illustrates the range of choices, healthy and unhealthy, available to people in our society today—as well as some of the diversity of our population.

Organization and Content: 23 Chapters to Better Health

Your Health Today is organized to support these themes and goals. We begin with an introductory chapter that presents foundational ideas, including the concepts of health and wellness, behavior change, health literacy, and health in a diverse society. The next five chapters, grouped together in Part 1 under the title Your Mind and Body, consider how people can cultivate optimal mental, physical, and spiritual health. The chapters in this part address both the genetic basis of health (Chapter 2, Your Family Health History) and some of the intangibles that contribute to wellness, such as an optimistic attitude (Chapter 3, Mental Health), a sense of meaning and purpose (Chapter 4, Spirituality), a balance between challenge and relaxation (Chapter 5, Stress), and time for rest and renewal (Chapter 6, Sleep).

Part 2, Your Lifestyle and Health, highlights the connection between lifestyle choices and health. The chapters in this part explore how everyday choices about food (Chapter 7, Nutrition) and physical activity (Chapter 8, Fitness) affect both current and long-term health and wellness. Chapters on managing weight (Chapter 9, Body Weight and Body Composition) and managing *ideas* about weight (Chapter 10, Body Image) add relevant concepts to this picture of lifestyle choice.

Part 3, Your Health at Risk, addresses individual choices that may put personal health at risk. Chapter 11 (Alcohol) examines issues such as college binge drinking, drinking and

driving, and the influence of culture and society on attitudes toward alcohol consumption. Chapter 12 (Drugs) explores current trends in drug use, the effects of drug abuse, and approaches to the drug problem. Chapter 13 (Tobacco) looks at smoking as both an individual and a societal health issue.

Part 4, Your Relationships and Sexuality, focuses on the interpersonal, social, and sexual aspects of health and wellness. Chapter 14 (Relationships) looks at the qualities that make relationships healthy, whether friendships, partnerships, or family relationships. Chapter 15 (Sexual Health) looks at the role of sexuality in relationships and in our society. Chapter 16 (Reproductive Choices) addresses contraception, pregnancy, and childbirth and considers how we can ensure healthy families.

In Part 5, Protecting Your Health, we turn our attention to disease prevention. We consider how individuals can protect themselves from everything from the common cold to sexually transmitted diseases (Chapter 17, Infectious Diseases) and from heart disease (Chapter 18, Cardiovascular Disease) to cancer (Chapter 19). We also consider health care options of all kinds (Chapter 20, Complementary and Alternative Medicine).

Finally, Part 6, Challenges to Your Health, highlights forces that affect the well-being of individuals, communities, society, and the world. We consider the threat of violence (Chapter 21), the effects of unintentional injury (Chapter 22), and the increasingly critical impact of human activities on the health of the planet (Chapter 23). In each chapter, we emphasize steps that individuals can take to avoid or prepare for these challenges, reduce their impact, and contribute to a healthier world.

What's New in the Second Edition of *Your Health Today?*

We've made substantial revisions to the second edition of *Your Health Today,* in content, features, and design. We've focused much more on the college population and the relevance of health topics to their lives. In many chapters, the text narrative and features have been streamlined to present concepts more clearly and concisely. At the same time, many new topics and issues have been added to ensure that the text is current and relevant to students. Every chapter includes new, expanded, or updated information on a wide range of topics. For a complete, chapter-by-chapter description of content changes in the second edition, visit the Online Learning Center at www.mhhe.com/teague2e.

NEW BOXES: REFLECTING TODAY'S HEALTH SCENE

Two new types of boxes have been added in this edition:

■ "Who's At Risk" boxes inform students about variations in health risks—ranging from risk for obesity to risk for unintended pregnancy—for different groups and population segments, based on current data and statistics from the CDC, the AHA, and other reliable organizations.

Information is presented in a variety of formats, including tables, graphs, maps, lists, and narratives, to accommodate different learning styles. A few "Who's At Risk" topics:

- Variations in Leading Causes of Death Among Americans
- Obesity Trends Among Adults in the United States
- College Students and Binge Drinking
- Cancer Incidence and Mortality by Race and Ethnicity
- Global Climate Change and Health

- "Public Health in Action" boxes highlight activities designed to target health issues at the population level, such as public service announcements like the "Brain on Drugs" ad and the "What a Difference a Friend Makes" campaign to reduce the stigma of mental illness. Inclusion of the public health perspective helps students see the big picture of health and health care in our society today. A few "Public Health in Action" topics:
  - Love Your Body Day
  - Recognizing and Treating PTSD
  - Globalization of the Western Diet
  - Campus Fire Safety
  - The Greening of College Campuses

A complete list of all the boxed features in the second edition follows the Table of Contents.

A NEW LOOK

The look of the second edition has been completely updated for today's students. Colors, images, and design elements have been chosen to give *Your Health Today* a contemporary appeal, and many new, current photos have been included to help students see the connection between health topics and their own lives.

Teaching Tools and Resources: A Complete Package for Instructors

ONLINE LEARNING CENTER
WWW.MHHE.COM/TEAGUE2E

The Online Learning Center includes a variety of resources to help you teach your course:

- The *Course Integrator Guide* includes lecture outlines, suggested activities, media resources, and Web links. It also describes the print and electronic supplements available with the text and shows how to integrate them into lectures and assignments for each chapter.

- The *Test Bank* includes multiple choice, true-false, short answer, and matching. It is available as a set of Word files and as a Computerized Test Bank with EZ Test computerized testing software. EZ Test provides a powerful, easy-to-use way to create printed quizzes and exams; it runs on both Windows and Macintosh systems. For secure online testing, exams created in EZ Test can be exported to WebCT, Blackboard, and EZ Test Online. EZ Test is packaged with a Quick Start Guide. Once the program is installed, you have access to the complete User's Manual, including Flash tutorials. Additional help is available at www.mhhe.com/eztest.

- A comprehensive set of **PowerPoint slides** provides a lecture tool you can use as is or expand to meet the needs of your course. The slides correspond to chapter content and cover key lecture points and images from the text and outside sources. For more classroom options, a complete **Image Bank** of illustrations from the text is also included on the Online Learning Center.

INSTRUCTOR'S VIDEO DVD-ROM

The videos included in this collection are designed to help you engage students in class discussions and promote critical thinking about personal health topics. The library contains student interviews and historical health videos on body image, depression, stress, genetics, spirituality, and many other topics. For each video clip, an Instructor's Guide is available to describe the objective of the clip, provide critical thinking questions to ask before the video is shown, and suggest follow-up discussion questions.

CLASSROOM PERFORMANCE SYSTEM

Classroom Performance System (CPS) brings interactivity into the classroom or lecture hall. It is a wireless response system that gives instructors and students immediate feedback from the entire class. The wireless response pads are essentially remotes that are easy to use and engage students. CPS is available for both Microsoft Windows and Macintosh computers. Suggested polling questions are included on the Online Learning Center.

PRIMIS ONLINE
WWW.MHHE.COM/PRIMIS/ONLINE

Primis Online is a database-driven publishing system that allows instructors to create content-rich textbooks, lab manuals, or readers for their courses directly from the Primis Web site. The customized text can be delivered in print or electronic (eBook) form. A Primis eBook is a digital version of the customized text sold directly to students as a file downloadable to their computers or accessed online by a password. *Your Health Today* can be customized using Primis Online.

Student Resources Available With *Your Health Today*

ONLINE LEARNING CENTER
WWW.MHHE.COM/TEAGUE2E

For students, the Online Learning Center offers learning and study tools that will help them get the most out of their course. Included are:

- Self-scoring chapter quizzes

- Flashcards and crossword puzzles (for learning key terms and definitions)

- Internet activities

- Web links

- Detailed chapter summaries

- Comprehensive sets of chapter review questions

DAILY FITNESS AND NUTRITION JOURNAL (ISBN 0-07-332567-8)

This logbook helps students track their diet and exercise programs. It can be packaged with any McGraw-Hill textbook for a small additional fee.

NUTRITIONCALC PLUS (ISBN 0-07-332865-0)

NutritionCalc Plus 3.0 is a suite of dietary self-assessment tools with an easy-to-use interface. It allows users to track their nutrient and food group intakes, energy expenditures, and weight control goals, and it generates a variety of reports and graphs for analysis, including comparisons with the Dietary Reference Intakes. The ESHA database includes thousands of ethnic foods, supplements, fast foods, and convenience foods. Users can also add foods to the database. NutritionCalc Plus is available on CD-ROM or in an Internet version. For more information, visit http://nutritioncalc.mhhe.com.

WELLNESS WORKSHEETS (ISBN 0-07-328253-7)

This collection of 120 assessments allows students to evaluate their health behaviors, attitudes, and knowledge and to implement successful behavior change. Topic areas include wellness and behavior change, stress management, psychological and spiritual wellness, intimate relationships and communication, sexuality, addictive behaviors and drug dependence, nutrition, physical activity and exercise, weight management, and consumer health. The worksheets are available online or packaged with the text.

A Note of Thanks

Many instructors and health experts reviewed the first edition of *Your Health Today*, and many others participated in symposia and focus groups. Their suggestions, knowledge, and insights have been invaluable in helping us develop the second edition. Please refer to the inside back cover of the text for a full listing of their names and academic affiliations.

We also want to thank the *Your Health Today* book team at McGraw-Hill for their contributions to this edition: Carlotta Seely, Kate Engelberg, and Sarah Hill, Developmental Editors; Joseph Diggins, Sponsoring Editor; Bill Minick, Marketing Manager; Christopher Johnson, Executive Editor; William Glass, Editorial Director; Leslie LaDow, Production Editor; Jeanne Schreiber and Amanda Kavanagh, Designers; Robin Mouat, Art Editor; Alex Ambrose and Jennifer Blankenship, Photo Researchers; Randy Hurst, Production Supervisor; Marty Moga, Text Permissions Coordinator; Amy Marks, Copy Editor; and Laura Iwasaki, Proofreader.

Michael Teague
Sara Mackenzie
David Rosenthal

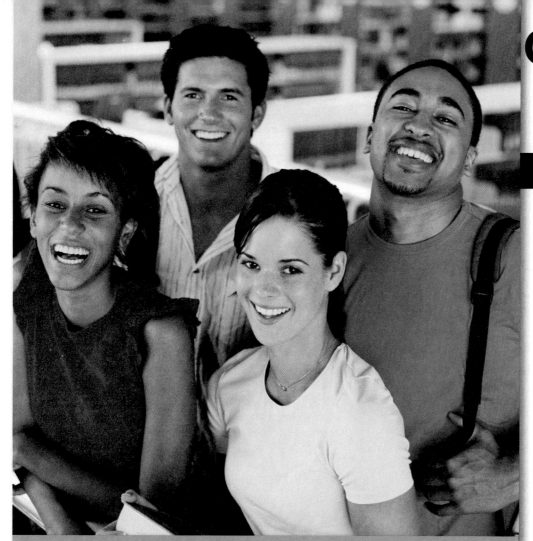

Ever Wonder...

- when ethnic minorities will make up more than half of the U.S. population?

- why health advice always seems to be changing?

- if your children's life expectancy will be longer or shorter than yours?

WWW

Your Health Today

www.mhhe.com/teague2e

Go to the Online Learning Center for *Your Health Today* for interactive activities, quizzes, flashcards, Web links, and more resources related to this chapter.

As individuals, we are all responsible for our own health. It's up to each of us to choose a healthy lifestyle—to be physically active, to eat a healthy diet, to get enough sleep, to make sure we see a doctor when we need to. Yet we do not live in a social vacuum. Our actions and choices are influenced by our environment—our families and friends, the community around us, and the larger society and culture in which we live. We are better able to make healthy choices when our environment supports those choices.

In this book we explore personal health in the context of the social and cultural environment. In addition to those personal actions we take as individuals to ensure our own health, this book also considers the social, economic, and environmental conditions under which people live. By taking all these factors into account, along with the biological and genetic endowment each person is born with, we hope to present a more complete picture of personal health than is given when individual behavior alone is considered.

Personal Health in Context

In this section we consider the meaning of the terms *health* and *wellness*, and we explore the factors that shape and influence our personal health.

HEALTH AND WELLNESS

Traditionally, people were considered "healthy" if they did not have symptoms of disease. In 1947 the World Health Organization (WHO) broke new ground by defining **health** as a state of complete physical, mental, and social well-being, not merely the absence of disease and infirmity. Physical health referred to the biological integrity of the individual. Mental health included emotional and intellectual capabilities, or the individual's subjective sense of well-being. Social health meant the ability of people to interact effectively with other people and the social environment.[1]

health
State of complete physical, mental, social, and spiritual well-being.

wellness
Process of adopting patterns of behavior that can lead to improved health and heightened life satisfaction; wellness has several domains and can be conceptualized as a continuum.

More recently, a spiritual domain has been added to the WHO definition, reflecting the idea that people's value systems or beliefs can have an impact on their overall health. Spiritual health does not require participation in a particular organized religion but suggests a belief in (or a searching for) some type of greater or higher power that gives meaning and purpose to life. Spiritual health involves a connectedness to self, to significant others, and to the community.

Wellness is a slightly different concept. It is generally defined as the process of adopting patterns of behavior that can lead to improved health and heightened life satisfaction. Like health, wellness is seen as encompassing several dimensions: physical, emotional, intellectual, spiritual, interpersonal or social, and environmental. Some definitions also include occupational health as one of the dimensions of wellness. These dimensions of wellness can be represented as a wheel (Figure 1.1).

Wellness may also be conceptualized as a continuum (Figure 1.2). One end of the continuum represents extreme illness and premature death; the other end represents wellness and optimal health. Historically, Western medicine has focused primarily on the illness side of the continuum, treating people with symptoms of disease. When an individual reaches the midpoint of the continuum, representing a state in which no symptoms of disease are present, traditional Western medicine has few tools to help this individual reach a state of wellness, or optimal well-being. More recently, approaches to health have focused on the wellness side of the continuum, seeking ways to help people live their lives fully, as whole people, with vitality and meaning.[2]

Although most people want to have good health, it typically is not an ultimate goal in and of itself. Usually, people desire good health in order to reach other goals—to be more productive, more attractive, more comfortable, more independent—in other words, to have a higher quality of life. In this sense, wellness and an optimal quality of life can be seen as an ultimate goal, with good health a means to attain it.[3]

HEALTH-RELATED BEHAVIOR CHOICES

How do you achieve good health and optimal wellness? A key role is played by your health-related behavior choices (or lifestyle choices)—those actions you take and decisions you make that affect your own individual health (and, possibly, the health of your immediate family members). They include choices concerning your physical, mental, emotional, spiritual, and social well-being—what you eat, how much exercise you get, whether you spend time developing

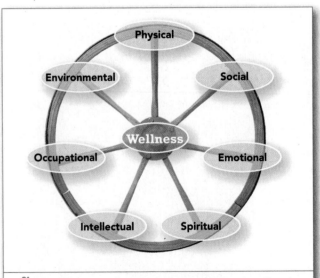

figure **1.1**   **Dimensions of health and wellness.**
Sources: Adapted from The World Health Report 2006: Working Together for Health, *by World Health Organization, 2006, Geneva, Switzerland;* Wellness Index: A Self-Assessment for Health and Vitality, *by J.W. Travis and S.R. Ryan, 2004, Berkeley, CA: Ten Speed Press (Celestial Arts).*

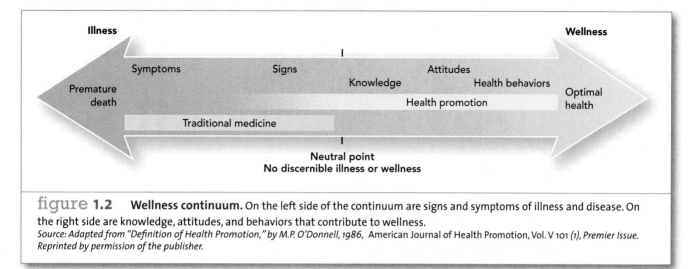

Illness   **Wellness**

Symptoms Signs Attitudes

Premature death Knowledge Health behaviors Optimal health

Health promotion

Traditional medicine

Neutral point
No discernible illness or wellness

figure 1.2 **Wellness continuum.** On the left side of the continuum are signs and symptoms of illness and disease. On the right side are knowledge, attitudes, and behaviors that contribute to wellness.
Source: Adapted from "Definition of Health Promotion," by M.P. O'Donnell, 1986, American Journal of Health Promotion, Vol. V 101 *(1), Premier Issue. Reprinted by permission of the publisher.*

meaningful relationships, and so on. For example, having an apple instead of a bag of chips is a healthy behavior choice, as is quitting smoking. Other examples are getting enough sleep, practicing safe sex, wearing a safety belt in a car, finding effective ways to manage stress, drinking alcohol in moderation if at all, and getting regular health checkups.

In the United States the focus on lifestyle behavior choices emerged in health education and policy in the second half of the 20th century. As infectious diseases were increasingly brought under control, a new pattern of disease became apparent: Chronic, degenerative illnesses such as cardiovascular disease, stroke, and cancer began to emerge as the leading causes of death. Health experts began to look not just at the listed causes of death (heart attack, for example) but at the "actual causes" or underlying factors in those deaths (such as obesity). Health experts shifted their attention to behavioral factors; they began to focus on preventing degenerative conditions by encouraging people to adopt healthier behaviors early in life and to take personal responsibility for their health.

It is in the realm of lifestyle choice that individuals have the most control over their health, and lifestyle choice is also the primary focus of much of *Your Health Today*. To make good health decisions, people need information, consumer skills, and strategies to transform unhealthy behaviors into healthy ones—all of which are provided by this text. As noted earlier, however, there is more to personal health than lifestyle choices, and we consider these aspects of health in more detail in the next section and throughout this text.

SOCIAL DETERMINANTS OF HEALTH

Health experts are concerned not just with individual behavior choice but also with what are known as the **social determinants of health**—the economic, social, cultural, and physical conditions that contribute to or detract from the health of individuals and communities.[4] These determinants include such factors as income and socioeconomic status, educational attainment and literacy, employment

social determinants of health
Societal conditions that affect health and can potentially be altered by social and health policies and programs.

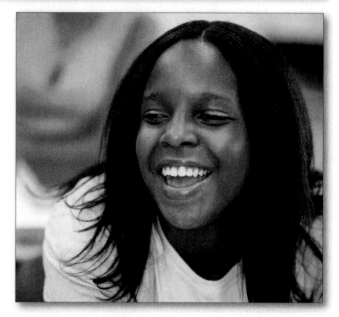

■ Qualities associated with wellness include self-confidence, optimism, a sense of humor, an active mind, vitality, and joy in life, among many others.

status and working conditions, housing and transportation, social support networks, and available health care services.[5] Also included are aspects of the physical environment, such as water and air quality, weather, and climate (Figure 1.3). Thus our personal health is affected by our living conditions—where we live, what our housing is like, what we do for a living, who our friends and peers are, what kind of health insurance we have (or don't have), and a host of other factors beyond the individual choices we make.

A model that addresses all the determinants of health is the *ecological view of health and wellness*. This model focuses on the complex interactions among individual behaviors; environmental factors; and genetic, or hereditary, factors. (The term *ecology* refers to all the patterns of inter-relationship between individuals and their environments.) According to the ecological view (Figure 1.4), health and wellness are determined by the following factors:

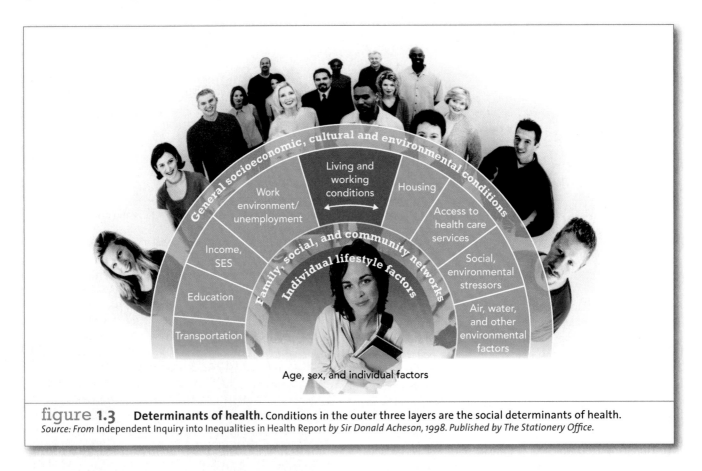

Age, sex, and individual factors

figure 1.3   **Determinants of health.** Conditions in the outer three layers are the social determinants of health.
Source: From Independent Inquiry into Inequalities in Health Report *by Sir Donald Acheson, 1998. Published by The Stationery Office.*

■ *Genetic factors* are the person's inherited genetic capabilities, limitations, and predispositions. (In this text, we discuss this aspect of health in Chapter 2). Although some diseases and health conditions are caused by a single gene, more often diseases with a genetic component are caused by the interaction of genes and the environment. The nature of this interaction depends largely on the behavior of the individual and his or her exposure to environmental risks.[6]

■ *Behavioral factors* are the patterns of behavior and health practices that protect a person or put him or her at risk. These are the individual health-related behavior choices the person makes, like exercising, eating a healthy diet, or smoking.[5]

■ *Environmental factors,* or social determinants of health, are factors external to the individual that can be modified to support or detract from health. They include factors in both the social environment and the physical environment. For example, in the social environment, health is influenced by the nature of social relationships in a school, neighborhood, or workplace, which in turn are shaped by values, norms, organizational support, peer support, and formal and informal social policies and structures. In the *built* physical environment, health is influenced by the kinds of housing, schools, streets, and sanitation systems that have been constructed. In the *natural* physical environment, health is influenced by air and water quality.[5]

Note that in the ecological model, the arrows indicating influence between genetics and behavior and between behavior and environment go both ways—all these determinants have reciprocal relationships with each other.

Both in the United States and worldwide, worse health outcomes are associated with poorer living conditions—with poverty; unemployment; poor housing; low educational attainment; environmental pollution; and other negative social, economic, and physical factors. Addressing these inequities is one of the goals of national and international health policies; this topic is discussed in more detail later in the chapter.

COMMUNITY HEALTH

Because of the complexity of the relationships among all the determinants of health, responsibilities for health and wellness extend beyond the individual. Issues, events, and activities related to the health of a whole community or population fall into the realms of community health and public health. **Community health** refers to activities directed toward bettering the health of the public or activities employing resources available in common to members of the community.[7] For example, a community may decide to create bike lanes on public streets to protect cyclists, encourage

community health
Issues, events, and activities related to the health of a whole community, as well as activities directed toward bettering the health of the public and/or activities employing resources available in common to members of the community.

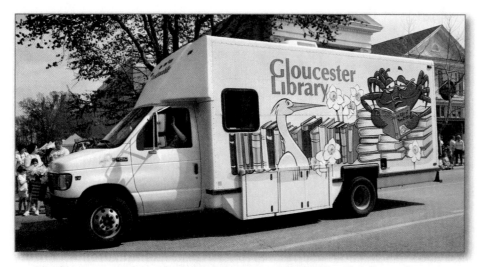

■ A healthy community provides services that support the health and wellness of community members. A bookmobile, like this one in Gloucester, Virginia, not only improves access to books but promotes values like reading and community participation.

people to be more physically active, and cut down on traffic and air pollution. A community may support the creation of a health clinic within its boundaries, or it may require builders to include green space or parks in their construction plans.

Such community actions interact with individual behaviors to promote or detract from a person's health. For example, consider the community that provides bike lanes on public streets. A person living in this community may be more likely to ride a bike to work than someone who lives in a community dominated by dangerous, traffic-clogged streets or highways. The cyclist experiences health benefits (a higher level of cardiorespiratory fitness, better weight management, better mental health) from increased physical activity that are not available to the person living in the community without bike lanes. Even though riding a bike to work is a lifestyle choice, it is a choice encouraged or dis-

couraged by the social and physical environment.

Similarly, a community may be able to prevent a toxic waste dump from being located within its boundaries through grassroots activism and political lobbying. Another community, with a lower level of political influence or socioeconomic power, may not be able to protect itself from such environmental hazards. A person living near a toxic dump, in a community with high levels of pollution, or in a dangerous neighborhood is not going to have the opportunity to attain the same level of wellness as someone living in a safer, healthier environment, no matter what lifestyle decisions the person makes.

The idea of community health extends beyond the traditional relationship between an individual and a health care professional to involve a host of agencies, organizations, and institutions working to promote people's health. Health promotion programs can be implemented in communities through a range of settings (home, school, worksite, health care facilities), by a variety of techniques (health education, environmental controls, health programs), and under the auspices of an array of sponsors (business, labor unions, volunteer agencies, hospitals, public schools, self-care groups).[8]

PUBLIC HEALTH

This concept of community health is formalized in the field of **public health**, which is the study and practice of health promotion and disease prevention at the population level.[9] Public health is both a branch of medicine and a focus of

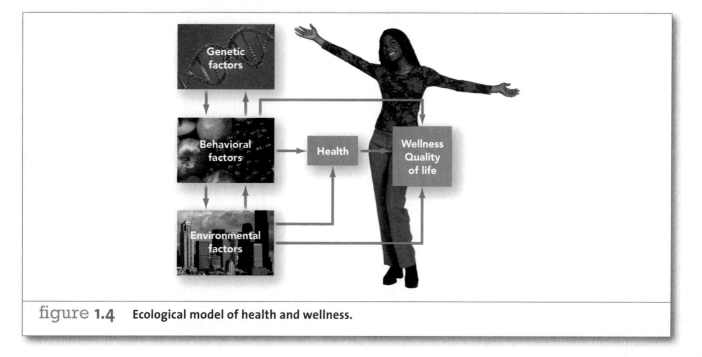

figure **1.4** **Ecological model of health and wellness.**

government action. In the United States the Public Health Service, led by the surgeon general, and the Centers for Disease Control and Prevention in Atlanta, Georgia, are responsible for public health nationwide. State, county, and city health departments are involved in public health measures at the state and local levels.

Some of the functions and activities of the public health system include preventing epidemics and the spread of infectious diseases, promoting healthy behaviors, preventing injuries, protecting against environmental hazards, responding to disasters and helping communities recover from them, and ensuring the accessibility and quality of health services. As noted above, the two broad goals of public health are disease prevention and health promotion. Whereas **disease prevention** focuses on defensive actions taken to ward off specific diseases and their consequences (such as administering flu shots to older adults), **health promotion** focuses on actions designed to maintain a current health state or advance to a more desirable state (such as publicizing cancer screening guidelines). Examples of public health measures include vaccination programs; educational campaigns about HIV/AIDS, smoking, or methamphetamine use; and laws and policies related to everything from fluoridation of water to food handling in restaurants. The key is the focus on the health of entire populations rather than of individuals. (See the box "Public Service Announcements.")

In previous eras, major public health efforts were aimed at such measures as purifying drinking water, improving sanitation systems, promoting food refrigeration and pasteurization, and increasing public awareness of the importance of hygienic practices. In the 19th and early 20th centuries, these efforts were largely responsible for the control of infectious diseases, the leading killers of the day. Today, public health concerns range from HIV/AIDS to childhood overweight to natural disasters like Hurricane Katrina. Increased attention is also being paid to the social determinants of health, mentioned earlier in the chapter, such as poverty, inequality, and low educational attainment. Public health experts are interested in addressing disparities in health among different segments of the population and promoting policies that improve the health of the whole population in an equitable way.

public health
The study and practice of health promotion and disease prevention at the population level.

disease prevention
Public-health-related actions designed to ward off or protect against specific diseases.

health promotion
Public-health-related actions designed to maintain a current healthy state or advance to a more desirable state.

Health in a Multicultural Society

As a nation of immigrants, the United States has always had a diverse population. As the 21st century unfolds, the U.S. population is rapidly becoming more diverse. According to the 2000 U.S. Census, approximately 30 percent of the pop-

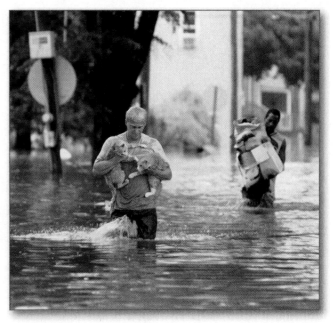

■ Heavy rains and floods forced the evacuation of communities throughout the Midwest in June 2008. Extreme weather, natural disasters, and other events that affect whole populations fall into the domain of public health.

ulation currently belongs to a racial or ethnic minority group.[10] This percentage is expected to increase to 50 percent by 2050. The primary minority groups in the United States, again according the U.S. Census Bureau, are African Americans (or Black Americans), Hispanic Americans, Native Americans, Asian Americans, and Pacific Islanders.[11] There is tremendous diversity within each of these groups as well: Asian Americans, for example, include people from China, Japan, Korea, Vietnam, Laos, Cambodia, the Philippines, and other countries. (Note that diversity also refers to differences among people in gender, age, sexual orientation, ability or disability, educational attainment, socioeconomic status, geographic location, and other characteristics.)

UNDERSTANDING CULTURAL TERMS

There are many different meanings of the term *culture*, but here the term is used in a sense articulated for a health promotion context.[12] According to this view, a **culture** is defined by five basic criteria: (1) a common language or common patterns of communication; (2) similarities in dietary practices; (3) common patterns of dress; (4) predictable socialization and relationship patterns; and (5) a common set of shared values and beliefs. As you can see in this definition, cultures help clarify acceptable and unacceptable behaviors, including health-related behaviors, in any given society.

culture
A group's shared, distinctive pattern of living, defined by a common language, similarities in dietary practices, common patterns of dress, predictable socialization and relationship patterns, and a common set of shared values and beliefs. (Note that many other definitions of culture exist.)

Public Health in Action

Public Service Announcements

"This is your brain. This is your brain on drugs. Any questions?"

This antidrug public service announcement (PSA), developed by the Partnership for a Drug-Free America, became one of the most widely viewed and best-known public health messages ever shown on television. First appearing in 1987, it has been frequently quoted, referenced, reenacted, and parodied on T-shirts, posters, and television shows, including *Roseanne, Beverly Hills 90210,* and *Saturday Night Live.* The message can now be viewed in the Museum of Broadcast Communications and the Smithsonian Institution. An interesting side note is that in the original ad, the lines were, "This is your brain. This is drugs. This is your brain on drugs. Any questions?" Popular memory has dropped the line, "This is drugs."

PSAs have become the medium for many health communication strategies that appear on radio, television, the Internet, and wirelesss communication systems as well as local print media like billboards. Targets of PSAs have ranged from smoking ("Tell No More Lies") to childhood obesity ("Don't Take It Lightly") to drug use ("Crystal Mess") to safety belts ("Click It or Ticket"). No matter what the topic, the objectives of PSAs are to increase awareness and knowledge, influence attitudes, and change behaviors.

With the growing diversity in our society, as well as growing disparities across diverse populations within our society, health officials are looking to PSAs as an increasingly important intervention for improving the health of the American people. Although broad messages that are relevant across most populations (like the "brain on drugs" ad) are believed to be effective, health officials are recommending more targeted ads that speak to specific populations. An analysis of 18 large-scale public health campaigns by the Institute of Medicine (a nonprofit advising organization under the National Academy of Sciences) found that mass health communication campaigns were more effective if they were designed to take into account multiple dimensions of their audience. These dimensions include economic context; community resources (including access to health services); and commonly held attitudes, norms, and self-efficacy beliefs.

More specifically, the Institute of Medicine analysis emphasized the importance of understanding the sociocultural contexts that shape behavior, including the belief systems, religious and cultural values, and group identity that serve as filters for information. The Institute's report recommended that members of targeted communities be included in decision making about public health campaigns. It also recommended that older media, such as print publications and the telephone, continue to be used to reach audiences that may not have the latest technology, while new technologies are used where access can be assumed. The report noted that without action, new computer technologies may exacerbate inequities in health care rather than reduce them.

For all their apparent simplicity, PSAs are not easily crafted. They require a multidisciplinary approach that relies on knowledge from many different fields: mass communication, behavior change theory, health communication theory, medicine, health care, marketing, technology, and social psychology. To these can now be added a deep understanding of the social and cultural circumstances of their target audiences.

Source: Speaking of Health: Assessing Health Communication Strategies for Diverse Populations, *Institute of Medicine, 2007, Washington, DC: The National Academies Press. Available at www.nap.edu.*

Ethnicity refers to the sense of identity individuals draw from a common ancestry, as well as from a common national, religious, tribal, language, or cultural origin. This identity nurtures a sense of social belonging and loyalty for people of common ethnicity. It helps shape how a person thinks, relates, feels, and behaves within or outside an ethnic group. Ethnicity is often confused with **race,** a term used to describe ethnic groups based on physical characteristics, such as skin color or facial features. Although classifying people by race has been convenient for social scientists, the fact is that biologically separate and distinct races do not exist within the human species. Genetic traits are inherited individually, not in clumps, groups, or "races." Thus it is more accurate to think of similarities and differences among people as a matter of culture or ethnicity.

In the United States we see many levels of **acculturation,** the degree to which an individual gives up the traits of one culture and adopts those of the dominant culture. Degree of acculturation, in addition to ethnic origin in general, can be a significant factor in personal health in the United States. Many people have a natural tendency to resist acculturation, holding on to traditional beliefs and rejecting mainstream health beliefs and practices. Miscommunication and misunderstanding pose significant challenges to the promotion

ethnicity
The sense of identity an individual draws from a common ancestry and/or a common national, religious, tribal, language, or cultural origin.

race
Term used in the social sciences to describe ethnic groups based on physical characteristics, such as skin color or facial features; race does not exist as a biological reality.

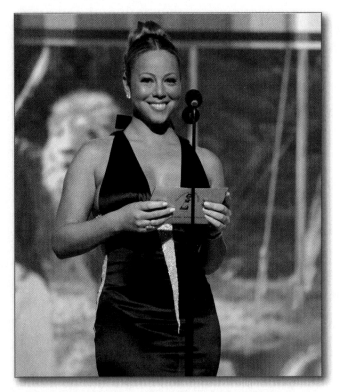

■ *Race* exists only as a social construct, not as a biological reality. People with biracial backgrounds—like Mariah Carey, whose mother was Irish American and whose father was Afro-Venezuelan—inherit a random mix of individual traits from each parent.

CULTURAL DIFFERENCES IN CONCEPTS OF ILLNESS AND HEALTH

One common and significant health-related belief in many non-Western cultures is that illness may result from an imbalance within a person or from an unbalanced or improper relationship between a person and his or her family, community, environment, or spiritual world. Such a view is incompatible with the Western medical model, which is based on the idea that illness and disease are caused by organic changes in the body or by pathogens like bacteria and viruses. In the Western model, health care is provided by medical specialists who use drugs, vaccines, and surgery to treat and cure illness.

Although these differences are profound, some common ground exists between the two models, and in recent years Western medicine has looked with more interest at the possibility that such factors as social support, interpersonal relationships, mind-body connections, and spiritual health play some role in health and illness. This interest has contributed to the growing emphasis on wellness in Western medicine. Complementary and alternative approaches to medicine are now well known in the United States and include acupuncture, chiropractic, therapeutic massage, relaxation techniques, herbal remedies, and many other practices. The term *complementary* is used to indicate that these practices can work with Western medical practices in some cases but shouldn't supplant Western practices that have proved successful, such as using vaccines to prevent polio and smallpox, antibiotics to treat sexually transmitted infections, and surgery to remove tumors. Complementary and alternative medicine is discussed in Chapter 20.

HEALTH CONCERNS OF ETHNIC MINORITY POPULATIONS

Over the past 100 years, advances in medical technology, lifestyle improvements, and environmental protections have produced significant health gains for the general U.S. population. These advances, however, have not produced equal health benefits for most of the country's ethnic minority populations.[13] Morbidity and mortality rates (rates of illness and death, respectively) for ethnic minority populations are disheartening. Many have higher rates of cancer, diabetes, cardiovascular disease, infant mortality, alcoholism, drug abuse, unintentional injury, and premature death than the general population does. Most also have significantly higher lifestyle risk factors, such as high-fat diets, lack of exercise, and exposure to carcinogens and other environmental toxins (see the box "Racial and Ethnic Health Disparities").

In line with the ecological model described earlier, many of these health problems can be attributed to social and economic conditions, including poverty, discrimination, and limited access to health information and resources. Different theories have been proposed to explain the mechanisms by which these social determinants affect health. According to the *risk exposure theory,* minority communities are more

of healthy lifestyles among ethnic populations. In some cases, individuals may not understand or adopt behaviors that would clearly be beneficial to them, such as taking medications according to directions. In other cases, U.S. health care practitioners may misunderstand or dismiss practices that are health enhancing in another culture, such as the participation and support of the entire extended family in medical decisions and treatments.

When misunderstandings occur between members of ethnic minority groups and health care practitioners, people on both sides may be guilty of **ethnocentrism,** the assumption that the beliefs and practices of one's own culture are true and correct. Standing in contrast to ethnocentrism is **ethnosensitivity,** an openness to and respect for cultural and ethnic differences in values, customs, and practices. Ethnosensitivity requires knowledge and understanding of other cultures, but it also requires awareness of one's own biases, prejudices, and stereotypes of other groups.[12]

acculturation
Degree to which an individual gives up the traits of a culture of origin and adopts the traits of a dominant culture.

ethnocentrism
Assumption that the beliefs and practices of one's own culture are true and correct.

ethnosensitivity
Openness to and respect for cultural and ethnic differences in values, customs, and practices.

Highlight on Health

Racial and Ethnic Health Disparities

How significant are racial and ethnic health disparities? Consider these examples:

- *Immunization.* Rates of immunization are lower among minorities (excluding Asian Americans, whose immunization rates are comparable to those of Whites).

- *Infant mortality.* Minorities have higher infant mortality rates than Whites. For example, African American infants are 2.5 times more likely to die before their first birthday than are White infants.

- *HIV/AIDS.* Although African Americans and Hispanics comprise 26 percent of the nation's population, they account for about 82 percent of pediatric AIDS cases and 69 percent of new HIV infections among adults.

- *Diabetes.* In comparison with Whites, American Indians, Alaskan Natives, African Americans, and Hispanic Americans are more likely to have type 2 diabetes.

- *Breast cancer.* Breast cancer death rates have declined steadily since 1996, but death rates remain higher for Black women than for White women.

- *Cervical cancer.* Women belonging to racial and ethnic minorities are less likely than White women to have Pap smear tests and to follow up on abnormal test results.

Given that racial and ethnic minorities comprise an ever-increasing proportion of the population, the number of people affected by health disparities will continue to increase unless culturally appropriate, community-driven programs to address these issues are implemented. One such program is Racial and Ethnic Approaches to Community Health (REACH), developed by the CDC in 1999. REACH 2010 is focusing community efforts to improve the health status of racial and ethnic minority groups.

Sources: Racial and Ethnic Approaches to Community Health (REACH 2010): Addressing Disparities in Health, *Centers for Disease Control and Prevention;* Atlanta, GA, retrieved from www.cdc.gov/nccdphd/publications/aag/reach.htm. Looking Through a Glass, Darkly: Eliminating Health Disparities, *Centers for Disease Control and Prevention, Atlanta, GA, retrieved from www/cdc/gov/pcd/issues/2006/jul/05_0209.htm.*

likely than White communities to be exposed to environmental health risks, such as toxic dump sites, crime, and liquor stores. According to the *resource deprivation theory,* the infrastructure needed to support healthy lifestyles, such as supermarkets and pharmacies, is less likely to be available in minority communities.[14]

Other theories focus on psychosocial and cultural factors. The *racial discrimination theory* suggests that minority populations are disproportionately exposed to racism, which may be a source of both chronic and acute stress. A growing body of research documents the relationship between stress and various health outcomes, including heart disease, breast cancer survival, chronic obstructive pulmonary disease, infant mortality, low birth weight, and depression. Racism may affect health even if it is not perceived as a stressor. Individuals may experience reduced access to goods, services, and opportunities as a result of *institutional racism.* Prejudice, bias, and stereotyping by health care providers may contribute to health disparities for minority populations.[14]

Reducing or eliminating health disparities among different cultural and ethnic populations in the Untied States is not only a critical challenge of the 21st century but also an explicit national health goal.

NATIONAL HEALTH GOALS: *HEALTHY PEOPLE 2010*

Healthy People 2010 is a set of national health goals aimed at improving the quality of life for all Americans.[15] The U.S. government issued the first *Healthy People* report in

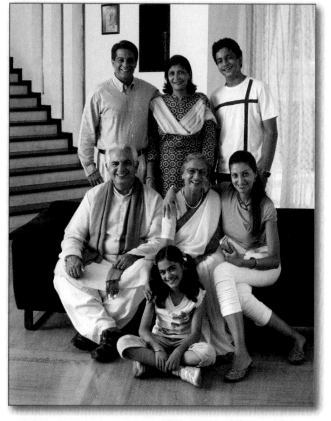

- Different degrees of acculturation are common in multigenerational immigrant families in the United States, as in this family from India.

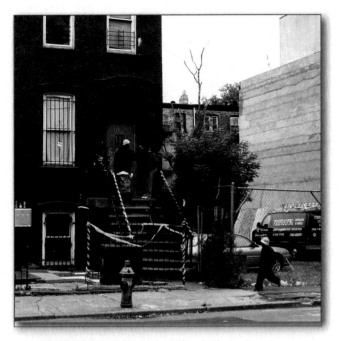

■ Health disparities between racial and ethnic groups are largely attributable to social and economic conditions. A poor neighborhood does not provide the same opportunities for a healthy life as a more affluent neighborhood.

1980 and has issued revised reports every 10 years since. The reports include targets for improvement in individual actions, such as using safety belts in motor vehicles, engaging in regular physical activity, and maintaining a healthy weight, as well as broad community health goals (Figure 1.5).

The current *Healthy People* report, *Healthy People 2010,* sets two broad goals:

■ Help individuals of all ages increase life expectancy and improve their quality of life

■ Eliminate health disparities among different segments of the population

The report includes a focus on "community response-ability," the ability of individuals and the community to unite to respond to both personal needs and challenges presented by the social and political environments. The vision of *Healthy People 2010* is healthy people in healthy communities. The identification of specific goals and objectives, with targets expressed as percentages of the population (for example, "Reduce the proportion of adults who use cigarettes from 21 percent to 12 percent"), helps focus the national health agenda and make health goals more concrete.

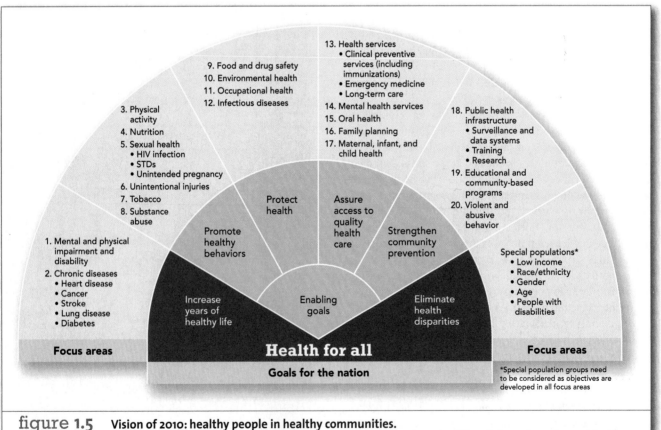

figure 1.5   **Vision of 2010: healthy people in healthy communities.**
Source: From Developing Objectives for Healthy People 2010, *Department of Health and Human Services, Office of Disease Prevention and Health Promotion, 1997, Washington, DC.*

Understanding Health-Related Behavior Change

It should be clear by now that good health depends on many interacting factors, ranging from individual lifestyle choices to government policies and even to global conditions. The area over which you have the most control, of course—and the primary focus of this text—is individual lifestyle choice. You have the opportunity to significantly enhance your health by eating healthy foods, getting enough exercise, not abusing alcohol and other drugs, and making other wise decisions about your life.

Interesting questions arise when we consider why people make choices that don't enhance their health and why people don't change behaviors they know are hurting them. (To evaluate some of your own lifestyle behaviors, see Part 1 of the Add It Up feature for Chapter 1 at the end of the book.) For example, it is nearly impossible to live in the United States and not know that smoking is bad for your health, yet millions of Americans continue to smoke. Why do people make poor choices and persist in them in the face of overwhelming evidence that their choices are incompatible with good health, a high level of wellness, and a long, vital life?

Psychologists have proposed many theories about health behavior choices and change. A major assumption underlying most of these models is that people usually gravitate toward unhealthy lifestyles. According to this assumption, most illnesses and cases of premature death are caused by unhealthy habits that people freely choose for themselves. If this is the case, then the challenge is to find ways to motivate people to change their habits and to help them overcome obstacles to change. The question is, What does it take to motivate people to change?

THE HEALTH BELIEF MODEL

One theory about health behavior change is the **Health Belief Model (HBM)**, developed in the 1950s in an effort to

Health Belief Model (HBM)
Model of behavior change that focuses on a person's knowledge and beliefs.

understand why people failed to take advantage of disease prevention or detection programs that were accessible and low cost, such as screening for tuberculosis.[16] The model was subsequently expanded and applied to a wide range of health behaviors, including smoking, exercising, using seat belts, using sunscreen, drinking and driving, changing sexual behavior to avoid HIV infection, and many others.

According to this model, people make decisions based on their *knowledge and perceptions* about a health problem and about the behavior recommended in relation to that problem. The following factors and questions are involved in making a health decision:

- *Perceived susceptibility.* Am I at risk for this problem?
- *Perceived severity.* Is the problem a serious threat?
- *Perceived barriers.* What are the costs and inconveniences associated with changing my behavior?
- *Perceived benefits.* What are the positive consequences of changing the behavior?
- *Perceived efficacy.* Am I capable of making the change?
- *Cues to action.* What external influences are promoting the new behavior?

Thus, according to the Health Belief Model, people will change an unhealthy behavior if they determine they are at risk for an illness, if the threat is serious, if the benefits of changing outweigh the costs, if they believe they *can* make the change, and if the environment supports the change. Unfortunately, although the model continues to be a valuable guide for health experts crafting health messages for the public, it has not proven to be an effective intervention tool for helping individuals change unhealthy behaviors. At least part of the reason may be that it focuses almost exclusively on cognitive factors (knowledge and beliefs).

THE TRANSTHEORETICAL MODEL

The **Transtheoretical Model (TTM),** developed in the 1990s, is a more popular and useful framework for understanding health behavior change, perhaps because it takes into account thinking, feelings, behaviors, relationships, and many other factors besides knowledge. The TTM is also known as the Stages of Change model.

Transtheoretical Model (TTM)
Model of behavior change that focuses on stages of change.

Stages of Change   The psychologists who developed this model, James Prochaska and Carlo DiClemente, realized that many individuals are ambivalent about making significant

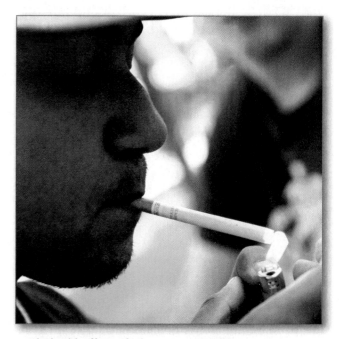

■ The health effects of tobacco use are well known, yet 20 percent of Americans continue to smoke.

health changes even when they know they should. Change is not a one-time event but rather a process that unfolds through a series of stages:[17]

- *Precontemplation.* The individual has no motivation to change and in fact does not realize or acknowledge that there is a problem. Precontemplators may just want other people to stop nagging them.
- *Contemplation.* The individual acknowledges that there is a problem and is thinking about making a change, often within the next six months. Contemplators may be trying to understand the problem and searching for solutions.
- *Preparation.* The individual is planning for change in the immediate future, usually the next month. People in this stage are focusing more on the solution than the problem and more on the future than the past.
- *Action.* The individual is implementing the behavior change. This stage is marked by the greatest commitment of time and energy.
- *Maintenance.* The new behavior has been in place for six months or more. The individual consolidates gains and works to prevent relapse. Maintenance is a long and ongoing process.

A sixth stage, termination, occurs for some types of behavior change. At this stage, the behavior is firmly entrenched as a part of a person's lifestyle and there is zero temptation to return to the old behavior. For some types of health problems, such as alcohol addiction, few people may reach termination. Instead, a lifetime of maintenance is required.

If a person is not ready to change, undertaking a health behavior change program is pointless and even counterproductive; failure and discouragement are the likely outcomes. For this reason, it is important to assess readiness for change at the outset. (A simple test of your own readiness for change is provided in the box "Assessing Your Stage of Change.")

Research suggests that most people have to try several times before they successfully change a behavior; four out of five people experience some degree of backsliding. **Relapse** is the rule rather than the exception in the process of behavior change. A person who relapses may cycle back to the contemplation or even the precontemplation stage. The stages of change are more like a spiral than a linear progression (Figure 1.6).[17, 18]

relapse
Backslide into a former health state.

processes of change
Broad strategies that inspire, motivate, and support behavior change.

Processes of Change The TTM identifies a number of **processes of change**—broad strategies that inspire, motivate, and support change. Each process is more appropriate or useful at some stages of change than at others. For example, in the precontemplation and contemplation stages, an important process of change is *consciousness raising*—learning more about the problem and its effects. In the action and maintenance stages, an important process of

Challenges & Choices

Assessing Your Stage of Change

Responding to four simple statements can help determine your readiness for behavior change as well as your stage of change for a chosen health behavior. First, choose a health area in which you think there might be room for improvement or a specific health behavior that you think you might like to change. Then respond yes or no to the following statements:

- ____ 1. I solved my problem more than six months ago.
- ____ 2. I have taken action on my problem within the past six months.
- ____ 3. I am intending to take action in the next month.
- ____ 4. I am intending to take action in the next six months.

Scoring: Answering no for all four statements means you are in the precontemplation stage. If you answered yes to statement 4 and no to the other three statements, you are in the contemplation stage. If you answered yes to statements 3 and 4 and no to statements 1 and 2, you are in the action stage. If you answered yes to statement 2 and no to statement 1, you are in the action stage. A yes answer to statement 1 means you are in the maintenance or, possibly, the termination stage.

It's Not Just Personal . . .
According to the U.S. Department of Health and Human Services, the leadng causes of premature death (death before age 65) involve behavior choice: (1) unhealthy behavior patterns, 40 percent; (2) genetic disposition, 30 percent; (3) social circumstances, 15 percent; (4) shortcomings in medical care such as health care access, 10 percent; and (5) environmental causes, 5 percent.

Sources: Adapted from Changing for Good: The Revolutionary Program That Exhibits Six Stages of Change and Shows You How to Free Yourself from Bad Habits, by J.O. Prochaska, J.C. Norcross, and C.C. DiClemente, 1994, New York: William Morrow; U.S. Department of Health and Human Services (www.hhs .gov/news/2002pres/prevent.html; retreived March 8, 2008).

change is *countering*—substituting a healthy behavior for an unhealthy one. Other common processes of change include the following:

- *Social liberation.* Making use of healthy alternatives offered by the environment
- *Emotional arousal.* Experiencing feelings about the problem behavior
- *Self-reevaluation.* Assessing your own thoughts and feelings about yourself and the problem
- *Commitment.* Committing to change or believing in your ability to change
- *Environment control.* Avoiding stimuli that trigger the problem behavior
- *Reward.* Rewarding yourself for making changes
- *Helping relationships.* Enlisting the help of others

A diagram showing which change processes are most useful in each stage of change is shown in Figure 1.7.

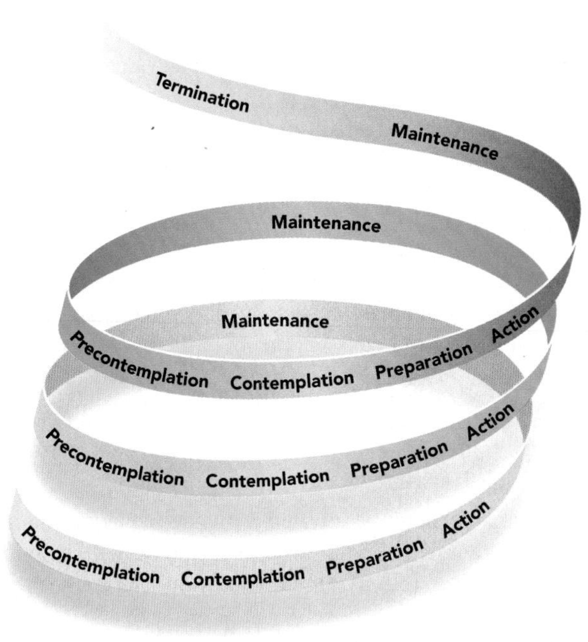

CREATING A BEHAVIOR CHANGE PLAN

Research has given us a great deal of information about how behavior change occurs. How can you use this information to change your own behavior? The first step is accepting responsibility for your health and making a commitment to change. Ask yourself these questions:

- *Is there a health behavior I would like to change?* It could be smoking, overeating, procrastinating, not getting enough exercise, or a host of other behaviors.
- *Why do you want to change this behavior?* There can be many reasons and motivations, but it's best if you want to change for yourself.

figure 1.6 **The stages of change: A spiral model.** *Source: Adapted from "In Search of How People Change," by J.O. Prochaska, C.C. DiClemente, and J.C. Norcross, 1992, American Psychologist 47 (9), pp. 1102–1114.*

- *What barriers are you likely to encounter?* Having a plan to deal with barriers will increase your chances of success.
- *Are you ready to change the behavior?* As noted earlier, beginning a behavior change plan when you haven't fully committed to it will likely result in relapse.

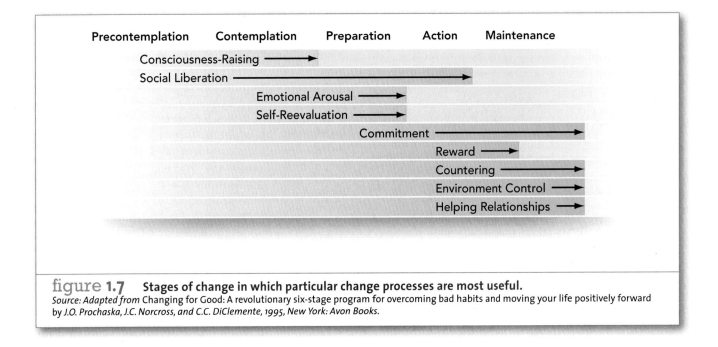

figure 1.7 **Stages of change in which particular change processes are most useful.**
Source: Adapted from Changing for Good: A revolutionary six-stage program for overcoming bad habits and moving your life positively forward *by J.O. Prochaska, J.C. Norcross, and C.C. DiClemente, 1995, New York: Avon Books.*

Although making an initial commitment is an important step, it isn't enough to carry you through the process of change. For enduring change, you need a systematic behavior change plan. Once you have identified a behavior you would like to change, assessed your readiness to change, and made a commitment to change, follow these seven steps:

1. Set goals that are specific, measurable, attainable, realistic, and timely (SMART goals). An example of a SMART goal might be, "I will increase my consumption of vegetables, especially dark green and orange vegetables, to 3 cups per day over the next four weeks, reaching my goal by October 30."

2. Develop action steps for attaining goals within a set time frame. For example, "I will include baby carrots in my lunch starting October 1."

3. Identify benefits associated with the behavior change. For example, "Eating more vegetables will help me lose weight, improve my complexion, and be healthier overall."

4. Identify positive enablers (skills, physical and emotional capabilities, resources) that will help you overcome barriers. An important capability is a sense of **self-efficacy**, the belief that you are competent to perform a specific task. Another capability might be the confidence that comes from having succeeded at behavior change in the past, along with skills that were used at that time. For example, "I was able to quit drinking so much soda last year. I think I'll be able to improve my diet now."

5. Sign a behavior change contract to put your commitment in writing. Ask a friend or family member to witness your contract to increase your commitment. Signing a behavior change contract is one of the most effective strategies for change. An example of a behavior change contract is provided in Part 2 of the Add It Up feature for Chapter 1 at the end of the book.

6. Create benchmarks to recognize and reward interim goals. Particularly when a goal is long term, it is useful to have rewards for short-term goals reached along the way. Reward yourself with something that particularly appeals to you (for example, buying a new CD, going to a movie).

7. Assess your accomplishment of goals and, if necessary, revise the plan.

Many lifestyle behaviors are established early in life and have significant pleasurable aspects. Eating fast food, for example, is a popular, convenient, inexpensive, socially acceptable way to fill up at lunch time. Many people are in the habit of grabbing a burger, fries, and a shake at one of the hundreds of thousands of fast-food restaurants that dot the American landscape. A person who wants to increase his or her consumption of dark green and orange

self-efficacy
Internal state in which the person feels competent to perform a specific task.

vegetables (as recommended by the 2005 *Dietary Guidelines for Americans*), however, will probably have to cut back on visits to the drive-through lane. Thus positive changes can and usually do entail losses as well, and an effective behavior change plan identifies and acknowledges both the pros and the cons of change.

Although behavior change theories offer valuable insights into the change process, they also have limitations. The major limitation of the behavior change approach is that it does not take into account health factors beyond the control of the individual,[18] primarily the kinds of social environmental factors described earlier in the chapter. In the case of fast food, these factors might include peer pressure, community resources, media messages, and broader societal norms. If eating fast food is the norm; if the college food court offers a variety of ethnic food choices but no fruit, milk, or whole grain products; or if the campus is peppered with commercial logos and brand names—then the individual will have fewer opportunities to make healthy choices.

Health Challenges in a Changing Society

We are inundated with health-related information, some reliable and some not. We are immersed in a culture that overwhelms us with unhealthy but attractive options at every turn. We are confronted with perplexing ethical, social, and political issues in association with the concept of health promotion. How do we meet these challenges?

BEING AN INFORMED CONSUMER

Part of taking responsibility for your health is learning how to evaluate health information, sorting the reputable and credible from the disreputable and unsubstantiated—in other words, becoming an informed consumer. Your successful navigation of the health marketplace requires that you develop **health literacy**—the ability to obtain, interpret, understand, and use health information. Among other things, health literacy includes having a basic understanding of medical research studies and a good sense of how to use health information technology.[19]

health literacy
The degree to which individuals have the capacity to obtain, process, and understand basic health information and services needed to make appropriate health decisions.

Developing Health Literacy   Three types of health literacy can be identified:[19]

- *Functional literacy.* Basic reading and writing skills that enable consumers to follow health messages
- *Interactive literacy.* Advanced literacy, cognitive, and interpersonal skills that enable consumers to navigate the health care system

■ *Critical literacy.* Critical thinking skills that enable consumers to evaluate information for credibility and quality, analyze relative health risks, and interpret health test results

Changes in our society have made all types of health literacy both more important and more difficult to achieve. One change is that our health care system has moved from a *paternalistic model,* in which physicians were regarded as authority figures who knew best and were beyond questioning, to a *partnership model,* in which more responsibility is placed on individuals for prevention, informed decision making, and self-management of health conditions. Another change is that consumers are faced with enormous amounts of health information, including conflicting media reports. A third change is that many more consumers come from diverse cultural backgrounds that include ideas about health and health care that may be incompatible with Western models. Their interpretation and use of health information may be filtered through their cultural belief systems and social norms.[20]

A particularly perplexing concept for many consumers is **health risk.** Many people define *health risk* as simply a probability or likelihood of an event. A more complete definition of health risk includes the probability of an exposure to a hazard that can result in negative consequences. Many factors contribute to an individual's health risk for a particular condition, including age, gender, family history, income, education, geographical location, and other factors that make the person unique.

health risk
Probability of an exposure to a hazard that can result in negative consequences.

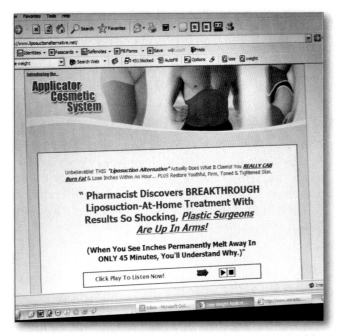

■ Health literacy includes the ability to critically analyze health messages and distinguish credible from outlandish claims. What do you think about this product's promise to "permanently melt away inches in 45 minutes"?

Health literacy requires the use of critical thinking—the mental process of analyzing information by examining evidence and drawing conclusions based on facts. If you apply your critical thinking skills and are still uncertain about a health message, it's always a good idea to consult with your physician, since he or she is likely to be aware of medical advances. The Institute of Medicine (www.iom.edu), a government organization, publishes an excellent guide called *Health Literacy: A Prescription to End Confusion.* In addition, many state governments provide readable, trustworthy health information and health advice networks.

Understanding Medical Research Studies Scientists use different types of research studies to explore and confirm relationships between risk factors and disease. Some types of studies—for example, *correlational studies*—suggest likely associations but do not establish cause-and-effect relationships. Other types of studies—*clinical* or *experimental studies*—are considered to establish cause-and-effect relationships. In clinical studies, researchers randomly assign matched participants to either a treatment group or a control group, apply a treatment to the first group and a *placebo* (a look-alike but ineffective treatment, such as a sugar pill) to the second, and after a period of time (usually a year or more) determine whether the treatment group has experienced a significant effect from the treatment in comparison with the control group. To be considered reliable, the same results must be obtained by other researchers replicating the study. Although they are considered to establish cause-and-effect relationships, clinical studies are often costly and time consuming.

When you read or hear about the results of a new research study in the news, ask yourself several questions about it:

■ Was it a clinical study? If not, the results are not likely to "prove" that something is caused by something else.

■ If it was a clinical study, were participants randomly assigned to groups?

■ Were large enough numbers of participants used to ensure that results weren't skewed?

■ Was it a *double-blind study*—that is, was researcher bias minimized by making sure the scientists were unaware of which group was receiving the treatment and which was receiving the placebo?

■ Was the study sponsored by an impartial research institute or government agency, or were there sponsors who stood to benefit from the results?

■ Has the study been replicated by other researchers?

■ Was the study published in a reputable, peer-reviewed medical or health journal?

The answers to all these questions and more affect how much credence you can put in the research results.

Consumer Clipboard

Evaluating Health Information on the Internet

Although many Web sites provide accurate health information, others contain incorrect information that can be dangerous. Ask yourself these five questions when trying to evaluate a Web site.

- *Who maintains and pays for the site?* Almost anyone can set up a health Web site. Reliable sites will tell you who their authors and sponsors are. This can help you understand the purpose of the site. Some sites provide information; others are designed to sell products or promote certain points of view.

- *How often is the site updated?* Information about medical conditions and treatments is always changing. A good Web site will clearly state when the site was last updated. Look for sites that update their pages often.

- *Does the site include a disclaimer?* Sites dispensing medical information or adivce should. Reputable sites

will tell you to always check with your physician or other medical provider for definite information on your particular situation.

- *Does the site promise "miracle" cures?* It may be tempting to believe promises of miracle cures. Unfortunately, most turn out to be untrue. Double-check information on other Web sites and *always* consult your physician before trying a new treatment for your condition.

- *Does the site subscribe to the principles of the Health on the Net Foundation?* The Health on the Net (HON) Foundation has established the HON Code of Conduct for medical and health Web sites. Sites that subscribe to the code must follow eight principles set by the foundation. Although there are many trustworthy sites that do not subscribe to the HON Code, this certification is one more way to judge the reliability of a site. A caution: The HON logo may appear on sites that are not certified. To verify certification, click on the HON logo. You should be directed to a page that includes the HON code number for the site.

Source: "Guide to Using Health Sites on the Web," State of Wisconsin Department of Health and Human Services, retrieved from www.dhfs.state.wi.us/guide/info/web.htm.

All reputable studies contribute to the body of scientific knowledge we now have. Correlational studies are like legal arguments built on circumstantial evidence, exploring possible relationships between risk factors and disease. Clinical studies can be used to confirm these relationships in more precisely controlled ways. Both types of studies help scientists put together the "big picture" and make useful health recommendations. Keep in mind that scientists typically consider individual studies stepping-stones in an ongoing search for answers to complex questions. Members of the lay public have a tendency to regard the results of a single study as conclusive and definitive, and many times, the media are guilty of creating or fostering this impression.[21]

Using Health Information Technology More than 70 million people use online technologies for researching health issues.[23] The range of uses for the Internet includes everything from accessing basic health information, to scheduling online chat sessions or consultations with health care professionals, to joining online support groups formed for people struggling with similar health concerns.[22]

The most important rule for consumers of health information on the Internet is that such information should support, not replace, a patient's relationship with his or her physician. When you do use the Internet to access health information, you need to use the same critical thinking skills that are called for in evaluating research study results. In general, you can rely on

- Web sites of large, stable, nonprofit organizations such as the American Heart Association and the American Cancer Society

- Web sites of government organizations and agencies like the National Institutes of Health, the Department of Health and Human Services, and the Centers for Disease Control and Prevention

- Web sites associated with educational institutions such as Harvard University, the University of California at Berkeley, and Johns Hopkins University.

For more advice from consumer advocates, see the box "Evaluating Health Information on the Internet."

FACING CURRENT HEALTH CONCERNS

Americans have more health challenges than learning to be critical consumers of health information. They are also faced with lifestyle decisions that affect their own health, their children's health, and ultimately the health of the nation (see the box "Variations in Leading Causes of Death Among Americans"). *Healthy People 2010* identifies the "leading health indicators" that reflect the top 10 current health concerns in the United States:[15]

- Physical activity
- Overweight and obesity
- Tobacco use
- Substance abuse
- Responsible sexual behavior
- Mental health
- Injury and violence

- Environmental quality
- Immunization
- Access to health care

As just one example, let's consider the problem of childhood overweight.

The Case of Childhood Overweight A major health concern confronting not just the American people but the people of many developed nations is that of childhood overweight. (Overweight is defined as having a body mass index of 25 to 29, and obesity is defined as having a body mass index of 30 or higher. Body mass index is a single number that represents height-to-weight ratio, as explained in Chapter 9.) The National Center for Health Statistics estimates that 64 percent of children and adolescents between 6 and 19 years of age are overweight.[23]

The health toll associated with being overweight at such a young age includes a greater risk for high blood pressure, high cholesterol, Type-2 diabetes, heart disease, and other debilitating illnesses. If the childhood overweight epidemic continues unabated, the life expectancy of today's children may be shortened by two to five years. This would be

Who's at Risk

Variations in Leading Causes of Death Among Americans

The leading causes of death for Americans overall are heart disease, cancer, and stroke, but the top 10 causes of death vary somewhat across racial/ethnic groups. For example, among American Indians and Hispanics, the third-leading cause of death is unintentional injury (accidents). Alzheimer's disease is among the top 10 for Whites and Asians but not for Blacks, American Indians, or Hispanics. Other variations can be seen in the following table. For the most part, variations in leading causes of death are a reflection of differences in social, economic, and cultural factors.

Ten Leading Causes of Death, 2004, by Race and Hispanic Origin

Rank (by number of deaths)	All Groups	White	Black/African American	American Indian/Alaska Native	Asian/Pacific Islander	Hispanic/Latino
1	Heart disease	Heart disease	Heart disease	Heart disease	Cancer	Heart disease
2	Cancer	Cancer	Cancer	Cancer	Heart disease	Cancer
3	Stroke	Stroke	Stroke	Unintentional injury	Stroke	Unintentional injury
4	Chronic lower respiratory diseases	Chronic lower respiratory diseases	Diabetes mellitus	Diabetes mellitus	Unintentional injury	Stroke
5	Unintentional injury	Unintentional injury	Unintentional injury	Stroke	Diabetes mellitus	Diabetes mellitus
6	Diabetes mellitus	Alzheimer's disease	Homicide	Liver disease	Pneumonia/ influenza	Liver disease
7	Alzheimer's disease	Diabetes mellitus	Kidney disease	Chronic lower respiratory diseases	Chronic lower respiratory diseases	Homicide
8	Pneumonia/ influenza	Pneumonia/ influenza	Chronic lower respiratory diseases	Suicide	Suicide	Chronic lower respiratory diseases
9	Kidney disease	Kidney disease	HIV/AIDS	Pneumonia/ influenza	Kidney disease	Pneumonia/ influenza
10	Septicemia (blood infection)	Suicide	Septicemia (blood infection)	Kidney disease	Alzheimer's disease	Perinatal conditions

Source: Health, United States, 2007, *by National Center for Health Statistics, 2007, Hyattsville, MD: National Center for Health Statistics.*

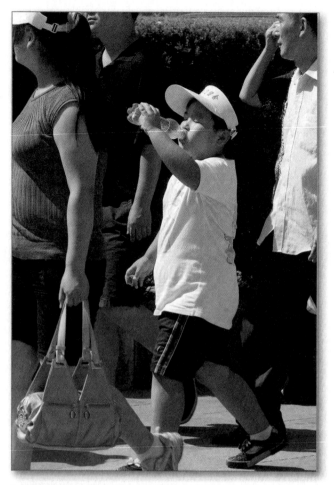

■ The obesity epidemic is a major public health concern. Overweight children are at increased risk for overweight and obesity in adulthood, conditions associated with a host of health problems and reduced life expectancy.

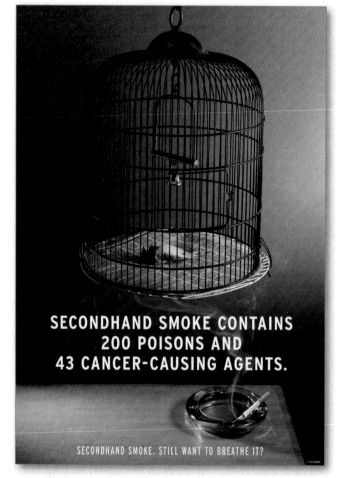

SECONDHAND SMOKE CONTAINS 200 POISONS AND 43 CANCER-CAUSING AGENTS.

SECONDHAND SMOKE. STILL WANT TO BREATHE IT?

■ Individuals may defend their right to choose unhealthy behaviors, but secondhand smoke makes smoking a public health concern.

the first time that life expectancy in the United States has ever decreased. Minority populations would be hardest hit, because they have higher overweight and obesity rates than the population overall and less access to medical services.[24]

Some scientists argue that such predictions should be treated with caution, since factors such as reduced smoking rates and improved medical care may more than offset the negative effects of childhood overweight on life expectancy. But the fact remains that the current rates of overweight and obesity are unprecedented. People who are overweight at age 40 are likely to die at least three years sooner than people who are not overweight, even if they lose weight at a later age. People who are obese at age 40 have an even greater reduction in life expectancy compared to people of normal weight; for men, the difference is 5.8 years, and for women, it's 7.1 years.[23]

Being overweight or obese may overtake smoking as the leading cause of preventable death, and some experts consider it even more worrisome, with health effects extending into every area of life. On an individual level, overweight and obesity cause immense suffering, especially for children; on a population level, the obesity epidemic is quickly becoming a public health crisis.[23]

Ethical Issues for Individuals and Society   If the leading causes of death in the United States are at least partially attributable to lifestyle behaviors such as smoking, inactivity, and poor diet, as is the prevailing view, and if it is in everyone's interest to reduce the incidence of heart disease, cancer, strokes, diabetes, and other chronic conditions in our society, then what are the implications in terms of individual rights and responsibilities? If you have the fundamental right to freely choose health-related behaviors, do you also have a responsibility to make wise choices? If you make poor choices, is your resulting poor health your own responsibility? And if your poor choices lead to illness or disability, should you be held responsible for the costs to society, medical or otherwise?[25]

In this context, personal choices have ethical implications for individuals, but increasingly, ethical issues are challenges faced by entire communities. As a free society, we respect the autonomy and integrity of the individual and do not dictate to people how they must behave in many situations. People who smoke, drink, take drugs, have unsafe sex, eat unhealthy foods, and do not exercise may not share the same vision that others have of how they should live. They may be gambling that the risk of long-term health consequences is worth taking

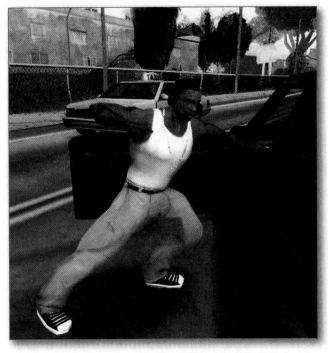

■ Do violent video games like "Grand Theft Auto" promote aggressive or violent behavior in the children, teens, and adults who play them? Should the government regulate or censor media violence?

in exchange for immediate enjoyment. They may not want to (or be able to) practice the kind of self-discipline required to change a long-standing or addictive behavior. They may be tired of being told what to do.

For these or other reasons, they may ignore even the most carefully crafted public health message aimed at educating people about a particular unhealthy behavior. If they get sick as a result of their unhealthy lifestyles, we often try not to blame them for their illness, even when their behavior has contributed to it, and we typically do not ask people to repay society for the costs of their illnesses.

Still, these considerations raise complex ethical and moral questions about responsibility and accountability. Should people who smoke have to pay more for health insurance? Should a man who has damaged his liver through alcohol abuse have the same eligibility for a transplant as a child with liver disease? Should a woman who uses cocaine during pregnancy be held criminally liable for the health effects on her child?

However we answer these questions, we cannot avoid the fact that public policies designed to promote personal health—for example, campaigns against smoking, drinking, and using drugs during pregnancy—have ethical, moral, social, and political implications.[26] In this book we discuss many of the social issues associated with health behaviors, such as state-imposed vaccination programs and actions taken by colleges to curb binge drinking.

In the future we can expect our society to face even more complex questions, largely as a result of technological

advances that have outpaced our ethics. Some of the issues we as a society will have to make decisions about include

■ Pornography on the Internet and Internet addiction. Although Internet addiction is not an official medical condition, users can build up a tolerance for Internet use and need more of it to be satisfied.

■ Censorship and violence in the media and the entertainment industry.

■ Use of DNA technology to repair genetic disorders in the womb, replace a child who has died, or clone a human being.

■ Harvesting of stem cells from embryos grown in laboratories to develop treatments for Parkinson's disease and other neurological disorders.

In addition, we need to decide to what extent we can use ethical and moral values, religious beliefs, and legal principles to help guide us through the many uncharted health issues that loom in the immediate future and, in some cases, are upon us today.

Looking Ahead   Clearly, we have many challenges, on both the personal and the community/societal level. We need to sort healthy options from unhealthy ones in a culture that sometimes overwhelms us with choice. We need to embrace responsibility in the areas in which we have power and accept those areas that are beyond our control. We need to work to build communities and a society that provide all people with the services and resources they need to live healthy lives. These challenges can seem daunting. But on the individual level, we do have the opportunity to make a difference every day—by making thoughtful decisions that support our own health.

Throughout this book we explore the relationship between good health and a variety of lifestyle behaviors and choices. In every chapter we attempt to summarize what is known and not known about healthy and unhealthy choices. Our intent is to provide useful information that will help you understand and assess the health risks in your life. Beyond this, we want to give you the tools to change and to make a difference. As you read the chapters, reflect on your current level of wellness in that area. Is there a behavior you would like to change? First, assess your readiness to change; then develop a plan for behavior change using the tips offered throughout the book pertaining to specific types of behavior. Our hope is that applying health information to your own life in this way will empower and inspire you.

We also hope you will find ways to use this information to make better decisions involving health for your family, friends, and community. As pointed out throughout this chapter, personal and community health are intertwined; the individual cannot be truly healthy without a supportive environment. A well-informed and educated citizenry understands health not only from a personal point of view but also from a broader social and cultural perspective.

You Make the Call

How Should Americans Describe Their Racial and Ethnic Identities?

If you are asked to identify your race and ethnicity on a form, what do you check? Guidelines from the Office of Management and Budget (OMB) have added complexity—some would say confusion—to this question. The OMB guidelines allow people to check more than one race on all federally required forms, including college financial aid forms. Previously, federal forms listed four racial groups—White, Black, American Indian or Alaska Native, and Asian or Pacific Islander—and two ethnic categories—Hispanic origin and not Hispanic origin. Respondents were asked to check just one box in each category.

Under the new guidelines, respondents can check more than one box, and some categories have been listed more than once under different names. For example, respondents have a choice of selecting "Black," "African American," or both, or "Hispanic," "Latino," or both. There are now 57 possible combinations that can be selected to represent a person's racial and ethnic identity.

One issue that has arisen under the new system is how to count people who identify with more than one race. Respondents who check both Black and White are counted as Mixed Race but not as Black or White. The same is true for respondents who check more than two boxes, such as Black, White, and Asian. Interracial marriages and partnerships, immigration, and a growing acceptance of multiple identities have made it difficult for people to place themselves in discrete categories. Many people, especially the children of multiracial and multiethnic partnerships, don't wish to identify with a particular race at all. The "Unhyphenated American" Web site encourages people to write in "Human" rather than checking a racial identifying category.

So what's the problem? Information from federal forms is used for a variety of purposes, including government-sponsored research and government funding of educational and health-related programs; the information is also used by business and industry. The main objection to the use of such a wide range of racial and ethnic categories is that specific groups will be undercounted, leading to the underfunding or elimination of programs aimed at minority populations. Whereas supporters of the new guidelines argue that they reflect the reality of an increasingly diverse society, opponents say they create more problems than they solve. What do you think?

PROS

- These changes are a long-overdue response to the diversity of American society. Change is necessary even though it evokes resistance and causes disruption.

- Historically, the American system of categorizing people by race and ethnicity was developed by Whites, the dominant group, to distinguish and subordinate other, non-White groups. In our increasingly diverse society, this alone is reason enough to dismantle the system of classifying people along strict racial lines.

- The arbitrary nature of racial and ethnic categories can be seen by looking at some of these historical categories. For example, Jews and Irish people were not considered to belong to the White race in some previous eras.

- Race is a socially constructed concept. People are a mixed bag of genetic traits that are inherited separately, not in racial groupings. The ancient Greeks classified people according to culture and language rather than by physical differences. As long as they spoke Greek and adopted Greek customs, they were considered Greek citizens.

- The American Medical Association and the National Institutes of Health have endorsed the new guidelines, saying they provide better information about the population and a more accurate way to track diseases based on genetic profiles.

- People should have the choice about how to describe themselves, and the new guidelines give them more options.

CONS

- Race is a powerful factor in determining which groups get resources and opportunities. Regardless of underlying philosophy, the use of so many categories leads to undercounting, underfunding, and continued discrimination against minority racial groups.

- Since 1900, the U.S. Census has used 26 different racial terms to identify groups. The ever-changing classification system on federal forms leaves the general public confused about which category or categories to check.

- The guidelines assume that Americans understand the concepts of race and ethnicity, which is not necessarily the case.

- Changing the classification system makes it difficult or impossible to compare current numbers with older ones, which in turn makes it difficult to track trends and understand how the population is changing.

Sources: "Demography's Race Problem," by David R. Harris, 2000, presented at the National Institute of Child Health and Human Development, retrieved from www.nichd.nih.gov/about/meetings/2001/DBS_planning/harris.cfm; "The Unhyphenated American," http://home.cinci.rr.com/justamerican/; "U.S. Proposal Offers Students Wider Way of Racial Identity," by E. Gootman, The New York Times, August 9, 2006; "Top 10 Facts About Race," retrieved from http://racerelations.about.com/od/thehierarchyofrace/tp/racematters.htm.

In Review

1. **How are health and wellness defined?** *Health* is defined by the World Health Organization as a state of complete physical, mental, social, and spiritual well-being, not just the absence of disease. *Wellness* is defined as the process of adopting patterns of behavior that lead to better health and greater life satisfaction, encompassing several dimensions: physical, emotional, intellectual, spiritual, interpersonal or social, environmental, and, in some models, occupational. Very often, people want to have good health as a means to achieving wellness, an optimum quality of life.

2. **What factors influence a person's health?** Individual health-related behavior choices play a key role in health, but economic, social, cultural, and physical conditions—referred to as the *social determinants of health*—are also important, along with the person's individual genetic makeup. Community health and public health actions are needed to ensure the personal health of individuals.

3. **What health-related trends are occurring in our society?** As the United States becomes more multiethnic and multicultural, concepts of health and wellness from other cultures are being integrated into Western health care. At the same time, advances in medicine and health care have not reached many minority groups in the United States. Eliminating health disparities among different segments of the population is one of the broad goals of the national health initiative Healthy People 2010.

4. **What is health-related behavior change?** The process of changing a health behavior (for example, quitting smoking, changing your diet) has been conceptualized in the Transtheoretical Model as unfolding over several "stages of change," from precontemplation to maintenance of new behavior. Many different strategies and techniques are needed to implement lasting behavior change.

5. **What health challenges do we face?** Health challenges for individuals include learning to be more informed consumers of health information and making lifestyle decisions that enhance rather than endanger their health. Health challenges for society include addressing health-related ethical issues and promoting health across all segments of the population.

WWW For a detailed summary of this chapter and a comprehensive set of review questions, visit the Online Learning Center at **www.mhhe.com/teague2e**.

Web Resources

Centers for Disease Control and Prevention: The CDC provides a national focus for disease prevention and control as well as for health promotion and education. Its Web site features health and safety topics and offers authoritative information for use in making health decisions.
www.cdc.gov

U.S. Food and Drug Administration: The FDA site provides information on the many products this government agency regulates, such as food, drugs, medical devices, biologics, and cosmetics. Its news section highlights hot topics in health.
www.fda.gov

National Health Information Center: A health information referral service, NHIC is designed to connect consumers and professionals who have health questions with the organizations best suited to answer them. Its database includes 1,400 organizations and government offices offering health information.
www.health.gov/nhic

National Institutes of Health: This Web site provides health information through its A–Z index, health hotlines, and databases. MEDLINEplus, a database associated with the National Library of Medicine, is a resource for finding and evaluating health information on the Web.
www.nih.gov

U.S. Department of Health and Human Services: This site offers a wide range of health information on topics such as diseases and conditions, safety and wellness, drug and food information, and disasters and emergencies. Its news section includes daily updates on statements and reports by the DHHS.
www.os.dhhs.gov

PART ONE

Your Mind and Body

"A healthy mind in a healthy body" is a well-known prescription for a happy life. How can you cultivate optimal mental, physical, and spiritual health? The chapters in Part I address both the genetic basis of health and some of the intangibles that contribute to wellness, such as a sense of meaning and purpose, an optimistic attitude, a balance between challenge and relaxation, and time for renewal. Together these chapters will help you get started on a path towards a higher quality of life.

Think It Over

- If you could design your own genetic makeup, what choices would you make?
- Is your life in good balance, or is it a work in progress?
- What does spirituality mean to you?
- Are you working to prevent stress, or are you reacting to it?
- Is getting a good night's sleep on your priority list?

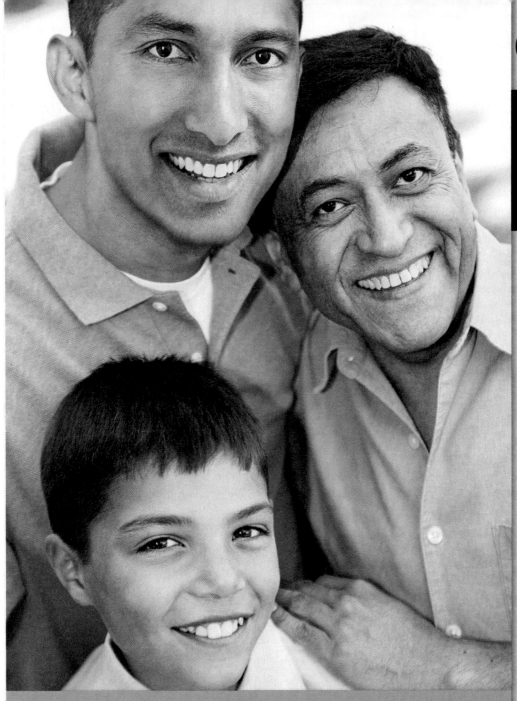

Your Family Health History Understanding Your Genetic Inheritance

Ever Wonder...

- if alcoholism can run in families?
- if sexual orientation could be genetic?
- what causes schizophrenia or Down syndrome?

WWW

Your Health Today

www.mhhe.com/teague2e

Go to the Online Learning Center for *Your Health Today* for interactive activities, quizzes, flashcards, Web links, and more resources related to this chapter.

23

It is perhaps the biggest inheritance you will ever receive. It gives you the potential to be tall or short; apple-shaped or pear-shaped; brown-eyed or blue-eyed; blonde, brunette, or bald. This inheritance may give you the athletic potential to climb to the top of the Olympic podium, grace you with a talent for languages, or require you to use a wheelchair for mobility each day. It gives you a unique bundle of strengths, vulnerabilities, and physical characteristics. It is your genetic makeup.

People have long been curious about what contribution their genetic inheritance makes to their overall makeup as individual human beings and what contribution their upbringing makes—the classic "nature versus nurture" debate. Are people the way they are as a result of their genetic endowment or because of experiences they have had? The answer isn't black and white. Who we are as individuals is the result of a complex, ongoing interaction among

- Our genetic inheritance
- Our lifestyle choices
- Environmental factors of many kinds

This last category includes everything from our prenatal environment, to our family and community, to our ethnic or cultural group, to our society and the world at large.

What we can say definitively about genetic inheritance is that it plays a key role in establishing some of the outside parameters of what a person can be and do in his or her life. You can think of genetic inheritance as a person's blueprint, or starting point. The blueprint is filled in and actualized over the course of the person's entire life.

Genetic inheritance is also the starting point for understanding your personal health. It is important for two reasons:

- If you know what special health risks you may have, such as a predisposition for heart disease, a particular type of cancer, or even alcoholism, you have the opportunity to make informed lifestyle choices.
- If you know of any genetic disorders you may be at risk for and you plan to have children, you have more options for addressing such risks, especially as advancing technology improves our ability to prevent and treat genetic disorders.

This chapter will help you understand your genetic inheritance and use that knowledge to enhance your health.

Your Family Health History

You do not have to be a scientist to realize that traits can be passed from one generation to the next. As with the color of your skin, hair, and eyes, some health traits are passed from one generation to the next. Your grandmother's history of colon cancer may mean you have inherited an increased risk for colon cancer from her side of the family. Your uncle's heart attack at age 40 may mean you have received an increased risk of heart disease from his side of the family. How can you take this information and organize it in a useful way?

CREATING A FAMILY HEALTH TREE

A **family health tree**, also called a genogram or genetic pedigree, is a visual representation of your family's genetic history. Creating a health tree can help you see your family's patterns of health and illness and pinpoint any areas of special concern or risk for you. It is a first step in taking into account the genetic aspect of your health.

To construct your family health tree, you need to assemble information concerning as many family members as you can. (A sample tree is shown in Figure 2.1.) The more detailed and extensive the tree, the easier it will be for you to see patterns. Basic information for each family member should include date of birth, major diseases, and age and cause of death for any deceased relatives. You might include additional data, such as the age of a family member when his or her disease was diagnosed, disabilities, major operations, aller-

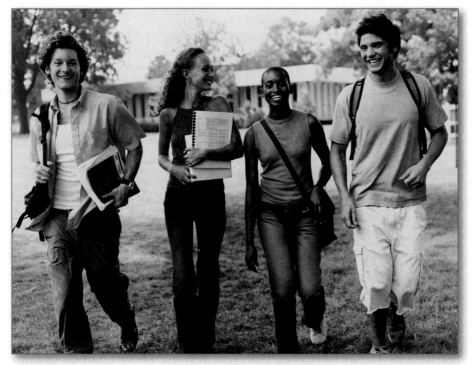

■ Genetic inheritance sets the stage for individual health, and lifetime experiences determine how that inheritance plays out. Each of these students has a unique genetic endowment that carries both limits and opportunities.

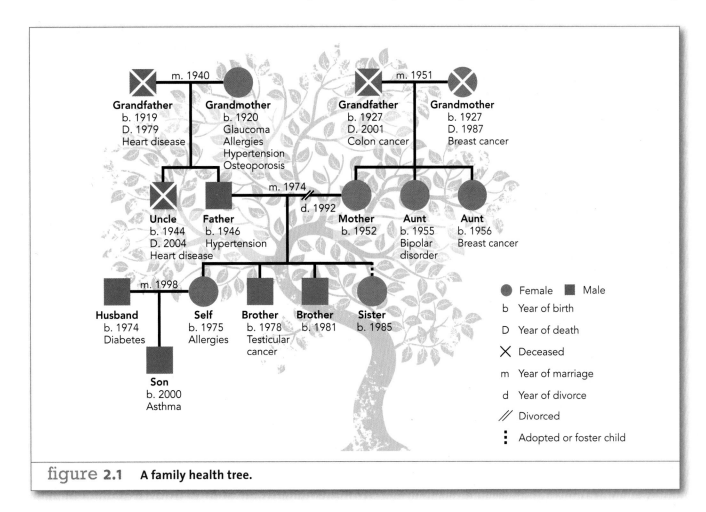

figure **2.1** **A family health tree.**

---

family health tree
Diagram illustrating the patterns of health and illness within a family; also called a genogram or genetic pedigree.

---

gies, lifestyle habits, reproductive problems, mental health disorders, or behavioral problems. Your tree should include parents, siblings, grandparents, cousins, aunts, and uncles. The Add It Up feature for this chapter at the end of the book provides detailed instructions on how to go about putting together your own family health tree.

Gathering family health information to construct a tree may not be an easy process. Only one-third of Americans report that they have tried to gather and write down this information. In recognition of the importance of the task, the U.S. surgeon general has launched a national public health campaign called the U.S. Surgeon General's Family History Initiative. As part of the initiative, Thanksgiving Day has been declared National Family History Day. When families gather, they are encouraged to discuss and record health problems that seem to run in the family.[1] Adopted individuals may not have the same access to their biological parents' health history. Several organizations can aid in the search for such information; see the Web Resources at the end of this chapter for a start.

WHAT CAN YOU LEARN FROM YOUR HEALTH TREE?

Certain patterns of illness or disease suggest that the illness is more likely to be genetically linked, as in the following instances:

- An early onset of disease is more likely to have a genetic component.
- The appearance of a disease in multiple individuals on the same side of the family is more likely to have a genetic correlation.
- A family member with multiple cancers represents a greater likelihood of a genetic association.
- The presence of disease in family members who have good health habits is more suggestive of a genetic cause than is disease in family members with poor health habits.

If you discover a pattern of illness or disease in your health tree, you may want to consult with your physician or a genetic counselor about its meaning and implications. You may want to implement lifestyle changes, have particular screening tests, or watch for early warning signs. Again, a pattern of illness does not automatically mean that you will be affected. The main use of a health tree is to highlight your personal health risks (such as a family history of diabetes) and strengths (such as a family tendency to be long-lived).

You and Your Genes: The Basics of Heredity

In the 1850s, two defining events (and people) shaped the path of modern genetics. Charles Darwin, after years of studying plants and animals around the world, noticed that how something looks or acts changes randomly. He called this *random variation in traits*. He observed that certain traits are favored in particular environments and can be passed to future generations in a process he labeled *descent with modification*. During the same period but unknown to Darwin, Gregor Mendel proposed that traits are passed from parents to offspring as discrete units. He determined the patterns of inheritance by breeding generations of garden peas. Neither Darwin nor Mendel understood how the units were passed to future generations, but we now know that the units of heredity are **genes**. So what are genes and how do they work?

gene
Sequence of DNA that encodes a protein or other functional product; the unit of heredity.

DNA AND GENES

Our bodies are made up of about 260 different types of cells, each performing different, specific tasks. Almost every cell in the body contains one nucleus that acts as the control center (only red blood cells have no nucleus). Within the nucleus is an entire set of genetic instructions stored in the form of tightly coiled, threadlike molecules

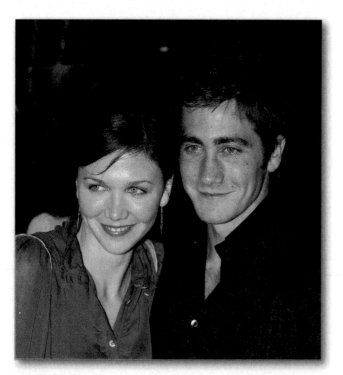

■ Family resemblance—like that between siblings Maggie and Jake Gyllenhaal—is just the most obvious indicator of all that family members share genetically.

called **deoxyribonucleic acid,** or **DNA**. If we were to uncoil the DNA (and magnify it thousands of times), we would find it consists of two long strands arranged in a double helix—a kind of spiraling ladder (Figure 2.2). DNA has four building blocks, or bases, called adenine (A), guanine (G), cytosine (C), and thymine (T). The two strands of DNA are held together with bonds between the building blocks; an A on one strand always connects to a T on the opposite strand, and a G on one strand connects to a C on the opposite strand. The consistent pairing is important—each strand is an image of the other (Figure 2.2).

deoxyribonucleic acid (DNA)
Nucleic acid molecule that contains the encoded, heritable instructions for all of a cell's activities; DNA is the genetic material passed from one generation to the next.

The complete set of DNA is called a person's **genome**. Within the nucleus, DNA is divided into 23 pairs of **chromosomes** (one set of each pair comes from each parent). One pair of chromosomes—the sex chromosomes—is slightly different and is labeled with an X or a Y rather than a number. Females have two X chromosomes; males have an X and a Y chromosome.

genome
The total set of an organism's DNA.

chromosome
Gene-carrying structure found in the nucleus of a cell, composed of tightly wound molecules of DNA.

DNA is the body's instruction book. The four bases are like a four-letter alphabet. Just as the letters in our 26-letter alphabet can be arranged to make thousands of words with different meanings, a series of thousands or millions of A-T-G-C combinations can be arranged to form a distinct message; this message is a gene. Each chromosome contains hundreds or thousands of genes located at precise points along the chromosome. Genes serve as a template and are transcribed into *RNA*, a temporary message that can travel out of the nucleus and is further translated into protein. Proteins, structures composed of amino acids arranged in a specific order, direct the activities of cells and functions of the body.

Although our cells contain the same full set of genes, most of the cells in our body become specialized—that is, they take on characteristic shapes or functions, such as skin, bone, nerve, or muscle. Genes turn on or off to regulate this activity in a process called **differentiation**. Once a cell is differentiated, it can no longer become other cell types (it is as if certain "chapters" of the DNA instruction book are locked shut). Unspecialized cells, called **stem cells**, are present in an embryo (embryonic stem cells) and are retained within tissues (adult stem cells).

differentiation
The process by which an unspecialized cell divides and gives rise to a specialized cell.

stem cell
An undifferentiated cell that is ca pable of giving rise to different types of specialized cells.

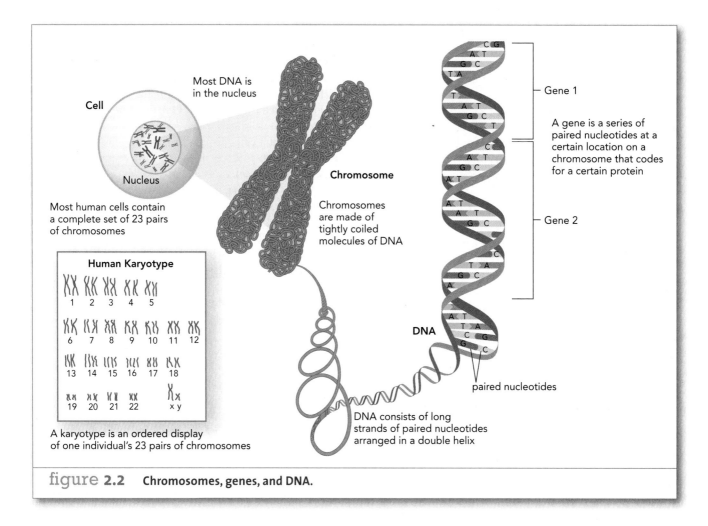

figure **2.2** **Chromosomes, genes, and DNA.**

Cell

Most human cells contain a complete set of 23 pairs of chromosomes

Nucleus

Most DNA is in the nucleus

Human Karyotype

1 2 3 4 5

6 7 8 9 10 11 12

13 14 15 16 17 18

19 20 21 22 x y

A karyotype is an ordered display of one individual's 23 pairs of chromosomes

Chromosome

Chromosomes are made of tightly coiled molecules of DNA

DNA

DNA consists of long strands of paired nucleotides arranged in a double helix

paired nucleotides

Gene 1

A gene is a series of paired nucleotides at a certain location on a chromosome that codes for a certain protein

Gene 2

THE HUMAN GENOME PROJECT

By the early 20th century, scientists had discovered chromosomes and genes and determined that DNA was the genetic material. In 1953 James Watson and Francis Crick discovered the shape and structure of DNA. By the 1980s DNA technology and knowledge reached such an advanced state that scientists began to think about the possibility of sequencing and mapping the location of all genes on the 23 chromosomes in the human genome. *Genetic sequencing* is the process of determining the order of the DNA bases (A-T-G-C) in human DNA. *Genetic mapping* is the process of determining the position of genes in relation to one another and their location on the chromosomes.

In 1990 the Human Genome Project (HGP) was launched, organized as an international, collaborative research consortium of 20 groups in six countries: China, France, Germany, Great Britain, Japan, and the United States. In 2003 the consortium announced that the sequencing of the human genome was complete. The project determined that the human genome contains approximately 2.85 billion bases and identified the sequence of 99 percent of the bases.[2]

Scientists expected humans to have some 100,000 genes, given our complexity as an organism. However, they were surprised to discover that a human has only 20,000 to 25,000 genes—the same number as a mouse.[3] Genes range in size from 2,000 to 2 million base-pairs. Another surprising finding was that only an approximate 2 percent of human DNA is used in protein-coding genes. The rest of the DNA used to be called "junk DNA." However, ongoing work of a related consortium suggests the story is more complicated. Genes may actually overlap one another and interact with genes on other chromosomes. The areas of DNA between genes, so-called junk DNA, are constantly being transcribed into RNA and contain signals and messages that are not well understood.[4]

The scientific implications of the HGP are vast, as are the potential applications in medicine and pharmaceuticals. There are also ethical, legal, and social implications of possessing such detailed genetic information about human beings. The HGP allows us to revisit age-old questions and assumptions, and it raises many new questions. For example, the HGP has allowed us to examine the relationship between race and genetics. Human genetic diversity occurs on a continuum with no clearly defined breaks between so-called racial groups. Thus the HGP has helped confirm that race is a sociocultural construct; it does not have a biological basis. Race categories are far too simple to describe the true genetic diversity of people.

As discussed in Chapter 1, health disparities between racial groups have little to do with genetic differences and more to do with culture, diet, socioeconomic status, health care access, education, and environment. However, population genetics (the study of the genetic makeup of large groups of people) does show us that some traits occur more frequently in populations from similar geographical areas of the world. Thus, until we can more clearly identify ancestral origin, race may sometimes still serve as an imperfect surrogate.[5] Other implications of genetic research are discussed in greater detail later in this chapter.

THE ROLE OF MUTATIONS

Individuals inherit one set of chromosomes from each parent and thus have two copies of each gene (excluding genes on the sex chromosome). The position of each gene is in a corresponding location on the same chromosome of every human. Every so often, changes occur in a gene; such a change is called a **mutation**. The change may involve a letter being left out (for example, a series A-T-G becomes A-G), an incorrect letter being inserted (for example, a series A-T-G becomes A-A-G), or an entire series of letters being left out, duplicated, or reversed. The location of the mutation determines the effect. If we go back to the analogy of the alphabet, consider what happens to the following sentence when a single letter change is made:

mutation
Alteration in the DNA sequence of a gene.

"When my brother came home, he lied."

If we change one letter to a "d," it can turn the sentence into nonsense:

"When my drother came home, he lied."

Or it can change the meaning entirely:

"When my brother came home, he died."

Something similar happens with a mutation in a gene. Many mutations are neither harmful nor beneficial (such as changes that lead to blue eyes or brown eyes). Other mutations may be harmful and cause disease. For example, in sickle cell disease (discussed later in the chapter), an adenine (A) is replaced by a thymine (T) in the gene for hemoglobin (a protein that carries oxygen in red blood cells). This single change at a crucial spot changes the gene's instructions and causes it to produce an altered form of hemoglobin that makes red blood cells stiff and misshapen.

While some mutations are harmful, other mutations can be beneficial or have no effect. The important thing about mutations is that they allow for human diversity. Alternative forms of the same gene are called **alleles**. Humans share 99.9 percent of the same DNA with one another. Slight differences in the remaining 0.1 percent account for all the genetic variation among humans in appearance, functioning, and health.[6]

allele
Alternate form of a gene.

Most characteristics (like height or skin color) are determined by the interaction of multiple genes at multiple sites on different chromosomes. However, some traits are determined by a single gene. To understand the relationship between genes and appearance, let's consider a single-gene trait. An individual inherits two alleles for each gene (one copy from mom, one copy from dad). The two alleles can be the same version of the gene or they may be different versions. If they are different, one version may be dominant over the other. This version is then said to be the *dominant allele*, since it will be expressed and will determine appearance. The other version is said to be a *recessive allele*—it is hidden by the dominant allele and is not expressed. A recessive allele is expressed only if both copies of the gene are the recessive version.

As an example, let's consider earlobe appearance. A single gene appears to determine whether earlobes are attached or detached. Each person has two copies of the "earlobe" gene. Let's call the two gene versions the "detached allele" and the "attached allele." The detached allele is dominant, meaning a single copy will make the earlobes appear detached (remember, if a dominant allele is present, it determines appearance). The attached allele is recessive, meaning two copies are required for the earlobes to appear attached.

This is an example of the simplest relationship between alleles. There are other possible relationships. Some alleles have incomplete dominance or codominance, meaning that both alleles affect appearance in varying degrees. Many traits

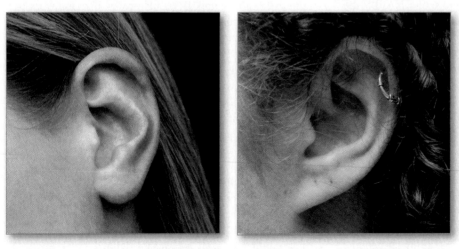

■ Earlobe appearance is an example of a trait determined by a single gene, with detached earlobes (left) dominant and attached earlobes (right) recessive. Most physical traits and conditions are determined by multiple genes interacting with each other and with environmental factors.

have more than two alleles. Most traits involve the interaction of multiple genes, each with multiple alleles.

THE INHERITANCE OF GENETIC DISORDERS

When genetic mutations occur, they can cause genetic disorders, as in the case of sickle cell disease. Genetic disorders are passed through families following certain rules or probabilities, so certain patterns in a family health tree can signal inherited disorders.

Sometimes a mutation in just one gene can cause a disease or disorder, called a **single-gene disorder**. Most disorders are caused by interactions among one or more genes and the environment; these are called **multifactorial disorders**. And some disorders are the result of alterations in entire chromosomes; these are called **chromosomal disorders.**

Single-Gene Disorders As with the innocuous characteristic of earlobe appearance, some diseases are caused by the alteration of a single gene. Although the diseases caused by single-gene mutations are rare, there are many different ones, and so, as a group, they affect a lot of people. They follow distinct patterns in family health trees depending on whether they are dominant or recessive disorders and whether they are on the **autosomal chromosomes** (chromosomes 1–22) or the **sex-linked chromosome** (chromosome X or Y).

In an *autosomal dominant disorder*, the gene is on one of the autosomal chromosomes and the disease allele is dominant, so only one copy of the disease allele is required for the disorder to be present. Thus, in a family health tree, males and females are affected equally, and the disease does not skip generations. People with an autosomal dominant disorder have a 50 percent chance of passing the condition on to their children. Hundreds of known autosomal dominant conditions exist (see the box "Sudden Death in Young Athletes").

In an *autosomal recessive disorder,* the gene is again on one of the autosomal chromosomes but the disease-causing allele is recessive, so two copies are required for a disease to be present. Thus, in a family health tree, again both males and females are affected equally, but the disease may skip generations. For a person to show signs of the disease, he or she must inherit two copies of the disease-causing allele. A person with one healthy allele and one abnormal allele will not have the disorder. This person is said to be a **carrier**, because he or she carries the abnormal gene but does not show signs of the disease. Each carrier has a 50 percent chance of passing the recessive allele on to his or her children. If two carriers have children, each child has a 25 percent chance of not receiving the disease-causing allele, a 50 percent chance of being a carrier, and a 25 percent chance of having the disease.

Sex-linked disorders follow slightly different patterns of inheritance. Most sex-linked disorders are caused by genes on the X chromosome. The Y chromosome is small and contains few genes and no known diseases. Therefore, sex-linked diseases are sometimes called *X-linked diseases*. Most are recessive. A female would need two copies of an abnormal allele for the disease to be expressed (females have two X chromosomes). If she has only one copy, she is a carrier. A male requires one copy of an abnormal allele to have the disease (males have one X and one Y chromosome). Thus X-linked diseases usually affect males.

Multifactorial Disorders Most genetic disorders are associated with interactions among multiple

single-gene disorder Disease caused by a mutation within one gene.

multifactorial disorder Disease caused by the interaction of genetic and environmental factors.

chromosomal disorder A disorder that is the result of alteration in an entire chromosome.

autosomal chromosome Any of the chromosomes (22 in humans) that do not contain genes that determine sex.

sex-linked chromosome Chromosome that includes genes that determine sex.

carrier A person who has one copy of an autosomal recessive mutation; this person shows no signs of the disease but may pass the disease on to his or her offspring.

■ Short-limb dwarfism, or achondroplasia, is an autosomal dominant, single-gene disorder that occurs in about 1 in 25,000 individuals of all ethnic groups. Mutations in a gene on chromosome 4 cause this disorder of bone development.

Highlight on Health

Sudden Death in Young Athletes

The sudden death of a high school or college athlete receives extensive media attention. Collapse and death on the playing field is catastrophic and hard to understand. Exercise and athletics are supposed to be healthy, not life-threatening.

The most common cause of these deaths is a heart condition called *hypertrophic cardiomyopathy*—a thickening of the heart muscle that increases the risk for fatal arrhythmias (abnormal heartbeats). This rare condition is inherited, often in an autosomal dominant pattern, and has been linked to mutations in 1 of 12 genes.

Each summer or early fall, thousands of athletes across the country schedule their sports physicals so that they can be screened for this condition. Hypertrophic cardiomyopathy often appears during adolescence or early adulthood. Athletes are asked if they experience symptoms such as breathlessness during exercise, chest pain, fainting spells, or rapid heart rate, and the physician or health care provider listens for a certain type of heart murmur. The physician or health care provider also asks the most important screening question: Is there a family history of hypertrophic cardiomyopathy or the sudden death from an unexplained cause in an athlete's family member?

If an abnormality is suspected, it should be evaluated fully prior to the athlete's starting training or competition, as the risk of sudden death is greatest during or immediately after exercise. If an abnormality is confirmed, the athlete may be fitted with a device that can reduce the risk of death if an arrhythmia occurs. The athlete will also need to consider modifying the type of sports in which he or she participates.

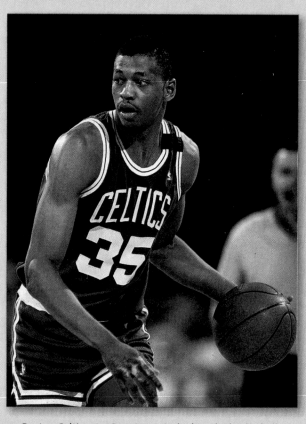

■ Boston Celtics star Reggie Lewis died on the basketball court on July 27, 1993, from sudden cardiac death, subsequently attributed to hypertropic cardiomyopathy. He was 27.

Sources: "Recommendations and Considerations Related to Preparticipation Screening for Cardiovascular Abnormalities in Competitive Athletes: 2007 Update. A Scientific Statement from the American Heart Association Council on Nutrition, Physical Activity, and Metabolism," by B.J. Maron, P.D. Thompson, M.J. Ackerman, et al., 2007, Circulation, 115, pp. 1643–1655.

genes and the interaction of those genes with environmental factors, such as tobacco smoke, pollution, and diet. These *multifactorial disorders* include heart disease, cancer, diabetes, obesity, schizophrenia, and a broad range of other disorders. Because so many diseases with a genetic component are multifactorial—they account for the majority of illnesses and deaths in the developed world—paying attention to the lifestyle and environmental factors that contribute to them is crucial. Figure 2.3 shows the relative contribution of genetic and environmental factors to a spectrum of common diseases.

To determine the relative contribution of genetic and environmental factors of a particular disease, researchers look at how often it occurs among family members of a person with that disease (by examining the family health tree) compared with how often it occurs in the general population. If a disease has a genetic link, it usually occurs more frequently among first-degree relatives (mother, father, brother, or sister) of a person with the illness than it does in the general population. These studies are called family or familial studies. Because family members often share environmental conditions as well as genes, familial studies don't necessarily provide clear-cut evidence that disorders are genetic.

More definitive findings come from twin studies. Because identical twins have the same set of genes, an illness with a significant genetic contribution should occur more frequently among them than among fraternal twins (who are only as closely genetically related as any siblings).[7]

Let's consider heart disease as an example of a multifactorial illness. Many environmental factors increase the risk for heart disease, including smoking tobacco, having a sedentary lifestyle, and being overweight. In addition, the first-degree relatives of someone suffering from heart disease have a sixfold increase in risk for heart disease over that of the general population, so it is clear that there are genetic risks as well. In families with a high risk for heart disease, there may be genetic mutations that elevate cholesterol, blood pressure, or risk of heart attack.[8, 9] Individuals

← Environmental				Genetic →
	Infections	Congenital heart disease	Diabetes	Schizophrenia
Trauma, poisoning	Teratogenic defects	Neural tube defects	Coronary heart disease	Single-gene disorders

figure **2.3** **Relative contribution of environmental and genetic factors in some common disorders.**
Source: Adapted from "Relative Contribution of Environment and Genetic Factors in Some Common Disorders," in ABC of Clinical Genetics, by Helen Kingston, 2nd Impression (revised), 1997, BMJ Publishing Group. Used by permission of Blackwell Publishing.

with this kind of genetic family history need to pay even more attention to lifestyle and environmental factors than do individuals without genetic risk.

Chromosomal Disorders In a chromosomal disorder, an entire chromosome may be added, lost, or altered. Many chromosomal disorders lead to fetal death or death in the first year of life. Because so much genetic information is involved, individuals with chromosomal abnormalities exhibit a broad set of symptoms, called a *syndrome,* ranging from characteristic physical traits to developmental delays to growth abnormalities.

In *Down syndrome,* the individual is born with an extra copy of chromosome 21. Down syndrome occurs in about 1 in every 800 live births. Risk increases with maternal age. Down syndrome can be diagnosed during pregnancy or shortly after birth. At birth, infants with Down syndrome have characteristic facial features that include low-set ears, a flat face, protruding tongue, and extra skin on the neck. A child with Down syndrome may take longer than usual to learn to walk and talk. They may also have other health problems such as heart disease, bowel problems, and an increased risk for infection.

Early diagnosis and improved health care have had a significant impact on the lives of children with Down syndrome. In 1965 a child with Down syndrome had a 50 percent chance of living to age 5. In comparison, a child born today with Down syndrome has an 80 percent chance of living to age 30 or beyond.[10, 11]

The Role of Genes in Health, Personality, and Behavior

How does genetic inheritance play out in a person's life? In this section we consider just a few examples of how individuals are shaped by their genes.

ETHNICITY AND GENETIC DISORDERS

Because of the way different human groups have moved around the planet over the course of human evolution, often remaining isolated from other groups for hundreds of generations, some genetic patterns occur more frequently in particular groups than in others (see the box "Ancestral Origin

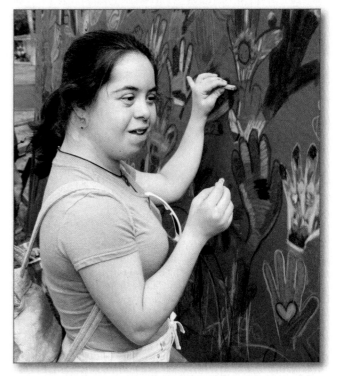

■ Down syndrome is an example of a disorder involving an entire chromosome, so many areas of functioning are affected. With improvements in treatment over the last 40 years, many individuals with Down syndrome lead satisfying and productive lives.

and Genetic Disorders"). Geneticists have used sophisticated DNA analysis to study the migration patterns of these different populations and their genetic make-up,[12] confirming that closely knit populations share genes. Thus individuals from such populations are more likely to have the same gene variants (alleles) than are individuals from other populations.

Put another way, the likelihood of sharing a genetic mutation with a partner from the same ethnic group is higher than with a partner from another ethnic group. Similarly, the risk of a child receiving the same genetic mutation from both parents is higher if both parents share the same ethnic background. The result is an increased frequency of certain inherited genetic disorders within particular ethnic groups. Sickle cell disease, Tay-Sachs disease, and cystic fibrosis are examples of this type of inheritance and highlight the importance of considering ethnicity in a family health tree.

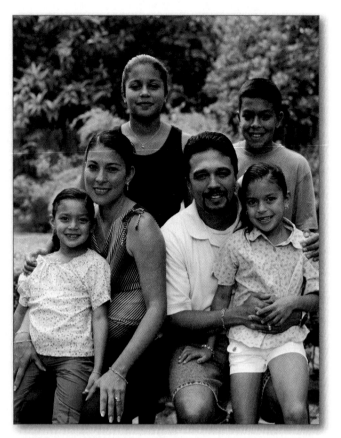

■ Certain genes, including those for genetic disorders, may be concentrated in particular ethnic groups as a result of evolutionary processes occurring over hundreds of generations. The members of this Hispanic family share some genetic traits with other people of Hispanic origin.

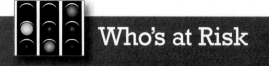

Who's at Risk

Ancestral Origin and Genetic Disorders

Some genetic variants or alleles are more likely to occur in people who trace their ancestry to a particular geographical region. Although these disorders can occur in any ethnic group or population, they occur with increased frequency in these groups.

Population group	Genetic disorder
African, African American, South or Central American, Caribbean Islander, Mediterranean, Indian, and Saudi Arabian	Sickle cell disease
Chinese and Southeast Asian	Beta thalassemia (a form of anemia)
Ashkenazi Jews (from eastern and central Europe)	Tay-Sachs disease Breast cancer gene (BRCA)
Southeast Asian, African, African American, Native American	Lactose deficiency
Southeast Asian	Acetaldehyde dehydrogenase deficiency (causes facial flushing when alcohol is consumed)
Scandinavian	Alpha-antitrypsin deficiency (a deficiency of an enzyme in the liver)
European Caucasian	Cystic fibrosis
Irish, northern European, Turkish	Phenylketonuria (PKU)

Sickle Cell Disease   An autosomal recessive disorder, sickle cell disease affects millions of people worldwide. It is most common in descendants of people who live or lived in Africa, South or Central America (especially Panama), the Caribbean islands, Mediterranean countries (such as Turkey, Greece, and Italy), India, and Saudi Arabia. As noted earlier, the disease is caused by a mutation in a gene that codes for a component of hemoglobin, the protein in red blood cells that carries oxygen (see the box "Living with Sickle Cell Disease").

About 1 in 400 African Americans has sickle cell disease, meaning that such individuals have two copies of the mutated gene. About 1 in 12 African Americans is a carrier, meaning that such individuals have one copy of the mutated gene.[13] Carriers usually do not experience symptoms, but some evidence of the disease can be seen in their blood under laboratory examination. The reason for the relatively high frequency of the sickle cell gene is that those who have it are less likely to die from malaria than are those without it. In areas where malaria has historically been a common cause of death, having the sickle cell gene is an advantage.

Tay-Sachs Disease   Another autosomal recessive disorder, Tay-Sachs disease occurs in people of Ashkenazi (eastern European) Jewish ancestry about 100 times more frequently

than in other populations. Between 1 in 27 and 1 in 30 people of Ashkenazi Jewish ancestry carry the mutated gene. Tay-Sachs disease is a fatal degenerative brain disorder. Children with Tay-Sachs disease seldom live more than a few years.

Carriers of the Tay-Sachs allele have a reduced level of a specific enzyme and can be identified by measuring the activity level of this enzyme or through DNA analysis. The widespread use of enzyme and DNA testing has made it rare for infants in the United States and Canada to be affected by Tay-Sachs disease. In fact, the incidence of Tay-Sachs disease in the Jewish population has been reduced by more than 90 percent.[14]

Cystic Fibrosis   Cystic fibrosis (CF) is another autosomal recessive disorder. It occurs much more frequently in White people of European descent than in people of other ethnic backgrounds. CF occurs in 1 of every 3,200 live births to Caucasians, 1 in 15,000 live births to African Americans, and 1 in 31,000 live births to Asian Americans.[15]

In cystic fibrosis a defective gene codes for a protein that causes the body to produce thick, sticky mucus that clogs the lungs, obstructs the pancreas, and interferes with digestion. The majority of patients are diagnosed before the age of 3. In the past, individuals with cystic fibrosis seldom survived childhood, but with advances in treatment, more are living into adulthood and even into their 50s and 60s. One promising treatment approach under active investigation is gene therapy, a technique discussed later in this chapter.

MENTAL DISORDERS

Many mental disorders are believed to have a genetic component, including schizophrenia, depression and bipolar disorder, and Alzheimer's disease.

Schizophrenia   A family link has long been suspected for schizophrenia, a mental disorder characterized by delusions (distortions in thought, not being able to determine what is real), hallucinations, disorganized speech, emotional withdrawal, and bizarre behavior. Most people who develop schizophrenia show signs by their late teens to late

20s. It affects about 1 percent of the population. Data from multiple studies are used to estimate the risk of developing schizophrenia. If a person has a sibling with the disorder, his or her risk is 8 to 10 percent. If a person has two parents with the disorder, his or her risk may be as high as 50 percent.[16]

Depression and Bipolar Disorder   Major depression and bipolar disorder also appear to have a genetic link. About 10 percent of the population will experience depression (characterized by fatigue, loss of energy, feelings of hopelessness and worthlessness, loss of interest and pleasure in daily activities, and thoughts of death or suicide) at some point in their lives. Women experience it at twice the rate of men. The first-degree relatives of a person with depression have two to three times the risk of developing depression compared to the general population.

Bipolar disorder, sometimes referred to as manic depression, is characterized by episodes of mania (euphoria, racing thoughts, excessive talkativeness, and inflated self-esteem) alternating with episodes of depression. The first-degree relatives of a person with bipolar disorder have nearly ten times the rate of the illness experienced by the general population.[17]

Challenges & Choices

Living With Sickle Cell Disease

Nearly 70,000 Americans are living with sickle cell disease. Most cases are diagnosed at birth through newborn screening. The diagnosis is important, because good health care helps people with the disorder live longer, more productive lives.

In sickle cell disease, a mutated gene causes red blood cells to become sickle-shaped (C-shaped) rather than round. The misshapen cells clump together and don't move easily through blood vessels. Clumps of cells can block blood flow to various parts of the body, causing pain, infections, and damage to organs, including the eyes, lungs, kidneys, and liver. A painful episode of blockage is called a sickle cell crisis.

Sickle cells also have a shorter lifespan than normal red blood cells (about 16 days compared to up to 120 days). This can lead to anemia, which can cause the person to feel tired, short of breath, and weak. The person may require blood transfusions if the anemia is severe.

Each person with sickle cell disease will have a different experience. Some have a very mild disease with rare crises, while others have frequent, severe crises requiring hospitalization. Regular medical care is important to reduce

pain, treat infections, provide vaccinations (for example, pneumonia and meningitis vaccines to reduce the risk of infections), and monitor for complications.

Individuals with sickle cell disease can make certain lifestyle choices that reduce the risk of problems:

- Eat a healthy diet and take a folic acid supplement to help make red blood cells
- Drink plenty of water throughout the day to stay hydrated
- Sleep regular hours and avoid stress
- Avoid extremes of hot and cold weather and high altitude
- Exercise regularly but avoid extreme exercise
- Report any signs of infection (such as a fever) immediately to your physician
- Get regular health checkups and keep vaccinations up to date

It's Not Just Personal . . .

In some areas of sub-Saharan Africa, an estimated 2 percent of children are born with sickle cell disease. An estimated 50 percent of these children will die by age 5 as a result of infection and anemia.

Sources: "What Is Sickle Cell Anemia?" National Heart, Lung, and Blood Institute, U.S. Department of Health and Human Services, National Institutes of Health, retrieved July 13, 2007, from www.nhlbi.nih.gov/health/dci/Diseases/Sca/SCA_WhatIs.html; "Sickle-Cell Anaemia," World Health Organization, 2005, retrieved July 8, 2007, from http://www.who.int/gb/ebwha/pdf_files/EB117/B117_34-en.pdf.

Alzheimer's Disease   The most common form of dementia, Alzheimer's disease is a mental disorder marked by a gradual mental deterioration that includes loss of thinking skills and memory. The disease usually begins imperceptibly, often with a decline in alertness and interest in life, and progresses to confusion, disorientation, agitation, and a loss of contact with reality. Eventually individuals lose the ability to walk, talk, or eat. Alzheimer's disease affects less than 1 percent of the population under age 65, but risk increases progressively with age, such that it affects 24 to 33 percent of people over age 85.

A gene called APOE has the strongest association with the usual form of Alzheimer's disease. Mutations in this gene increase a person's risk of developing Alzheimer's disease by two- to threefold. In a less common form called early-onset familial Alzheimer's disease, the individual exhibits symptoms of the disease before age 65. Three genes are associated with early-onset Alzheimer's; they are inherited in an autosomal dominant manner. The child of an individual with one of these genetic mutations would have a 50 percent chance of early-onset familial Alzheimer's disease.[18]

PERSONALITY AND BEHAVIOR

Currently, researchers are studying the genetic contribution to personality and behavior, looking at such characteristics as shyness, aggressiveness, sensation seeking, depression, and intelligence, to name a few.

Personality   One way to define *personality* is the sum of the mental, emotional, social, and physical characteristics of an individual. This unique, dynamic organization of characteristics influences your behavior and responses to the environment—how you communicate, react to others, and express emotions. It influences how much you exercise, study, work, play, sleep, eat, and engage in a host of other behaviors. In other words, your personality is what makes you uniquely you.

The foundation of personality is temperament, defined as a disposition that is present at birth, remains stable across the lifespan, and has a pervasive influence on a person's behavior. As the individual grows and develops and interacts with the environment, temperament is shaped into personality. Temperament seems to be the raw material for the formation of personality, and the core traits of temperament appear to be inherited.[19]

Three broad aspects of temperament are observably different across individual infants:

- *Sociability* is an individual's style of reaction to the environment. Some infants tend to withdraw from social contact, while others are eager to interact. Differences in sociability may account for shyness and introversion in some adults and friendliness and extraversion in others.
- *Reactivity* or *emotionality* is the tendency to become aroused in response to the environment. In addition, there may be differences in the tendency to experience positive emotions (happiness, joy) versus negative emotions (fear, anger). This difference may underlie optimistic versus pessimistic outlooks in adults.

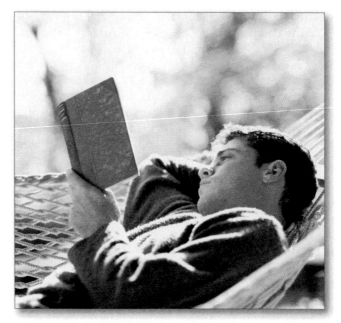

■ Personality traits like shyness or introversion may be based in core traits of temperament, which appear to be inherited and enduring across a lifetime. Differences in such traits contribute to human diversity.

- *Activity level* is the amount of response to the environment an individual puts out, in terms of intensity and speed of activity. Some infants and children are highly active and others are less so; these differences persist into adult life.

Although temperament is enduring, personality is the result of a person's life experiences. Further, no temperament type or personality style is more desirable or worthwhile than any other. The differences we observe in infants and subsequently in children, adolescents, and adults are all part of the rich diversity of the human species.

Sexual Orientation   The precise genes involved in sexual orientation have not been identified, but twin and family studies show it is at least partially heritable. Other biological factors appear to also play a role, including birth order (with the number of older brothers increasing the likelihood of male homosexual orientation), prenatal factors, and brain development. Sexual orientation appears to exist on a continuum, ranging from heterosexuality (emotional and sexual attraction to people of the other sex), to bisexuality (attraction to people of both sexes), to homosexuality (attraction to people of the same sex). It appears that factors influencing sexual orientation are different for men and women.[20]

Addiction   Also known as *dependence*, addiction involves a pathological need for a substance (or activity), usually with increasing amounts of the substance required to achieve the desired effect and unpleasant withdrawal symptoms occurring without it. Addiction to alcohol and other substances is widespread in U.S. society. Although family and environmental factors play a role in addiction, there is also clearly a genetic component. Research suggests that addiction may involve genes that lead to greater sensitivity to alcohol and

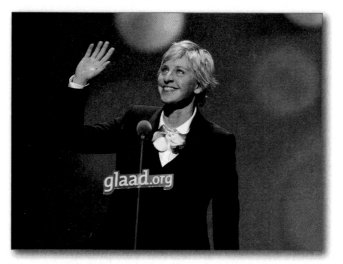

■ Sexual orientation appears to be at least partly genetic. Social and cultural factors can make it hard for people to realize they may be gay, as was the case for Ellen DeGeneres. The comedienne and talk show host has said she questioned her sexual orientation well into adulthood.

drugs, more motivation to use them, more craving for them, and greater loss of control despite negative consequences.

Of all forms of dependence, alcoholism has been the most widely studied. The tendency to become addicted to alcohol has been found to run in families. Individuals with one alcoholic parent have a higher likelihood of being alcoholics themselves, and the risks are even higher if both parents are alcoholic. When children of alcoholic parents are adopted into nonalcoholic families, their rates of alcoholism are closer to those of their biological parents than to those of their adoptive parents.[21, 22]

Ironically, the most clearly identified genes with a role in alcoholism are genes that protect against it. Three gene variations have been identified that affect the way alcohol is metabolized. These genetic variations are found at higher frequencies in Asian and Southeast Asian populations. For people with these variations, even small amounts of alcohol cause an extremely unpleasant reaction known as flushing syndrome, which includes flushing of the skin, racing heart, nausea, and headache. These effects are a deterrent to alcohol use.[22]

Environmental factors also play a critical role in the development of alcoholism, as evidenced, for example, by the fact that the great majority of children of alcoholics do not become alcoholics themselves. Environmental factors include family dynamics, psychological and personality characteristics, ethnic and cultural customs, social expectations, and a host of others.

Diagnosing and Managing a Genetic Condition

People who have or are at risk for genetic disorders have many more options than they did in the past. The first step is genetic counseling.

GENETIC COUNSELING

The purpose of genetic counseling is to help individuals and families understand the role of genetics in a particular disorder, evaluate their risks, learn about the diagnostic tests available, and discuss treatment options. In the past, genetic counseling typically took place after a genetic disorder was diagnosed. Today, as technology improves and expands, genetic counseling is often offered before a disorder is diagnosed. (See the box "Should You See a Genetic Counselor?" for more information on this topic.)

Many people who see a genetic counselor and learn about their risks decide not to be tested, partly because of the potential consequences of such testing. In some cases, there is no treatment for a genetic disorder. In other cases, people are worried about privacy issues and how their genetic information may be used. Some of these issues are discussed later in this chapter.

GENETIC TESTING

Several different types of genetic testing are available, categorized as diagnostic tests, predictive tests, carrier tests, prenatal screening tests, and newborn screening tests.

Diagnostic Tests   When an individual shows signs of an illness, a genetic test may help confirm or exclude the possibility of certain diseases. For example, if a 35-year-old man shows symptoms of dementia, a genetic test can be performed to confirm or exclude the presence of a gene mutation associated with early-onset familial Alzheimer's disease. In this situation, when the genetic test helps to confirm a diagnosis, it is called a diagnostic test.

Predictive Tests   If an individual is currently healthy but has a family history of a genetic disorder, a genetic test may be given to assess the individual's risk for developing the disease in the future. Such predictive tests are further divided into two types: presymptomatic and predispositional. **Presymptomatic tests** are for a genetic mutation that if present will *ensure* the eventual development of the disorder (that is, the mutation is inherited in an autosomal dominant pattern). **Predispositional tests** are for a genetic mutation that if present *increases the risk* for a genetic disorder but does not ensure the development of the disorder. These tests are associated with multifactorial diseases (those involving the interaction of a gene or genes with environmental factors).

Both types of predictive tests create challenges for the individuals and families who consider them. Although a presymptomatic test confirms the presence of a genetic mutation that will lead to a genetic disorder, it does little to predict when symptoms will appear or how severely

presymptomatic test
Test designed to detect a mutation that if present ensures the eventual onset of symptoms.

predispositional test
Test designed to detect a mutation that if present increases the risk of developing a disease.

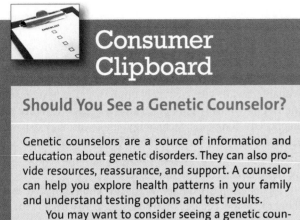

Consumer Clipboard

Should You See a Genetic Counselor?

Genetic counselors are a source of information and education about genetic disorders. They can also provide resources, reassurance, and support. A counselor can help you explore health patterns in your family and understand testing options and test results.

You may want to consider seeing a genetic counselor if

- You have a family history of a genetic condition
- Your family health tree shows a pattern suggesting for a genetic condition
- You have been diagnosed with a genetic disorder
- You know or suspect you may be a carrier of a genetic disorder
- You and your partner are having trouble getting pregnant
- You or your partner have had several miscarriages
- Prenatal screening or a diagnostic test has revealed a fetal abnormality

The National Society of Genetic Counselors is a good place to start if you are trying to find a counselor. At their Web site, www.nsgc.org, you can search by ZIP code and the distance you are willing to travel. You can search for the genetic specialty area you are interested in, such as infertility, cancer, or cardiac disease.

affected the individual will be. The predispositional tests raise even more questions at this early stage of genetic knowledge, because there is less certainty about how the presence or absence of a genetic mutation will affect a person. Both types of test, but particularly predispositional tests, have implications for society and social policy, because the leading causes of disease and disability, including cancer, heart disease, and other chronic conditions, are multifactorial in origin.

Carrier Tests   If a healthy individual has a genetic mutation for a disorder that is inherited in an autosomal recessive or X-linked recessive manner, the individual is said to be a carrier, as discussed earlier. If a genetic test is available to look for that recessive gene, it is called a carrier test. A carrier test may be offered to a healthy individual with a family member who has a certain genetic disorder or who has been identified as a carrier. Carrier tests are also offered to individuals in certain racial and ethnic groups that are known for having high carrier rates for disorders such as sickle cell disease, Tay-Sachs disease, and cystic fibrosis.

Prenatal Screening Tests   As part of prepregnancy planning or during routine pregnancy care, women are assessed in some manner for their risk of genetic or chromosomal diseases. If either member of a couple has a family history of a genetic disease or belongs to a population with a high incidence of an autosomal recessive disease, the couple is counseled on the risks and benefits of genetic screening. Women are also routinely offered a blood test called a *triple screen* during the early part of pregnancy. This test cannot diagnose a genetic condition but can suggest an increased risk for a neural tube defect (problem with the spinal cord) or chromosomal abnormality. In the case of an abnormal result, the woman will be referred on for an ultrasound and a test to assess fetal chromosomes (*amniocentesis* or *chorionic villus sampling*). As the risk for chromosomal abnormalities increases with age, pregnant women over age 35 are routinely offered testing to evaluate fetal chromosomes.

Although prenatal screening is commonplace today, the results can create a challenging situation for the prospective parents. For example, amniocentesis can tell them that their fetus has Down syndrome, but it cannot tell them how functional the child will be. Many children who have a genetic disease lead happy, productive lives with their own unique limitations and challenges. Genetic testing during pregnancy does, however, allow parents time to prepare for the upcoming birth.

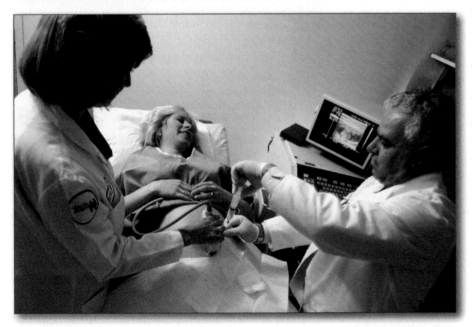

■ Amniocentesis is a prenatal screening procedure in which fluid is drawn from the amniotic sac to test for genetic disorders, birth defects, and fetal health problems.

Newborn Screening Tests Newborn screening for phenylketonuria (PKU) is a model of successful genetic testing. Screening began in the 1960s for this autosomal recessive mutation. A child with two copies of the mutated gene is unable to process an amino acid called phenylalanine, which is in many foods. If a child with PKU consumes too much phenylalanine, toxic chemicals build up that cause seizuers and severe mental retardation. If the condition is detected at birth and the child is placed in a diet that restricts phenylalanine, the child can develop normally. At present, all states require newborn screening for PKU.

Newborn screening has expanded since the initial introduction of PKU screening. The American College of Medical Genetics has identified 29 core treatable conditions for which it recommends all newborns be screened. In the United States, each state can determine which of the tests it will offer; as of 2007, 90 percent of babies live in states that require screening for at least 21 of the 29 conditions. However, that means that roughly 10 percent of babies are still not having the benefit of being screened for easily identifiable, treatable conditions.[23]

MANAGEMENT AND TREATMENT

Treatments are available for a number of genetic disorders. They include dietary modification, medications, environmental adaptations, and gene therapy.

Dietary Modification Some genetic disorders can be fully or partially treated through dietary modification, whether restriction, exclusion, or supplementation.

- *Restriction* is called for when a common food is toxic to a person with a genetic mutation, as in the case of phenylketonuria.

- *Exclusion* is required when a person has a life-threatening reaction to a particular food, as in certain food allergies. Some people are allergic to even minuscule amounts of shellfish or peanuts, and these foods have to be completely excluded from their diet.

- *Supplementation* is helpful for some genetic disorders. In cystic fibrosis, for example, the fat-soluble vitamins A, D, E, and K are poorly absorbed, so individuals with this disorder benefit from taking vitamin supplements.

Medications For some genetic disorders, drugs can decrease symptoms or prevent serious complications. For instance, people with hemophilia, who are missing a blood-clotting factor, can take a synthetic form of the factor. People at high risk of colon cancer due to hereditary colon polyps can take anti-inflammatory medicines to decrease the risk.

Environmental Adaptations Avoiding harmful environmental factors can be effective in managing many genetic disorders. People with albinism, for example, have an increased risk of skin cancer because they lack normal pigment in the skin, hair, and eyes; they have to avoid sun exposure more than others must. Individuals with a genetic predisposition for diabetes can lower their risk for the disorder by maintaining a healthy weight.

Gene Therapy Although the treatments just described have helped people with genetic diseases to live better lives, they do not eliminate or cure the genetic disease. In 1972 scientists proposed replacing defective genes with healthy ones, which would treat or eliminate the cause of disease rather than simply treating symptoms of disease.[24] In theory, the healthy gene, once inserted into a cell, would provide the instructions for the cell to produce the protein that the defective gene was unable to produce.

Scientists optimistically envision a future in which heart disease or cancer can be cured by injections of healthy DNA. Remember, however, that cells are microscopic and DNA is even smaller. The minuscule section of DNA that makes up the healthy gene must be collected and then somehow inserted into the cell without destroying the cell. The healthy gene then must incorporate itself into the cell's DNA in such a way as to function.

Many challenges arise during this process. A major challenge is delivering the healthy gene to the cells where it is needed. One technique is to remove cells from a patient, insert the healthy gene in the cells, grow the cells in a culture dish, and then place them back into the patient. The cells studied are usually stem cells. Another technique is to use a virus to carry a healthy gene into a cell that has an abnormal gene. Viruses function by injecting their genetic material into host cells and getting the host cell to incorporate the virus's genes into its own DNA and replicate the virus. Scientists can exploit a virus's ability to infect cells by putting a healthy gene into a virus. When the virus is injected into the patient, it releases the healthy, desired gene into the cells, which theoretically then start replicating the healthy gene. The gene, in turn, starts encoding the protein needed for the cell to do its job (Figure 2.4).

Gene therapy via viral transport is still in an early research stage and is not ready to be widely used. Aside from potentially fatal immune responses, other problems associated with viral transport need to be solved, including how to ensure that the healthy gene will work once it is inside the cell and how to transport a gene that is larger than a virus.

Implications of Genetic Research for Individuals and Society

Genetic research has conferred benefits on individuals, families, and society (see "Disease Outbreaks and Genetics"). At the same time, it has raised troubling issues. In this section we consider both aspects of our advancing genetic knowledge and technology.

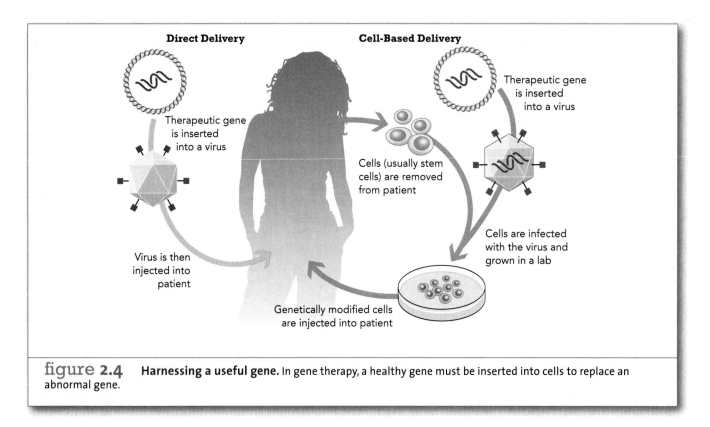

figure 2.4 **Harnessing a useful gene.** In gene therapy, a healthy gene must be inserted into cells to replace an abnormal gene.

MEDICAL ADVANCES AND CURES

The face of medicine will probably change dramatically in the next few decades, with genetic diagnosis and treatment becoming part of routine health care. Some people envision a day when the family health tree will be replaced by a personal genetic profile, created by mapping and sequencing all of an individual's genes. Physicians could then provide personalized recommendations for lifestyle choices and medical screenings based on individual risk, rather than broad public health recommendations.

Research on genes and the proteins they produce may also expand and be applied to more and more genetic diseases. Research on gene therapy for cystic fibrosis, for example, has already had some success in depositing healthy genes that produce the proteins needed for normal lung function in the damaged airway cells of CF patients.

Another line of research is under way in muscle wasting diseases, such as muscular dystrophy. In the most common form of this disease, Duchenne muscular dystrophy, a defective gene leads to the absence of a protein, dystrophin, that protects muscles against the damage caused by everyday use. As muscle fibers are injured and die, patients become increasingly weak and debilitated. A similar loss of muscle occurs in natural aging but over a much longer period of time. Researchers have experimented with injecting synthetic genes that produce a muscle growth factor into muscle cells to hasten repair. Such therapies could have applications not only in curing muscular diseases but in slowing down or preventing muscle loss in older adults.

As promising as these prospects are, some gene therapies may be subject to misuse. An example is *gene dop-*

ing. Athletes wishing to build muscle and increase strength beyond what they can accomplish through training may someday be able to use the techniques developed to treat muscular dystrophy.[25] Unlike the effects of performance-enhancing drugs, gene therapy could be confined to the muscle into which the gene was injected and would be virtually untraceable. If such genetic enhancement were to become common practice, the climate of athletics and sport would undoubtedly be quite different from what it is today.

ISSUES IN GENETIC SCREENING AND TESTING

Other issues arise in the context of genetic screening and testing. The understanding of genes and genetic disorders has far outpaced treatments and cures. Most people don't want to know they have a defective gene that might cause them harm if there is nothing they can do about it. Thus, in many instances, testing is not recommended even when a defective gene can be identified, as in the case of the gene for Alzheimer's disease. In such cases, genetic information may cause alarm and anxiety without, as yet, offering hope for a treatment or cure.

Further issues arise in the context of prenatal screening. Some physicians have reservations about offering tests because they feel it puts pressure on parents to consider abortion as an option. Offering prenatal screening for certain non-life-threatening conditions, such as deafness, may convey the idea that these conditions are diseases. Another issue for physicians is the concern that parents may sue them for malpractice if they fail to offer a particular screening test, especially if offering the test becomes standard practice in some states.

Public Health in Action

Disease Outbreaks and Genetics

- A girl in New York is admitted to the hospital with bloody diarrhea.
- An elderly man in Oregon visits his health clinic with diarrhea and dehydration.
- Three college students in Texas are evaluated at their student health center for fevers and diarrhea.

What do these people have in common? And what does it have to do with genetics?

It is possible that all of these people ate food contaminated with a disease-causing bacteria, such as *E. coli* 0157:H7, *Shigella*, *Salmonella*, or *Listeria*. Each of these bacteria can cause bloody diarrhea, fever, and severe illness. In the past, when food was locally produced and eaten, it was easier to identify outbreaks of food-borne infections—everyone who was ill might have eaten at the same restaurant or church social. With current food production practices—foods being prepared and packaged in one location and then distributed widely across the United States or world—it is much more difficult. These individuals with diarrhea may have eaten the same brand of peanut butter or prepack-

aged salad mix. The physicians involved in their care may do a great job caring for each individual, but they would not be aware of the other cases and thus not be able to prevent more people from becoming infected.

How can we know if cases of foodborne illness are past of a widespread outbreak? This is where genetics comes in. Bacteria have DNA and genes. As an example, let's consider *Shigella*. There are different *Shigella* strains, slightly different subtypes that arise due to genetic mutations. If each person was infected from the same source, we would expect their *Shigella* subtypes to look genetically very similar. If they were unrelated infections, the *Shigella* subtypes would be different.

In response to changing patterns of food distribution and with the increasing understanding of genetics, a program was initiated in the 1990s to aid in detecting foodborne disease outbreaks. PulseNet, a national network of laboratories and public health agencies, performs genetic testing of food-borne disease-causing bacteria. Using DNA technology, the laboratories will "fingerprint" the bacteria and send the information to a database at the Centers for Disease Control and Prevention. DNA patterns that come in from around the country are compared. If the number of submitted samples increases, and the samples have a similar DNA fingerprint, the bacteria may have come from the same source and an outbreak may be occuring. A computer alert activates health agencies so that they can evaluate cases for possible links. Ill people are interviewed to determine if they have eaten similar foods.

If a common food is identified, public health personnel can go to homes, collect samples of food, and test to see if bacteria with the same DNA profile are found. If so, further illness can be prevented through recall of contaminated food and warnings issued to the general public not to eat that product. Inspectors can also backtrack to see where in the preparation and distribution process food was contaminated in order to pervent further disease outbreaks.

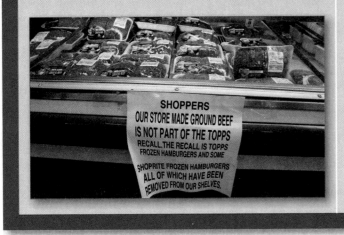

> SHOPPERS
> OUR STORE MADE GROUND BEEF
> IS NOT PART OF THE TOPPS
> RECALL. THE RECALL IS TOPPS
> FROZEN HAMBURGERS AND SOME
> SHOPRITE FROZEN HAMBURGERS
> ALL OF WHICH HAVE BEEN
> REMOVED FROM OUR SHELVES.

Source: PulseNet, U.S. Department of Health and Human Services, Centers for Disease Control and Prevention, retrieved July 24, 2007, from www.cdc.gov/pulsenet/.

ISSUES OF PRIVACY AND DISCRIMINATION

Another area of concern is the possibility of discrimination based on genetic information. Individuals who undergo genetic testing may find that they are not the only ones interested in detailed genetic information about themselves; employers and health insurance companies may also be interested in that information.

In the workplace, genetic testing has two potentially beneficial uses: It can be used to determine whether an employee is at increased risk for developing a disease if exposed to specific factors in the work environment, and it can be used to monitor a worker's genetic make-up for changes during his or her employment, thus helping to identify hazardous materials and increase worker safety. Neither of these has been shown to be clearly

useful.[26] The down side of genetic testing in the workplace is that employers may use the information to withhold promotions or refuse to hire a person—for example, someone who appears to be at risk for developing a disease or disability.

Genetic information is also of interest to insurance companies, who use information about risk for disease to help determine whom to cover and how much to charge for health insurance. There have been many cases in which people were denied health insurance because of genetic information. In response, recommendations have been made by different organizations to prohibit health insurers from using genetic information to limit or deny coverage.

Currently the Health Insurance Portability and Accountability Act (HIPAA), enacted in 1996, provides federal protection against genetic discrimination in health insurance. HIPAA prohibits group health plans from using past or current medical conditions, including genetic information, as a basis for denying or limiting an individual's coverage. It also states that genetic information in the absence of a current diagnosis may not be considered a preexisting condition. These protections apply only to employer-based and commercially issued group health insurance, however. No similar law exists for individuals seeking health insurance on their own.[27]

In response to gaps in the current protections, a majority of states have proposed genetic nondiscrimination bills, and federal legislation, the Genetic Information Nondiscrimination Act of 2008, has been passed by Congress and awaits consideration by the president.[28] In Canada, human rights laws and insurance laws are believed to offer some protection against genetic discrimination. However, there remains an absence of statutes and regulations that specifically address genetic testing information.[29]

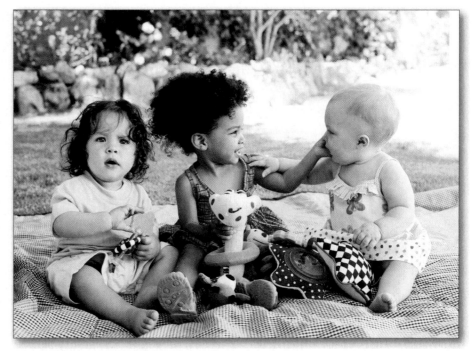

■ If parents were able to select the traits they want in their children, what would they select? How would it affect the human species as a whole?

EUGENICS

Yet another area of concern associated with genetic information is *eugenics*, the practice of selective breeding, or controlling a group's reproductive choices, in an attempt to improve the human species. A popular idea in the late 19th century, eugenics was carried to an extreme by the Nazis during World War II, and it continues to occur in troubled places around the world under the guise of ethnic cleansing.

Genetic testing and genetic screening during pregnancy has paved the way for a potential new eugenics movement. When this technology is used by parents to reduce the risk of their child facing a debilitating disease, many (but not all) are comfortable. However, the technology could also be used to allow parents to select the traits they want in their child—high intelligence, athletic ability, physical appearance, and so on. Although this kind of eugenics may be different in the sense that parents are making decisions about their children's and family's future rather than hav-

ing standards imposed on them by a state, such practices may change how we as a society view qualities and flaws in appearance, personality, and the other varied dimensions of human difference.[30]

GENETICS, LIFESTYLE CHOICES, AND PERSONAL HEALTH

We conclude this chapter by reiterating the point we made at the outset: Genetics is simply the starting point of personal health. It determines potential but not outcome. Healthy genes do not guarantee a healthy life, nor does a genetic defect lead inevitably to a life of disability. Our genes are only one part of our overall wellness profile; other significant factors include individual lifestyle choices, socioeconomic factors, and sociocultural factors.

If you choose to explore your personal genetics, either by completing a family health tree or by having genetic tests done (for one of the reasons discussed in this chapter), keep in mind that this information is best used in helping you decide how to balance your health choices. Knowledge of your unique strengths and weaknesses, genetic and otherwise, can help you assess the risks and benefits of your actions and make the decisions that are right for you.

You Make the Call

Should Embryonic Stem Cell Research Be Supported?

Scientists believe that stem cells have the potential for a wide range of applications, including treatment of diabetes, many cancers, and genetic and neurological diseases like Parkinson's disease and Alzheimer's disease. However, the source of stem cells to be used in research is a subject of debate. Of further debate is whether federal funds should support such research.

Stem cells, undifferentiated cells with the potential for unlimited division, can be derived from either embryonic or adult sources. Embryonic stem cells come from human embryos, usually supplied by fertility clinics. In the process of infertility treatment, fertilized eggs are allowed to develop in culture for 4–5 days to the blastocyst stage (a ball of 70–100 cells). It is common for extra blastocysts to be created and frozen until a couple decides to use them (by implantation into the uterus), donate them (for use by another infertile person), destroy them, or donate them for research purposes. If a person or couple elects to donate the embryo for research, cells from the blastocyst are allowed to grow, producing millions of embryonic stem cells—referred to as an embryonic *stem cell line*.

Adult stem cells are found in many tissues and organs in the adult body. They differ in several ways from embryonic stem cells:

- Embryonic stem cells can differentiate into all cell types in the body, but adult stem cells are generally limited to the cells types of their tissue of origin thus are less versatile.

- Embryonic stem cells can be grown relatively easily in culture, creating millions of cells. Adult stem cells are rare, their isolation is difficult, and they are more difficult to culture in large numbers.

- Many scientists believe embryonic stem cells have greater potential than adult stem cells because of their greater versatility.

What is the controversy about? Opponents of embryonic stem cell research believe that it is unacceptable to destroy human embryos in pursuit of any goal, no matter how noble. President George W. Bush referred to embryonic stem cell research as "crossing a fundamental moral line" by sanctioning the destruction of human embryos that "have at least a potential for life." In 2001 the Bush administration restricted federal funding of stem cell research to adult stem cell lines and embryonic stem cell lines that existed prior to that date.

Supporters argue that while embryos represent the potential for human life, there are people already alive who are suffering from diseases and who could benefit from this research. They point out that according to most definitions, pregnancy begins when a blastocyst implants in the lining of the uterus, usually about a week after fertilization; until this point, the cluster of cells cannot really be considered potential human life. Proponents further claim that the existing embryonic stem cell lines are insufficient for the research that could be done, and they dispute the number of usable lines. They also point out that adult stem cells do not have the vast potential of embryonic stem cells.

In addition, supporters warn that without a nationally sanctioned embryonic stem cell research program, other countries will outpace the United States, making advances in medicine and technology and luring U.S. scientists to their labs. They also argue that a nationally sanctioned research program would impose uniform standards on researchers who may be working now with few constraints. A January 2007 public opinion poll indicated that 61 percent of Americans support the use of embryonic stem cells in medical research, while 31 percent oppose it.

Embryonic stem cell research might hold out hope for millions, but opponents question the moral and ethical cost. What do you think?

PROS

- Embryonic stem cell research may eventually lead to therapies that could be used to treat diseases that afflict millions of people.

- Embryonic stem cells are derived from excess embryos created in the course of infertility treatment. Individuals must eventually decide the fate of their excess embryos, and many people are willing to donate them for research purposes.

- Adult stem cell research has resulted in therapeutic treatments. Scientists believe embryonic stem cells hold even greater promise.

- If federal funding is restricted, states and private organizations may proceed in a less regulated fashion.

CONS

- There are already more than 60 human embryonic stem cell lines in existence, and federal funds can be used for research on these lines.

- Using adult stem cell lines does not involve the moral dilemma associated with use of human embryos.

- Current federal guidelines are intended to provide a uniform national policy.

- If scientists are allowed to create new embryonic stem cell lines, there may be an incentive for the creation of embryos specifically for this purpose.

Sources: "Public Opinion Snapshot: Solid Backing for Embryonic Stem Cell Research," Center for American Progress, 2007, retrieved February 14, 2008, from www.americanprogress.org/issues/2007/03/opinion_ stem_cells.html; "Stem Cell Basics," National Institutes of Health, 2006, retrieved February 14, 2008, from http://stemcells.nih.gov/info/basics.

In Review

1. **Why is it important to know your family health history and understand your genetic inheritance?** There are two broad reasons: (1) to identify any areas where you may have an inherited predisposition for a health problem so that you have the opportunity to make informed lifestyle choices and (2) to know if your unborn children are at increased risk for any genetic diorders so that you have the opportunity to address issues associated with those disorders.

2. **How do genes affect your health?** Although some diseases and disorders are caused by a single gene, most genetic disorders are multifactorial; that is, they are associated with interactions among several genes and interactions of genes with environmental factors, such as tobacco smoke, diet, and air pollution. Even if you have a genetic predisposition for a disease, you may never get that disease if the environmental factors are not present.

3. **Why do some genetic disorders occur more frequently in certain ethnic or racial groups?** Because of the way different human populations have migrated around the globe over hundreds of generations, certain mutations and genetic patterns have become concentrated in certain groups. Often, a mutation that causes a disorder has persisted in the gene pool because it also provides some advantage in a particular environment.

4. **What are the benefits and potential pitfalls of genetic research and its applications?** Some experts foresee a day when every individual will have a personalized genetic profile that will allow physicians to provide highly customized medical treatment and lifestyle recommendations, rather than broad public health recommendations. The main concern about this possibility is that genetic information may be used to dicriminate against people in employment and insurance situations.

WWW For a detailed summary of this chapter and a comprehensive set of review questions, visit the Online Learning Center at **www.mhhe.com/teague2e**.

Web Resources

Access Excellence Resource Center: Associated with the U.S. Department of Health and Human Services, this national educational program provides health, biology, and life sciences information. It offers answers to questions such as the following: What are genes? What is genetic testing? How do gene mistakes occur? www.accessexcellence.org

Child Welfare Information Gateway: This is a good place to start if you are looking for information about your biological parents. www.childwelfare.gov

Gene Tests: This site offers authoritative information on genetic testing and its use in the diagnosis and management of disease and genetic counseling. Funded by the National Institutes of Health, it promotes the appropriate use of genetic services in patient care and personal decision making. www.genetests.org

Genetics Society of America: This organization includes more than 4,000 scientists and educators in the field of genetics. Through its journal *Genetics*, it publishes information on advances in genetics. www.genetics-gsa.org

Gene Watch UK: Featuring developments in genetic technologies from the perspective of public interest, environmental protection, and animal welfare, this group explores topics ranging from genetically modified crops and foods to genetic testing in humans. www.genewatch.org

National Human Genome Research Institute: The leader of the Human Genome Project for the National Institutes of Health, this institute continues to do research in genetics aimed at improving human health and fighting diseases. www.genome.gov

National Society of Genetic Counselors: This society offers FAQs about genetic counselors, such as: What is a genetic counselor? How do I find a genetic counselor near me? What can you expect on a first visit to a genetic counselor? www.nsgc.org

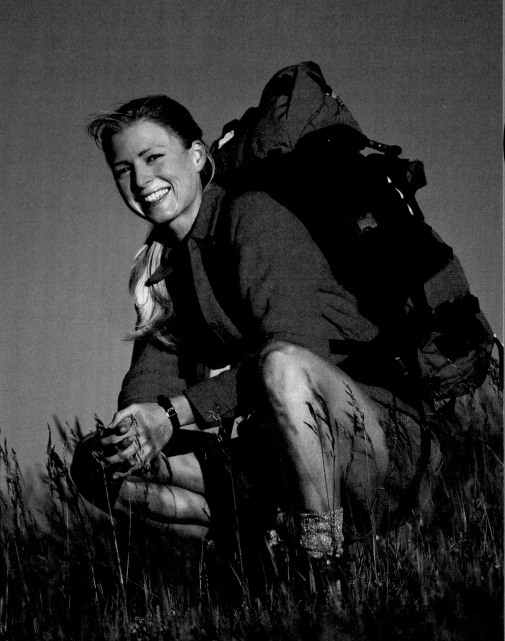

Chapter 3

Mental Health
Creating
a Balance

Ever Wonder...

- what it means to be "mentally healthy," as opposed to "mentally ill"?

- if you have ever been clinically depressed or were just feeling down?

- if you could benefit from psychotherapy?

WWW

Your Health Today

www.mhhe.com/teague2e

Go to the Online Learning Center for *Your Health Today* for interactive activities, quizzes, flashcards, Web links, and more resources related to this chapter.

Mental health encompasses several aspects of overall health and wellness. It can include the emotional, psychological, cognitive, interpersonal, and/or spiritual aspects of a person's life. It includes the capacity to respond to challenges, frustrations, joys, and failures in ways that allow continued growth and forward movement in life. The key to mental health and happiness is not freedom from adversity in life—no one goes through life without some experience of loss, pain, guilt, or regret—but rather the ability to respond to adversity in adaptive, effective ways. A mentally healthy person is able to deal with life's inevitable challenges without becoming impaired or overwhelmed by them.

The majority of people are mentally healthy, but many experience emotional or psychological difficulties at some point in their lives, and mental disorders are fairly common. More than 26 percent of the adult American population—more than 57 million people, or one in four Americans—are affected by a diagnosable mental disorder in a given year.[1] An estimated 50 percent of Americans experience some symptoms of depression during their lifetime. Many people have symptoms of more than one mental disorder at a given time, such as depression, anxiety, and substance abuse. Mental disorders are the leading cause of disability for people aged 15–44 in both the United States and Canada.

What Is Mental Health?

Like physical health, mental health is not just the absence of illness but also the presence of many positive characteristics and traits. In this section we consider a variety of ways in which mental health and mentally healthy people can be conceptualized.

POSITIVE PSYCHOLOGY AND CHARACTER STRENGTHS

Psychologists have long been interested in such positive human characteristics as optimism, attachment, love, and emotional intelligence, but in recent years this interest has coalesced in the **positive psychology** movement. Rather than focusing on mental illness and problems, positive psychologists focus on positive emotions, character strengths, and conditions that create happiness—in short, "what makes life worth living."[2] By investigating such topics as gratitude, forgiveness, awe, inspiration, hope, curiosity, humor, and happiness, positive psychologists strive to understand the full spectrum of human experience. (For more on these topics, see Chapter 4.)

positive psychology
Area of interest within the field of psychology that focuses on positive emotions, character strengths, and conditions that create happiness.

One outcome of this research has been the identification of a set of character strengths and virtues that "enable human thriving" and that are endorsed by nearly all cultures across the world.[3] The six broad virtues are wisdom, courage, humanity, justice, temperance, and transcendence. Under each virtue are particular strengths that meet numerous other criteria. For example, they contribute to individual fulfillment and satisfaction, they are valued in their own right and not as a means to an end, they do not diminish others, and they are deliberately cultivated by individuals and societies. The most commonly endorsed strengths are kindness, fairness, authenticity, gratitude, and open-mindedness. The character strengths and virtues are described in Table 3.1. Which ones are your top strengths? How can you use them more often in your daily life?

CHARACTERISTICS OF MENTALLY HEALTHY PEOPLE

People who are described as mentally healthy have certain characteristics in common (often expressions of the character strengths and virtues):

- They have high **self-esteem** and feel good about themselves.
- They are realistic and accepting of imperfections in themselves and others.
- They are altruistic; they help others.
- They have a sense of control over their lives and feel capable of meeting challenges and solving problems.

self-esteem
Sense of positive regard and valuation for oneself.

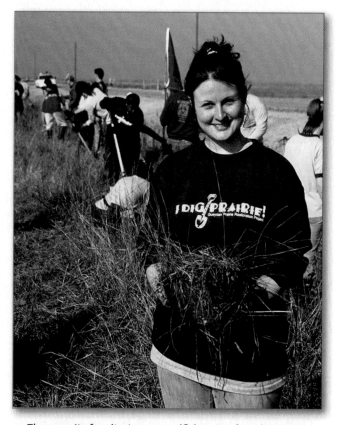

■ The capacity for altruism—unselfish caring for others—is associated with psychological health. These volunteers are working to restore native habitats in Louisiana, showing their concern for the earth and for future generations.

Table 3.1	Classification of 6 Virtues and 24 Character Strengths	
Virtue and Strength	**Definition**
1. Wisdom and knowledge	**Cognitive strengths that entail the acquisition and use of knowledge**
Creativity	Thinking of novel and productive ways to do things
Curiosity	Taking an interest in all of ongoing experience
Open-mindedness	Thinking things through and examining them from all sides
Love of learning	Mastering new skills, topics, and bodies of knowledge
Perspective	Being able to provide wise counsel to others
2. Courage	**Emotional strengths that involve the exercise of will to accomplish goals in the face of opposition, external or internal**
Authenticity	Speaking the truth and presenting oneself in a genuine way
Bravery	Not shrinking from threat, challenge, difficulty, or pain
Persistence	Finishing what one starts
Zest	Approaching life with excitement and energy
3. Humanity	**Interpersonal strengths that involve "tending and befriending" others**
Kindness	Doing favors and good deeds for others
Love	Valuing close relations with others
Social intelligence	Being aware of the motives and feelings of self and others
4. Justice	**Civic strengths that underlie healthy community life**
Fairness	Treating all people the same according to notions of fairness and justice
Leadership	Organizing group activities and seeing that they happen
Teamwork	Working well as a member of a group or team
5. Temperance	**Strengths that protect against excess**
Forgiveness	Forgiving those who have done wrong
Modesty	Letting one's accomplishments speak for themselves
Prudence	Being careful about one's choices; *not* saying or doing things that might later be regretted
Self-regulation	Regulating what one feels and does
6. Transcendence	**Strengths that forge connections to the larger universe and provide meaning**
Appreciation of beauty and excellence	Noticing and appreciating beauty, excellence, and/or skilled performance in all domains of life
Gratitude	Being aware of and thankful for the good things that happen
Hope	Expecting the best and working to achieve it
Humor	Liking to laugh and tease; bringing smiles to other people
Religiousness	Having coherent beliefs about the higher purpose and meaning of life

Source: From Character Strengths and Virtues: A Handbook and Classification, *by C. Peterson and M. Seligman, 2004, Washington, DC: American Psychological Association.*

- They demonstrate social competence in their relationships with others, and they are comfortable with other people and believe they can rely on them.
- They are not overwhelmed by fear, love, or anger; they try to control irrational thoughts and levels of stress.
- They are optimistic; they try to maintain a positive outlook.
- They have a capacity for intimacy; they do not fear commitment.
- They are creative and appreciate creativity in others.
- They take reasonable risks in order to grow.
- They bounce back from adversity.

THE SELF-ACTUALIZED PERSON

Many of these healthy characteristics are found in the self-actualized person. The concept of **self-actualization** was developed by Abraham Maslow in the 1960s as a model of human personality development in his "hierarchy of needs" theory (Figure 3.1). Maslow proposed that once people meet their needs for survival, safety and security, love and belonging, and achievement and

self-actualization
In Maslow's work, the state attained when a person has reached his or her full potential.

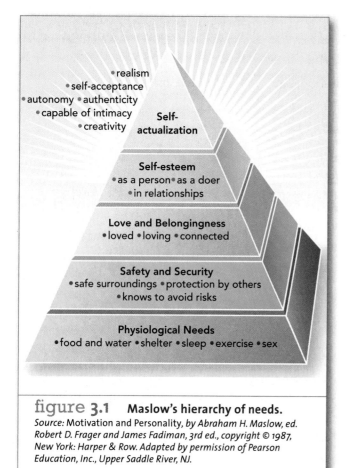

figure 3.1 Maslow's hierarchy of needs.

Source: Motivation and Personality, *by Abraham H. Maslow, ed. Robert D. Frager and James Fadiman, 3rd ed., copyright © 1987, New York: Harper & Row. Adapted by permission of Pearson Education, Inc., Upper Saddle River, NJ.*

self-esteem, they have opportunities for self-exploration and expression that can lead them to reach their fullest human potential. According to Maslow, a self-actualized person is realistic, self-accepting, self-motivated, creative, and capable of intimacy, among other traits. Those who reach this level achieve a state of transcendence, a sense of a well-being that comes from finding purpose and meaning in life. To assess your own progress toward self-actualization, see the Chapter 3 Add It Up feature at the back of the book.

OPTIMISM, SELF-EFFICACY, AND RESILIENCE

A key characteristic of mentally healthy people is *optimism.* People with an "optimistic explanatory style"—the tendency to see problems as temporary and specific rather than permanent and general—seem to have better physical and mental health than more pessimistic people do.[4] Optimistic people react to failures as things they can do something about, as challenges and opportunities for learning and growth. Pessimistic people tend to attribute failure to personal defects and react with discouragement and a sense of defeat. (Of course, you also need to be realistic and recognize your own limitations; a person who disregards all the incoming information provided by successes and failures will end up only with more disappointment.)

Related to optimism is *self-efficacy,* a general sense that you have some control over what happens in your life.

Mentally healthy people have a basic belief that they can guide their own lives and take unexpected events in stride, adapt, and move on.

This ability to bounce back from adverse events is known as **resilience**, and it is another characteristic of mentally healthy individuals. People who can respond flexibly to life's challenges and redirect their energies toward positive actions tend to be more successful in life. Our lives will always have moments of adversity and vulnerability and be filled with challenging situations. Individuals who are resilient learn ways to respond to these events and situations. Resilience involves patterns of thinking, feeling, and behaving that contribute to a balanced life based on self-esteem, satisfying relationships, and a belief that life is meaningful. Resilience research over the past two decades has suggested that most children, even those growing up in very difficult and challenging situations, not only survive but are able to build very positive lives for themselves. These children were found to be able to overcome adversity because of the protective factors or buffers that were also part of their lives.[5]

resilience
Ability to bounce back from adversity.

EMOTIONAL INTELLIGENCE

Intelligence is commonly thought of as a person's general capacity for reasoning, solving problems, and performing other mental functions accurately and efficiently. As such, intelligence can be measured by tests like the Stanford-Binet Intelligence Test, which gives a person a score referred to as an intelligence quotient (IQ). If you score above 100 on this test, you are considered to be of above-average intelligence; if you score below 100, you are considered below average.

The concept of intelligence was expanded by psychologist Howard Gardner, who argued that the traditional definition of intelligence does not encompass all the abilities human beings are known to have.[6] In his theory of **multiple intelligences**, Gardner proposed eight different types of intelligence: linguistic, logical-mathematical, naturalist, spatial, bodily-kinesthetic, musical, interpersonal, and intrapersonal. Additional intelligences have also been proposed, such as spiritual intelligence. Although Gardner's theory has been criticized for lack of empirical support, it has been widely accepted by educators and applied in classrooms.[7]

multiple intelligences
In Gardner's work, the many areas in which intelligence can be manifested, such as logical-mathematical, spatial, and interpersonal.

emotional intelligence
In Goleman's work, the kind of intelligence that includes an understanding of emotional experience, self-awareness, and sensitivity to others.

The concept of intelligence was further expanded by psychologist Daniel Goleman to include the idea of **emotional intelligence**. Goleman argued that such qualities as self-awareness, self-discipline, persistence, and empathy are much more important to success in life than IQ. People who are emotionally intelligent have an ability to (1) recognize, name, and understand their emotions, (2) manage their emotions and control their moods, (3) motivate themselves, (4) recognize and respond to emotions in others, and (5) be socially competent.[8] The last ability involves skills in understanding relationships, cooperating, solving problems, resolving conflicts, being assertive at communicating, and being considerate and compassionate.[9]

Whereas qualities such as resilience and optimism pertain more to internal characteristics, emotional intelligence involves how you relate to others. Like many of the other characteristics of mentally healthy people, emotional intelligence can be learned and improved. Many groups, workshops, and self-help books assist people in learning how to control impulses, manage anger, recognize emotions in themselves and others, and respond more appropriately in social situations.

ENHANCING YOUR MENTAL HEALTH

Several other factors appear to be related to the development of mental health:

- A supportive social network
- Good communication skills
- Healthy lifestyle patterns

Social support—family ties, friendships, and involvement in social activities—is one of the primary ingredients in a mentally healthy life. These social connections can provide a sense of belonging, support in difficult times, and a positive influence when you drift toward unhealthy behaviors.

Communication skills are necessary for negotiating relationships of all kinds. The ability to be assertive—to communicate what you want clearly and appropriately without violating other people's rights—is an important part of healthy communication. Another is the ability to be an effective listener. Tips on improving your communication skills are provided in Chapter 14.

Like physical health, mental health depends on a healthy lifestyle—eating well, exercising, getting enough sleep, and so on. But it is also improved by participating in activities that challenge you mentally, emotionally, socially, and physically. Consider some of the suggestions in the box "Taking Healthy Risks."

The Brain's Role in Mental Health and Illness

Human beings have always experienced mental disturbances: Descriptions of conditions called "mania," "melancholia," "hysteria," and "insanity" can be found in the literature of many ancient societies. It wasn't until the 18th and 19th centuries, however, that advances in anatomy, physiology, and medicine allowed scientists to identify the brain as the organ afflicted in cases of mental disturbance and to propose biological causes, especially damage to the brain, for mental disorders. Since then, other explanations have been

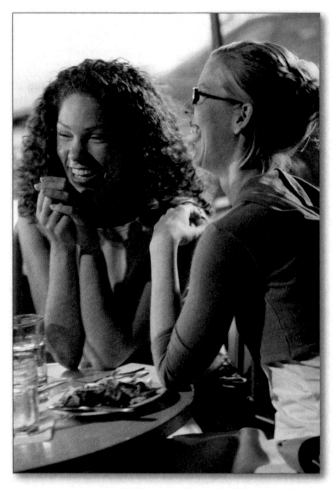

■ Having a strong social support system—including friends to laugh and cry with—is an important ingredient in the maintenance of psychological health.

proposed, involving, for example, psychological factors, sociocultural and environmental factors, and faulty learning. Debate over the roles of these various categories of causal factors continues to this day. Although it is clear that mental disorders are best understood as the result of many factors interacting in complex ways, the central role of the brain in mental health and mental illness is beyond doubt. Mental illnesses are diseases that affect the brain.[10]

ADVANCES IN KNOWLEDGE AND UNDERSTANDING OF THE BRAIN

The human brain has been called the most complex structure in the universe.[11] This unimpressive-looking organ is the central control station for human intelligence, feeling, and creativity.

Since the 1980s, knowledge of the structure and function of the brain has increased dramatically. In fact, the 1990s were called the "decade of the brain" because of the advances made in understanding how the brain works. Most of these discoveries were made possible by advances in imaging technologies, such as computerized axial tomography (CAT scans), positron emission tomography (PET scans), magnetic resonance imaging (MRIs), and functional MRIs (fMRIs).

Research has also expanded in the physiology of the brain and the function of **neurotransmitters.** These brain chemicals are responsible for the transmission of signals from one brain cell to the next. There are dozens of neurotransmitters, but four seem to be particularly important in mental disorders: norepinephrine (active during the stress response; see Chapter 5); dopamine (implicated in schizophrenia); serotonin (implicated in mood disorders); and gamma aminobutyric acid, or GABA (implicated in anxiety).[11] Neurotransmitter imbalances are believed to be involved in a variety of mental disorders. Many drugs have been developed to correct these imbalances, such as the class of antidepressants that affect levels of serotonin and includes Prozac.

neurotransmitters
Brain chemicals that conduct signals from one brain cell to the next.

THE TEENAGE BRAIN

One surprise that recent brain research produced is that the brain continues to change and grow through adolescence into the early 20s. Previously, scientists thought that brain development was completed in childhood, and in fact, 95 percent of the structure of the brain is formed by the age of 6. Scientists discovered, however, that a growth spurt occurs in the **frontal cortex**—the part of the brain where "executive functions" such as planning, organizing, and rational thinking are controlled—just before puberty. During adolescence, these new brain cells are pruned and consolidated, resulting in a more mature, adult brain by the early to mid-20s.

frontal cortex
The part of the brain where the executive functions of planning, organizing, and rational thinking are controlled.

Challenges & Choices

Taking Healthy Risks

What risks have you taken in your life? Were they healthy or unhealthy? The kind of risks that are unhealthy are those that involve potentially dangerous consequences, such as taking drugs, having unprotected sex, running away from home, or defying authority just for the sake of defiance. The kind of risks that are healthy force you to reach beyond your comfort zone to grow as a person. They can push you mentally, emotionally, and spiritually. Here are some examples of healthy risks. Try taking one today.

- Stand up for something you believe in.
- Say no to someone instead of going along.
- Confront someone who is expressing sexist or racist views.
- Run for class office.
- Run for public office.
- Address the city council on an issue you care about.
- Take up a new sport, one you've been afraid to try.
- Sign up for a marathon or cycling event to raise money for a charity, even if you don't believe right now that you can complete the event.
- Assert your right to get what you want in an intimate relationship.
- Call or talk to someone you have been admiring from afar.

It's Not Just Personal . . .

In 2007 more than 2,300 cyclists participated in the seventh annual AIDS/Lifecycle ride from San Francisco to Los Angeles. Cyclists on the 7-day, 500-mile ride raised more than $11 million for HIV services and prevention. In other events, amateur runners, walkers, swimmers, cyclists, and triathletes have raised millions of dollars for research on breast cancer, leukemia and lymphoma, cystic fibrosis, and a host of other serious diseases. These fund-raising events are made possible by people taking risks and stretching beyond their comfort zones.

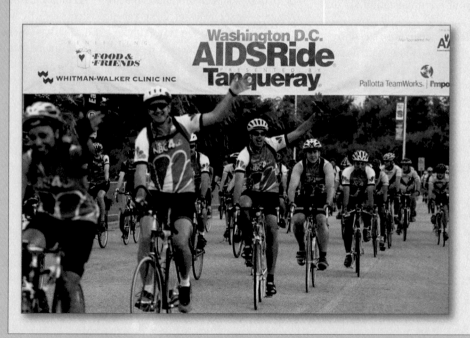

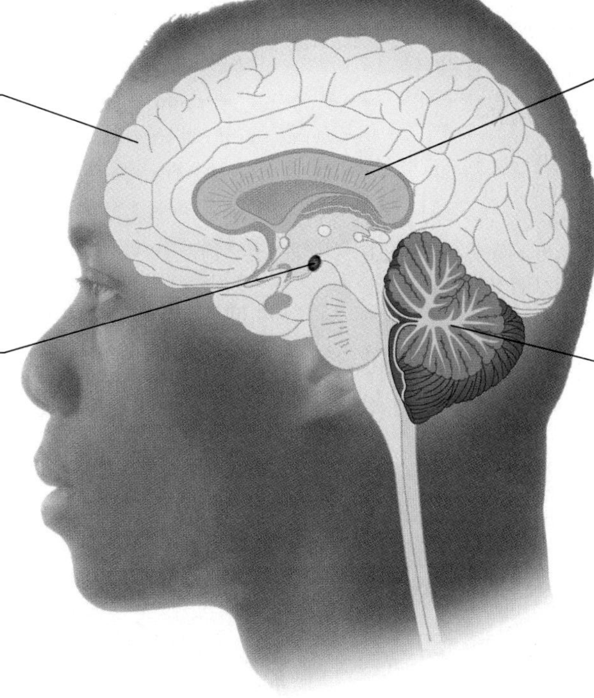

Frontal cortex
Controls planning, organizing, rational thinking, working memory, judgment, mood modulation. Undergoes rapid growth just before puberty, followed by pruning and consolidation during adolescence.

Amygdala
Controls emotional responses and instinctual, "gut" reactions. Adolescents appear to rely more heavily on this part of the brain to interpret situations than adults do. As they mature, the center of brain activity shifts to the frontal cortex.

Corpus callosum
Relays information between the two hemispheres of the brain and is believed to play a role in creativity and problem solving. Grows and changes significantly during adolescence.

Cerebellum
Long known to be involved in motor activity and physical coordination; now understood to coordinate thinking processes, including decision making and social skills. Undergoes dynamic growth and change during adolescence.

figure **3.2**   **The teenage brain.**
Sources: Adapted from "Adolescent Brains Are Works in Progress," by S. Spinks, 2005, Frontline, www.pbs.org; "Teenage Brain: A Work in Progress,"
2001, National Institute of Mental Health, NIH Publication No. 01-4929, www.nimh.nih.gov.

One implication of these findings is that the impulsivity, emotional reactivity, and risk-taking behavior that are more typical of adolescence than of adulthood may be caused in part by a still-maturing brain rather than (or in addition to) hormonal changes or other factors. Figure 3.2 shows the teenage brain and describes how its functions may differ from those of the adult brain.

Another implication is that because structural changes are taking place in the brain through adolescence and into early adulthood, the activities that teenagers engage in can have lifelong effects. The brain cells and connections that are used for academics, music, sports, language learning, and other productive activities—or, alternatively, for watching television and playing video games—are the ones that are more likely to be hardwired into the brain and survive.[11]

Some experts have disputed these conclusions about the teenage brain. They argue that the differences seen in brain images are not necessarily the *cause* of erratic or impulsive teen behaviors, and they point out that adolescents in other cultures are often fully ready to regulate and be responsible for their behavior. In addition, some research has indicated a relationship between impulsive, risk-taking teen behavior and exposure to movies, television, and video games. More research is needed to sort out the effects of biological versus cultural influences on teen behavior.[12]

MENTAL DISORDERS AND THE BRAIN

Although all behavior, both normal and abnormal, is mediated in some way by the brain and the nervous system, mental disorders that are caused specifically by some pathology in the brain are rare. These disorders are referred to as *cognitive disorders*; an example is Alzheimer's disease. More commonly, mental disorders are caused by complex interactions of biological factors (such as neurotransmitter levels, genetics), psychological processes, social influences, and cultural factors, especially those affecting a person during early childhood. Although evidence of mental disorders like depression or schizophrenia can be found in the brain, and although many disorders can be treated with drugs that act on the brain, neither of these facts means that mental disorders originate in the brain.

diathesis-stress model
A model of mental illness in which a diathesis (a predisposition or vulnerability) exists, but a stressor (a precipitating event) is needed to trigger the onset of illness.

Influences on the Development of Mental Health and Illness

How does a person become mentally healthy or mentally ill? One model of mental illness, called the **diathesis-stress model,** proposes that a person may have a particular predisposition or vulnerability (diathesis) for an illness, but an event (stressor) must occur to trigger the illness itself. For example, a person may have a genetic predisposition for depression, but the illness appears only if the person experiences a trauma.

PROTECTIVE FACTORS AND RISK FACTORS

Many factors come into play in the diathesis-stress model. *Protective factors* serve to buffer the person from threats to psychological well-being; *risk factors* increase the individual's chances for mental health problems. Both protective factors and risk factors occur at the levels of the individual, the family, and the community and environment:

- Individual factors include genetic traits or predispositions, conditions attributable to prenatal influ-

ences, and any other inborn characteristics such as temperament.

- Family factors include quality of parenting, family dynamics, and other interpersonal relationships in early childhood.

- Community and environmental factors include schools; neighborhoods; community resources and opportunities; and social, economic, and cultural factors.

For an overview of protective factors and risk factors at the individual, family, and community levels, see Tables 3.2 and 3.3. The more risk factors children are exposed to, the more likely they are to develop mental health problems. When sufficient numbers of protective factors are present, however, they seem to moderate the impact of those factors that place children at risk.

ERIKSON'S THEORY OF PSYCHOSOCIAL DEVELOPMENT

Another way to think about influences on the development of mental health and mental illness is Erik Erikson's **theory of**

Table 3.2	Protective Factors for Mental Health
Individual Protective Factors	Active, easy, outgoing temperament
	Positive responsiveness to others
	Sense of humor
	High intelligence
	Problem-solving skills
	Emotional regulation
	Verbal/communication skills
	Self-efficacy
	Hopefulness
	Recognized talents/accomplishments
	Social skills
	Self-confidence
	Strong, positive ethnic identity
	Religious faith/affiliation/participation
	Educational aspirations
	Sense of direction or purpose
Family Protective Factors	Competent parenting
	Authoritative parenting style
	High but realistic expectations of child
	Educational attainment
	Involved in schools
	Family cohesion, marital harmony
	Socioeconomic advantages
	Religious faith/affiliation/participation
	Children have family/household duties
Community/ Environmental Protective Factors	Adequate resources for child care, health care
	Good schools
	Community cohesion, stability
	Availability of prosocial role models, norms
	Supportive friends, neighbors
	Employment opportunities
	Opportunities for involvement in community activities

Source: Adapted from "Resilience in Ecosystemic Context," by M. Waller, 2001, American Journal of Orthopsychiatry, 71 (3), pp. 290–297.

Table 3.3	Risk Factors for Mental Health Problems
Individual Risk Factors	Physical health problem or disability
	Difficult temperament
	Learning problem or attention difficulty
	Poor social skills
	Poor verbal/communication skills
	Poor impulse control
	Lack of self-efficacy
	Sensation seeking
	Aggressiveness
	Antisocial tendencies
	Tolerance for deviant roles, norms
Family Risk Factors	Low parental attachment
	Poor parenting (for example, inconsistent, too many or too few rules)
	Family conflict
	Low educational attainment
	Socioeconomic disadvantages
	Isolation, lack of social connections
	Emotional disturbance/psychological problem in parent
	Physical/emotional/sexual abuse
	Parental alcohol or drug abuse
Community/ Environmental Risk Factors	Poverty
	Negative peer influence
	Neighborhood disorganization
	Poor housing
	Poor schools
	Lack of employment opportunities
	Failure to achieve at school
	Criminal activity/violence

Source: Adapted from "Resilience in Ecosystemic Context," by M. Waller, 2001, American Journal of Orthopsychiatry, 71 (3), pp. 290–297.

Table 3.4	Erikson's Stages of Development		
Age	**Challenge**	**Important People**	**Basic Strength**
Birth–18 months	Trust vs. mistrust	Mother or other primary caregiver	Hope
18 months–3 years	Autonomy vs. shame and self-doubt	Parents	Will
3–6 years	Initiative vs. guilt	Family	Purpose
6–12 years	Industry vs. inferiority	Neighborhood and school	Competence
Adolescence	Identity vs. identity confusion	Peers	Fidelity
Young adulthood	Intimacy vs. isolation	Close friends, intimate partners	Love
Middle adulthood	Generativity vs. self-absorption	Work associates, children, community	Care
Older adulthood	Integrity vs. despair	Humankind	Wisdom

Source: Adapted from The Life Cycle Completed, *extended version, by E. Erikson, copyright © 1997 by Joan M. Erickson. Copyright © 1982 by Rikan Enterprises Ltd. New York: W. W. Norton & Company.*

theory of psychosocial development
Erikson's theory that personality development proceeds through a series of eight life stages.

psychosocial development. Erikson proposed that development proceeds through a series of eight life stages, each shaped by the interaction of internal, biological drives, on the one hand, and external, social and cultural forces, on the other.

According to this theory, individuals face predictable challenges at particular periods or stages in their lives. If they meet these challenges more or less successfully, they develop "ego strengths" and continue growing in healthy ways. If they are unable to meet the challenges successfully, their psychological, emotional, and social growth may be blocked, it may be harder to meet later challenges, and they may not reach their fullest potential.

For example, the challenge of infancy, according to Erikson, is to develop *trust,* a sense that you can rely on someone to provide for your needs and that the world is a safe place. When this challenge is successfully negotiated as a result of loving and responsive parenting, the individual develops the capacity for hope. When the challenge is not so successfully met—for example, as a result of unresponsive or inattentive parenting—the person develops an inclination more toward mistrust than trust and may, in adulthood, have difficulty trusting people in interpersonal and intimate relationships.

Similarly, the challenge of early childhood (age 18 months to 3 years) is to develop a sense of *autonomy,* the feeling that you are a separate person, can stand on your own feet, and can assert your will. This stage is embodied by a 2-year-old telling her parents "No!" at every turn simply to assert her personhood. When parents are able to understand and accept this behavior as age-appropriate and to set limits with love, the individual develops a sense of will power. When this stage is not so successfully negotiated, perhaps because parents cannot tolerate the child's assertiveness, the individual may instead become more inclined toward shame and doubt.

Each of the eight life stages in Erikson's theory has a characteristic challenge or set of tasks that must be mas-

tered, as shown in Table 3.4. Failure to master a particular challenge does not mean that a person is condemned to a lifetime of distress—in fact, it is important to develop a healthy balance of qualities at each stage. However, Erikson's theory does suggest that if a person has difficulty mastering one challenge, the challenges that follow will be more difficult to negotiate. It further suggests that difficulties later in life may be traced to the stage at which the person insufficiently mastered a particular psychosocial task. This would be an area the person might benefit from addressing in psychotherapy.

In old age, Erikson proposed a ninth life stage, "very old age," which he called *gerotranscendence.* This stage, reached by some people in their 80s and 90s, is characterized by a circumscribed sense of time and space (limited perhaps to "today" or "this week" and to the movements allowed by one's physical capabilities), feelings of connection with the universe, and an understanding of death as "the way of all living things."[13] It can be expected that, with lifespan lengthening and the population aging, an increasing number of Americans will have some experience of gerotranscendence.

Mental Disorders

Mental health is determined not by the challenges a person faces but by how the person responds to those challenges. The challenges themselves come in a range of intensities—from being turned down for a date to the death of a loved one—and people's responses also vary in how well they work in allowing the person to maintain an overall sense of balance and well-being.

HOW DO EVERYDAY PROBLEMS DIFFER FROM MENTAL DISORDERS?

In general, a mental disorder is diagnosed on the basis of the amount of distress and impairment a person is experiencing. According to the *Diagnostic and Statistical Manual of*

Mental Disorders (DSM-IV-TR), a **mental disorder** is a pattern of behavior in an individual that is associated with distress (pain) or disability (impairment in an important area of functioning, such as school or work) or with significantly increased risk of suffering, death, pain, disability, or loss of freedom.[14] Deciding when a psychological problem becomes a mental disorder is not easy. Nevertheless, a basic premise of the *DSM-IV-TR* is that a mental disorder is qualitatively different from a psychological problem that can be considered normal, and it can be diagnosed from a set of symptoms.

> **mental disorder**
> According to the *DSM-IV-TR*, a pattern of behavior in an individual that is associated with distress (pain) or disability (impairment in an important area of functioning, such as school or work) or with significantly increased risk of suffering, death, pain, disability, or loss of freedom.

Some of the most common experiences that people struggle with in life, especially during the college years, are feeling sad and discouraged. These feelings can occur in response to disappointment, loss, failure, or other negative events, or they can occur for no apparent reason. Usually such experiences don't last too long; people recover and go on with their lives. If the feelings *do* go on for a long time and are painful and intense, the person may be experiencing depression.

Similarly, worries, fears, and anxieties are common during the college years. Individuals have stresses to deal with, such as grades, relationships, and learning how to live on their own without parental guidance or support. They may be feeling homesick and lonely, or they may be having problems sleeping. Most people gradually make their way, learning who they are and how they want to relate to other people. Some people, however, may develop anxiety disorders or stress-related disorders. They may, for example, experience panic attacks or be overwhelmed with fears and worries.

People experience many emotional difficulties in the course of daily living that are not a cause for alarm. At the same time, it is important to be able to recognize when a person needs professional help. Far too often, people struggle with mental disorders without knowing that something is wrong or that treatments are available. They don't realize that their problems may be causing them unnecessary distress and that professional treatment can help. (See the box "Reducing the Stigma of Mental Illness.")

Public Health in Action

Reducing the Stigma of Mental Illness

In 2008 the Substance Abuse and Mental Health Services Administration (SAMHSA) of the U.S. Department of Health and Human Services launched a campaign to challenge and reduce the stigma associated with mental illness on college campuses. The effort is designed to reach 18- to 25-year-olds and to encourage them to support friends with mental health problems. Materials created specifically for college students were distributed on more than 200 campuses nationwide.

The incidence of mental health problems in this age group is the highest of any segment of the adult population, yet they are the least likely to get help. According to the National College Health Assessment Report, more than half of the students surveyed on U.S. college campuses said they felt hopeless, more than a third reported being "so depressed it was difficult to function," and about 10 percent said they had seriously considered suicide in the past year. Suicide is the second leading cause of death for college students, according to the Centers for Disease Control and Prevention. One of the premises of the campaign is that young people will be more likely to seek mental health services if there is more social acceptance of such treatment.

The campaign, called "What a Difference a Friend Makes," emphasizes the important role of friends in recovery from mental illness: "Friends can make a difference by offering reassurance, companionship, and emotional strength." The "What a Difference" brochure provides information on mental illness, myths and facts about mental illness, and guidelines on how to help a friend. In a public service announcement (PSA) for television, young adults are shown talking with a friend who was recently diagnosed with bipolar disorder. The PSA explains that bipolar disorder is a mental health problem that typically begins in the mid-20s and that affects a person's moods, energy levels, and thoughts. The ad also reports that half of all people experiencing a mental health problem reach out to family and friends first.

The ad campaign was developed by SAMSHA and the Advertising Council and distributed, with the help of several nonprofit organizations, in the form of brochures delivered to campus bookstores, program manuals for peer educators, television and radio ads, and other outreach materials. The time for airing the ads was donated by the media. The college campaign was an extension of the National Mental Health Anti-Stigma Campaign, launched in 2006. Anti-stigma campaigns are spreading and are now under way in several states. The aim of all such programs is to counter stigma and discrimination, reduce barriers to treatment, educate people about recovery, and emphasize the importance of quality, accessible mental health services available in the community.

Sources: "SAMHSA and Ad Council Debut National Mental Health Anti-Stigma Campaign on College Campuses," Substance Abuse and Mental Health Services Administration, 2008, retrieved May 5, 2008, from www.samhsa.gov/newsroom/advisories/0803273627.aspx; "What a Difference a Friend Makes," Substance Abuse and Mental Health Services Administration, retrieved May 5, 2008, from www.samhsa.gov.

Highlight on Health

Symptoms of Depression

A person who experiences five or more of the following symptoms (including the first and second symptoms listed) for a 2-week period may be suffering from depression:

- Depressed mood, as indicated by feelings of sadness or emptiness or such behaviors as crying.
- Loss of interest or pleasure in all or most activities.
- Significant weight loss or weight gain or a change in appetite.

- Insomnia, hypersomnia, or other disturbed sleep patterns.
- Agitated or retarded (slow) body movement.
- Fatigue or loss of energy.
- Feelings of worthlessness or excessive guilt.
- Diminished ability to think, impaired concentration, or indecisiveness.
- Recurrent thoughts of death, ideas about suicide, or a suicide plan or attempt.

Source: Reprinted with permission from Diagnostic and Statistical Manual of Mental Disorders, *4th ed., Text Revision (DSM-IV-TR), copyright © 2000, American Psychiatric Association.*

MOOD DISORDERS

Also called depressive disorders or affective disorders, mood disorders include major depressive disorder, dysthymic disorder, and bipolar disorder (formerly called manic depression). They are among the most common mental disorders around the world.

People of all ages can get depressed, including children and adolescents, but the average age at onset for major depressive disorders is the mid-20s. In any one year, more than 18 million adults in the United States—about 9.5 percent of the adult population—suffer from a depressive illness. Of

these individuals, a significant number will be hospitalized, and many will die from suicide.[15] Women are at significantly greater risk for depression than men, experiencing depressive episodes twice as frequently.

In many of these situations, the illness goes undiagnosed, and people struggle for long periods of time. About two-thirds of depressed individuals seek help, but many are undertreated, meaning that they don't get enough medication or they don't see a therapist on a regular basis. Many medications for depression take up to 4 weeks to begin to have an effect, and some people conclude they aren't working and stop taking them.

Major Depressive Disorder Symptoms of **depression** include depressed mood, as indicated by feelings of sadness or emptiness or by behaviors such as crying, a loss of interest or pleasure in activities that previously provided pleasure, fatigue, feelings of worthlessness, and a reduced ability to concentrate (see the box "Symptoms of Depression"). If a person experiences one or more episodes of depression (characterized by at least five of the nine symptoms listed) lasting at least 2 weeks, he or she may be diagnosed with *major depressive disorder*.

depression
Mental state characterized by a depressed mood, loss of interest or pleasure in activities, and several other related symptoms.

Dysthymic Disorder Low-grade, chronic depression that goes on for 2 years or more may be diagnosed as *dysthymic disorder*. Individuals with this disorder have a generally depressed mood and may have a poor appetite, disturbed sleep patterns, low self-esteem, low energy, poor concentration and difficulty making decisions, and/or feelings of hopelessness.

Bipolar Disorder A person with *bipolar disorder* experiences one or more manic episodes, often but not always alternating with depressive episodes. A *manic episode* is a distinct

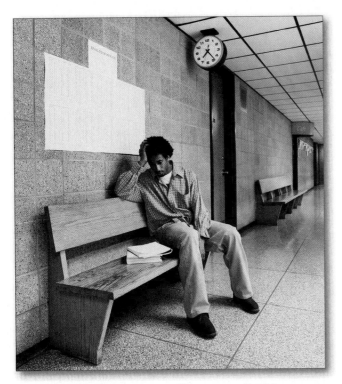

- Feelings of sadness, guilt, worthlessness, and hopelessness can be signs of depression, a treatable mental disorder.

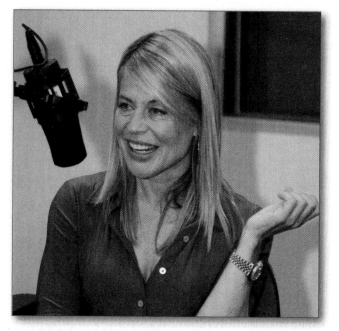

■ Actress Linda Hamilton, who portrayed Sarah Connor in the *Terminator* movies, is one of many talented people who have talked and written about their struggles with bipolar disorder.

period during which the person has an abnormally elevated mood (see the box "Symptoms of a Manic Episode"). Individuals experiencing manic episodes may be euphoric, expansive, and full of energy, or, alternatively, highly irritable. They may be grandiose, with an inflated sense of their own importance and power; they may have racing thoughts and accelerated and pressured speech. They may stay awake for days without getting tired or wake from a few hours of sleep feeling refreshed and full of energy. People experiencing a manic episode typically are not aware they are ill.

Bipolar disorder occurs equally in men and women, with an average age at onset of about 20. Family and twin studies offer strong evidence of a genetic component in this disorder.

ANXIETY DISORDERS

Along with depression, anxiety disorders are the most common mental disorders affecting Americans. Almost 19 million Americans between the ages of 18 and 54—more than 13 percent of all people in this age group—have an anxiety disorder.[15]

Many of these disorders are characterized by a **panic attack,** a clear physiological and psychological experience of apprehension or intense fear in the absence of a real danger.

panic attack
Clear physiological and psychological experience of apprehension or intense fear in the absence of a real danger.

Symptoms include heart palpitations, sweating, shortness of breath, chest pain, and a sense that one is "going crazy." There is a feeling of impending doom or danger and a strong urge to escape. Panic attacks usually occur suddenly and last for a discrete period of time, reaching a peak within 10 minutes.[16]

Panic disorder is characterized by recurrent, unexpected panic attacks along with concern about having another attack. The attacks may be triggered by a situation, or they may "come out of nowhere" (see the box "Symptoms of Panic Disorder"). Twin studies and family studies indicate a genetic contribution to this disorder. First-degree relatives of persons with panic disorder are eight times more likely to develop the disorder than the general population.[16]

panic disorder
Mental disorder characterized by recurrent, unexpected panic attacks along with concern about having another attack.

A *specific phobia* is an intense fear of an activity, situation, or object, exposure to which evokes immediate anxiety. Examples of common phobias are flying, heights, specific animals or insects (dogs, spiders), and blood. Individuals with phobias realize their fear is unreasonable, but they cannot control it. Usually they try to avoid the phobic situation or object, and if they can't avoid it, they endure it with great distress. Often the phobia interferes with their lives in some way.

Agoraphobia is characterized by anxiety about being in situations where escape may be difficult or embarrassing, or where help might not be available in case of a panic attack. Such situations may include being in a crowd, on a bus,

Highlight on Health

Symptoms of a Manic Episode

A person who experiences the following symptoms may be having a manic episode:

■ A distinct period of abnormally and persistently elevated, expansive, or irritable mood lasting at least 1 week.

■ During this period, three or more of the following symptoms are present:
  - Inflated self-esteem or grandiosity.
  - Decreased need for sleep.
  - More talkative than usual.
  - Flighty ideas or sense that thoughts are racing.
  - Distractability.
  - Increase in goal-directed activity or psychomotor agitation.
  - Excessive involvement in pleasurable activities with a high potential for painful consequences (such as shopping sprees, sexual indiscretions).

Source: Reprinted with permission from Diagnostic and Statistical Manual of Mental Disorders, *4th ed., Text Revision (DSM-IV-TR), copyright © 2000, American Psychiatric Association.*

Highlight on Health

Symptoms of Panic Disorder

A person who experiences the following symptoms may be suffering from panic disorder:

- Recurrent, unexpected panic attacks.

- One or more of the following in the month after an attack:

  - Persistent concern about having another attack.

  - Worry about what the attack means (for example, losing control, having a heart attack, going crazy).

  - A significant change in behavior related to the attacks.

Source: Reprinted with permission from Diagnostic and Statistical Manual of Mental Disorders, 4th ed., Text Revision (DSM-IV-TR), *copyright © 2000, American Psychiatric Association.*

on a bridge, in an open space, or simply outside the home. Individuals with untreated agoraphobia usually try to structure their lives in such a way as to avoid these situations; in extreme cases, they may not leave their home for years.

A *social phobia* involves an intense fear of certain kinds of social or performance situations, again leading the individual to try to avoid such situations. If the phobic situation is public speaking, individuals may be able to structure their lives so as to avoid all such situations. However, some social phobias involve simply conversing with other people. This is different from shyness; individuals with this disorder experience tremors, sweating, confusion, blushing, and other distressing symptoms when they are in the feared situation.

Excessive and uncontrollable worrying, usually far out of proportion to the likelihood of the feared event, is known as *generalized anxiety disorder*. Adults with this disorder worry about routine matters such as health, work, and money; children with the disorder worry about their competence in school or sports, being evaluated by others, or even natural disasters.

Obsessive-compulsive disorder is characterized by persistent, intrusive thoughts, impulses, or images that cause intense anxiety or distress. For example, the person

may have repeated thoughts about contamination, persistent doubts about having done something, or a need to have things done in a particular order. To control the obsessive thoughts and images, the person develops compulsions—repetitive behaviors performed to reduce the anxiety associated with the obsession. For example, a woman might be plagued with worries about whether she locked the door, and she returns to the house or gets up out of bed numerous times to check.

ADDICTION

Addiction—dependence on a substance or a behavior—is classified as a mental disorder. The key characteristic of addiction is continued, compulsive use of the substance or involvement in the behavior despite serious negative consequences. Individuals with a substance addiction may spend a great deal of time trying to obtain the substance, give up important parts of their lives to use it, and make repeated, unsuccessful attempts to cut down or control their use.

addiction
Dependence on a substance or a behavior.

A person with *physiological dependence* on a substance experiences *tolerance*, reduced sensitivity to its effects such that increased doses are needed to give the same high, and *withdrawal*, uncomfortable symptoms that occur when substance use stops. Tolerance and withdrawal are indicators that the brain and body have adapted to the substance. Even without physiological dependence, the person can experience *psychological dependence*.

Typically, a person begins by using a substance to reduce pain or anxiety or to produce feelings of pleasure, excitement, confidence, or connection with others. With repeated use, users can come to depend on being in this altered state, and without the drug, they may feel worse than they did

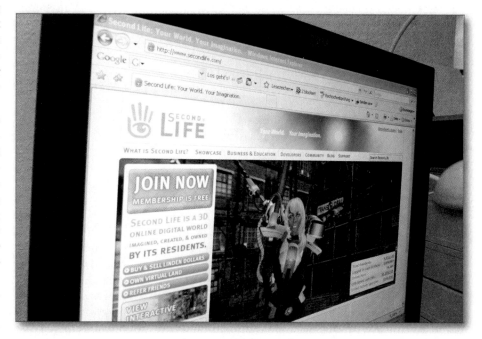

■ Internet addiction is promoted by games like "Second Life," a virtual world with millions of "residents" from around the world.

before they ever took it. Although most people don't think they will become addicted when they start, gradually the substance takes over their lives.

Although addiction is usually associated with drug use, many experts now extend the concept of addiction to other areas in which behavior can become compulsive and out of control, such as gambling. Research has established that drugs cause addiction by operating on the "pleasure pathway" in the brain and changing brain chemistry (see Chapter 12 for details of this process). Some scientists speculate that compulsive behaviors may follow the same pathway in the brain, causing feelings of euphoria along with a strong desire to repeat the behavior and a craving for the behavior when it stops.

Compulsive or pathological gambling is the best known of these behavioral disorders, but people can also be addicted to Internet use, sex, shopping, eating, exercising, or other activities (Figure 3.3). The key component in these conditions is that the person feels out of control and powerless over the behavior. Both psychotherapy and self-help groups are available to assist individuals struggling with these troubling behavior patterns.

SCHIZOPHRENIA AND OTHER PSYCHOTIC DISORDERS

Psychotic disorders are characterized by delusions, hallucinations, disorganized speech or behavior, and other signs that the individual has lost touch with reality. The most common psychotic disorder is **schizophrenia**. A person with schizophrenia typically has disorganized and disordered thinking and perceptions, bizarre ideas, hallucinations (often voices), and impaired functioning.[17] The symptoms are sometimes so severe that the person becomes socially, interpersonally, and occupationally dysfunctional.

schizophrenia
A psychotic disorder in which a person has disorganized and disordered thinking and perceptions, bizarre ideas, hallucinations (often voices), and impaired functioning.

The number of people reported with schizophrenia is relatively small, approximately 1–2 percent of the adult population.[14] It occurs worldwide, but it can manifest differently in different cultures because the content of delusions can be culture specific. Age at onset is usually the early 20s for men and the late 20s for women.

Schizophrenia has a strong genetic component. First-degree relatives of individuals with schizophrenia have a risk for the disorder 10 times higher than that of the general population.[14] All of the brain scanning and visualizing technologies reveal abnormalities in the brains of people with schizophrenia. Studies indicate that these abnormalities are present before the onset of symptoms, suggesting that this illness is the result of problems in brain development, perhaps even occurring prenatally.

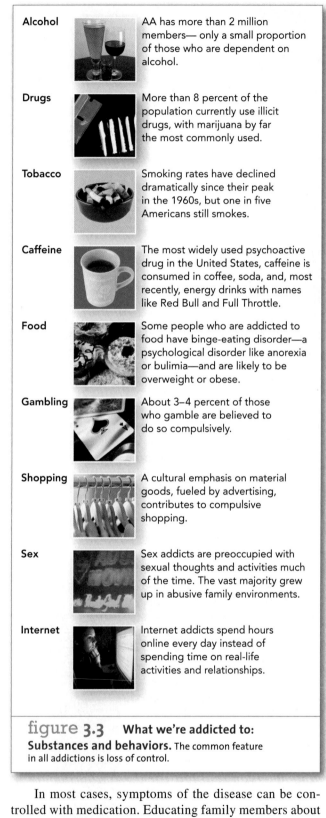

Alcohol	AA has more than 2 million members— only a small proportion of those who are dependent on alcohol.
Drugs	More than 8 percent of the population currently use illicit drugs, with marijuana by far the most commonly used.
Tobacco	Smoking rates have declined dramatically since their peak in the 1960s, but one in five Americans still smokes.
Caffeine	The most widely used psychoactive drug in the United States, caffeine is consumed in coffee, soda, and, most recently, energy drinks with names like Red Bull and Full Throttle.
Food	Some people who are addicted to food have binge-eating disorder—a psychological disorder like anorexia or bulimia—and are likely to be overweight or obese.
Gambling	About 3–4 percent of those who gamble are believed to do so compulsively.
Shopping	A cultural emphasis on material goods, fueled by advertising, contributes to compulsive shopping.
Sex	Sex addicts are preoccupied with sexual thoughts and activities much of the time. The vast majority grew up in abusive family environments.
Internet	Internet addicts spend hours online every day instead of spending time on real-life activities and relationships.

figure 3.3   What we're addicted to: Substances and behaviors. The common feature in all addictions is loss of control.

In most cases, symptoms of the disease can be controlled with medication. Educating family members about the illness can help them better understand the cycle of the illness and the importance of medications. Another key is *case management*, an approach to treatment in which a multidisciplinary team of people is involved to ensure that all aspects of a person's life are addressed.

MENTAL DISORDERS AND SUICIDE

A major public health concern, particularly among young people, suicide is the second leading cause of death among college students. According to the National College Health Assessment (fall 2007), approximately 45 percent of college students have been so depressed that they could not function. About 10 percent of students seriously considered suicide, and almost 2 percent attempted to kill themselves in the past year.[18]

Among high school students, 16.9 percent had seriously considered attempting suicide in the past 12 months; over 22 percent of females and 12 percent of males reported having serious suicidal thoughts. Overall, during the past 12 months, 13 percent of high school students had made a plan, 8.4 percent had attempted suicide, and 2.3 percent of those surveyed had to receive treatment from a doctor or nurse for injuries sustained during a suicide attempt.[19]

Overall, women in U.S. society are more likely than men to attempt suicide, but men are four times more likely to succeed, probably because they choose more violent methods, usually a firearm. In the United States, firearms are used in 55–60 percent of all suicides. Women tend to use less violent methods for suicide, but in recent years they have begun to use firearms more frequently (see the box "Suicide Rates by Age, Sex, Race, and Ethnicity").

What Leads a Person to Suicide?   Individuals contemplating suicide are most likely experiencing unbearable emotional pain, anguish, or despair. As many as 90 percent of those who commit suicide are suffering from a mental disorder, often depression. Studies indicate that the symptom linking depression and suicide is a feeling of hopelessness. Depression and alcoholism may be involved in two-thirds of all suicides. Substance abuse is another factor; the combination of drugs and depression can be lethal. People experiencing psychosis are also at risk.

Besides mental disorders and substance abuse, other major risk factors associated with suicide are a family history of suicide, serious medical problems, and access to the means, such as a gun or pills. The most significant risk factor, however, is a previous suicide attempt or a history of such attempts (see the box "Risk Factors for Suicide").

Sometimes, vulnerable individuals turn to suicide in response to a specific event, such as the loss of a relationship or job, an experience of failure, or a worry that a secret will be revealed. Other times there is no apparent precipitating event, and the suicide seems to come out of nowhere. However, suicide is always a process, and certain behavioral signs indicate that a person may be thinking about suicide:

- Comments about death and threats to commit suicide.
- Increasing social withdrawal and isolation.
- Intensified moodiness.
- Increase in risk-taking behaviors.
- Sudden improvement in mood, accompanied by such

Who's at Risk

Suicide Rates by Age, Sex, Race, and Ethnicity

Suicide is the 11th leading cause of death in the United States, accounting for more than 31,000 deaths per year (about 1.3 percent of all deaths). This compares with nearly 700,000 deaths from heart disease and more than 550,000 deaths from cancer. Suicide rates vary by sex, race, ethnicity, and age, as shown in the following table. Data are for 2005, the latest year available. The population segment with the highest suicide rate is white males over 65.

Group	Rate (number of suicides per 100,000 people)
All	
Nation	11.0
Sex	
Males	17.7
Females	4.5
Race/Ethnicity	
Whites	12.3
White males	19.7
White females	5.0
Blacks/African Americans	5.1
Black males	8.7
Black females	1.8
Hispanics/Latinos	5.1
Native Americans	12.4
Asian/Pacific Islanders	5.2
Age Group	
Teens, young adults, age 15–24	10.0
Older adults, age 65+	14.7

Source: "USA Suicide: 2005 Official Final Data," American Association of Suicidology, 2008, retrieved March 16, 2008, from www.suicidology.org/associations/1045/files/2005datapgs.pdf.

behaviors as giving away possessions. (The person may have made the decision to commit suicide.)

How to Help   If you know someone who seems to be suicidal, it is critical to get the person help. All mentions of suicide should be taken seriously. It is a myth that asking a person if he or she is thinking about suicide will plant the seed in the person's mind. Ignoring someone's sadness and depressed mood only increases the risk. Encourage the person to talk, and ask direct questions:

- Are you thinking about killing yourself?
- Do you have a plan?

- Do you have the means?
- Have you attempted suicide in the past?

Encourage the person to get help by calling a suicide hotline or seeking counseling. Do not agree to keep the person's mental state or intentions a secret. If he or she refuses to get help or resists your advice, you may need to contact a parent or relative or, if you are a student, share your concern with a professional at the student health center. Do not leave a suicidal person alone. Call for help or take the person to an emergency room.

If you have thought about suicide yourself, we encourage you to seek counseling. Therapy can help you resolve problems, develop better coping skills, and diminish the feelings that are causing you pain. It can also help you see things in a broader perspective and understand that you will not always feel this way. Remember the saying, suicide is a permanent solution to a temporary problem.

SELF-INJURY

Self-injury, sometimes known as self-harm, self-mutilation, or self-injurious behavior, is defined as any intentional injury to one's own body. Specific behaviors include cutting, burning, scratching, branding, picking, hair pulling, and head banging. Self-injurious behaviors are sometimes mistaken for suicide attempts. Individuals who self-injure often have a history of physical and/or sexual abuse as well as coexisting problems such as substance abuse and eating disorders.

There is evidence that the incidence of self-injury is increasing, particularly among adolescents.[20] It has been estimated that between 12 and 35 percent of college students have engaged in at least one incident of self-injury.[21] Many of the college students reporting self-injurious behaviors had never been in therapy for any reason and only rarely disclosed their behaviors to anyone.[22] The disorder seems to be

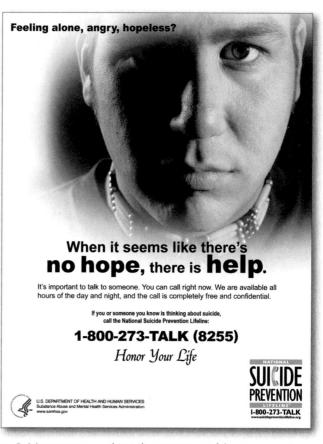

Feeling alone, angry, hopeless?

When it seems like there's **no hope,** there is **help.**

It's important to talk to someone. You can call right now. We are available all hours of the day and night, and the call is completely free and confidential.

If you or someone you know is thinking about suicide, call the National Suicide Prevention Lifeline:

1-800-273-TALK (8255)

Honor Your Life

U.S. DEPARTMENT OF HEALTH AND HUMAN SERVICES
Substance Abuse and Mental Health Services Administration
www.samhsa.gov

SUICIDE PREVENTION LIFELINE
1-800-273-TALK
www.suicidepreventionlifeline.org

- Raising awareness about the symptoms of depression and suicidal thinking—and about the availability of help—is a major public health goal.

equally prevalent among men and women, and the behavior does not appear to be limited by race, ethnicity, education, sexual orientation, socioeconomic status, or religion.

The Internet has recently become a place where people who injure themselves can find a safe forum to discuss personal stories, voice opinions, and give and receive support. However, caution is advised because participation in these message boards may also expose vulnerable adolescents to a subculture in which self-injury may be normalized and even reinforced.[23] A variety of treatments can help people who injure themselves, including family therapy and medications.

Treating Mental Disorders

More than 250 different models of psychotherapy exist for the treatment of mental disorders, and many different drugs can be prescribed. Most of the mild and moderate mental disorders are readily treatable with therapy and, if needed, medications.

PSYCHOTHERAPY

The key feature of most forms of **psychotherapy** (or *counseling*) is the development of a positive inter-

psychotherapy
Treatment for psychological problems usually based on the development of a positive interpersonal relationship between a client and a therapist.

Highlight on Health

Risk Factors for Suicide

A number of factors place adolescents at risk for suicide. The following list highlights the leading predictors.

- Suicidal thoughts
- Psychiatric disorders
- Drug and/or alcohol abuse
- Previous suicide attempts
- Access to firearms
- Recent loss or stressful situation
- Feelings of hopelessness
- Family history of suicide

personal relationship between a person seeking help (the client or patient) and a therapist, a trained and licensed professional who can provide that help. Most therapy models agree on the central importance of this interpersonal relationship between client and therapist.

For convenience, therapies can be grouped into broad categories reflecting underlying theories. Some commonly used categories are psychodynamic, behavioral, and cognitive-behavioral (see the box "Counseling Services on Campus").

Therapies based on the psychodynamic model are founded on theories originally developed by Sigmund Freud and subsequently adapted and modified by a host of later theorists. Psychodynamic therapies search for the origin of psychological problems and maladaptive behaviors in the client's past, such as in early relationships and family dynamics. Through active conversation, the therapist tries to clarify distortions and challenge defenses, helping the client gain insight. Through the therapeutic relationship, the therapist attempts to provide the client with corrective emotional experiences. Psychodynamic therapies can be helpful for dealing with deep-rooted or long-standing problems.

Behavioral therapies are based on the view that problems arise from faulty learning and that new, healthy behaviors can be instilled through behavior modification and other types of training. Therapy focuses on changing the behavior in the present, not on uncovering the cause of the maladaptive behavior in the past. Behavioral therapies are more effective with well-defined problems, such as phobias or sexual dysfunctions, than with vague or pervasive problems like depression.

Cognitive-behavioral therapies incorporate the role of thinking and thought patterns into the causes of psychological problems, focusing on how faulty and illogical thinking can influence emotions, motivation, and behavior. Therapy attempts to challenge and correct distorted thoughts and change how people think about themselves and others. This approach has gained adherents because it has proven effective in the treatment of many disorders, including depression, anxiety disorders, eating disorders, and even some more severe disorders.

Although most therapists espouse a particular theoretical orientation, many take an eclectic approach; that is, they feel comfortable using ideas from a variety of different theories and approaches. For example, a therapist with a psychodynamic approach may conceptualize a client's issues in terms of early needs and interpersonal relationships, but if the client is struggling with anxiety or depression, he or she may use cognitive-behavioral techniques to help resolve that problem and move the client forward.

Consumer Clipboard

Counseling Services on Campus

Counseling services on campus vary greatly. At small schools the staff may consist of just one professional, but at large universities there is typically a team of psychologists, social workers, nurse practitioners, and usually at least one psychiatrist. At many colleges the services fall somewhere in between.

If you're trying to decide whether you need professional help, ask yourself these questions:

- Am I feeling sad (homesick, lonely) a lot of the time?
- Am I having trouble studying for exams?
- Am I having more difficulty than usual with concentration?
- Do I have increased feelings of inadequacy?
- Am I feeling overwhelmed?
- Is this problem interfering with my everyday life?
- Have my friends and family asked if there's a problem?
- Have I lost interest in doing the things I usually like to do?
- Am I avoiding friends because of the problem?

Many colleges provide free psychological assessments, short-term counseling, and referrals. If you decide that you need help, consider these points:

- *Do I want to work with a professional counselor, or would another approach be better for me?* There may be support groups on campus that offer the chance to share your problems with peers. This may help put your problem in perspective, and it may be all the help you need. If you have ties to a religious organization, you may want to seek pastoral counseling in the local community.
- *Will my insurance cover mental health counseling?* Your college tuition, fees, or health insurance may cover some mental health services. However, if you choose to go off campus for counseling or treatment, those services may not be covered by your college benefits. If you are covered by health insurance through your parents, you will need to check with that insurance company about coverage.
- *Do I want my family to know that I'm in counseling?* Different schools have varying policies on this matter. If you're over 18 and don't want your parents notified about your counseling, most schools will leave that up to you. If you're considered to be at risk for suicide, though, most counselors will encourage you to inform your parents about the counseling.

Source: Adapted from "The Dorms May Be Great, But How's the Counseling?" by M. Duenwald, October 26, 2004, New York Times, p. D1.

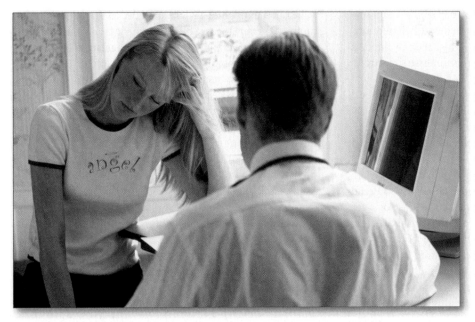

■ Counseling can help a struggling individual explore her thoughts and feelings in a safe environment and gain relief from symptoms like anxiety and depression.

What should you expect if you decide to try therapy? You can expect to be treated with warmth, respect, and an open, accepting attitude. The therapist will try to provide you with a safe place to explore your feelings and thoughts. At the end of the first session, the therapist will probably propose a plan for treatment, such as a series of ten sessions or a referral to another professional.

MEDICATIONS

Until the 1950s few effective medications for the symptoms of mental illness existed. Since that time, discoveries and breakthroughs in drug research have revolutionized the treatment of mental disorders. Today the symptoms of many serious disorders can be treated successfully with drugs.

The symptoms of schizophrenia and other psychotic disorders, especially delusions and hallucinations, can be treated with *antipsychotics*. Many of these drugs work by blocking the action of the neurotransmitter dopamine in the brain. Symptoms of mood disorders can be relieved with any of several different types of *antidepressants*, most of which act on the neurotransmitters serotonin and norepinephrine. The first antidepressants to be developed, in the 1950s, were a group called monoamine oxidase (MAO) inhibitors. They were followed, in the 1960s, by a group that caused fewer side effects, the tricyclics. In the 1990s another group with even fewer side effects was developed, selective serotonin reuptake inhibitors (SSRIs). Three SSRIs—Prozac, Zoloft, and Paxil—are among the most frequently prescribed drugs in the United States today. The most frequently prescribed drugs overall are antidepressants.

Symptoms of anxiety disorders can be reduced with antianxiety drugs (or *anxiolytics*). Benzodiazepines, the most widely used antianxiety drugs, are believed to act on the neurotransmitter GABA, which has a role in the inhibition of anxiety in the brain during stressful situations. Commonly prescribed antianxiety medications include Valium, Xanax, and Ativan. Besides the medications mentioned here, hundreds of other drugs are used to treat a wide array of symptoms and disorders.

If you seek help for a psychological problem from your physician or from a psychiatrist, your treatment is more likely to begin with medication than if you see a clinical psychologist, social worker, marriage and family counselor, school counselor, or other licensed therapist who is not also a medical doctor (Table 3.5). Treatment is also likely to begin with medication if you are experiencing acute symptoms of depression, anxiety, or another mental disorder. Medications can help stabilize the condition so that you can make decisions and obtain benefits from psychotherapy.

Table 3.5	Selected Mental Health Practitioners		
Practitioner	**Degree***	**License****	**Focus of Treatment**
Psychiatrist	MD, OD	Psychiatrist	Biomedical approach; prescription medication; psychotherapy
Clinical psychologist	PhD, PsyD	Psychologist	Psychotherapy; assessment
Counseling psychologist	PhD	Psychologist	Psychotherapy; assessment
Clinical social worker	MSW	LCSW*	Case management; psychotherapy
Psychotherapist, mental health counselor	MS, MA	LMFT, LPC**	Psychotherapy for "moderate" problems, adjustment difficulties, and the like; family counseling; couples counseling
School psychologist	PhD, EdD	Psychologist	Psychotherapy, assessment, psychoeducation within school environment

* *EdD:* doctor of education; *MA:* master of arts; *MD:* doctor of medicine; *MS:* master of science; *MSW:* master of social work; *OD:* doctor of osteopathy; *PhD:* doctor of philosophy; *PsyD:* doctor of psychology.

** *LCSW:* licensed clinical social worker; *LMFT:* licensed marriage and family therapist; *LPC:* licensed professional counselor.

The use of medications has increased dramatically in recent years. Between 1987 and 1997, for example, more people were treated for depression with medications than with psychotherapy, even though many studies have shown that therapy can be just as effective as medications.

The use of drugs has also increased for children and adolescents diagnosed with mental disorders, a controversial issue in our society. The controversy was highlighted in 2004 when a study showed that certain antidepressants increased the risk of suicidal thinking and behavior in adolescents.[24] The FDA directed manufacturers of all antidepressants to include "black box" warnings to physicians and parents on their labels.

More recent studies have indicated that antidepressants also significantly increase the risk of suicidal thoughts and behaviors in young adults aged 18–24, usually during the first 1–2 months of treatment. This effect is not seen in adults older than 24. In adults aged 65 and older, antidepressants apparently reduce the risk of suicide. The FDA has proposed that the warnings on antidepressants be updated to include young adults.[25]

The increase in the use of drug treatments is due not just to improvements in the drugs themselves but also to the growing use of managed health care in the United States. Insurance companies often prefer to pay for medications, which tend to produce faster, more visible, and more verifiable results, than for psychotherapy, which may last for months or years and produce results that are less objectively verifiable. Although drugs can be extremely effective at reducing pain and misery, they treat only the symptoms of mental disorders. For understanding the root causes of problems and changing maladaptive patterns of thinking, feeling, and behaving, some form of psychotherapy is usually needed.

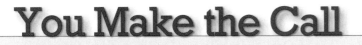

You Make the Call

Should Teachers and Administrators Be Responsible for Recognizing Mental Health Problems in Students?

On Friday, November 1, 1991, a physics student in a PhD program at the University of Iowa shot and killed three faculty members, one administrator, and a fellow physics student and permanently paralyzed a student employee. The student, Gang Lu, then killed himself. Lu was upset that he had not won a dissertation prize. In news reports following the murders, Lu was described as being extremely bright and capable but having a very bad temper and psychological problems.

On Tuesday, April 20, 1999, two students at Columbine High School in Littleton, Colorado, carried out a shooting rampage, which killed 12 students and a teacher and wounded 24 others, before committing suicide. Three years earlier, one of the students, Eric Harris, had begun a blog that included instructions on how to make bombs and expressed threats of violence against other students and teachers. The county sheriff's office was notified of the site, but no action was taken. In 1998 Harris and his friend Dylan Klebold were caught with stolen computer equipment and sentenced to juvenile diversion. They attended anger management classes, and Harris started seeing a psychiatrist. He was prescribed antidepressants and was taking them at the time of the shootings.

On April 16, 2007, Seung-Hui Cho killed 33 people and wounded 25 before killing himself at Virginia Tech University in Blacksburg, Virginia. Cho had been accused of stalking two female students in 2005 and was declared mentally ill by a Virginia special justice. An English professor

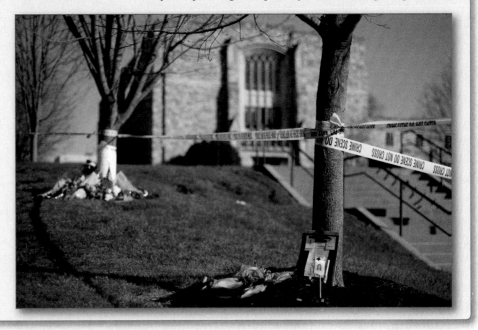

Continued…

Continued...

had found Cho's writing so disturbing that she asked to have him removed from her creative writing class to protect the other students. During Cho's time at Virginia Tech, at least one professor had recommended that he seek counseling.

On February 14, 2008, Steven Kazmierczak, a graduate of Northern Illinois University, killed 5 students and injured 16 others when he entered a lecture hall and opened fire. Kazmierczak was seeing a psychiatrist and reportedly taking Xanax (for anxiety), Ambien (for insomnia), and Prozac (for depression). He had discontinued the Prozac about 3 weeks before the shooting, and his subsequent behavior was described as erratic.

Four separate incidents, with one striking thing in common—people in authority, including mental health professionals, were aware of how troubled these individuals were. Although treatment was recommended, mandated, or even in progress, tragedies still occurred.

Some observers believe that faculty and administrators should have recognized the students' mental health problems and done more to prevent the shootings. They believe people in authority should be proactive about intervening when they see red flags suggesting a person is mentally disturbed. They argue that such individuals should be required to participate in mental health treatment or be expelled from school. They also argue that counselors in college counseling centers should breach confidentiality if they believe a client poses a threat to other students. (State laws vary regarding the circumstances that justify or require breaking client-therapist confidentiality.)

Opponents respond that such a hypervigilant attitude would have a chilling effect on free speech and could result in civil rights violations for some eccentric but harmless individuals. They point out that mass killings, though tragic and catastrophic, are very rare and proposed measures are an overreaction. They also argue that it's unrealistic and unfair to place the responsibility for recognizing mental illness on untrained persons. What do you think?

PROS:

- The safety of students and staff should be the highest priority of any college administration. Schools should be safe havens.

- Those who have the most contact with troubled individuals—faculty and other students—are most likely to be able to recognize a dangerous individual. The more people who report such an individual, the more likely that person is to get help.

- Even if some innocent or harmless people are embarrassed or feel harassed, it's worth it to prevent mass killings.

CONS:

- Free speech and protection of civil rights should be the highest priority of college administrations. Encouraging students and faculty to identify persons they view as a threat could create a climate of suspicion, reminiscent of a witch hunt.

- Students and professors are not qualified to make mental health assessments; most of their referrals are likely to be inappropriate.

- Harmless individuals who are identified as threats or who are forced to get an assessment will be needlessly harassed, stigmatized, and traumatized.

- If client-therapist confidentiality can be breached, individuals who need treatment and could benefit from it—for example, by talking about their anger instead of acting on it—would be less likely to seek help.

In Review

1. **What is mental health?** Mental health is usually conceptualized as the presence of many positive qualities, such as optimism, a sense of self-efficacy, and resilience (the ability to bounce back from adversity). Some specific approaches include positive psychology's focus on "character strengths and virtues," Maslow's self-actualization model, and Goleman's concept of emotional intelligence.

2. **What causes mental illness?** There are many theories, but a general explanation is offered by the diathesis-stress model. This model proposes that a person with a mental illness most likely has a genetic predisposition and that life stressors trigger the onset of symptoms. A variety of protective factors and risk factors at the individual, family, and environmental levels increases or decreases a person's vulnerability to mental illness.

3. **What are the most common mental disorders?** The most common are the mood disorders—depression, dysthymia, and bipolar disorder—and the anxiety disorders—panic disorder, phobias, generalized anxiety disorder, and others. Addiction, whether to a substance or a behavior, is classified as a mental disorder. Schizophrenia is a relatively rare but severe disorder.

4. **What leads a person to commit suicide?** Most people who commit suicide are suffering from a mental disorder, often depression, and are experiencing feelings of hopelessness. Alcohol or other substance abuse is often involved. Frequently, there are warning signs, such as comments about death, social withdrawal, and a sudden improvement in mood when the person has made the decision. All mentions of suicide should be taken seriously, and a suicidal person should never be left alone.

5. **How is mental illness treated?** The two broad approaches to treatment are medications and psychotherapy. Both are effective.

www For a detailed summary of this chapter and a comprehensive set of review questions visit the Online Learning Center at **www.mhhe.com/teague2e.**

Web Resources

American Psychiatric Association (APA): This organization offers a helpful fact sheet series and a Let's Talk Facts pamphlet series, both designed to dispel myths about mental illness. The Web site also includes information about mental health treatment and related insurance issues.
www.psych.org

American Psychological Association (Help Center): This Web site features articles and information on many topics, such as work/school issues, family and relationships, and health and emotional wellness. It also offers free brochures on topics such as counseling help and the warning signs of mental problems.
http://helping.apa.org

National Alliance for the Mentally Ill (NAMI): NAMI is a nonprofit organization for people affected by severe mental illness. Its Web site focuses on informing yourself about mental health issues, finding support, and taking action.
www.nami.org

National Institute of Mental Health (NIMH): This division of the National Institutes of Health focuses on dispensing health information to the public and sponsoring research on mental health and illness. Its authoritative information ranges from breaking news to explanations of common mental disorders.
www.nimh.nih.gov

National Mental Health Association (NMHA): This organization's resource center offers brochures on mental health and referrals to treatment centers, support groups, and other national organizations. Answers to frequently asked questions about mental health are especially helpful.
www.nmha.org

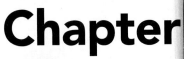

Chapter 4

Spirituality
Finding
Meaning
in Life and
Death

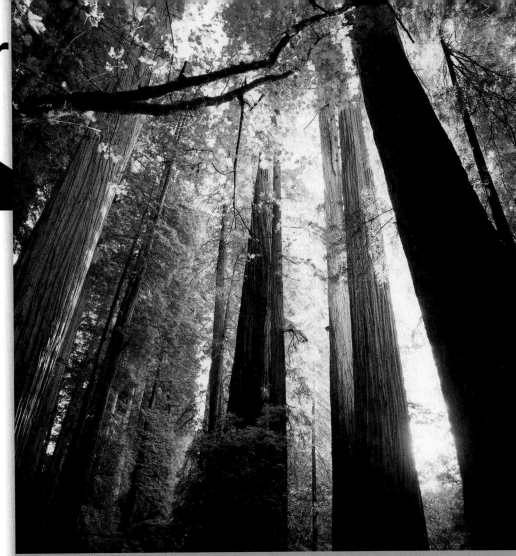

WWW

Your Health Today

www.mhhe.com/teague2e

Go to the Online Learning Center for *Your Health Today* for interactive activities, quizzes, flashcards, Web links, and more resources related to this chapter.

Ever Wonder...

- if you can be spiritual without belonging to an organized religion?

- if praying for yourself or someone else can have an effect on health?

- what meditation is all about?

Someone once said that the longest journey is the journey inward. The spiritual journey is deeply personal and individual. It may begin as a yearning for connection with what is universal and timeless or a belief in a power in the universe that is greater than oneself. It often involves a search for meaning and purpose or a desire for a more intense participation in life. Many people now believe that spiritual health enhances their psychological and physical well-being, and they pursue spiritual wellness as one of the important dimensions of total wellness.

It seems that all people in all times have experienced spiritual aspirations. Worldwide, there are more than 20 major religions and thousands of other forms of spiritual expression. In the spirit of modern genetics, some scientists have been searching for a biological basis for human spirituality—a gene or genes that would account for our spiritual experiences and yearnings—and one researcher, Dean Hamer of the National Cancer Institute, believes he has found such a gene.[1] No matter what the role of biology, however, spiritual experience and expression are clearly the product of complex interactions between individuals and their cultures.

What Is Spirituality?

Because spirituality may involve different paths for different people, it has been defined in many ways. In health promotion literature, **spirituality** is commonly defined as a person's connection to self, significant others, and the community at large. Many experts also agree that spirituality involves a personal belief system or value system that gives meaning and purpose to life.[2] For some individuals this personal value system may include a belief in and reverence for a higher power, which may be expressed through an organized religion. For others the spiritual dimension is nonreligious and centers on a personal value system that may be reflected in activities such as volunteer work. In either case, spirituality provides a feeling of participation in something greater than oneself and a sense of unity with nature and the universe.

spirituality
The experience of connection to self, others, and the community at large, providing a sense of purpose and meaning.

SPIRITUALITY IN EVERYDAY LIFE

All of us have questions about our existence: Am I connected to something, or am I alone, isolated, and cut off? Is my life guided by my values, or am I drifting without a moral compass? What gives my life meaning? Searching for answers to these questions is part of life's spiritual journey.

Connection to Self and Others   Being connected to yourself involves knowing who you are, developing self-awareness, and building self-esteem. Growth in these areas is an incremental process in which you develop a reservoir of inner strengths through such practices as becoming more compassionate or learning to be a better listener.

Spirituality also includes being responsible for yourself and taking charge of your life. Your spiritual health affects your capacity for love, compassion, joy, forgiveness, altruism, and fulfillment. It can be an antidote to stress, cynicism, anger, fear, anxiety, self-absorption, and pessimism.

Connection with significant others through positive relationships is also essential to spiritual health and growth. Healthy relationships involve a balance between closeness and separateness and are characterized by mutual support, respect, good communication, and caring actions. Having strong personal relationships improves self-esteem and gives greater meaning to life.[3]

Connection with the community includes enjoying constructive relationships at school, in the workplace, or in the neighborhood. Several studies have demonstrated links between social connectedness and positive outcomes for individual health and well-being.[4] Evidence shows that social participation and engagement are related to the maintenance of cognitive function in older adulthood and to lowered mortality rates. In general, the size of a person's social network and his or her sense of connectedness are inversely related to risk-related behaviors such as alcohol and tobacco consumption, physical inactivity, and behaviors leading to obesity.[5]

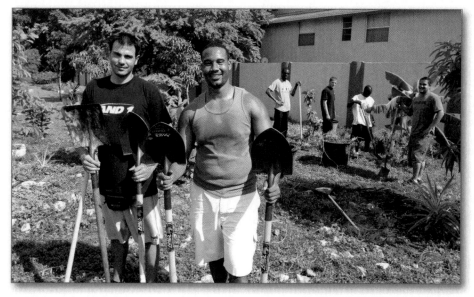

■ Participating in activities that reinforce feelings of connectedness with others is a way of enhancing spirituality in everyday life. These Florida men are volunteering during "Hands On Miami" Day.

A Personal Value System   Another aspect of spirituality involves developing a personal **value system**, a set of guidelines for how you want to live your life. *Values,* the criteria for judging what is good and bad, underlie moral principles and behavior. Your value system shapes who you are as a person, how you make decisions, and what goals you set for yourself. When you develop a way of life that makes sense and enables you to navigate the world effectively, the many choices you face each day become much less complex and easier to handle. Your value system becomes your map, providing a structure for decision making that allows flexibility and the possibility of change.

value system
Set of criteria for judging what is good and bad that underlies moral decisions and behavior.

Meaning and Purpose in Life   Why am I here? This question has been asked by people all over the world, in all eras, and at all stages of life. For young people, the answer may involve developing relationships and connections. For adults, the answer may be caring for others. For older adults, it may be working for a healthier planet. Positive psychology contributes the idea that meaning in life comes from using one's personal strengths to serve some larger end.

HAPPINESS AND LIFE SATISFACTION

The study of happiness is part of the positive psychology movement, with its focus on what makes life worth living (see Chapter 3). Surveys indicate that happiness is typical rather than unusual—9 out of 10 Americans report being very happy or pretty happy.[6] According to one poll, wealth, education,

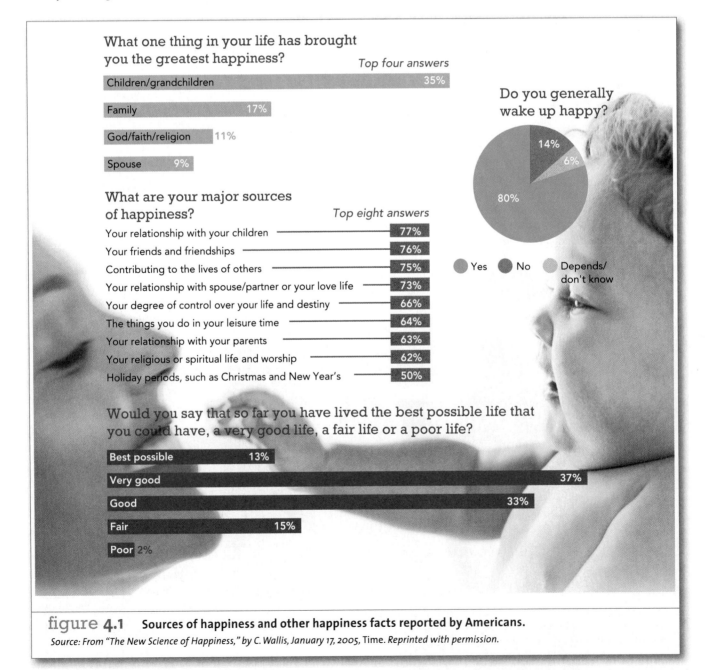

figure 4.1   **Sources of happiness and other happiness facts reported by Americans.**
Source: From "The New Science of Happiness," by C. Wallis, January 17, 2005, Time. Reprinted with permission.

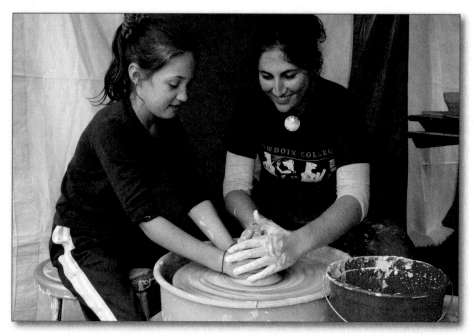

■ Engagement in meaningful activities—such as sharing one's expertise and passion with a younger person—is a major sourse of happiness and satisfaction for most people.

IQ, and youth have little impact on happiness; instead, the top source of happiness is connections with family and friends (Figure 4.1).[7] Other sources of happiness include contributing to the lives of others, having a sense of control over one's life, and having a religious or spiritual life.

In their research, positive psychologists have found that happiness involves three components: positive emotion and pleasure (savoring sensory experiences); engagement (depth of involvement with family, work, romance, and hobbies); and meaning (using personal strengths to serve some larger end).[8] The happiest people are those who orient their lives toward all three, but the latter two—engagement and meaning— are much more important in giving people satisfaction and happiness.

Happiness research has found that people can increase their level of happiness by practicing certain "happiness exercises":[8]

■ *Three Good Things in Life.* Write down three things that went well each day and their causes every night for a week.

■ *Using Signature Strengths in a New Way.* Using the classification of character strengths and virtues (see Table 3.1), take the inventory of your character strengths and identify your top five strengths, your "signature strengths." Use one of these top strengths in a new and different way every day for a week.

■ *Gratitude Visit.* Write a letter of gratitude and then deliver it in person to someone who has been especially kind to you but whom you have never thanked properly.

Research found that two of these exercises—Three Good Things and Using Signature Strengths in a New Way— increased happiness and decreased depressive symptoms for 6 months. The Gratitude Visit caused large positive changes for 1 month.

Related research has identified other ways to increase happiness and life satisfaction, including performing acts of kindness, savoring life's joys, and learning to forgive (see the box "Steps to a More Satisfying Life"). Positive psychologists say that happiness exercises give meaning to life by helping people feel more connected to others. Almost everyone feels happier when they are with other people, even those who think they want to be alone.

The down side is that people may have a happiness "set point," determined largely by genetics. That is, no matter what happens in life, people may have a tendency to return to their norm. The notion that people can increase their happiness reinforces Western cultural biases about how individual initiative and a positive attitude can solve complex problems.[7] In addition, because happiness research focuses on internal processes, little or no attention is paid to the very real sources of unhappiness in people's lives that are connected to their social and economic circumstances.

Enhancing Your Spirituality

How do you build a spiritual life? Greater connectedness and meaning can be found through a variety of practices, especially if they are done on a regular basis.

MEDITATION

Human beings are engaged in a constant inner monologue, reviewing the past, commenting on the present, and speculating about the future. This inner chatter can keep us from being fully present in our lives. **Meditation** is a way to slow your racing thoughts and quiet your mind by focusing on a word, an object (such as a candle flame), or a process (such as breathing). With practice, meditation can help you become calmer as you go about your daily routines. There are many ways to meditate, but all involve introspection and attention to your inner life.

meditation
Technique for quieting the mind by focusing on a word, an object (such as a candle flame), or a process (such as breathing).

If you are interested in trying meditation as a way to build a spiritual life, follow the guidelines in the box "Learning to Meditate." Although meditation may not appeal to everyone, the practice can offer many benefits. It is widely used in stress management and stress reduction programs. Proponents claim that meditation provides deep relaxation, promotes health, increases creativity and intelligence, and brings inner happiness and fulfillment.

Mindfulness is both a form of meditation and the practice of living fully in the moment. By learning to be conscious of your thoughts as they pass by— observing them, not judging them— you develop your ability to control

mindfulness
Awareness and acceptance of living fully in the moment.

and stop habitual, impulsive, or undesirable reactions. You become more capable of responding in a "thoughtful" and "mindful" way rather than becoming overwhelmed with negative emotions or self-criticism.[9] As you learn to focus on the present moment, you can be more in touch with your life as it is happening.

When people learn to live fully in the moment, they sometimes experience a phenomenon known as **flow**, a feeling of being completely absorbed in an activity and a moment. In this state, people forget themselves, lose track of time, and feel as if they have become one with what they are doing. Writers describe times when words seem to come through them; athletes

flow
Pleasurable experience of complete absorption and engagement in an activity.

refer to being "in the zone." Flow has been described as one of the most enjoyable and valuable experiences a person can have.[10] When you learn to be mindful and live in the moment, you are more likely to experience flow in your daily activities.

Mindfulness is celebrated by the noted Vietnamese monk Thich Nhat Hanh in these words:

> Our true home is in the present moment.
> To live in the present moment is a miracle.
> The miracle is not to walk on water.
> The miracle is to walk on the green Earth in the
>   present moment,
> To appreciate the peace and beauty that are
>   available now.[11]

JOURNALING

Another approach to building a spiritual life is *journaling*. As you record your feelings, thoughts, breakthroughs, and desires in a private journal, you will begin to understand yourself more clearly. Psychologist James Pennebaker has found that writing about emotional upheavals can improve

Challenges & Choices

Steps to a More Satisfying Life

Want to be happier? Here are some practical suggestions, based on research findings by psychologist Sonia Lyubomirsky and other positive psychologists:

1. *Count your blessings.* Keep a gratitude journal in which you write down three to five things for which you are grateful once a week.

2. *Practice acts of kindness.* Being kind to others has many positive effects, including a greater sense of connection with the people around you.

3. *Savor life's joys.* Pay attention to moments of pleasure and wonder; keep a store of such memories so that you can call on them in less happy times.

4. *Thank a mentor.* Express your appreciation to those who have been kind to you.

5. *Learn to forgive.* Write a letter of forgiveness to anyone who has hurt or wronged you. Letting go of anger and resentment allows you to move on.

6. *Invest time and energy in friends and family.* Strong personal relationships are the biggest factor in life satisfaction.

7. *Take care of your body.* Practicing good self-care— getting enough sleep, exercising, smiling and laughing—makes your daily life more satisfying.

8. *Develop strategies for coping with stress and hardship.* For some people, religious faith offers help. For others, secular beliefs—even "this too shall pass"—serve as coping tools.

It's Not Just Personal . . .

Research has found that happiness has more benefits than just feeling good. Happy people have better health, are more successful, and are more engaged with their community. The cause-and-effect relationship goes both ways.

Sources: *"Positive Psychology Progress: Validation of Interventions,"* by M. Seligman, T. Steen, N. Park, and C. Peterson, 2005, American Psychologist, 60 (5): pp. 410–421; *"The New Science of Happiness,"* by C. Wallis, January 17, 2005, Time.

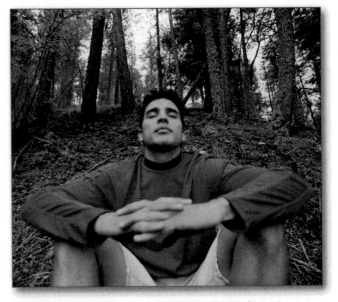

■ Meditation is a calming and centering spiritual practice.

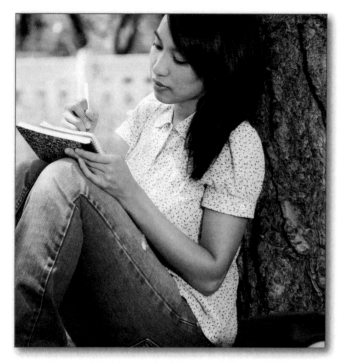

■ Journaling offers a way to explore your feeelings, deepen your self-understanding and discover what is important to you.

Challenges & Choices

Learning to Meditate

Meditation is an ancient technique with modern adaptations. Various forms of meditation have been developed, but their common goals are to calm the mind, raise awareness, and increase attention to what is happening in the present moment. Here are some guidelines for a type of meditation in which you focus on your breathing:

■ Sit in a comfortable place—on a pillow on the floor or in a chair, for example—in a quiet room where you won't be disturbed. Close your eyes.

■ Breathe deeply. Feel the breath as it enters your nostrils and fills your chest and abdomen; then release it.

■ Focus your attention on your breathing and awareness of the moment. Try to be silent and still.

■ Remain passive and relaxed as your thoughts come and go, noticing them without judging them. At first, your mind will fill with memories, worries, and random thoughts. Let go of the thoughts and feelings and return to the awareness of breath. Eventually, you will be able to concentrate for longer periods of time, and these periods of concentration may be accompanied by feelings of great tranquility.

Meditate for brief periods of time each day. Start out with 5 minutes and gradually build up to 15 minutes or more. Make a commitment to continue meditating for 3 months; you will not experience any changes or benefits unless you practice. Experiment until you find a place, time, and approach that works for you. If you would like more information about techniques, contact a meditation center, consult a teacher or book, search online, talk with more experienced meditators, or listen to a tape.

It's Not Just Personal . . .
People all over the world, of all spiritual and secular persuasions, practice meditation. Types of meditations include transcendental, mindfulness, mantra (chanting), zazen (sitting), walking, and chakra, among many others.

physical and mental health. He suggests writing about any of the following:

■ Something that you are thinking or worrying about too much.

■ Something that you are dreaming about.

■ Something that you feel is affecting your life in an unhealthy way.

■ Something that you have been avoiding for days, weeks, or years.[12]

The more honest you are, the better. Don't censor yourself as you write; just let your thoughts flow. Try to move beyond the superficial telling to asking yourself, Why am I feeling this way?

Journaling is an effective way to learn about who you are and where you have been. Listening to your inner dialogue may offer you a sense of peace and a positive outlook on your experiences. In some cases, journaling can be painful, stirring up emotions that may be difficult to handle on your own. If you find yourself feeling overwhelmed, consider contacting a professional for counseling.[13]

RETREAT

A *retreat* is a period of seclusion, solitude, or group withdrawal for prayer, meditation, or study. Retreats are intended to reenergize your life and restore your zest for living. A spiritual retreat might offer a balance of activities that encourage growth, foster learning, and restore energy, so that when you return to your normal surroundings, you may live life to the fullest in a purposeful way.

Many kinds of facilities offer retreats, workshops, and programs for spiritual growth, but you can use your home for a retreat as well. Set aside a weekend and plan to give up all social events, phone calls, errands, television, newspapers, Internet, and all nonessential housework. Then prepare for exploration. You might meditate, journal, draw, write poetry, take walks to enjoy the beauty of nature, listen to music, read—whatever you want to do that you find deepening and centering. At their best, retreats stimulate the mind, enhance self-awareness, and refresh the spirit. They provide food for the body, mind, and spirit.

THE ARTS

Scholar Joseph Campbell once asserted, "The goal of life is rapture. Art is the way we experience it. Art is the transforming experience." Experiencing the arts—whether sculpture, painting, music, poetry, literature, theater, storytelling, dance, or some other form—is another way to build a spiritual life. Experiencing great art can inspire you, through felt experience, to think about the purpose of life and the nature of reality.[14] By engaging your heart, mind, and spirit, art can give you fresh insights, challenge preconceptions, and trigger inner growth.

When you enjoy and appreciate the arts, you embrace diverse cultures past and present and frequently discover in them the universal themes of human existence—love, loss, birth, death, isolation, community, continuity, change. When you express yourself creatively, you may be able to experience a spiritual connection between your inner core and the natural world beyond yourself. Both experiences—art appreciation and artistic expression—can be transforming. If the visual or performing arts are not part of your life right now, try to schedule time to visit a museum or attend a concert. Make notes or sketches in a journal reflecting on your experiences. Doing so may stimulate new spiritual connections in your life.

LIVING YOUR VALUES

Building a spiritual life also means bringing your deepest beliefs and intentions into the world—that is, living your values (see the box "Understanding Your Personal Values"). Can you articulate what is most important to you in life? Are you living and acting in accordance with it? Try writing a "purpose statement" that will remind you of who you truly are and why you believe you are here on earth. Then ask yourself, Do I stay "on purpose" in my daily interactions and activities? Commit your purpose statement to memory, and read or recite it daily. It may be "to live and learn" or "to know my higher being and teach and express love."

Adopting a new habit, such as putting your best intentions into practice, takes time and work. Experts say that you have to continue to take action for 60 to 90 days to make a behavior change stick. As Aristotle understood almost 2,500 years ago, "We are what we repeatedly do. Excellence is not an act, then, but a habit."

One way to create new habits is to develop rituals—routines or practices, often symbolic, that you follow regularly. Another way to change an old habit or build a new one is through supportive relationships. Anyone who has had a workout buddy, attended Alcoholics Anonymous, or prayed with a group on retreat is familiar with the powerful effect of acting in concert with others. In a 2-year study of 200 people who made New Year's resolutions, psychologist John Norcross found that those individuals most likely to persist beyond 6 months were those with social support.[15]

Health Benefits of Spirituality

According to a CBS News poll, 80 percent of Americans believe that prayer holds the power to heal,[16] and according to a 2004 study, one-third of Americans use prayer, in addition to conventional medical treatments, for health concerns.[17]

The connection between spirituality and health is gaining serious attention from the medical and scientific communities.[18] Hundreds of studies have been conducted on spirituality and health, and more than half the nation's medical schools now offer courses on spirituality and medicine, whereas only three did 20 years ago. The National Institutes of Health plans to spend millions of dollars over the next several years on "mind-body" medicine.[19] The pursuit is not without its skeptics, however, and the connection between spirituality and health remains an area of controversy and debate.

PHYSICAL BENEFITS

Can prayer cure cancer or slow its progression? Can it lower blood pressure? Does spirituality speed healing after accidents or help people recover from surgery? Do religious people live longer?

There are no definitive answers to these questions, but a majority of

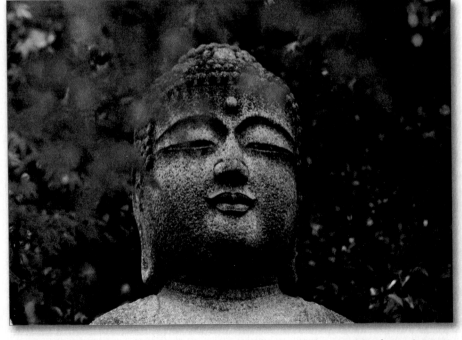

■ Contemplating the serene face of the Buddha can be an artistic or a spiritual experience or both. This statue is in the Golden Pavilion in Kyoto, Japan.

350 studies of physical health and 850 studies of mental health suggest a direct relationship between religious involvement and spirituality, on the one hand, and better health outcomes, on the other.[20] Research has found that religious involvement and spirituality are associated with lower blood pressure, decreased risk of substance abuse, less cardiovascular disease, less depression, less anxiety, enhanced immune function, and longer life.[21] Meditation and prayer in combination with traditional medical treatments are reported to relieve medical problems such as chronic pain, depression, anxiety, insomnia, and premenstrual syndrome.[22] There are enough positive results to spur further inquiry.

One of the most consistent research findings is that spiritually connected persons stay healthier and live longer than those who are not connected.[21, 23] An important reason for this outcome is that people who are religious or spiritually connected generally have healthier lifestyles. They smoke less, drink less alcohol, have better diets, exercise more, and are more likely to wear seat belts and to avoid drugs and unsafe sex. However, these factors don't seem to account for all of the health-related benefits of religious and spiritual commitment. Studies find that the positive differences in death rates persist even after controlling for factors such as age, health, habits, demographics, and other health-related variables.[21]

Another explanation for better health among people who are spiritually involved is that they react more effectively to health crises. People who are religious or spiritual seem to

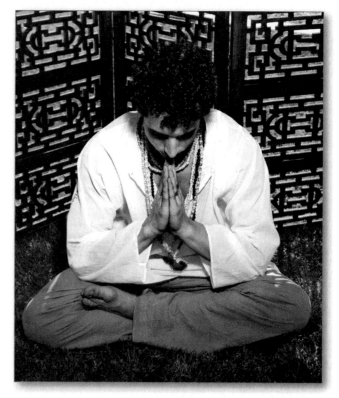

■ Spiritual commitment is associated with physical and mental health, but the association may have more to do with psychosocial factors than with spiritual beliefs or practices.

Challenges & Choices

Understanding Your Personal Values

Many people are unaware of their core values and the guiding principles by which they live their lives. We seldom think through our values until we are faced with a difficult choice, and even then we may make a choice without being aware of our values. For inspiration we can look to people who stood up for their values despite enormous pressure to conform and foreseeable negative consequences. A prime example is Rosa Parks, who sparked the civil rights movement when she refused to sit in the back of the bus.

How would you articulate your own core values? Consider the following list of major life values:

achievement	family
autonomy	financial well-being
compassion	freedom
connectedness	health
creativity	home
education	honesty
integrity	relationships
learning	service
love	social justice
personal growth	spirituality
prestige	status

Which of these (or others) are most important and meaningful to you? What guiding principles can you derive from them? How can you embody them in your life?

It's Not Just Personal . . .
Societies as well as individuals operate from core values and principles. Some core values of American society, as expressed in such documents as the Declaration of Independence and the U.S. Constitution, include life, liberty, the pursuit of happiness, justice, popular sovereignty, the common good, truth, diversity, and patriotism. How do your personal values line up with these societal values?

be more willing than those who are not spiritually connected to alter their health habits, to be proactive in seeking medical treatment, and to accept the support of others. People who have strong ties to a religious group or another community segment may receive help and encouragement from that community in times of crisis.[24] Friends may transport them to the doctor and to church, shop for them, prepare meals, arrange child care, and encourage them to get appropriate medical treatment.

MENTAL BENEFITS

People who are spiritually involved tend to enjoy better mental health as well as physical health. One reason may be that religious people tend to be more forgiving, and recent research has linked forgiveness with lower blood pressure, less back pain, and overall better personal health.[25]

In addition, spiritual practices such as meditation, prayer, and worship seem to promote positive emotions such as hope, love, contentment, and forgiveness, which can result in lower levels of anxiety. This in turn may help to minimize the stress response, which suppresses immune functioning.[26–28] Many people may even turn to religion in times of stress.[29] Studies have also shown that prayer and certain relaxation techniques, such as meditation, yoga, and hypnotherapy, reduce the secretion of stress hormones and their harmful side effects.

Depression may also be mediated by spiritual involvement. Some studies indicate that people who are religiously involved suffer less depression and recover faster when they are depressed.[30, 31] Religious people are also less likely to consider suicide.[19]

Studies have shown that spiritual connectedness appears to be associated with high levels of *health-related quality of life*, the physical, psychological, social, and spiritual aspects of a person's daily experience. Spiritual connectedness is especially important when a person is coping with serious health issues such as cancer, HIV infection, heart disease, limb amputation, or spinal cord injury.[21] This positive relationship persists even as physical health declines with serious illness.[32]

A DIFFERENT VIEW

Although the majority of studies indicate that spiritual connectedness has health benefits, many studies have found no relationship between health and spirituality. Some researchers have even suggested that spirituality can have negative outcomes for physical and mental health. For example, several studies indicate that when people experience

a spiritual conflict in association with a health crisis, there is a negative impact on their health status.[21, 33–36] And one study concluded that people who knew they were receiving intercessory prayer (prayer by strangers) may have experienced increased anxiety and more complications than those who were unsure they were being prayed for.[37] It seems that the connection between spirituality and health can have both positive and negative implications and needs more study (see the box "Spirituality and Health").

Spirituality and Community Involvement

Many believe that people can develop their spirituality by participating in their communities in a positive way. Unpaid work directly promotes community well-being through the services provided, whether that means caring for an elderly relative or working on a community project. It also has indirect benefits by building the social networks that contribute to optimal well-being.

service learning
Form of education that combines academic study with community service.

SERVICE LEARNING

One way that people can connect classroom activities to community service and community building is through **service learning.** The purpose of integrating community service with academic study is to enrich learning, teach civic responsibility, and strengthen communities. Students are encouraged to take a positive role in their community, such as by tutoring, caring for the environment, or conducting oral histories with senior citizens. All of these activities are

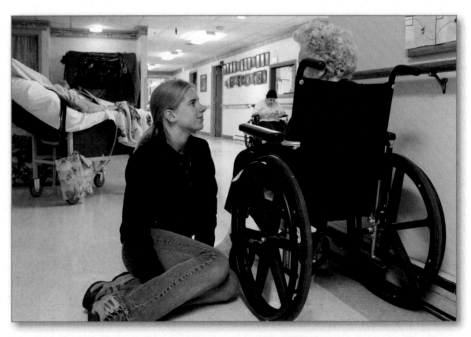

■ Some people find connection, meaning , and spiritual fulfillment through service to others.

Who's at Risk

Spirituality and Health

Do people with spiritual or religious beliefs and practices have better health outcomes than people without such beliefs and practices? Many research studies have been conducted to investigate various aspects of this question, with contradictory and inconsistent results. The findings of a few of them are described here:

- A combination of frequent religious attendance, prayer, Bible study, and strong beliefs predicted a faster recovery from depression.[a]

- Frequency of religious attendance in African Americans with sickle cell disease was associated with significantly lower levels of pain, but prayer/Bible study and intrinsic religiosity were not related to pain levels.[b]

- Patients with advanced cancer, particularly African American and Hispanic patients, reported a significantly higher quality of life if either the religious community or the medical system provided spiritual support.[c]

- Cardiac patients who received intercessory prayer (prayer by strangers) fared no better than patients who did not receive such prayer.[d]

- Religious struggles and negative religious coping (for example, "questioning God's love") were correlated with higher risk of death in hospitalized older adults.[e]

- People who attended religious services had a lower prevalence of hypertension than nonattendees.[f]

- Neither self-reported spirituality, frequency of church attendance, nor frequency of prayer was associated with recovery from heart attack.[g]

- An increase in religiosity/spirituality after a diagnosis of HIV infection was correlated with slower disease progression after 4 years.[h]

Sources:

a "Religion and Remission of Depression in Medical Inpatients with Heart Failure/Pulmonary Disease," by H.G. Koenig, 2007, Journal of Nervous and Mental Disease, 195, 389–395.

b "Religiosity/Spirituality and Pain in Patients With Sickle Cell Disease," by M.O. Harrison et al., 2005, Journal of Nervous and Mental Diseases, 193, 250–257.

c "Religiousness and Spiritual Support Among Advanced Cancer Patients and Associations With End-of-Life Treatment Preferences and Quality of Life," by T.A. Balboni et al., 2007, Journal of Clinical Oncology, 25, 555–560.

d "Music, Imagery, Touch, and Prayer as Adjuncts to Interventional Cardiac Care," by M.W. Krucoff et al., 2005, Lancet, 366, 211–217.

e "Religious Struggles as a Predictor of Mortality Among Medically Ill Elderly Patients," by K.I. Pargament et al., 2001, Archives of Internal Medicine, 161, 1881–1885.

f "Frequency of Attendance at Religious Services, Hypertension, and Blood Pressure: The Third National Health and Nutrition Examination Survey," by R.F. Gillium and D.D. Ingram, 2006, Psychosomatic Medicine, 68, 382–385.

g "Spirituality, Religion, and Clinical Outcomes in Patients Recovering From an Acute Myocardial Infarction," by J.A. Blumenthal et al., 2007, Psychosomatic Medicine, 69, 501–508.

h "An Increase in Religiousness/Spirituality Occurs After HIV Diagnosis and Predicts Slower Disease Progression Over 4 Years in People With HIV," by G. Ironson, R. Stuetzie, and M.A. Fletcher, 2006, Journal of General Internal Medicine, 21, 562–568.

meant to teach people how to extend themselves beyond their enclosed world, taking a risk to get involved in the lives of others. In this way they learn about caring and taking care of—two particularly important concepts for personal growth.

VOLUNTEERING

Volunteering is another way to be connected with other people. Volunteers may experience a "helper's high," similar to a "runner's high."[38] Research shows that people who give time, money, and support to others are likely to be more satisfied with their lives and less depressed.[39]

Not all kinds of volunteering have the same effect, however. One-on-one contact and direct involvement significantly influence the effect of volunteering on the volunteer.[40] Working closely with strangers appears to increase the potential health benefits of the experience. Liking the volunteer work, performing it consistently, and having unselfish motives further increase the feelings of helper's high and the health benefits associated with it.[41] Simply donating money or doing

volunteer work in isolation does not seem to have the same positive effect.

Just as the high of helping may create enjoyable immediate benefits, the calm of helping may result in significant long-term health benefits. For example, volunteering may reduce the negative health effects of living with high levels of stress for long periods of time. Those who have experienced a helper's high have noted specific improvements in their physical well-being. These improvements included a reduction in arthritis pain, lupus symptoms, asthma attacks, migraine headaches, colds, and episodes of the flu. Volunteering may even result in longer life for the volunteer.[42, 43]

SOCIAL ACTIVISM AND THE GLOBAL COMMUNITY

Some people connect with their communities—local, national, and global—through social activism. A social cause, such as overcoming poverty or fighting illiteracy, can unite people from diverse backgrounds for a common good. Many people find it meaningful to participate in global citizenship by joining organizations such as those described in the box "Global Activism."

Highlight on Health

Global Activism

Many organizations help individuals put their values into practice in the world. Here are a few:

- Amnesty International is a worldwide movement of people who campaign for internationally recognized human rights—physical and mental integrity, freedom of conscience and expression, and freedom from discrimination.
- Doctors Without Borders delivers emergency aid to victims of armed conflict, epidemics, and natural and human-made disasters and to others who lack health care due to social or geographical isolation. Each year, more than 2,500 volunteer doctors, nurses, other medi-

cal professionals, logistics experts, water/sanitation engineers, and administrators provide medical aid in more than 80 countries.
- Greenpeace focuses on the most crucial worldwide threats to the planet's biodiversity and environment. Greenpeace has been campaigning against environmental degradation since 1971, bearing witness in a nonviolent manner.
- The Earth Charter Initiative is an international organization dedicated to building a sustainable world based on respect for nature, universal human rights, economic justice, and peace. A basic premise of the Earth Charter is that these attributes must be cultivated at the local community level before they can emerge at the national and global levels.

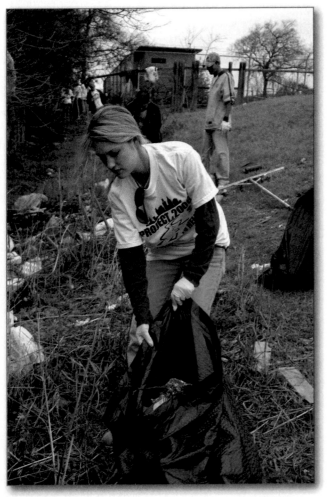

- Volunteering in an environmental cleanup is a way to live your values

If you are interested in social activism, look for ways to participate through your school, your religious community, or groups you locate on the Internet. When you volunteer for such an organization, you commit yourself to building a foundation for a better world, making a contribution through service to others, and creating opportunities for mutual understanding.

How is spirituality related to community involvement? Some claim that when we attend to our inner life, we nurture our compassionate responses to human need and develop a passion for social justice. Others believe that contributing to community welfare and striving for justice are the ways to a rich inner life.

Some people turn away from social activism because they think it's "just politics." We hear news stories that use catchphrases associating traditional values with the religious right and social justice with the liberal left. Any action can be cloaked in the guise of religiosity, and distinguishing politics with a religious flavor from the practice of authentic spiritual values can be difficult. The former is designed to manipulate people's feelings for political gain; the latter has no hidden agenda or ulterior motive.

The question for the individual is, How can I best put my passion into action while respecting the beliefs of others? Some social activists have transcended their religious and social conditioning and become universal spiritual beings, ready to serve all. Both Mahatma Gandhi and the Reverend Martin Luther King, Jr., developed an integrated worldview and worked to create global community.

NATURE AND THE ENVIRONMENT

The impulse that propels people to the mountains or seashore for their holidays is the same impulse that drives pilgrims to sites of religious importance—the need to reconnect with

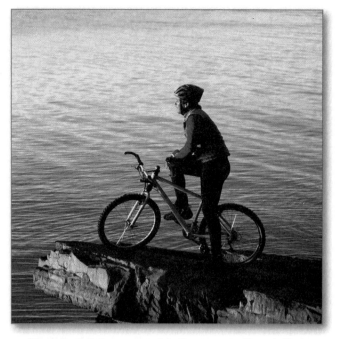

■ "The miracle is to . . . appreciate the peace and beauty that are available now." (Trich Nhat Hahn)

the natural world. Many cultures in history, including many Native American cultures, did and do have a strong spiritual connection to nature or "Mother Earth." These cultures promote reverence for the universe, which results in a strong spiritual connection to nature.

Some people combine ecological, ethical, and spiritual interests and beliefs into what has been called *eco-spirituality.* They may participate in retreats or periods of reflection to deepen their connections to the earth. They may advocate respect for the sacredness of creation and the concept of tending (caring for, nurturing, and participating in nature). Daily activities that incorporate environmental values might include recycling, composting, and walking or riding a bike instead of driving. As with volunteerism and social activism, when you are environmentally active, the benefits flow back to you, sustaining your spirituality and adding meaning to life.

Death and Dying

Death and dying have great spiritual significance for people of all cultures. In one study, 89 percent of Americans described a "good death" as one that included making peace with God.[45] Many also included prayer and discussing the meaning of death in their description of a good death.

When someone you love dies, the experience is extremely personal, yet it is one that you also share with others. Life and death are part of the cycle of existence and the natural order of things. Many report that because of their personal faith, they do not fear death, since they know that their lives have had meaning within the context of a larger plan.

STAGES OF DYING AND DEATH

In 1969 Elisabeth Kübler-Ross published *On Death and Dying,* one of the first books to propose a set of stages that people go through when they believe they are in the process of dying.[44] The five stages are (1) denial and isolation, (2) anger, (3) bargaining, (4) depression, and (5) acceptance. Over time, further study has shown that these stages are not linear—individuals may experience them in a different order or may return to stages they have already gone through—nor are they necessarily universal—individuals may not experience some stages at all.

Many believe that life is full of transitions, with death being the last. A shared sense of mortality can be the basis for feeling connected with other human beings. Recently, health care professionals have begun to describe ways to *live* with an illness rather than simply looking at the diagnosis as the point at which one begins to prepare for death. As medical care has improved, many individuals diagnosed with cancer or HIV infection have recovered or lived with the disease for many years. The critical thing to remember is that one need not go on a "death watch" after a diagnosis; usually, there is time to repair relationships, to build memories, and to review one's life. The dying person may find comfort and strength in talking through the process with family and friends or with a spiritual advisor (see the box "The Hospice Movement: In Search of the Good Death").

Research has found that terminally ill persons derive strength and hope from spiritual and religious beliefs. In fact, terminally ill adults report significantly greater religious involvement and depth of spiritual perspective than do healthy adults. Studies suggest that, unrelated to belief in an afterlife, religiously involved people at the end of life are more accepting of death than those who are less religiously involved. In addition, religious involvement and spirituality are associated with less death anxiety.[21]

HEALTHY GRIEVING

Grief is a natural reaction to loss. Besides the loss of loved ones to death, we grieve many kinds of losses throughout our lives: divorce, relocation, traumatic experiences, loss of health and mobility, and even expected life transitions such as having the last child leave home. Grief is often expressed by feelings of sadness, loneliness, anger, and guilt. These feelings are part of the process of healing, since we do not begin to feel better until we have acknowledged and felt sorrow over our loss.

Physical symptoms of grief may include crying and sighing, aches and pains, sleep disturbances, headaches, lethargy, reduced appetite, and stomach upset. The intense emotions you feel at the time of a loss can have a negative impact on immune system functioning, reducing your ability to fight off illness. Studies have shown that surviving spouses may have increased risk for heart disease, cancer, depression, alcoholism, and suicide.[46, 47] Everyone has higher risk for disease after the loss of a loved one, but those who are more resilient may cope with the loss better.

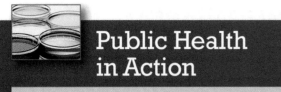

Public Health in Action

The Hospice Movement: In Search of the Good Death

As they think about end-of-life issues, many people hope for a "good death." By this, most people mean that they have peace of mind, are with family members and friends, and do not have pain. The development of the **hospice** movement has helped people move closer to this ideal.

Originally, the term *hospice* referred to a place of shelter for weary and sick travelers, often returning from religious pilgrimages. Today, hospice care is intended for people who no longer respond to cure-oriented medical treatment. Hospice is not a place but a concept of care. The goal is to improve the quality of life in a patient's last days by providing *palliative care*—pain management, comfort, and attention to the person's physical, spiritual, emotional, and social needs. Hospice programs also provide support for family members, including help with caring for their loved one. The hospice team—social workers, nurses, physicians, counselors, and volunteers—normalizes the dying process as part of life and works to support patients throughout the process.

> **hospice**
> Program that provides care for the terminally ill and their loved ones.

Eighty percent of hospice care is provided in the patient's home, a family member's home, or a nursing home. To be eligible for hospice care, an individual must be certified by a physician to have a life expectancy of 6 months or less. Hospice care is available 24 hours a day, 7 days a week. A team member will visit the home whenever needed and appropriate. Sometimes, a person's health improves and he or she leaves the hospice program but is eligible to return if a downturn in health occurs.

The modern hospice movement was founded by Dr. Cicely Saunders, a British physician, in the 1960s, and the first hospice in the United States opened in New Haven, Connecticut, in 1974. Today there are more than 3,200 hospice programs in the United States, collectively providing end-of-life care for almost 1 million people. According to the Hospice Foundation of America, more than 95,000 people volunteer for hospice annually, giving more than 5 million hours of care. A goal of Healthy People 2010 is to increase the percentage of the population with access to the continuum of long-term care services, including hospice care.

Source: What Is Hospice? *Hospice Foundation of America, retrieved May 6, 2008, from www.hospicefoundation.org.*

Bereavement after the loss of a loved one typically involves four phases:

- *Numbness and shock.* This phase occurs immediately after the loss and lasts for a brief period. The numbness protects you from acute pain.

- *Separation.* As the shock wears off, you start to feel the pain of loss, and you experience acute yearning and longing to be reunited with your loved one.

- *Disorganization.* You are preoccupied and distracted; you have trouble concentrating and thinking clearly. You may feel lethargic and indifferent. This phase can last much longer than you anticipate.

- *Reorganization.* You begin to adjust to the loss. Your life will never be the same without your loved one, but your feelings have less intensity and you can reinvest in life.

If you experience the death of a loved one, it is important to take care of yourself while you are grieving. There is no right or wrong way to grieve and no specific timetable. Friends who suggest that it's time to move on need to understand that you are on your own journey and cannot be rushed. You need to give yourself permission to feel the loss and take time to heal. Some people seem to cope better if they talk about the death rather than internalizing their feelings. During the grieving process it is vital that you eat a balanced diet, exercise regularly, drink plenty of fluids, and get enough rest. Keeping a journal and talking about the person who has died can also be part of the healing process. Finally, you should not hesitate to ask friends for support, since having a nurturing social network is particularly helpful in coping with loss.

If intense grief persists for more than a year, or if you find yourself losing or gaining weight or not sleeping, consult a health professional to get a treatment referral. Treatment options might include support groups, family therapy, individual counseling, or a psychiatric evaluation.

RITUALS AROUND DEATH

Beliefs about death and rituals for marking the loss of loved ones vary across cultures. In some cultures, mourners have wakes and parties that last for days; in others, they sing and play music; in still others, they cover mirrors so they cannot see what they look like during times of grief.

Many rituals that surround death and dying are actually for the living, to help people cope with the loss of a loved one. Rituals help mourners move through the emotional work of grieving. When a person has been important to us, we never forget that person or lose the relationship. Instead, we find ways of "emotionally relocating" the deceased person in our lives, keeping our bonds with them while moving on. Cultural rituals can facilitate this process.

END-OF-LIFE DECISIONS

Many people dread a situation in which they or those they trust will have no say in decisions about their end-of-life treatment.[44] To avoid this situation, they can make known

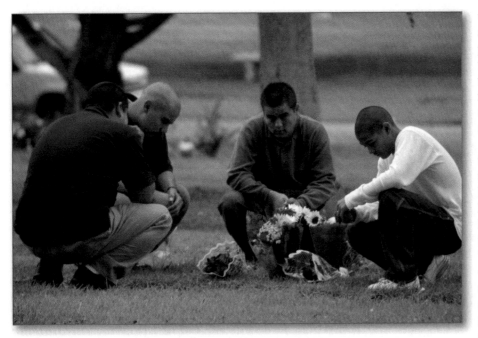

■ Spiritual beliefs and rituals can help people deal with grief and pain when a loved one dies.

with family members, close friends, a spiritual advisor, and health care professionals. Such decisions must take into account the patient's values, the most common ones being family and interpersonal relationships, spiritual beliefs or religion, and independence.[48, 49]

Beyond medical decisions, there are also practical concerns to take care of at the end of life. People need to let their loved ones know whether they want to be buried or cremated, whether they want to donate their organs (see the box "Considering Organ Donation"), what kind of funeral or memorial service they prefer, and who will administer their financial and legal affairs, among other issues. There are also profound emotional issues to work through, including the grief of both the dying person and the loved ones who will be left behind.

their preferences through the use of formal legal documents that grant a **durable power of attorney for health care (DPOAHC)** to someone they trust. These directives, which may be called *living wills* or *advance directives,* may cover any issue the patient considers important.

A common concern is whether life-sustaining treatment should be withdrawn when there is no hope of recovery. These decisions should be made in supportive consultation

durable power of attorney for health care (DPOAHC)
Formal legal power to make health care decisions for someone who is no longer able to do so for himself or herself.

LIFE AFTER DEATH

Belief in an afterlife is a tenet of most faith traditions. Although some investigators say no proof of life after death exists, other researchers argue that there is empirical evidence from individuals who have been resuscitated following a near-death experience.[50, 51] It would be comforting to know that there is some afterlife and that we will be reunited with our loved ones in another state of existence. However, such comforts cannot be provided by science; they remain in the realm of faith and belief.

Consumer Clipboard

Considering Organ Donation

Have you ever noticed that on the reverse side of your driver's license there's an option for organ donation? You may have told yourself you'd think about that decision later. Although every day 70 people in the United States receive an organ transplant, 16 people die because of a shortage of donated organs, so it's worth thinking about now.

■ *Who can be an organ donor?* If you're in good physical condition, you can be an organ donor. Age doesn't matter, but if you're younger than 18, you'll need the consent of a parent or guardian.

■ *Which organs are most commonly transplanted?* Transplant procedures commonly involve the kidney, cornea, heart, liver, lung, pancreas, and bone marrow, but successful transplantation of other organs has been done on a limited basis.

■ *If I have a preexisting medical condition, can I still donate?* Determination of suitability for donation is made at the time of donation. Organs are tested for infectious diseases, including HIV. The final decision is based on a combination of factors, including the donor's general health and the urgency of the recipient's need.

■ *Are there any negative consequences for the donor?* Donating an organ will not disfigure your body. Organ

Continued...

Continued...

removal involves a standard surgical procedure. You can still have a funeral, including an open-casket service.

- *Who pays for organ donation?* All costs associated with organ or tissue donation are paid for by the recipient, not the donor. This is usually done through the recipient's insurance plan.

- *How are organs distributed for donation?* Patients are matched to organs based on several factors, such as blood and tissue type, medical urgency, time on the waiting list, and geographical location.

- *If I decide to become an organ donor, what do I need to do?* Simply indicate that you intend to be an organ and tissue donor on your driver's license. Another step, though, is to discuss your decision with family members and loved ones, because your family may be asked to sign a consent form before the donation can be carried out. It's also a good idea to record your wishes about organ donation in legal documents related to end-of-life decisions.

Sources: Adapted from U.S. Government Advisory Committee on Organ Transplantation, 2005, www.organdonor.gov; "The Ultimate Gift: 50 Years of Organ Transplants," by L.K. Altman, December 21, 2004, New York Times, p. F1.

You Make the Call

Do You Have the Right to Choose?

Ethical questions about the right to die have become more prominent since the 1975 case of Karen Ann Quinlan. She was brought to the hospital in a coma and subsequently declared to be in a persistent vegetative state. After many years of court battles, her parents were finally granted their request to have her life support discontinued. Since then, similar cases have been fought in the public spotlight, including the case of Terri Schiavo, who was taken off life support in 2005 after 2 years in a persistent vegetative state.

It is now generally acknowledged that patients have the right to refuse life-sustaining treatment, and all states authorize written advance directives by means of which individuals can state their wishes. More controversial than withdrawing treatment is the practice of actively hastening a person's death, referred to as *active euthanasia* or *physician-assisted suicide*. In this case, a physician helps a terminally ill patient administer a lethal dose of drugs to himself or herself.

Oregon is currently the only state that permits physician-assisted suicide. The Oregon Death with Dignity Act requires that a patient be terminally ill with less than 6 months to live, be judged mentally competent by two physicians, and make two oral requests and one written request at least 2 weeks apart. Since its passage, more than 200 people have taken advantage of the provisions of the bill. The legality of the act was upheld by the U.S. Supreme Court in 2006.

Proponents of physician-assisted suicide, sometimes referred to as the right to die, believe that individuals have the right to choose how they will die, just as they have the right to choose how they will live. The rights of patients to refuse life support and to sign do-not-resuscitate orders are currently protected, and they are not so different from the right to actively choose how and when to die, according to this view.

Opponents of the right to die argue that human life is unconditionally valuable and that allowing physician-assisted suicide opens the door to abuse. They believe that if more attention were paid to palliative care at the end of life, people would not need to request physician-assisted suicide.

Do terminally ill people have the right to end their lives on their own terms, or is assisted suicide a violation of our cultural values? You make the call.

PROS

- Although life should be protected, people should be allowed to die with dignity when they are terminally ill or in unbearable pain. It is the humane thing to do.

- Loss of autonomy and control are among the most feared aspects of dying. Allowing people the right to die lets them maintain their sense of personal identity until the end of their lives.

- Medical and financial resources are used keeping people alive who want to die. These resources could be freed up for other uses if terminally ill patients were allowed to choose to die.

CONS

- Life is unconditionally valuable, and commitment to life is a value of virtually all societies. Physician-assisted suicide undermines this value, legitimizes suicide, and gives "permission" to more people to commit suicide.

- The vow to "do no harm" is part of the physician's oath. Any compromise in this commitment would undermine the public's faith in the medical profession.

- The practice opens the door to abuse. Some people may feel pressured to end their lives to relieve financial or emotional strains on their families, and in some cases, family members may apply such pressure.

- If attention is paid to pain management and palliative care, people can live out their days and die a natural death. Pain should be managed and depression treated so that people don't feel the need to end their lives.

In Review

1. **How is spirituality defined?** Spirituality is often defined as a person's connection to self, others, and the community at large. It usually involves a personal belief system or a value system that gives meaning and purpose to life. It provides a feeling of participation in something greater than oneself and a sense of unity with nature and the universe.

2. **How does a person build a spiritual life?** Anyone can develop a regular spiritual practice. Examples include meditation, mindfulness, journaling, retreat, experiencing the arts, and developing a daily routine that embodies one's values. Some people develop their spirituality through community involvement, such as volunteering or social activism, and others find their spiritual connection in nature.

3. **What health benefits are associated with spirituality?** Spiritually connected people tend to enjoy better mental and physical health than those who do not describe themselves as spiritually connected, although the reasons for these differences are a matter of debate. Spiritual connectedness appears to be related to higher levels of health-related quality of life—the physical, psychological, social, and spiritual aspects of a person's daily experiences.

4. **What kinds of experiences are associated with death and dying?** Death is a natural part of the cycle of existence, but most people experience anxiety when facing the prospect of their own death or the death of a loved one. People with spiritual beliefs tend to derive strength and hope from their beliefs and may be more accepting of death. Hospice care can make the end of life a more comfortable and peaceful experience.

WWW For a detailed summary of this chapter and a comprehensive set of review questions, visit the Online Learning Center at **www.mhhe.com/teague2e**.

Web Resources

American Meditation Institute for Yoga Science and Philosophy: As an introduction, this Web site describes a systematic procedure for meditation. For those interested in learning meditation, the organization advocates finding a qualified teacher for personal instruction.
www.americanmeditation.org

A Campaign for Forgiveness Research: This organization is dedicated to promoting forgiveness around the world as a way of improving the human condition. The site features myths and truths about forgiveness and offers ways to make forgiveness a part of your life.
www.forgiving.org

Hospice Foundation of America: Focusing on hospice as a concept of care, this site describes the growth of the hospice movement and explains its goals. Hospice is presented as a unique source of comfort for patients and families facing death.
www.hospicefoundation.org

Organ Donation: This official U.S. government Web site for organ donation and transplantation describes the myths and facts associated with organ donation. It features a donor card that you can sign and carry.
www.organdonor.gov

Chapter

5

Stress
Managing
Pressure

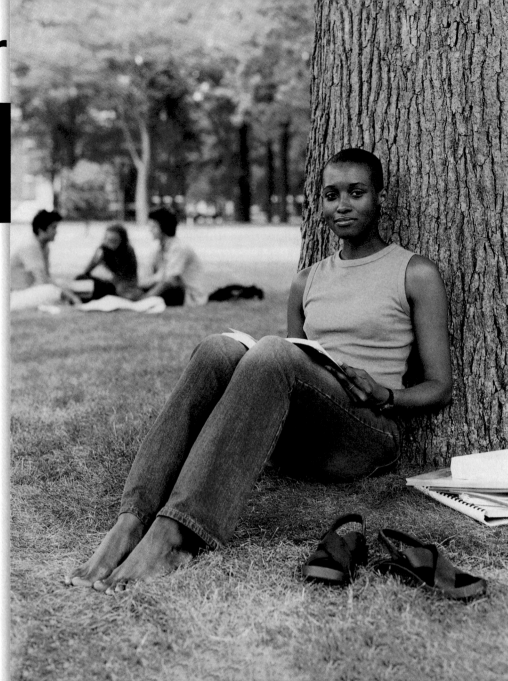

Your Health Today

www.mhhe.com/teague2e

Go to the Online Learning Center for *Your Health Today* for interactive activities, quizzes, flashcards, Web links, and more resources related to this chapter.

Ever Wonder...

- what's going on in your body when you feel stressed out?

- if stress can have long-term health effects?

- if there are better ways to handle stress than by eating, drinking, and smoking?

Stress is a fact of life; you experience varying levels of stress throughout the day as your body and mind continually adjust to the demands of living. We often think of stress as negative, as an uncomfortable or unpleasant pressure—for example, to complete a project on time or to deal with a traffic ticket—but stress can also be positive. When you get a promotion at work or when someone throws you a surprise birthday party, you also experience stress.

A survey conducted by the American Psychological Association in 2007 found that one-third of Americans report regularly experiencing extremely high levels of stress, and one in five report that they experienced these levels on 15 or more days per month.[1] Three-fourths report experiencing physical and psychological symptoms of stress, including fatigue, headaches, upset stomach, muscle tension, teeth grinding, irritability, nervousness, and feeling like crying. Nearly half of Americans say their stress levels have increased over the past 5 years (see the box "Stress in America").

Such statistics only reinforce the need to manage the stress in our lives and to reduce its negative impact on our

Who's at Risk

Stress in America

All segments of the population apparently experience unhealthy levels of stress on a regular basis, but the experiences vary across gender, age, income, and other dimensions.

Gender

Women experience more stress than men as well as more physical symptoms of stress.

	Women	Men
Percentage who report experiencing extreme stress	35	28
Percentage who report being concerned about their level of stress	54	50
Percentage who report their stress levels have increased over the last 5 years	50	46
Percentage who report experiencing physical symptoms of stress (sleep, overeating, using prescription medications)	82	71
Number of nights per month lying awake	8	7

Age

Younger adults are less stressed than adults in midlife, but they handle stress in less healthy ways.

	18–34 years	35–54 years	55+ years
Percentage who report extreme levels of stress	29	39	25
Percentage who report relationships as top stressor	80	83	73
Percentage who report workload as stressor	83	81	69
Percentage who report money and housing costs as stressors	80	81	64
Percentage who report smoking more cigarettes due to stress	73	68	57

	18–34 years	35–54 years	55+ years
Percentage who report skipping a meal due to stress	42	38	28
Percentage who report lying awake at night due to stress	52	49	44

Income

People with lower incomes handle stress less effectively and have more symptoms than do people with higher incomes.

	Household income less than $50,000	Household income $50,000 or more
Percentage who report managing stress poorly	24	15
Percentage who report physical symptoms of stress	80	74
Percentage who report psychological symptoms of stress	77	68

Marital status

Stress affects personal relationships, more so for singles than for married people.

	Single	Married
Percentage who say stress has a negative impact on their social life	48	34

Region

People on the coasts have a harder time handling stress than do people in the South and Midwest.

	East	Midwest	South	West
Percentage who report managing stress poorly	21	15	15	22

Source: Data from Stress in America, *by American Psychological Association, 2007, Washington, DC: American Psychological Association.*

well-being. When excessive stress is unavoidable, having a repertoire of stress management techniques to fall back on is invaluable.

What Is Stress?

Events or agents in the environment that cause us stress are called **stressors.** They can range from being late for class to having a close friend die, from finding a parking space to winning the lottery. Your reaction to these events is called the *stress response;* this concept is discussed at length in the next section. Stressors disrupt the body's balance and require adjustments to return systems to normal. **Stress** can be defined as the general state of the body, mind, and emotions when an environmental stressor has triggered the stress response.

Different people respond differently to stressors, depending on such variables as personality factors, past experiences, overall level of wellness, and different ways of thinking about the stressful event. These variables can be thought of as mediating the stress response, making the same situation stressful for one person and not stressful for another. For example, one person may find public speaking exciting and asking someone for a date excruciating. Another person may be terrified of public speaking and relaxed about asking for a date. We discuss such differences later in the chapter.

Because there is so much variation in individual responses to stressors, stress may be thought of as a *transaction* between an individual and a stressor in the environment, mediated by personal variables that include the person's perceptions and appraisal of the event.[2] When faced with a stressor, you evaluate it without necessarily realizing you are doing so: Is it positive or negative? How threatening is it to my well-being, my self-esteem, my identity? Can I cope with it or not? When you appraise an event as positive, you experience *eustress,* or positive stress. When you appraise it as negative, you experience *distress.*

THE STRESS RESPONSE

Regardless of the nature of the stressor and the individual's appraisal of it, all stressors elicit the **stress response** (also known as the **fight-or-flight response**), a series of physiological changes that occur in the body in the face of a threat. All animals, it appears—humans included—need sudden bursts of energy to fight or flee from situations they perceive as dangerous.

The stress response is carried out by the branch of the nervous system known as the *autonomic nervous system,* which controls involuntary, unconscious functions like breathing, heart rate, and digestion. The autonomic ner-

stressors
Events or agents in the environment that cause stress.

stress
The general state of the body, mind, and emotions when an environmental stressor has triggered the stress response.

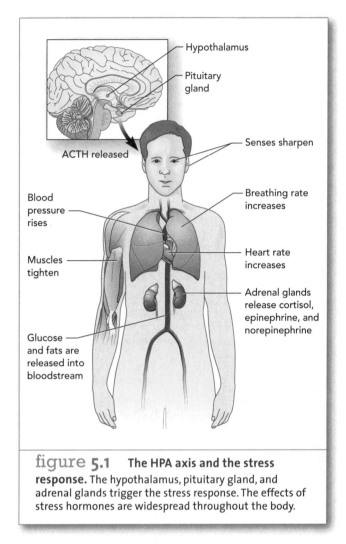

figure **5.1**   **The HPA axis and the stress response.** The hypothalamus, pituitary gland, and adrenal glands trigger the stress response. The effects of stress hormones are widespread throughout the body.

vous system has two branches: The *sympathetic branch* is responsible for initiating the stress response, and the *parasympathetic branch* is responsible for turning off the stress response and returning the body to normal.

The stress response begins when the cerebral cortex (in the front of the brain) sends a chemical signal to the hypothalamus, which sends a signal to the pituitary gland. The pituitary gland sends adrenocorticotropic hormone (ACTH) to the adrenal glands, which release the hormones cortisol, epinephrine (adrenaline), and norepinephrine (noradrenaline) into the bloodstream. Glucose and fats are released from the liver and other storage sites to provide energy. The hypothalamus, pituitary gland, and adrenal glands together are known as the *HPA axis.* They govern many hormonal activities and serve as a feedback loop that turns off the stress response when the threat is over (Figure 5.1).

As stress hormones surge through your body, your heart rate, breathing rate, muscle tension, metabolism, and blood

**stress response
or fight-or-flight
response**
Series of physiological changes that activate body systems, providing a burst of energy to deal with a perceived threat or danger.

pressure all increase. Your hands and feet get cold as blood is directed away from your extremities into the larger muscles that can help you run or fight. Your pupils dilate to sharpen your vision, your hearing becomes sharper, your lungs take in more oxygen, and your liver begins to convert glycogen to glucose for instant energy to fuel your muscles (Figure 5.2). All this happens in an instant.

The challenge that elicits this chain of events does not have to be an actual threat or danger, as noted earlier. You may be about to go onstage, walk down the aisle, or even play in a pick-up basketball game. No matter what the challenge, your body reacts by becoming more aroused and alert. You may be able to do things you would not have believed possible as a result of your acute concentration.

THE RELAXATION RESPONSE

When a stressful event is over—you decide the situation is no longer dangerous, or you complete your task—the parasympathetic branch of the autonomic nervous system takes over, turning off the stress response.[3] Heart rate, breathing, muscle tension, and blood pressure all decrease. The body returns to **homeostasis,** a state of stability and

homeostasis
State of stability and balance in which body functions are maintained within a normal range.

balance in which functions are maintained within a normal range. The term **relaxation response** has been used to describe this process, and we discuss it in more detail later in this chapter.

ACUTE STRESS AND CHRONIC STRESS

According to evolutionary biology, the fight-or-flight response served an important function for our ancestors. Today, most of us do not live in such dangerous environments, but this innate response to threat is still essential to our survival, warning us when it is time to fight or flee. Although the fight-or-flight response requires a great deal of energy—which is why you often feel so tired after a stressful event—your body is equipped to deal with short-term, **acute stress** as long as it does not happen too often and as long as you can relax and recover afterward.

relaxation response
Series of physiological changes that calm body systems and return them to normal functioning.

acute stress
Short-term stress, produced by the stress response.

A problem occurs, however, when the stress response occurs repeatedly or when it persists without being turned off. In these instances, the stress response itself becomes damaging. Many people live in a state of **chronic stress,** in

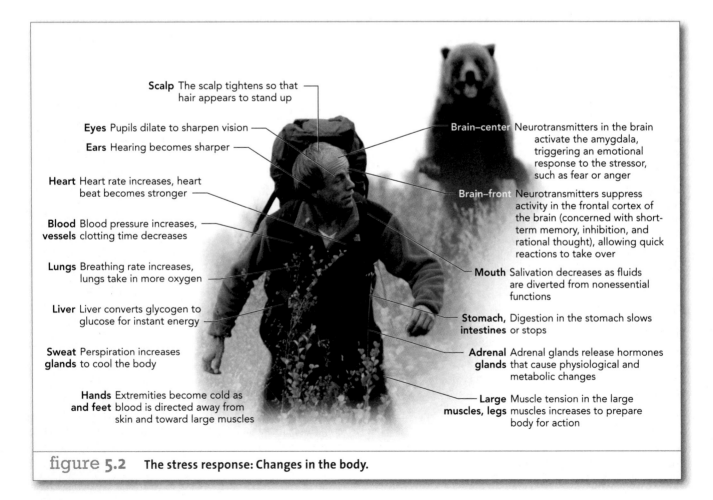

figure **5.2**   **The stress response: Changes in the body.**

which stressful conditions are ongoing and the stress response continues without resolution. Chronic stress increases the likelihood that the person will become ill or, if already ill, that her or his defense system will be overwhelmed by the disease. Prolonged or severe stress has been found to weaken the immune system, strain the heart, damage memory cells in the brain, and contribute to physical illnesses such as heart disease, arthritis, and diabetes. Sources of chronic stress include everything from financial worries, relationship concerns, and loneliness to poverty, crowding, and discrimination. In these situations, reducing and managing levels of stress are critical.

chronic stress
Long-term, low-level stress in which the stress response continues without resolution.

Stress and Your Health

Researchers have been looking at the relationship between stress and disease since the 1950s. One of the first scientists to develop a broad theory of stress and disease was Hans Selye,[4] who in turn drew from the work of Walter Cannon. Early in his career, Selye studied the effects of an ovarian extract on the body. During his experiments, he had a difficult time injecting his lab rats with the extract, mishandling them and sometimes accidentally dropping them on the floor. He later realized that the physiological changes he observed in the rats could not have been due to the extract; instead, he theorized, they were a result of the stress the rats experienced because of his poor technique.

General Adaptation Syndrome (GAS)
Selye's classic model used to describe the physiological changes associated with the stress response. The three phases are alarm, resistance, and exhaustion.

THE GENERAL ADAPTATION SYNDROME

Selye developed what he called the **General Adaptation Syndrome (GAS)** as a description and explanation of the physiological changes that he observed and that he believed to be predictable responses to stressors by all organisms. The process has three stages (Figure 5.3):

- *Alarm.* The body experiences the stress response. During this stage, immune system functioning is suppressed, and the person may be more susceptible to infections and illness.
- *Resistance.* The body works overtime to cope with the added stress and to stay at a peak level.
- *Exhaustion.* The body can no longer keep up with the demands of the stressor.

Without a period of rest and relaxation, the immune system breaks down, and the body is vulnerable to serious stress-related disorders.

SYMPTOMS OF STRESS

Since the time of Selye's work, researchers have concluded that almost every system in the body can be damaged by stress[5] (see the box "Symptoms of Stress"). According to the American Medical Association, stress plays a role in 80–85 percent of all human illness and disease.[6] For example, stress-triggered changes in the lungs increase the symptoms of asthma and other respiratory conditions. Stress appears to inhibit tissue repair, which increases the likelihood of bone fractures and is related to the development of osteoporosis (porous, weak bones). Stress can lead to sexual problems, including failure to ovulate and amenorrhea (absence of menstrual periods) in women and sexual dysfunction and loss of sexual desire in both men and women. Some suggest that high levels of stress can even speed up the aging process.[7]

STRESS AND THE IMMUNE SYSTEM

Since Selye's time, research has definitively shown that stress decreases immune function. One study demonstrated a strong relationship between levels of psychological stress and the possibility of infection by a common cold virus. Other studies have found that both brief and long-term stressors have an impact on the function of the immune system.[8] Stressors as diverse as taking exams, experiencing major life events, and providing long-term care for someone with Alzheimer's disease affect the immune system. Scientists still do not fully understand why the stress response suppresses immune function or whether there is an evolutionary explanation for this suppression.

STRESS AND THE CARDIOVASCULAR SYSTEM

The stress response causes heart rate to accelerate and blood pressure to increase. When heart rate and blood pressure do not return to normal, as occurs in chronic stress, the person can experience elevated levels for long periods of time. Chronic hypertension (high blood pressure) makes blood vessels more susceptible to the development of atherosclerosis, a

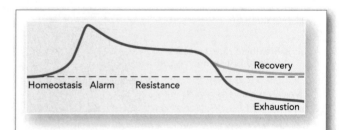

figure 5.3   **General Adaptation Syndrome.** Selye's model describes the physiological response to stress. In the alarm stage, the body's fight-or-flight response is activated, accompanied by reduced immune system functioning. In the resistance stage, the body uses energy to adjust to the continued stress. After prolonged exposure to stress, the body may become totally depleted, leading to exhaustion, illness, and even death.

Highlight on Health

Symptoms of Stress

Cognitive Symptoms

Anxious thoughts
Fearful anticipation
Poor concentration
Memory problems
Continual worry
Trouble thinking clearly
Loss of sense of humor
Lack of creativity

Emotional Symptoms

Feelings of tension
Irritability
Restlessness
Worries
Inability to relax
Depression
Crying
Lack of meaning in life and pursuits
Loneliness
Quick temper

Behavioral Symptoms

Avoidance of tasks
Sleep problems
Fidgeting
Tremors
Grinding teeth
Strained facial expression
Clenched fists
Changes in drinking, eating, or smoking behaviors
Procrastination
Increased drive to be with, or withdraw from, others

Physical Symptoms

Stiff or tense muscles
Sweating
Tension headaches
Feeling faint
Feeling of choking
Difficulty swallowing
Stomachache, nausea, or vomiting
Diarrhea or constipation
Frequent or urgent urination
Heart palpitations
Backaches
Fatigue

Social Symptoms

Change in the quality of relationships

Source: Stress Management: Techniques for Preventing and Easing Stress, *by H. Benson, 2006, Cambridge, MA: Harvard Medical School Press.*

disease in which arteries are damaged and clogged with fatty deposits. Both hypertension and atherosclerosis increase the risk of heart attack and stroke. Overall stress levels are typically higher for individuals who have suffered heart attacks.

Sudden severe stress can cause heart failure in some people who do not have heart disease. The condition, called *stress-induced cardiomyopathy,* is believed to occur when the heart muscle is temporarily "stunned" by a huge burst of adrenaline and cannot contract properly. The condition is reversible and causes no permanent heart damage, but it resembles a heart attack and requires medical treatment. Ninety-five percent of those experiencing the condition are women, and most are middle-aged.[9]

STRESS AND THE GASTROINTESTINAL SYSTEM

Some 66 percent of people surveyed in one study reported that stress affected their gastrointestinal functioning, with most describing diarrhea as their most significant problem.[10] Another 49 percent of those who were surveyed reported that stress caused some type of abdominal pain.[11] Although not conclusive, evidence suggests that gastrointestinal problems can be stress related. More specifically, conditions such as acid reflux, indigestion, and stomach pain all seem to be more common in people who have higher levels or more frequent occurrences of stress. Irritable bowel syndrome (IBS) may be an example of individual response differences to the gastrointestinal tract by stress. When IBS patients are under stress, food seems to move more slowly through the small intestine in those individuals who are constipated; the opposite was true for those who suffer from diarrhea.

For a long time, stress was commonly believed to cause stomach ulcers. Research suggests, however, that ulcers may be caused or exacerbated by a bacterial infection that irritates the stomach lining. While not causing ulcers, stress may contribute to their development.

STRESS AND MENTAL HEALTH

Both acute and chronic stress can contribute to psychological problems and the development of psychological illnesses, including anxiety disorders and depression (see Chapter 3). In *acute stress disorder,* for example, a person develops symptoms after experiencing a severely traumatic event, such as an assault or a natural disaster. Symptoms can include a feeling of numbness, a sense of being in a daze, amnesia, flashbacks, increased arousal and anxiety, and impairment in functioning. If such symptoms appear 6 months or more after the traumatic event, the person may have *post-traumatic stress disorder* (PTSD), a condition characterized by a sense of numbness or emotional detachment from people, repeated reliving of the event through flashbacks and/or nightmares, and avoidance of things that might be associated with the trauma (see the box "Recognizing and Treating PTSD"). Years may pass after the trauma before PTSD symptoms appear.[13]

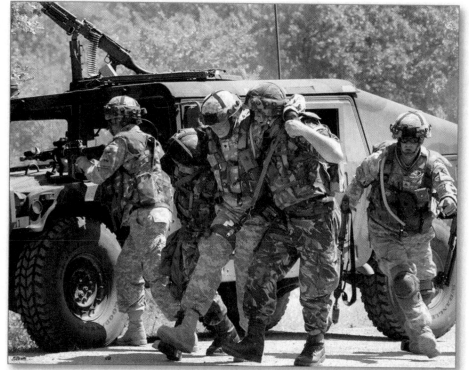

■ The stress and trauma of combat can lead to post-traumatic stress disorder in some individuals. Veterans of the conflicts in Iraq and Afghanistan have a wide range of mental health services available to them, but the stigma associated with accessing those services keeps many from getting effective treatment.

An example of a less severe stress-related disorder is *adjustment disorder,* in which a response to a stressor (such as anxiety, worry, social withdrawal) continues for a longer period than would normally be expected.

Low-level, unresolved chronic stress can also be a factor in psychological problems. Stress can diminish wellness and reduce the ability to function at the highest level even without an identifiable disorder. Symptoms such as irritability, impatience, difficulty concentrating, excessive worrying, insomnia, and forgetfulness, like physical symptoms, can be addressed with stress management techniques.

Mediators of the Stress Response

Different people respond differently to stressors. Among the factors that may play a role in these differences are past experiences and overall level of wellness. Also critical are personality traits, habitual ways of thinking, and inborn or acquired attitudes toward the demands of life.

PERSONALITY FACTORS

In the 1970s two cardiologists, Meyer Friedman and Ray Rosenman, described and named the **Type A behavior pattern.**[14] Type A individuals tend to be impulsive, need to get things done quickly, and live their lives on a time schedule. They seem to be guided by the perception that they are responsible for everything that goes on in their lives; they are hard driving, achievement oriented, and highly competitive. They tend to be impatient, easily angered, and hostile. They set unrealistic goals and are easily bored. Some estimates are that more than 40 percent of the population of the United States and possibly half of all men might be Type As.

Individuals who fit this description are prime candidates for stress-related illnesses. The relationship between Type A personality traits and heart disease has been known for some time. More recently, there have been indications that a Type A personality can mean increased risk for a number of other diseases, including peptic ulcers, asthma, headaches, and thyroid problems.

However, not all the characteristics of this personality seem to be harmful. Many Type As are achievement oriented and successful and yet remain healthy. According to recent research, a key culprit is **hostility,** defined as an ongoing accumulation of irritation and anger. Hostile individuals are generally cynical toward others, frequently express anger, and display aggressive behaviors.[15] Research has indicated that hostility, by itself, is related to coronary heart disease, and it may also contribute to premature death.

Type A behavior pattern
Set of personality traits originally thought to be associated with risk for heart disease. Type A individuals are hard driving, competitive, achievement oriented, and quick to anger; further research has identified hostility as the key risk factor in the pattern.

hostility
Ongoing accumulation of irritation and anger.

Public Health in Action

Recognizing and Treating PTSD

Many soldiers returning from Vietnam experienced a set of symptoms we now call post-traumatic stress disorder (PTSD). At the time, it seemed these Vietnam vets had isolated cases of severe combat stress. Now we know that many combat veterans have this reaction, and it is not hard to imagine that the soldiers coming home from World Wars I and II with what was referred to as "shell shock" also had PTSD. Today the U.S. government attempts to provide education, information, and screening for PTSD for veterans of the wars in Iraq and Afghanistan.

PTSD is also common among people in the general population who have experienced severe trauma (for example, from assault, rape, domestic violence, child physical or sexual abuse, terrorist attacks, or natural disasters). Sometimes described as a form of chronic emotional injury, the disorder is recognized as a major public health problem. An estimated 10 million American children and adults are affected by PTSD, with women more at risk than men.

PTSD is characterized by a specific set of symptoms: reexperiencing the trauma (flashbacks, nightmares, intrusive thoughts), increased arousal (hypervigilance, exaggerated startle response, irritability), avoiding reminders of the trauma, and emotional numbing. Other symptoms include depression, anxiety, withdrawal and isolation, substance abuse, and difficulty functioning. It isn't clear why some people recover and others develop PTSD, but it is likely that the strong emotions associated with the traumatic event cause changes in the brain that produce the symptoms.

The National Center for PTSD was created within the Department of Veterans Affairs (VA) in 1989 to address the needs of veterans with military-related PTSD. The mission of the center is to "advance the clinical care and social welfare of U.S. veterans through research, education, and training on PTSD and stress-related disorders." The VA has also established three medical "centers of excellence" providing care for veterans with PTSD through more than 200 specialized treatment programs. The goal of these programs is to reduce the impact of trauma on veterans while also providing models of care that can be used for others with PTSD.

A public information campaign to inform the general public about PTSD through television public service announcements (PSAs) has been sponsored by four organizations, the Dart Center for Journalism and Trauma, the National Center for PTSD, the National Center for Victims of Crime, and Gift from Within, an international organization for survivors of trauma and victimization. The PSAs, designed to run in the weeks leading up to the anniversary of September 11, inform viewers about the symptoms of PTSD. The ads direct viewers to a Web site (www.ptsdinfo.org) that provides accurate medical information and links to organizations with information about coping. The PSAs can be viewed at www.giftfromwithin.org/html/psa.html.

Many people recover from trauma by practicing self-help and self-care following the event. Positive coping strategies include the following:

- Using natural supports (talking with family, friends, and coworkers about the event) but proceeding at one's own pace.

- Learning more about PTSD so as not to feel alone, weak, or "crazy."

- Talking with other trauma survivors for support.

- Mobilizing the resources that are available, such as talking with a doctor.

- Practicing relaxation techniques, exercising, and volunteering in the community.

- Increasing positive distracting activities but not at the expense of directly coping with the trauma.

- Maintaining a balanced, healthy lifestyle.

When these strategies are not helping, or when a trauma survivor is using negative coping actions such as drinking, taking drugs, withdrawing, or engaging in self-destructive behaviors, he or she is urged to seek help from a mental health professional. Several types of treatment are available, including cognitive-behavioral therapy, exposure therapy, group therapy, and medication. Veterans are encouraged to contact the VA, and others are encouraged to seek a referral from their physician or to look up mental health services in the phone book. Although time, patience, and understanding are needed, it is possible to find relief from the devastating symptoms of PTSD.

Sources: "What Is PTSD?" National Center for Posttraumatic Stress Disorder, retrieved May 31, 2008, from www.ncptsd.va.gov; "Self-Care and Self-Help Following Disasters," National Center for Posttraumatic Stress Disorder, retrieved May 31, 2008, from www.ncptsd.va.gov; "Trauma PSAs Offer Help as 9/11 Reminders Trigger Emotional Reactions," Gift from Within, retrieved May 31, 2008, from www.giftfromwithin.org; "Coping With a Traumatic Event," Centers for Disease Control and Prevention, retrieved June 2, 2008, from www.bt.cdc.gov/masscasualties/copingpub.asp.

Friedman and Rosenman also described a constellation of personality traits they labeled Type B. In contrast to the Type A personality, the Type B personality is less driven and more relaxed. Type Bs are more easygoing and less readily frustrated. All other things being equal, Type Bs are less susceptible to coronary heart disease. However, their personalities do not necessarily mean that they experience less stress in their lives. For example, if a Type B ends up in a Type A job, he or she may become overwhelmed by the competitiveness and pace needed to be successful.[14]

COGNITIVE FACTORS

Until you decide that an event is actually a threat and/or beyond your ability to cope, it remains merely a potential stressor. Experts suggest that people create their own distress with their habitual thinking patterns—illogical thinking, unrealistic expectations, and negative beliefs.[2] For example, a person may think she has to get straight As in order to be a worthy human being. If she gets a B, she will experience much more stress than if she had more realistic expectations about herself and was more self-forgiving. Her ideas can transform a relatively neutral event into a stressor.

Other common illogical ideas and unrealistic expectations are "life should be fair," "friends should be there when you need them," "everyone I care about has to love and approve of me," and "everything has to go my way." When everyday experiences don't live up to these ideas, people who hold them end up feeling angry, frustrated, disappointed, or demoralized. (For more on cognitive distortions, see the box "Challenge Your Thinking.") With a more realistic attitude, they can take things in stride and reduce the frequency and intensity of the stress response. This doesn't mean they should have unrealistically low expectations. When expectations are too low, people may

Starting college is a major life transition with unique stressors. Individuals with the qualities of resilience and hardiness are able to take the challenges in stride and respond with energy and excitement.

experience underachievement, depression, resignation, and lowered self-esteem. The goal is a realistic balance.

RESILIENCE AND HARDINESS

Just as resilience is a factor in mental health, it is also a factor in the ability to handle stress. Research has led to a better understanding of resilient or stress-resistant people. As noted in Chapter 3, they appear to share an optimistic explanatory style and assume troubles are temporary rather than permanent.[16] Stress-resistant people also seem to focus on immediate issues and explain their struggle in positive and helpful ways. For example, a poor grade on one exam might motivate the stress-resilient person to study harder, using the grade as motivation. A person who is not so resilient may react to a poor grade by feeling like a failure and giving up.

Another line of research has developed the concept of **hardiness,** an effective style of coping with stress. Researchers have studied people who were exposed to a great deal of stress but never seemed to become ill as a result.[17, 18] The researchers suggest that positive ways of coping with stress may buffer the body from its effects. They call this style *hardiness* and have suggested that people high in hardiness are more resistant to illness.

hardiness
Effective style of coping with stress, characterized by a tendency to view life events as challenges rather than threats, a commitment to meaningful activities, and a sense of being in control.

These researchers found three particular traits in those who stayed healthiest:

■ *Challenge.* Perceiving the demands of life as a challenge and responding with energy and excitement.

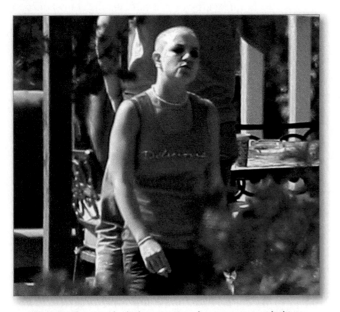

Many performers lack the emotional resources needed to handle the stress of celebrity and constant media attention. Britney Spears apparently succumbed to the pressures in her life in 2007 when she shaved her head and engaged in other erratic behaviors.

- *Commitment.* Participating in and being committed to meaningful activities.
- *Control.* Having a sense of being able to gain important information, make decisions, and be in control.

Having a sense of control may be especially critical in avoiding illness and responding to stressful situations. In sum, these researchers found that people who demonstrate an ability to see life as a challenge, who are committed to what they do, and who believe they are in control tend to do better.

Sources of Stress

Contemporary life presents us with nearly limitless sources of stress, ranging from major life events to our interpersonal relationships to some of our own feelings. In this section we describe some of these stressors, along with a variety of tips for handling them.

LIFE EVENTS

Can stressful life events make people more vulnerable to illness? Thomas Holmes and Richard Rahe, medical researchers at the University of Washington, observed that individuals frequently experienced major life events before the onset of an illness. They proposed that life events—major changes and transitions that force the individual to adjust and adapt—may precipitate illness, especially if several such events occur at the same time.[19] Holmes and Rahe developed a scale of stressful life events and compared it to the onset of illnesses. From this work they developed the Holmes-Rahe Social Readjustment Scale, a list of life events that require the individual to adjust and adapt to change. The higher a person's score on the scale, the more likely that person is to experience symptoms of illness.

The most stressful event on this scale is the death of a spouse, followed by such events as divorce, separation, a personal injury, and being fired from a job. Less stressful events on the scale include moving, going on vacation, experiencing a change in sleeping habits, and dealing with a minor violation of the law. An adaptation of the Social Readjustment Scale for college students, the Student Stress Scale, is presented in the Add It Up feature at the back of the book. Fill it out to find out what your stress level is and how likely you may be to experience stress-related health problems in the near future.

DAILY HASSLES

Surprisingly, everyday hassles can also cause health problems. In fact, daily hassles are related to subsequent illness and disease to a greater degree than are major life events.[20] Daily hassles include arguments, car problems, deadlines, traffic jams, long lines, money worries, and so on. All of these events can lead to a state of chronic, low-level stress, especially if they pile up and you don't have a period of recovery.

Challenges & Choices

Challenge Your Thinking

Distorted thinking can increase your stress levels unnecessarily. Learning to recognize your negative thinking patterns, challenging them, and replacing them with healthier, more balanced ways of thinking can be an effective stressbuster. If you notice a distorted thought, try to examine it logically. For example, is it really likely that not getting one job offer means you'll never get a job you want? Or that not having a date this weekend means you'll never find the right romantic partner? It takes vigilance and practice to take the power out of habitual thinking patterns, but the effort is worth it. Your stress levels will go down and your sense of well-being will go up!

Common Patterns of Distorted Thinking

- Focusing on the negative; filtering out the positive.
- Magnifying the bad things; minimizing the good things.
- Catastrophizing—expecting the worst.
- Overgeneralizing—creating expectations based on one incident.
- Blaming others for everything; blaming yourself for everything.
- Personalizing—thinking everything going on around you is about you.
- Mind reading—assuming you know what others are thinking and feeling without checking it out with them.
- Being perfectionistic—thinking you have to be perfect and it's not okay to make a mistake.
- Thinking in black and white—thinking if it's not one way, it's the other, when really there are always shades of gray; seeing only options 1 and 10 and missing all the options in between.

It's Not Just Personal ...

Several forms of psychotherapy use cognitive strategies to help treat depression, anxiety, and other psychological problems. Aaron Beck's cognitive therapy and Albert Ellis's rational emotive behavior therapy focus on improving psychological functioning and quality of life by dealing with strongly entrenched irrational beliefs and thinking patterns.

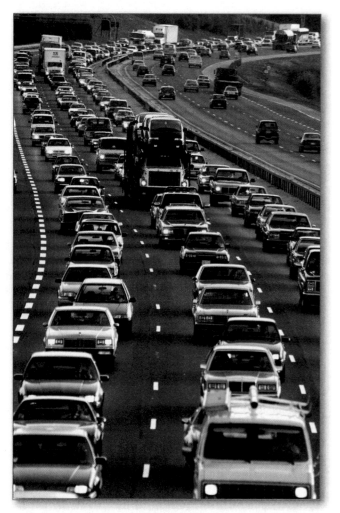

■ Daily hassles like commuting in heavy traffic may be even more stressful than major life events. Time pressures and worries about gas prices add to the stress.

COLLEGE STRESS

College students experience a great deal of life change, and some studies even suggest that the college years may be the most stressful time in people's lives.[21, 22] In one survey of college students, stress was identified as the top health concern, with 34 percent of respondents reporting that stress affected their academic performance.[23] Considering the health effects of stress, it should not be surprising that colds, mononucleosis, and sexually transmitted diseases are familiar on college campuses.

Besides the effect of this major life transition, common sources of stress for college students include academic work, exams and grades, sleep deprivation, worries about money, relationship concerns, and uncertainty about their futures. The pressure of college may be growing even more intense, particularly for young women. In one survey, 30 percent of first-year students described themselves as frequently feeling overwhelmed. Women were nearly twice as likely to feel this way as men.[24]

Rising tuition costs also appear to affect stress levels of many students. A record number of students say they have to work to afford college, and again, women in greater numbers describe themselves as feeling the pressure to work. Concern about the economy and being successful also has an impact on students.

College officials indicate that although more young people are going to college, they might also be less prepared to deal with college stressors and expectations. Almost all college students describe themselves as being depressed during their college experience, although the depression is often moderate and of a short duration. These episodes are often related to specific stressors such as difficulties in a relationship, poor grades, and general adjustment concerns. When the intensity of the situation increases or the student is unable to find support, symptoms such as changes in appetite or increases in risk-taking behaviors, self-injurious behaviors, and smoking may appear.

For reentry or older students entering college for the first time, there can be additional stressors. Many are trying, to balance work, family, and school. Other stressors include paying for school and family, reducing their time with friends, doubting their ability to do well in school, and believing they cannot retain information as well as they might have when they were younger. Like all students but perhaps with a bit more intensity, reentry students fear failing and what that might mean.

Many college students adopt habits to deal with stress that are ineffective, counterproductive, and ultimately unhealthy:

■ *Use of tobacco.* Two-thirds of smokers report that they smoke more when they are under stress.[1] The chemicals in tobacco can make a smoker feel both more relaxed and more alert. However, nicotine is highly addictive, and smoking causes a host of health problems. Tobacco use is the leading preventable cause of death in the United States.

■ *Use and abuse of alcohol.* Moderate use of alcohol can lower inhibitions and create a sense of social ease and relaxation, but drinking provides only temporary relief without addressing the sources of stress. Heavy drinking and binge drinking carry risks of their own, including the risk of addiction. All too often, what began as a solution becomes a new problem.

■ *Use and abuse of other drugs.* Like alcohol, illicit drugs alter mood and mind without solving problems, and they often cause additional problems. For example, stimulants like methamphetamine and cocaine increase mental alertness and energy, but they can induce the stress response and disrupt sleep. Opiates like oxycodone (OxyContin) and hydrocodone (Vicodin) can relieve pain and anxiety, but tolerance develops quickly, making dependence likely. Marijuana can cause panic attacks, and even caffeine raises blood pressure and levels of stress hormones.

■ *Use of food to manage feelings.* Many people overeat or eat unhealthy foods when they feel stressed. According to one survey, the top "comfort foods" are candy, ice cream, chips, cookies and cakes, fast food, and pizza, in that order.[1] Other people eat less or skip meals in response to stress. For most of us, eating is a pleasurable, relaxing experience, but using food to manage feelings and stress can lead to disordered eating patterns as well as overweight and obesity.

Other approaches to stress management popular with college students are listening to music, socializing with friends, going to movies, and reading. Though not unhealthy, these sedentary activities need to be balanced with more active stress management techniques, such as walking or exercising.

Colleges usually offer resources to help students deal with stress, and at some major universities 40 percent of all undergraduates visit the counseling center. However, a sign that not enough students are getting the help they need is the fact that suicide is the second leading cause of death on college campuses. More effort must be made to reach and educate students about stress reduction and stress management techniques, including time management, relaxation techniques, exercise, and good nutrition.

JOB PRESSURE

Occupational pressure appears to be the leading stressor for American adults; 74 percent report that work is a significant source of stress.[1] Half of employees report that they have left or considered quitting a job because of workplace stress, and more than half say they are less productive at work because of stress.[1] Job pressure contributes to many stress-related illnesses, including cardiovascular disease,[1] and may be related to the incidence of back pain, fatigue, muscular pain, and headaches. The costs are high in terms of dollars and worker performance, seen in accidents, absenteeism, turnover, reduced levels of productivity, and insurance costs.

Jobs can be stressful because they are too complex or difficult, too easy, boring, repetitive, unsafe, or environmentally stressful (noisy, too hot or cold, and so on). What seems to make a job particularly stressful is the combination of a great deal of responsibility and a lack of control over how to fulfill that responsibility.[2] Some of the most stressful occupations are law enforcement, teaching, and health care.

Over the past century many jobs have become physically easier, but expectations have grown that people will work more. Managers and professionals seem to work the longest days and are subject to associated stresses.[25] They bring work home and thus never really leave the job. Four out of ten Americans report that they don't take all of their allotted vacation time.[1] Many people who want to be successful become *workaholics,* never taking a break from work and setting themselves up for burnout.

Burnout is an adverse, work-related stress reaction with physical, psychological, and behavioral components.[26] The symptoms of burnout include increasing discouragement and pessimism about work; a decline in motivation and job performance; irritability, anger, and apathy on the job; and physical complaints.[27]

People who find themselves in danger of burnout can help themselves by evaluating whether they are really in the right work environment. If they decide they want to stay, they can take steps to improve their lives and protect their health. For example, they can speak up about what they can and cannot do, delegate some of their responsibilities to others, build a physical activity break into their workday, and make it a priority to maintain a balance between work and family.

burnout
Adverse work-related stress reaction with physical, psychological, and behavioral components.

MONEY AND FINANCIAL WORRIES

Financial worries are the second leading stressor for Americans, after work. Three-quarters of Americans report that money is a significant source of stress; they worry especially about housing costs.[1] In a survey of 30,000 college students, one in three students indicated that his or her financial situation was causing physical and/or mental stress.[28]

Many people experience financial stress because their income is not equal to their expenditures. Familiar sources of financial stress are fear of running short of money before the end of the month, carrying too much debt, reduced employment or unemployment, no savings to cover medical emergencies, and unexpected home or car repairs.

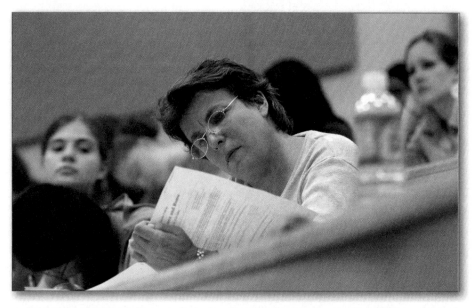

■ Returning or reentry college students experience their own stressors, including worries that they may not measure up, concerns about fitting in, and the need to balance school, work, and family obligations.

One of the best ways to relieve financial stress is to plan ahead. Being willing to follow a budget and make the lifestyle changes necessary to live within available funds may be the key to relief from financial stress. Simplifying your life, shedding those items and events that you can live without, can be liberating. Having some savings is reassuring, and experts recommend that people put money in a savings account every month before they use their money any other way, in effect "paying themselves" first. That money is then available if an emergency arises. Finding ways to ensure financial peace of mind is an excellent stress reduction technique.

FAMILY AND INTERPERSONAL STRESS

Families have to continuously adapt to a series of life changes and transitions. The birth of a baby places new demands on parents and siblings, and families must adapt as a teenager moves through adolescence to adulthood and leaves home. A family may be disrupted by death or divorce, and in fact, a growing number of children spend part of their lives in single-parent households, blended family units, or stepfamily systems.

Families may become weakened by these experiences, or they may become stronger and more resilient. Studies have identified a number of protective factors that make families resilient across the life cycle. These factors are associated with the family's ability to manage transitions and changes over time and with family harmony and balance. For example, resilient families tend to eat meals together, celebrate birthdays and other special family events, and have confidence that they can work through almost any challenge.

Relationships of all kinds have the potential to be stressful, including intimate partnerships. Many experts agree that the key to a successful relationship is not finding the perfect partner but being able to communicate effectively with the partner you have. Whereas poor communication skills can cause interactions to escalate into arguments and fights (or deteriorate into cold silences), thoughtful communication and conflict resolution techniques can resolve issues before they become problems.

OTHER SOURCES OF STRESS

Beyond life events, daily hassles, school, work, finances, and relationships, there are still more sources of stress in our lives.

Time Pressure, Overload, and Technology   Most of us experience some degree of time pressure in our lives. Many people find that they have more and more to do, despite time-saving devices, and want to compress more activity into less time. Multitasking is common—people talk on the phone while driving, answer e-mail while eating lunch, take laptops on vacation. The rush to do things quickly and use time well ultimately increases levels of stress.

Many people do not see their overstuffed schedules as a problem. Instead, they go to time management classes to learn how to squeeze more activities into the time they have. Although planning and good use of time are effective stress management techniques, there are limits to how much a person can do. Many times the solution is not to use time more effectively but to do less. Many "stressed out" people are not poor stress managers; they are simply overloaded with responsibilities. Sometimes, learning to say no to others' requests is the best way to handle time management issues.

Most new technologies are designed to save time and improve life, but they can also be sources of stress. We feel pressure to learn them and master them; once they are widely accepted, we find we are expected to use them to get more done in less time. Further, they often let us down at critical moments, as anyone can attest who has broken into a sweat when a computer crashes or a PowerPoint presentation fails to work as expected.

With each new technological innovation—e-mail, the Internet, voice mail, DVDs, mp3 players, camera phones, and on and on—we are faced with the choice of mastering it or ignoring it. Learning a new technology can be both fun and frustrating, as well as time consuming. Choosing to ignore a new tech-

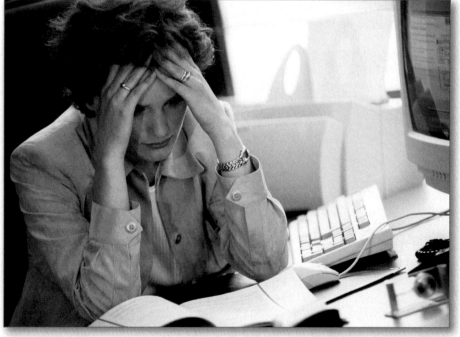

■ Work overload and time pressure are major sources of stress and stress-related illnesses, including headaches, stomachaches, and depression.

nology can raise the fear of being left behind in a fast-paced world. Both are stressful.

Anger Sometimes the source of stress is within the individual. Unresolved feelings of anger can be extremely stressful. The idea that blowing off steam, or venting, is a positive way to deal with anger is generally not the case. Releasing anger in an uncontrolled way often reinforces the feeling and may cause it to escalate into rage.[2] Venting can create anger in the person on the receiving end and hurts relationships. Suppressing anger or turning it against oneself is also unhealthy, lowering self-esteem and possibly fostering depression.

If you find yourself in a situation in which you are getting angry, take a time-out, remove yourself from the situation physically, and take some deep breaths. Examine the situation and think about whether your reaction is logical or illogical and whether you could see it another way. Look for absurdity or humor in the situation. Put it in perspective. If you cannot avoid the situation or reduce your reaction, try some of the stress management strategies and relaxation techniques described later in this chapter.

Trauma The effect of traumatic experiences has received a great deal of study. The events of September 11, 2001, and military service in Iraq and Afghanistan are frequently cited as traumatic events of the highest order. Human beings are not equipped to deal effectively with events of this magnitude. They overwhelm our ability to cope and destroy any sense of control, connection, or meaning. They shake the foundations of beliefs about the safety and trustworthiness of the world.

Some people develop post-traumatic stress disorder (PTSD) in response to trauma, as described earlier in this chapter. Although the triggering event may be overwhelming, often it alone is not sufficient to explain the occurrence of PTSD. Many people who are exposed to a traumatic event never develop PTSD. For example, fewer than 40 percent of those with war zone experience in Vietnam developed PTSD.[28] Again, this is evidence of the role of mediating factors in the individual experience of stress.

Societal Issues Intolerance, prejudice, discrimination, injustice, poverty, pressure to conform to mainstream culture—all are common sources of stress for members of modern society. Exposure to racism and homophobia, for example, can cause

■ Racism, sexism, and hate speech are major sources of stress for members of minorities in the United States. Members of the Rutgers University women's basketball team called a news conference to express their sadness and anger after radio show host Don Imus referred to them as "nappy-headed hos" in April 2007. Although Imus's show was promptly canceled because of this statement, he was back on-air with a different network by the end of the year.

distrust, frustration, resentment, negative emotions such as anger and fear, and a sense of helplessness and hopelessness. Experiencing racism has been associated with both physical and mental health-related symptoms, including hypertension, cardiovascular reactivity, depression, eating disorders, substance abuse, and violence.

Similar effects are seen in lesbians, gay males, bisexuals, and transgendered individuals when they are the targets of prejudice and homophobia.[30] These individuals often have higher rates of school-related problems, substance abuse, criminal activity, prostitution, running away from home, and suicide than do their nongay peers.

Managing Stress

The effects of unrelieved stress on the body and mind can range from muscle tension to a pervasive sense of hopelessness about the future, yet life without stress is unrealistic if not impossible. The solution is to find effective ways to manage stress.

CHOOSING AN APPROACH TO STRESS MANAGEMENT

There are many different ways to manage stress, but not all of them appeal to everyone. What works for someone else may not be helpful or comfortable for you. For example, some individuals feel comfortable with meditation, while others need a more active stress reduction method and might choose exercise. As you review the methods described in the following pages, consider how they might fit with your personality and lifestyle. Experiment with a few methods—and try something new—before you settle on something you think will work for you. Whatever methods you choose, we recommend practicing them on a regular basis. They will become second nature to you and part of your everyday life. They will be available during stressful moments and may even be activated naturally.

Sometimes stressful events and situations are overwhelming, and your resources and coping abilities are insufficient to support you. These times call for professional help. Don't hesitate to visit your college counseling center or avail yourself of other resources if you find that you need more support.

STRESS REDUCTION STRATEGIES

Any activity that decreases the number or lessens the effect of stressors is a stress reduction technique. Although you might not think of avoidance as an effective coping strategy, sometimes protecting yourself from unnecessary stressors makes sense. For example, try not listening to the news for a few days. You'll find that world events continue as always without your participation. If certain people in your life consistently trigger negative feelings in you, try not seeing them for a while. When you do see them, you may have a better perspective on your interpersonal dynamics. If you have too many activities going on in your life, assert your right to say no to the next request for your time. Downscaling and simplifying your life are effective ways of alleviating stress.

Time Management   One of the most difficult tasks of adult life is using time well—finding a balance between the things you have to do and the things you want to do. Sometimes people spend time in a frenzy of activity but end up achieving little. Often they spend time on the wrong tasks and never get to the things that matter. They may be over-committed and overscheduled; they may procrastinate or always be running late. All of these time-related behaviors and outcomes are stressful.

Time management is the topic of seminars and books, and some experts have devoted their entire careers to helping people learn how to manage their time. Here, we focus on two key points: planning and prioritizing. In time management, it has been noted that typically 80 percent of unfocused effort generates only 20 percent of results. The remaining 20 percent of effort produces 80 percent of results. In other words, people spend most of their time on the wrong tasks. You may be focusing on the wrong tasks if

- You're spending time on things you are not very good at
- The tasks are taking much longer than you expected

You may be focusing on the right tasks if

- You're engaged in activities that advance your overall purpose in life

- You're doing things you have always wanted to do or that make you feel good about yourself
- You're working on tasks you don't like, but you're doing them knowing they relate to the bigger picture[31]

To make sure you focus on the things that matter to you, think about your goals in life and what you want to achieve. Are they worthy of your time? Obviously, you need time for sleeping, working, studying, and so on, but remember to allow yourself time for maintaining wellness through such activities as relaxing, playing, and spending time with family and friends. A global picture of your goals and priorities provides a framework and perspective that can give you a sense of control and reduce stress.

When you want to manage your time on the everyday level, keep a daily "to do" list and prioritize the items on it. Write the items down, because it's stressful to just keep them in your head! As you look at the list, assign each task a priority:

- Is it something you must get done today, such as turning in a paper?
- Is it something you would like to get done, such as catching up on the week's reading?
- Is it something that can wait until tomorrow, such as buying a new pair of jeans?

Then organize the items into these three categories. Complete the tasks in the first category first, before moving on to tasks in the other two categories. This approach will help you be more purposeful, organized, and efficient about the use of your time, giving you more of a sense of control in your life.

In the course of evaluating your goals and prioritizing your daily tasks, you may find that you have too many

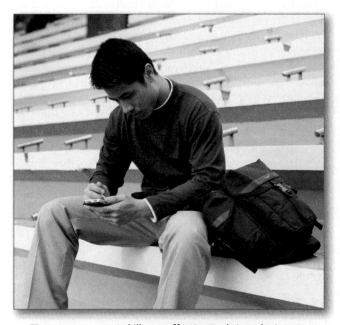

- Time management skills are effective tools in reducing stress. Keeping a daily planner can help you stay organized and on track throughout your day.

commitments, an issue discussed earlier in the chapter. Try thinking about this issue in terms of your commitments to yourself: How can you best honor and take care of yourself? If you are stressed out because you are breaking your commitments, you have three choices:

■ Don't make the commitments (lower your expectations).

■ Keep the commitments (get busy and work efficiently to wrap them up).

■ Reframe the commitments (constantly review and make intelligent choices about what you can and should be doing at any particular moment).

Trying to do more than you have time for and doing the wrong things in the time you have are stressful. Managing your time well is a key to reducing stress.

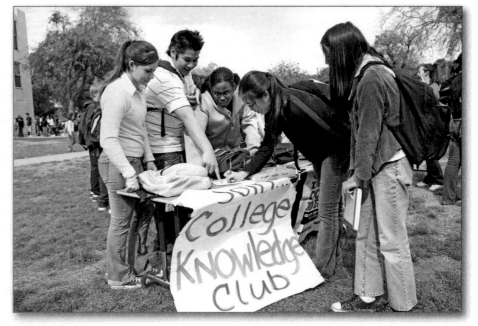

■ Getting involved in college clubs and activities helps you build a social support network that you can rely on in times of stress.

Social Support Another key to reducing stress, just as it is a key to mental health and to a meaningful spiritual life, is social support. Numerous studies show that social support decreases the stress response hormones in the body. Dr. Dean Ornish points out that people who have close relationships and a strong sense of connection and community enjoy better health and live longer than do those who live in isolation. People who suffer alone suffer a lot.[32]

Many people lack the sense of belonging and community that was provided by the extended family and closer-knit society of our grandparents' day. You may have to consciously create a social support system to overcome isolation and loneliness and buffer yourself from stress. The benefits make the effort worthwhile. They include a shoulder to lean on and an ear to listen when you need support. Communicating about your feelings reduces stress and helps you to work through problems and feel better about yourself.

The best way to develop a support system is to give support to others, establishing relationships and building trust:

■ Cultivate a variety of types of relationships.

■ Stay in touch with your friends, especially when you know they're going through a hard time, and keep your family ties strong.

■ Find people who share your interests and pursue activities together, whether it's hiking, dancing, or seeing classic movies. You may want to join a group with a goal that interests you, such as a church group, a study group, or a book club.

■ Try to get involved with your community and participate in activities that benefit others.

■ Maintain and improve your communication skills—both listening to other people's feelings and sharing your own.

When you have a network of relationships and a community to belong to, you will be able to cope with the stress of life more effectively. And when you need support, you will have a connection that can be reciprocated comfortably.

A Healthy Lifestyle A healthy lifestyle is an essential component of any stress management program. A nutritious diet helps you care for your body and keeps you at your best. Experts recommend emphasizing whole grains, vegetables, and fruits in the diet and avoiding excessive amounts of caffeine. Getting enough sleep is also essential for wellness, as are opportunities for relaxation and fun. (See the box "Dietary Supplements and Stress.")

Exercise is probably the most popular and most effective stress buster available. It has a positive effect on both physical and mental functioning and helps people withstand stress. Regular exercisers are also less likely to use smoking, drinking, or overeating as methods for reducing their levels of stress.[32] A growing body of evidence suggests that getting regular exercise is the best thing you can do to protect yourself from the effects of stress.

RELAXATION TECHNIQUES

If you are in a state of chronic stress and the relaxation response does not happen naturally, it is in your best interest to learn how to induce it. Relaxation techniques seem to have an effect on a number of physiological functions, including blood pressure, heart rate, and muscle tension. Here we describe just a few of the many techniques that have been developed.

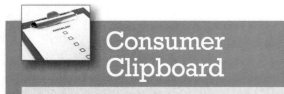

Consumer Clipboard

Dietary Supplements and Stress

Are there dietary supplements that can enhance immune system functioning over the long term, in response to chronic stress? Claims are made for several products, but so far none is without problems.

The herbal supplement kava (also known as kava kava), for example, is advertised as relieving anxiety, stress, and insomnia. It is made from the root of the pepper plant and has been used ceremonially for thousands of years by Pacific Islanders. Although kava may have sedative and pain-relieving properties, reports from several European countries have linked kava to cases of liver toxicity, including hepatitis, cirrhosis, and liver failure, and it is now banned in the United Kingdom. People in the United States with any kind of liver problem should talk to their health care provider before taking kava.

Other dietary supplements advertised as stress relievers are also problematic. The hormone supplement DHEA is promoted as relieving stress, since in its natural state it counteracts the stress hormone cortisol. However, it isn't clear whether taking DHEA in a supplement form has the same effect. B-complex vitamins are often advertised as stress busters because stress saps the body of B vitamins. But if you're not deficient in this vitamin, taking more of it won't help you. Similarly, zinc, which supports the immune system, is promoted as a stress reliever, but any direct connection between supplemental zinc and stress relief has not been proven.

The bottom line is that any product you take for stress acts on the symptoms of stress, not the causes. To reduce your stress levels, try one of the stress management strategies or relaxation techniques described in the chapter. And if you do decide to try a dietary supplement—consult with your health care provider first.

Deep Breathing   One relaxation tool that is simple and always available is breathing. When you feel yourself starting to experience the stress response, you can simply remember to breathe deeply. As you learn to be aware of breathing patterns and practice slowing that process, your mind and body will begin to relax. Breathing exercises have been found to be effective in reducing panic attacks, muscle tension, headaches, and fatigue.

To practice deep breathing, inhale through your nose slowly and deeply through the count of 10. Don't just raise your shoulders and chest; allow your abdomen to expand as well. Exhale very slowly through your nose or through gently pursed lips and concentrate fully on your breath as you let it out. Try to repeat this exercise a number of times during the day even when you're not feeling stressed. Once it becomes routine, you can use it to help you relax before an exam or in any stressful situation.

Progressive Relaxation   Progressive muscle relaxation is based on the premise that deliberate muscle relaxation will block the muscle tension that is part of the stress response, thus reducing overall levels of stress. Progressive relaxation has provided relief when used to treat such stress-related symptoms as neck and back pain and high blood pressure.

To practice progressive muscle relaxation, find a quiet place and lie down in a comfortable position without crossing your arms or legs. Maintain a slow breathing pattern while you tense each muscle or muscle group as tightly as possible for 10 seconds before releasing it. Begin by making a fist with one hand, holding it, and then releasing it. Notice the difference between the tensed state and the relaxed state, and allow your muscles to remain relaxed. Continue with your other hand, your arms, shoulders, neck, and so on, moving around your entire body. Don't forget your ears, forehead, mouth, and all the muscles of your face.

If you take the time to relax your body this way, the technique will provide significant relief from stress. You will also find that once your body learns the process, you will be able to relax your muscles quickly on command during moments of stress.

Visualization   Also called *guided imagery*, visualization is the mental creation of visual images and scenes. Because our thoughts have such a powerful influence on our reactions, simply imagining a relaxing scene can bring about the relaxation response.34 Visualization can be used alone or in combination with other techniques such as deep breathing and meditation to help reduce stress, tension, and anxiety.

To try visualization, sit or lie in a quiet place. Imagine yourself in a soothing, peaceful scene, one that you find particularly relaxing—a quiet beach, a garden, a spot in the woods. Try to visualize all you would see there as vividly as you can, scanning the scene. Bring in your other senses; what sounds do you hear, what scents do you smell? Is the sun warm, the breeze gentle? If you can imagine the scene fully, your body will respond as if you were really there. Commercial tapes are also available that use guided imagery to promote relaxation, but because imagery is personal and subjective, you may need to be selective in finding a tape that works for you.

Yoga   The ancient practice of yoga is rooted in Hindu philosophy, with physical, mental, and spiritual components. It is a consciously performed activity involving posture, breath, and body and mind awareness. In the path and practice of yoga, the aim is to calm the mind, cleanse the body, and raise awareness. The outcomes of this practice include a release of mental and physical tension and the attainment of a relaxed state.

The most widely practiced form of yoga in the Western world is hatha yoga. The practitioner assumes a number of different postures, or poses, holding them while stretching, breathing, and balancing. They are performed slowly and gently, with focused attention. Yoga stretching improves flexibility as well as muscular strength and endurance. For yoga to be effective, the poses have to be performed correctly. If you are interested in trying yoga, we recommend that you begin by taking a class with a certified instructor. There are also commercial videos that can get you started.

T'ai Chi   T'ai chi is a form of Chinese martial arts that dates back to the 14th century. Central to this method is the concept of *qi,* or life energy, and practicing t'ai chi is said to increase and promote the flow of *qi* throughout the body. T'ai chi combines 13 postures with elements of other stress-relieving techniques, such as exercise, meditation, and deep breathing. Research has shown that t'ai chi is beneficial in combating stress, although exactly how it works is unclear. You can take t'ai chi classes in a group setting, although these are not as widely available as yoga classes. Using instructional videos to learn t'ai chi is another option.

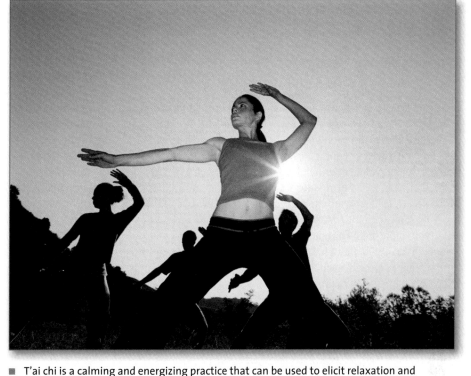

■ T'ai chi is a calming and energizing practice that can be used to elicit relaxation and manage stress.

Biofeedback   Biofeedback is a kind of relaxation training that involves the use of special equipment to provide feedback on the body's physiological functions. You receive information about your heart rate, breathing, skin temperature, and other autonomic nervous system activities and thus become more aware of exactly what is happening in your body during both the relaxation response and the stress response. Once you have this heightened awareness, you can use relaxation techniques at the first sign of the stress response in daily life. Biofeedback can be used to reduce tension headaches, chronic muscle pain, hypertension, and anxiety.[35] If you are interested in trying biofeedback, check with your school to see if the special equipment and training are available.

Affirmations   The literature is clear that when people have an optimistic attitude and a positive view of themselves, they are less likely to suffer the negative effects of stress. **Affirmations** are positive thoughts that you can write down or say to yourself to balance the negative thoughts you may have internalized over the course of your life. Repeatedly reciting such negative, distorted thoughts can increase stress levels. Although they may seem silly to some people, affirmations can help you shift from a negative view of yourself to a more positive one. The more often you repeat an affirmation, the more likely you are to believe it.

affirmations
Positive thoughts that you can write down or say to yourself to balance negative thoughts.

To create affirmations for yourself, think about areas of your life in which you would like to see improvements, such as health, self-esteem, or happiness, and then imagine what that change would look like. Here are some examples:

■ I make healthy choices for myself.

■ I am the right weight for me.

■ The more grateful I am, the more reasons I find to be grateful.

■ I love and accept myself.

■ I attract only healthy relationships.

■ I have abundant energy, vitality, and well-being.

■ I can open my heart and let wonderful things flow into my life.

We have provided just a sampling of stress reducing techniques; there are many others. Many people develop their own relaxation strategies, such as listening to soothing music, going for walks in a beautiful natural setting, or enjoying the company of a pet. Whatever your preferences, learn to incorporate some peaceful moments into your day, every day. You will experience an improved quality of life today and a better chance of avoiding stress-related illness in the future.

You Make the Call

Should Stress Reduction Programs Be Covered by Health Insurance?

Imagine this scene: You lead a stressful, complex life, and lately you have been experiencing a lot of anxiety. You find it hard to unwind at the end of the day and even harder to fall asleep. You've been feeling tense and nervous, and you realize it's time to get a better handle on your stress level. So the next time you see your regular physician, you mention that you sometimes feel overwhelmed by the stress in your life.

Your physician's first response is to offer some medication you could take to reduce anxiety. You're not sure you want to take drugs, though, so you ask if she can recommend some other approach, such as a stress management program. She says there are such programs, and in fact the clinic has a biofeedback training program, but it is not covered by your health insurance plan. She also mentions yoga classes and meditation groups—again, not covered by your insurance plan.

This is a fairly common scenario in many medical offices. Physicians often advise their patients to quit smoking, lose weight, exercise more, and engage in other health promotion activities that will improve their overall quality of life and reduce their effects on the health care system later in their lives. Numerous programs exist that help people make these difficult lifestyle changes. Some are commercial programs, and some are part of health promotion activities offered by clinics, hospitals, and other health care facilities. Most of them are not covered by health insurance.

The health promotion industry argues that getting people involved in taking care of their own health can result in improved quality of life and a reduction in overall health care costs. Recently, with overweight and obesity identified as major health problems for the nation, some have

suggested that health insurance companies should cover the cost of weight loss programs. Given the cost to the nation of stress-related illnesses and injuries, a similar case can be made for the coverage of stress reduction programs.

Insurance companies argue that their mandate is to pay medical expenses for people who are sick, not cover the cost of health promotion activities for people who are well. They also argue that most health promotion programs have not been proven effective by broad-based, high-quality research; most have not been studied at all. Without a research base, they cannot distinguish an effective stress reduction program from an ineffective one.

Decisions about these issues will affect public policy concerning coverage of health promotion and wellness activities in the future. What do you think?

PROS

- Participation in a stress reduction program can improve a person's quality of life.

- Individuals in such programs may get sick less often and may be at lower risk for chronic diseases such as cancer and heart disease. They may use the health care system less frequently.

- Such programs may contribute to a reduction in overall health care costs for the nation.

CONS

- Health insurance should cover only treatments for illness.

- Health promotion/stress reduction programs have not been proven to be effective.

- It is a slippery slope: If we cover these programs, where will it stop?

In Review

1. **What is stress?** Stress is defined as a general state of the body, mind, and emotions when an environmental stressor has triggered the stress response. It can be thought of as a transaction between an individual and a stressor, mediated by personal variables that include the person's perceptions and appraisal of the event. The stress response, also known as the fight-or-flight response, is the set of physiological changes that occurs in the body in the face of a threat.

2. **How does stress affect your health?** The body is equipped to deal with episodes of short-term, acute stress, provided they don't occur too often or last too long, but low-level, chronic stress takes a toll on the body, negatively affecting the immune system, the cardiovascular system, the gastrointestinal system, and mental health. Experiences of extreme stress or trauma can lead to post-traumatic stress disorder (PTSD).

3. **What accounts for different people's responses to stress?** The stress response can be mediated by personality factors such as hostility, by cognitive factors such as illogical ideas and unrealistic expectations, and by traits such as resilience and hardiness.

4. **What are the sources of stress in most people's lives?** Stress can be caused by major life events and by daily hassles, college students experience unique stressors. Other common sources of stress are job pressures, financial worries, interpersonal issues, time pressure and work overload, anger, trauma, and experiences of discrimination, injustice, and poverty.

5. **What are the main approaches to managing stress?** Stress can be managed by using stress reduction strategies such as time management and eliciting social support; by maintaining a healthy lifestyle that includes a balanced diet, exercise, and adequate sleep and that excludes self-medicating with alcohol, drugs, and tobacco; and by practicing relaxation techniques. These techniques include deep breathing, progressive relaxation, visualization, yoga, t'ai chi, biofeedback, and affirmations.

WWW For a detailed summary of this chapter and a comprehensive set of review questions, visit the Online Learning Center at **www.mhhe.com/teague2e**.

Web Resources

American Institute of Stress: This organization is a clearinghouse for information on all stress-related topics. Its monthly newsletter, *Health and Stress*, presents the latest advances in stress research and related health issues.
www.stress.org

Harvard Mind-Body Medical Institute: Highlighting the work of Herbert Benson, M.D., author of *The Relaxation Response*, this organization presents information on mind-body basics and wellness. It offers ways to deal with stress in everyday life.
www.mbmi.org

Medical Basis for Stress: This site presents practical approaches to dealing with stress in all aspects of life. It offers tips related to nutrition and exercise,

checklists to keep you on track, and rules to live by to reduce your stress level.
www.teachhealth.com

National Institute of Mental Health (NIMH): This organization takes a scientific approach to various mental health topics, including stress. Its breaking news feature and its highlights section are of particular interest.
www.nimh.nih.gov

National Institute for Occupational Safety and Health (NIOSH): A valuable resource for information about stress at work, this site focuses on understanding the influence of organizations and psychosocial factors on stress, illness, and injury. It also aims to find ways of redesigning jobs to create safer and healthier workplaces.
www.cdc.gov/niosh/topics/stress

Chapter 6

Sleep Renewal and Restoration

Ever Wonder...

- if sleeping in on weekends makes up for the sleep you lost during the week?

- if taking stimulant drugs to stay up late could harm your health?

- why it sometimes takes so long to fall asleep?

Your Health Today

www.mhhe.com/teague2e

Go to the Online Learning Center for *Your Health Today* for interactive activities, quizzes, flashcards, Web links, and more resources related to this chapter.

College students often have a reputation for missing early morning classes or falling asleep in class. It doesn't necessarily mean that they've been out partying. Most young adults have a **circadian rhythm**—an internal daily cycle of waking and sleeping—that tells them to fall asleep later in the evening and to wake up later in the morning than older adults. These circadian rhythms, accompanied by a demanding college environment, make college students vulnerable to chronic sleep deprivation. Most adults need about 8 hours of sleep each night, but the typical college student sleeps only 6 to 7 hours a night on weekdays.

circadian rhythm
Daily 24-hour cycle of physiological and behavioral functioning.

Unfortunately, sleeping in on the weekends does not fully recapture lost sleep. Colleges and universities are exploring ways to help their sleep-deprived students. Duke University, for example, has eliminated classes that start before 8:30 a.m. Other colleges and universities are including programs on sleep and health as part of summer orientation for freshmen.

According to the 2005 Sleep in America Poll[1] conducted by the National Sleep Foundation (NSF), many Americans are not sleeping enough to sustain optimum health. Of the poll's respondents—adults aged 18 to 54—71 percent reported sleeping less than 8 hours on weekdays, and nearly 30 percent said they slept less than 7 hours. On average, the respondents reported sleeping about 6.8 hours on weekdays and 7.4 hours on weekends.[1, 2] Many people are unaware of the vital role that adequate sleep plays in good health.

Sleep and Your Health

sleep
Period of rest and recovery from the demands of wakefulness; a state of unconsciousness or partial consciousness from which a person can be roused by stimulation

Sleep is commonly understood as a period of rest and recovery from the demands of wakefulness. It can also be described as a state of unconsciousness or partial consciousness from which a person can be roused by stimulation (as distinguished from a coma, for example). We spend about one-third of our lives sleeping, a fact that in itself indicates how important sleep is.

HEALTH EFFECTS OF SLEEP

Sleep is strongly associated with overall health and quality of life. During the deepest stages of sleep, restoration and growth take place. Growth hormone stimulates the growth and repair of the body's tissues and helps to prevent certain types of cancer. Natural immune system moderators increase during deep sleep to promote resistance to viral infections. When sleep time is deficient, a breakdown in the body's health-promoting processes can occur.

Sleep deprivation and sleep disorders are often associated with serious physical and mental health conditions, including these:

- Cardiovascular diseases (congestive heart failure, hypertension, heart attacks, strokes)
- Metabolic disorders (diabetes mellitus)
- Endocrine disorders (osteoporosis)
- Immunological disorders (influenza)
- Respiratory disorders (asthma, bronchitis)
- Mental health disorders (depression, suicide)
- Overweight and obesity (the mechanism for this connection is still unknown)

Sleeping less than 7 hours—sometimes called *short sleep*—increases the risk for negative health outcomes in both men and women. (Sleeping 10 hours or more—*long sleep*—has not been found to have negative health outcomes.) Studies strongly support the conclusion that sufficient quantity and quality of sleep are as vital to a healthy lifestyle as are good nutrition and exercise.[3–6]

SLEEP DEPRIVATION

Sleep deprivation refers to sleep of shorter duration than the average basal need of 7 to 8 hours. Most of us know what it feels like when we don't get enough sleep—we feel drowsy, our eyes burn, we find it hard to pay attention. The effects of sleep deprivation can be much more serious than this, however. Studies have shown that individuals with severe sleep deprivation (staying awake for 19 to 24 hours, for example) score worse on performance tests and alertness scales than do people with a blood alcohol concentration (BAC) of 0.1 percent—legally too drunk to drive.

sleep deprivation
Lack of sufficient time asleep, a condition that impairs physical, emotional, and cognitive functioning.

Sleep deprivation has effects in all domains of functioning. Heightened irritability, lowered anger threshold, frustration, nervousness, and difficulty handling stress are some of the emotional effects. Reduced motivation may affect school and job performance, and lack of interest in socializing with others may cause relationships to suffer. Performance of daily activities is affected, as is the brain's ability to learn new material. Reaction time, coordination, and judgment are all impaired. Individuals who are sleep deprived may experience microsleeps—brief episodes of sleep lasting a few seconds at a time—which increase their risk of being involved in accidents.[4, 7–11]

sleep debt
The difference between the amount of sleep attained and the amount needed to maintain alert wakefulness during the daytime, when the amount attained is less than the amount needed.

Sleeping less than you need causes a **sleep debt**.[12] Your sleep debt accumulates over time, so that sleeping 1 hour less than you need every night for a week, for example, feels to your body like staying up all night. College students are especially vulnerable to building up a sleep debt, such as by pulling an all-nighter to prepare for an exam. (See the box "Study and Stimulants: Taking a Risk.") Many college students and others who build up a sleep debt during the week—nightshift workers, for example—try to cancel the debt by sleeping more on the weekends. This "solution," however, can actually worsen sleep deprivation during the week by disrupting sleep structure.[3, 13, 14] Getting the same sufficient amount of sleep each night strengthens sleep structure.

How can you tell if you are getting enough sleep? A prime symptom of sleep deprivation is daytime drowsiness. If you feel alert during the day, you are probably getting enough sleep. If you are sleepy in sedentary situations such as reading, sitting in class, or watching television, you may be sleep deprived. Another measure of sleep deprivation is how long it takes you to fall asleep at night. A well-rested person will need 15 to 20 minutes to fall asleep.[3] If you fall asleep the instant your head hits the pillow, there is a good chance that you are sleep deprived.

What Makes You Sleep?

Over the course of the day, your body undergoes rhythmic changes that help you move from waking to sleep and back to waking. These *circadian rhythms* are maintained primarily by two tiny structures in the brain, the *suprachiasmic nuclei* (SCN), located directly behind the optic nerve in the hypothalamus (Figure 6.1). This internal "biological clock" controls body temperature and levels of alertness and activity. These controls are active in the daytime, increasing wakefulness, and inactive at night, allowing the body to relax and sleep. They are also less active in the early afternoon. In addition, the SCN control the release of certain hormones. They signal the pineal gland to release **melatonin**, a hormone that increases relaxation and sleepiness, and they signal the pituitary gland to release growth hormone during sleep, to help repair damaged body tissues.

melatonin
A hormone that increases relaxation and sleepiness, released by the pineal gland during sleep.

Also important in maintaining circadian rhythms are external, environmental cues, especially light. Neurons in the SCN monitor the amount of light entering the eyes, so that as daylight increases, the SCN slow down the secretion of melatonin and begin to be more active.[12] This process keeps your sleep/wake cycles generally synchronized with the changing lengths of day and night. The process is sensitive to artificial light as well as natural light, and even relatively dim lights in the evening (for example, from a lamp or a computer screen) may delay your biological clock from inducing sleepiness.

Challenges & Choices

Study and Stimulants: Taking a Risk

When an exam is coming up or a paper is due, many college students reach for some kind of caffeine product to stay awake—whether standards like coffee, Coke, or Mountain Dew; the newer energy drinks like Red Bull, Jolt, Venom, or Adrenaline Rush; or items like caffeinated gum, caffeinated lip balm, or NoDoz. Although caffeine increases alertness and decreases feelings of fatigue, consuming too much can cause anxiety, irritability, a racing heart rate, sleep disruption, and a caffeine crash when the drug wears off. Experts advise not consuming more than 300 mg of caffeine per day.

A growing number of students are turning to a different source when they want to keep going without sleep—stimulant medications prescribed for conditions such as attention deficit/hyperactivity disorder (ADHD), chronic fatigue, and depression. Among the more commonly abused of these drugs are Ritalin, Adderall, and Provigil. These medications work by affecting the levels of different neurotransmitters in the brain, including dopamine, serotonin, and norepinephrine. They can cause irregular heartbeat, high blood pressure, high body temperature, seizures, heart attacks, and strokes. They can also be psychologically and physically addictive, and their long-term effects are not known.

Some college administrators are concerned that students may fake symptoms of ADHD to obtain prescription stimulants for their own use, to share with friends, or to sell. On some campuses, physicians won't prescribe them. Many students resist the message that stimulant drugs can be dangerous. They say the drugs help them focus better, give them an extra edge, and help them meet the time demands of active social lives and academic schedules. Health experts warn that the risks aren't worth it.

It's Not Just Personal...
Although time pressure is a reality of college life, the key to healthier study and sleep habits is better time management. Some colleges are offering time management workshops to help their students avoid all-nighters and the need for stimulant drugs.

Sources: Data from "Seven Percent of College Students Have Used Prescription Stimulants for Nonmedical Purposes," 2005, www.news-medical.net; Wasting the Best and the Brightest: Substance Abuse at America's Colleges and Universities, *National Center on Addiction and Substance Abuse, Columbia University, March 2007, New York: Columbia University; "Performance and Alertness of Caffeine, Dextroamphetamine, and Modafinil During Sleep Deprivation," by N.J. Wesenton, D. William, S. Kilgore, and T.J. Balkin, 2005,* Journal of Sleep Research, 14 (3), p. 225.

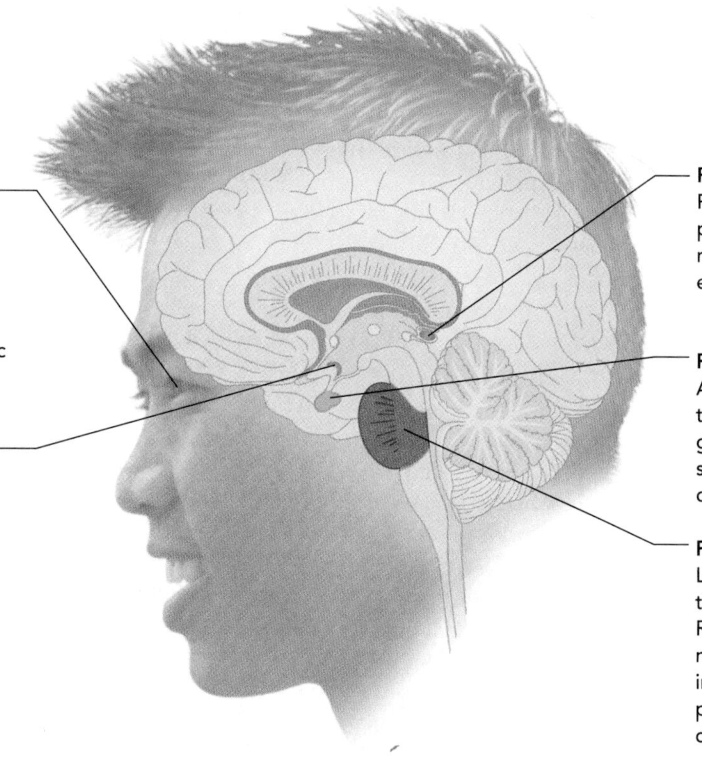

Retina (eye)
The job of the retina at the back of the eye is to sense changes in light levels during day and night. Once nerves in the retina are stimulated, the signal is sent through the optic nerve to the hypothalamus.

Suprachiasmic nuclei (SCN)
These two tiny neural structures are located in the hypothalamus and function as a master biological clock. By monitoring levels of light entering the eyes and managing body temperature, hormone release, and metabolic rate, the SCN control falling asleep and awakening.

Pineal gland
Regulated by the SCN, the pineal gland releases melatonin, a hormone that elicits drowsiness and sleep.

Pituitary gland
Also regulated by the SCN, the pituitary gland releases growth hormone during sleep to help repair damaged body tissues.

Pons
Located in the brain stem, the pons is active during REM sleep, when it signals nerves in the spine to immobilize the body to prevent movement during dreams.

figure **6.1**   **Brain structures involved in sleep and waking.**

The biological clock operates even without the cues of daylight or darkness, though not in perfect synchrony with a 24-hour day. Without the stimulation of light and dark, human beings would have a daily cycle several minutes longer than 24 hours. Every morning your body resets your biological clock to adjust to the next 24-hour period.[3] Your body easily tolerates a 1-hour adjustment. However, when bedtimes and awakening times differ greatly from their established norms, the adjustment is more difficult. Working night shifts and flying across several time zones, for example, can play havoc with your biological clock.[12, 15]

The Structure of Sleep

Studies have revealed that sleep consists of distinct stages in which muscle relaxation and nervous system arousal vary, as do types of brain waves and levels of neural activity. The brain cycles into two main states of sleep: non–rapid eye movement sleep, divided into four stages, and rapid eye movement sleep.

NREM SLEEP

You spend about 75 percent of your sleep time in **non–rapid eye movement (NREM) sleep,** a time of reduced brain activity with four stages.

Stage 1 of NREM sleep is a transitional, light sleep—a relaxed or half-awake state. Your heart rate slows and your breathing becomes shallow and rhythmic. This stage may last from 10 seconds to 10 minutes and is sometimes accompanied by visual imagery. People awakened in stage 1 often deny that they were asleep.[12, 16]

In stage 2, your brain's activity slows further, and you stop moving. This lack of movement decreases muscle tension and brain stem stimulation so that sleep is induced. Stage 2 lasts about 10 to 20 minutes and represents the beginning of actual sleep. You are no longer consciously aware of your external environment. People awakened in stage 2 readily admit that they were asleep.[12, 16]

During stages 3 and 4 your blood pressure drops, your heart rate and respiration slow, and the blood supply to your brain is minimized. If you were suddenly awakened during stage 4, referred to as *deep sleep*, you would feel momentarily groggy. You usually spend about 20 to 40 minutes at a time in deep sleep, and most of your deep sleep takes place in the first third of the night.[12, 16]

non–rapid eye movement (NREM) sleep
Type of sleep characterized by slower brain waves than are seen during wakefulness as well as other physiological markers; divided into four stages of increasingly deep sleep.

REM SLEEP

Rapid eye movement (REM) sleep begins about 70 to 90 minutes after you have fallen asleep. As you enter this stage, your breathing and heart rate increase, and brain wave activity becomes more like that of a waking state. REM sleep is characterized by noticeable eye movements, usually lasting between 1 and 10 minutes. During this period you are most likely to experience your first dream of the night. Although dreams may occur in all stages of sleep, they generally happen in REM sleep.[3, 12, 17]

rapid eye movement (REM) sleep
Type of sleep characterized by brain waves and other physiological signs characteristic of a waking state but also characterized by reduced muscle tone, or sleep paralysis; most dreaming occurs during REM sleep.

When you dream, there are periods when you have no muscle tone and your body cannot move, except for your eyes, diaphragm, nasal membranes, and erectile tissue (such as penis or clitoris).[3] This state is referred to as *REM sleep paralysis*, If you were not immobilized, there is a danger that you would act on—or act out—your dreams. REM sleep is sometimes called *paradoxical sleep*, because the sleeper appears peaceful and still but is in a state of physiological arousal.

Dreams and dreaming have long intrigued people in every part of the world. Probably the best-known theory of dreams in Western culture is that of Sigmund Freud, who believed that the purpose of dreaming was the gratification of unconscious desires. By dreaming about them in disguised, symbolic form while we are sleeping, we fulfill wishes we would find unacceptable during waking life. At the opposite pole is a theory proposed in the 1970s that dreams are the product of random neural activity that goes on during REM sleep. According to this theory, dreams have little or no meaning.[3]

Still, many people believe that dreams do have some meaning and relevance to daily life, often reflecting changes or shifts in emotions. By examining your dreams, according to this view, you may gain insight into the mental and emotional processes you are applying to problems or events in your life.

Besides giving us time to dream, REM sleep also appears to give the brain the opportunity to "file" important ideas and thoughts in long-term storage, that is, in memory. This reorganization and consolidation may account for the fact that we are able to solve problems in our dreams. Scientists further believe that creative and novel ideas are more likely to flourish during REM sleep, because we have easier access to memories and emotions. Because ideas are filed in long-term storage during REM sleep, memory may be impaired if sleep time is insufficient. As a result of such memory impairment, the ability to learn new skills is also impaired. Performance in learning a new skill does not improve until an individual has had 6 hours of sleep; performance improves even more after 8 hours of sleep.[3, 18, 19]

REM rebound effect
Increase in the length and frequency of REM sleep episodes that are experienced when a person sleeps for a longer time after a period of sleep deprivation.

The importance of REM sleep to the brain is demonstrated by what is called the **REM rebound effect**. If you get inadequate sleep for several nights, you will have longer and more frequent periods of REM sleep when you have a night in which you can sleep longer.[19]

SLEEP CYCLES

After your first REM period, you cycle back and forth between REM and NREM sleep stages. These cycles repeat themselves about every 90 to 110 minutes until you wake up. Typically, you experience four or five sleep cycles each night. After the second cycle, however, you spend little or no time in NREM stages 3 and 4 and most of your time in NREM stage 2 and REM sleep (Figure 6.2). After each successive cycle, the time spent in REM sleep doubles, lasting from 10 to 60 minutes at a time.[3, 12, 17]

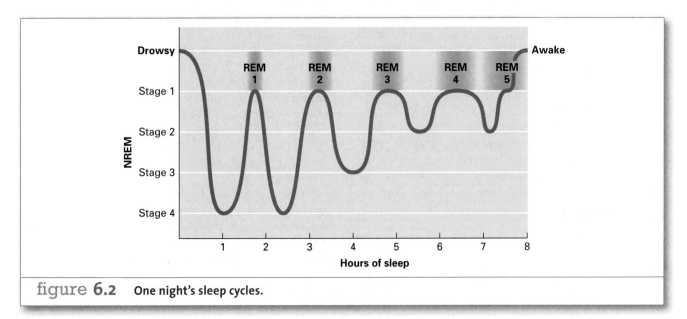

figure **6.2**   One night's sleep cycles.

The sleep cycle pattern changes across the lifespan, with children and young adolescents experiencing large quantities of NREM stages 3 and 4 sleep (deep sleep). Sleep needs are constant across adulthood, but as people get older, high-quality sleep may become more elusive, and older adults may experience less deep sleep and REM sleep and more NREM stage 1 sleep and wakefulness.[3] The production of melatonin and growth hormone declines with age, and the body temperature cycle may become irregular. All of these changes decrease total nighttime sleep.[20]

Medical conditions also affect sleep in older adults. Sleep is disrupted by such conditions as arthritis, heartburn, osteoporosis, Parkinson's disease, heart and lung diseases, dementia, incontinence, and cancer, as well as by some of the drugs used to treat these conditions. Additionally, sleep disorders are more common in middle and later life (see the next section).

However, many healthy older individuals have few or no sleep problems.[21] Some experts believe sleep problems are caused more by lifestyle choices—changes in diet, lack of exercise, decreased mental stimulation, daytime naps, and going to bed too early—than by biological changes. Older adults who maintain healthy lifestyle practices may still be able to get a good night's sleep.

There are also some gender differences in sleep cycles. Some of these differences begin as early as 6 months of age. Although the structure of sleep is essentially the same for men and women, women tend to have more slow-wave sleep (NREM stages 3 and 4) than men do and to experience more

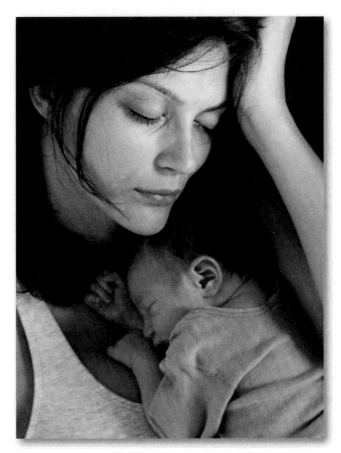

■ Women are more likely than men to get insufficient sleep. New mothers are particularly at risk for sleep deprivation.

Public Health in Action

Women and Sleep

According to the National Sleep Foundation's 2007 Sleep in America poll, sleep deprivation is a public health problem for women:

■ 60 percent of the women polled said they do not get enough sleep most nights of the week.

■ 43 percent said daytime drowsiness interferes with their daily activities.

■ 72 percent of working mothers and 68 percent of single working women reported symptoms of insomnia.

■ 74 percent of stay-at-home mothers reported symptoms of insomnia at least a few nights a week.

■ 27 percent reported driving while drowsy, and 10 percent did so with a child in the car.

Poor sleep affects mood and quality of life. About 55 percent of women reported they felt unhappy, sad, or depressed in the last month, and 35 percent said they had recently felt hopeless about the future. Many women sacrifice healthy activities to meet daily time demands. Sleep, mentioned by 52 percent of respondents, topped the list of activities women reported sacrificing:

Sleep	52 percent
Exercise	48 percent
Time spent with family and friends	39 percent
Healthy eating	37 percent
Sexual activity	33 percent

Many women are not practicing good sleep habits. For example, the National Sleep Foundation's poll found that women typically spend the last hour before bedtime doing household chores, working in front of the computer, or watching television. Sleep experts recommend that stressful activities be avoided in the presleep hour and that the lights be dimmed (no television or computer screens). Women experiencing sleep problems should consult their family doctor or a sleep specialist. Tips for improving sleep are provided later in this chapter.

Sources: "Sleep in America" Poll, National Sleep Foundation, 2007, Washington, DC: National Sleep Foundation; "No Rest for the Weary," by B. Kantrowitz, 2007, Newsweek, May 7, retrieved February 25, 2008, from www.newsweek.com/id/36400.

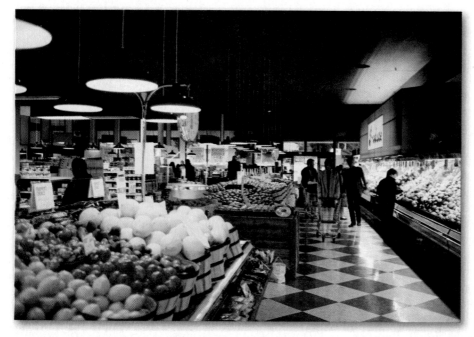

■ Supermarkets that are open 24 hours a day provide a haven for people with insomnia.

30, and 35 percent were older than 65.[1] Clinical symptoms of insomnia include (1) taking longer than 30 minutes to fall asleep, (2) experiencing five or more awakenings per night, (3) sleeping less than a total of 6½ hours as a result of these awakenings, and/or (4) experiencing less than 15 minutes of deep/slow-wave sleep.[23]

According to the NSF, insomnia can be caused by stress, anxiety, medical problems, poor sleep environment, noisy or restless partners, and schedule changes (due to travel across time zones or shift work, for example).[1] For adult women, more than half of whom report symptoms of insomnia during any given month, additional causes may include depression, headaches, effects of pregnancy, premenstrual syndrome, menopausal hot flashes, and overactive bladder. Often the person with insomnia has become distressed by his or her inability to fall asleep, which increases arousal and makes it even harder to fall asleep. In time, the bedroom, bedtime, or sleep itself becomes associated with frustration instead of relaxation, and a vicious cycle sets in.

Chronic insomnia is difficult to treat, but individuals may be able to break the cycle and experience relief through such approaches as improving their sleep habits and sleeping environment and using relaxation techniques such as deep breathing and massage. See the section "Getting a Good Night's Sleep" later in this chapter for more strategies and tips on dealing with insomnia.

Sleep Apnea Also known as breathing-related sleep disorder, **sleep apnea** is a condition characterized by periods of nonbreathing during sleep. Some health experts estimate that almost 40 percent of the U.S. population have some form of sleep apnea and that half of those afflicted may have a severe condition. Some 80 to 90 percent of these cases are undiagnosed. The condition occurs in all ethnic, age, and socioeconomic groups, although men are more at risk for developing sleep apnea than women are.[1, 24, 25]

Scientists have distinguished two main types of sleep apnea, central sleep apnea and obstructive sleep apnea. In *central sleep apnea*, a rare condition, the brain fails to regulate the diaphragm and other breathing mechanisms correctly. In *obstructive sleep apnea*, by far the more common type, the upper airway is obstructed during sleep.[3] Individuals with obstructive sleep apnea are frequently overweight

sleep apnea
Sleep disorder characterized by periods of nonbreathing during sleep; also known as breathing-related sleep disorder.

---

insomnia. Men have more REM periods. Men and women also tend to have some differences in habits and behaviors related to sleep. For example, women tend to get less sleep than they need in order to feel alert during the week, and men tend to get more sleep than they need (see the box "Women and Sleep"). However, men and women get about the same amount of sleep on the weekends.[22]

Sleep Disorders

The National Institutes of Health estimate that at least 40 million Americans suffer from long-term sleep disorders each year; another 20 million experience occasional sleep problems (see the box "Sleep Disorders"). Because many sleep disorders are undiagnosed or not reported to physicians, many people who are chronically exhausted may not know why. Sleep disorders can be divided into dyssomnias and parasomnias.

DYSSOMNIAS

Sleep disorders associated with difficulty in falling asleep or staying asleep or with excessive sleepiness—the timing, quality, and quantity of sleep—are labeled **dyssomnias**.

dyssomnias
Sleep disorders in which the timing, quality, and/or quantity of sleep are disturbed.

insomnia
Sleep disorder characterized by difficulty falling or staying asleep.

Insomnia In a poll conducted by the National Sleep Foundation (NSF), 75 percent of adults reported experiencing one or more symptoms of **insomnia**—defined as difficulty falling or staying asleep—at least a few nights a week.[3] About 5 percent of these people were younger than

Who's at Risk

Sleep Disorders

- Sleepwalking is more common among children aged 5 to 12 than among adults. It usually disappears during adolescence.

- More men than women report snoring, and more men experience sleep apnea. The population most likely to experience sleep apnea is middle-aged overweight men. People with this disorder stop breathing while asleep.

- Insomnia is more common among women than men. Women also have higher rates of depression, a condition that can cause insomnia.

- People with a family history of narcolepsy are 60 times more likely to develop the disorder than are people without such a history. A person with this disorder suffers "sleep attacks" at inappropriate times throughout the day.

- According to the 2005 National Sleep Foundation poll, one in four African Americans is at high risk for obstructive sleep apnea. Asians and Hispanics may also be at high risk for this condition.

- Native American, African American, and Hispanic women have less deep sleep duration than White women.

- Older adults are at particular risk for sleep disruption if they consume alcohol. The ability to metabolize alcohol slows after age 50, causing higher levels of alcohol to remain in the blood and brain than when the same amount of alcohol is consumed at younger ages.

Sources: "Sleep in America" Poll, National Sleep Foundation, 2005, Washington, DC: National Sleep Foundation; "Sleep Problems and Ethnicity," The Merck Manual of Medical Information (2nd home ed.), retrieved from http://sleepdisorders.ifetips.com/faq.120860/ohow-does-ethnicity-effect-the-prevalence-0; "Prevalence and Risk of Sleep Apnea in the U.S. Population," by D.M. Hiestand, P. Britz, M. Goldman, and B. Phillips, 2006, in American College of Chest Physicians, 130, pp. 780–786.

and have an excess of bulky soft tissue in the neck and throat. When the muscles relax during sleep, the tissue can block the airway (Figure 6.3).

In obstructive sleep apnea, the individual stops breathing many times during sleep, often for as long as 60 to 90 seconds. The person's breathing pattern is usually characterized by periods of loud snoring (when the airway is partially blocked), alternating with periods of silence (when the airway is completely blocked), punctuated by sudden loud snores or jerking body movements as the person awakens for a few seconds and gasps for air. The individual is usually not aware of this pattern of snoring and gasping, although bed partners and other members of the household often are. The chief complaint of those with obstructive sleep apnea is daytime sleepiness, not nighttime awakening.

Obstructive sleep apnea is a potentially dangerous condition; occasionally, it is even fatal. It is frequently seen in association with high blood pressure, and it can increase the risk of heart disease and stroke. Oxygen saturation of the blood decreases and levels of carbon dioxide rise when a person stops breathing, increasing the likelihood that heart and blood vessel abnormalities may occur. If sufficient oxygen is not delivered to the brain, death may occur during sleep.[3, 24, 26, 27]

In children, sleep apnea is usually associated with enlarged tonsils. In adults, obstructive sleep apnea occurs most often in overweight, middle-aged men, although it becomes almost equally common in women after menopause. It is associated with larger neck circumferences (greater than 17 inches in men and 16 inches in women).

People with the disorder often smoke, use alcohol, and/or sleep on their backs. There is sometimes a family history of sleep apnea, suggesting a genetic link.

If sleep apnea is not severe, it can be addressed with a variety of behavioral strategies. They include losing weight, forgoing alcoholic nightcaps or sedatives, avoiding allergens, not smoking, using a nasal decongestant spray, using a firm pillow and mattress, and not sleeping on the back. In addition, adjustable mouthpieces are available that extend the lower jaw, adding room to the airway. They are expensive, however, and may not be covered by health insurance.[3, 28]

In cases of severe sleep apnea, one treatment option is a continuous positive airway pressure (CPAP) machine. Through a comfortable mask, a CPAP machine gently blows slightly pressurized air into the patient's nose. Other treatment options include surgery to cut away excess tissue at the back of the throat and a new technique called *samnoplasty* that involves shrinking tissue in the back of the throat with radio-frequency energy.[3, 29]

Narcolepsy   The neurological disorder **narcolepsy** is characterized by frequent, irresistible "sleep attacks," in which the individual unintentionally falls asleep in inappropriate situations, such as while driving a car. A person with narcolepsy experiences excessive daytime sleepiness, falls asleep for 10 to 20 minutes, and awakes feeling refreshed. Within 2 to 3 hours, however, the person once again feels sleepy.

narcolepsy
Sleep disorder characterized by frequent, irresistible "sleep attacks."

Narcolepsy affects about 3 to 6 people in 10,000. Nearly 80 percent of cases of narcolepsy are not diagnosed. A person who has a relative with narcolepsy has a 3 percent chance of developing this disorder—a risk 60 times greater than that of someone with no family history of narcolepsy. If a person has one parent with narcolepsy, the odds are 1 in 20 that the person will have the disorder. Narcolepsy occurs as early as age 3 but usually does not begin until puberty, which suggests that maturation of the brain may play an important role in onset.[3, 23]

There is no cure for narcolepsy, but symptoms may be reduced by taking a 10- to 20-minute nap every 2 hours throughout the day, avoiding alcohol and sleeping pills, and getting sufficient sleep on a regular basis.[30] Stimulant medications such as amphetamines have been used to treat pervasive daytime sleepiness.

Restless Legs Syndrome   As the name suggests, **restless legs syndrome (RLS)** is a sleep disorder characterized by disagreeable sensations in the limbs, usually the legs. These uncomfortable and sometimes painful feelings, such as creeping, tingling, or burning, create an almost irresistible urge to move the legs. Discomfort is relieved by vigorously stretching and crossing the legs and, sometimes, walking about for a short time. The symptoms and the individual's responses to them can delay and disturb sleep, leading to daytime sleepiness. Sleep experts estimate that about 4 percent of the population have this syndrome.[23] Taking iron and vitamin E supplements may help reduce RLS symptoms. Avoiding late-night alcohol and engaging in moderate exercise are also encouraged.

restless legs syndrome (RLS)
Sleep disorder characterized by disagreeable sensations in the limbs, usually the legs.

Other Dyssomnias   In **hypersomnia,** a person experiences excessive daytime sleepiness despite an adequate amount of sleep at night. Individuals with this disorder may require up to 12 hours of sleep a night. In some cases of hypersomnia there is a family history of the disorder and evidence of nervous system dysfunction.[3]

In **circadian rhythm sleep disorder,** the person's internal sleep/wake cycle is out of sync with the sleep/wake demands of the environment. In one subtype of this disorder, individuals seem unable to delay or advance their internal clocks to match the clock time of their occupations or of society in general. In the delayed phase type, individuals naturally go to sleep later at night than is commonly accepted and have a hard time getting up in the morning. In the advanced phase type, people fall asleep early in the evening and wake up early in the morning. Other subtypes

hypersomnia
Sleep disorder characterized by excessive daytime sleepiness despite an adequate amount of sleep at night.

circadian rhythm sleep disorder
Condition in which a person's internal sleep/wake cycle is out of sync with the sleep/wake demands of the environment.

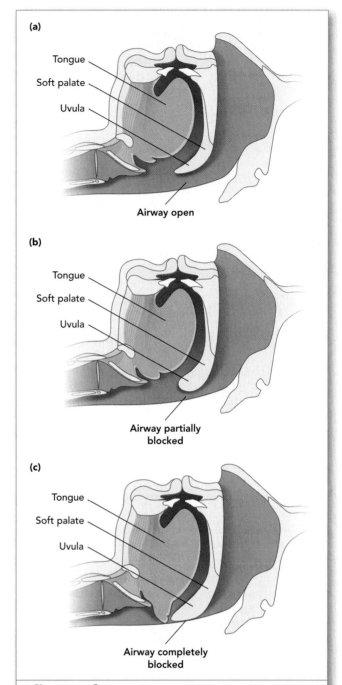

(a)

Tongue
Soft palate
Uvula

Airway open

(b)

Tongue
Soft palate
Uvula

Airway partially blocked

(c)

Tongue
Soft palate
Uvula

Airway completely blocked

figure 6.3   **Obstructive sleep apnea.**
(a) Normally, the airway is open during sleep. (b) When the muscles of the soft palate, tongue, and uvula relax, they narrow the airway and cause snoring. (c) If these structures collapse on the back wall of the airway, they close the airway, preventing breathing. The efforts of the diaphragm and chest cause the blocked airway to become even more tightly sealed. For breathing to resume, the sleeper must rouse enough to cause tension in the tongue, which opens the airway.

are *jet lag type,* in which there is a discrepancy between the person's internal clock and the sleep/wake cycle of the time zone to which the person has traveled, and *shift work type,* in which the person's internal clock is mismatched with the requirements of night-shift work. In general, circadian rhythm disturbances are not disorders except in the context of environmental demands and to the extent that they cause the individual distress.[3, 23]

sleep paralysis
An episode of immobility while awake, caused when REM sleep intrudes during the transition from sleep to waking.

Sleep paralysis is an awareness of being awake accompanied by head-to-toe immobility, including an inability to utter a sound or word. The condition occurs when an episode of REM sleep intrudes during the transition from sleep to waking. Episodes of sleep paralysis may last anywhere from 30 seconds to several minutes. They may be accompanied by tingling sensations and "waking dreams" with a hallucinatory quality.

PARASOMNIAS

Whereas dyssomnias involve the timing, quality, or quantity of sleep, **parasomnias** involve physiological functioning or behavior during sleep. Body systems become activated as if the person were awake, usually during specific stages of sleep.

parasomnias
Sleep disorders in which physiological functioning or behavior during sleep is disturbed.

sleepwalking disorder
Sleep disorder in which a person rises out of an apparently deep sleep and acts as if awake.

Sleepwalking Disorder People with **sleepwalking disorder** rise out of an apparently deep sleep and act as if they are awake. They do not respond to other people while in this state, or, if they do, it is with reduced alertness. For example, they may answer a question or acquiesce to a request to return to bed, but they do so automatically, often with a blank stare. Sleepwalking takes place during slow-wave (stages 3 and 4) NREM sleep and therefore usually occurs during the first third of the night's sleep. Episodes typically last less than 10 minutes.[3] If sleepwalkers are awakened, they are often confused for several minutes; if they are not awakened, they may return to bed and have little or no memory of the episode the next day.

Sleepwalking usually begins between the ages of 5 and 12 and disappears in most cases during adolescence. It rarely starts in adulthood; adults who sleepwalk usually did so as children. Although there may be a genetic link to sleepwalking, most sufferers do not have a family history of this disorder. Episodes may be brought on by excessive sleep deprivation, fatigue, stress, illness, and the use of sedatives.[3, 23]

Nocturnal Eating Disorder A person with **nocturnal eating disorder** rises from bed during the night and eats and drinks while asleep. About three quarters of people with this disorder are female. The person may consume bizarre concoctions but has no memory of these experiences in the morning. Fifty percent of people suffering from this disorder binge eat without awakening. Although they may binge up to six times a night, they do not experience indigestion or feelings of fullness after the binge.[3, 5]

Distinct from nocturnal eating disorder is a newly identified sleep disorder, **night eating syndrome,** in which affected persons binge eat late at night, have difficulty falling asleep, repeatedly awaken during the night and eat again, and then eat very little the next day. Some people with night eating syndrome consume more than 50 percent of their daily calories at night. Sleep experts estimate that the syndrome's frequency is about 1.5 percent in the general population and up to 10 percent among obese people seeking treatment for their weight. Treatments include medications and behavior management techniques.[3, 5]

nocturnal eating disorder
Sleep disorder in which a person rises from bed during the night and eats and drinks while asleep.

night eating syndrome
Condition in which a person eats excessively during the night while awake.

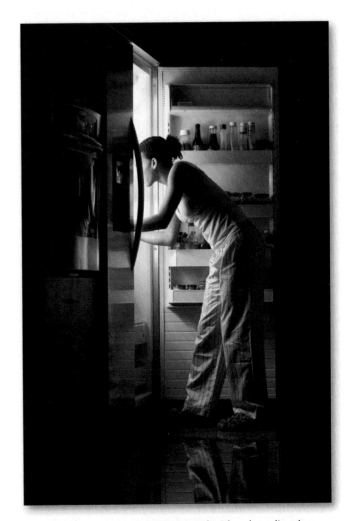

■ Night-time eating can be associated with a sleep disorder. People with nocturnal eating disorder binge eat without waking up; people with night eating syndrome consume a large portion of their daily calories during the night.

Nightmare Disorder   A person with **nightmare disorder** experiences vivid, often frightening dreams during REM sleep. Nightmares commonly occur in the middle to late part of the sleep night, when REM sleep periods become longer. They may be accompanied by sleep talking and body movements. Typically, the dreamer awakens from the nightmare, is fully alert, and can recount the dream, which usually involves imminent danger or threat. About 50 percent of very young children experience nightmares, beginning between the ages of 2 and 5. Although nightmares typically disappear completely by age 7, they can continue into adulthood. Only about 1 percent of the adult population experiences recurrent nightmares, but adults who do should consult a sleep specialist.[3, 23]

nightmare disorder
Sleep disorder in which a person experiences vivid, often frightening dreams during REM sleep.

Nightmare disorder is different from *sleep terror disorder,* or *night terrors.* In this disorder, the individual awakens from deep NREM sleep, usually with a scream or cry, and is difficult to orient. The person does not remember a dream or nightmare but is physiologically aroused, with rapid breathing, pounding heart, sweating, skin flushing, and other signs of extreme fear. Sleep terror disorder is seen in both children and adults and occurs more often when there is a family history of the disorder, indicating a genetic link. Many people with sleep terror disorder experience superhuman power. For example, individuals with severely limited movement caused by multiple sclerosis can jump out of bed with great speed and strength.[12]

REM Behavior Disorder   In **REM behavior disorder,** which occurs most often in older adults,[23] the inhibition of muscle movement that normally occurs during REM sleep does not take place. As a result, individuals get up and act out their dreams, often injuring themselves in the process. They are easily awakened and can recount the dream they were having. The disorder can occur as a result of Parkinson's disease, brain stem damage, alcoholism, or the use of hallucinogenic drugs. Men are more likely than women to have REM behavior disorder. Scientists are not sure why. Sleep experts recommend that the bedroom be structured for safety to protect the individual from injury.[3] In addition, medications have been shown to be effective in treating the disorder.

REM behavior disorder
Sleep disorder in which muscle movement is not inhibited during REM sleep, allowing the person to move around while dreaming.

Sexsomnia   Sexsomnia involves masturbating, fondling another person, or actual intercourse with a nonconsenting person while asleep. Most people who experience sexsomnia have no memory of the event. An intriguing legal question is whether a person committing a sexual assault while asleep has committed a crime. The judicial system has been inconsistent in its decisions concerning sexsomnia and sexual assaults. Curbing alcohol use and maintaining a regular sleep cycle are prevention factors. This condition is one of the remote side effects of the sleep drug Ambien.[12]

Evaluating Your Sleep

How can you tell if you have a sleep problem? First, get a sense of your general level of daytime sleepiness by taking the **sleep latency** test (a measure of how long it takes you to fall asleep) in Part 1 of the Add It Up feature for Chapter 6 at the end of the book. Next, check to see if you have any symptoms of a sleep disorder by completing Part 2 of the Add It Up feature. Then take a look at the various behavior change strategies in the next section of the chapter and make any appropriate improvements. Of course, the most basic recommendation is to make sure you are getting enough hours of sleep every night. If you still experience a sleep problem after following these recommendations, you may want to consult your physician. If the problem is serious enough, your physician may refer you to a sleep clinic or lab or a sleep disorder specialist.

sleep latency
Amount of time it takes a person to fall asleep.

Multiple Sleep Latency Test
Test of sleep latency, administered as an index of daytime sleepiness and usually given five times in a sleep clinic.

If you are referred to a sleep clinic or lab, you may be asked to monitor your sleeping habits at home by keeping a sleep diary for a week or more. You will record the times you go to bed, awaken during the night, and wake up in the morning, as well as what and when you eat in the evening, any alcohol, tobacco, or drugs you consume, and so on. Alternatively, you may be evaluated at the lab. You may take a **Multiple Sleep Latency Test,** in which you lie down in a dark room and are told not to resist sleep. This test, repeated five times during the day, measures sleep latency as an index of daytime sleepiness.

Getting a Good Night's Sleep

What is the best way to ensure healthy sleep patterns over the course of the lifespan? In this section we provide several strategies and tips that will help you get a good night's sleep.

ESTABLISHING GOOD SLEEP HABITS

Several habits and behaviors concerning when and where you sleep and what you do before you sleep can help you sleep better and solve sleep problems.

Maintain a Regular Sleep Schedule   Try to get about 8 hours of sleep every night, 7 days a week. With a regular sleep schedule, you fall asleep faster and awaken more easily, because you are psychologically and physiologically conditioned for sleep and waking. Most students have an irregular sleep schedule.[6] As noted earlier, such a schedule throws off your internal biological clock and disrupts the structure of sleep.

Create a Sleep-Friendly Environment Your bedroom should be a comfortable, secure, quiet, cool, and dark place for inducing sleep. Your mattress should be hard enough to allow you to get into a comfortable sleep position. If it is too hard, however, it may not provide an adequate cushion to prevent painful pressure on your body.[3]

Noise can reduce restful sleep. Research on people who live near airports has found that excessive noise may jog individuals out of deep sleep and into a lighter sleep. Street noises have a similar effect. Noise levels above 40 decibels (about as loud as birds singing) can disturb sleep. College residence halls and apartment complexes often have noise levels that exceed 40 decibels. Earplugs and earphones can reduce noise levels by as much as 90 percent.

If it isn't possible to eliminate noise, try creating *white noise,* a monotonous and unchanging sound such as that of an air conditioner or a fan. Noise generators that create soothing sounds such as falling rain, wind, and surf have been proven effective in protecting sleep.[5, 28]

Temperature is important too. You sleep best when the temperature is within your specific comfort zone. A tem-

perature below or above that zone often causes fragmented sleep or wakefulness. The ideal is usually 62° F to 65° F. Generally, temperatures above 75° F and below 54° F cause people to awaken.[3]

Finally, don't expect to get a good night's sleep if you cannot lie down. Research has shown that people sleeping in an upright position have poorer quality sleep than those sleeping in a horizontal position. The amount of slow-wave sleep a person experiences in a sitting position is almost zero. If you fall asleep while standing up, your body begins to sway so that you quickly awaken. Perhaps the brain operates in a similar fashion when you are sleeping in a seated position. With your body mainly upright, your brain may interpret this position as not sufficiently safe to allow deep sleep.[3]

Avoid Caffeine, Nicotine, and Alcohol Caffeine, a stimulant, disrupts sleep, whether it comes in coffee, tea, chocolate, or soda. It enters your bloodstream quickly, reaches a peak in about 30 to 60 minutes, and may take up to 6 hours to clear your blood system. A single cup of coffee may double the amount of time it takes an average adult to fall asleep. It may also reduce the amount of slow-wave or deep sleep by half and quadruple the number of nighttime awakenings.[12] Avoiding caffeine intake 6 to 8 hours before going to bed may improve sleep quality.

Like caffeine, nicotine is a stimulant that can disrupt sleep. People who smoke a pack of cigarettes a day have been shown to have sleep problems. Brain wave pattern analysis indicates that they do not sleep as deeply as non-smokers. Smoking also affects the respiratory system by causing congestion in the nose and swelling of the mucous membranes lining the throat and upper airway passages. These physiological factors increase the likelihood of snoring and aggravate the symptoms of sleep apnea. They also decrease oxygen uptake, which leads to more frequent awakenings.[3, 31, 32]

Alcohol induces sleepiness and reduces the amount of time it takes to fall asleep, but it causes poorer sleep and restlessness later in the night. Even if consumed 6 hours before bedtime, alcohol can increase wakefulness in the second half of the night, probably through its effect on serotonin and norepinephrine, neurotransmitters that regulate sleep. Because alcohol is a depressant, it prevents REM sleep from occurring until most of the alcohol has been absorbed. After absorption, vivid dreams are more likely. Sleep experts call this an *alcohol rebound effect,* in which the body seems to be trying to recover REM sleep that was lost earlier.

Additionally, alcohol can aggravate sleep disorders such as obstructive sleep apnea and trigger episodes of sleepwalking, sleep-related eating disorders, and REM behavior disorder. The impact of alcohol on sleep apnea is of particular concern; it can even be deadly. Alcohol consumption makes throat muscles even more relaxed than during normal sleep; it also interferes with the ability to awaken.[32, 33]

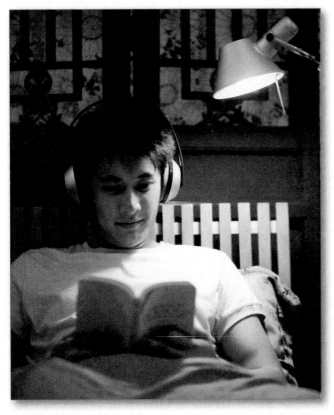

■ One key to getting a good night's sleep is creating a pleasant environment and establishing a relaxing bedtime routine.

Highlight on Health

Critters in Your Bed and Bedroom

Dust mites are extremely common bedroom pests. A typical used mattress may have as many as 100,000 to 10 million microscopic dust mites inside, and 10 percent of the weight of a 2-year-old pillow may be made up of dust mites and their droppings. If not controlled, dust mites can spread throughout the house. To control dust mites, follow these precautions:

- Replace pillows frequently.
- Use synthetic rather than down pillows.
- Vacuum your mattress thoroughly, or cover it with a plastic case that can be wiped with a damp cloth.
- Wash your bed linens weekly in hot water (at least 130° F).
- Vacuum the bedroom carpet frequently.
- Choose hardwood floors over carpet.

Bed bugs are another bedroom pest. For unknown reasons, many cities have recently experienced an upsurge in bed bug infestations. Bed bugs are small, brownish, flattened insects that feed on the blood of animals. Adults are about 1/4 inch long. They are active primarily at night and during the day prefer to hide in the tiny crevices provided by the mattress, box spring, bed frame, or headboard. Their bites, usually on the arms or legs, cause welts and itching that are often mistaken for mosquito bites. Professional pest control may be needed to control a bed bug problem.

Another bedroom pest is the brown recluse spider, found primarily in the central midwestern states southward to the Gulf of Mexico. This spider is about 3/8 inch long and is sometimes referred to as a fiddleback or violin spider because of the faint violin-shaped marking on its back. The brown recluse is not an aggressive spider; people are usually bitten when they accidentally crush, handle, or disturb it, as can happen if it has crawled into bedding. Most bites leave only a small reddish mark, but in some cases the bite can cause a deep, painful wound that can blister, enlarge, and cause a general systemic reaction that includes agitation, itching, fever, chills, nausea, vomiting, or shock. Children, older adults, and people with immune suppression disorders are more vulnerable to systemic reactions.

To prevent bites by the brown recluse or any other spider, follow these precautions:

- Inspect bedding and towels before use.
- Move your bed away from the wall.
- Shake out clothing and shoes before getting dressed.
- Dust and vacuum regularly.
- Eliminate clutter in closets.
- Seal and caulk crevices where spiders can enter your home.
- Wear gloves when handling cardboard boxes, firewood, or rocks.

Many commercial pesticide products are effective for spider control, but if the problem is widespread, you may need to use a pest management company. [35, 36, 37, 38]

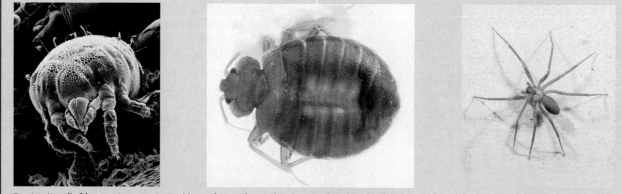

Dust mites (left) are microscopic. Bed bugs (center) are about 1/4 inch in length. The brown recluse spider (right) is about 3/8 inch in length.

Get Regular Exercise but Not Close to Bedtime Regular exercise during the day or early evening hours may be beneficial for sleep. Exercising within 3 hours of going to bed, however, is not recommended, because exercise stimulates the release of adrenaline and elevates core body temperature. It takes 5 to 6 hours for body temperature to drop enough after vigorous exercise for drowsiness to occur and deeper sleep to take place.[3, 34]

Manage Stress and Establish Relaxing Bedtime Rituals Stress increases physiological arousal and can adversely affect sleep patterns. Stress management and reduction techniques, such as those described in Chapter 5, can be used to help induce sleepiness. For example, keep a worry book by your bedside and record bothersome thoughts and problems in it that keep you awake at night. Once you've written them down, tell yourself you'll work on them during daylight hours, and then let go of them. Use your notes to focus energy and attention on these problems over the course of the next few days.

It can also be helpful to develop a bedtime ritual, such as reading, listening to soothing music, or taking a warm (but not too hot) bath; your mind and body will come to associate bedtime with relaxation and peacefulness. Avoid stressful or stimulating activities before bedtime, such as working or paying bills, and dim the lights to let your internal clock know that drowsiness is appropriate. Experiment until you find a method of calming down and relaxing at bedtime that works for you.

If you do have a hard time falling asleep, don't stay in bed longer than 30 minutes. Get up, leave the room, and listen to soothing music or read until you feel sleepy.

Avoid Eating Too Close to Bedtime

Try not to eat heavy meals within 3 hours of bedtime, particularly meals with high fat content. When you are lying down, the force of gravity cannot assist the movement of food from the stomach into the small intestine to complete digestion, and you may experience acid indigestion, or heartburn. Also avoid caffeinated beverages, citrus fruits and juices, tomato-based products, and pasta sauce, because these foods can temporarily weaken the esophageal sphincter. When weakened, this sphincter allows stomach contents to move back into the esophagus, a condition known as *acid reflux*. If you have acid reflux, try raising the head of your bed 6 to 8 inches, which will allow gravity to help empty stomach contents into the small intestine. Tilting the bed is more effective than elevating the upper body with pillows. For those who are overweight, moderate weight loss may reduce discomfort, because excessive stomach fat can cause abdominal pressure that contributes to heartburn.[3, 5]

Be Smart About Napping

The typical North American adult takes one or two naps a week, and about a third of adults nap more than four times a week. On the other hand, about a fourth never take a nap. If you are a napper, sleep experts recommend naps of only 15 to 45 minutes, which can be refreshing and restorative. If you nap longer than 45 minutes, your body is able to enter stage 4 deep sleep. It is more difficult to awaken from this stage, and you are more likely to feel groggy.[3, 35]

If you know you will be going to bed later than usual, you may want to take a "preventive nap" of 2 to 3 hours. Research suggests that people who take preventive naps increase their alertness by about 30 percent over that of people who do not nap. Napping 15 minutes every 4 hours until you attain 2 hours of preventive napping is also recommended. This short nap strategy has been effectively used by physicians and law enforcement officers, who must perform in emergency situations for long hours.[35]

Get Rid of Dust Mites and Other Bedroom Pests

Dust mites are microscopic insects that feed on dead skin cells. They live primarily in pillows and mattresses. Dust mite droppings become airborne and are inhaled while people are sleeping, causing allergic reactions and asthma in sensitive individuals. If you experience itchy or watery eyes, sneezing, wheezing, congestion, or difficulty breathing in your bedroom, the culprit may be dust mites. For guidelines on preventing and controlling dust mites, and for information on other bedroom pests, see the box "Critters in Your Bed and Bedroom."

Consider Your Bed Partner Snoring is a major disrupter of partners' sleep, and body movement during sleep can also be a problem for partners. Avoiding alcohol before bedtime, using nasal sprays, sleeping on your side, and using a humidifier may help reduce snoring.

Men tend to thrash around in bed more than women do, and older couples tend to move in less compatible ways than do younger couples. A mattress with low motion transfer may help prevent sleep disruption caused by a partner's movement. Sleep can also be disrupted if a partner has a different sleep schedule or has a sleep disorder. If your partner's sleep habits create a problem for you, encourage your partner to improve his or her sleep habits or to see a sleep disorder specialist. As a last resort, you or your partner may have to sleep in a different bed or room.

USING SLEEP AIDS

Because sleep is so influential in your daily functioning, and because sleep problems are so common, it should not be surprising that many people resort to sleep aids of one kind or another to help them get a good night's sleep. About 15 percent of adults use a prescription sleep medication and/or an over-the-counter sleep aid to help them sleep a few nights a week.[36]

Prescription Medications Safe and effective sleep medications are those that can be taken at higher doses, are not addictive, do not produce serious side effects, and wear off quickly so that you are not drowsy the next day. Sleep experts disagree about whether today's sleep medications meet these criteria.[3] No sleep medication should be used over a long period without physician consultation.

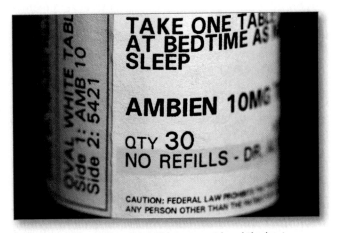

■ Ambien belongs to a class of drugs considered the best prescription sleep aids, but use of this medication is associated with unusual side effects, including eating, driving, and having sex while asleep.

The most frequently prescribed, longer acting sleep medications are the benzodiazepines Restoril, Dalmon, and Doral. These drugs induce sleep but suppress both deep sleep and REM sleep. Their effects can last from 3 to 24 hours, and daytime side effects include decreased memory and intellectual functioning. People quickly build tolerance to long-lasting benzodiazepines, which are addictive and lose their effectiveness after 30 nights of consecutive use. There are some shorter acting benzodiazepines on the market that do not suppress deep sleep and REM sleep.[34]

A new category of sleep medications is the imidazopyridines. The National Sleep Foundation considers these drugs the best prescription sleeping aids.[34] One drug in this category, zolpidem, sold under the trade name Ambien, has become the best-selling prescription sleep aid in the United States, but it has been associated with some disturbing side effects (see the box "Sleep Aids and Bizarre Behaviors").

Over-the-Counter Medications   Nonprescription, or over-the-counter, medications can be useful for treating transient or short-term insomnia, such as may occur under conditions of great stress or trauma. They should be discontinued once the cause of the problem has been eliminated, ideally within 2 weeks. The recommended maximum use is 4 weeks.

Many over-the-counter sleep products contain antihistamine, a type of drug developed to treat allergies. The effects of antihistamines are general throughout the body; besides drowsiness, they cause dehydration, agitation, and constipation. Additionally, you can quickly develop tolerance to antihistamines, and when you stop taking them, you may experience **rebound insomnia**—insomnia that is worse than what you experienced before you started taking the medication.[34] Rebound insomnia can be avoided by gradually reducing the dose.

rebound insomnia
Insomnia that occurs after a person stops taking sleep medication and that is worse than it was before the medication was started.

Complementary and Alternative Products and Approaches   Complementary and alternative products and approaches to sleep problems include herbal products, dietary supplements, and aromatherapy. The herbal product most commonly used for insomnia is valerian, which has a tranquilizing or sedative effect. Hops is another product currently receiving attention as a possible sleep aid. Both are widely available in health food stores. Herbal products can interact with other medications and drugs, including caffeine and alcohol; it is strongly recommended that you consult with your physician before trying any herbal remedies.

Melatonin is a dietary supplement that has been marketed as a sleep aid, but health experts are divided on its effectiveness. As noted earlier in this chapter, melatonin is a hormone naturally secreted by the pineal gland in response to darkness. It lowers body temperature and causes drowsiness. Most experts agree that the 3-milligram dose of synthetically produced melatonin available in health food

stores is too high and that a dose of 0.1 milligram is as effective as a higher dose.[34, 36] Potential side effects, interactions with drugs, and long-term health effects of melatonin supplements have not been studied extensively. Caution is advised, because some studies have reported increased risk of heart attack, infertility, fatigue, and depression with melatonin use.

Consumer Clipboard

Sleep Aids and Bizarre Behaviors

Sleep medications commonly have such side effects as next-day drowsiness, dizziness, headaches, confusion, agitation, and even hallucinations. More bizarre reactions are said by drug manufacturers to be "remote," defined as fewer than one episode per 1,000 users. But in recent years, there have been reports of people eating, cooking, and driving in their sleep after taking Ambien, a sleep aid.

A study by the Minnesota Regional Sleep Center found that thousands of Ambien users have experienced sleep-eating and sleep-driving behaviors. Sexsomnia—engaging in sexual behavior while asleep—is also associated with Ambien. Scientists believe that sleep-aid medications may suppress the brain's arousal system and cause these and other bizarre behaviors.

Another condition associated with sleep medications is "traveler's amnesia." Sleep aids typically cause temporary amnesia, lasting for a few hours after the drug is taken. Temporary memory loss is usually not a problem, because the user is asleep. But when a sleep medication is taken by someone who is traveling, the person may have to wake up before the drug has worn off. Many people in this situation have found they have amnesia for the hours when the drug was still active.

The side effects of sleep medications can vary, depending on the person's general health, drug tolerance, and other medications. Most of these sleep medications, however, have not been tested for long-term use, and the U.S. Food and Drug Administration has requested that manufacturers use stronger language on their labels warning of potential risks. Some physicians question the value of these drugs, since users fall asleep faster than nonusers by only about 15 to 20 minutes.

If you use sleep aids, consult with your physician or pharmacist about proper dosage and possible side effects. Sleep medications should not be crushed or chewed, and alcohol should not be used in combination with sleep aids.

Sources: A Good Night's Sleep, by L.J. Epstein, 2007, New York: McGraw-Hill; "Ambien Linked to 'Sleep Eating'," by D. DeNoon, retrieved from www.webmd.com/content/Article/120/113595.htm?pagenumber=3.

In aromatherapy, certain essential oils, such as jasmine and lavender, are used to induce relaxation and sleepiness. Aromatherapists believe these oils relieve insomnia by reducing stress, enhancing moods, and easing respiratory or muscular problems, but no strong scientific evidence supports these claims.[39] Aromatherapy oils may be applied to the skin by full body massage, or a drop may be placed on the wrist or at the base of the throat so the scent is inhaled during sleep. Scented sprays can be used on bed linens, but aromatherapy candles should not be used when you are sleeping. Aromatherapy products are generally available in health food stores. If you are interested in trying this approach, however, it is recommended that you consult a trained aromatherapist before making any purchases.

* * *

As noted, it is not surprising that people go to great lengths to get enough high-quality sleep. Nothing is so refreshing and restorative as a good night's sleep, giving us a fresh perspective and renewed energy for facing the demands of the day. Shakespeare called sleep the "balm of hurt minds, chief nourisher in life's feast." Sleep, he wrote, "knits up the ravell'd sleeve of care." Conversely, almost nothing is so distressing as being unable to avail ourselves of the respite provided by sleep. Chronic sleep deprivation can interfere with physical, emotional, and cognitive functioning and leave us fatigued, depressed, and more susceptible to illness and disease. As with so many other facets of lifestyle, good sleep habits and practices, established early in life, can help you maintain wellness in both younger and older adulthood.

You Make the Call

Should Drowsy Drivers Be Criminally Liable for Crashes They Cause?

Maggie McDonnell, a 20-year-old college student from Washington Township, New Jersey, was killed in July 1997 when the car she was driving was hit head-on by a van that had crossed three lanes of traffic. The driver of the van told police he had not slept in 30 hours and had smoked crack cocaine a few hours before the crash. He was charged with vehicular homicide.

At the time, conviction for vehicular homicide under New Jersey law required driver recklessness. A person who drove while knowingly fatigued and caused a fatal crash could be charged only with careless driving. The jury was not allowed to consider driver fatigue as a factor in this case. The first trial ended in a deadlock on the charge of vehicular homicide, and the second trial ended in acquittal. The driver was fined $200 and received two points on his driving record.

In 2003, New Jersey passed the first statute to specifically cite driver fatigue as a factor that could be considered under the charge of vehicular homicide. New Jersey's Drowsy Driving Act, called Maggie's Law, explicitly allows a jury to find a driver reckless if he or she was awake for 24 hours prior to causing a fatal crash. Maggie's Law prevents the defense from using an inadequate law as a tool to defend the guilty. A motorist violating the law can be charged with vehicular homicide, punishable by up to 10 years in prison and a fine of $150,000.

Since Maggie's death, the number of criminal prosecutions and civil suits involving driver-fatigue crashes has increased. A Virginia man who killed two people when he fell asleep at the wheel received a 5-year jail sentence. This sentence exceeded state sentencing guidelines. McDonald's Corporation paid $400,000 to the family of a victim killed

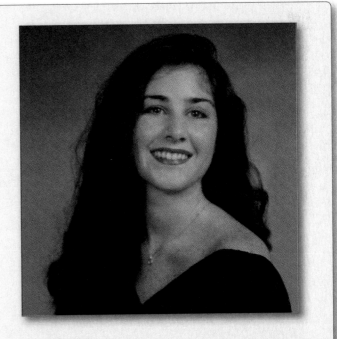

by a teenage McDonald's employee in Oregon who had only 7 hours of sleep in the previous 48 hours due to his work and school schedule. The accident occurred when the employee was driving home from work. The Los Angeles City Council approved a $16 million settlement to the family of a woman permanently disabled by a city maintenance truck when the driver fell asleep at the wheel.

In 2002, a bill named Maggie's Law: National Drowsy Driving Act of 2002 was introduced in the U.S. House of Representatives. Although it never became law, the bill would have encouraged states and communities to develop traffic safety programs to reduce crashes related to driver fatigue and sleep deprivation, to create a driver's education curriculum,

Continued...

Continued...

to standardize reporting of fatigue-related crashes on police report forms, and to implement countermeasures such as continuous shoulder rumble strips and rest areas.

Many states besides New Jersey have passed laws making driver drowsiness a form of recklessness under the vehicular homicide charge. Proponents of these measures claim that stringent laws with severe consequences are needed to get sleep-deprived drivers off the roads, but opponents argue that the measures are unnecessary, ineffective, and difficult to enforce. What do you think?

PROS

- Up to 60 percent of adults who drive say they have driven their vehicles while feeling drowsy, and 37 percent of adults report falling asleep while driving. An estimated 60 million Americans are operating vehicles each day without adequate sleep. These people need to be held responsible for the outcomes of their choices.

- Driving fatigue has been underestimated as a factor in driving performance. The National Highway Traffic Safety Administration conservatively estimates that 100,000 police-reported crashes are the direct result of driver fatigue each year, resulting in 1,550 deaths and 71,000 injuries.

- Investigation of driver fatigue can be improved with new technology. States may mandate that cars come equipped with eyelid-measuring devices. Post-crash investigators could use this information to determine if a driver involved in a crash was significantly impaired by drowsiness.

CONS

- Most police officers are not trained to properly investigate driver drowsiness accidents. This lack of training makes it difficult to collect sufficient evidence for prosecution and wastes taxpayers' money on cases that can't be won.

- The point of New Jersey's Drowsy Driving Act was to make driver drowsiness akin to driving while intoxicated. Research suggests similarities between these two conditions, but it is much more difficult for a police officer to detect driver fatigue than to detect intoxication. A driver involved in a crash or pulled over for erratic driving may experience an adrenaline rush that masks fatigue symptoms.

- It is easy for people to lie about how many hours they have been awake in order to avoid prosecution.

- Under this law, people with diagnosed sleep disorders that can cause daytime drowsiness, such as sleep apnea or narcolepsy, could be punished for having conditions they can't help and could be held liable for outcomes for which they are not really responsible.

Sources: "Testimony of the Impact of Driver Fatigue. Report Before the Subcommittee on Highways and Transit, Committee on Transportation and Infrastructure," June 27, 2002, retrieved from www.drowsydriving.org; "A Place to Crash: The Dangers of Driving While Drowsy," by A. Dalton, retrieved June 1, 2008, from www.legalaffairs.org/printerfriendly.msp?id=843; "Sleep in America" Poll, National Sleep Foundation, 2006, Washington DC: National Sleep Foundation.

In Review

1. **How does sleep impact your health?** Quantity and quality of sleep are strongly associated with overall health and quality of life. Adequate sleep gives the body time for repair, recovery, and renewal. Sleep deprivation is associated with a wide range of health problems, ranging from cardiovascular disease to depression to overweight and obesity.

2. **What makes you sleep?** Sleep is induced by the activity of a specific set of structures in the brain, in combination with environmental cues such as darkness. Humans have a circadian rhythm slightly longer than 24 hours; every morning the body resets this biological clock to adjust to the next 24-hour cycle.

3. **What is the structure of sleep?** Every night, people cycle through several stages of sleep, characterized by different brain waves, different states of muscle relaxation, and different nervous system activity. Non-REM sleep includes stages of deep sleep, whereas REM sleep includes dreaming and brain activity related to the consolidation of learning and memory.

4. **What are sleep disorders?** Problems associated with falling or staying asleep are classified as dyssomnias; they include insomnia, sleep apnea, narcolepsy, and restless leg syndrome. Problems associated with behavior during sleep are classified as parasomnias; examples are sleepwalking, nocturnal eating disorder, nightmare disorder, and a disorder sometimes associated with sleep medications, sexsomnia.

5. **How can you enhance the quality of your sleep?** The key to a good night's sleep is establishing good sleep habits, such as maintaining a regular sleep schedule, creating a sleep-friendly environment, and avoiding stimulants late in the day. Sleep aids, whether prescription, over the counter, or herbal, can help with situational sleep problems but shouldn't be used over the long term.

WWW For a detailed summary of this chapter and a comprehensive set of review questions, visit the Online Learning Center at **www.mhhe.com/teague2e.**

Web Resources

American Academy of Sleep Medicine: This professional organization focuses on the advancement of sleep medicine and sleep research. Its Web site offers links to several sleep resources, such as journals and other sleep organizations.
www.aasmnet.org

American Sleep Apnea Association: This organization focuses on increased understanding of sleep apnea disorders. It is dedicated to reducing injury, disability, and death from sleep apnea and to enhancing the well-being of those affected by this common disorder.
www.sleepapnea.org/asaa.html

National Sleep Foundation: From the basics of getting a good night's sleep to understanding sleep problems and disorders, this site offers helpful information. It features interactive sleep quizzes, brochures, and a variety of tools for better sleep.
www.sleepfoundation.org

SleepNet: If you want to locate a sleep lab, take a sleep test, understand sleep terms, and learn about sleep disorders, this site is the place to visit. It highlights various sleep problems, offering clear explanations, and features related readings.
www.sleepnet.com

Sleep Research Society: This organization is dedicated to scientific investigation of all aspects of sleep and sleep disorders. It promotes the exchange of knowledge pertaining to sleep.
www.sleepresearchsociety.org

PART TWO

Your Lifestyle and Health

Think It Over

- How much attention do you pay to what you eat every day?
- Where does physical fitness fall in your list of priorities?
- Have you been the same weight for most of your adult life, or is your weight increasing over time?
- If you could change one thing about your appearance today, what would it be?

"Tell me what you eat and I will tell you what you are," wrote a French philosopher—or, in plain language, "You are what you eat." How do your everyday food choices, along with your everyday choices about physical activity, affect your health and wellness? Diet and exercise are the areas in which you have the most control and the greatest opportunity for change. The chapters in Part 2 show you how to make daily lifestyle decisions that will help you look, feel, and be healthier.

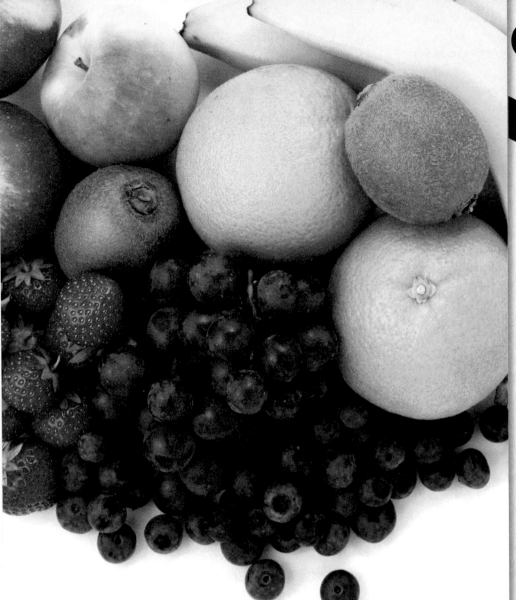

Nutrition
Healthy
Food
Choices

Ever Wonder...

- what the nutritional content of a fast-food meal is?

- if organic food is better for you than conventional food?

- where empty plastic water bottles end up?

WWW

Your Health Today

www.mhhe.com/teague2e

Go to the Online Learning Center for *Your Health Today* for interactive activities, quizzes, flashcards, Web links, and more resources related to this chapter.

Your day begins with a bagel spread with cream cheese and a jolt of caffeine from freshly brewed coffee. Mid-morning hunger pangs are relieved by an energy bar and an energy drink. Lunch at the local fast-food place includes a cheeseburger, fries, and a soda. Another energy bar in mid-afternoon, accompanied by a bottle of water, tides you over to dinner. Still, you're so hungry when you get to the campus food court that you overindulge, downing several soft tacos with salsa, shredded lettuce, and sour cream. Late-night studying is supported by the consumption of popcorn, cookies, and another energy bar. Welcome to college dining!

Unfortunately, healthy dining can be a challenge in a culture that promotes the consumption of fast foods and convenience foods in shopping malls, sports arenas, airports, and college dining halls. Many people have acquired a taste for the high-calorie, full-fat, heavily salted foods so plentiful in our environment. It *is* possible to choose a healthy diet, however, and this chapter will help you see how.

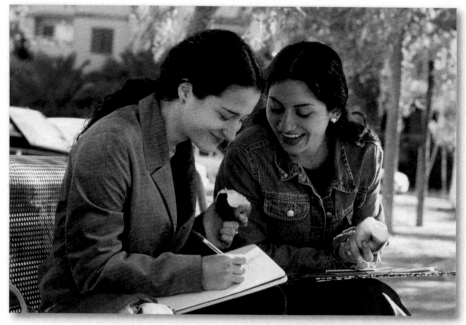

■ College life often offers limited opportunities for healthy eating. Students may have to go out of their way to make sure they get healthy foods like fresh fruit.

Understanding Nutritional Guidelines

As discussed in Chapter 1, society has a vested interest in the good health of its citizens. A natural outcome of this is that both governmental and nongovernmental organizations support scientific research in nutrition and have developed several different kinds of guides to healthy eating.

In 1997 the National Academies' Food and Nutrition Board introduced the **Dietary Reference Intakes (DRIs),** a set of recommendations designed to promote optimal health and prevent both nutritional deficiencies and chronic diseases like cancer and cardiovascular disease. The DRIs, developed by American and Canadian scientists, encompass four kinds of recommendations. The *Estimated Average Requirement (EAR)* is the amount of nutrients needed by half of the people in any one age group, for example, teenage boys. Nutritionists use the EARs to assess whether an entire population's normal diet provides sufficient nutrients. The EARs are used in nutrition research and as a basis on which recommended dietary allowances are set.

The **Recommended Dietary Allowance (RDA)** is based on information provided by the EARs and represent the average daily amount of any one nutrient an individual needs to protect against nutritional deficiency. If there is not enough information about a nutrient to set an RDA, an *Adequate Intake (AI)* is provided. The *Tolerable Upper Intake Level (UL)* is the highest amount of a nutrient a person can take in without risking toxicity.

In 2002 the Food and Nutrition Board introduced another measure, the **Acceptable Macronutrient Distribution Range (AMDR).** These ranges represent intake levels of essential nutrients that provide adequate nutrition and that are associated with reduced risk of chronic disease. If your intake exceeds the AMDR, you increase your risk of chronic disease. For example, the AMDR for dietary fat for adult men is 20–35 percent of the calories consumed in a day. A man who consumes more than 35 percent of his daily calories as fat increases his risk for chronic diseases.

Whereas the DRIs are recommended intake levels for individual nutrients, the *Dietary Guidelines for Americans,*

Dietary Reference Intakes (DRIs)
An umbrella term for four sets of dietary recommendations: Estimated Average Requirement, Recommended Dietary Allowances, Adequate Intake, and Tolerable Upper Intake Level; designed to promote optimal health and prevent both nutritional deficiencies and chronic diseases.

Recommended Dietary Allowance (RDA)
The average daily amount of any one nutrient an individual needs to protect against nutritional deficiency.

Acceptable Macronutrient Distribution Range (AMDR)
Intake ranges that provide adequate nutrition and that are associated with reduced risk of chronic disease.

Dietary Guidelines for Americans
Set of scientifically based recommendations designed to promote health and reduce the risk for many chronic diseases through diet and physical activity.

published by the U.S. Department of Agriculture (USDA) and the U.S. Department of Health and Human Services, provide scientifically based diet and exercise recommendations designed to promote health and reduce the risk of chronic disease. The *Dietary Guidelines,* first published in 1980 and revised every 5 years, is the cornerstone of U.S. nutrition policy. The most recent version was published in 2005.

To translate DRIs and the *Dietary Guidelines* into healthy food choices, the USDA also publishes **MyPyramid**, a graphic nutritional tool that can be customized depending on your calorie needs. Also developed by the USDA, the **Daily Values** are used on food labels and indicate how a particular food contributes to the recommended daily intake of major nutrients in a 2,000-calorie diet.

MyPyramid
Graphic nutritional tool developed to accompany the 2005 *Dietary Guidelines for Americans.*

Daily Values
Set of dietary standards used on food labels to indicate how a particular food contributes to the recommended daily intake of major nutrients in a 2,000-calorie diet.

Before we explore how you can use these tools to choose a healthy diet, we take a look at the major nutrients that make up our diet. For each nutrient, we include general recommendations for intake based on either the DRIs or the AMDRs.

Types of Nutrients

As you engage in daily activities, your body is powered by energy produced from the food you eat. Your body needs the **essential nutrients**—water, carbohydrates, proteins, fats, vitamins, and minerals—contained in these foods, but not only to provide fuel. They are also needed to build, maintain, and repair tissues; regulate body functions; and support the communication among cells that allows you to be a living, sensing human being.

essential nutrients
Chemical substances used by the body to build, maintain, and repair tissues and regulate body functions. They cannot be manufactured by the body and must be obtained from foods or supplements.

These nutrients are referred to as "essential" because your body cannot manufacture them; they must come from food or from nutritional supplements. People who fail to consume adequate amounts of an essential nutrient are likely to develop a nutritional deficiency disease, such as scurvy from lack of vitamin C or beri-beri from lack of vitamin B_1. Nutritional deficiency diseases are seldom seen in developed countries because most people consume an adequate diet.

We need large quantities of *macronutrients*—water, carbohydrates, protein, and fat—for energy and important functions like building new cells and facilitating chemical reactions. We need only small amounts of *micronutrients*—vitamins and minerals—for regulating body functions.

When food is *metabolized*—chemically transformed into energy and wastes—it fuels our bodies. The energy provided by food is measured in kilocalories, commonly shortened to *calorie.* One **kilocalorie** is the amount of energy needed to raise the temperature of 1 kilogram of water by 1 degree centigrade. The more energy we expend, the more kilocalories we need to consume. We get the most energy from fats, 9 calories per gram of fat. Carbohydrates and protein provide 4 calories per gram. In other words, fats provide more calories than do carbohydrates or proteins, a factor to consider when planning a balanced diet that does not lead to weight gain.

kilocalorie
Amount of energy needed to raise the temperature of 1 kilogram of water by 1 degree centigrade; commonly shortened to *calorie.*

WATER—THE UNAPPRECIATED NUTRIENT

You can live without the other nutrients for weeks, but you can survive without water for only a few days. We need water to digest, absorb, and transport nutrients. Water helps regulate body temperature, carries waste products out of the body, and lubricates our moving parts.[1]

The right *fluid balance*—the right amount of fluid inside and outside each cell—is maintained through the action of substances called **electrolytes,** mineral components that carry electrical charges

electrolytes
Mineral components that carry electrical charges and conduct nerve impulses.

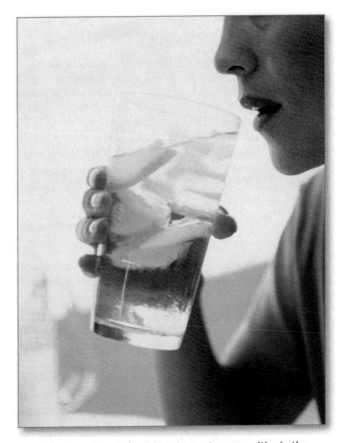

■ Water is an essential nutrient. In most communities in the United States, the quality and safety of tap water are equal or superior to the quality and safety of bottled water.

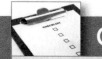

Consumer Clipboard

Bottled Water: Healthy or Hype?

Drinking bottled water is a healthy choice, right? Yes and no. Drinking water keeps you hydrated, which is especially important during moderate to vigorous physical activity and when the weather is hot. But in most parts of the country you can fill a reusable bottle with tap water and get water of the same quality as the expensive kind you purchase—if not better.

Many people assume bottled water is purer and safer than tap water, but for the most part the water supply in the United States is well regulated and very safe. The Environmental Protection Agency (EPA) sets standards for water quality and inspects water supplies for bacteria and toxic chemicals. (Some bottled water is drawn from municipal water supplies, including Coca-Cola's Dasani and Pepsi's Aquafina, despite ads and labels showing pristine springs and snowy mountain peaks.) You can check the quality of your community's water supply at the National Tap Water Quality Database (www.ewg.org/tapwater/yourwater).

In contrast, bottled water is regulated by the FDA only if it is shipped across state lines. About 70 percent is bottled and sold within the same state, so it is exempt from FDA inspection. Bottled water has been found to contain contaminants, and health experts warn that it lacks fluoride, which is added to most water supplies and prevents tooth decay.

What about water that's been enhanced with vitamins, minerals, and other nutrients? Although they offer a colorful and flavorful alternative to plain water, they add little nutritional value to the typical American diet, since the average American adult consumes 100 percent of the DRI for most vitamins. They do pack a wallop when it comes to added sugars, however. A 20-ounce bottle of Vitaminwater, for example, has 32.5 grams of sugar (two heaping tablespoons) and 125 calories, about the same as a soft drink. In 2007 the company that produces Vitaminwater, Glaceau, was bought by Coca-Cola.

Aside from their effect on health, bottled waters have a huge impact on the environment. About 1.5 million tons of plastic are used in the manufacture of water bottles for global consumption every year, creating 1.5 million tons of plastic garbage. Although plastic bottles can be recycled, 80 percent of them are thrown out and end up in landfills or in the world's oceans. According to Food and Water Watch, about 47 million gallons of oil are used to produce the bottles, in addition to the gasoline expended in transporting the bottles to market. Some bottled water producers pump water from springs, depleting underground aquifers and disrupting ecosystems.

Consuming bottled water is hard on your wallet as well. Tap water is estimated to cost about $0.0015 per gallon, compared to $1.25 per gallon for bottled water, a thousand-fold cost difference. Americans spent more than $7 billion for bottled water in 2002, and sales are increasing at a phenomenal rate. No wonder food industry giants Coca-Cola, Pepsi, and Nestle are staking their claim in the bottled water business and multinational corporations are purchasing groundwater rights around the world.

The Sierra Club urges consumers to use containers they can fill with tap water when away from home. If there is a problem with water quality or taste, they suggest buying a water filter for your tap water, still a much less expensive option than bottled water. They also urge people to advocate for good public management of municipal water systems and to monitor unusual land purchases near natural springs. The Sierra Club points out that safe and affordable water is a natural resource that many feel is a basic human right—not a commodity.

Sources: "5 Reasons to Not Drink Bottled Water," Light Footstep, 2007, retrieved April 4, 2008, from http://lightfootstep.com; "Corporate Water Privatization: Bottled Water Campaign," Sierra Club, 2004, retrieved April 4, 2008, from www.sierraclub.org/committees/cac/water/bottled_water; "Is Vitaminwater Good for You?" Scienceline, 2007, retrieved April 4, 2008, from http://scienceline.org/2007/12/03/ask-intagaliata-vitaminwater.

and conduct nerve impulses. Electrolytes include sodium, potassium, and chloride. Water, in combination with a balanced diet, replaces electrolytes lost daily through sweat.[2]

Your water needs vary according to the foods you eat, the temperature and humidity in your environment, your activity level, and other factors (see the box "Bottled Water: Healthy or Hype?"). Adults generally need 1 to 1.5 milliliters of water for each calorie spent in the day. If you expend 2,000 calories a day, you require 2 to 3 liters—8 to 12 cups—of fluids.[3] Heavy sweating increases your need for fluids. You obtain fluids not only from the water you drink but also from the water in foods, particularly fruits such as oranges and apples. Caffeinated beverages and alcohol are not good sources of your daily fluid intake because of their dehydrating effects, although some recent research suggests that the water in such beverages may offset these effects to some extent.[3]

CARBOHYDRATES—YOUR BODY'S FUEL

Carbohydrates are the body's main source of energy.[3] They fuel most of the body's cells during daily activities; they are used by muscle cells during high-intensity exercise; and they are the only source of energy for brain cells, red blood cells, and some other types of cells. Athletes in particular need to consume a high-carbohydrate diet to fuel their high-energy activities.

Carbohydrates are the foods we think of as sugars and starches. They come almost exclusively from plants (the exception is lactose, the sugar in milk). Most of the carbohydrates and other nutrients we need come from grains, seeds, fruits, and vegetables.[2]

Simple Carbohydrates Carbohydrates are divided into simple carbohydrates and complex carbohydrates. **Simple carbohydrates** are easily digestible carbohydrates composed of one or two units of sugar. Six simple carbohydrates (sugars) are important in nutrition: glucose, fructose, galactose, lactose, maltose, and sucrose. Glucose is the main source of energy for the brain and nervous system. Sugars are absorbed into the bloodstream and travel to body cells, where they can be used for energy. Glucose also travels to the liver and muscles, where it can be stored as **glycogen** (a complex carbohydrate) for future energy needs.

simple carbohydrates
Easily digestible carbohydrates composed of one or two units of sugar.

glycogen
The complex carbohydrate form in which glucose is stored in the liver and muscles.

When you eat a food containing large amounts of simple carbohydrates, sugar enters your bloodstream quickly, giving you a burst of energy, or a "sugar high." It is also absorbed into your cells quickly, leaving you feeling depleted and craving more sugar. Foods containing added sugar, such as candy bars and sodas, have an even more dramatic effect. Consumption of sugar has been linked to the epidemic of overweight and obesity in the United States and to the parallel increase in the incidence of diabetes, a disorder in which body cells cannot use the sugar circulating in the blood.

Complex Carbohydrates The type of carbohydrates called **complex carbohydrates** is composed of multiple sugar units and includes starches and dietary fiber. **Starches** occur in grains, vegetables, and some fruits. Most starchy foods also contain ample portions of vitamins, minerals, proteins, and water. Starches must be broken down into single sugars in the digestive system before they can be absorbed into the bloodstream to be used for energy or stored for future use.

complex carbohydrates
Carbohydrates that are composed of multiple sugar units and that must be broken down further before they can be used by the body

starches
Complex carbohydrates found in many plant foods.

The complex carbohydrates found in whole grains are often refined or processed to make them easier to digest and more appealing to the consumer, but the refining process removes many of the vitamins, minerals, and other nutritious components found in the whole food. Refined carbohydrates include such foods as white rice, white bread and other products made from white flour, pasta, and sweet desserts. Like sugar, refined carbohydrates can enter the bloodstream quickly and just as quickly leave you feeling hungry again. Whole grains (such as whole wheat, brown rice, oatmeal, and corn) are preferred because they provide more nutrients, slow the digestive process, and make you feel full longer (see the box "Good Carbs, Bad Carbs, and Glycemic Response"). The consumption of whole grains is associated with lowered risk of diabetes, obesity, heart disease, and some forms of cancer.[4]

The RDA for carbohydrates is 130 grams for males and females aged 1 to 70 years. The AMDR for carbohydrates is 45–65 percent of daily energy intake, which amounts to 225 to 325 grams in a 2,000-calorie diet (even though only about 130 grams per day are enough to meet the body's needs). In the typical American diet, carbohydrates do contribute about half of all calories, but most of them are in the form of simple sugars or highly refined grains. Instead, carbohydrates should come from a diverse spectrum of whole grains and other starches, vegetables, and fruits.[5] The Food and Nutrition Board recommends that no more than 25 percent of calories come from added sugars, and many health professionals recommend only 10 percent.[3]

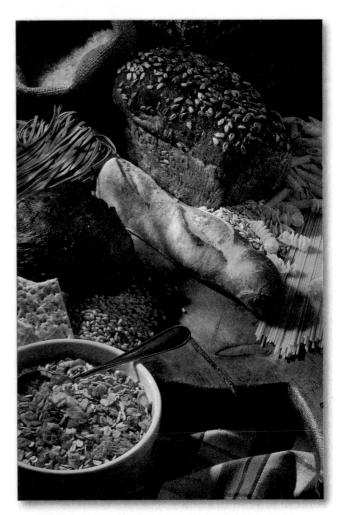

■ Nutrition experts recommend that 45 to 65 percent of your daily calories come from carbohydrates. Whole grains are favored over refined products because of their higher nutrient value.

Fiber   **Dietary fiber,** a complex carbohydrate found in plants, cannot be broken down in the digestive tract. A diet rich in dietary fiber makes stools soft and bulky. They pass through the intestines rapidly and are expelled easily, helping to prevent hemorrhoids and constipation.[6, 7] Some foods contain **functional fiber,** natural or synthetic fiber that has been added to increase the healthful effects of the food. **Total fiber** refers to the combined amount of dietary fiber and functional fiber in a food.

Dietary fiber that dissolves in water, referred to as *soluble fiber,* is known to lower blood cholesterol levels and can slow the process of digestion so that blood sugar levels remain more even. Dietary fiber that does not dissolve in water, called *insoluble fiber,* passes through the digestive tract essentially unchanged. Because it absorbs water, insoluble fiber helps you feel full after eating and stimulates your intestinal wall to contract and relax, serving as a natural laxative.

The RDAs for fiber are 25 grams for women aged 19 to 50 and 38 grams for men aged 14 to 50 (or 14 grams of fiber for every 1,000 calories consumed). For people over 50, the RDA is 21 grams for women and 30 grams for men.[1] The typical American diet provides only about 14 or 15 grams of fiber a day. If you want to increase the fiber in your diet, it is important to do so gradually. A sudden increase in daily fiber may cause bloating, gas, abdominal cramping, or even a bowel obstruction, particularly if you fail to drink enough liquids to easily carry the fiber through the body.[2]

Fiber is best obtained through diet. Pills and other fiber supplements do not contain the nutrients found in high-fiber foods.[2] Excessive amounts of fiber (generally 60 grams or more per day) can decrease the absorption of important vitamins and minerals such as calcium, zinc, magnesium, and iron.[2] Fruits, vegetables, dried beans, peas and other legumes, cereals, grains, nuts, and seeds are the best sources of dietary fiber.

dietary fiber
A complex carbohydrate found in plants that cannot be broken down in the digestive tract.

functional fiber
Natural or synthetic fiber that has been added to food.

total fiber
Combined amount of dietary fiber and functional fiber in a food.

Challenges & Choices

Good Carbs, Bad Carbs, and Glycemic Response

When you eat "good carbs"—carbohydrates that are not processed and that contain fair amounts of fiber—your blood sugar gradually increases and insulin is released from the pancreas to allow body cells to use the sugar for energy. When you eat "bad carbs"—carbohydrates that are refined or processed—sugar surges into your bloodstream and insulin is released rapidly, causing the sugar to be stored in muscles and fat cells. High levels of insulin in the blood can lead to a variety of biochemical processes that set the stage for diabetes and heart disease, as well as a rapid return to a hunger state.

The *glycemic index* (GI) was developed to predict the body's *glycemic response*—the blood sugar response to different foods. Foods are given a GI value and rated low (below 55), intermediate (55–69), or high (above 69), using a standard reference point of 100 (white bread). You might think that nutritionists would recommend using the index as a guide to healthy eating, but the picture is more complicated than that. First of all, your body's glycemic response to a food also depends on how much carbohydrate it contains and how much of it you eat. For example, carrots have a high GI but contain little carbohydrate and hardly affect blood sugar. Another measure, the *glycemic load* (GL), was developed to give a more accurate idea of the body's response to a food. GL is the GI multiplied by the amount of carbohydrates in a serving, then divided by 100.

To make matters even more complicated, the GI of a food can change depending on how the food is prepared, how ripe the food is, and how GI is measured. Some high-GI foods are good sources of nutrients (for example, carrots, bananas, raisins). Your body's glycemic response can also vary depending on your body composition and how much exercise you get. Finally, the GI refers to the effect of a single food on blood sugar levels, but meals usually contain several foods, all with their own GIs, and it is difficult to estimate the combined effect.

The bottom line is that the GI works best as a general tool, not a strict dietary guide. The American Diabetes Association and the American Heart Association do not recommend using the GI or GL for weight loss programs. In general, avoid the "bad carbs"—soft drinks, white potatoes (including french fries), white bread, sweets, and refined cereals—especially if you have a family history of diabetes or heart disease. Eating more "good carbs"—fruits, vegetables, and whole grains—supports good nutrition and a healthy weight.

It's Not Just Personal . . .
The World Health Organization (WHO) has predicted that rates of diabetes will increase worldwide by 60 percent between 1995 and 2030. In some countries, rates increased by more than that percentage in the 10 years from 1995 to 2005. Countries with the highest rates of increase are India, China, and the United States.

PROTEIN—NUTRITIONAL MUSCLE

Your body uses **protein** to build and maintain muscles, bones, and other body tissues. Proteins also form enzymes that in turn facilitate chemical reactions. Proteins are constructed from 20 different amino acids. Amino acids that your body cannot produce on its own, nine in all, are called **essential amino acids;** they must be supplied by foods. Those that can be produced by your body are called nonessential amino acids.

Food sources of protein include both animals and plants. Animal proteins (meat, fish, poultry, milk, cheese, and eggs) are usually a good source of **complete proteins,** meaning they are composed of ample amounts of all the essential amino acids. Vegetable proteins (grains, legumes, nuts, seeds, and other vegetables) provide **incomplete proteins,** meaning they contain small amounts of essential amino acids or some, but not all, of the essential amino acids. If you do not consume sufficient amounts of the essential amino acids, body organ functions may be compromised.

People who eat little or no animal protein may not be getting all the essential amino acids they need. One remedy is to eat plant foods with different amounts of incomplete proteins. For example, beans are low in the essential amino acid methionine but high in lysine, and rice is high in methionine and low in lysine. In combination, beans and rice form *complementary proteins.* Eating the two together at one meal or over the course of a day provides all the essential amino acids.[3] The matching of such foods is called *mutual supplementation.*

The AMDR for protein is 10–35 percent of daily calories consumed.[5] The need for protein is based on body weight: The larger your body, the more protein you need to take in. A healthy adult typically needs 0.8 grams of protein for every kilogram (2.2 pounds) of body weight, or about 0.36 grams for every pound.[8] At the upper end of the AMDR range, the percentages provide a more than ample amount of protein in the diet.

protein
Essential nutrient made up of amino acids, needed to build and maintain muscles, bones, and other body tissues.

essential amino acids
Amino acids that the body cannot produce on its own.

complete proteins
Proteins composed of ample amounts of all the essential amino acids.

incomplete proteins
Proteins that contain small amounts of essential amino acids or some, but not all, of the essential amino acids.

FATS—A NECESSARY NUTRIENT

fats
Also known as lipids, fats are an essential nutrient composed of fatty acids and used for energy and other body functions.

Fats are a concentrated energy source and the principal form of stored energy in the body. The fats in food provide essential fatty acids, play a role in the production of other fatty acids and vitamin D, and provide the major material for cell membranes and for the myelin sheaths that surround nerve fibers. They assist in the absorption of the fat-soluble vitamins (A, D, E, and K) and affect the texture, taste, and smell of foods. Fats provide an emergency reserve when we are sick or our food intake is diminished.

Types of Fat Fats, or lipids, are composed of fatty acids. Nutritionists divide these acids into three groups—saturated, monounsaturated, and polyunsaturated—on the basis of their chemical composition. **Saturated fats** remain stable (solid) at room temperature; **monounsaturated fats** are liquid at room temperature but solidify somewhat when refrigerated; **polyunsaturated fats** are liquid both at room temperature and in the refrigerator. Liquid fats are commonly referred to as oils.

Saturated fatty acids are found in animal sources, such as beef, pork, poultry, and whole-milk dairy products. They are also found in certain tropical oils and nuts, including coconut and palm oil and macadamia nuts. Monounsaturated and polyunsaturated fatty acids are found primarily in plant sources. Olive, safflower, peanut, and canola oils, as well as avocados and many nuts, contain mostly monounsaturated fat. Corn and soybean oils contain mostly polyunsaturated fat, as do many kinds of fish, including salmon, trout, and anchovies.

saturated fats
Lipids that are the predominant fat in animal products and other fats that remain solid at room temperature.

monounsaturated fats
Lipids that are liquid at room temperature and semisolid or solid when refrigerated.

polyunsaturated fats
Lipids that are liquid at room temperature and in the refrigerator.

Cholesterol Saturated fats pose a risk to health because they tend to raise blood levels of **cholesterol,** a waxy substance that can clog arteries, leading to cardiovascular disease. More specifically, saturated fats raise blood levels of low-density lipoproteins (LDLs), known as "bad cholesterol," and triglycerides, another kind of blood fat. Unsaturated fats, in contrast, tend to lower blood levels of LDLs, and some unsaturated fats (monounsaturated fats) may also raise levels of high-density lipoproteins (HDLs), known as "good cholesterol."[9]

cholesterol
A waxy substance produced by the liver and obtained from animal food sources; essential to the functioning of the body but a possible factor in cardiovascular disease if too much is circulating in the bloodstream.

Cholesterol is needed for several important body functions, but too much of it circulating in the bloodstream can be a problem. The body produces it in the liver and also obtains it from animal food sources, such as meat, cheese, eggs, and milk. It is recommended that no more than 300 milligrams of dietary cholesterol be consumed per day. The effects of cholesterol on cardiovascular health are discussed in detail in Chapter 18.

Trans Fats Another kind of fatty acid, **trans fatty acid,** is produced through **hydrogenation,** a process whereby liquid vegetable oils are turned into more solid fats. Food manufacturers use hydrogenation to prolong a food's shelf life and change its texture. Peanut butter is frequently hydrogenated, as is margarine. With some hydrogenation, margarine becomes semisoft (tub margarine); with further hydrogenation, it becomes hard (stick margarine).[10]

Trans fatty acids (or trans fats) are believed to pose a risk to cardiovascular health similar to or even greater than that of saturated fats, because they tend to raise LDLs and lower HDLs. Foods high in trans fatty acids include baked and snack foods like crackers, cookies, chips, cakes, pies, and doughnuts, as well as deep-fried fast foods like french fries.[11] In packaged foods, the phrase "partially hydrogenated vegetable oil" in the list of ingredients indicates the presence of trans fats. In 2006 the FDA began requiring that trans fat be listed on nutrition labels if a food contains more than 0.5 grams, and many food manufacturers and restaurants have stopped using trans fats in their products. Some cities, including Philadelphia and New York City, have enacted laws to ban or phase out the use of trans fats in restaurants.

trans fatty acids
Lipids that have been chemically modified through the process of hydrogenation so that they remain solid at room temperature.

hydrogenation
Process whereby liquid vegetable oils are turned into more solid fats.

Omega-3 and Omega-6 Fatty Acids   Unlike trans fats, two kinds of polyunsaturated fatty acids—omega-3 and omega-6 fatty acids—provide health benefits. **Omega-3 fatty acids,** which contain the essential nutrient alpha-linolenic acid, help slow the clotting of blood, decrease triglyceride levels, improve arterial health, and lower blood pressure. They may also help protect against autoimmune diseases such as arthritis.[10] **Omega-6 fatty acids,** which contain the essential nutrient linoleic acid, are also important to health, but nutritionists believe that Americans consume too much omega-6 in proportion to omega-3.[12] They recommend increasing consumption of omega-3 sources—fatty fish like salmon, trout, and anchovies; vegetable oils like canola, walnut, and flaxseed; and dark green leafy vegetables—and decreasing consumption of omega-6 sources, mainly corn, soybean, and cottonseed oils.

omega-3 fatty acids
Polyunsaturated fatty acids that contain the essential nutrient alpha-linolenic acid and that has beneficial effects on cardiovascular health.

omega-6 fatty acids
Polyunsaturated fatty acids that contain linoleic acid and that has beneficial health effects.

Although the USDA recommends two servings of fish per week, there are concerns about contamination with mercury and other industrial pollutants, which can accumulate in the tissue of certain types of fish. Mercury may cause fetal brain damage, and high levels of mercury may damage the hearts of adults. Polychlorinated biphenyls (PCBs) and dioxin may be associated with cancer. In 2004 the FDA and the EPA issued a joint warning stating that pregnant women, women planning to become pregnant, nursing mothers, and young children should consume no more than 12 ounces of fish and shellfish per week, should avoid certain types of fish (king mackerel, golden bass, shark, and swordfish), and should vary the kinds of fish they eat. (For more information, see the EPA fish advisory site at www.epa.gov/waterscience/fish.)

Dietary Recommendations for Fat   How much of your daily caloric intake should come from fat? The AMDR is 20–35 percent.[5] It is recommended that Americans get about 30 percent of their calories from fats and only about one third of that (10 percent) from saturated fats. Most adults need only 15 percent of their daily calorie intake in the form of fat, whereas young children should get 30–40 percent of their calories from fat to ensure proper growth and brain development, according to the American Academy of Pediatrics. A tablespoon of vegetable oil per day is recommended for both adults and children.[3] The American Heart Association recommends limiting consumption of saturated and trans fat to no more than 10 percent of total daily calories; in a 2,000-calorie diet, that's about 22 grams.

These recommendations are designed to help improve cardiovascular health and prevent heart disease. On average, fat intake in the United States is about 34 percent of daily calorie intake.[3] You can limit your intake of saturated fat by

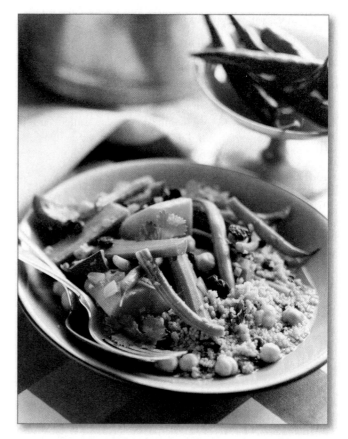

■ You can reduce your risk of chronic diseases by building your diet around colorful meals that include whole grains, legumes, two or more vegetables, and small quantities of chicken or fish.

selecting vegetable oils instead of animal fats, reducing the amount of fat you use in cooking, removing all visible fat from meat, and choosing lean cuts of meat over fatty ones and poultry or fish over beef. Limit your consumption of fast-food burgers and fries, since these foods are loaded with saturated fats.

minerals
Naturally occurring inorganic micro-nutrients, such as magnesium, calcium, and iron, that contribute to proper functioning of the body.

MINERALS—A NEED FOR BALANCE

Minerals are naturally occurring inorganic substances that are needed by the body in relatively small amounts. Minerals are important in building strong bones and teeth, helping vitamins and enzymes carry out many metabolic processes, and maintaining proper functioning of most body systems.

Our bodies need 20 essential minerals. We need more than 100 milligrams daily of each of the six *macrominerals*—calcium, chloride, magnesium, phosphorous, potassium, and sodium. We need less than 100 milligrams daily of each of the *microminerals,* or *trace minerals*—chromium, cobalt, copper, fluorine, iodine, iron, manganese, molybdenum, nickel, selenium, silicon, tin, vanadium, and zinc. Other minerals are present in foods and the body, but no requirement has been found for them. Table 7.1 provides an overview of key vitamins and minerals.

A varied and balanced diet provides all the essential minerals your body needs, so mineral supplements are not recommended for most people.[2] (Exceptions are listed in the next section.) These insoluble elements can build up in the body and become toxic if consumed in excessive amounts.

Iron provides an illustration of this need for balance. If your body is deprived of iron, you cannot make enough

Table 7.1	Key Vitamins and Minerals		
		Adult Daily DRI*	
Vitamins/Minerals	**Food Sources**	**Men**	**Women**
Vitamin A	Liver, dairy products, fish, dark green vegetables, yellow and orange fruits and vegetables	900 µg	700 µg
Vitamin C	Citrus fruits, strawberries, broccoli, tomatoes, green leafy vegetables, bell peppers	90 mg	75 mg
Vitamin D	Vitamin D–fortified milk and cereals, fish, eggs	5 µg	5 µg
Vitamin E	Plant oils, seeds, avocados, green leafy vegetables	15 mg	15 mg
Vitamin K	Dark green leafy vegetables, broccoli, cheese	120 µg	90 µg
Vitamin B₁ (thiamine)	Enriched and whole-grain cereals	1.2 mg	1.1 mg
Vitamin B₂ (riboflavin)	Milk, mushrooms, spinach, liver, fortified cereals	1.3 mg	1.1 mg
Vitamin B₆	Fortified cereals, meat, poultry, fish, bananas, potatoes, nuts	1.3 mg	1.3 mg
Vitamin B₁₂	Fortified cereals, meat, poultry, fish, dairy products	2.4 µg	2.4 µg
Niacin	Meat, fish, poultry, peanuts, beans, enriched and whole-grain cereals	16 mg	14 mg
Folate	Dark green leafy vegetables, legumes, oranges, bananas, fortified cereals	400 µg	400 µg
Calcium	Dairy products, canned fish, dark green leafy vegetables	1,000 mg	1,000 mg
Iron	Meat, poultry, legumes, dark green leafy vegetables	8 mg	18 mg
Magnesium	Wheat bran, green leafy vegetables, nuts, legumes, fish	420 mg	320 mg
Potassium	Spinach, squash, bananas, milk, potatoes, oranges, legumes, tomatoes, green leafy vegetables	4,700 mg	4,700 mg
Sodium	Table salt, soy sauce, processed foods	1,500 mg	1,500 mg
Zinc	Fortified cereals, meat, poultry, dairy products, legumes, nuts, seeds	11 mg	8 mg

* For a complete listing, see the Web site of the Food and Nutrition Board (www.iom.edu/CMS/3788.aspx).

Source: "Dietary Reference Intakes," Food and Nutrition Board, Institute of Medicine of the National Academies, retrieved April 2, 2008, from www.iom.edu/CMS/3788/21370.aspx.

hemoglobin for new blood cells, resulting in anemia. Too much iron, however, damages tissue and organs, including the heart.[13]

VITAMINS—SMALL BUT POTENT NUTRIENTS

Vitamins are organic substances needed by the body in small amounts. They serve as catalysts for releasing energy from carbohydrates, proteins, and fats; they aid chemical reactions in the body; and they help maintain components of the immune, nervous, and skeletal systems.

Our bodies need at least 11 specific vitamins: A, C, D, E, K, and the B-complex vitamins—thiamine (B_1), riboflavin (B_2), niacin, B_6, folic acid, and B_{12}. Biotin and pantothenic acid are part of the vitamin B complex and are also considered important for health. Choline, another B vitamin, is not regarded as essential.

Four of the vitamins, A, D, E, and K, are fat soluble (they dissolve in fat), and the rest are water soluble (they dissolve in water). The fat-soluble vitamins can be stored in the liver or body fat, and if you consume larger amounts than you need, you can reach toxic levels over time. Excess water-soluble vitamins are excreted in the urine and must be consumed more often than fat-soluble vitamins. Most water-soluble vitamins do not cause toxicity, but vitamins B_6 and C can build to toxic levels if taken in excess. Toxicity usually occurs only when these substances are taken as supplements.

More than half the people in the United States take vitamin and mineral supplements. The food supplement industry markets these products as a kind of insurance against nutritional deficiencies, but for most people they are unnecessary.[3, 14] Specific groups for whom vitamin and/or mineral supplements may be recommended include

- People with nutrient deficiencies
- People with low energy intake (less than 1,200 calories per day)
- Individuals who eat only foods from plant sources
- Women who bleed excessively during menstruation
- Individuals whose calcium intake is too small to preserve strength
- People in certain life stages (infants, older adults, women of childbearing age, and pregnant women)

Taking supplements to enhance your energy level or athletic performance or to make up for perceived inadequacies in your diet is not recommended.[3] Instead, try to adopt a healthy diet that provides needed nutrients from a variety of foods. Many foods provide, in one serving, the same amounts of nutrients found in a vitamin supplement pill. For a concise overview of recommended daily intakes of the macronutrients and micronutrients, see Table 7.2.

vitamins
Naturally occurring organic micronutrients that aid chemical reactions in the body and help maintain healthy body systems.

Table 7.2 | Overview of Recommended Daily Intakes

Nutrient	Recommended Daily Intake
Water	1–1.5 ml per calorie spent; 8–12 cups of fluid
Carbohydrates	AMDR: 45–65% of calories consumed
Added sugars	No more than 10–25% of calories consumed
Fiber	14 g for every 1,000 calories consumed; 21–25 g for women, 30–38 g for men
Protein	AMDR: 10–35% of calories consumed; 0.36 g per pound of body weight
Fat	AMDR: 20–35% of calories consumed
Saturated fat	No more than 10% of calories consumed
Trans fat	As little as possible
Minerals	
6 macrominerals	More than 100 mg
14 trace minerals	Less than 100 mg
Vitamins	
11 essential vitamins	Varies

OTHER SUBSTANCES IN FOOD: PHYTOCHEMICALS

One promising area of nutrition research is **phytochemicals,** substances that are naturally produced by plants. In the human body, phytochemicals may keep body cells healthy, slow down tissue degeneration, prevent the formation of carcinogens, reduce cholesterol levels, protect the heart, maintain hormone balance, and keep bones strong.[15]

phytochemicals
Substances that are naturally produced by plants to protect themselves and that provide health benefits in the human body.

Antioxidants Every time you take a breath, you inhale a potentially toxic chemical that could damage your cell DNA: oxygen.[16] If you breathed 100 percent oxygen over a period of days, you would go blind and suffer irreparable damage to your lungs. The process of oxygen metabolism in the body produces unstable molecules, called **free radicals,** which can damage cell structures and DNA. The production of free radicals can also be increased by exposure to certain environmental elements, such as cigarette smoke and sunlight, and even by stress. Free radicals are believed to be a contributing factor in aging, cancer, heart disease, macular degeneration, and other degenerative diseases.[1]

free radicals
Unstable molecules that are produced when oxygen is metabolized and that damage cell structures and DNA.

antioxidants
Substances in foods that neutralize the effects of free radicals.

Antioxidants are substances in foods that neutralize the effects of free radicals. Antioxidants are found primarily in fruits and vegetables, especially brightly colored ones (yellow, orange, and dark green), and in green tea. Vitamins E and C are antioxidants, as are some of the precursors to vitamins, such as beta carotene.

Most nutritionists do not recommend supplements as a source of antioxidants because of the potential toxic effects of vitamin megadoses.[15] The best source is whole foods. The top antioxidant-containing foods and beverages have been identified as blackberries, walnuts, strawberries, artichokes, cranberries, brewed coffee, raspberries, pecans, blueberries, cloves, grape juice, unsweetened baking chocolate, sour cherries, and red wine. Also high in antioxidants are brussels sprouts, kale, cauliflower, and pomegranates.

Phytoestrogens *Phytoestrogens* are plant hormones similar to human estrogens but less potent. Research suggests that some phytoestrogens may lower cholesterol and reduce the risk of heart disease. Other claims—that they lower the risk of osteoporosis and some types of cancer and reduce menopausal symptoms like hot flashes—have not been supported by research.

Phytoestrogens have been identified in more than 300 plants, including vegetables of the cabbage family such as brussels sprouts, broccoli, and cauliflower. Phytoestrogens are also found in plants containing lignins (a woody substance like cellulose), such as rye, wheat, sesame seed, linseed, and flax seed, and in soybeans and soy products. Foods containing phytoestrogens are safe, but, as with all phytochemicals, research has not established the safety of phytoestrogen supplements.[3, 17]

Phytonutrients *Phytonutrients* are substances extracted from vegetables and other plant foods and used in supplements. For example, lycopene is an antioxidant found in tomatoes that may inhibit the reproduction of cancer cells in the esophagus, prostate, or stomach.[18] A group of phytochemicals known as *bioflavonoids* are believed to have a benefical effect on the cardiovascular system.

To date, the FDA has not allowed foods containing phytochemicals to be labeled or marketed as agents that prevent disease. Nutritionists do not recommend taking phytochemical supplements.[19] In 2007 the FDA announced that manufacturers of all dietary supplements, including vitamins and herbs, must evaluate the identity, purity, strength, and composition of their products and accurately label them so that consumers know what they are buying. Manufacturers must comply with the new rules by 2010.[21]

National campaigns such as "Reach for It" in Canada and "Eat 5 a Day" in the United States encourage consumers to select fruits and vegetables high in phytochemicals. Because different fruits and vegetables contain different phytochemicals, a color-coded dietary plan has been developed that helps you take full advantage of all the beneficial phytochemicals available (Figure 7.1).

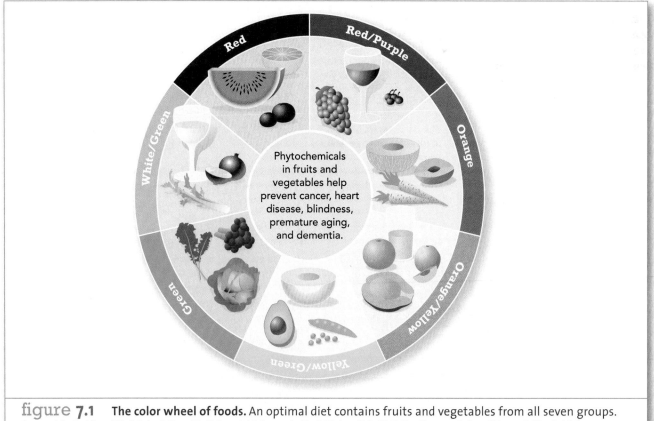

figure **7.1   The color wheel of foods.** An optimal diet contains fruits and vegetables from all seven groups.
Source: Adapted from What Color Is Your Diet? *Copyright © 2001 by David Heber, M.D., Ph.D. Used by permission of HarperCollins Publishers.*

Planning a Healthy Diet

Knowing your daily nutritional requirements in grams and percentages is not enough; you also need to know how to translate DRIs, RDAs, and AMDRs into healthy food choices and appealing meals. In this section we look at several tools that have been created to help you do that.

THE 2005 *DIETARY GUIDELINES FOR AMERICANS*

The 2005 *Dietary Guidelines* is designed to address two major concerns:

- The role of poor diet and a sedentary lifestyle in the major causes of disease and death
- The role of these same factors in the increase in overweight and obesity

Key areas addressed by the *Dietary Guidelines* are described in Table 7.3.[20]

MYPYRAMID

Like earlier food pyramid guides, MyPyramid is based on the familiar food groups (grains, vegetables, fruit, milk, meat and beans) and has some similar messages—for example, eat more of some foods than others, eat a variety of foods, practice moderation, and so on (Figure 7.2). But MyPyramid also highlights physical activity (represented by the person climbing the steps), gradual improvement (setting small, reachable goals, as captured in the slogan "Steps to a Healthier You"), and, especially, personalization.

You can go to the MyPyramid Web site (www.mypyramid.gov) and use interactive tools to assess your current diet, calculate your calorie needs, develop a customized food plan, and learn strategies for achieving a healthy weight. For example, the feature Inside the Pyramid provides in-depth information on the food groups, including portion sizes, and many practical tips on food choices. MyPyramid Tracker allows you to keep a detailed daily record of everything you eat and drink for up to a year. You can estimate your calorie requirements based on your sex and age at three activity levels, as shown in Table 7.4. The activity levels are defined as

- *Sedentary.* A lifestyle that includes only the light physical activity associated with typical day-to-day life.
- *Moderately active.* A lifestyle that includes physical activity equivalent to walking about 1.5 miles per day at 3–4 miles per hour.
- *Active.* A lifestyle that includes physical activity equivalent to walking more than 3 miles per day at 3–4 miles per hour.

The MyPyramid Plan provides specific serving recommendations (in cups, ounce-equivalents, and other specific measurements) for each of 12 different calorie levels, from

Table 7.3	2005 *Dietary Guidelines for Americans:* Key Messages
Adequate Nutrients Within Calorie Needs	Consume a variety of nutrient-dense foods and beverages while choosing foods that limit the intake of saturated and trans fats, cholesterol, added sugars, salt, and alcohol.
	Meet recommended intakes within energy needs by adopting a balanced eating pattern, such as MyPyramid or the DASH Eating Plan.
Food Groups to Encourage	Consume a sufficient amount of fruits and vegetables—in a 2,000-calorie diet, 2 cups of fruit and 2 1/2 cups of vegetables per day—without exceeding energy needs.
	Choose a variety of fruits and vegetables each day; select from five vegetable subgroups (dark green, orange, legumes, starchy vegetables, and other vegetables) several times a week.
	Consume 3 or more ounce-equivalents of whole-grain products per day, with the rest of the recommended grains coming from enriched or whole-grain products.
	Consume 3 cups of fat-free or low-fat milk or equivalent milk products.
Fats	Consume less than 10 percent of calories from saturated and trans fats and less than 300 mg/day of cholesterol, and keep trans fat to less than 1 percent of total calories.
	Keep total fat intake between 20 and 35 percent of calories, with most fats coming from sources of monounsaturated and polyunsaturated fatty acids, such as fish, nuts, and vegetable oils.
	When selecting and preparing meat, poultry, dry beans, and milk or milk products, make choices that are lean, low fat, or fat free.
Carbohydrates	Choose fiber-rich fruits, vegetables, and whole grains often.
	Choose and prepare foods and beverages with little added sugars or caloric sweeteners.
Sodium	Consume less than 2,300 mg of sodium per day (approximately 1 teaspoon of salt).
	Choose and prepare foods with little salt. At the same time, consume potassium-rich foods, such as fruits and vegetables.

Source: Dietary Guidelines for Americans, *U.S. Department of Agriculture and U.S. Department of Health and Human Services, 2005, retrieved from www.health.gov/dietaryguidelines.*

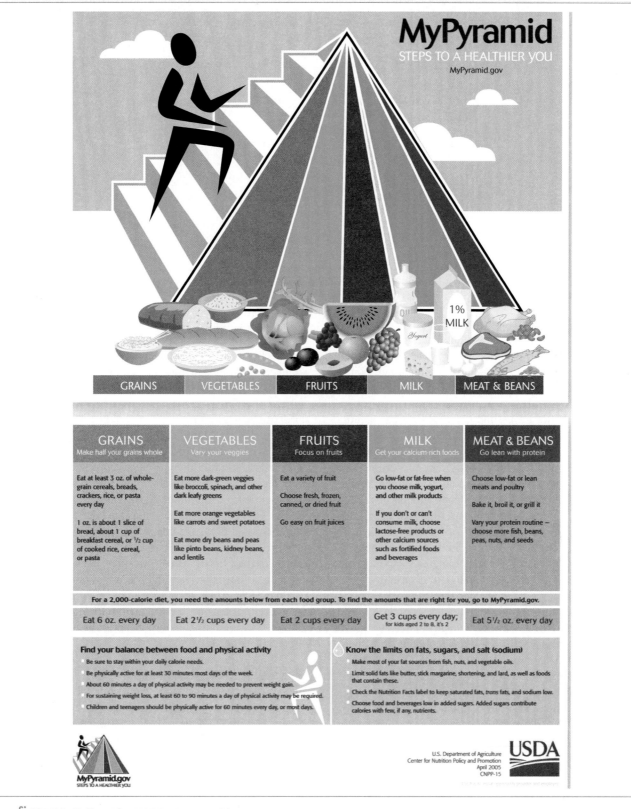

figure **7.2**   **The USDA MyPyramid**. Released in 2005, this chart emphasizes whole grains, a variety of vegetables, and a balance between food and physical activity. Specific pyramids for 12 different calorie levels are available at www.MyPyramid.gov.
Source: MyPyramid, 2005, U.S. Department of Agriculture, Center for Nutrition Policy and Promotion.

Table 7.4	Estimated Calorie Requirements at Three Activity Levels, by Age and Gender			
			Activity Level*	
Gender	Age (years)	Sedentary	Moderately Active	Active
Female	14–18	1,800	2,000	2,400
	19–30	2,000	2,000–2,200	2,400
	31–50	1,800	2,000	2,200
	51+	1,600	1,800	2,000–2,200
Male	14–18	2,200	2,400–2,800	2,800–3,200
	19–30	2,400	2,600–2,800	3,000
	31–50	2,200	2,400–2,600	2,800–3,000
	51+	2,000	2,200–2,400	2,400–2,800

Source: Dietary Guidelines for Americans, U.S. Department of Agriculture and U.S. Department of Health and Human Services, 2005, retrieved from www.health.gov/dietaryguidelines.

1,000 to 3,200 calories per day. Figure 7.2 shows the recommendations for a 2,000-calorie diet. The graphic also includes short statements summarizing important points from the *Dietary Guidelines,* such as "Eat more orange vegetables like carrots and sweet potatoes."

The *Dietary Guidelines* and MyPyramid differ significantly from current eating patterns in the United States (and, increasingly, the rest of the world—see the box "Globalization of the Western Diet"). Specifically, they encourage more consumption of whole grains, vegetables, legumes, fruits, and low-fat milk products and less consumption of refined grain products, total fats, added sugars, and calories. They emphasize foods high in **nutrient density**—proportion of vitamins and minerals to total calories. Especially in a lower calorie diet, the goal is that all the calories consumed provide nutrients (as opposed to the "empty calories" in sodas, sweets, and alcoholic beverages). Otherwise, you reach your maximum calorie intake without having consumed the nutrients you need.

nutrient density
The proportion of nutrients to total calories in a food.

If you choose nutrient-dense foods from each food group, you may have some calories left over—your discretionary calorie allowance—that can be consumed as added fats or sugars, alcohol, or other foods. At the 2,000-calorie level, your discretionary calorie allowance is 267 calories.

The DASH Eating Plan The other eating plan recommended by the *Dietary Guidelines* is the DASH Eating Plan, originally developed to reduce high blood pressure. (DASH stands for Dietary Approaches to Stop Hypertension.) The DASH plan is similar to MyPyramid, but it also has a nuts, seeds, and legumes group. For more information, visit www.nhlbi.nih.gov/health/public/heart/hbp/dash/new_dash.pdf.

Recommendations for Specific Population Groups The *Dietary Guidelines* also includes recommendations, where relevant, for specific population groups, including children and adolescents, older adults, pregnant and breastfeeding women, overweight adults and children, and people with chronic diseases or special medical problems. For example, women of childbearing age and women in the first trimester of pregnancy are advised to consume adequate synthetic folic acid daily in addition to eating foods rich in folate. Individuals with hypertension, African Americans, and middle-aged and older adults are advised to consume no more than 1,500 milligrams of sodium per day. Special pyramids have been developed for children (MyPyramid for Kids) and for women who are pregnant or breastfeeding (MyPyramid for Pregnancy and Breastfeeding.)

Other Eating Plans and Pyramids The food pyramid concept has been extended to a variety of other food preferences and ethnic diets. The term *diet* in this context includes the concept of cuisine, a particular style of preparing food, and *food way,* the food habits, customs, beliefs, and preferences of a certain culture.[4]

The Mediterranean pyramid was developed from the diet typical of the region in southern Europe, including Italy and Greece, where rates of cardiovascular disease and some kinds of cancer are lower than in Northern Europe and North America.[3] Like MyPyramid, the Mediterranean pyramid emphasizes grains, fruits, and vegetables, but it also recommends daily servings of beans, legumes, and nuts and foods that are high in protein, fiber, and fats. In addition, it encourages the use of olive oil over other oils.

The Latin American pyramid was developed by the Latino Nutrition Coalition to combat high rates of obesity, Type-2 diabetes, and heart disease in the Latin American population. It is designed to encourage Latinos (and others who want to enjoy Latino food) to eat healthier by maintaining traditional Latin American cooking. This diet emphasizes grains (including maize and quinoa), fruits (including tropical fruits like mango and papaya), vegetables, and plant sources of protein. You can learn more about the food plan and find meal ideas and shopping tips at www.latinonutrition.org.

The Asian food pyramid draws from the cuisines of South and East Asia. Like the Latin American pyramid, it emphasizes grains, fruits, vegetables, and plant sources of protein. At the base of the pyramid are rice and rice products, noodles, breads, millet, corn, and other minimally refined grains. Meat is at the top of the pyramid, to be consumed only monthly or, if more often, in small amounts. Dairy products that are consumed on a daily basis should also be consumed in small to moderate amounts. For more on this diet, visit www.oldwayspt.org/asian_pyramid.html.

PLANNING A VEGETARIAN DIET

The 2005 *Dietary Guidelines for Americans* provides some direction for vegetarian choices, and several pyramids have been developed for vegetarian diets. The vegetarian pyramid has a bread, cereal, rice, and pasta group at the base and vege-table and fruit groups above that. It also has a milk, yogurt, and cheese group but allows 0–3 servings to accommodate those vegetarians who do not eat dairy products. Instead of a meat, fish, and poultry group, it has a dried beans, nuts, seeds, eggs, and meat substitutes group. This group includes soy products (for example, tofu, tempeh), legumes, and peanut butter. Vegetarians using this pyramid should also adopt the recommendations included in the 2005 *Dietary Guidelines* (such as making sure foods in the bread group are whole grain).

Vegetarian diets may offer protection against obesity, heart disease, high blood pressure, diabetes, digestive disorders, and some forms of cancer, particularly colon cancer,[22] depending on the type of vegetarian diet followed. Some research suggests that vegetarians live longer than nonvegetarians. Despite the potential benefits of vegetarian diets, however, vegetarians need to make sure that their diets provide the energy intake and food diversity needed to meet dietary guidelines.[5] (See the box "Vegetarian Diet Planning.")

Public Health in Action

Globalization of the Western Diet

Dietary and physical activity patterns have changed significantly at different times in human history. The term *nutrition transition* refers to the shifting of broad patterns of diet, nutrition, physical activity, and health. For example, when humans relied on hunting and gathering for food, they were very physically active and their diet was high in carbohydrates and fiber and low in fat, especially saturated fat (meat from wild animals contains more polyunsaturated fat than meat from domesticated animals). With the development of agriculture and the domestication of animals, diets and activity patterns changed.

In the 19th century, most people had a physically active lifestyle and consumed a diet based on whole foods. In the 20th century, there was a shift toward a sedentary lifestyle and a diet high in calories, fat (particularly saturated fat), refined carbohydrates, and sugar and low in fiber. This pattern, often referred to as the Western diet, is typical of most high-income societies and is accompanied by increased risk for obesity and chronic and degenerative diseases like diabetes and heart disease. For example, 4 of the 10 leading causes of death in the United States are linked to diet.

The Western diet is now spreading to the developing world, bringing with it the same health risks that plague the developed nations. One element in this modern nutrition transition is increased food importation from the developed world, so that traditional diets are giving way to diets high in fats and sugar. At the same time, many farmers in developing countries who fed their families from subsistence crops now grow a single cash crop for export. Another element is internal development as a result of economic reforms, as is the case in China. With growing per capita income in China has come soaring consumption of high-fat foods As the Western diet takes hold in developing countries, rates of obesity and related diseases rise.

The societal costs for overweight populations are enormous, since obesity decreases productivity, shortens lifespan, and increases morbidity and mortality rates. The world's growing disease burden is disproportionately suffered by developing nations and especially their poorest citizens. As high-fat diets become more available, the poor have access to a richer diet. Whereas the elite can choose to adopt healthy lifestyles, the poor have fewer choices and less access to nutrition education. Thus, overweight, which used to be a sign of wealth and prosperity, becomes a sign of poverty. The World Health Organization and the United Nations' Food and Agriculture Organization are actively seeking solutions to these problems.

Some experts are looking to the emergence of another dietary pattern, one that draws more on plant foods and less on animal foods, particularly red meat. This pattern relies on behavior change aimed at preventing degenerative diseases and prolonging healthy life. To be successful, this modern nutrition transition will have to incorporate the traditions of different cultures worldwide. In some places, this shift is under way, fueled by consumers. A large-scale shift, however, will require significant support from government policies.

Sources: "What Is the Nutrition Transition?" University of North Carolina, Carolina Population Center, Nutrition Transition Program, retrieved April 3, 2008, from www.cpc.unc.edu/projects/nutrans/whatis.html; "The Nutrition Transition and Obesity," Food and Agriculture Organization of the United Nations, retrieved April 3, 2008, from www.fao.org/FOCUS/E/obesity/obes2.htm.

DAILY VALUES AND FOOD LABELS

Daily Values are another set of standards, based on a variety of dietary guidelines and used on the food labels on packaged foods. Food labels are regulated by the FDA (labeling of meat and poultry products is regulated by the USDA).[23] The information in the Nutrition Facts panel on a food label tells you how that food fits into a 2,000-calorie-a-day diet that includes no more than 65 grams of fat (30 percent of total calories) (Figure 7.3).

The top of the label lists serving size and number of servings in the container. The second part of the label gives the total calories and the calories from fat. A quick calculation will tell you whether this food is relatively high or low in fat. Look for foods with no more than 30 percent of their calories from fat.

The next part of the label shows how much the food contributes to the Daily Values established for important nutrients, expressed as a percentage. The bottom part of the label, which is the same on all food labels, contains a footnote explaining the term "% Daily Value" and shows recommended daily intake of specified nutrients in a 2,000- and a 2,500-calorie diet.

Packaged foods frequently display food descriptors and health claims, which are also regulated by the FDA to help consumers know what they are getting. For example, the term *light* can be used if the product has one-third fewer calories or half the fat of the regular product. To find out more about common nutritional claims, visit the FDA Web site.

Current Consumer Concerns

The food-related topics that you are likely to hear about in the media are consumer issues and concerns, such as the problems associated with soft drinks, high-sodium diets, and fast foods.

OVERCONSUMPTION OF SOFT DRINKS

Americans consume an average of 25 pounds of sugar per person each year, about 32 teaspoons daily. Sugar is believed to promote and maintain obesity, cause and aggravate diabetes, increase the risk of heart disease, and cause dental decay, gum disease, osteoporosis, and kidney stones. It should be noted, however, that scientific evidence suggests that moder-

Highlight on Health

Vegetarian Diet Planning

Vegetarian diets can be healthy if they are carefully designed to include adequate amounts of all the essential nutrients. Vegetarians need to pay careful attention to the following nutrients:

- **Protein**   Some vegetarians can get their protein from dairy products, eggs, fish, or poultry. Vegans (vegetarians who eat no animal products whatsoever) can get all the essential and nonessential amino acids by eating a variety of plant foods—whole grains, legumes, seeds and nuts, and vegetables—and consuming foods from two or more of these categories over the course of a day. Soy protein provides all the essential amino acids and can be the sole protein source in a diet.

- **Iron**   Good plant sources of iron are prune juice, dried beans and lentils, spinach, dried fruits, molasses, brewer's yeast, and enriched products, such as enriched flour. Cooking in iron cookware (cast-iron pans) also provides iron in the diet.

- **Vitamin B$_2$, riboflavin**   Good sources of this vitamin are dairy products, nutritional yeast, leafy green vegetables (collard greens, spinach), broccoli, mushrooms, and dried beans.

- **Vitamin B$_{12}$**   This vitamin is found naturally only in animal sources, so it is particularly important for vegans to make sure it is present in their diets. It can be found in some fortified (not enriched) breakfast cereals, fortified soy beverages, some brands of nutritional (brewer's) yeast, and other foods (check the labels), as well as vitamin supplements.

- **Vitamin D**   This vitamin is found in eggs, butter, and fortified dairy products. Sunlight transforms a provitamin into a substance that the body can use to make vitamin D. Vegans who don't get much sunlight may need a vitamin D supplement (but supplementation should not exceed the RDA).

- **Calcium**   Calcium is plentiful in dairy products, molasses, leafy green vegetables like kale and mustard greens, broccoli, tofu and other soy products, and some legumes. (The calcium in some foods, including spinach, chocolate, and wheat bran, is poorly used in the body.) Studies show that vegetarians absorb and retain more calcium from foods than nonvegetarians do.

- **Zinc**   Good plant sources of this essential mineral are legumes, whole grains, soy products, peas, spinach, and nuts. It is also abundant in dairy products and shellfish. Take care to select supplements containing no more than 15–18 milligrams of zinc. Supplements containing 50 milligrams or more may lower HDL ("good") cholesterol in some people.

- **Calories**   Plant foods have fewer calories than animal foods; vegetarians should make sure they are consuming enough calories to meet their bodies' energy needs.

Source: Adapted from "Vegetarian Diets," American Heart Association, 2004, www.americanheart.org.

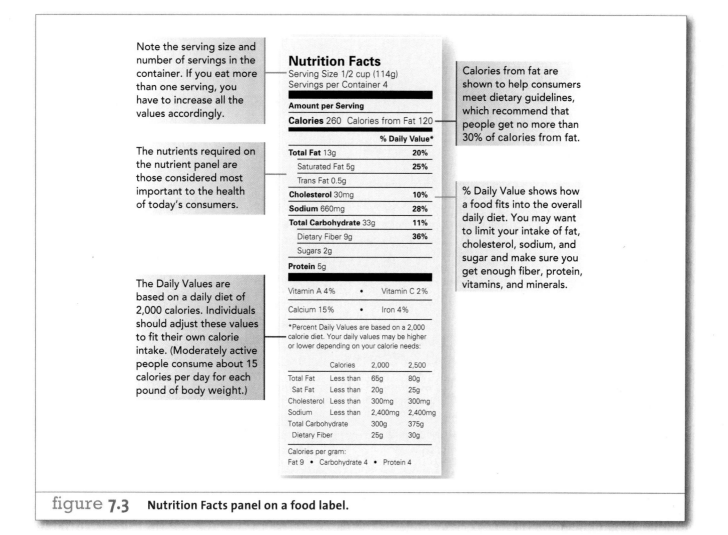

Note the serving size and number of servings in the container. If you eat more than one serving, you have to increase all the values accordingly.

The nutrients required on the nutrient panel are those considered most important to the health of today's consumers.

The Daily Values are based on a daily diet of 2,000 calories. Individuals should adjust these values to fit their own calorie intake. (Moderately active people consume about 15 calories per day for each pound of body weight.)

Calories from fat are shown to help consumers meet dietary guidelines, which recommend that people get no more than 30% of calories from fat.

% Daily Value shows how a food fits into the overall daily diet. You may want to limit your intake of fat, cholesterol, sodium, and sugar and make sure you get enough fiber, protein, vitamins, and minerals.

Nutrition Facts
Serving Size 1/2 cup (114g)
Servings per Container 4

Amount per Serving

Calories 260 Calories from Fat 120

	% Daily Value*
Total Fat 13g	**20%**
Saturated Fat 5g	**25%**
Trans Fat 0.5g	
Cholesterol 30mg	**10%**
Sodium 660mg	**28%**
Total Carbohydrate 33g	**11%**
Dietary Fiber 9g	**36%**
Sugars 2g	
Protein 5g	

Vitamin A 4%	•	Vitamin C 2%	
Calcium 15%	•	Iron 4%	

*Percent Daily Values are based on a 2,000 calorie diet. Your daily values may be higher or lower depending on your calorie needs:

	Calories	2,000	2,500
Total Fat	Less than	65g	80g
Sat Fat	Less than	20g	25g
Cholesterol	Less than	300mg	300mg
Sodium	Less than	2,400mg	2,400mg
Total Carbohydrate		300g	375g
Dietary Fiber		25g	30g

Calories per gram:
Fat 9 • Carbohydrate 4 • Protein 4

figure 7.3   **Nutrition Facts panel on a food label.**

ate levels of sugar (no more than 10 percent of total calories) pose no health risk.[3, 5, 24]

Much of this sugar comes from soft drinks. These beverages represent the largest contributor of daily calories, about 7 percent of calories consumed. For teenagers, they account for 13 percent of calories consumed daily. Consumption of soft drinks doubled from the mid-1970s to the mid-1990s and increased further in the decade that followed. Soft drinks account for one in every four beverages consumed in the United States. Some experts attribute the surge in overweight and obesity among American children and adults largely to the increase in the consumption of soft drinks.

Equally important is the decreased consumption of milk, which is a major source of calcium, protein, vitamin A, and vitamin D, as well as decreased consumption of orange juice and other fruit juices.[25, 26] Soft drinks contain about the same number of calories as milk and juice but none of the nutrients. Diet soft drinks don't contain sugar, but like regular soft drinks, they fill you up without providing any nutrients (Figure 7.4).

Soft drinks also contain relatively high levels of caffeine, which is mildly addictive and can lead to nervousness, irri-

tability, insomnia, and bone demineralization. Although soft drink manufacturers claim that caffeine is added for its flavoring effects, its primary effect is to stimulate the central nervous system.[26] Nutritionists recommend limiting soft drinks in the diet and drinking low-fat milk and water instead.

HIGH-SODIUM DIETS

Another current concern is the amount of sodium consumed in our diets. Sodium is an essential nutrient, but we need only about 500 milligrams per day—about 1/10 of a teaspoon. Although many foods contain sodium, we get most of our sodium—about 90 percent—from salt (which is made up of sodium and chloride). The recommended upper limit for salt is 2,400 milligrams per day, about 1 teaspoon, and the 2005 *Dietary Guidelines* recommends no more than 2,300 milligrams per day.

Salt may be a factor in causing hypertension (high blood pressure) in some "salt-sensitive" people. Even people who are not salt sensitive can benefit from reducing the salt in their diets.[3]

Many packaged foods, convenience foods, fast foods, and restaurant foods are heavily salted, primarily to enhance

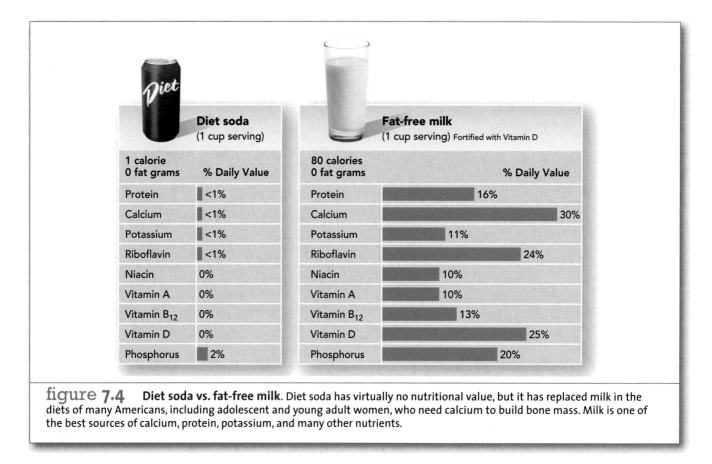

Diet soda (1 cup serving)		Fat-free milk (1 cup serving) Fortified with Vitamin D	
1 calorie 0 fat grams	**% Daily Value**	**80 calories 0 fat grams**	**% Daily Value**
Protein	<1%	Protein	16%
Calcium	<1%	Calcium	30%
Potassium	<1%	Potassium	11%
Riboflavin	<1%	Riboflavin	24%
Niacin	0%	Niacin	10%
Vitamin A	0%	Vitamin A	10%
Vitamin B_{12}	0%	Vitamin B_{12}	13%
Vitamin D	0%	Vitamin D	25%
Phosphorus	2%	Phosphorus	20%

figure 7.4   **Diet soda vs. fat-free milk.** Diet soda has virtually no nutritional value, but it has replaced milk in the diets of many Americans, including adolescent and young adult women, who need calcium to build bone mass. Milk is one of the best sources of calcium, protein, potassium, and many other nutrients.

flavor. At one nationwide restaurant chain, for example, an order of grilled baby back ribs has between 3,300 and 5,300 milligrams of sodium, depending on the preparation and sauce. At the same chain, an order of chicken tacos has 4,400 milligrams of sodium, and an order of steak fajitas has more than 3,000 milligrams of sodium.[27] Canned soups, lunch meats, pickles, soy sauce, teriyaki sauce, catsup, mustard, salad dressing, and barbecue sauce are also high in sodium (see the box "Food, Diet, and Health").

You can reduce the amount of salt in your diet by emphasizing whole foods, like grains, vegetables, and fruits, which are naturally low in sodium. Remove the salt shaker from your table, and don't use salt in cooking. When buying packaged foods, read the labels to check for salt content, and look for descriptors such as "reduced sodium" or "low sodium." (For more guidelines on grocery shopping, see the box "Shopping Tips for College Students" on p. 138.) Highly salted food is an acquired taste; if you use less salt, you will gradually rediscover the natural taste of the food. Although scientists have found substitutes for sugar, substitutes for salt are much more elusive, since it has a distinct taste. Potassium is a salty substance that has been used as a salt substitute, but some people find it too bitter.

FOOD ALLERGIES AND FOOD INTOLERANCES

Food allergies occur when the immune system overreacts to specific proteins in food; they affect about 7 percent of children and 2 percent of adults. More than 200 food ingredients can cause an allergic reaction, but eight foods are responsible for 90 percent of food allergies—milk, eggs, peanuts, tree nuts, fish, shellfish, soy, and wheat. Allergic reactions to these foods cause 30,000 emergency room visits each year and 150 to 200 deaths.[28] The Food Allergen Labeling and Consumer Protection Act of 2004 requires that these allergens be clearly identified on all packaged foods below the list of ingredients.

Typical symptoms of allergic reactions include skin rash, nasal congestion, hives, nausea, and wheezing. Most children eventually outgrow food allergies, except for allergies to peanuts, nuts, and seafood.[3] Generally, people suffer temporary discomfort, but approximately 30,000 people each year in the United States have an *anaphylactic shock* reaction to a food they have eaten—the throat swells enough to cut off breathing.[2] A person experiencing this type of allergic reaction needs immediate medical attention.

Most food reactions are not caused by allergies, however; most are caused by food intolerances.[3] These are less severe than allergies and can be triggered by almost any food. The most common culprits are lactose, sulfur-containing additives in preservatives (used, for example, in dried fruits and red wine), and monosodium glutamate (a flavor enhancer). Lactose intolerance, a condition that results from an inability to digest the milk sugar lactose, is especially prevalent.

There is no treatment or cure for food allergies or intolerances. If you experience these reactions, the best you can do is try to avoid the offending food.[3] It can be especially hard to avoid allergenic foods when eating out, because restaurants are not required to reveal this information. Many health experts are now calling for menu labeling by restaurants, not only for health reasons but also for personal, cultural, and religious reasons. For example, McDonald's has been sued in class action suits brought by vegetarian groups and Muslim associations for flavoring french fries with small amounts of meat, milk, and wheat products without informing customers.[29]

ENERGY BARS AND ENERGY DRINKS

Energy bars are a convenient source of calories and nutrients for people with busy schedules or intense exercise regimens. Luna Bars, Power Bars, and Balance Bars are examples of these convenience foods. Some energy bars claim to have all the amino acids, dietary fiber, and other nutrients to meet 100 percent of the DRIs. Most are low in saturated and trans fats and contain up to 5 grams of fiber. They are better for you than candy bars and other snack foods high in saturated fat, but they can also be high in calories and sugar. Healthier alternatives are whole foods like fruits and vegetables, with their abundant vitamins, minerals, and phytochemicals. If you do buy energy bars, check the labels for calories, total fat, saturated fat, protein, fiber, and sugar and choose the healthiest ones.[30]

Energy drinks are marketed by the sports supplement industry as a source of instant energy, improved concentration and memory, and enhanced physical performance. They have names like Red Bull, Speed Stack, Full Throttle, and Cell Tech. Energy drinks are not considered a health risk if

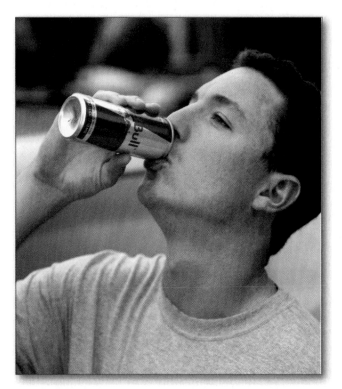

■ Energy drinks provide a brief burst of alertness, typically fueled by caffeine and usually followed by a crash. Most energy drinks carry a long list of cautions.

Who's at Risk

Food, Diet, and Health

■ People with low incomes generally cannot afford healthier foods. They tend to rely more on processed foods than on fresh foods. The migration of supermarkets to the suburbs and the lack of transportation in low-income communities may contribute to malnutrition among these populations.

■ About half of all African American and Latino children born in the year 2000 are expected to develop diabetes at some time in their lives. A healthy diet and a healthy body weight are essential in preventing this disease. On average, a child with diabetes at age 10 will have his or her life expectancy reduced by 17 to 26 years.

food security
Having enough food at all times to support an active, healthy lifestyle.

■ **Food security** is defined as having enough food at all times to support an active, healthy life. It is estimated that about 4 percent of the population do not have enough food to eat. About two-thirds of households with incomes below the poverty line experience food insecurity.

■ About 3 percent of households with children report food insecurity. Children in these households experience not having enough to eat an average of 5.5 days during the month. Children in food-insufficient households experience more headaches, stomachaches, and infections. Malnutrition impairs cognitive development in children and decreases social interaction due to low energy levels.

■ Women in food-insecure households consume less than two-thirds of the DRI for calories, calcium, iron, vitamin E, magnesium, and zinc. Pregnant women experiencing food insecurity are at higher risk for providing inadequate nutrition for the fetus.

■ About 33 percent of the general population are heavy consumers of sugar. Individuals who consume high levels of sugar tend to have a higher calorie intake and lower nutrient intake than those who consume low levels of sugar.

Sources: Perspectives in Nutrition, *by G.M. Wardlaw, J.S. Hampal, and R.A. DiSilvestro, 2006, New York: McGraw-Hill; "Neighborhood Characteristics Associated With the Location of Food Services Places," by K. Morland, S. Wing, A.D. Roux, and C. Poole, 2002, in* Race, Ethnicity, and Health, *ed. T.A. LaVeist, San Francisco: Jossey-Bass; "Food Insecurity and Hunger. LET: Health Disparities Module," www.epi.umn.edu/let/nutri/disparities/ insecure.shtm;* Liquid Candy, *by M.F. Jacobson, 2005, Washington, DC: Center for Science in the Public Interest.*

consumed in recommended amounts, but there are no long-term studies on their side effects, if any.

In addition to water, sodium, and glucose, many energy drinks contain caffeine and a variety of dietary supplements, such as ginseng, guarana, and B vitamins. Caffeine can stimulate mental activity and may increase cardiovascular performance, but consumption should not exceed 300 milligrams per day. Caffeine levels above 400 milligrams are likely to produce negative effects, including loss of focus, racing heart rate, nausea, and anxiety. For most other additives, little or no empirical research either supports their effectiveness or details their potential dangers. The FDA does not monitor energy drinks, but it is beginning to take an interest in doing so.

If you consume energy drinks, your maximum intake should be two 20-ounce cans a day. Consuming more than 20 ounces an hour can cause an increase in arterial pressure and in blood sugar levels. Energy drinks should not be consumed immediately after a vigorous workout or in combination with alcohol. They should not be consumed by pregnant women, children, young teens, older adults, or people with cardiovascular disease, glaucoma, or sleep disorders. The bottom line, according to many health experts, is that the risks associated with energy drinks outweigh any perceived benefits.[31]

FAST FOODS

Americans eat out more than four times a week, and every day, one in four Americans eats fast food.[32] Fast-food meals tend to be high in calories, fat, sodium, and sugar and low in vitamins, minerals, and fiber. A single fast-food meal can approach or exceed the recommended limits on calories, fat, saturated fat, and sodium for a whole day's meals (Figure 7.5).

Challenges & Choices

Shopping Tips for College Students

- Make a shopping list before you go to the store. Better yet, make a menu for the week and buy all the things you need on one trip.

- Take a quick inventory of the food in your kitchen when making your list. You may already have many of the items you need. If you have coupons, keep them with your shopping list. They can reduce your grocery bill significantly.

- Eat something before you go to the store. Grocery stores thrive on impulse buying and are designed to take advantage of the powers of smell and sight. Almost every food looks good when you're hungry.

- Know your budgetary limits and check prices when you're shopping. Read the unit price (usually posted on the shelf below the item) and not just the package price. Unit prices will tell you cost per pound or ounce. Compare this information with similar food items, which are usually nearby on the shelf.

- Concentrate your shopping around the periphery of the store, where you'll find produce, meat, dairy products, and bakery sections. Limit your forays into the middle of the store to find beans, whole grains, cereals, pasta, and other nutrient-dense items.

- Read labels and look for foods that are minimally processed. Be sure to look at the serving size so that you'll know if the information applies to less than the whole container.

- In the produce aisle, look for brightly colored fruits and vegetables.

- In the bread aisle, look for products with the word "whole" in the first ingredient on the ingredient list (whole wheat, whole grain).

- In the snack aisle, choose pretzels, rice cakes, baked corn or potato chips, and popcorn over regular potato chips. Another healthy, inexpensive choice is peanut butter.

- Choose fresh vegetables over frozen and frozen over canned. Canned vegetables are loaded with sodium.

- Choose olive, canola, or safflower oil; if you use mayonnaise, get a light or low-fat version.

- In the dairy section, choose low-fat or fat-free milk, cottage cheese, yogurt, and cheese. Choose tub margarine over stick margarine or butter. Consider trying a soy product.

- Soup is very high in sodium. Look for low-salt versions, and try bean or lentil soup for fiber, folate, and protein.

- At the meat counter, choose lean cuts of beef and skinless poultry (or remove the skin yourself at home). Put meat in a plastic bag to catch leaks. To ensure food safety, buy meats and frozen foods last.

- Watch the scanner to make sure the register rings up the same price you saw on the shelf. If not, ask the cashier to check the price.

It's Not Just Personal . . .

Some studies suggest that grocery store loyalty cards (discount cards) may not actually save you money. Stores that issue these cards may have higher prices overall than stores without them. There are also privacy issues, since stores can track your purchases via your discount card.

Sources: "Cut Three Hundred or More Off your Grocery Bill" by D.L. Montaldo, http://couponing.about.com/cs/grocerysavings/a/groceryshoptips.htm; Restaurant Confidential, by M.F. Jacobson and J.G. Hurley, 2002, New York: Workman; "Smart Food Shopping," by C. Palumbo, 2007, retrieved April 3, 2008, from www.foodfit.com/healthy/archive/healthy/About_dec01.asp.

Many fast-food restaurants (and restaurants in general) are offering healthier choices these days, though, so if you know what to order, it's possible to make healthy choices:

- Don't supersize or order extra-large servings. Standard size orders are already very large.

- Go easy on sauces, toppings, and condiments like sour cream, guacamole, tartar sauce, mayonnaise, and gravy.

- Order grilled chicken or fish on a whole wheat roll, but have them hold the "special sauce."

- Order a salad with dressing on the side or a fat-free dressing. A dinner salad without dressing may have about 150 calories, but a Caesar salad with dressing may have almost 1,000 calories.

- Order a baked potato with vegetables instead of butter or sour cream.

- Instead of a soda, order orange juice, low-fat milk, or a glass of iced water.

- Instead of pie or cake, order yogurt and fruit.

The least healthy options are fried fish or fried chicken sandwiches, chicken nuggets, croissants and pastries, onion rings, and large fries. Most fast-food restaurants will give

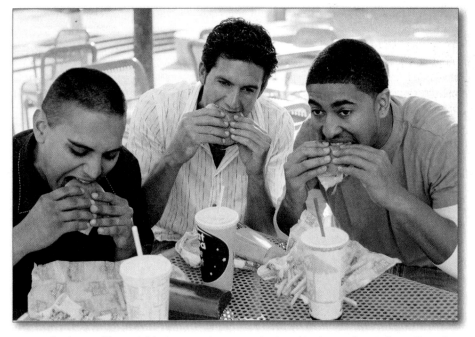

■ Fast food is readily available, inexpensive, convenient, and tasty—and sometimes the only option. Even at fast food restaurants, though, some choices are healthier than others.

you a nutritional brochure if you ask for it, or it may be posted; choose the healthiest options.

Food Safety and Technology

Although the FDA is charged with monitoring the safety of the U.S. food supply, consumers, too, need to learn to distinguish between safe and unsafe foods and understand key elements of food safety, including organic and natural foods, functional foods, foodborne illness, and genetically modified foods.

ARTIFICIAL SWEETENERS

Artificial sweeteners are just one type of food additive—substances that are added to food to maintain or improve nutrient value, aid in food preparation, and/or improve taste or appearance.[3] Currently, about 2,800 different additives are approved by the FDA, which requires that they be effective, detectable, measurable, and safe.

Artificial sweeteners enable people to enjoy a sweet taste in foods and beverages without consuming sugar. One sweetener, saccharin, was associated with bladder cancer in animal studies in 1977. The FDA proposed banning it but withdrew the proposal because of public opposition. The FDA has set the acceptable daily intake (ADI) for saccharin at 5 milligrams per kilogram (2.2 pounds) of body weight,[3] and excessive consumption is probably not safe.

Another sweetener, aspartame, has undergone rigorous study. It is marketed as Nutrasweet, Equal, and Spoonful. Many products contain it, including Diet Pepsi and Diet Coke. In the United States, the ADI of aspartame is 50 milligrams

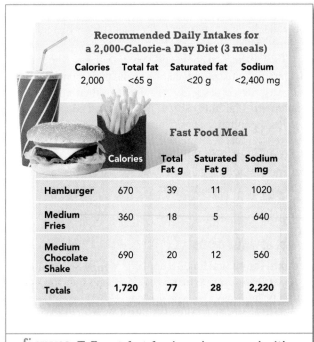

Recommended Daily Intakes for a 2,000-Calorie-a Day Diet (3 meals)

Calories	Total fat	Saturated fat	Sodium
2,000	<65 g	<20 g	<2,400 mg

Fast Food Meal

	Calories	Total Fat g	Saturated Fat g	Sodium mg
Hamburger	670	39	11	1020
Medium Fries	360	18	5	640
Medium Chocolate Shake	690	20	12	560
Totals	1,720	77	28	2,220

figure **7.5** **A fast-food meal compared with recommended daily intakes.**

per kilogram of body weight; in Canada, it is 40 milligrams per kilogram.[3] This means a 150-pound person would have to consume 97 packets of Equal or 20 cans of diet soft drinks a day to exceed the ADI. The typical person consumes less than 5 milligrams of aspartame per kilogram of body weight per day.[33]

Aspartame contains phenylalanine and should be avoided by people with phenylketonuria (PKU), an inherited metabolic disorder (see Chapter 2). Generally, artificial sweeteners are considered safe.[3] Still, they should be consumed only in moderation and as part of a well-balanced diet.

ORGANIC FOODS

Plant foods labeled "organic" are grown without synthetic pesticides or fertilizers,[2] and animal foods labeled organic are from animals raised on organic feed without antibiotics or growth hormone. Organic foods appeal to health- and environment-conscious consumers.[34] They tend to be more expensive than foods grown using conventional methods, however, and consumers cannot always determine exactly how some foods were grown.

The USDA regulates the use of terms related to organic foods on the labels of meat and poultry products. The label "100% organic" means that all contents are organic; "organic" means that contents are at least 95 percent organic; "made with organic ingredients" means the contents are at least 70 percent organic. Food manufacturers who comply with the

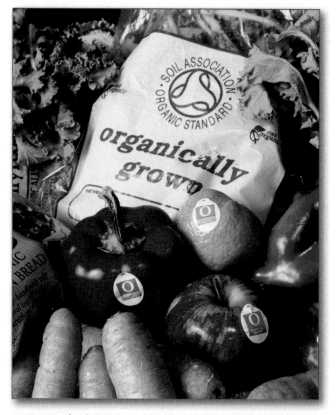

■ Organic foods aren't necessarily healthier, but organic farming is better for the environment. Many consumers are now choosing organic, locally grown produce and other foods.

USDA standards can place the seal "USDA Organic" on their labels.

The USDA's National Organic Program (NOP) is responsible for certifying organic food agencies, which, in turn, send inspectors to organic farms and food processors. The NOP has a staff of about 10 people to monitor more than 20,000 organic farms and food processors. Unfortunately, insufficient resources make it difficult for the NOP to ensure that organic standards are upheld.

Although it seems that organic foods ought to be healthier and safer than foods grown conventionally, no research has demonstrated that this is the case. Conventional food products do contain pesticide residues that can be toxic at high doses, but research has not documented ill effects from them at the levels found in foods, nor is there any evidence that people who consume organic food are healthier than those who don't.[3]

What has been documented is that organic farming is beneficial to the environment. It helps maintain biodiversity of crops; it replenishes the earth's resources; and it is less likely to degrade soil, contaminate water, or expose farm workers to toxic chemicals. As multinational food companies get into the organic food business, however, consumers should look for foods that are not only organic but also locally grown. The average food item currently travels at least 1,500 miles to its destination, consuming massive amounts of oil for transportation. Locally grown food tastes better, keeps money in the local economy, and cuts down on the consumption of processed food. The burgeoning popularity of farmers' markets is a sign of growing interest in locally grown food.

A disadvantage of organic foods is that they may place consumers at higher risk of contracting foodborne illnesses. If you purchase organic food, buy only the amount you need immediately, store and cook the food properly, and wash organic produce thoroughly before eating it.[3, 35]

Some experts recommend that consumers who want to buy organic fruits and vegetables spend their money on those that carry higher pesticide residues than their conventional counterparts (the "dirty dozen"): apples, bell peppers, celery, cherries, imported grapes, nectarines, peaches, pears, potatoes, red raspberries, spinach, and strawberries. Fruits and vegetables that carry little pesticide residue whether grown conventionally or organically include asparagus, avocados, bananas, broccoli, cauliflower, corn, kiwi, mangoes, onions, papaya, pineapples, and peas.[35]

FUNCTIONAL FOODS

The term **functional foods** is applied to foods that do more than provide nutrients; they may also help prevent chronic diseases and provide other health benefits.[36] The term is most commonly used to describe foods to which ingredients have been added to improve their health benefits. Functional foods include

functional food
Foods that may help prevent disease, usually because health-promoting ingredients have been added to them.

cereals with added vitamins and minerals, orange juice with added calcium, and various foods with added soy protein or fiber. The FDA allows functional foods to make research-based health claims on their labels, such as "Proven to significantly reduce cholesterol" or "Reduces the risk of heart disease."

The FDA does not have full regulatory authority over herbs, however, nor does it review general claims like "Boosts energy" or "Enhances mood." Foods touted as "liquid vitamins" or sold under names such as "St. John's Wort Tortilla Chips" or "Kava Kava Corn Chips" should be viewed with some skepticism. Claims that herbally fortified foods improve memory, lift moods, melt away pounds, or soothe joint pain are not supported by scientific evidence.[37]

FOODBORNE ILLNESSES

The Centers for Disease Control and Prevention (CDC) estimates that 76 million people get sick every year from foodborne illness, 325,000 are hospitalized, and 5,000 die.[38] Foodborne illnesses may be caused by food intoxication or by food infection; both types are commonly referred to as *food poisoning.*

Food intoxication occurs when a food is contaminated by natural toxins or by microbes that produce toxins. Botulism is an example of food intoxication. When food has been contaminated with the botulism bacterium and then improperly prepared or stored, the bacterium releases a dangerous and potentially fatal toxin. Warning signs of botulism poisoning are double vision, weak muscles, difficulty swallowing, and difficulty breathing.[3] Immediate medical treatment is needed.

food intoxication
A kind of food poisoning in which a food is contaminated by natural toxins or by microbes that produce toxins.

food infection
A kind of food poisoning in which a food is contaminated by disease-causing microorganisms, or pathogens.

Food infection is caused by disease-causing microorganisms, or pathogens, that have contaminated the food. The more commonly contaminated foods are ground beef, chicken, turkey, salami, hot dogs, ice cream, lettuce and other greens, sprouts, cantaloupe, and apple cider.

Common Food Pathogens Three of the most common pathogens that cause food infection are *Escherichia coli (E. coli)*, salmonella, and campylobacter. *E. coli* occurs naturally in the intestines of humans and animals. Raw beef, raw fruits and vegetables, leafy greens, sprouts, and unpasteurized juices and cider are the foods most commonly contaminated by it. A 2007 nationwide outbreaks of *E. coli* infection was traced to packaged spinach and lettuce grown in California and contaminated by domestic animals and wildlife.

One strain, *E. coli* O157:H7, is especially dangerous because it can cause *hemolytic uremic syndrome (HUS)*, which can lead to kidney failure, a potentially fatal condition. The CDC estimates that *E. coli* O157:H7 causes nearly 73,000 illnesses each year in the United States and kills 250

to 500 people.[39] Young children and older adults are particularly at risk. *E. coli* is a hearty microbe, thriving in moist environments for weeks and on kitchen countertops for days.

Salmonella enteritis can contaminate raw eggs, poultry and meat, fruits, and vegetables, and other foods. Eggs containing salmonella enteritis are the number-one cause of food poisoning outbreaks in the nation. The best way to prevent salmonella infection is to thoroughly cook eggs, chicken, and other foods to kill the bacterium. Avoid eating raw or undercooked eggs, such as in raw cake batter or cookie dough, salad dressings, and eggnog.[38]

Campylobacter occurs in raw or undercooked poultry, meat, and shellfish, in unpasteurized milk, and in contaminated water. Campylobacter from contaminated poultry can spread when juices from packages spill onto kitchen surfaces and other foods; it can also be spread by hand.[40] Campylobacter and salmonella together cause 80 percent of the illnesses and 75 percent of the deaths associated with meat and poultry practices.[40]

Food poisoning causes flu-like symptoms such as diarrhea, abdominal pain, vomiting, fever, and chills. More serious complications can include rheumatoid arthritis, kidney or heart disease, meningitis, HUS, and death. Some symptoms are cause for immediate medical attention:

- Bloody diarrhea or pus in the stool
- Fever that lasts more than 48 hours
- Faintness, rapid heart rate, or nausea when standing up suddenly
- Significant drop in the frequency of urination[38, 41]

Although only about 20 percent of food poisoning cases occur at home, the best defense against foodborne illness is the use of safe food practices in your own kitchen (Figure 7.6).[42]

Food Irradiation Many government regulations are in place to ensure that the food supply is safe. A relatively new approach to safety is **food irradiation,** a process in which food is passed through a chamber containing radioactive rods that emit powerful gamma rays. These eliminate almost all microbiological threats, with the exception of the pathogens that cause botulism, hepatitis, and bovine spongiform encephalitis (mad cow disease).

food irradiation
Process that exposes food to gamma rays to destroy contaminants.

The American Dietetic Association Scientific Position on food irradiation is that it is an effective way to protect consumers from foodborne illness.[43] There is disagreement, however, on the safety of irradiation. One fear is that radiation may destroy nutrients and cause people to develop nutrient deficiencies. The FDA argues that the loss of nutrients is minimal. Another fear is that the health effects of irradiated foods are not completely understood. Some studies have found chromosomal abnormalities, impaired fertility, and depressed immune responses in animals on diets containing

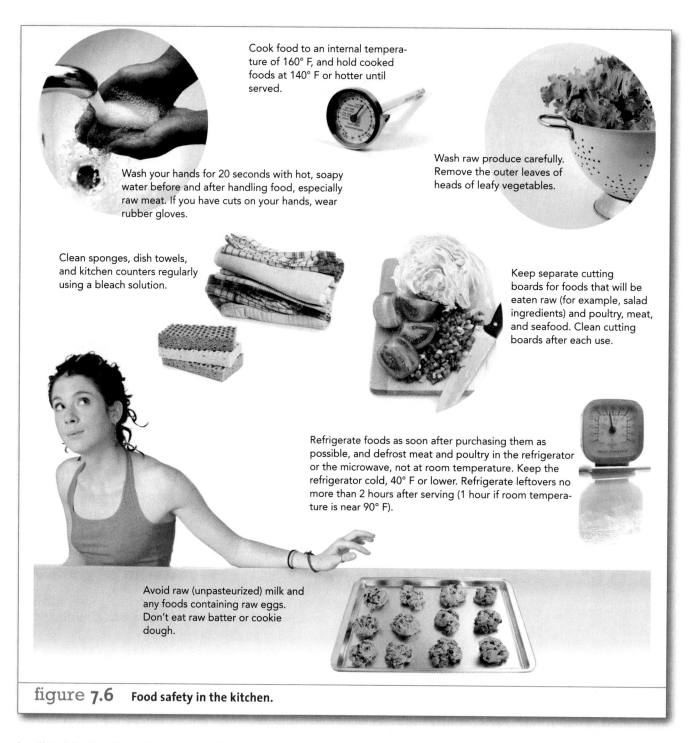

Cook food to an internal temperature of 160° F, and hold cooked foods at 140° F or hotter until served.

Wash your hands for 20 seconds with hot, soapy water before and after handling food, especially raw meat. If you have cuts on your hands, wear rubber gloves.

Wash raw produce carefully. Remove the outer leaves of heads of leafy vegetables.

Clean sponges, dish towels, and kitchen counters regularly using a bleach solution.

Keep separate cutting boards for foods that will be eaten raw (for example, salad ingredients) and poultry, meat, and seafood. Clean cutting boards after each use.

Refrigerate foods as soon after purchasing them as possible, and defrost meat and poultry in the refrigerator or the microwave, not at room temperature. Keep the refrigerator cold, 40° F or lower. Refrigerate leftovers no more than 2 hours after serving (1 hour if room temperature is near 90° F).

Avoid raw (unpasteurized) milk and any foods containing raw eggs. Don't eat raw batter or cookie dough.

figure **7.6**   **Food safety in the kitchen.**

irradiated foods, although research on humans has not produced the same findings.

A third fear is that radioactive substances used to irradiate food may endanger food plant workers, the general population, and the environment. Food industrialists who support food irradiation advocate strict safety regulations and enforcement to limit radiation exposure.[3]

GENETICALLY MODIFIED FOODS

Farmers, scientists, and breeders have long been tinkering with the genetic makeup of plants and animals to breed organisms with desirable traits, a process known as *selective breeding*. Compared to modern techniques, however, selective breeding is slow and imprecise. Using biotechnology to produce **genetically modified (GM) organisms** is a faster and more refined process. Genetic modification involves the addition, deletion, or reorganization of an organism's genes in order to change that organism's protein production. Research on genetic modification in agriculture has focused on three areas:

genetically modified (GM) organisms
Organisms whose genetic makeup has been changed to produce desirable traits.

- New strains of crops and animals with improved resistance to disease and pests (for example, corn plants that resist blights)

- Strains of microorganisms that produce specific substances that occur in small amounts or not at all in nature (for example, bovine somatotropin, a growth hormone used in cattle to produce more meat)

- Crops that resist destruction by herbicides (for example, soybean plants that can survive herbicides used to kill weeds)

Many crops have already been genetically modified, and 60 percent of processed foods currently sold in supermarkets contain one or more GM ingredients.[44]

Proponents of GM crops and animals say we must develop new agricultural technologies that increase crop and animal productivity and support food growers and producers economically while not harming the environment. They see genetic modification as a promising agricultural technology that may meet these needs, and many in the food and biotechnology industries have hailed the benefits of GM organisms.[44]

On the other hand, a growing number of consumers, animal rights supporters, national consumer watchdog organizations, and environmentalists have expressed concerns about GM foods. They fear that agriculture driven by biotechnology without restraint will destroy natural ecosystems, create new viruses, increase cruelty to animals, and reduce biodiversity.[44] They have called for all foods containing GM ingredients to be labeled.

The safety of food products produced by biotechnology is assessed by the FDA's new National Center for Food Safety and Technology. To date, the center has held that GM foods do not require any special safety testing—nor do they have to be labeled as GM foods—unless they differ significantly from foods already in use.[3, 38]

The American Dietetic Association and many other scientific organizations support the FDA position on GM foods, citing the potential benefits. For biotechnology in agriculture to achieve the objectives of ensuring safe, abundant, and affordable food, however, it must be accepted by the public. Surveys suggest that consumers are not well informed about this technology but are cautiously optimistic about its potential benefits in food production and processing.[44]

* * *

North Americans enjoy the safest and most nutritious food supply in the world. We also enjoy immense choice in what we eat. With choice comes responsibility—the responsibility to be informed, to make wise decisions, to consume foods that promote health and prevent disease. After reading this chapter, you have sufficient information to make nutrition choices that support your own lifelong health and, by extension, the well-being of society at large. We encourage you to make those healthy choices!

You Make the Call

Who Is Responsible for What We Eat?

In 2000 a class action suit was filed against McDonald's Corporation on behalf of New York children, claiming that McDonald's food contributed to or caused obesity, diabetes, high blood pressure, and heart disease. The plaintiffs accused McDonald's of five wrongdoings: (1) deception of the public through marketing its food as nutritious and encouraging consumers to "supersize" their orders; (2) targeting children in marketing campaigns such as "Mighty Kids' Meals"; (3) selling food high in calories, fat, sugar, and sodium; (4) failing to warn consumers of unhealthy ingredients in its food; and (5) acting negligently in marketing food products that are psychologically and physiologically addictive (sugar).

A federal judge dismissed the case in 2003 as overly vague in its allegations, but more suits were brought against McDonald's and other fast-food corporations. Lawyers for McDonald's warned Congress that if such cases were allowed to proceed, the fast-food industry would be paralyzed by an avalanche of frivolous lawsuits. Congress agreed and proposed the Personal Responsibility in Food Consumption Act of 2005. This act bans frivolous lawsuits against food and beverage manufacturers, marketers, distributors, advertisers, sellers, and trade associations for claims of injuries associated with a person's weight gain, obesity, or any health condition associated with weight gain or obesity. The act was passed by the House of Representatives but not by the Senate, so it has never gone into effect.

Proponents of laws like the Personal Responsibility in Food Consumption Act assert that individuals have to take responsibility for their lifestyle choices. They argue that it is common knowledge that fast food is high in calories, fat, sodium, and sugar. A person consuming fast food in copious amounts knows or should know that it can lead to obesity and associated health disorders. This view has been expressed by the Center for Consumer Freedom.

Opponents of such laws argue that society shares responsibility for shielding citizens from harm. They point out that if corporations engage in deceptive advertising and manipulative marketing techniques, individuals can hardly be expected to uncover the deception. According to this view, which has been articulated by the Center for Science in the Public Interest, a consumer activist organization, legislation is needed to control these practices. What do you think?

PROS

- The food and beverage industries are a significant part of the U.S. economy and should not be encumbered by frivolous lawsuits.

- A person's weight gain, obesity, or health condition is associated with a multitude of factors, including genetics and lifestyle behaviors under control of the individual. People are not forced to supersize their food orders.

- Parents have responsibility for their children. The lawsuits against McDonald's imply that the television cannot be turned off and that parents have no control over their children, both of which are false assumptions.

- Most Americans reject efforts to limit their choices. In one survey, 72 percent of Americans agreed with the statement "When I go out to a restaurant, I like to order what I really want, whether it's healthy or not."

CONS

- Overweight and obesity, especially in children, is a public health crisis with staggering medical, economic, and personal costs. Placing personal responsibility on the individual for the obesity epidemic has not worked. The United States has a long history of implementing legislative and regulatory action to protect the public when personal responsibility falls short. Seat belt laws are an example.

- The food industry has a history of pressuring legislators to pass favorable laws and rulings. It's not surprising that fast-food corporations would not want to help consumers understand what they are eating.

- Children watch an estimated 50 days of television every year, during which time they view 10,000 food ads. Many of the ads target children with cartoon characters promoting sugary cereals and other unhealthy foods. Parents cannot possibly counter these ads in favor of healthy foods.

- Food companies stand to profit when people eat larger portions. Marketing campaigns take advantage of people's natural desire to get more for their money. A study by the American Institute for Cancer Research found that two-thirds of subjects completely consume whatever is on their plate regardless of serving size. Thus corporate greed and desire for profits are causing consumers harm.

- Americans in poor neighborhoods have 2.5 times the exposure to fast-food restaurants as people living in wealthier neighborhoods. This discrepancy partially explains health disparities for racial and ethnic groups.

Sources: Food Fight, *by K.D. Brownell, 2004, New York: McGraw-Hill; "Personal Responsibility in Food Consumption Act of 2005," Food Consumer Organization, retrieved from www.foodconsumer.org; "Restaurants: Latest Target Under Scrutiny by Activists in the Name of 'The Public Interest'," by B. Hyde, retrieved August 19, 2006, from www.consumerfreedom.com/oped_detail.cfm?oped=129.*

In Review

1. **What are the categories of nutrients?** The macronutrients are water, carbohydrates, proteins, and fats. The micronutrients are vitamins and minerals. A balanced diet includes adequate intake of all the nutrients, primarily from nutrient-rich foods (as opposed to dietary supplements). Whole foods and especially plant foods contain additional important substances, such as antioxidants.

2. **How do you plan a healthy diet?** The *Dietary Guidelines for Americans* translates the findings of nutritional research into daily dietary recommendations, and MyPyramid customizes these recommendations to the individual, based on activity levels and calorie needs. Many other sets of guidelines are available as well, including pyramids for vegetarians and for those who want to follow ethnic diets.

3. **What are the main nutrition-related concerns currently affecting our society?** Americans overall do not eat a very healthy diet compared to what is recommended, and overweight and obesity are significant problems. The American diet tends to include too many calories; too much sugar, salt, and fat; and too few vegetables, fruits, and whole foods. Current concerns include the overconsumption of soft drinks, high-sodium diets, and the prevalence of fast food.

4. **What are the main food safety–related issues?** The main safety issue is foodborne illness, typically caused by pathogens such as *E. coli* and salmonella. The American food supply is safe overall, but increasing centralization of food production and distribution creates the conditions for widespread outbreaks of foodborne illness from a single source of contamination. Other safety-related issues of interest to consumers include the use of artificial sweeteners, food irradiation, and genetically modified foods. Consumers are becoming increasingly interested in organic and locally grown foods.

 For a detailed summary of this chapter and a comprehensive set of review questions, visit the Online Learning Center at **www.mhhe.com/teague2e**.

Web Resources

American Heart Association, Face the Fats: This site provides information about dietary fats and includes an interactive feature, My Fats Translator, that guides consumers in understanding their fat intake.
www.americanheart.org/facethefats

Center for Science in the Public Interest: This advocacy organization focuses on nutrition and health, food safety, alcohol policy, and sound science.
www.cspinet.org

FDA Center for Food Safety and Applied Nutrition: This resource offers a wide range of information—from food and nutrition topics in the news to legal issues related to food safety.
http://vm.cfsan.fda.gov

Food Allergy and Anaphylaxis Network: Featuring information on common food allergens, this site offers practical approaches to living with food allergies.
www.foodallergy.org

Food Safety: This is an excellent resource for food news and safety alerts, consumer advice, and topics related to children and teens.
www.foodsafety.gov

National Institutes of Health, Office of Dietary Supplements: This government site provides reliable information on popular dietary supplements.
www.ods.od.nih.gov

Nutrition.gov: A gateway to reliable information on nutrition, from the U.S. government.
www.nutrition.gov

USDA, MyPyramid: This official site offers a wealth of information and interactive tools for using MyPyramid to improve your diet.
www.mypyramid.gov

Chapter

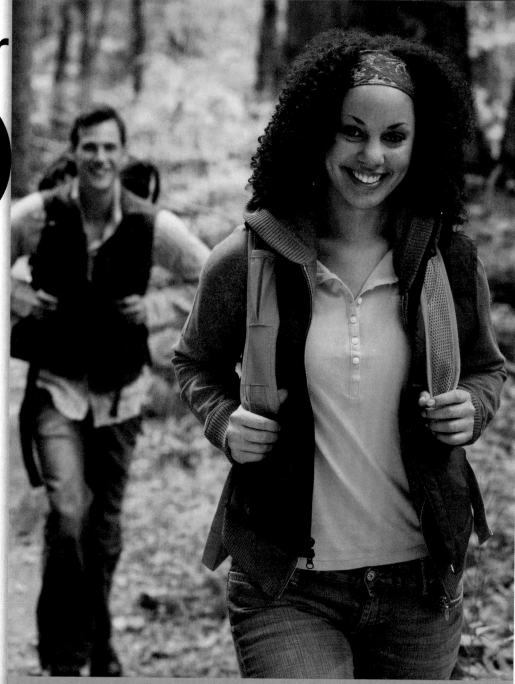

8

Fitness
Physical
Activity
for Life

WWW

Your Health Today

www.mhhe.com/teague2e

Go to the Online Learning Center for *Your Health Today* for interactive activities, quizzes, flashcards, Web links, and more resources related to this chapter.

Ever Wonder...

- how much exercise you should be getting?
- if you can wash your running shoes in the washing machine?
- how long it takes to burn off the calories from a burger and fries?

You are jogging through the airport to make a flight on another concourse on your way home for winter break. Your Nike iPod Sport Kit shoe is blaring your favorite song into your earbuds when a voice suddenly interrupts the music: "5 minutes completed. 0.30 miles. Pace, 5 miles per hour. Calories burned, 45." The Nike iPod shoe is just one of many new devices designed to motivate the general public to exercise, particularly young adults.

Unfortunately, Americans need a lot of motivation. Although many public health campaigns are aimed at Americans' sedentary habits, the fact is that most people don't exercise. Of all those adults who hear the message about exercise, 20 percent become believers and 80 percent tune it out. According to the U.S. surgeon general, at least 50 percent of American adults do not get enough physical activity for health benefits.[1] (See the box "Exercise and Health.")

The good news is that there are simple and enjoyable ways to build physical activity into your lifestyle and to increase the amount of exercise you get. This chapter will show you now.

What Is Fitness?

In the context of *fitness*, you are considered to be in good health if you have sufficient energy and vitality to accomplish daily living tasks and leisure-time physical activities without undue fatigue. **Physical activity**—activity that requires any type of movement—is an important part of good health. Any kind of physical activity is better than no activity at all, and benefits increase as the level of physical activity increases, up to a point. Too much physical activity can make you susceptible to injury. **Exercise** is structured, planned physical activity, often carried out to improve fitness.

physical activity
Activity that requires any type of movement.

exercise
Structured, planned physical activity, often carried out to improve fitness.

physical fitness
Ability of the body to respond to the physical demands placed upon it.

skill-related fitness
Ability to perform specific skills associated with various sports and leisure activities.

health-related fitness
Ability to perform daily living activities with vigor.

Physical fitness, in general, is the ability of the body to respond to the physical demands placed upon it. When we talk about *fitness,* we are really talking about two different concepts: skill-related fitness and health-related fitness.[2] **Skill-related fitness** refers to the ability to perform specific skills associated with various leisure activities or sports. Components of skill-related fitness include agility, speed, power, balance, coordination, and reaction time.

Health-related fitness refers to the ability to perform daily living activities (like shopping for

Who's at Risk

Exercise and Health

- The prevalence of leisure-time physical activity among children and adults has declined in the past decade. In 2005 about 24 percent of adults reported no leisure-time physical activity. About one in four older adults is classified as sedentary.

- Less than half of all adults in the United States meet Centers for Disease Control and Prevention/American College of Sports Medicine aerobic/endurance activity recommendations for health, with 50.7 percent of men and 47.9 percent of women meeting the objectives. Caucasian adults (51.1 percent) are more likely than Hispanics (44 percent) or African Americans (41.8 percent) to meet the objectives.

- The prevalence of strength training among Caucasian adults is 23.1 percent; among African Americans, 22.9 percent; and among Hispanics, 15 percent. These prevalence rates fall far below the Healthy People 2010 goals of 30 percent of all adults.

- Men are more likely than women to participate in strength training, with 21.9 percent of men and 17.5 percent of women participating. Muscle strength decreases significantly for men between the ages of 50 and 70 years and even more dramatically after age 80. For women, muscle strength losses begin to accelerate in their early 20s.

- Only 17 percent of adults walk when the trip distance is 1 mile or less. Only 31 percent of children and adolescents walk to school when the trip distance is 1 mile or less. Less than 3 percent of children and adolescents bike to school when the trip distance is 2 miles or more. Many communities are actively designing environments that will encourage walking and biking short distances.

- Communities are using point-of-decision prompts to encourage people to take the stairs rather than escalators and elevators. Both obese and nonobese people have been positively influenced by these prompts. Obese people are more likely than nonobese people to use the stairs, particularly when the prompt signs link stair climbing to weight loss and other health benefits.

Sources: The Guide to Community Preventive Health Services, *by S. Zara, P.A. Briss, and K.W. Harris, 2005, New York: Oxford University Press;* "Physical Activity and Public Health: Updated Recommendation for Adults from the American College of Sports Medicine and the American Heart Association," *by W.L. Haskell, L. I-Min, R.R Pate, et al., 2007, Circulation, 116 (9), pp. 1081–1093.*

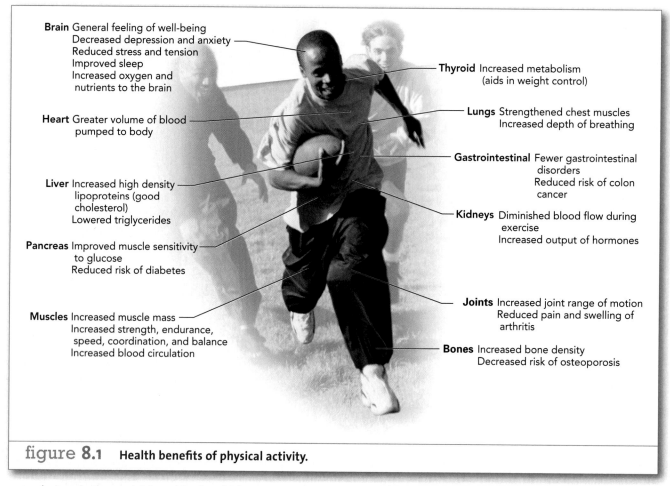

Brain General feeling of well-being
Decreased depression and anxiety
Reduced stress and tension
Improved sleep
Increased oxygen and
nutrients to the brain

Heart Greater volume of blood
pumped to body

Liver Increased high density
lipoproteins (good
cholesterol)
Lowered triglycerides

Pancreas Improved muscle sensitivity
to glucose
Reduced risk of diabetes

Muscles Increased muscle mass
Increased strength, endurance,
speed, coordination, and balance
Increased blood circulation

Thyroid Increased metabolism
(aids in weight control)

Lungs Strengthened chest muscles
Increased depth of breathing

Gastrointestinal Fewer gastrointestinal
disorders
Reduced risk of colon
cancer

Kidneys Diminished blood flow during
exercise
Increased output of hormones

Joints Increased joint range of motion
Reduced pain and swelling of
arthritis

Bones Increased bone density
Decreased risk of osteoporosis

figure **8.1**   **Health benefits of physical activity.**

groceries) and other activities with vigor.[2] The components of health-related fitness are cardiorespiratory fitness, musculoskeletal fitness, and body composition. Musculoskeletal fitness, in turn, includes muscular strength, muscular endurance, and flexibility.

BENEFITS OF PHYSICAL ACTIVITY AND EXERCISE

Why should you be physically active? Your answers to this question may include having fun, looking good, feeling good, and other excellent answers. Beyond these, however, is another reason to be physically active: People who are active are healthier than those who are not.[3] There are benefits in the domains of physical, cognitive, psychological, emotional, and spiritual health, among others. An overview of the health benefits associated with physical activity is presented in Figure 8.1.

Physical Benefits of Exercise   One benefit of physical activity is a longer lifespan: people with moderate to high levels of physical activity live longer than people who are sedentary. Physical activity and exercise are associated with improved functioning in just about every body system, from the cardiorespiratory system to the skeletal system to the immune system. A sedentary lifestyle, on the other hand, has been associated with 28 percent of deaths from the leading chronic diseases, including cancer, heart disease, osteoporosis, diabetes, high blood pressure, and

obesity.[4–11] Results from just a few research studies are shown in Figure 8.2.

Cognitive Benefits of Exercise   Although there is no compelling evidence that short-term exercise training significantly improves cognitive functioning,[12] some research has suggested positive effects. For example, evidence suggests that fit individuals process information more quickly than do less fit individuals of the same age. Other research has shown that aerobic fitness may prevent or slow down the loss of cognitive functions associated with advancing age.[13] However, generalizations about the influence of exercise on cognitive performance must be viewed with caution. Improvements as a result of physical activity may have more to do with overall feelings of well-being than with specific cognitive functions (see the box "Exercising Your Brain").

Psychological and Emotional Benefits of Exercise Moderate-to-intense levels of physical activity have been shown to influence mood, decrease the risk of depression and anxiety, relieve stress, and improve overall quality of life.[15] Although biological explanations have been proposed for the improved sense of well-being associated with physical activity, better explanations are improved self-esteem, improved quality of sleep, more opportunities for social interaction, and more effective physiological responses to stress.

Challenges & Choices

Exercising Your Brain

The benefits of mental activities (chess, bridge, crossword puzzles) for brain function are well established. Animal studies and some human studies are now beginning to show that physical activity is beneficial to the brain as well. Exercise stimulates the growth of new brain cells in the hippocampus (the part of the brain where learning is centered) and in the frontal cortex (the center for decision making, planning, and other executive functions). Exercise encourages brain cells to branch out, join together, and communicate with each other in new ways, and it prompts nerve cells to form denser, more interconnected webs that enable the brain to operate more quickly and efficiently.

Because the brain is not fully developed until early adulthood, exercise is vital to optimal brain development and function. In children and young adults up to about age 25, exercise facilitates the enlargement of the hippocampus and the development of the frontal lobes. Some states cite the importance of exercise for brain development in pushing for mandatory daily physical education up until ninth grade.

Exercise may also help prevent cognitive disorders like Alzheimer's disease in older adults. Some studies found that inactive individuals were twice as likely to develop Alzheimer's disease as those who participated in aerobic exercise at least 30 minutes a day three times a week. Research has particularly focused on the benefits of walking and running and has found that even nonstrenuous walking can improve learning, concentration, and abstract reasoning.

A unique system of mental exercise called neurobotics has been developed by Lawrence Katz to help the brain manufacture the nutrients that strengthen, preserve, and grow new brain cells. These exercises are designed to shape daily routines in unexpected ways. An example is using your nondominant hand to control your computer mouse or to brush your teeth. The awkwardness and discomfort you feel reflect the brain's attempt to learn a new skill. Challenging your brain in such ways strengthens neural connections and even creates new ones.

It's Not Just Personal . . .

American society is entrenched in sedentary activity fueled by video games, television, and computers. Children today spend about 5 hours a day in sedentary activities. Almost half of people aged 12 to 21 do not participate in vigorous physical activity on a regular basis. Encouraging children and teens to be more active is vital not just for physical functioning but for mental functioning as well.

Sources: "Stronger, Faster, Smarter," by M. Carmichael, March 26, 2007, Newsweek, pp. 38–55; "On Your Marks," by A. Kuchment, March 26, 2007, Newsweek, pp. 56–59; "While You Wait: The Cost of Inactivity," 2005, Nutrition Action Newsletter, 32 (10), pp. 3–6; "Exercise and the Brain," Society for Neuroscience, retrieved from www.sfn.org.

The magnitude of a person's "cardiovascular reactivity" to stress—increased heart rate, blood pressure, and so on—can be mitigated by exercise. If you are physically fit, your body is conditioned to react more calmly to stressful situations. Exercise can also help you deal with stressful situations by providing a temporary distraction, increasing your feelings of control or commitment, and providing a sense of success in doing something that is important to you.[16]

Spiritual Benefits of Exercise   When you exercise, you are taking charge of your life and taking care of yourself. Exercising and being physically active give you the opportunity to connect with yourself, with other people, and with nature in deep and immediate ways. As you jog through a park, cycle on a bike path, hike in a natural area, or cross-country ski on a wilderness trail, you may find yourself feeling refreshed and reinvigorated both by a sense of physical well-being and by the natural scene around you. Thus, exercise enhances your feelings of self-esteem and mastery as well as your connection to yourself and something beyond yourself.

GUIDELINES FOR PHYSICAL ACTIVITY AND EXERCISE

Many leading health organizations publish physical activity and exercise guidelines aimed at achieving a variety of health goals. A widely accepted set of guidelines aimed at promoting and maintaining health and preventing chronic diseases and premature mortality was updated and issued jointly by

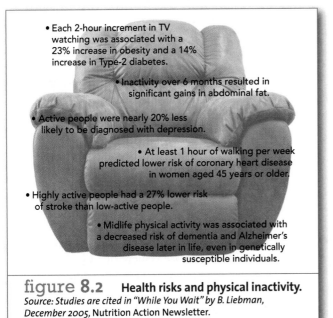

- Each 2-hour increment in TV watching was associated with a 23% increase in obesity and a 14% increase in Type-2 diabetes.
- Inactivity over 6 months resulted in significant gains in abdominal fat.
- Active people were nearly 20% less likely to be diagnosed with depression.
- At least 1 hour of walking per week predicted lower risk of coronary heart disease in women aged 45 years or older.
- Highly active people had a 27% lower risk of stroke than low-active people.
- Midlife physical activity was associated with a decreased risk of dementia and Alzheimer's disease later in life, even in genetically susceptible individuals.

figure 8.2   **Health risks and physical inactivity.**
Source: Studies are cited in "While You Wait" by B. Liebman, December 2005, Nutrition Action Newsletter.

Table 8.1 | Metabolic equivalents (METs) of Common Physical Activities

Light	METs	Moderate	METs	Vigorous	METs
Slow walking	2.0	Walking 3.0 mph	3.3	Walking 4.5 mph	6.3
Canoeing	2.5	Cycling leisurely	3.5	Cycling moderately	5.7
Golf with cart	2.5	Golf, no cart	4.4	Jogging 7 mph	11.5
Croquet	2.5	Table tennis	4.0	Tennis singles	8.0
Fishing–sitting	2.5	Slow swimming	4.5	Moderate swimming	8.0
Billiards	2.5	Boat sailing	3.0	Volleyball	8.0
Darts	2.5	Ballroom dance	4.5	Basketball	8.0
Playing cards	1.5	Calisthenics	4.0	Competitive soccer	10.0
Walking the dog	3.0	Tennis doubles	5.0	Rope skipping	12.0

Note: MET values can vary due to many factors, including skill level, body weight, body fat, and environmental conditions.

the American College of Sports Medicine (ACSM) and the American Heart Association (AHA) in 2007. The report recommends a minimum of 30 minutes of moderate-intensity aerobic (endurance) activity 5 days per week or 20 minutes of vigorous-intensity aerobic activity 3 days a week for all healthy adults aged 18 to 65. Moderate-intensity activity is defined as activity that noticeably accelerates the heart rate; an example is a brisk walk. Vigorous-intensity activity causes rapid breathing and a substantial increase in heart rate, as exemplified by jogging. The recommended activity is in addition to the light activities associated with daily living.[17]

Combinations of moderate-intensity activity and vigorous-intensity activity may be used to meet the recommendation. For example, you may walk briskly on a flat surface for 30 minutes 2 days a week and jog for 20 minutes 2 days a week. You can accumulate your 30 minutes per day in shorter bouts of at least 10 minutes. These are minimum recommendations; exercise levels beyond the minimum can confer additional health benefits, such as the prevention of unwanted weight gain.[17] In general, people with disabilities should follow the same recommendations as people without disabilities. The ACSM/AHA guidelines also include recommendations for improving muscular strength and endurance; we describe these recommendations later in the chapter.

If you want to combine moderate- and vigorous-intensity exercise to meet the recommendations, you can estimate your energy expenditure during exercise using a measure called a MET (metabolic equivalent). One MET represents a person's energy expenditure while sitting quietly. Activities with intensities of less than 3–4 METs are considered low intensity; activities with intensities of 3–6 METs are considered moderate intensity; and activities with intensities above 6 are considered vigorous intensity. Examples of several common physical activities classified as light, moderate, and vigorous intensity and their METs are shown in Table 8.1.

To apply this concept, let's assume you want to walk at 3 miles per hour (3.3 METs, as shown in Table 8.1) for 30 minutes on a flat surface 5 days a week to meet the minimum aerobic recommendation for health. You can determine the MET minutes of this activity as follows:

$$3.3 \times 30 \times 5 = 495 \text{ accumulated MET minutes}$$

If you chose to jog at 5 miles per hour (8 METs) for 20 minutes 3 days a week, your accumulated MET minutes would be 480 ($8 \times 20 \times 3 = 480$). If you chose to walk for 30 minutes 2 days a week and jog 20 minutes 2 days a week, your combination activity MET minutes would be 518 ($3.3 \times 30 \times 2 = 198$ plus $8 \times 20 \times 2 = 320$).

Using MET minutes for various activities allows you to combine moderate- and vigorous-intensity activities to meet or exceed the minimum goal for physical activity. The minimum goal when combining moderate and vigorous activities is in the range of 450 to 750 MET minutes per week. This recommendation is based on the MET moderate activity range of 3 to 5 for 150 minutes a week ($3 \times 150 = 450$, $5 \times 150 = 750$). If you are just beginning a physical activity program to meet this aerobic goal, start on the lower end of the MET minute range.[18]

Components of Health-Related Fitness

Fitness training programs can improve each of the components of health-related fitness—cardiorespiratory fitness, musculoskeletal fitness (muscular strength, muscular endurance, and flexibility), and body composition.

The key to fitness training is the body's ability to adapt to increasing demands by becoming more fit—that is, as a general rule, the more you exercise, the fitter you become. The amount of exercise, called *overload,* is significant, however. If you exercise too little, your fitness level won't improve. If you exercise too much, you may be susceptible to injury. When you are designing an exercise program, you need to think about four different dimensions of your exercise sessions that affect overload: frequency (number of sessions per week), intensity (level of difficulty of each exercise session), time (duration of each exercise session), and type (type of exercise in each exercise session). You can remember these dimensions with the acronym FITT.

CARDIORESPIRATORY FITNESS

cardiorespiratory fitness
Ability of the heart and lungs to efficiently deliver oxygen and nutrients to the body's muscles and cells via the bloodstream.

Cardiorespiratory fitness is the ability of the heart and lungs to efficiently deliver oxygen and nutrients to the body's muscles and cells via the bloodstream. This should be at the center of any fitness program. It is developed by activities that use the large muscles of the body in continuous movement, such as jogging, running, cycling, swimming, cross-country skiing, and aerobic dance.

Cardiorespiratory Training Benefits of cardiorespiratory training are an increase in the oxygen-carrying capacity of the blood, improved extraction of oxygen from the bloodstream by muscle cells, an increase in the amount of blood the heart pumps with each heartbeat, and increased speed of recovery back to a resting level after exercise. Cardiorespiratory training improves muscle and liver functioning and decreases resting heart rate, resting blood pressure, and heart rate at any work level. The average resting heart rate of a fit person ranges from 55 to 65 beats per minute. A person who is not fit has to work 20–30 percent harder just to meet the minimal energy needs for everyday activities.

How do you go about developing a cardiorespiratory training program to improve your level of fitness? Start by using the FITT acronym (frequency, intensity, time, and type of activity).

Frequency In general, you must exercise at least twice a week to experience improvements in cardiorespiratory functioning. The ideal frequency for training is three times per week. Interestingly, several studies have suggested that running four or five times per week provides either no greater benefits or only slightly greater benefits than running three times per week.[16] Exercising five or six times a week is appropriate if weight control is a primary concern.[19]

Intensity A certain level of vigor in exercise is necessary to condition the cardiorespiratory system, but finding the right level of intensity can be tricky. The in-between point at which you are stressing your cardiorespiratory system for optimal benefit but not overdoing it is called the **target heart rate (THR) zone.** The most accurate way to calculate your THR, the heart rate reserve method, is shown in the box "Calculating Your Target Heart Rate Zone Using the Heart Rate Reserve Method." The ACSM recommends that people set their THR at 55–90 percent of their MHR—that is, that they exercise at 55 percent to 90 percent of their maximum heart rate.

target heart rate (THR) zone
Range of exercise intensity that allows you to stress your cardiorespiratory system for optimal benefit without overloading the system.

Another way to determine your target heart rate is using the maximum heart rate formula. The formula is 220 (MHR) minus your age times your desired intensity. For example, if you are 20 and want to work out at 60–80 percent intensity, you would subtract 20 from 220 and multiply by 0.60 and 0.80. Your target heart rate zone would be 120 to 160. The Harvard Health Studies recommend a more precise maximum heart rate formula: 208 minus (0.7 × age in years) times intensity.

Time Generally, exercise sessions should last from 15 to 60 minutes; 30 minutes is a good average to aim for. Duration and intensity of exercise have an inverse relation with each other, so that a shorter, higher intensity session can give your cardiorespiratory system the same workout as a longer, lower intensity session, all other things being equal. For example, you can achieve significant cardiorespiratory improvements by exercising from 5 to 10 minutes at a 90 percent

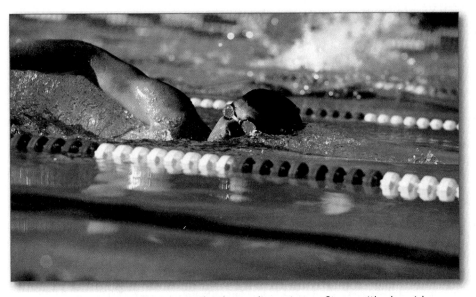
■ Swimming is an excellent way to develop cardiorespiratory fitness with a low risk of injury. Cardio training can include any form of exercise that involves continuous movement by the large muscles of the body.

THR intensity level. This practice, however, is not advisable for older adults or sedentary people. It is used primarily by those interested in elite athletic competition.[20]

Type of Activity There are two types of aerobic exercise: (1) exercises that require sustained intensity with little vari-

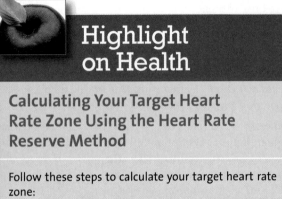

Highlight on Health

Calculating Your Target Heart Rate Zone Using the Heart Rate Reserve Method

Follow these steps to calculate your target heart rate zone:

1. To determine your resting heart rate (RHR), take your pulse at the carotid (neck) or radial (wrist) artery while you are at rest. Use your middle finger or forefinger or both when taking your pulse; do not use your thumb, since it has a pulse of its own. Take your pulse for 15 seconds and multiply by 4.

2. To determine your maximum heart rate (MHR), subtract your age from 220.

3. To determine your THR objective, use the maximal **heart rate reserve (HRR)** formula, which is considered the most accurate method. Heart rate reserve is the difference between your maximum heart rate and your resting heart rate. The THR is usually 60–80 percent for young adults and 55–70 percent for older adults. Here is the HRR formula:

> **heart rate reserve (HRR)**
> Difference between maximum heart rate and resting heart rate.

$$THR = X\% (MHR - RHR) + RHR$$

Example: Serena is 20 years old and just starting a cardiorespiratory training program. Her THR goal is 60–80 percent, and she has a resting heart rate of 70. For a 60 percent threshold, the THR would be calculated as follows:

$$0.6 (200 - 70) + 70 =$$

$$0.6 (130) + 70 = 78 + 70 = 148$$

For an 80 percent threshold, the THR would be calculated as follows:

$$0.8 (200 - 70) + 70 =$$

$$0.8 (130) + 70 = 104 + 70 = 174$$

Thus, Serena's THR is between 148 and 174.

ability in heart rate response, such as running and rowing, and (2) exercises that involve "stop and go" activities and do not maintain continuous exercise intensity, such as basketball, soccer, and tennis. Stop and go activities usually have to be done for a longer period of time than do sustained intensity activities before they confer cardiorespiratory benefits. Both types of activity can be part of a cardiorespiratory training program.

Training Progression To receive the maximum benefit from exercise, you need to adjust your level of activity by altering duration and intensity every so often. As a general rule, it takes people between the ages of 20 and 29 2 weeks to adapt to a cardiorespiratory activity workload. Older people need to add 10 percent to adaptation time for each decade after age 30. A 20-year-old, for example, can expect to adjust activity workload every 2 weeks. A 70-year-old would adjust workload about every 3 weeks (40 percent longer is about 6 days). After you have obtained a satisfactory level of cardiorespiratory fitness and are no longer interested in increasing your conditioning workload, you can maintain your fitness level by continuing the same level of workout.

Developing Your Own Program To develop your own regular cardiorespiratory training program, start out slowly to avoid injury and gradually build up your endurance. If you have any known medical conditions, or if you have been sedentary and are over the age of 40, see your physician for a checkup before starting. To ensure that you will stick with your program, select activities that you enjoy and that are compatible with the constraints of your schedule, budget, and lifestyle. Whether you choose running, swimming, cycling, a team sport, or another aerobic activity, try to build sessions of at least 30 minutes duration into your schedule three times a week. If you make these sessions part of your life, they can be the foundation of a lasting fitness program.

MUSCULAR STRENGTH AND ENDURANCE

Health-related fitness also includes muscular strength and muscular endurance. Benefits of improved muscular fitness are increased lean body mass, which helps prevent obesity; increased bone mineral density, which prevents osteoporosis; improved glucose metabolism and insulin sensitivity, which prevents diabetes; and decreased anxiety and depression, which improves quality of life.[21] Muscular fitness improves posture, prevents or reduces low back pain, enables you to perform the tasks of daily living with greater ease, and helps you to look and feel better.[22, 23]

Muscular fitness has two main components: muscular strength and muscular endurance. **Muscular strength** is the capacity of a muscle to exert force against resistance. It is primarily dependent on how much muscle mass you have. Your muscular strength is measured by how much you can lift, push, or pull in a single,

> **muscular strength**
> Capacity of a muscle to exert force against resistance.

all-out effort. **Muscular endurance** is the capacity of a muscle to exert force repeatedly over a period of time, or to apply and sustain strength for a period lasting from a few seconds to a few minutes.

muscular endurance
Capacity of a muscle to exert force repeatedly over a period of time.

Strength Training Muscular strength and endurance are developed by strength training, also known as weight training or resistance training. This is a type of exercise in which the muscles exert force against resistance, such as free weights (dumbbells, barbells) or exercise resistance machines.

Intensity and Duration: The Strength-Endurance Continuum
The same exercises develop both strength and endurance, but their intensity and duration vary. To develop strength, you need to exercise at a higher intensity (greater resistance or more weight) for a shorter duration; to develop endurance, you need to exercise at a lower intensity for a longer duration. Duration is measured in terms of repetitions—the number of times you perform the exercise (for example, lift a barbell). If you lift a heavy weight a few times (for example, 1 to 5 repetitions), you are developing strength. If you lift a lighter weight more times (for example, 20 repetitions), you are developing endurance.

Frequency and Type of Activity Two to three resistance training sessions a week are sufficient for building muscle strength and endurance. The primary muscle groups targeted in resistance training are the deltoids (shoulders), pectorals (chest), triceps (back of upper arms), biceps (front of upper arms), quadriceps (front of thighs), hamstrings (back of thighs), gluteus maximus (buttocks), and abdomen. Other areas to exercise are the upper back, the lower back, and the calves. Whether you choose free weights or weight machines, try to exercise every muscle group during your strength training sessions.

When you participate in one activity or sport to improve your performance in another, or when you use several different types of training for a specific fitness goal, you are **cross training.** For example, you might lift weights, run, and cycle on different days of the week. Two key advantages of cross training are that you avoid the boredom of participating in the same exercise every day and you reduce the risk of overuse injuries.

cross training
Participation in one sport to improve performance in another, or use of several different types of training for a specific fitness goal.

Breathing and Safety Oxygen flow is vital for preventing muscle fatigue and injury during resistance training. Inhale when your muscles are relaxed and exhale when you initiate the lifting or push-off action. Never hold your breath while performing resistance exercises.

Gender Differences in Muscle Development The amount of muscle that can be developed in the body differs by gen-

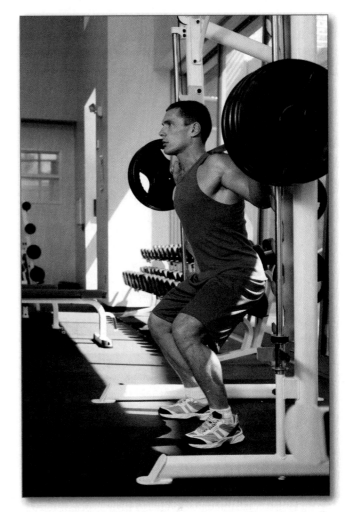

■ Muscular strength and endurance, important components of a fitness program, are developed by weight training, using either weight machines (shown here), free weights, or the weight of the body (as in calisthenics).

der. Muscle mass growth is influenced by the male sex hormone testosterone, and although women do produce this hormone, they do so at levels that are only about 10 percent of the levels seen in men. Women can increase muscle mass through strength training programs, but the increase will be less than that achieved by men.[22]

There is also a wide range of individual variability in both men and women. Regardless of gender, some people can make significantly more improvements than others can.[23] Body type (*somatotype*) plays a role in some of these differences. People with a *mesomorphic* body type (stocky, muscular) gain muscle more easily than those with an *ectomorphic* body type (tall, thin) or *endomorphic* body type (short, fat). Both men and women with mesomorphic bodies have higher levels of testosterone, and thus a greater ability to build muscle, than do those with the other two body types.

Training for Muscular Power In addition to strength training, there are many other ways of developing the physical capabilities of the body. The amount of work that can be performed in a given period of time is known as **muscular power.** Power is determined by the amount and quality of muscle; it requires great strength and the ability to

muscular power
Amount of work performed by muscles in a given period of time.

produce that strength quickly. You can train for muscular power by performing any exercise faster.

One type of exercise program developed specifically for muscular power is *plyometrics,* a program that trains muscles to reach maximum force in the shortest possible time. A muscle that is stretched before contracting will contract more forcefully and rapidly. You can experience this effect by crouching and immediately jumping. You can jump higher than if you initiate the movement from a crouched position.[24]

Core-Strength Training   Another type of training is **core-strength training,** also called *functional strength training,*

core-strength training
Strength training that conditions the body torso from the neck to the lower back.

which conditions the body torso from the neck to the lower back. The objectives of core-strength training are to lengthen the spine, develop balance, reduce the waistline, prevent back injury, and sculpt the body without bulking it up. Scientific evidence in support of these claims is

sparse. Exercise experts, however, argue that training programs increase muscle mass, and metabolic expenditure provides health benefits.[25]

Probably the most popular core-body training program being taught in health clubs today is Pilates ("pi-**lah**-teez"), an exercise system developed in the 1920s by physical trainer Joseph Pilates. The exercises, performed on special apparatus, are based on the premise that the body's "powerhouse" is in the torso, particularly the abdomen. Exercises are taught by trained instructors and are tailored to the individual.

Many other core-body training programs are currently popular. Remember to use your critical thinking skills when investigating any commercial product, whether an exercise system, a particular type of equipment, or a health club.

Gaining Weight and Muscle Mass Safely   When people want to gain weight it is usually to improve appearance, health, or performance. Gaining weight simply by eating more is not a productive strategy, because the weight gain will be nearly all fat. The goal is to increase muscle tissue with little or no increase in body fat stores. The healthy way to attain such a gain is through physical activity, particularly strength training, combined with a high-calorie diet. Some people, especially athletes, attempt to gain muscle tissue by using drugs, dietary supplements, or protein supplements. Most of these substances are expensive and ineffective; some are dangerous, and some are illegal.

Drugs and Dietary Supplements   People who use performance-enhancing drugs and dietary supplements may enhance their athletic performance by building bigger

muscles, but they also may be heading for health problems that can shorten their lives. Unfortunately, any discussion of the risks and benefits of these substances is clouded by a lack of scientific data. Scientists often don't know who is using them, what the effects of different doses are, how long they can be taken before causing side effects, or what happens when they are taken with other drugs.[26] An overview of some of the major performance-enhancing drugs and dietary supplements, along with their possible benefits and side effects, is shown in Table 8.2.

Protein Supplements   The sports and fitness industry is experiencing a boom in protein supplements.[27] The protein in these products is from natural protein sources, such as soy, eggs, milk, or chicken. Other substances, such as purified amino acids, are often added. Commercial protein supplements are expensive and do not carry all the nutrients of natural fuels. They can serve as a convenient adjunct to a balanced diet for people who are too busy to obtain enough protein in their diet, but most Americans, including athletes, get more than enough protein their diets.

Training Programs for Weight Gain   The best way to gain muscle tissue, as noted earlier, is through a weight training program combined with a high-calorie diet. Gaining a pound of muscle and fat requires consuming about 3,000 extra calories.[28] To build muscle, you need to consume 700–1,000 calories a day above energy needs or take in sufficient calories to support both the added activity energy requirements and the formation of new muscle.[27] A gain of a half pound to a pound a week is a reasonable goal. Your primary exercise activity to gain muscle should be weight training.

Developing a Strength Training Program   Besides their recommendations for aerobic exercise, the ACSM and AHA also issue guidelines for a strength training program. They recommend doing strength training 2 to 3 nonconsecutive days a week, performing 8 to 10 exercises (working all the major muscle groups), and using sufficient resistance to fatigue the muscles. Do one or more sets of 8 to 12 repetitions for each exercise. When you can do three sets of 12 repetitions, increase the weight.

Strength training can be a safe and effective form of exercise if appropriate guidelines are followed:

- Warm up by gently stretching, jogging, or lifting light weights.

- Do not hold your breath or hyperventilate. As you are lifting, breathe rhythmically.

- To protect your back, hold weights close to your body. Do not arch your back. Weight belts may prevent arching.

- When using resistance training machines, always check to make sure the pins holding weights are in place. When using free weights, make sure collars are tight.

- Lift weights with a slow, steady cadence through a full range of motion. Do not jerk the weight to complete a repetition.

Table 8.2 | Selected Performance-Enhancing Drugs and Dietary Supplements and Their Effects

Substance or Dietary Supplement	Effects	Side Effects
Anabolic steroid, testosterone	Promotes muscle growth by improving ability of muscle to respond to training and improving recovery.	Masculinization of females; feminization of males; acne; mood swings; sexual dysfunction.
Human growth hormone	Promotes muscle growth.	Widened jaw line and nose, protruding eyebrows, buck teeth; increased risk of high blood pressure, congestive heart failure.
Ephedrine	Boosts energy, promotes weight loss (stimulates metabolism).	High blood pressure; irregular heartbeat; increased risk of stroke and heart attack.
Androstenedione (Andro)	Promotes muscle growth.	Decreased good cholesterol (HDL); increased levels of estrogen, promotes breast enlargement in men; increased risk of pancreatic cancer; may significantly increase testosterone levels in women (little known about Andro effects in women).
Dehydroepiandrosterone (DHEA)	May promote muscle growth.	Body hair growth; liver enlargement; aggressive behavior; long-term health effects not known.
Creatine monohydrate	May increase performance in brief high-intensity exercises; promotes increased body mass when used with resistance training.	Diarrhea; dehydration and muscle cramping; muscle tearing; long-term health effects not known.
Chromium picolinate	May build muscle tissue, facilitate burning of fat, and boost energy.	Chromium buildup with large doses and possible liver damage and other health problems; long-term health effects not known.

Sources: "The Physiological and Health Effects of Oral Creatine Supplementation," American College of Sports Medicine, 2000, Medicine and Science in Sports and Exercise, 32, pp. 706–717; "Dietary Supplements and the Promotion of Muscle With Resistance Exercise," by R.B. Kreider, 1999, Sports Medicine, 27, pp. 97–110; "How Effective Is Creatine?" by C. Nelson, 1998, Sport Medicine Digest, 73, pp. 73–81; The Ergogenic Edge: Pushing the Limits of Sports Performance, by M.H. Williams, 1998, Champaign, IL: Human Kinetics.

- Always use a spotter when working out with free weights.
- Allow at least 48 hours between training sessions if you will be exercising the same muscle groups.

If you join a health or fitness center, it will probably offer an orientation session to introduce you to the equipment, programs, and staff. These facilities usually employ fitness professionals who are certified and work as personal trainers. Many personal trainers work independently as well. Personal trainers can help you assess your current fitness, set realistic goals, and develop a safe and effective strength training program.

FLEXIBILITY

Another important component of musculoskeletal fitness is **flexibility,** the ability of joints to move through their full range of motion. Good flexibility helps you maintain posture and balance, makes movement easier and more fluid, and lowers your risk of injury. It is a key factor in preventing low back pain and injury.

Flexibility is affected by factors that you cannot change, such as genetic endowment, gender, and age, and by factors that you can change, such as physical activity patterns. A common misconception is that flexibility declines steadily once a person reaches adulthood. Flexibility does seem to be highest in the teenage years, and aging is accompanied by a shortening of tendons and an increased rigidity in muscles and joints. However, there is also strong evidence that much of the loss of flexibility that results from aging can be reduced by stretching programs.[20]

flexibility
Ability of joints to move through their full range of motion.

Types of Stretching Programs Medical and fitness experts agree that stretching the muscles attached to the joints is the single most important part of an exercise program designed to promote flexibility, reduce muscle tension, and prevent injuries. However, stretching done incorrectly can cause more harm than good. Thus, understanding the right stretching techniques and progressing gradually are keys to a successful program.

In *passive stretching,* a partner applies pressure to your muscles, typically producing a stretch beyond what you can do on your own. If you can totally relax your muscle fibers, the use of pressure by another person can help prevent the problem of partial contraction of muscle fibers. Passive stretching is often used by physical therapists. There is a danger, however, of forcing a stretch beyond the point of normal relaxation of the muscles and tendons, causing tearing and injury. For this reason, passive stretching should be limited to supervised medical situations and persons who cannot move by themselves.[29]

In *static stretching,* you stretch until you feel tightness in the muscle and then hold that position for a set period of time without bouncing or forcing movement. After you have held the stretch for 30 to 60 seconds, the muscle tension will seem to decrease, and you can stretch farther without pain. Static stretching lengthens the muscle and surrounding tissue, reducing the risk of injury. Static stretching is the kind of stretching done in hatha yoga and is the type recommended for general fitness purposes.

In *ballistic stretching,* the muscle is stretched in a series of bouncing movements designed to increase the range of motion. As you bounce, receptors in the muscles, called *muscle spindles,* are stretched. Ballistic stretching is used by experienced athletes, but because it can increase vulnerability to muscle pulls and tears, it is not recommended for most people.

Proprioceptive neuromuscular facilitation (PNF) is a therapeutic exercise that causes a stretch reflex in muscles. It is used primarily in the rehabilitation of injured muscles.[30]

Developing Your Own Flexibility Program   The ACSM recommends that stretching exercise be done for all the major joints, including the neck, shoulders, upper back and trunk, hips, knees, and ankles. Stretching should be done a minimum of 2 to 3 days a week and ideally 5 to 7 days a week. Stretch to a point of mild discomfort (not pain) and hold the stretch for 15 to 30 seconds. Do two to four repetitions of each stretch.

Stretching can be part of your warm-up for your cardio-respiratory or resistance training program as long as these stretches are gentle, slow, and steady. To prevent injury, warm up first with 5 to 10 minutes of brisk walking, marching in place, or calisthenics. This warm-up will increase your heart rate, raise your core body temperature, and lubricate your joints. You will experience the greatest improvement in flexibility, however, if you do your stretching exercises after your other exercise, when your muscles are warm and less likely to be injured by stretching.

BODY COMPOSITION

The final component of health-related fitness we consider here is **body composition**—the relative amounts of fat and fat-free mass in the body. Fat-free mass includes muscle, bone, water, body organs, and other body tissues. Body fat includes both fat that is essential for normal functioning, such as fat in the nerves, heart, and liver, and fat stored in fat cells, usually located under the skin and around organs. The recommended proportion of body fat to fat-free mass, expressed as *percent body fat,* is 21–35 percent for women and 8–24 percent for men.

body composition
Relative amounts of fat and fat-free mass in the body.

The relative amount of body fat has an effect on overall health and fitness. Too much body fat is associated with overweight and obesity and with a higher risk for chronic diseases like heart disease, diabetes, and many types of cancer. A greater amount of fat-free mass, on the other hand, gives the body a lean, healthy appearance. The heart and lungs function more efficiently without the burden of extra weight. Because muscle tissue uses energy at a higher metabolic rate than does fat tissue, the more muscle mass you have, the more calories you can consume without gaining weight.

We discuss body composition in more detail in Chapter 9 on body weight. Here, the basic message is that you can control body weight, trim body fat, and build muscle tissue by incorporating more physi-

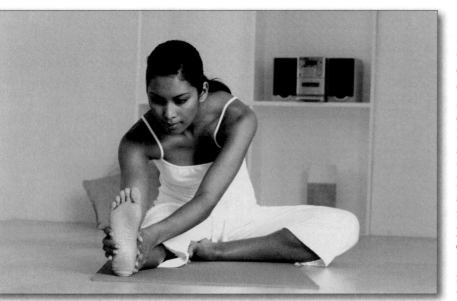

■ Developing flexibility through stretching exercises should be part of a regular fitness program. Stretching is most beneficial and effective when the muscles are warm, as they are after a workout.

Table 8.3	Summary of Physical Activity Recommendations for Adults	
Aerobic (Endurance) Activity	30 minutes of moderate-intensity aerobic activity 5 days per week. OR 20 minutes of vigorous-intensity aerobic activity 3 days per week. OR A combination of moderate- and vigorous-intensity physical activity that meets the recommendation.
Muscle-Strengthening Activity	8 to 10 exercises that stress the major muscle groups on 2 or more nonconsecutive days per week. Do one or more sets of 8 to 12 repetitions for each exercise using sufficient resistance to fatigue the muscles.
Flexibility	Stretching exercise for all major joints, at least 2 to 3 days per week, ideally 5 to 7 days per week. Stretch to the point of tension, hold for 15 to 30 seconds, and repeat 2 to 4 times.
Weight Management	To prevent unhealthy weight gain, 60 minutes of moderate- to vigorous-intensity physical activity most days of the week. To sustain weight loss, 60 to 90 minutes of moderate-intensity physical activity every day of the week.

Sources: Adapted from "Physical Activity and Public Health: Updated Recommendations for Adults from the American College of Sports Medicine and the American Heart Association," by W.L. Haskell et al., 2007, Medicine & Science in Sports & Exercise, 39, pp. 1423–1434; Dietary Guidelines for Americans, 2005, USDA and USDHHS, 2005, retrieved April 10, 2008, www.health.gov/dietaryguideline; ACSM's Guidelines for Exercise Testing and Prescription, American College of Sports Medicine, 2006, Philadelphia: Lippincot Williams and Wilkins.

cal activity into your daily life. Use the stairs rather than taking the elevator, walk or ride your bike rather than driving, and if you drive, park your car at the far end of the parking lot.

Beyond such simple steps to increase physical activity, plan to incorporate regular exercise into your life as well. According to the 2005 *Dietary Guidelines for Americans* and the National Academies' Institute of Medicine, prevention of unhealthy weight gain requires about 60 minutes of moderate- to vigorous-intensity activity on most days of the week. Adults who have lost substantial amounts of weight need 60 to 90 minutes of moderate-intensity physical activity daily in order to maintain the weight loss.[17, 31] If you work toward these goals, you will see improvements not only in your body composition but also in many other areas of your life.

For a summary of physical activity recommendations for adults, see Table 8.3.

Improving Your Health Through Moderate Physical Activity

As noted earlier, exercise does not have to be vigorous to provide health benefits. There are many simple, easy, and enjoyable ways to use physical activity to obtain health benefits.

MAKING DAILY ACTIVITIES MORE ACTIVE

How do you spend most of your time? To find out exactly, use a personal time sheet to record all of your activities on a typical day. The more specific you can be, the better. At the end of the day, add up the minutes you spent being active (walking to class, for example) and the minutes you spent being inactive (watching television, driving, and so on).

After determining your time spent in activity versus inactivity, look at the sedentary activities in your day. How can you make them more active? Try getting up to change the TV channel instead of using the remote, or walk around, stretch, or do sit-ups during commercials. Ride your bike to class instead of taking the bus, take the stairs instead of the elevator at the library, or walk around while checking your cell phone messages.

You can also turn light activity into moderate activity by cranking up the intensity. For example, when you are standing in line, stretch or do isometric exercises (such as contracting and relaxing your abdominal muscles). Increase your pace while cycling, walk briskly instead of strolling, take the stairs two at a time.

Why is it important to move from light to moderate activities? Consider that an order of french fries contains about 400 calories. If you are sitting and watching television, it will take you 308 minutes, or more than 5 hours, to use up that many calories. If you are walking briskly or jogging slowly, it will take you about an hour.

WALKING FOR FITNESS

Walking is the most popular physical activity in North America,[32] and it has many health benefits. Results from the Harvard Nurses' Health Study indicate that women who walk 1 hour a week have half the risk of cardiovascular disease experienced by those who are sedentary. Women who do moderate or vigorous physical activity at least 4 hours a week reduce their risk of premature death by 25–35 percent.[33] Thus,

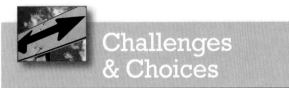

Challenges & Choices

Walking for Fitness

If you have been completely sedentary, begin a walking program with 10 minutes of walking a day. Gradually work up to 30 minutes a day, most days of the week. If you want to lose weight by walking, you will need to walk from 45 to 60 minutes a day, most days of the week. To improve your cardiovascular functioning, walk briskly (at a pace of 4–4.5 mph). In urban areas, a general rule of thumb is to count 12 average city blocks as 1 mile. If you are counting your steps, 80 steps a minute is considered a leisurely pace, 100 steps a minute is considered a brisk pace, and 120 steps a minute is considered a fast pace. The following are some guidelines for getting the most out of walking:

- Schedule your daily walk as you would an appointment. Plan it for a time of day when you're most likely to make it a permanent habit.

- Increase your walking time gradually. Don't increase duration by more than 10–20 percent a week.

- After you have walked for a couple of weeks, focus on quicker steps. As you do so, bend your arms 90 degrees at the elbow and move them when you walk. Moving your arms increases your caloric expenditure.

- Stretch at the end of your walk or after warming up. Adding 4 minutes of stretching to your daily walk can have a beneficial effect on your muscles, joints, and bones.

- Don't ignore or exercise through pain. If the pain is severe, see a physician. Pain that is not serious should be treated by rest, ice, compression, and elevation; massage may also help. Discontinue walking up or down hills if doing so causes pain.

It's Not Just Personal . . .

Although walking can be done by almost anyone almost anywhere, studies have shown that people walk more if there is a park, trail, school track, or other facility nearby. They also walk more if they have a destination, such as a hardware store or grocery store, within walking distance. Some experts argue that more businesses and recreational facilities need to be located in residential areas to encourage people to make walking trips from home.

as with other activity, increasing the pace and/or duration of walking results in greater health benefits. For tips on walking, see the box "Walking for Fitness."

Experts at the Shape Up America! program found that people could control their weight if they walked 10,000 steps each day.[34] Walking 10,000 steps (about 5 miles) expends between 300 and 400 calories, depending on body size and walking speed—well above the recommended 150 calories a day. Walking 10,000 steps a day 5 days a week expends the optimal 2,000 calories per week recommended for preventing premature death.

You can count your steps with a pedometer, a pager-sized device worn on the belt or waistband centered over the hipbone. Pedometers that convert activities into calories expended are not accurate, because they do not factor in activity intensity.

If you are interested in counting your steps, first determine how many steps you typically take each day. Record the number of steps you take every day for 7 days. Most inactive people take between 2,000 and 4,000 steps a day. Then, to set a reasonable goal, plan to increase this number by about 500 steps at a time. If you typically take 5,000 steps a day, set a

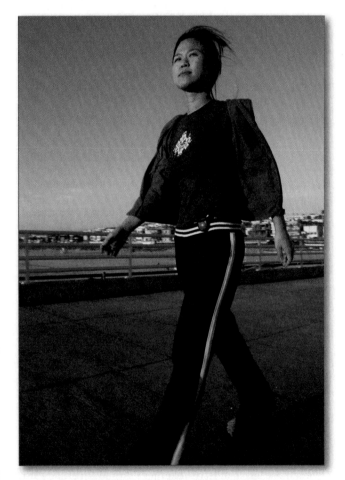

■ Counting steps with a pedometer is one way to move toward fitness. Walking 10,000 steps a day confers health benefits and helps people control their weight.

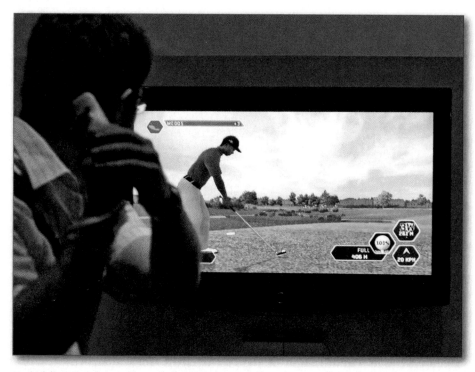

■ A visitor at an interactive entertainment convention plays a golf simulation game on a Nintendo Wii console. Exercise gaming is the latest in consumer-oriented approaches to fitness.

ness-oriented video games. The game Kung Fu allows the player to execute kung fu movements to battle animated fighters. A tiny video camera captures the player's every move. The Nintendo Wii lets players make the moves involved in various recreational activities and sports. Some fitness clubs have incorporated Wii workout stations into circuit training programs. Users punch, run, and jump with the station's movement-sensation controller. During one 30-minute workout, the user can expend 75 to 125 calories.

Many health experts welcome this new generation of video games as a positive step by the "sedentary entertainment industry." The games do have their downside, though. They can be expensive, they may limit social interaction, and they may send a message that being fit requires technology. Fitness video games should not be considered a substitute for active outdoor play and physical activity. They can best be viewed as part of an overall strategy to encourage children, teens, and adults to become more active.[3, 6]

goal of 5,500 steps. Once you achieve 5,500 steps, raise your goal by 500 steps, and continue until you reach 10,000 steps.[35] This is an easy and painless way to add physical activity to your day and to move from light to moderate activity levels.

TAKING THE STAIRS

Climbing stairs is an excellent activity for improving leg strength, balance, and fitness. Stair climbing is twice as taxing to your heart and lungs as brisk walking on a level surface. A Harvard Health Alumni study found that men who climb an average of eight flights of stairs a day experience 33 percent lower mortality than men who are sedentary. Always make sure the stairs are safe before taking them, though.[33, 36]

If you have access to stair-climbing machines at your fitness center, they also provide a good workout. Dual-action climbers exercise your legs, arms, and heart. This equipment provides a moderate- to high-intensity workout with low impact on your joints. An elliptical trainer is a cross between a bicycle, a stair-climber, and a cross-country skiing machine; as one foot moves forward and up, the other foot moves down and back. You also move your arms against resistance. More elaborate elliptical machines allow you to pedal backward against resistance to work on buttock muscles.[36] If you don't have access to exercise machines, just take the stairs.

EXERCISE GAMING

A recent trend in the video game industry is the development of games that include physical activity (see, for example, eyetoy.com and reebok.com). Dance Dance Revolution, introduced in 2001, spurred the development of more fit-

Special Considerations in Exercise and Physical Activity

Special considerations have to be taken into account to ensure health and safety in exercise and physical activity, to accommodate the effects of certain environmental conditions, and to make exercise appropriate for particular populations.

HEALTH AND SAFETY PRECAUTIONS

Injuries and illness associated with exercise and physical activity are usually the result of either excessive exercise or improper techniques. In this section we look at several considerations related to health and safety:

Warm-Up and Cool-Down Proper warm-up before exercise helps to maximize the benefits of a workout and minimize the potential for injuries. Muscles contract more efficiently and more safely when they have been properly warmed up.

Suggested warm-up activities include light calisthenics, walking or slow jogging, and gentle stretching of the specific muscles to be used in the activity. You can also do a low-intensity version of the activity you are about to engage in, such as hitting tennis balls against a wall before a match. Your warm-up should last from 5 to 10 minutes.

Consumer Clipboard

Running Shoe Prescription

More than 30 million runners develop injuries each year; 20–30 percent of these injuries require medical care. Proper shoe selection and maintenance can reduce running-related injuries by as much as 56 percent.

Shoe Selection

■ Buy shoes from a running specialty store or reputable Internet vendor to guarantee a high-quality shoe. Running magazines typically provide a list of specialty stores.

■ Feet swell by the end of the day, so have your shoes fitted in the evening. Make sure there is one-half inch between your longest toe and the end of the shoe toe. Wear running socks when trying on the shoes and insert orthotics if you use these devices.

■ Buy two pairs of running shoes. Running shoes need to be replaced after about 400–600 miles. Switching shoes each run can extend the life expectancy of the midsoles for both pairs of shoes.

■ Ask the store to allow you to run in the shoes for a short distance before buying. Select your shoes by fit, not by the size on the shoe box. Most runners use running shoes that are two sizes larger than their street shoes. Women's shoes are usually narrower than men's shoes, and the heel is slightly smaller, but about

25 percent of women runners have feet that conform more comfortably to the shape of men's shoes.

■ Look at your old exercise shoes. If there are wear spots on the forefoot and you experience knee pain, you may need running shoes with anti-pronation capabilities (that is, they keep your foot from turning in or out). If the wear pattern is on the outside of the forefoot, you can probably select a neutral shoe that has adequate cushioning and flexibility. It is important to have a shoe that feels natural on the foot while you are running.

Shoe Care

■ Use your shoes only for running to preserve the motion control and cushioning of your shoes.

■ Untie your shoes before taking them off. Kicking off tied shoes can damage the heel counter.

■ Do not run in wet shoes; a wet midsole has 40–50 percent less shock-absorbing capability. Let wet shoes dry naturally. Excessive heat will degrade shoe components.

■ Never wash your shoes in the washing machine; it destroys the shoe shape.

■ Running shoes lose 30–50 percent of their shock-absorbing capability after about 250 miles of use. Unused shoes sitting on the shelf will lose a significant amount of shock-absorbing capability after 1 to 2 years.

Sources: "What Every Runner Should Know About Shoes," 2005, Physician and Sports Medicine, 33 (1), pp. 23–24; Running: Getting Started, by J. Galloway, 2005, United Kingdom: Meyer & Meyer Sport.

A minimum of 5 to 10 minutes should also be devoted to cool-down, depending on environmental conditions and the intensity of the exercise program. Pooling of blood in the extremities may temporarily disrupt or reduce the return of blood to the heart, momentarily depriving your heart and brain of oxygen. Fainting or even a coronary abnormality may result. If you continue the activity at a lower intensity, the blood vessels gradually return to their normal smaller diameter.

Walking, mimicking the exercise at a slower pace, and stretching while walking are all excellent cool-down activities. Never sit down, stand in a stationary position, or take a hot shower or sauna immediately after vigorous exercise.

Fatigue and Overexertion   Fatigue is generally defined as an inability to continue exercising at a desired level of intensity. The cause of fatigue may be psychological—for example, depression can cause feelings of fatigue—or physiological, as when you work out too long or too hard, do an activity you're not used to, or become overheated or dehydrated. Sometimes fatigue occurs because the body cannot

produce enough energy to meet the demands of the activity. In this case, consuming enough complex carbohydrates to replenish the muscle stores of glycogen may solve the problem. Athletes need to eat a high-carbohydrate diet to make sure they have enough reserve energy for their sport.[37]

Overexertion occurs when an exercise session has been too intense. Warning signs of overexertion include (1) pain or pressure in the left or midchest area, jaw, neck, left shoulder, or left arm during or just after exercise; (2) sudden nausea, dizziness, cold sweat, fainting, or pallor (pale, ashen skin); and (3) abnormal heartbeats, such as fluttering, rapid heartbeats or a rapid pulse rate immediately followed by a very slow pulse rate. These symptoms are similar to signs of a heart attack. If you experience any of these symptoms, consult a physician before exercising again.

Soft Tissue Injury   Injuries to soft tissue (muscles and joints) include tears, sprains, strains, and contusions; they usually result from a specific activity incident, such as a bicycle crash. Some injuries, known as overuse injuries, are caused by the cumulative effects of motions repeated many

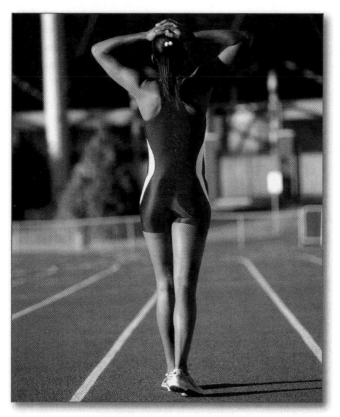

■ Cooling down after vigorous exercise gives the cardiovascular system time to return to normal. Cool down by walking or continuing your exercise activity at a much lower intensity.

times. Tendinitis and bursitis are examples of overuse injuries. (For tips on preventing running-related injuries, see the box "Running Shoe Prescription.")

Soft tissue injuries should be treated according to the R-I-C-E principle: rest, ice, compression, and elevation. Immediately stop doing the activity, apply ice to the affected area to reduce swelling and pain, compress it with an elastic bandage to reduce swelling, and elevate it to reduce blood flow to the area. Do not apply heat until all swelling has disappeared. When you no longer feel pain in the area, you can gradually begin to exercise again. Don't return to your full exercise program until your injury is completely healed.

EFFECTS OF ENVIRONMENTAL CONDITIONS ON EXERCISE AND PHYSICAL ACTIVITY

Certain environmental conditions require adjustment of physical activity and exercise workload. Environmental conditions of particular concern are altitude, heat and cold, and air pollution.

Altitude Traveling too quickly to elevations above 6,000–8,000 feet causes altitude sickness, or acute mountain sickness (AMS), in about 7 percent of men and 22 percent of women.[38] Symptoms of AMS include cough, headache, difficulty breathing, rapid heartbeat, general malaise, weakness and nausea, loss of appetite, and difficulty sleeping. These symp-

toms occur as the body adjusts to the lower oxygen content of the air, which probably results in accumulation of carbon dioxide in body tissues and leakage of fluids into the brain. It is not clear why men and women are affected differently.

If you are going to be in a situation that puts you at risk for AMS, the best prevention strategy, besides acclimation over a period of 1 to 2 weeks, is adjustment of physical activity workload and nutrition.[39] Your initial activity should be less intense and shorter in duration than your activity at lower altitudes. To prevent dehydration, increase your fluid intake from water, instant fruit drinks, reconstituted powdered milk, hot chocolate, and soup. To prevent glycogen depletion, eat small, frequent meals, and consume at least 60 percent of your calories from carbohydrates, since they are better tolerated than fat is at higher altitudes.[37]

Heat and Cold Heat disorders can be caused by impaired regulation of internal core temperature, loss of body fluids, and loss of electrolytes (Table 8.4).[27] Two strategies for preventing excessive increases in body temperature are skin wetting and hyperhydration. Skin wetting involves sponging or spraying the head or body with cold water. This strategy cools the skin but has not been shown to effectively decrease core body temperature.[27]

Hyperhydration is taking in extra fluids shortly before participating in physical activity in a hot environment.[40] This practice is recommended by the ACSM and may improve cardiovascular function and temperature regulation during physical activity in conditions of excessive heat.[41]

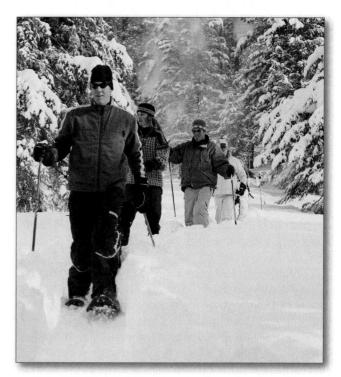

■ High altitude and cold weather are two environmental conditions that affect your ability to follow your usual exercise routine. Adjusting activity load, nutrition, hydration, and clothing are recommended as sensible adaptations.

Table 8.4 | Heat-Related Disorders

Heat Disorder	Cause	Symptoms	Treatment
Heat cramps	Excessive loss of electrolytes in sweat; inadequate salt intake.	Muscle cramps.	Rest in cool environment; drink fluids; ingest salty food and drinks; get medical treatment if severe.
Heat exhaustion	Excessive loss of electrolytes in sweat; inadequate salt and/or fluid intake.	Fatigue; nausea; dizziness; cool, pale skin; sweating; elevated temperature.	Rest in cool environment; drink cool fluids; cool body with water; get medical treatment if severe.
Heat stroke	Excessive body temperature.	Headache; vomiting; hot, flushed skin (dry or sweaty); elevated temperature; disorientation; unconsciousness.	Cool body with ice or cold water; give cool drinks with sugar if conscious; get medical help immediately.

Source: Adapted from Nutrition for Health, Fitness and Sport, 7th ed., by M.H. Williams, 2007, New York: McGraw-Hill.

If you are going to be exercising in very hot conditions, you can hyperhydrate by drinking a pint of water (16 ounces) when you get up in the morning, another pint 1 hour before your activity, and a final pint 15 to 30 minutes before exercising. Plan to consume from 4 to 8 ounces of fluid every 15 minutes during your exercise. After exercise, consume 24 ounces of water for every pint you lose.[27]

Water intoxication (hyponatremia) may be a problem for people who hydrate too much before exercising. Excess water causes an electrolyte imbalance and tissue swelling, which can result in irregular heartbeat, fluids entering the lungs, and pressure on the brain and nerves. If not treated, seizures, coma, and death may result. Treatment includes restricting water intake and administering a salt solution. The adult kidney can handle about 15 liters of fluid intake a day, so water intoxication is rare.[42]

Exercising in excessive cold also puts a strain on the body. Symptoms of **hypothermia** (dangerously low body temperature) include shivering, feelings of euphoria, and disorientation.[41] Core body temperature influences how severe these symptoms are and whether the hypothermia is considered mild, moderate, or severe. To stay warm, dress in several thin layers of clothes and wear a hat and mittens. If cold air bothers your throat, breathe through a scarf.

hypothermia
Low body temperature, a life-threatening condition.

Many people do not take in sufficient fluid when exercising outside during the winter. Fluid losses during the winter can be very high, since cold, dry air requires the body to humidify and warm the air, resulting in the loss of significant amounts of water. An effective strategy is to consume needed fluids 1.5 to 2 hours before exercising and to drink more fluids just before exercising.

Air Pollution   If you live and exercise in a large city, air pollution can be a concern. Pollution can have an irritating effect on the airways leading to your lungs,[43] causing coughing, wheezing, and shortness of breath. To minimize the effect of air pollution, exercise early in the morning before motor vehicle pollution has its greatest impact. If possible, exercise in areas with less motor vehicle traffic, such as parks. Pay attention to smog alerts, and move your exercise indoors when air pollution is severe.

EXERCISE FOR SPECIAL POPULATIONS

In this section we look briefly at special exercise considerations for children and adolescents, people with disabilities, and older adults.

Exercise for Children and Adolescents   To obtain the direct and indirect health benefits of fitness, children should get 60 minutes of exercise a day. Children have smaller hearts and lungs and less blood volumes than adults, so they should not be expected to perform physically like adults.[44] The cardiovascular system does not fully mature until late in the teen years. This means that children's hearts deliver less oxygen to working muscles. The musculoskeletal and reproductive systems are rapidly maturing and are vulnerable to lifelong damage.[44] Children are also more vulnerable to overheating than adults, so they need to be properly hydrated.

A serious concern is the incidence of sudden death in adolescents engaged in strenuous physical activities and competitive sports programs. About 12 young athletes die each year from heart disease while participating in vigorous sports.[45] Most of these deaths are thought to be caused by congenital heart defects, such as an abnormally enlarged heart, that go undetected until an incident occurs. (See Chapter 2 for more on sudden death in young athletes.) Health insurance companies usually will not cover sophisticated screening for heart defects for children, since the tests have not proven to be cost effective.[45]

New guidelines issued by the American Heart Association (AHA) urge parents, coaches, and physicians to be vigilant for symptoms that may indicate a heart defect.[45] These symptoms include fainting episodes, sudden chest pain during exercise or at rest, high blood pressure, and irregular or high heart rate at rest or during exercise. The AHA also recommends that a family history of heart disease or unexplained death be considered in evaluating whether children should be involved in vigorous physical activity.[45]

Exercise for Persons With Disabilities Physical activity and exercise are especially beneficial for persons with disabilities and chronic health problems. Immobility or inactivity may aggravate the original disability and increase the risk for secondary health problems, such as heart disease, osteoporosis, arthritis, and diabetes. The ACSM stresses the importance of physical activity for people with disabilities for two reasons: (1) to counteract the detrimental effects of bed rest and sedentary living patterns and (2) to maintain optimal functioning of body organs or systems.[11]

Not too long ago, regular physical activity was missing in the lives of many people with disabilities.[46] The reasons for this absence included lack of knowledge about the importance of physical activity, limited access to recreation sites and difficulty with transportation, a low level of interest, and the lack of exercise facilities and resources designed to accommodate people with disabilities.

Laws have strengthened the rights of persons with disabilities and fostered their inclusion in programs and facilities providing physical activity opportunities. Increased visibility and positive images of people with disabilities engaging in physical activity, such as in the Special Olympics and wheelchair basketball, have also helped raise awareness.[46]

Exercise for Older Adults When the ACSM and AHA issued their physical activity recommendations for adults in 2007, they also issued a companion report with recommendations for older adults—men and women aged 65 or older and adults aged 50 to 64 with clinically significant chronic conditions and/or functional limitations.[47] Older adults are the least physically active of any age group and generate the highest medical costs. The report states that by following the recommendations, older adults can reduce the risk of chronic disease, premature death, functional limitations, and disabilities.

The aerobic activity recommendations for older adults are the same as for adults, but the recommended intensity of aerobic activity takes into account the wide variation in aerobic fitness among older adults. Intensity of activity is gauged on a 10-point scale of perceived exertion, with sitting at 0 and all-out effort at 10. Moderate-intensity activity, which produces noticeable increases in heart rate and breathing is a 5 or 6 on this scale. Vigorous-intensity activity, which produces large increases in heart rate and breathing, is a 7 or 8.

Exercises to develop muscular strength and endurance are also recommended. They should be performed on 2 or more nonconsecutive days of the week, focusing on 8 to 10 exercises for the major muscle groups and using a weight that allows 10 to 15 repetitions for each exercise. Unlike the recommendations for adults, the recommendations for older adults include flexibility exercises, performed at least 2 days per week for at least 10 minutes. For those

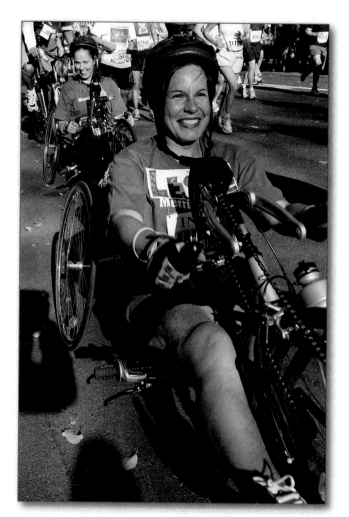

■ Having a disability does not mean a person can't exercise or be fit. Exercise counters the effects of immobility and inactivity, improves all body functions, and enhances self-esteem for individuals with disabilities as well as for people in the general population.

older adults at risk for falls, exercises that maintain or improve balance should also be performed 2 days per week.

Physical activity is an effective antidote to many of the effects of aging.[47, 48] It is never too late to become more active. The ACSM has concluded that older adults generally respond to increased physical activity and receive health and fitness benefits similar to those of young adults.[20] These benefits include improvements in cardiorespiratory endurance, lean body mass, muscular strength and endurance, flexibility, balance, postural stability, motor agility, and mental and psychological functioning.

Physical Activity for Life

The most significant drop in physical activity occurs in the last few years of high school and the first year of college.[3] The decline accelerates again after college graduation. In young adulthood 40 percent of men and 30 percent of women continue to participate in various physical

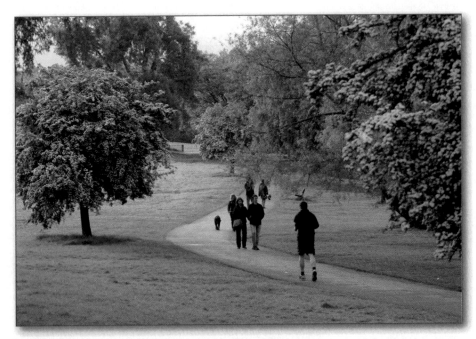

■ When communities provide spaces for physical activity and improve access to those spaces, people respond by becoming more active. Thus, public policy and community planning play important roles in the physical fitness of community members.

activities.[1] Certain key factors help people make physical activity a lifetime pursuit. In this section we consider two of them—commitment to change and social and community support.

MAKING A COMMITMENT TO CHANGE

Let's consider exercise in terms of the Transtheoretical Model (refer to Chapter 1 for an explanation of this stages of change model). In the precontemplation and contemplation stages, the biggest challenges for most people are barriers to exercise.[49] Common barriers to active lifestyles cited by adults are inconvenience, lack of self-motivation, lack of time, fear of injury, the perception that exercise is boring, lack of social support, and lack of confidence in one's ability to be physically active. (To find out what your barriers are, see the Add It Up feature for Chapter 8 at the end of the book.) If you are in the precontemplation or contemplation stage and feel overwhelmed by these or other barriers, see the box "Strategies for Overcoming Barriers to Physical Activity."

In the preparation stage, self-assessment is critical. Ask yourself these four questions: (1) What physical activities do I enjoy? (2) What are the best days and times for me to participate in physical activities? (3) Where is the best place to pursue these activities? and (4) Do I have friends and/or family members who can join in my physical activities? In making specific preparations, you need to take into account your current level of fitness and your previous experiences in various physical activities. This information about yourself will help you develop an exercise program that you can commit to and maintain.

In the action stage, a key component is goal setting. Your goals should be based on the benefits of physical activity, but they should also be specific and reasonable. Achievable and sustainable goals are essential for exercise compliance. Include both short-term and long-term goals in your plan, and devise ways to measure your progress. Build in rewards along the way.

When you have been physically active almost every day for at least 6 months, you are in the maintenance stage. One key to maintaining an active lifestyle is believing that your commitment to physical activity can make a difference in your life. People who establish a personal stake in physical activity are more likely to maintain an active lifestyle. When exercise has become entrenched as a lifelong behavior—when it's as much a part of your day as eating and sleeping—you are in the termination stage.

Which stage are you in right now? If you are in an early stage, you probably do not have sufficient commitment to follow through on an exercise plan. To make any change, you must want to change. Work on overcoming barriers and gaining more information about the health benefits of physical activity and the problems associated with a sedentary lifestyle. Knowledge is one of the best predictors of a commitment to healthy living.[46] Being a mentor to friends and family members can also help you become or stay motivated to make exercise a lifelong habit. Remember, the more active you are, the more health benefits you will receive.

USING SOCIAL AND COMMUNITY SUPPORT

A network of friends, coworkers, and family members who understand the benefits of exercise and join you in your activities can make the difference between a sedentary and an active lifestyle. Family and friends are not enough, however; activity-friendly communities are also instrumental in promoting physical activity. Many communities have paths, trails, sidewalks, and safe streets that encourage people to become physically active.[51, 52] There are community programs that encourage parents to walk their children to school, that promote "mall walking" (walking at shopping malls), and that sponsor biking and walking days (see the box "Creating Activity-Friendly Communities").

What can you do to encourage community planning that promotes physical activity? In existing communities, you can advocate for new growth designed around public transportation hubs and for bicycle lanes incorporated into

Highlight on Health

Strategies for Overcoming Barriers to Physical Activity

Lack of time

- Identify available time slots. Monitor your daily activities for 1 week. Identify at least three 30-minute time slots you could use for physical activity.
- Add physical activity to your daily routine: Walk or ride your bike to work or shopping, organize school activities around physical activity, walk the dog, or park farther away from your destination.
- Make time for physical activity. Walk, jog, or swim during your lunch hour; take fitness breaks instead of coffee breaks.
- Select activities requiring minimal time, such as walking, jogging, or stair climbing.

Social influence

- Explain your interest in physical activity to friends and family. Ask them to support your efforts.
- Invite friends and family members to exercise with you. Plan social activities involving exercise.
- Develop new friendships with physically active people. Join a group, such as the YMCA.

Lack of energy

- Schedule physical activity for times in the day or week when you feel energetic.
- Convince yourself that physical activity will increase your energy level; then try it.

Lack of willpower

- Plan ahead. Make physical activity a regular part of your schedule and write it on your calendar.
- Invite a friend to exercise with you on a regular basis, and write the dates on both your calendars.
- Join an exercise group or class.

Fear of injury

- Learn how to warm up and cool down safely.

- Learn how to exercise appropriately considering your age, fitness level, skill level, and health status.
- Choose activities involving minimum risk.

Lack of skill

- Select activities requiring no new skills, such as walking, climbing stairs, or jogging.
- Exercise with friends who are at the same skill level as you.
- Find a friend who is willing to teach you new skills.
- Take a class to develop new skills.

Lack of resources

- Select activities that require minimal equipment, such as walking, jogging, or calisthenics.
- Identify inexpensive, convenient resources available in your community, such as park and recreation programs.

Weather conditions

- Develop a set of regular activities that are always available regardless of weather (indoor cycling, aerobic dance, indoor swimming, calisthenics, stair climbing, rope skipping, dancing).
- Think of outdoor activities that depend on weather conditions (cross-country skiing, outdoor swimming, outdoor tennis) as "bonuses"—extra activities possible when weather and circumstances permit.

Family obligations

- Trade babysitting time with a friend, neighbor, or family member who also has small children.
- Exercise with your children. Go for a walk together, play tag or other running games, get an aerobic dance or exercise tape for kids.
- Hire a babysitter and look at the cost as an investment in your physical and mental health.
- Jump rope, do calisthenics, ride a stationary bicycle, or use other home gymnasium equipment while the kids are playing or sleeping.
- Try to exercise when the kids are not around (during school hours or their nap time).
- Encourage exercise facilities to provide child care.

Source: "Physical Activity for Everyone: Making Physical Activity Part of Your Life," Centers for Disease Control and Prevention, 2005. www.cdc.gov.

new and redeveloped streets. As a citizen and taxpayer, you can vote on local growth measures and become active in local chapters of organizations such as New Urbanism and Smart Growth America.[53, 54] Taking political action can work. In 2002, for example, New Jersey voters and antisprawl lobbyists were

rewarded with an executive order against sprawl from their governor, which preserved open areas and focused expansion and redevelopment on existing urban and suburban areas.[55, 56]

When making personal choices about where to live and work, look at a map of the immediate area and think about

Public Health in Action

Creating Activity-Friendly Communities

Physical activity levels are influenced by diverse factors that go beyond individual motivation, knowledge, and behavior. The Centers for Disease Control and Prevention (CDC) established the Task Force on Community Preventive Services to investigate how lifestyles are affected when changes are made in the physical environment, social networks, organizational norms and policies, and laws through environmental and policy initiatives. Among the Task Force's findings, compiled in the 2005 *Guide to Community Preventive Services*, were that community-wide campaigns to increase physical activity are effective and that creating or improving access to places for physical activity increases the percentage of people who exercise.

A related CDC program, the Active Community Environments Initiative (ACES), promotes walking, bicycling, and the development of accessible recreational and park facilities. The program draws on the expertise of several disciplines, especially public health, urban design, and transportation. The underlying idea is that activity-friendly environments play a vital role in promoting physical activity. Some ACES activities include

- Development of the Kids-Walk-to-School program.
- Promotion of National and International Walk-to-School Day.
- Partnership with the National Park Service's Rivers, Trails, and Conservation Assistance Program to facilitate the development of close-to-home parks and recreational facilities.
- Collaboration with an Atlanta-based study to assess the relationship among land use, transportation, air quality, and physical activity.
- Collaboration with the Environmental Protection Agency on a national study that surveyed attitudes of the American public toward the environment, walking, and bicycling.

In partnership with ACES, some communities have increased the safety of walking and biking by developing or improving bike lanes, and others have promoted walking by designing sidewalks and streets to ensure continuity and connectivity. Studies have found that these efforts may increase physical activity by well over 100 percent.

ACES also promotes social support in community settings. Examples include setting up buddy systems and sponsoring walking groups. Studies have found that social support in community settings can increase the time spent being physically active by 44 percent and the frequency of physical activity by 20 percent. Enhanced access to places for physical activity combined with informational outreach activities (seminars, forums, workshops, counseling, referrals to physicians for risk assessment) can be especially effective in getting people to exercise more. Studies examining this strategy found a median increase of about 48 percent in the number of people exercising three times or more a week.

Sources: The Guide to Community Preventive Services, *by S. Zaza, P.A. Briss, and K.W. Harris, 2005, New York: Oxford University Press; "Physical Activity Resources for Health Professionals: Active Environments: ACES-Active Community Environments Initiative," Centers for Disease Control and Prevention, retrieved from www.cdc.gov/nccdphp/dnpa/physical/health/_professionals/active_environments/aces.*

how communities you're considering are planned. How close are recreational areas? What types of places are within a 10-minute walking radius of home and work? Will living in this community help to make you more active and physically fit? Taking such questions into consideration will give you more opportunities to make physical activity and exercise a natural part of your life.

The key message of this chapter is that physical activity is a natural, enjoyable, sometimes thrilling, frequently challenging part of human life. It is a part of life that children instinctively embrace but that adults may have lost touch with living in a fast-paced, sedentary culture. We encourage you to get up, get moving, and get back in touch with the lifelong pleasures of physical activity.

You Make the Call

Is "Fitness for Life" Physical Education the Right Direction?

Elementary school students juggle balls, rings, and pins. Middle school students propel push scooters through an obstacle course lined with balloons, hoops, nets, rings, and mats. High school students play a modified version of volleyball with a rubber chicken. All of these activities are part of a kinder, gentler physical education promoting fitness for life. Today's physical education classes bear little resemblance to the competitive, military-style fitness classes of the past.

As early as the mid-1700s, Benjamin Franklin argued that schools needed to provide running, leaping, wrestling, and swimming activities for children. Physical education in schools, however, did not become a national priority until the 1950s, when a much-publicized study reported that 58 percent of American children could not pass a muscular fitness test, compared with only 9 percent of Austrian, Italian, and Swiss youth. In 1956 the Eisenhower administration established the President's Council on Youth Fitness (changed to the President's Council on Physical Fitness and Sports in the Johnson administration) and developed the President's Youth Fitness Test. The test consisted of a series of fitness skills, including pull-ups, sit-ups, the standing long jump, the shuttle run, the 50-yard dash, the softball throw, and the 600-yard run.

The President's Youth Fitness Test conferred an official status on school physical education (PE) programs, and fitness levels greatly improved throughout the 1960s. But, beginning in the early 1970s, a series of events reversed the status of school PE programs. In 1972, the federal law known as Title IX established the right of girls to the same physical education opportunities as boys, which led to coed PE classes except in cases where contact sports like football and basketball were being played. Although equal rights were served, PE classes changed to accommodate the different physical capabilities of males and females and the coed population.

A second event was a national decline in reading and math scores, which led to the redirection of funds supporting PE into academic programs. Physical education classes grew so large that logistical and equipment problems became common. School boards and local and state governments have continued to slash funds for PE programs over the past three decades (despite concerns over a youth overweight and obesity crisis). Although PE has declined in importance, competitive sports have become a priority in many school districts. As a result of these and other changes, PE programs have become oriented more toward leisure activities and fitness for life skills and less toward exercise, physical fitness, and sports skills.

Some physical educators say that fitness for life and leisure activities do not meet the health-related physical fitness demands of youth. They are calling for a return to physical education programs that place a premium on physical fitness activities. Proponents of the kinder, gentler type of physical education say that a wellness orientation promotes lifelong physical activity and teaches students self-discipline. What do you think?

PROS

- A focus on fitness for life and leisure activities encourages cooperation over competition and movement over intimidation, thus contributing to students' healthy development and eliminating the terrors that old-fashioned PE classes held for many students.

- Physical fitness is more than cardiorespiratory fitness and weight management; PE classes also need to provide students with relief from stress, opportunities for socialization, and ways to enhance self-esteem.

- Leisure activities such as Frisbee golf, Tae-Bo, and kickboxing are enjoyable activities that students will pursue throughout their lives.

- School fitness centers that provide various cardiovascular machines and weight training equipment are used by students before and after school. Wellness-oriented physical education facilitates this use.

CONS

- Fitness scores on the President's Youth Fitness Test have dropped significantly in the past decade.

- In light of current concerns about overweight and obesity among American children and teenagers, a return to the rigorous physical education programs of the past would seem to make sense.

- The orientation toward fitness for life and leisure activities makes physical education seem trivial and irrelevant, both to students and to the public. Only about 26 percent of high school students in the United States have a daily PE class; only 40 percent of high school students are enrolled in PE of any kind; and 75 percent of high school seniors get no physical education at all.

- As further evidence of the decline in status of physical education, only seven states require elementary schools to employ a certified physical education instructor; in all the other states, classroom teachers are responsible for physical education.

Sources: Active Community Environments Init iative (ACES) Project, Centers for Disease Control and Prevention, 2000, www.cdc.gov; "Gym Class Struggle," by A. Singer, April 24, 2000, Sports Illustrated, pp. 82–96; "Adolescent Participation in Sports and Adult Physical Activity," by T. Tammelin, S. Nayha, A.P. Hills, and M.R. Jarvelin, 2003, American Journal of Preventive Medicine, 24 (1), pp. 22–28.

In Review

1. **What is fitness?** Physical fitness is generally defined as the ability of the body to respond to the demands placed upon it. Skill-related fitness is the ability to perform specific skills associated with recreational activities and sports; health-related fitness is the ability to perform daily living activities with vigor. Physical activity is activity that requires any kind of movement; exercise is structured, planned physical activity.

2. **What are the components of health-related fitness?** The most important component is cardiorespiratory fitness; other components are musculoskeletal fitness (muscular strength, muscular endurance, and flexibility) and body composition.

3. **What are the benefits of physical activity and exercise?** Physical activity and exercise confer benefits in every domain of wellness, ranging from improved cognitive functioning to relief from depression to better cardiovascular health. Inactivity is a leading preventable cause of premature death from such causes as cardiovascular disease and cancer. Of all the positive health-related behavior choices you can make, exercising may be the easiest, most effective, and most important.

4. **How much should you exercise?** A widely accepted set of guidelines aimed at promoting and maintaining health and preventing chronic disease, issued jointly by the American College of Sports Medicine and the American Heart Association, calls for a minimum of 30 minutes of moderate-intensity aerobic activity 5 days a week or 20 minutes of vigorous-intensity activity 3 days a week. Activity should also be included for muscle strengthening, flexibility, and weight management.

5. **What special exercise-related considerations and precautions are important for health and safety?** It's important to warm up and cool down before and after exercise, to avoid fatigue and overexertion, to take proper care of injuries, and to take environmental conditions into account. Everyone can benefit from exercise, as long as they follow any relevant special guidelines, such as those for older adults and people with disabilities.

www For a detailed summary of this chapter and a comprehensive set of review questions, visit the Online Learning Center at **www.mhhe.com/teague2e**.

Web Resources

Adult Fitness Test: The President's Council on Physical Fitness and Sports developed this adult fitness test. The test consists of three components for aerobic fitness, muscular strength, and flexibility. You can enter your test results online to see where you rank among people of the same age based on percentile.
www.adultfitnesstest.org

Aerobics and Fitness Association of America: In addition to training and certification of fitness professionals, this organization offers information on exercise, health and safety, lifestyle, and nutrition.
www.afaa.com

American College of Sports Medicine: ACSM presents various health and fitness topics, with expert commentary and tips for maintaining a lifestyle of physical fitness, through its e-newsletter and brochures.
www.acsm.org

American Council on Exercise: This site offers health and fitness information, including core stability training, healthy recipes, fitness fact sheets, and what to look for in a health club.
www.acefitness.org

Centers for Disease Control and Prevention, Body and Mind: This child-dedicated site provided by the CDC lets children play games, take quizzes, and construct their own fitness calendars.
www.bam.gov.

National Center for Chronic Disease Prevention and Health Promotion: Look here for CDC recommendations on physical activity, information on measuring physical activity intensity, and strength training for older adults.
www.cdc.gov/nccdphp/dnpa

The National Center on Physical Activity and Disability: This site features information on lifetime sports, competitive sports, and exercise and fitness for individuals with disabilities.
www.ncpad.org

Shape Up America! Fitness Center: This site features a variety of ways to improve your fitness and lose weight, offering assessment tools, tips on motivation, and ways to design an improvement program that matches your individual needs and goals.
www.shapeup.org/fitness.html

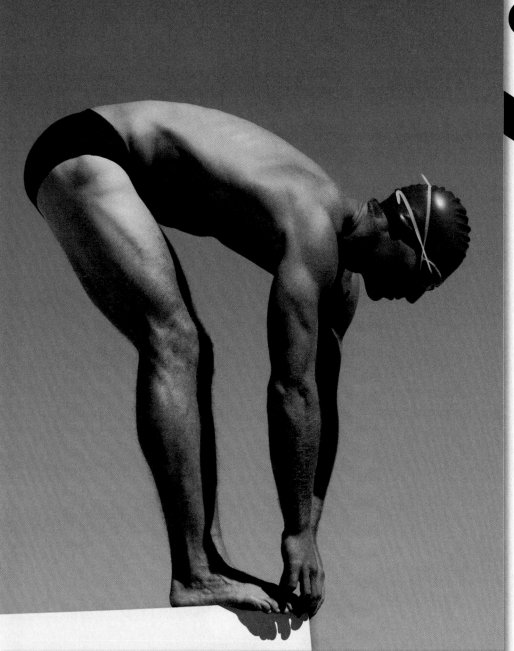

Ever Wonder...

- if diets work?
- if being overweight can run in families?
- what is causing the so-called obesity epidemic in America?

WWW

Your Health Today

www.mhhe.com/teague2e

Go to the Online Learning Center for *Your Health Today* for interactive activities, quizzes, flashcards, Web links, and more resources related to this chapter.

Overweight and obesity are increasingly worrisome problems in the United States and around the world. Among American adults, 66 percent meet the criteria for overweight and 34 percent meet the criteria for obesity.[1] **Overweight** is defined as body weight that exceeds the recommended guidelines for good health; **obesity** is body weight that greatly exceeds the recommended guidelines.

overweight
Body weight that exceeds the recommended guidelines for good health.

obesity
Body weight that greatly exceeds the recommended guidelines for good health, as indicated by a body mass index of 30 or more.

In 1991 four states reported a prevalence rate of obesity greater than 15 percent, and no states reported prevalence greater than 20 percent. Sixteen years later, in 2007, only Colorado reported a prevalence rate less than 20 percent (see the box "Obesity Trends Among Adults in the United States").[2] If these trends continue, all Americans could be overweight within a few generations. Worldwide, an estimated 300 million people are obese; rates vary tremendously by country, ranging from less than 5 percent in parts of China, Japan, and certain African countries to more than 75 percent in urban Samoa.[3]

No sex, age, state, racial group, or educational level is spared from the problem of overweight, although the problem is worse for the young and the poor. Rates of overweight and at-risk for overweight are increasing among children between 6 and 19 years of age, with 16.3 percent currently overweight and 32 percent at-risk for overweight.[4] (The CDC does not apply the term *obese* to children.) The trend is particularly worrisome because an elementary school child who is overweight has an 80 percent likelihood of being overweight at age 12; a person who is obese at age 18 faces odds 28 to 1 against maintaining a healthy adult weight.[5]

What Is a Healthy Body Weight?

How much should you weigh? The answer to this question depends on who is asking and why. If you are a 16-year-old varsity wrestler getting ready for your competition weigh-in, your coach and the wrestling weight classes may influence your weight goals. If you are an 18-year-old girl comparing yourself with the fashion models you see daily in magazines, your goals may be determined by a media-generated cosmetic ideal. If you are a 50-year-old woman wondering whether you should be concerned about the 25 pounds you gained last year, you may be more interested in health goals for weight and fitness.

There is no ideal body weight for each person, but there are ranges for a healthy body weight. A healthy body weight is defined as (1) an acceptable body mass index (explained in the following sections); (2) a fat distribution that is not a risk factor for illness; and (3) the absence of any medical conditions (such as diabetes or hypertension) that would suggest a need

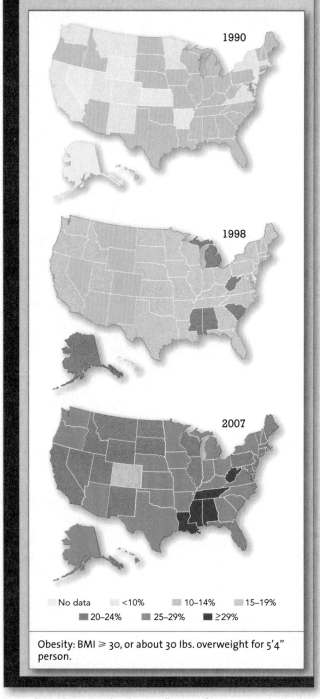

Who's at Risk

Obesity Trends Among Adults in the United States

Rates of obesity have soared since 1990 and especially since 2000. Multiple factors—some known, some still to be identified—account for this trend.

1990

1998

2007

No data   <10%   10–14%   15–19%
20–24%   25–29%   ≥29%

Obesity: BMI ≥ 30, or about 30 lbs. overweight for 5'4" person.

Source: "U.S. Obesity Trends 1985–2007," Centers for Disease Control and Prevention, Behavioral Risk Factor Surveillance System, 2008, retrieved from www.cdc.gov/nccdphp/dnpa/obesity/trend/maps.

for weight loss.[6] If you currently meet these criteria, you will want to focus on maintaining your current weight. If you don't meet them, you may need to lose weight or gain weight.

BODY MASS INDEX

Body mass index (BMI) is a measure of your weight relative to your height; it correlates with total body fat. BMI is used to estimate the health significance of body weight. You can use a table to determine your BMI (see Table 9.1) or calculate it using the following formula:

> **body mass index (BMI)**
> Measure of body weight in relation to height.

$$BMI = \frac{\text{weight in kg}}{(\text{height in meters})^2} \ OR \ \frac{\text{weight in pounds}}{(\text{height in inches})^2} \times 703 \ (\text{conversion factor})$$

There appears to be a U-shaped relationship between BMI and risk of death. The lowest risk of death is in the 18.5 to 25 range. As such, the National Institutes of Health and the World Health Organization use the following guidelines for adult BMI categories:[2, 3]

	BMI
Underweight	Less than 18.5
Healthy weight	18.5 to 24.9
Overweight	25 to 29.9
Obese	$\geqslant$30

A different measure is used to define overweight in children and adolescents. For these age groups, BMI is plotted using growth charts (for either boys or girls), and a percentile ranking is determined (percentile indicates the relative position of BMI compared to other children of the same sex and age). The following guideline is used for children and adolescents:[7]

	BMI
Underweight	Less than 5th percentile
Healthy weight	5th to less than 85th percentile
At risk of overweight	85th to less than 95th percentile
Overweight	Greater than 95th percentile

There are some limitations to using the BMI to calculate risk of disease. BMI estimates body fat but does not actually calculate it. As such, BMI may incorrectly estimate risk for some people. In athletes or others with a muscular build, BMI may overestimate body fat (and risk). In the elderly or others who have lost muscle mass, BMI may underestimate body fat (and risk). Similarly, at the same BMI, women tend to have a higher percentage of body fat than men.

BODY FAT PERCENTAGE

Body composition is measured in terms of percentage of body fat. There are no clear, accepted guidelines for healthy body fat ranges, although ranges of 11–20 percent have been used for men and 17–30 percent for women. Some body fat is essential to healthy function; the lower healthy range may be 5–10 percent for male athletes and 15–20 percent for female athletes. Below a certain body fat threshold, hormones cannot be produced and problems can occur, such as infertility, lack of menstruation, depression, and abnormal appetite.

At each level of BMI, there are differences in body fat percentage for certain groups. Women on average have 10–12 percent more body fat than men. African American men average slightly lower body fat percentage than White men, and Asian men average slightly higher body fat percentage than White men. As people get older, body fat percentage increases at each level of BMI.[8, 9]

Because body fat percentage is considered an important component in judging the need for weight reduction, it may be measured as part of a physical examination. Several methods exist to measure body fat percentage. The most accurate methods are expensive and require special equipment. They include weighing a person underwater (immersion), in a chamber using air displacement to measure body volume (Bod Pod), or using a type of X-ray called dual energy X-ray absorptiometry (DXA). Two simpler but slightly less reliable methods are measuring thickness of skin and fat in several locations of the body (skinfold measurement or caliper testing) and sending a weak electrical current through parts of the body and measuring the electrical resistance of tissue to calculate body fat (bioelectroimpedence).

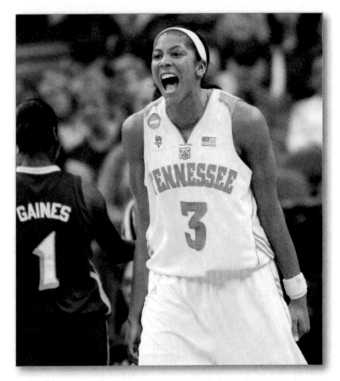

■ BMI can be an inaccurate indicator of healthy body weight and fat percentage in athletes with a high proportion of muscle tissue. This is not the case for Candace Parker, star player for the NCAA champion Lady Vols of the University of Tennessee. At 6 feet, 4 inches and 172 pounds, Parker has a BMI of 21, well within the healthy range.

Table 9.1 | Body Mass Index (BMI)

Find your height in the lefthand column and look across the row until you find the number that is closest to your weight. The number at the top of that column identifies your BMI. The darkest shaded area represents healthy weight ranges.

BMI	18	19	20	21	22	23	24	25	26	27	28	29	30	31	32	33	34
Height																	
4'10"	86	91	96	100	105	110	115	119	124	129	134	138	143	148	153	158	162
4'11"	89	94	99	104	109	114	119	124	128	133	138	143	148	153	158	163	168
5'0"	92	97	102	107	112	118	123	128	133	138	143	148	153	158	163	168	174
5'1"	95	100	106	111	116	122	127	132	137	143	148	153	158	164	169	174	180
5'2"	98	104	109	115	120	126	131	136	142	147	153	158	164	169	175	180	186
5'3"	102	107	113	118	124	130	135	141	146	152	158	163	169	175	180	186	191
5'4"	105	110	116	122	128	134	140	145	151	157	163	169	174	180	186	192	197
5'5"	108	114	120	126	132	138	144	150	156	162	168	174	180	186	192	198	204
5'6"	112	118	124	130	136	142	148	155	161	167	173	179	186	192	198	204	210
5'7"	115	121	127	134	140	146	153	159	166	172	178	185	191	198	204	211	217
5'8"	118	125	131	138	144	151	158	164	171	177	184	190	197	203	210	216	223
5'9"	122	128	135	142	149	155	162	169	176	182	189	196	203	209	216	223	230
5'10"	126	132	139	146	153	160	167	174	181	188	195	202	209	216	222	229	236
5'11"	129	136	143	150	157	165	172	179	186	193	200	208	215	222	229	236	243
6'0"	132	140	147	154	162	169	177	184	191	199	206	213	221	228	235	242	250
6'1"	136	144	151	159	166	174	182	189	197	204	212	219	227	235	242	250	257
6'2"	141	148	155	163	171	179	186	194	202	210	218	225	233	241	249	256	264
6'3"	144	152	160	168	176	184	192	200	208	216	224	232	240	248	256	264	272
6'4"	148	156	164	172	180	189	197	205	213	221	230	233	246	254	263	271	279
6'5"	151	160	168	176	185	193	202	210	218	227	235	244	252	261	269	277	286
6'6"	155	164	172	181	190	198	207	216	224	233	241	250	259	267	276	284	293

Underweight	Healthy Weight	Overweight	Obese
(<18.5)	(18.5–24.9)	(25–29.9)	(≥30)

Source: Adapted from "Body Mass Index Table," National Heart, Lung, and Blood Institute, retrieved from www.nhlbi.nih.gov/guidelines/obesity/bmi_tbl.htm.

BODY FAT DISTRIBUTION

Not only the amount but also the distribution of body fat is important in determining your health risk. Fat carried around and above the waist is abdominal fat and is considered more "active" than fat carried on the hips and thighs. Abdominal fat (also called *central obesity*) is a disadvantage because it breaks down more easily and enters the bloodstream more readily. A large abdominal circumference or waist circumference (more than 40 inches for a man, more than 35 inches for a woman) is associated with high cholesterol levels and higher risk for heart disease, stroke, diabetes, hypertension, and some types of cancer.

Waist-to-hip ratio is another way to judge the location of body fat. You can calculate your ratio by dividing your waist measurement by your hip measurement (say your waist is 30 inches and your hips are 35 inches; 30 divided by 35 equals 0.86). For men, a ratio of less than

waist-to-hip ratio
Ratio between the circumference of the waist and the circumference of the hips, used as a measure of overweight and obesity.

0.80 (pear shape) is considered low risk, 0.81 to 0.99 is considered moderate risk, and 1.00 or more (apple shape) is considered high risk. For women, a ratio of less than 0.70 (pear shape) is considered low risk, 0.71 to 0.89 is considered moderate risk, and 0.9 or more (apple shaped) is considered high risk.

Obese men tend to accumulate abdominal fat, whereas obese women tend to accumulate fat on the hips and thighs. However, women have a change in body fat distribution at the onset of menopause, with fat shifting to the abdomen. This shift coincides with an increased risk of heart disease for women.

HEALTH ISSUES RELATED TO OVERWEIGHT AND OBESITY

Overweight and obesity are associated with serious health problems. Obese people are four times more likely than people with a healthy weight to die before reaching their expected lifespan. They have an increased risk for high blood pressure, diabetes, elevated cholesterol levels, coronary heart disease, stroke, gallbladder disease, osteoarthritis (a type of arthritis caused by excessive wear and tear on the joints), sleep apnea (interrupted breathing during sleep), lung problems, and certain cancers, such as uterine, prostate, and colorectal (see the box "Diabetes and Obesity"). Women who are obese before pregnancy are at increased risk of having a baby with a birth defect.[10] Obesity is also a component of *metabolic syndrome,* a condition associated with a significantly increased risk for cardiovascular disease and the development of Type-2 diabetes (see Chapter 18). There has been some controversy over the number of annual deaths attributable to overweight and obesity; estimates range from 112,000 to 365,000.[11]

What Factors Influence Your Weight?

There is no simple answer to why Americans are getting fatter. Many factors contribute to this trend, both individual and environmental. You may look to other family members, for example, and think that it is your genes that make you overweight. Unless you are adopted, however, the people who gave you your genes also taught you how to eat, chose your neighborhood, and influenced your educational status and perhaps your occupation.

Highlight on Health

Diabetes and Obesity

The rise in obesity in the United States has been paralleled by a rise in rates of diabetes. As obesity increasingly becomes an issue among children and adolescents, so does a disease that previously was rare in this age group.

Diabetes is a disease in which the levels of glucose circulating in the bloodstream are too high. Normally the pancreas produces the hormone insulin in response to rising glucose levels. Insulin binds to receptors in body cells, allowing glucose to enter the cells to be used for energy and keeping blood levels of glucose fairly stable. Without insulin, levels of glucose in the bloodstream rise, setting the stage for such health complications as heart disease, kidney failure, blindness, sexual dysfunction, and others.

There are two forms of diabetes. In Type-1 diabetes, little or no insulin is produced by the pancreas and has to be provided by injection or a pumping device. Type-1 diabetes is not related to obesity, and levels of this form of the disease appear to be remaining fairly stable. Type-1 diabetes is sometimes referred to as juvenile-onset diabetes, because the average age at onset is 14. In Type-2 diabetes, body cells become resistant to the effects of insulin. The pancreas produces insulin at normal or even higher than normal levels, but the body's cells do not respond, causing blood glucose levels to rise. Type-2 diabetes is sometimes called adult-onset diabetes because, previously, the average age at diagnosis was 40.

Type-2 diabetes is by far the more common form of the disease; 90–95 percent of people with diabetes have Type-2. Numerous factors contribute to its prevalence: There is a genetic component, and the disease runs in families, but there is also a lifestyle component. Obesity, high caloric intake, and low levels of exercise are important factors. In fact, the onset of Type-2 diabetes can be delayed and early Type-2 diabetes can be treated by intensive lifestyle change, including nutritional education, a low-fat, lower calorie diet with a goal of 5–7 percent weight loss, and 150 minutes of exercise per week.

The onset of Type-2 diabetes is usually gradual. Symptoms include excessive thirst, frequent urination, and fatigue. In rare cases, the first symptoms are nausea, vomiting, and confusion. If you are overweight and have a family history of diabetes, you should have your blood glucose level checked by your physician on a regular basis. Early diagnosis and lifestyle changes can prevent or delay the onset of the disease.

Sources: "Changes in the Incidence of Diabetes in U.S. Adults 1997–2003," by L.S. Geiss, L. Pan, B. Cadwell, et al., 2006, American Journal of Preventive Medicine, *30(5), pp. 371–377.*

■ Genes and hormones play a role in overweight and obesity—as do family, social, cultural, and other environmental factors. These can include favorite family and ethnic foods, mealtime rules and traditions, and the kinds of restaurants and grocery stores available in the community.

GENETIC AND HORMONAL INFLUENCES

If neither of your parents is obese, you have a 10 percent chance of becoming obese. The risk increases to 80 percent if both of your parents are obese. Adopted children also tend to be similar in weight to their biological parents, and twin studies support a genetic tendency toward obesity. These findings have led to the search for genes associated with obesity. It appears that for most people, obesity is a multifactorial disease; that is, it results from a complex interaction among multiple genes and the environment. Each gene can increase a person's susceptibility to obesity, and, together, multiple genes can further increase risk.

Genetic mutations that increase risk for obesity usually cause an increase or a decrease in the level of a hormone or in the body's responsiveness to the hormone. For example, *leptin* is an appetite-suppressing hormone produced by fat cells themselves. An increase in fat cells or energy stores produces an increase in leptin, which leads to a decrease in appetite and an increase in energy expenditure.

Another hormone, *ghrelin*, is nicknamed the "hunger hormone." It is produced primarily in the stomach in response to certain triggers. If you eat meals at scheduled times (say 7 a.m., 1 p.m., and 7 p.m.), your blood levels of ghrelin will increase as those hours approach and make you feel hungry. If you see or smell food, your ghrelin level probably increases.

Nearly two dozen other hormones identified thus far play a role in appetite and energy expenditure. They act in the brain to influence when to start or finish eating; to monitor external cues for food, such as smells, sights, and texture; to monitor internal cues, such as body fat stores, glucose level, free fatty acids, and stomach fullness; and to adjust metabolic rate. It is a complex interaction that is not yet fully understood. If you are maintaining your current weight, the interaction of hormones controls your daily calorie intake to within 10 calories (a single potato chip) of balanced food intake and energy expenditure.[12]

Some medical conditions can be associated with weight gain. Thyroid disorders are a prime example. The thyroid gland, located in the neck, produces a hormone that is involved in metabolism. If the gland becomes less active, metabolism slows and weight is gained. If the gland is overactive, metabolism speeds up and weight can be inappropriately lost.

Except in rare cases of a single gene mutation, genetics alone does not fully explain obesity. The rapid rise in obesity since the 1980s is too sudden to be due to genetics. The hormonal controls of appetite and energy expenditure evolved at a time when food was rare and result in a drive to eat if food is available. By looking at groups that have moved from one country to another, we can see that they change their weight but not their genes (at least not for the first few generations). Consider the Pima Indians in the American Southwest. They have a significant obesity problem and 20 times the rate of diabetes seen in Whites in the Southwest. When American Pima Indians are compared with Mexican Pima Indians, the results are startling. The average American Pima woman has a BMI of 35.5, compared with the average Mexican Pima woman's BMI of 26.3. The average American Pima man has a BMI of 33.3, compared with the average Mexican Pima man's BMI of 23.8.[13]

Japanese immigrants to the United States have a similar pattern. Among Japanese men from 45 to 49 years of age, the percentages of obesity are 4 percent in Japan, 12 percent in Hawaii, and 14 percent in California. Genes are slow to change, requiring generations and hundreds of years. Environmental influences, such as abundant food and a sedentary lifestyle, can produce such effects in a much shorter period.

GENDER AND AGE

Most of us develop our eating patterns from our families during childhood. Poor childhood eating habits are believed to be a major cause of the recent surge in overweight and obesity. There are several crucial times in your life when you may change these patterns, a critical one being the first time you leave home for college or to live independently. Take advantage of this opportunity to evaluate the eating habits you learned at home and make changes if they are needed.

During puberty, boys and girls undergo significant hormonal changes that alter their respective body compositions. Female hormones begin preparing girls for childbearing with increases in body fat, especially on the hips, buttocks, and thighs. Before puberty, a girl of a healthy weight will have approximately 12 percent body fat. After puberty, the healthy range can increase to up to 25 percent body fat.

In contrast, a boy's hormones in late adolescence are geared more toward muscle development. Before puberty, a boy of healthy weight has approximately 12 percent body fat; after puberty, he levels out at approximately 15 percent body fat. In addition to experiencing the hormonal influences of puberty on body composition, the average adolescent girl is less physically active than are her male peers, an additional pressure toward increased body fat percentage. Physical activity levels for both boys and girls are declining in adolescence.[14]

Between the ages of 20 and 40, both men and women gain weight. Married men weigh more than do men who have never been married or were previously married but are currently unmarried. For women, these are the years in which pregnancy typically occurs. Weight gain is a normal part of pregnancy. The majority of women will lose most of this weight within a year of delivery. However, about 15–20 percent of women continue to maintain significant weight a year after delivery, partly as a result of changes in lifestyle associated with childrearing.[15]

As people enter their 50s, both women and men can have potentially serious problems with weight gain. Men tend to see an increase in abdominal fat. Women in their late 40s and early 50s undergo significant hormonal changes and shifts in body fat distribution.

At the age of 60 and beyond, weight tends to decline. This loss can be attributed to a number of causes, including decreased calorie needs, less muscle tissue, and less body mass. These changes give older adults thinner limbs. During these years, weight-bearing exercise, such as walking, becomes critical to maintain body mass and bone strength.

FOOD ENVIRONMENTS

The new term *obesogenic environment* has been coined to highlight the fact that our chances of becoming obese are significantly influenced by our environment.

Food Choices   In general, unhealthy foods are more available, more convenient, more heavily advertised, and less expensive than healthy foods, especially in low-income neighborhoods. In these communities, fast-food outlets and small food markets dominate the retail food landscape, providing consumers with less healthy foods at higher prices. In more affluent neighborhoods, where supermarkets predominate, low-fat and whole-grain foods are much more readily available, along with diverse fruit and vegetable choices.

One study found that supermarkets were four times more likely to be located in affluent rather than low-income communities. The presence of supermarkets (in contrast to convenience stores) has been associated with lower rates of obesity. Obesity rates are highest among the poorest and least educated segments of the population.[16, 17]

Eating Out   In the 1950s eating out was a rare event; today it has become a part of daily life. Forty-eight percent of adults report eating out daily. Twenty-one percent of households use some form of take-out food or food delivery service daily.[17] This trend is most likely related to the increased number of dual-career households and single-parent households, and the convenience and accessibility of fast foods. Foods served in restaurants and fast-food outlets tend to be higher in fat and total calories and lower in fiber than are foods prepared at home. Increased reliance on fast foods is associated with weight gain.[18] For ideas on eating out without going overboard, see the box "Tips for Eating Out."

Larger Portions   Serving size has increased steadily both inside and outside the home. The largest increases in serving size have occurred in fast-food restaurants and may be due to "supersized" pricing strategies. Serving sizes of other foods have increased as well. Bagels and muffins used to weigh 2–3 ounces; now the standard is 4–7 ounces. In 1916 Coca-Cola was sold in 6.5-ounce bottles; in 1950 it was offered in

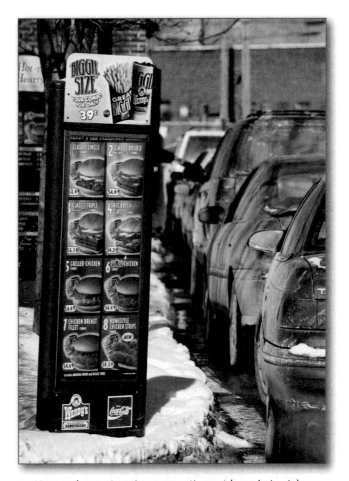

■ More and more Americans are eating out (or ordering in) on a daily basis, and many are getting their meals in the drive-through lane. This major cultural shift is one of the factors implicated in the current overweight and obesity phenomenon.

10- and 12-ounce bottles; now it is common to find Coke in 20- or 32-ounce bottles.[18, 19]

The impact of supersizing on the caloric bottom line is dramatic. When confronted with large serving sizes in restaurants or prepackaged foods, people eat more. The larger the portion of food, the worse we become at estimating how much we are eating. (See Figure 9.1 for some visual images of portion sizes.) Paying attention to package labeling, dividing prepackaged food into smaller serving sizes, and using visual cues can help with more appropriate serving sizes.[20]

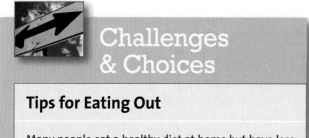

Challenges & Choices

Tips for Eating Out

Many people eat a healthy diet at home but have less success in restaurants, college dining halls, and food courts. Try these tips to maintain control the next time you eat out.

- Increase the proportion of plant-based foods in your diet. Take larger servings of vegetables and fruits and smaller servings of meat, cheese, and eggs.

- Include two vegetables in your meal or a vegetable and a salad.

- Choose whole-wheat bread, brown rice, or whole-grain cereals. Whole-grain foods are more filling.

- Have fresh fruit or yogurt for dessert instead of cake or ice cream.

- Drink water instead of soda or juice.

- Control your portion size by taking smaller servings. Don't go back for seconds.

- Eat slowly and savor the taste of your food.

- Stop eating when you first feel full rather than waiting until you feel stuffed.

- Share large portions or take some home for another meal. Don't feel obligated to eat everything on your plate.

- Don't skip meals—you'll only be inclined to eat quickly and more at the next meal.

It's Not Just Personal . . .
Eating out has become a way of life. Americans consume about 30 percent of their calories in restaurants and spend almost half of every food dollar on food eaten outside the home. The restaurant industry is one of the nation's largest businesses.

Source: Data from "The Way We Eat Now," by C. Lambert, May–June 2004, Harvard Magazine.

LIFESTYLE INFLUENCES ON WEIGHT

Before the mid-1900s, most of the population would never have considered exercise to be a necessity for health, because their daily lives involved regular physical activity. Our current lifestyle has become so mechanized, and sedentary, however, that many of us can go through a regular day spending almost no energy on physical activity. In addition, 60 percent of adults engage in little or no leisure-time physical activity.[18]

The Automobile   Surveys show that 25 percent of all trips in the United States are less than 1 mile, and yet 75 percent of these trips are taken by car. Less than 30 percent of children living within a mile of their school walk to school.[21] Increased time spent in the car each day increases the risk of obesity.[22]

Safety considerations and community structure are factors likely to influence transportation (and transportation options are likely to influence community structure). Consider a hypothetical suburbanite on a typical workday: She gets up and gets into her car (opening and closing the garage door with an automatic opener), drives a 20- to 45-minute commute to work, parks near her building, takes the elevator to the office, and sits at a computer all day, only to reverse the path at night. Should we be surprised that we are out of shape and gaining weight? People are beginning to see the connection between community design—the so-called built environment—and

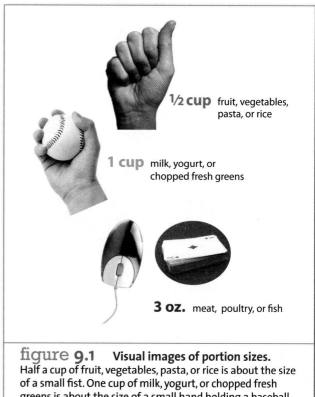

figure 9.1   **Visual images of portion sizes.**
Half a cup of fruit, vegetables, pasta, or rice is about the size of a small fist. One cup of milk, yogurt, or chopped fresh greens is about the size of a small hand holding a baseball. Three ounces of meat, poultry, or fish is about the size of a computer mouse or a deck of cards.

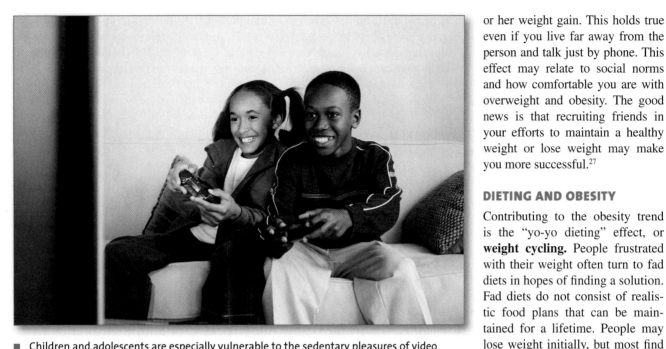

■ Children and adolescents are especially vulnerable to the sedentary pleasures of video games, television, and computers. They need adult role models who appreciate and can demonstrate the different kind of pleasure provided by physical activity.

health. People who live in neighborhoods that are designed to favor walking (with sidewalks, green space, and reliable public transportation) have lower rates of obesity than do people who live in less walkable communities.[22, 23]

Television Watching television continues to be the leading form of sedentary entertainment. In 2005–2006, the average U.S. household spent 8 hours and 14 minutes a day watching television or, on average, 4 hours and 35 minutes per person.[24] Studies have found an association between television watching and overweight in children, youth, and adults.[25, 26]

Television is thought to influence obesity patterns in two ways. First, sitting in front of the television takes minimal energy. Second, food intake increases during viewing in response to food advertisements. Candy, snacks, packaged foods, soft drinks, and alcohol are the most commonly advertised items. In addition, people often eat mindlessly while watching TV, oblivious of how much they are consuming.[18]

Computers Computers and other technological advancements have further altered the activity level of children and adults. Talking to friends, playing games, and shopping online are just a few computer activities that would previously have involved some physical activity. In addition, people who sit long hours at a computer for their work are at increased risk of gaining weight due to little energy expenditure.

Friends and Weight Your social network appears to have an influence on your weight. If your friends gain weight, you are more likely to gain weight. The more strongly you identify a person as a friend, the more likely you are to match his

or her weight gain. This holds true even if you live far away from the person and talk just by phone. This effect may relate to social norms and how comfortable you are with overweight and obesity. The good news is that recruiting friends in your efforts to maintain a healthy weight or lose weight may make you more successful.[27]

DIETING AND OBESITY

Contributing to the obesity trend is the "yo-yo dieting" effect, or **weight cycling.** People frustrated with their weight often turn to fad diets in hopes of finding a solution. Fad diets do not consist of realistic food plans that can be maintained for a lifetime. People may lose weight initially, but most find it difficult to maintain the harsh restrictions, returning to their previous patterns. With rapid weight loss on a highly restrictive diet, the body can enter starvation mode, with decreased basal metabolism. When a person goes off the restrictive diet, he or she rapidly gains back the weight lost and sometimes gains even more before the body's metabolism readjusts.

weight cycling
Repeated cycles of weight loss and weight gain as a result of dieting; sometimes called yo-yo dieting.

THE STRESS RESPONSE

In response to stress, our bodies release several hormones, including adrenaline and cortisol. Fat cells release fatty acids and triglycerides in response to these hormones and increase the amount of circulating glucose. These responses are vital in enabling the body to handle acute stress, especially physical stress. But when stress is chronic, the constant presence of these hormones can influence fat deposits, increasing the amount of fat deposited in the abdomen. The stress response also affects eating patterns. Adrenaline is an appetite suppressant, whereas cortisol stimulates the appetite.

The Key to Weight Control: Energy Balance

The relationship between the calories you take in and the calories you expend is known as **energy balance.** If you take in more calories than you use through metabolism and movement (a positive energy balance),

energy balance
Relationship between caloric intake (in the form of food) and caloric output (in the form of metabolism and activity).

you store these extra calories in the form of body fat. If you take in fewer calories than you need (a negative energy balance), you draw on body fat stores to provide energy. Energy in must equal energy out in order to maintain your current weight. If you adjust one or the other side of the equation, you will gain or lose weight (Figure 9.2).

ESTIMATING YOUR DAILY ENERGY REQUIREMENTS

In Chapter 7 we discussed energy intake, the calories-in side of the energy equation. Here we are more interested in energy expenditure, the calories-out side. Components of energy expenditure include the thermic effect of food, adaptive thermogenesis, basal metabolic rate, and physical activity. Each of the components of energy expenditure is influenced by genetics, age, sex, body size, fat-free mass, and intensity and duration of activity.

thermic effect of food
Estimate of the energy required to process the food you eat.

The **thermic effect of food** is an estimate of the energy required to process the food you eat—chewing, digesting, metabolizing, and so on. The thermic effect of food is generally estimated at 10 percent of energy intake. If, for example, you ingested 2,500 calories of food during a day, you would burn approximately 250 calories processing what you ate. *Adaptive thermogenesis* takes into account the fact that your baseline energy expenditure varies with changes in the environment, such as in response to cold, or with physiological events, such as trauma, overeating, and changes in hormonal status.

basal metabolic rate (BMR)
Rate at which your body uses energy for basic life functions, such as breathing, circulation, and temperature regulation.

Basal metabolic rate (BMR) is the rate at which the body uses energy to maintain basic life func-

tions, such as digestion, respiration, and temperature regulation. About 60–70 percent of energy consumed is used for these basic metabolic functions. BMR is affected by several factors, including age, gender, and weight (Table 9.2).

After the age of 25, BMR decreases by 2–3 percent per decade. The decreases with age are due to changes in body composition, loss of muscle, and hormonal changes that affect metabolism. Endurance and strength-building activities can help preserve lean muscle tissue and counter this trend.

Table 9.2	Factors Affecting Basal Metabolic Rate
Factor	**Effect on BMR**
Age	BMR decreases 2–3% per decade after age 25.
Height	Tall, thin people have higher BMRs.
Growth	Children and pregnant women have higher BMRs.
Stress	Stress from disease and medications can raise BMR.
Environmental temperature	Heat and cold raise BMR.
Fasting/starvation	Lower BMR.
Malnutrition	Lowers BMR.
Smoking	Raises BMR.
Caffeine	Raises BMR.
Body composition	Lean tissue turns toward fat at a 2–3% rate per decade after age 25, lowering BMR.

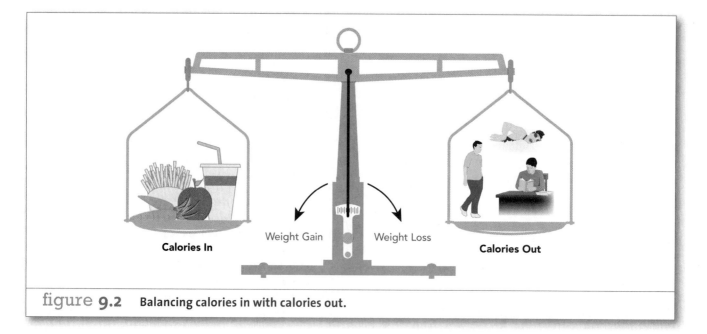

Calories In   Weight Gain   Weight Loss   Calories Out

figure **9.2**   **Balancing calories in with calories out.**

Between 10 and 30 percent of the calories consumed each day are used for physical activity, depending on level and duration of activity. Physical activity influences the energy balance in two ways: Exercise itself burns calories, and exercise increases muscle mass, which is associated with a higher BMR.

You can estimate your daily energy expenditure by considering (1) the thermic effect of food, (2) the energy spent on basal metabolic rate, and (3) the energy spent on physical activities. The effects of adaptive thermogenesis on basal metabolic rate are usually not taken into account except in extreme situations, such as severe injury or prolonged illness. To estimate your daily energy expenditure, complete the Add It Up activity for Chapter 9 at the end of the book.

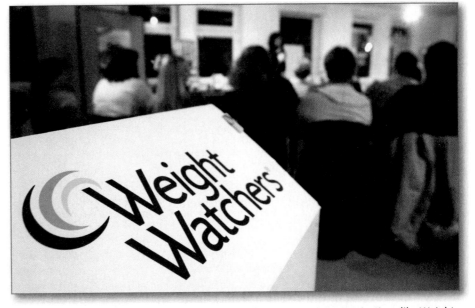

■ People who participate in well-established weight management organizations like Weight Watchers have a reasonable rate of success in losing pounds and maintaining the weight loss. Weight Watchers offers nutritional education, social support and structure, and prepared foods.

ADJUSTING YOUR CALORIC INTAKE

Dietary guidelines recommend that if you are trying to lose weight, a reasonable weight loss of 1 pound to 2 pounds per week is a healthy goal. Because a pound of body fat stores about 3,500 calories, you will need to decrease your total calorie intake for the week by about 3,500 calories in order to lose 1 pound per week. Weight loss beyond these guidelines tends to include loss of lean tissue like muscle. Additionally, diets too low in calories may not provide enough nutrients. If you are trying to increase your weight, you will need to increase your total calorie intake for the week by 3,500 calories in order to gain 1 pound per week. (Note that these are estimates.)

Reducing your intake of fat is also important. A high fat intake leads to higher caloric intake and is linked with obesity. High-carbohydrate foods also have a greater thermic effect than do high-fat foods. Thus it takes more energy to process a high-carbohydrate diet, and less of the food's energy is available for storage as fat.

Are There Quick Fixes for Overweight and Obesity?

Time is a major issue for most Americans, and most of us would love a quick and easy way to stay at a healthy body weight. How healthy are fad diets? Are they worth the money? And do they work?

THE DIET INDUSTRY

Americans pay an estimated $55.4 billion for the diet industry's quick fixes.[28] Two prominent players in this field are

fad diets and weight management organizations. Remember to be skeptical of unrealistic promises and to use your critical thinking skills when considering a diet or weight loss program. Some programs have been around for years, while others seem to come and go. For a comparison of several programs, see Table 9.3.

Fad Diets Every year, "new and improved" fad diets seduce consumers despite the fact that their safety and effectiveness are often unproven. No matter what the latest title, fad diets follow a pattern of altering the balance of carbohydrates, protein, and fat with the goal of promoting weight loss.

Most dieticians and physicians encourage people to monitor energy balance and eat a diet that emphasizes complex carbohydrates rather than trying fad diets. When evaluating a diet, consider if the food plan is something you can live with for the long haul. If the diet is too drastically different from your current eating patterns, chances are you will not be able to stick with it. If the diet calls for completely eliminating certain foods, requires specific food combinations, or claims that certain foods will "burn away fat"—beware. No scientific data exist to support these claims. For some other tips, see the box "Myths and Misconceptions About Weight Gain and Weight Loss."

Weight Management Organizations Weight management organizations offer group support, nutrition education, dietary advice, exercise counseling, and other services. Some of these organizations are associated with hospitals or university wellness programs, and others are commercial. Weight Watchers, Take Off Pounds Sensibly (TOPS), and Overeaters Anonymous are three well-known weight management

Table 9.3 | A Comparison of Selected Diets and Weight Management Organizations

Diet/Organization	Theory	Pros and Cons
Volumetrics (self-help book)	Focus on low-energy-dense foods (vegetables, soup broth, nonfat milk) in place of high-energy-dense foods (chips, cookies, candy, nuts, oils) Includes physical activity	Emphasis on lifelong eating patterns Low drop-out rate* Recipes may be time-consuming to prepare
Weight Watchers (commercial organization)	Point exchange system (calorie counting equivalent) Earn or spend points with exercise and food Weekly behavioral component (group support), weigh-ins, and physical activity recommendations	Low drop-out rate* 4.6-pound weight loss at 1 year**
Jenny Craig (commercial organization)	Restrict calorie intake Prepackaged meals only Individual behavioral counseling and exercise recommendations	Expensive due to meals Minimal time for food prep Average drop-out rate* 14-pound weight loss at 1 year***
Slim-Fast (commercial products)	Meal replacement system – 1 to 2 meals a day are replaced with 400-calorie drink or bar	Convenient, minimal time involvement High drop-out rate* Reported "as effective as calorie-control diet"
Atkins (self-help book)	Low-carbohydrate diet No restriction on proteins or fats	Requires total calorie restriction for weight loss Average drop-out rate* 4.6-pound weight loss at 1 year**
Ornish (self-help book)	Low-fat diet Bans on meat, fish, oils, alcohol, sugar, white flour	Drastic diet change for most people Average drop-out rate* 3.3-pound weight loss at 1 year**
TOPS (nonprofit organization)	Group-format weekly sessions teaching skills for healthy eating and exercise Low-calorie diet emphasis Encourages exercise	Nonprofit No recent published data on weight loss or retention
Overeaters Anonymous (self-help organization)	12-step program Weekly sessions emphasizing healthy eating and physical, emotional, and spiritual recovery Assigned sponsor	May be beneficial for binge eaters or others with emotional issues attached to eating No published data on weight loss or retention

*Drop-out rate: low drop out = more than 50% continue at 1 year; average drop out = approximately 50% continue at 1 year; high drop out = less than 50% continue at 1 year.

**Independent study trials confirm weight loss amounts listed.

***Recent small randomized trial evaluating Jenny Craig versus control.

Sources: "Comparison of Atkins, Ornish, Weight Watchers and Zone Diets for Weight Loss and Heart Disease Risk Reduction: A Randomized Trial," by M.L. Daninger, J.A. Gleason, J.L. Griffith, et al., 2006, Journal of the American Medical Association, 293 (1), pp. 43–53; "Systematic Review: An Evaluation of Major Commercial Weight Loss Programs in the United States," by A.G. Tsai and T.A. Wadden, 2005, Annals of Internal Medicine, 142 (1), pp. 56–67; "Randomized Trial of a Multifaceted Commercial Weight Loss Program," by C.L. Rock, B. Pakiz, S.W. Flat, et al., 2007, Obesity, 15, pp. 939–949.

organizations. TOPS and Overeaters Anonymous are free and provide group support. Weight Watchers is a commercial program. TOPS focuses on teaching. Overeaters Anonymous may be more suitable for binge eaters or others with emotional issues related to weight.[29] (See Table 9.3.)

THE MEDICAL APPROACH

Because obesity is a major risk factor for many health conditions, health centers are involved in helping people find solutions. We consider here three medical strategies used to treat obesity: very-low-calorie diets, diet drugs, and surgical procedures.

Consumer Clipboard

Myths and Misconceptions About Weight Gain and Weight Loss

Myth Skipping meals is an effective way to lose weight.

Reality People who skip meals tend to be heavier than people who eat smaller, regular meals four to five times a day. Eating smaller meals throughout the day may help control appetite.

Myth Eating snacks late at night causes you to gain weight.

Reality How much you eat is the critical factor in determining whether you gain, lose, or maintain weight. Eating late at night in and of itself does not alter risk if total calorie intake is not increased.

Myth Certain foods, such as grapefruit and cabbage, can burn fat.

Reality No foods can burn fat. Some substances, such as caffeine, may increase metabolism in the short term.

Myth Nuts should be avoided if you are trying to lose weight as they are high in fat.

Reality Nuts are high in fat and calories, but they are also a good source of protein, fiber, and minerals. Nuts are a healthy choice if consumed in small quantities.

Myth Doing multiple sets of leg lifts every day will help "spot reduce" large thighs.

Reality Spot reducing (targeting a particular body location with exercises) does not work. Fat distribution is determined by genetics, hormones, and total body fat. Weight training may help improve muscle definition, but it won't reduce fat in a specific area unless it contributes to reduction in total body fat.

Myth You have to avoid fast foods if you want to lose weight.

Reality No food or restaurant is inherently "bad." The key is moderation. When eating at a fast-food restaurant, order grilled foods or a salad, drink water instead of soda, don't supersize your meal, and don't eat there every day.

Myth A vegetarian diet is a guaranteed way to lose weight.

Reality Although you may lose weight on a vegetarian diet, you can also gain weight on it if you make poor choices. Avoiding meat does not inherently cause weight loss. A vegetarian diet needs to be well planned to ensure balanced calories and adequate nutrients.

Myth Liquid diets are a good, long-term way to lose weight.

Reality Liquid diets or other food replacement systems can be effective for short-term weight loss, but they are difficult to stick with in the long term.

Source: Adapted from Weight Loss and Nutrition Myths *(NIH Publication No. 04-4561), March 2004, updated August 2006, retrieved August 16, 2007, from www.win.niddk.nih.gov/publications/myths.htm#dietmyths.*

Very-Low-Calorie Diets (VLCDs) An aggressive option for patients with high health risks because of obesity, VLCDs require a physician's supervision. These diets provide a daily intake of 800 calories or less and *must* be monitored closely.

VLCDs are used for moderately to severely obese patients (people with BMIs greater than 30) who are highly motivated but have not had success with more conservative plans. Patients with BMIs of 27 to 30 with medical conditions that could improve with rapid weight loss are also candidates. Weight loss after a 26-week program averages 20 percent of the patient's initial weight. However, maintaining weight loss is challenging.

Prescription Drugs Because of the expense, potential for side effects, and need for medical supervision, weight loss drugs are intended for people who are at least 30 percent over their healthy body weight. There are currently three categories of weight-loss drugs: appetite suppressants, thermogenic drugs, and fat-blocking drugs.

Appetite Suppressants Amphetamines were once the most widely prescribed appetite suppressant. The continuous use of amphetamines curbs the appetite for about 3 months, but after that time, higher doses are needed and can cause dangerous side effects. Amphetamines also have addictive potential, so their prescription use in weight control has been discontinued.

Drugs that increase the levels of dopamine, serotonin, and norepinephrine in the brain have been shown to have weight loss potential. Fenfluramine (part of the popular diet combination Phen-fen) was an effective medication in this category of drug. Fenfluramine was widely prescribed as an aid to weight loss in the 1990s, but when evidence linked it to an increased risk of heart valve abnormalities and primary pulmonary hypertension, the drug was removed from the market. Phenteramine (the other component of the Phen-fen combination) is still used alone but is not as effective at producing weight loss without fenfluramine.

Sibutramine is an appetite suppressant that results in a weight loss of 3–8 percent when used as an adjunct to lifestyle modification. Rimonabant is another drug used in Europe but not yet approved for use in the United States due to safety issues.[30, 31]

Thermogenic Drugs Thermogenic drugs function as a stimulant to the body, increasing the BMR to produce the same effect as increased energy expenditure. Ephedrine and caffeine fall into this category. These drugs can cause shakiness, dizziness, and sleeping difficulties. Currently, no thermogenic drugs are approved for weight loss.

Fat-Blocking Drugs This category of drugs reduces the absorption of dietary fat by the body. The breakthrough drug in this area is Orlistat, which works by inhibiting the enzymes that break down fat in the stomach and intestines. Digestion of fat is reduced by about 30 percent; the undigested fat passes through the body. The use of Orlistat leads to an average weight loss of 8–10 percent of initial body weight within 6 months. With continued use, the weight loss is maintained at 2 years. Orlistat also has a positive effect on blood cholesterol levels. The FDA has recently approved an over-the-counter version in lower strength with the trade name Alli.

A drawback is that dietary fat is only part of the obesity equation; total caloric intake is also important. In addition, Orlistat has some bothersome side effects, including stomach cramps, gas, and fecal incontinence (leaking stool). The reduction in fat absorption also leads to a loss of fat-soluble vitamins and beta-carotene.[30]

Surgical Options Surgery is never a first-line approach to obesity. The National Institutes of Health has determined that surgical therapy should be considered for patients with a BMI of 40 or greater and a history of failed medical treatments for obesity, or for patients with a BMI of 35 or greater with other illnesses or risk factors.

Gastric surgeries to treat obesity alter the anatomy of the stomach and intestines and are said to be either *restrictive* or *malabsorptive* (or both). A restrictive surgery makes the stomach smaller and therefore limits the amount of food a person can consume at one sitting. A malabsorptive surgery bypasses part of the intestines and thus less food is absorbed after a meal.

Typical weight loss after gastric surgery ranges from 44 pounds to 110 pounds. Most people have significant improvement in or resolution of diabetes, hypertension, and other obesity-related conditions. As with any surgical procedure, side effects can occur at the time of surgery or after surgery.[32]

Nonprescription Diet Drugs and Dietary Supplements
Popular over-the-counter diet drugs and dietary supplements include diet teas, bulking products, starch blockers, diet candies, sugar blockers, and benzocaine. Safety concerns have arisen over the use of these drugs and supplements. One example is ephedra, a stimulant found in many over-the-counter weight loss supplements. Ephedra can cause cardiac arrhythmia (abnormal heart rhythm) and even death by constricting blood vessels while increasing the heart rate and speeding up the nervous system. In February 2004, the FDA banned dietary supplements containing ephedra because of the association of this drug with heart attack, stroke, hyper-tension, and heat stroke. Again, consumers need to always use their critical thinking skills when considering the use of any product, including herbal supplements, to help them lose weight.

THE PROBLEM OF UNDERWEIGHT

The prevalence of obesity often obscures the problem of underweight. A sudden, unintentional weight loss without a change in diet or exercise level may signify an underlying illness and should prompt a visit to a physician. Depression, substance abuse, eating disorders, thyroid disease, infections, and cancer can all be associated with unexpected weight loss.

However, some people just have difficulty keeping on weight. In this situation, calorie intake is inadequate for energy output. To gain weight, the person needs to change the energy balance. Calories can be increased by eating more frequent meals and increasing servings of healthy, more energy-dense foods, such as nuts, fish, or yogurt. Adding protein powders or nutritional supplements to the diet as snacks is another option. The pattern of physical activity can also be changed, so that aerobic exercise is reduced and weight training is increased.

The Size Acceptance Movement

The size acceptance movement started in response to the frustration felt by many people in attempting to lose weight. The approach seeks to decrease negative body image and to encourage self-acceptance. The focus is on how people who are large can be healthy. The movement is based on six basic tenets:[33, 34]

1. Good health is a state of physical, mental, and social well-being. All people can achieve good health through eating a variety of foods, being physically active, and appreciating their bodies as they are.

2. People come in a variety of shapes and sizes. This should be viewed as a positive characteristic of the human race.

3. There is no ideal body size, body shape, BMI, or body composition that everyone should strive to achieve.

4. Self-esteem and body image are strongly linked. Helping people feel good about their bodies and about who they are can help them achieve and maintain healthy behaviors.

5. Each person is responsible for taking care of his or her body.

6. Appearance stereotyping is wrong. No matter what their weight, all people deserve equal treatment in employment and respectful treatment by health professionals.

Perhaps in response to the size acceptance movement, or perhaps in response to the increasing number of overweight and obese people, language is beginning to change

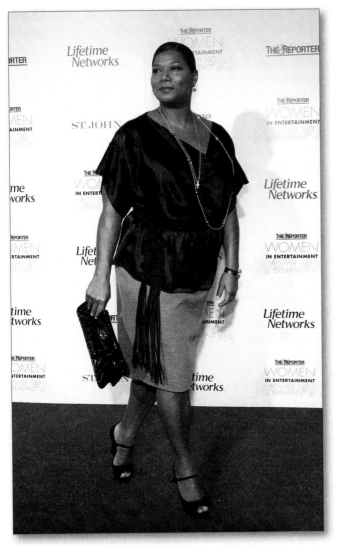

■ Singer and actress Queen Latifah has consistently celebrated her body size and exuded confidence about her personal appearance.

in the direction of greater acceptance of overweight. The movement has also had some political impact: Several states have passed laws against weight discrimination.

The size acceptance movement has made strides in changing health approaches from weight loss to weight management. However, pleas by the size acceptance movement should not obscure the fact that obesity is a serious medical problem. The goal is to find a balanced approach that combines personal acceptance with promotion of a healthy body composition.

Achieving a Healthy Body Weight and Body Composition for Life

Overweight and obesity are long-term problems and require long-term solutions. Both individuals and society have roles to play in reversing this trend.

TASKS FOR INDIVIDUALS

If your genetics or behavioral history predisposes you to being overweight or underweight, you can improve your overall health through moderate lifestyle changes. The emphasis should be on a healthier lifestyle, with these components:

■ A balanced diet emphasizing fruits, vegetables, and whole grains in appropriate portion sizes.

■ A goal of 30 to 60 minutes of moderate-intensity physical activity every day. This can be divided into smaller sections of time throughout the day (more physical activity may be necessary if you are aiming to lose weight, less if you are aiming to gain weight).

■ A goal of overall health improvement through targeted improvement in selected areas, such as blood pressure, cholesterol level, and blood sugar level.

■ Inclusion of peer support.

■ Self-acceptance of body size.

■ Follow-up evaluation by a health professional, as needed.

Set Realistic Goals Drastic diet changes and quick-fix solutions are unlikely to last for long. The key to long-term weight management is making reasonable, moderate changes that fit in with your life, culture, and tastes. Consider each of the following areas:

■ *Variety.* A diet that includes all food groups is easier to maintain than one that excludes food groups.

■ *Proportionality and balance.* Eat more of nutrient-dense foods and less of high-fat foods and foods with empty calories.

■ *Moderation.* Limit portion size of foods. When shopping for home, buy smaller packages of foods or divide foods into single-serving sizes; when eating out, split an entrée with a friend, order an appetizer instead of an entrée, or take half your order home.

■ *Gradual change.* Make small, sustainable changes, such as switching from regular soda to diet soda or from whole milk to low-fat milk.[35, 36]

Get Active Physical activity enhances weight maintenance and weight loss achieved through dietary changes. Even if your weight does not change, the addition of exercise to a daily routine confers health benefits for all people. Simple lifestyle changes that increase physical activity and that you can incorporate into your daily routine are the best way to guarantee long-term success. More vigorous activity will help even more, but make it something you can really enjoy. Exercise does not have to be brutal to be good for you.

Manage Behavior Many behavior management tools are available to help you learn new eating and activity patterns. The following strategies may help get you started:

■ *Stimulus control.* Identify environmental cues associated with unhealthy eating habits. Become conscious of when, where, and why you are eating. For example, if you live in a dorm and eat at night in your room when you study, you may not be aware of how many calories you are consuming.

■ *Self-supervision.* Keep a log of the foods you eat and the physical activity you do. Schedule time for exercise and plan time for healthy eating.

■ *Social support and positive reinforcement.* Recruit others to join you in your healthier eating and exercising habits. Exercise together, encourage each other, and plan non-food rewards for reaching goals.

■ *Stress management.* Use relaxation techniques, exercise, and problem-solving strategies to handle stresses in your life, instead of overeating or skipping meals.

■ *Cognitive restructuring.* Moderate any self-defeating thoughts and emotions, redefine your body image, and be realistic about weight loss or gain.

TASKS FOR SOCIETY

Changes in social policies are also needed to combat the obesity epidemic.

Promote Healthy Foods The U.S. surgeon general has asked that all schools reduce junk food and promote healthy, balanced meals. Schools can limit access to candy and soda, and municipalities can provide better access to healthy foods, through such means as community gardens and equitable supermarket distribution. Federal, state, and local governments can provide financial incentives, such as loan guarantees and reduced property taxes, for supermarkets and small stores that provide healthy foods. They can also provide assistance with zoning approval and building permits.

Food subsidies and pricing strategies are a broad-based intervention that can alter eating patterns. Lowering the price of low-fat, nutritious food would increase the rates at which people would buy them. However, in the 15-year period from 1985 to 2000, the cost of fruits and vegetables increased 117 percent, while the cost of soft drinks increased just 20 percent.

Support Active Lifestyles Through Community Planning Suburbanization and a cultural focus on cars play a major role in Americans' decreased physical activity. As a society, we need to consider ways to encourage a more active lifestyle (see the box "Can Community Gardens Help Reduce Obesity?"). Community planning can incorporate ideas to encourage physical activity, such as walking areas and parks in all communities, increased public transportation, showering and changing room facilities in workplaces to encourage biking or walking to work, and flexible work hours to reduce stress and encourage activity.

Support Consumer Awareness In a free society we avoid restricting the media and advertising, but consumers can become more conscious of their effects on eating patterns. Advertising is a supply-and-demand industry. If consumers don't buy the products depicted in ads, or if they complain about the content of ads, food manufacturers will eventually respond.

Parents can also limit children's exposure to media and advertising by limiting television viewing time. When children are encouraged to reduce TV time, they have a more positive attitude toward physical activity. Limiting TV time will also decrease exposure to junk food advertising and decrease the amount of food consumed in front of the television set.[37]

Encourage Health Insurers to Cover Obesity Prevention Programs Health insurance companies have been slow to cover all preventive health care, and prevention of obesity is no exception. Although conclusive evidence shows that obesity is associated with risks of multiple medical conditions, few insurance plans currently cover health visits for obesity education or treatment. With concern about health care and health care costs rising, we may see changes in the future. Employers and educational institutions can push legislators to make preventive medicine a priority for insurance companies.

Obesity is considered a chronic degenerative condition, which may help individuals, insurers, and health care providers move away from the "quick fix" mentality.

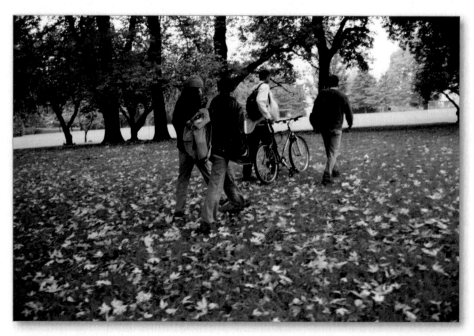

■ Building physical activity into your routine in small ways every day is one key to weight management and weight loss maintenance.

As with any chronic condition, the focus has to be on sustainable changes. Programs that combine nutritional education, exercise education, and lifestyle modification may help promote healthier, more sustainable weight loss.

Although the American girth has grown steadily in the recent past, this trend does not have to continue. People can successfully manage their weight by establishing careful eating habits and integrating physical activity and exercise into their daily routines. A healthy energy balance is the key to attaining lifelong weight control goals. Our communities and society need to support and encourage individuals in making these lifestyle changes.

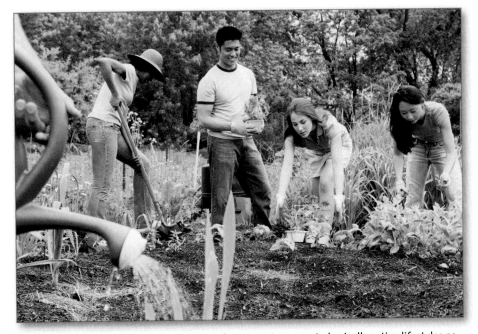

■ Community gardens are being promoted as a way to support physically active lifestyles as well as social involvement and healthy eating.

Public Health in Action

Can Community Gardens Help Reduce Obesity?

The United States has a long history of community gardening, dating back to World War II, when people came together to grow food for the war effort in "victory gardens." The 1970s saw a resurgence of interest in community gardening in response to environmental concerns. Currently an effort is under way to revitalize the community garden movement in urban settings to combat inequities in access to healthy foods for low-income and urban populations. The USDA Community Food Projects Grant was established to promote food security in low-income neighborhoods, and one-third of the project's funds are designated for setting up community gardens. New York and Tennessee have laws in place to protect and encourage the conversion of vacant city land to vegetable gardens. Seattle has an ambitious, comprehensive plan to create one community garden for every 2,500 households. The Edible Schoolyard Project in Berkeley, California, has established a vegetable garden at a local elementary school where children learn to grow fresh foods and then prepare them on-site.

How might community gardens impact the current obesity trends? People with garden plots eat more fruits and vegetables than those who do not have them. Gardening provides a leisure-time recreational activity that is physically active; it includes walking to a neighborhood plot, cultivating the land, picking vegetables, and weeding. Youth garden programs can help young children learn new skills and build self-esteem, and they encourage children to try fruits and vegetables they may never have eaten before. Communal gardening may also help reduce feelings of isolation and stress as people get to know their neighbors, develop a sense of community, and gain access to nutritious foods. Take a look at your own community and see what is being done. Could you help start the next garden?

Source: "Community Design for Healthy Eating: How Land Use and Transportation Solutions Can Help," by Barbara McCann, 2006, Robert Wood Johnson Foundation, retrieved August 11, 2007, from www.rwjf.org/files/publications/other/communitydesignhealthyeating.pdf.

You Make the Call

Should Employers Have Weight Loss Contests?

Weight loss challenges are popping up at workplaces across the country, with catchy names based on the TV show "The Biggest Loser." Employers offer money or prizes for the male and female employee who loses the most weight in a defined period of time. Employers are interested in employees' weight because of the medical complications associated with obesity and the rising cost of health insurance. Employers adopting these weight loss challenges say they can improve employee general health, increase productivity, and reduce absenteeism. They also point to the benefits for employees, for whom a work-based challenge may be helpful because a significant portion of the day is spent at work. The support of colleagues in exercising, making dietary changes, and identifying nonfood rewards may also be helpful.

Opponents of weight loss challenges say that drawing attention to obesity and focusing on individual behavior change may enhance bias and discrimination against overweight employees. Clear patterns of stigmatization and bias already exist in employment settings. Studies show that employers are less likely to hire overweight applicants than average weight applicants and that they judge overweight applicants to be significantly less neat, productive, ambitious, disciplined, and determined, all other factors being equal. Once hired, overweight individuals continue to experience bias. They have been shown to get lower wages for the same job performed by nonobese employees, and they are less likely to be promoted than their nonobese colleagues.

Opponents suggest that employers can better promote employee health through interventions that focus less on individuals with certain characteristics and more on the general health and wellness of the entire workforce. Employers can offer flexible work hours, allowing employees time for exercise or time to use alternative forms of transportation, such as bicycling. They can promote healthy food choices by providing vending machines with fresh fruit and low-fat snacks. The work facility can be adapted to provide safe, accessible stairs, secure bike storage, and on-site showering and changing facilities. These systemwide options would not target specific individuals.

Proponents argue that overweight and obese people know they have a health problem and need help from any source. Opponents believe weight loss contests in the workplace are inappropriate and counterproductive. What do you think?

PROS

■ Obesity is a major health concern, and obese employees are likely to cause higher health care costs for employers and insurance companies.

■ A significant part of most people's day is spent at work; colleagues can provide social support for individual behavior change.

■ Workplace challenges are fun and reduce the stigma associated with obesity.

CONS

■ Bias and discrimination against overweight employees already exist in the workplace; focusing on individual behavior change may further increase negative attitudes and stigmatization.

■ Overweight and obesity have multiple causes, including genetics and cultural factors that may be beyond the control of the individual. Workplace weight loss challenges assume that anyone can lose weight if he or she tries hard enough, an assumption that fails to take into account all the determinants of health.

■ The workplace focus should be on systems that enhance the health of all employees, not just certain easily identifiable individuals.

Source: "Bias, Discrimination, and Obesity," by R. Puhl and K.D. Brownell, 2001, Obesity Research, 9 (12), pp. 788–805.

In Review

1. **What are the current trends in overweight and obesity?** These two conditions, defined in general terms as body weight that exceeds or greatly exceeds the recommended guidelines, have been increasing exponentially among Americans as well as among people in many developed countries. Two-thirds of Americans meet the criteria for overweight, and one-third meet the criteria for obesity. Overweight and obesity are risk factors for a wide range of serious health problems.

2. **How is healthy body weight defined?** Healthy body weight can be defined by an acceptable body mass index (a measure of weight relative to height), by a pattern of body fat distribution that is not a risk factor for illness, or by the absence of a medical condition that suggests a need for weight loss (for example, diabetes, hypertension). People who don't meet these criteria could probably benefit from losing weight.

3. **What causes a person to be overweight?** Influences on weight include genetic and hormonal factors, gender and age, "obesogenic environments," and lifestyle behaviors (for example, eating out, supersizing, sedentary living). Weight is also influenced by "yo-yo dieting" and by the frequency with which a person experiences the stress response.

4. **What is the best way to manage body weight?** The key to weight control is balancing energy intake (calories) with energy output (physical activity and exercise). Fad diets usually don't work, and consumers who join weight management organizations often regain the weight they lose. Medical approaches, including surgery, are available for people with serious health risks due to obesity. The best approach is making long-term, moderate lifestyle changes that include a balanced diet, daily physical activity, realistic goals, social support, and stress management. Communities can help by promoting healthy foods and planning activity-friendly environments.

WWW For a detailed summary of this chapter and a comprehensive set of review questions, visit the Online Learning Center at **www.mhhe.com/teague2e**.

Web Resources

American Diabetes Association: Highlighting diabetes prevention, this organization offers information about weight loss and exercise through its healthy recipes, tip sheets, and brochures.
www.diabetes.org

Ask the Dietitian/Overweight: The Q&As on this site focus on real-life weight issues, offering tips on motivation, dealing with setbacks, and the challenges of lifetime weight management.
www.dietitian.com

Calorie Control Council: This site offers an online calorie counter, an exercise calculator, and a BMI calculator. Healthy recipes and a guide to effective weight control are also offered.
www.caloriecontrol.org

U.S. Consumer Gateway/Health: Dieting and Weight Control: This site takes you to several government resources on weight loss and weight management, including guidelines on diet, how to lose weight safely, and finding a weight loss program that will work for you.
www.consumer.gov

Weight-Control Information Network (WIN): An information service of the National Institute of Diabetes and Digestive and Kidney Diseases, WIN features government publications and other resources on weight control for adults, children, and pregnant women.
http://win.niddk.nih.gov

Chapter 10

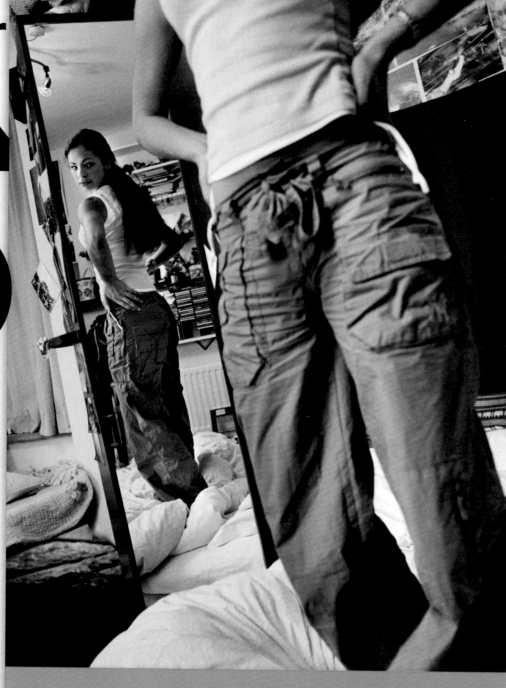

Body Image
Viewing Yourself

Ever Wonder...

- where you get your ideas about personal appearance and beauty?

- if it's possible to exercise too much?

- what you can do if you think a friend has anorexia or bulimia?

How do you evaluate your appearance? Such evaluations usually reflect societal and cultural values and ideals as conveyed by family, peers, language, advertising, and the media. Very often, cultural ideals are far removed from most people's natural appearance, and for some, the discrepancy can produce feelings of inadequacy, dissatisfaction, and self-criticism. For others, it can lead to a resolve to reach the ideal, no matter how unrealistic the goal or unhealthy the means. And for a few, it leads to a quest for perfection that results in psychological illness.

Chapter 9 focused on the current problem of overweight and obesity, and we explored ways to achieve and maintain a healthy body weight and body composition. This chapter considers the other side of the coin—our society's obsession with thinness and dieting and the corresponding prevalence of eating disorders. The message about attaining a healthy body weight has to be balanced with a message about developing a healthy body image, setting realistic goals, and maintaining emotional well-being.

What Shapes Body Image?

Like all ideas, values, attitudes, and beliefs, **body image**—the mental representation that a person has of his or her own body, including perceptions, attitudes, thoughts, and emotions—is strongly influenced by culture. American culture places a premium on appearance, especially for women but increasingly for men. Every day we see hundreds of images and messages about how we should look, whether we are reading a magazine, seeing a movie, noticing ads in public places, or watching television in the privacy of our homes. The advertising industry and the media are relentless in selling the American consumer an image of the ideal body, and many of us buy into what they are selling. The message of the media is powerful.

body image
Mental representation that a person has of his or her own body, including perceptions, attitudes, thoughts, and emotions.

WOMEN AND BODY IMAGE

For girls and women, beauty has long been held up as a desirable trait. Pioneering English feminist Mary Wollstonecraft pointed out back in 1792 that women would submit to anything to reach the ideal of beauty, even giving up the right to think for themselves. Repeated cycles of feminist thinking and activism over the last two centuries have attempted to change the

message society sends to women and to free women from their obsession with the body.

Current Cultural Messages   Today, women have more educational and occupational opportunities than ever before, and they fulfill a broad range of valued roles in society. Despite progress in areas of women's rights, however, our culture still tells women that their most important job is to be beautiful. From infancy onward, when baby girls are described as "delicate," "soft," and "pretty," females are encouraged to define themselves in terms of their bodies. The female body is portrayed by the media as an object of desire, and this objectification reinforces women's focus on their appearance. The media place a heavy emphasis on women's physical attributes rather than on their abilities, performance, or accomplishments.

Since the 1950s, what is held to be the ideal female body in U.S. culture has been getting thinner. It is well known that actresses and beauty queens of the 1940s and 1950s had much more ample proportions, as exemplified by the curvaceous Marilyn Monroe. The 1960s brought a trend toward thin, boyish figures that persists to this day.

Many girls and women aspire to the weight and shape of the super-thin fashion model. Unfortunately, the average fashion model is thinner than 98 percent of all American women. Models represent a tiny subset of the population but provide an unattainable goal for millions.[1] For some tips on critically evaluating media messages, see the box "Media Literacy."

It is not surprising, then, that women experience high levels of dissatisfaction with their bodies. Magazines directed toward young women contain 10 times as many articles and advertisements that emphasize thinness as do magazines directed toward young men. These magazines can leave

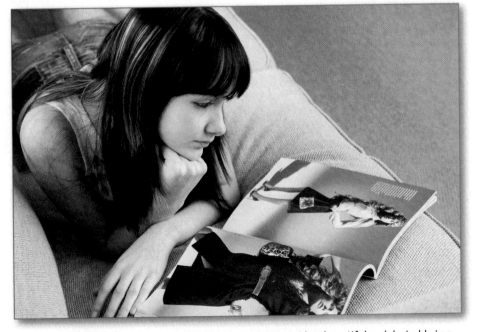

■ Girls get many of their ideas about what our society considers beautiful and desirable in a woman from the media, especially fashion magazines. Unrealistic hopes and dreams set some girls on a course toward disordered eating.

women feeling inadequate, preoccupied with a desire to be thin, unhappy with their own bodies, and afraid of becoming fat. Studies show that after women view media images of thin women, they are less satisfied with their own bodies than they are after viewing images of average-sized women.[2–4]

Belief in the thin ideal and body dissatisfaction can lead to dieting. This combination increases the risk for disordered eating behaviors, such as severe **calorie restriction** or getting rid of calories by **purging**. Disordered eating can progress further into an eating disorder. Eating disorders occur most often in cultures in which female attractiveness is linked with being thin. However, not all women develop eating disorders. Other factors to be considered are genetics, self-esteem, and cultural support.[4]

Effects of Puberty Eating disorders are most likely to develop during adolescence. As noted in Chapter 9, hormonal changes cause increases in body fat in girls, especially on the hips, buttocks, and thighs. The percentage of body fat in healthy girls increases from about 12 percent to about 25 percent during puberty. Given the cultural emphasis on thinness, many girls become concerned about their bodies at this time.

However, girls are concerned even before puberty. By sixth grade, twice as many girls as boys consider themselves fat, even though they are not overweight by objective standards. Sixth-grade girls are more likely to want to lose weight to become thin, whereas boys are more likely to want to gain weight, especially in the upper body, to become more muscular.

calorie restriction
A reduction in calorie intake below daily needs.

purging
Using self-induced vomiting, laxatives, or diuretics to get rid of excess calories that have been consumed.

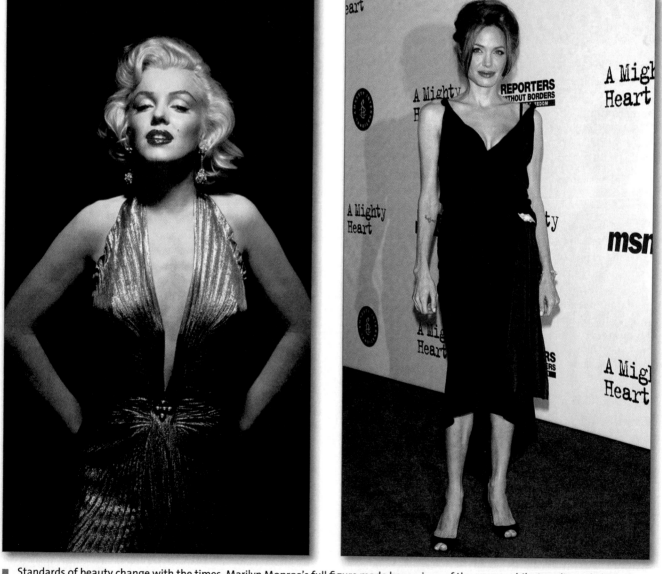

■ Standards of beauty change with the times. Marilyn Monroe's full figure made her an icon of the 1950s, while Angelina Jolie's waif-like proportions more closely match today's thin ideal.

MEN AND BODY IMAGE

Male body image has been less affected by cultural expectations and the media than female body image has. Historically, men have been judged by achievement and strength more than by looks. Media and advertising have promoted a masculine image that emphasizes power, performance, and choice for men, focusing on action and performance rather than on appearance. Correspondingly, men are generally more satisfied with their body size and appearance than women are.

However, men are not immune to body image concerns. They are increasingly drawn into the world of beauty and appearance. Hair, skin, and grooming products directed toward men are making male use of beauty products acceptable, although they are given a manly aura. Words like *musk, wood, spice*, and *surf* are used to describe scents, and product names are chosen to suggest power ("Brut," "The Baron").

The marketing of the male body image has created an environment in which a man's physique is becoming as important as his possessions and accomplishments. As with women, the ideal male body shape has become more unrealistic, distorted, and extreme. Men's magazines publish more advertisements and articles about changing body shape rather than weight loss. Today's male models have trimmer waists and bulkier biceps than in the past. The evolution of G.I. Joe action figures mirrors society's changing male image. In 1964 G.I. Joe had the physique of an average man in reasonably good shape. By 1992 he had a build that most men could not attain without the use of anabolic steroids. The exposure to highly muscled male images in magazines has been shown to leave male college students more depressed and less satisfied with their own bodies, compared with male college students not exposed to such images.[5]

For some men, this unrealistic message about supersized bodies can lead to a condition known as **muscle dysmorphia** (or muscle dysmorphic disorder; sometimes referred to as "bigorexia"). Men with this condition perceive themselves as being insufficiently massive or muscular in appearance, no matter how bulked up they really are. (Muscle dysmorphia is discussed in more detail in a later section of this chapter.) Some observers suggest that supermuscularity may be one way men believe they can distinguish themselves in a world of increasing gender equality.[6, 7]

muscle dysmorphia
Disorder in which a person perceives his body to be underdeveloped no matter how highly developed his muscles really are.

About 10 percent of eating disorders are diagnosed in men. However, a recent study found a surprisingly higher proportion of men reporting anorexia nervosa and bulimia nervosa—nearly one in four cases.[8, 9] Much speculation exists about why eating disorders occur less often among men. Perhaps the earlier societal focus on male accomplishments rather than physique is protective. As men buy into the cultural quest for physical perfection and pursue unrealistic

Consumer Clipboard

Media Literacy

Media images and advertisements for consumer products—from clothes to cosmetics to food to cars—are everywhere. These images and ads are a form of communication created by an industry with something to sell. They have been carefully crafted to convey values, reflect a point of view, and sell a product or an idea. They are designed to make you feel a certain way when you view them. What "reality" do the messages ask you to believe? How accurate is this reality? What message is being left out or goes untold? These are some of the important factors to consider in developing media literacy.

Once you become conscious of all the images around you and what they are designed to make you think and feel, you can gain control over whether you want to buy into the image or message being sold. To protect your self-esteem and body image, it's important to carefully filter media images and understand what the advertiser wants you to believe. Then decide if you want to believe the message. Here are some points to consider:

- What is the product or service being advertised?
- Who created the advertisement? Who paid for it? Who profits from it?
- What does the advertisement directly claim the product will do?
- What are the messages or persuasive techniques asking you to believe about the product? Commonly used persuasive techniques include symbols, flattery, fear, humor, power, and sex.
- How has the imagery been altered or enhanced? Has it been edited, colored, airbrushed, lightened, or darkened? To what end?
- What values are being promoted? What meaning does that have for you? How might it mean something different to people of another age, race, ethnicity, or religion?
- What does the ad make you think or feel about yourself? Does it make you feel good about yourself, or does it make you feel inadequate and somehow lacking? The latter is the best indicator that the message is designed to manipulate your feelings and induce you to buy a product.

goals, they may have increasing feelings of inadequacy and body dissatisfaction. This may lead to further increases in dieting and body-building. Men appear to report dieting for different reasons than those of women. Men are shape oriented rather than weight oriented; they focus on the upper

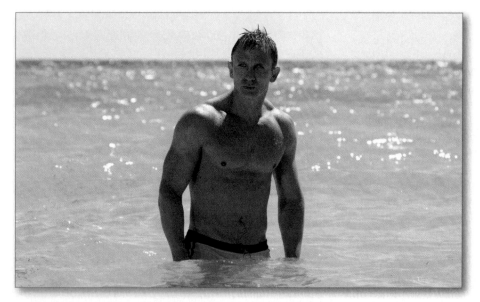

■ The marketing of the male body image has made physique an increasingly important part of male attractiveness in our society. Boys and men are coming under pressure to attain the kind of muscle development seen in actors like Daniel Craig.

body rather than the lower body; and they usually diet for a specific reason, such as sports performance.

Eating disorders among men may have been underdiagnosed because they have been considered a female problem. The current criteria for diagnosing anorexia nervosa include the cessation of menstrual periods. Obviously this excludes men from the diagnosis. With an increasing recognition of disordered eating among men, the criteria will need to change to more accurately include all affected groups.

Another factor thought to be important in the lack of recognition of eating disorders among men is that it remains a social taboo for men to publicly discuss their anxiety about their bodies. Thus men are secretive about their body dissatisfaction and their drive to bulk up.

ETHNICITY AND BODY IMAGE

Body satisfaction is also affected by one's ethnicity or cultural group. Historically, White women have been reported as experiencing greater body dissatisfaction and eating disturbance than women in other ethnic groups. Ethnic minorities were believed to have less cultural pressure to be thin. However, among women, it appears that differences between ethnic groups in fear of fatness, body dissatisfaction, dieting, and pressure to be thin have diminished to the point that White, Black, Asian, and Hispanic women report similar concerns.[10]

Among men, Blacks report more positive body image than Whites. Hispanics appear similar to Whites but may be affected by degree of acculturation. Native Americans report slightly greater body image concerns than White men. Among Asian men, findings have been inconsistent, perhaps because of the array of cultural groups considered "Asian." Interestingly, non-White males do appear to engage in more extreme weight loss strategies and binge eating than do White males.[11] As patterns of disordered eating change, education and treatment programs also have to change to respond to the needs, perceptions, and values of diverse groups.[12]

SPORTS AND BODY IMAGE

Participation in sports confers many health and fitness benefits, including higher levels of self-esteem in both boys and girls. Sports may provide protection against eating disorders by promoting a focus on performance rather than on appearance.[7] However, participation in sports also carries pressure, both from oneself and from coaches, teammates, and parents. High-level athletes often succeed because they have high expectations of themselves, accompanied by varying degrees of perfectionism and compulsiveness. Athletes often learn to disregard signals from their bodies, including pain, during training. Parents and coaches can directly and indirectly encourage disordered eating by commenting on appearance or performance when a young athlete has lost weight. They can also

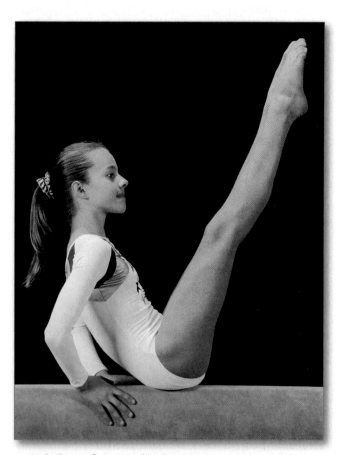

■ Body dissatisfaction and body image issues are particularly common in sports and activities that place a premium on a lean body, such as gymnastics, dance, and track.

indirectly foster disordered eating by not recognizing patterns of rapid weight loss.

In some sports, such as wrestling, dance, gymnastics, swimming, cycling, distance running, and horse racing, a premium is placed on leanness. The risk for eating disorders appears to be greatest for athletes competing at elite levels, such as college teams. Women who compete in nonelite sports that do not emphasize leanness have the least risk of developing eating disorders.[13, 14]

Eating Disorders

eating disorders
Conditions characterized by severely disturbed eating behaviors and distorted body image; eating disorders jeopardize physical and psychological health.

Eating disorders are chronic illnesses that jeopardize physical and mental health; they can be life threatening. The key characteristic of eating disorders is a severe disturbance in eating behavior. A second characteristic is a distorted body image. What begins as a diet takes on a life of its own, turning into self-induced starvation or repeated cycles of binging and purging.

The most extreme forms of disturbed eating behavior are anorexia nervosa and bulimia nervosa, both of which are classified as psychiatric disorders in the American Psychiatric Association's *Diagnostic and Statistical Manual of Mental Disorders* (*DSM-IV-TR*). Binge-eating disorder currently falls into a category called "eating disorder not otherwise specified." It shares features with other eating disorders and is considered an area in which further research is needed.

Eating disorders occur primarily among people in Western industrialized countries. They occur in every ethnic, cultural, and socioeconomic group. They appear to become more prevalent when food is abundant and has taken on symbolic meanings, such as comfort, love, belonging, fun, and control. They are also more common where being attractive is related to being thin (see the box "Eating Disorders").

The frequency of eating disorders appears to be directly related to rates of dieting. In the last 30 years, the number of diagnosed cases in the United States has doubled. Of course, not all people who diet have eating disorders. In fact, using the strict criteria proposed by the *DSM-IV-TR*, about 0.5–0.9 percent of women and 0.1–0.3 percent of men have anorexia; 1.1–2.8 percent of women and 0.1–0.5 percent of men have bulimia; and 3.3–3.5 percent of women and 0.8–2 percent of men have binge eating disorder.[9]

disordered eating behaviors
Abnormal eating patterns (for example, vomiting, use of laxatives, extreme dieting) that may not fit the rigid diagnostic rules for anorexia or bulimia but affect quality of life.

More common and widespread than eating disorders are **disordered eating behaviors,** such as restrictive dieting and binging and purging, which are not as severe or frequently practiced as those associated with diagnosed disorders. These behaviors may occur in response to emotional stress, an upcoming athletic event, concern about personal appearance, and so on. They may or may not develop into a full-blown eating disorder. The rates of disordered eating in the general population are not known but are thought to be much higher than the rates of diagnosed eating disorders.

FACTORS CONTRIBUTING TO EATING DISORDERS

Many factors most likely contribute to the development of eating disorders, and much about the process remains unknown. Why the widespread cultural ideals and beliefs promoting thinness and dieting for women and extreme muscularity for men become an overvalued, ruling passion for some is not totally clear. Exposure to the thin ideal, social pressure to conform, and recognition of a discrepancy between the ideal and one's own body can certainly lead to body dissatisfaction and have been shown to increase risk for eating disorders. However, this can't be the entire story, because the social pressures to be thin (or muscular) are pervasive and spreading globally and yet only a fraction of

Who's at Risk

Eating Disorders

- Eating disorders occur in any age group, from late childhood through older adulthood, but they are most common during the teens and early 20s.

- Although the incidence is increasing among men, eating disorders remain more common in women.

- A personal or family history of eating disorders, substance abuse, depression, anxiety, obesity, or obsessive-compulsive disorder is associated with an increased risk of eating disorders.

- Frequent dieting is associated with the onset of eating disorders.

- Life transitions can trigger emotional stress and a sense of loss of control; eating disorders are more likely to occur during these times.

- Overly controlling or critical family relationships can increase the risk for eating disorders.

- Frequent exposure to media messages promoting a thin body size and shape can increase the risk for eating disorders.

- Sports that emphasize thin body type or weight restrictions may increase the risk for eating disorders.

- Gay men may have an increased risk for eating disorders; lesbians do not appear to be at higher risk than heterosexual women.

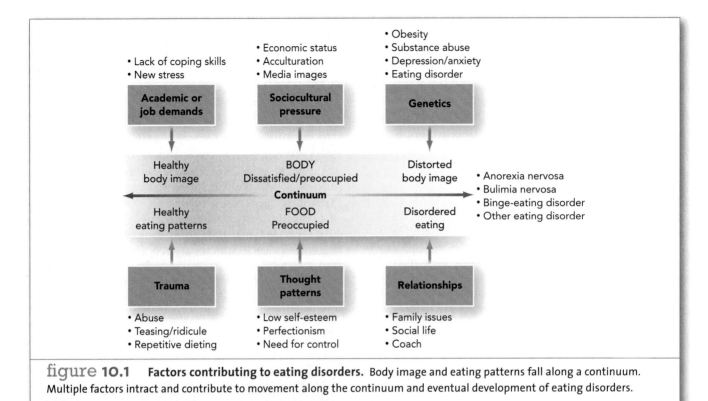

figure **10.1** **Factors contributing to eating disorders.** Body image and eating patterns fall along a continuum. Multiple factors intract and contribute to movement along the continuum and eventual development of eating disorders.

women and men go on to develop eating disorders. Other factors play a role.

Eating disorders and other associated traits run in families. A family history of eating disorders, depression, substance abuse, anxiety, obsessive-compulsive disorder, or obesity increases the risk for anorexia and bulimia. Most likely, genes predispose an individual and then certain experiences or characteristics further contribute to the development of eating disorders.[4, 15]

Gender is clearly a risk factor for eating disorders, with female gender increasing risk. Sexual orientation may alter risk for males, with gay and bisexual men at greater risk than heterosexual men. Gay and bisexual men aim to attract men and thus may be subject to the same pressures as heterosexual women. They may place greater value on physical appearance than do heterosexual men. Gay women appear to have the same rates of eating disorders as heterosexual women.[16]

The connection between eating disorders and depression and anxiety disorders is complicated. People with anorexia and bulimia frequently report symptoms of depression and anxiety. A history of depression appears to increase risk for eating disorders, but it can be difficult to diagnose depression in a person with anorexia because the starvation process produces similar symptoms, including changes in sleep patterns, a decline in energy level, and decreased interest in activities. Certain characteristics or thought patterns are associated with eating disorders, including the following:

- Low self-esteem
- Self-critical attitude

- Belief in the importance of thinness
- Black-and-white thinking
- Feelings of emptiness
- Need for power and control
- Difficulty expressing feelings
- Lack of coping skills
- Lack of trust in self or others
- Perfectionism

Not all of these patterns must be present, and many of these are found in people with anxiety disorders or depression but not eating disorders. Factors thought to increase risk for eating disorders are shown in Figure 10.1.

DIAGNOSING EATING DISORDERS

As recently as the 1980s the terms *anorexia nervosa* and *bulimia nervosa* were virtually unknown to the general public. Today, disturbed eating patterns have become common. In one study, 80 percent of eighth-grade girls thought that starving and purging are acceptable weight control methods.[17] Detecting when someone with disordered eating makes the transition to having an eating disorder is difficult. Guidelines have been developed, but disordered eating and eating disorders occur on a continuum, as shown in Figure 10.1. In this section we review the most common eating disorders and their diagnostic criteria.

anorexia nervosa
Eating disorder marked by distortion of body image and refusal to maintain a minimally normal body weight.

Anorexia Nervosa The word *anorexia* is of Greek origin: *an,* which means "lack of," and *orexis,* which means "appetite." However, most people with **anorexia nervosa** do not have a lack of appetite; they are more likely to be obsessed with food. At the same time, they are starving themselves and appear ultrathin or emaciated. Criteria for anorexia nervosa are as follows:[18]

- Refusal to maintain body weight at or above a minimally normal weight for age and height (usually less than 85 percent of expected body weight).
- Intense fear of gaining weight or becoming fat, even though underweight.
- Disturbance in the way in which one's body weight or shape is experienced, undue influence of body weight or shape on self-evaluation, or denial of the seriousness of the current low body weight.
- Amenorrhea—the absence of at least three consecutive menstrual cycles.

Some people with anorexia control their weight by severely restricting calories, and others engage in binge-eating and purging behavior. To get a sense of how anorexia plays out in a person's life, see the box "Alexis: A Case of Anorexia Nervosa."

Bulimia Nervosa The word *bulimia* is of Latin origin and means "hunger of an ox." People with **bulimia nervosa** consume a huge amount of food at one sitting and then use an inappropriate method to get rid of the calories they have consumed, either by purging or through excessive exercise. People with bulimia are usually neither underweight nor overweight, but they have a disturbed perception of body size and image. Binge-eating and purging behaviors are usually socially isolating. Criteria for bulimia nervosa are as follows:[18]

bulimia nervosa
Eating disorder marked by distortion of body image and repeated episodes of binge eating, usually followed by purging in the form of self-induced vomiting, misuse of diuretics or laxatives, excessive exercising, or fasting.

- Recurrent episodes of binge eating, characterized by both (1) eating, in a discrete period of time (for example, 2 hours), an amount of food that is definitely larger than most people would eat in that period of time, and (2) a sense of lack of control during the episode—a feeling that one cannot stop eating or control what or how much one is eating.
- Recurrent inappropriate compensatory behavior to prevent weight gain, such as self-induced vomiting; misuse of laxatives, diuretics, enemas, or other medications; fasting; or excessive exercise.
- The episodes occur, on average, at least twice a week for 3 months.

Highlight on Health

Alexis: A Case of Anorexia Nervosa

Alexis was the top runner on her high school cross-country team. She was recruited by several colleges and decided on a school in the Midwest. The summer before her freshman year, she increased her mileage in order to be prepared for the fall season.

When she arrived on campus and began running with the team, she was surprised by how good the other women were. She was used to being able to lead at practice and to being the top runner. Now she found herself struggling to keep up. A month into the season, her shins were beginning to bother her at the end of long runs. She didn't want to tell anyone because she was worried she would be told to cut back on her mileage.

Alexis began to perceive the other women on the team as much thinner than herself, and she began to think, I'm sure I can run faster if I just lose a few pounds. She decided she would drink only water as a beverage and cut all sweets and carbohydrates from her diet. She was pleased when she quickly lost about 10 pounds, taking her from a body mass index (BMI) of 19.8 to a BMI of 18.2.

At the same time, Alexis was beginning to struggle in her classes. She was feeling tired much of the time. During lectures, her mind would wander to how much she had eaten the day before, when she could eat today, and how that would impact her workouts with the team. Her roommate began to notice that Alexis was more withdrawn and no longer wanted to go out for movies or dinner. Alexis didn't want to be around her teammates because she worried they thought she did not deserve to be on the team.

In November, Alexis had to stop running because her shins were so painful. She felt like a failure and was sure that no one wanted her on the team. Her solution was to lose more weight so that she could get faster and prove herself. She cut back on her food intake by not allowing herself anything to eat after 3 p.m. By the time she went home for winter break, she had lost another 10 pounds and had a BMI of 16.7.

Alexis's parents were shocked when they saw her and took her to see the counselor she had seen for depression during her junior year of high school. The counselor told her she needed to see a physician immediately. Alexis initially did not want to go but eventually agreed. The physician diagnosed her with anorexia and explained the dangers of the condition. Working together, the physician, the counselor, and Alexis's family members helped her understand that she had a psychological illness that needed to be addressed immediately. She agreed to take the winter quarter off so that she could receive treatment.

Highlight on Health

Sophie: A Case of Bulimia Nervosa

Sophie, a 22-year-old college senior, spent the fall quarter in a travel abroad program in France. She had a good time and found it hard to return to campus. Her parents now expected her to focus on completing her business degree, graduating in June, and getting a job. Sophie felt guilty because her time in Europe made her want to travel more after graduation, and she was no longer so sure she wanted to go into business.

To complicate matters further, her boyfriend had broken up with her a month after her return. She had been hoping they were going to be making future plans together. She did not understand why he had broken up with her, but she began to think it might be because of the 10 pounds she had gained in France. She thought they might get back together if she just lost a little weight.

She decided she needed to try harder with the diet she had used in the past. However, after a month, she began to feel that she did not have enough self-control. She was doing pretty well sticking to the diet during the day, but a few times a week she would go out with friends, have a few drinks, and skip dinner. When she got home to her apartment later at night, she would feel depressed about being alone and start to eat whatever was in the fridge. On these evenings, she could consume several thousand calories within an hour. Then she would feel disgusted with herself and depressed that she was never going to get back together with her boyfriend. She was still using the laxatives she had begun to use in France, but after these binges, she started making herself throw up.

This continued for several months until she began to have almost constant pain in her abdomen and heartburn most evenings. She would also occasionally notice flecks of blood in her vomit. She decided to go to the student health clinic because of the pain. In the clinic, the nurse practitioner noticed her enlarged salivary glands and puffy face as well as the calluses on her hand and asked if she was making herself vomit. Reluctantly, Sophie told her what had been going on for nearly 7 months. The nurse practitioner told Sophie she had bulimia and needed treatment. She advised Sophie to have some blood work and tests done, and she recommended an intensive counseling program that was offered at the medical center near campus. After some discussion, Sophie began to recognize that she had lost control of her behavior, and she agreed to the treatment plan.

- Self-evaluation is unduly influenced by body shape and weight.

To get a sense of bulimia, see the box "Sophie: A Case of Bulimia Nervosa."

Binge-Eating Disorder   Disordered eating patterns can also cause obesity. **Binge-eating disorder** has increasingly been recognized as a psychological disturbance that is associated with obesity. This disorder involves binge-eating behaviors without vomiting or purging. About 10 percent of patients in weight loss clinics are believed to have binge-eating disorder. One quarter of patients seeking treatment are male. Prevalence in the community is 3.5 percent among women and 2 percent among men.[7, 19]

binge-eating disorder
Eating disorder marked by binge-eating behavior without the vomiting or purging of bulimia.

People with binge-eating disorder are not just a subset of obese people. They have body weight and shape concerns, emotional distress, and disordered eating patterns similar to those of people with anorexia or bulimia. They are more likely to have depression and more fluctuations in weight than other obese persons.[20] Treatment may need to be different from other obesity treatment programs. Emphasizing patterns of eating and putting less emphasis on dieting can be important.[17] Criteria for binge-eating disorder are as follows:[18]

- Recurrent episodes of binge eating, as defined for bulimia.
- The episodes are associated with (1) eating much more rapidly than usual, (2) eating to the point of feeling uncomfortably full, (3) eating large amounts of food when not feeling hungry, (4) eating alone because of being embarrassed by how much one is eating, (5) feeling disgusted with oneself, depressed, or guilty about overeating.
- Marked distress about binge eating.
- The binge eating occurs, on average, at least 2 days a week for 6 months.
- The binge eating is not associated with the regular use of inappropriate compensatory behaviors (purging, fasting, excessive exercise) and does not occur exclusively during the course of anorexia or bulimia.

To get a sense of binge-eating disorder, see the box "Zach: A Case of Binge-Eating Disorder."

HEALTH CONSEQUENCES OF EATING DISORDERS

Eating disorders have serious health implications; some short-term problems, such as heart rate abnormalities, can even lead to death. Long-term problems can cause significant disability. Although anorexia and bulimia often overlap, they are associated with slightly different medical problems.

Health Effects of Anorexia   Anorexia nervosa carries the highest death rate of all psychiatric diagnoses—10 percent, according to most studies.[21] Death is usually due to cardiac arrest, electrolyte imbalance, or suicide. The signs and symptoms of anorexia are due to starvation and are shown in Figure 10.2.

Most of the complications are reversible if the person receives enough calorie replacement. However, some complications do not appear to be reversible, most notably, bone loss. Decreased bone calcium (osteoporosis) is one of the most serious long-term effects of severe calorie restriction. Peak bone density is reached during the adolescent years. After that it remains relatively stable until the middle 30s, when it starts a slow decline. Thus, low calcium intake in the teens and early 20s has a long-term negative effect on the bones. Studies of bone density in 20- to 25-year-old women with anorexia have shown them to have the bone strength of 70- to 80-year-old women.[17]

Health Effects of Bulimia   Bulimia is associated more with electrolyte imbalance than with starvation. Bulimia can also be deadly due to low potassium, cardiac arrest, or suicide. The signs and symptoms of bulimia are shown in Figure 10.3.

Health Effects of Binge-Eating Disorder   The health consequences of binge-eating disorder are related primarily to obesity. As discussed in Chapters 8 and 9, obesity is a degenerative chronic health condition that often significantly shortens the lifespan. Diseases associated with overweight and obesity include cardiorespiratory disease, diabetes, high blood pressure, gallbladder disease, osteoarthritis, sleep apnea, and certain cancers.

TREATING EATING DISORDERS

Aside from osteoporosis, most medical conditions associated with anorexia and bulimia are reversible. Keys to recovery appear to be early intervention, lower incidence of purging behavior, the support and participation of family members and loved ones, and lack of other diagnosed psychological problems. When patients with anorexia receive appropriate treatment, as many as 76 percent recover fully and 86 percent recover partially.[17] A person is considered to have recovered when weight is restored to within 15 percent of recommended weight. In women, recovery includes the return of regular menstruation, and in men, the return to a normal testosterone level.

Recognizing the Problem   The first step toward treatment is the recognition that there is a problem. People with eating disorders often deny that they are ill and refuse treatment.[15] At the heart of many eating disorders is a desire to have a sense of control over one's life, and treatment involves both weight gain and a perceived loss of this control. Health care providers may face the dilemma of wanting to respect a patient's autonomy and wishes and at the same time wanting to provide effective treatment for a potentially life-threatening illness.

Friends, roommates, parents, and others who are close to those with eating disorders may also deny that there is

a problem or fail to recognize it, because dieting, exercise, and preoccupation with food are so much an accepted part of our culture. (See the boxes "Do You Know Someone With Anorexia?" and "Do You Know Someone With Bulimia?") Treatment is most effective when the patient and family members all recognize the problem and are involved in treatment decisions.

Components of Treatment   Ideally a pattern of food obsession or body image preoccupation can be detected by the individual or by friends and family at an early point. Local campus resources may be sufficient to address unhealthy thought patterns, identify sources of stress, and teach healthier coping mechanisms. Many campuses have a health center, counseling facilities, food and nutritional services, recreational facilities, and student groups that may be of sufficient help in an early phase on the disordered eating continuum.

Highlight on Health

Zach: A Case of Binge-Eating Disorder

Zach, a 21-year-old man who was working part-time and going to college, felt a lot of pressure to succeed. He was the first member of his family to attend college, and his parents bragged about him to everyone they knew. Sometimes, however, Zach felt depressed and unable to cope, and then he would find comfort by staying in his apartment and "pigging out." He might eat an entire large pizza in one sitting, followed by an entire box of cookies or a whole cake. Sometimes he wouldn't even bother to heat up his dinner in the microwave; he would just eat it cold. Zach frequently ate until he got so full it was unpleasant, even painful. He felt guilty and ashamed after these binges, but he couldn't seem to stop himself.

Zach had always been slightly overweight, but during his junior year in college he gained 25 pounds in 3 months. He began to feel disgusted with himself and his body and started avoiding people he knew. He noticed how much harder it was to move around and how fast his heart would beat after the slightest exertion. Zach wanted to lose weight but did not believe he had the ability to diet or to stop his food binges. He particularly worried about developing diabetes, which ran in his family, and it was this worry that finally brought him to a weight management program at his college wellness center. By working with experts to develop a sensible exercise and nutrition program, Zach began to take steps to bring his weight back under control.

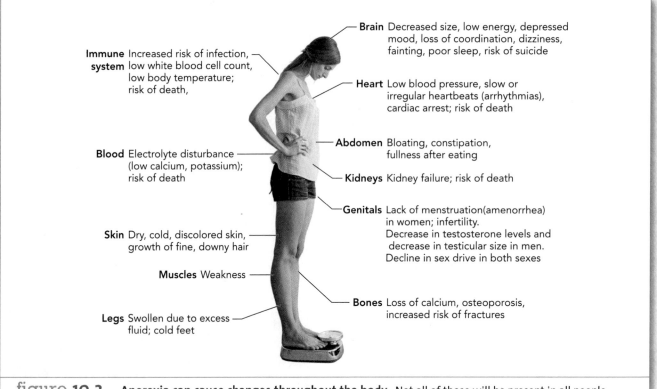

Immune system Increased risk of infection, low white blood cell count, low body temperature; risk of death,

Blood Electrolyte disturbance (low calcium, potassium); risk of death

Skin Dry, cold, discolored skin, growth of fine, downy hair

Muscles Weakness

Legs Swollen due to excess fluid; cold feet

Brain Decreased size, low energy, depressed mood, loss of coordination, dizziness, fainting, poor sleep, risk of suicide

Heart Low blood pressure, slow or irregular heartbeats (arrhythmias), cardiac arrest; risk of death

Abdomen Bloating, constipation, fullness after eating

Kidneys Kidney failure; risk of death

Genitals Lack of menstruation(amenorrhea) in women; infertility. Decrease in testosterone levels and decrease in testicular size in men. Decline in sex drive in both sexes

Bones Loss of calcium, osteoporosis, increased risk of fractures

figure 10.2   **Anorexia can cause changes throughout the body.** Not all of these will be present in all people with the disease.

Challenges & Choices

Do You Know Someone With Anorexia?

A person with anorexia will usually deny that he or she is too thin. If you think someone you know has anorexia, you might want to ask someone at your school health center for advice on what to do. Signs of anorexia include the following:

Physiological Signs
- Large weight loss in a short period of time.
- Others as illustrated in Figure 10.2.

Behavioral Signs
- Fasting or severe dieting.
- Cutting food into tiny bites, counting bites of food, or preparing food for others but refusing to eat.
- Expressing an intense fear of becoming fat despite being painfully thin.
- Staying away from situations where food is available, such as parties.

- Maintaining a harsh, no-excuses exercise regimen.
- Dressing in layers to hide weight loss.
- Binging or purging (vomiting; using laxatives, enemas, or diuretics).

Psychological Signs and Attitude Shifts
- Mood swings.
- Perfectionism.
- Insecurity about abilities despite competence.
- Tendency to judge self-worth by what he or she eats or does not eat.
- Tendency to be withdrawn.

It's Not Just Personal . . .
Studies conducted by the National Association of Anorexia and Associated Eating Disorders indicate that 20 percent of people with anorexia will die prematurely as a result of the disorder. The death rate associated with anorexia is 12 times higher than the death rate from all causes for females aged 15–24.

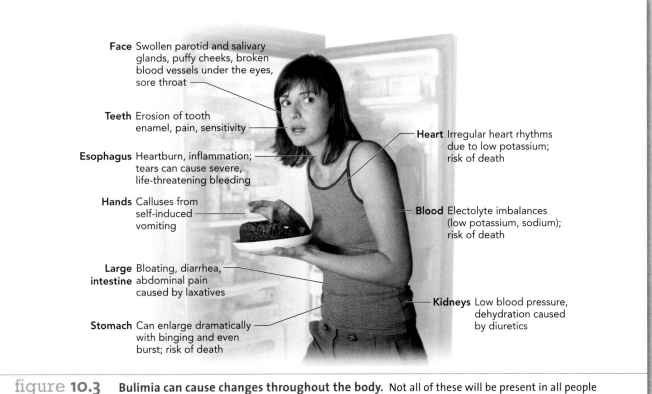

Face Swollen parotid and salivary glands, puffy cheeks, broken blood vessels under the eyes, sore throat

Teeth Erosion of tooth enamel, pain, sensitivity

Esophagus Heartburn, inflammation; tears can cause severe, life-threatening bleeding

Hands Calluses from self-induced vomiting

Large intestine Bloating, diarrhea, abdominal pain caused by laxatives

Stomach Can enlarge dramatically with binging and even burst; risk of death

Heart Irregular heart rhythms due to low potassium; risk of death

Blood Electolyte imbalances (low potassium, sodium); risk of death

Kidneys Low blood pressure, dehydration caused by diuretics

figure **10.3**   **Bulimia can cause changes throughout the body.** Not all of these will be present in all people with the disease.

Challenges & Choices

Do You Know Someone With Bulimia?

A person with bulimia is usually of normal weight. Signs of bulimia include the following:

Physiological Signs
- Yo-yo weight fluctuations within a 10- to 15-pound range.
- Others as illustrated in Figure 10.3.

Behavioral Signs
- Binging.
- Being secretive about food; stealing or hiding food.
- Talking constantly about food or weight.
- Avoiding restaurants, planned meals, or social events with food present.
- Putting oneself down for eating too much.
- Leaving the table and going to the bathroom right after a meal.

- Vomiting; using laxatives, enemas, or diuretics.
- Taking diet pills.
- Maintaining a harsh, no-excuses exercise regimen.
- Expressing an intense fear of becoming fat despite being of normal weight.

Psychological Signs and Attitude Shifts
- Mood swings that include depression, sadness, guilt, or self-loathing.
- Harsh self-criticism.
- Need for the approval of others.
- Self-worth based on weight.

It's Not Just Personal . . .

It is estimated that 10 percent of college-age women suffer from bulimia. About 10 percent of those with bulimia are men. An estimated 10 percent of individuals with bulimia will die from complications of the disorder, including cardiac arrest.

multimodality team
Group of health care providers working together to ensure that all areas of a patient's health are addressed.

However, if an individual has progressed farther along the continuum to a full-blown eating disorder, treatment often involves a multidisciplinary or **multimodality team**. This group of health care providers with different expertise—physician, psychiatrist, psychologist, social worker, nutritionist, nurses—work together to address all areas of a patient's health. Sometimes this requires referral from campus services to a center that specializes in the treatment of eating disorders.

If severe weight loss or another medical abnormality has occurred, hospitalization may be required while adequate nutrition is restored. During the weight gain phase of treatment, the focus is simply on getting patients to gain enough weight so that the symptoms of starvation will improve. While patients are in a physical crisis, they may find it hard to work on long-term change. If patients do not appear to be in imminent danger, they can usually be treated while living at home.

Once weight is stabilized, the second phase of treatment—including psychotherapy, behavioral relearning and modification, and nutritional rehabilitation and education—can be initiated. Because eating disorders are psychiatric illnesses, the most important part of treatment (aside from weight gain for severely anorexic patients) is psychotherapy. Once the patient has acknowledged that there is a problem, therapy focuses on such issues as low self-esteem and overemphasis on body image and body weight. For bulimia, the use of cognitive behavioral therapy has been effective; this approach focuses on changing specific behaviors and the thought patterns that maintain the behaviors. Nutritional education includes information about healthy eating patterns, normal weight, and nutritional needs. Treatment for eating disorders often involves the entire family.

Because an eating disorder is a chronic illness, part of treatment is learning how to maintain self-esteem, a positive body image, and healthy eating patterns for life. A goal of treatment is to teach the person to recognize self-destructive patterns of behavior and to develop better coping skills.

In some cases, medications, particularly antidepressants, may be used as a component of treatment. During the weight gain phases of anorexia treatment, antidepressants do not appear to be beneficial, but they do seem to be somewhat helpful in reducing relapses during the weight maintenance phase. In the treatment of bulimia, the use of antidepressants leads to a rapid decrease in the binge-purge cycle.[15, 22]

Body Dysmorphic Disorder

Many of us look at our bodies and see things we'd like to change. For some people, however, the pattern of seeing faults becomes an obsession that significantly interferes with their lives. A key feature of **body dysmorphic disorder** is a preoccupation with a defect in appearance. The preoccupation can be about a wholly imagined defect or exaggerated

concern about a slight defect. Criteria outlined for body dysmorphic disorder are as follows:[18]

■ Preoccupation with an imagined defect in appearance. If a slight physical anomaly is present, the person's concern is markedly excessive.

■ The preoccupation causes significant distress or impairment in social, occupational, or other important areas of functioning.

■ The preoccupation is not better accounted for by another mental disorder (such as anorexia).

body dysmorphic disorder
Preoccupation with an imagined or exaggerated defect in appearance.

The perceived fault can be in any part of the body. The person may worry about acne, wrinkles, skin color, baldness, facial or body asymmetry, or the size or shape of any body part, such as nose, eyebrows, ears, breasts, muscles, and so on. Concern about the perceived defect causes the person distress, and behaviors linked to the defect interfere with the normal activities of living. A person with body dysmorphic disorder may spend hours in front of the mirror (or may, alternatively, avoid mirrors). He or she may spend a good part of every day thinking about the defect and may avoid relationships or social situations out of embarrassment and self-consciousness.

MUSCLE DYSMORPHIA

Earlier we mentioned muscle dysmorphia, a subcategory of body dysmorphic disorder. This condition, sometimes called bigorexia or reverse anorexia, occurs in men who believe they appear thin even though their muscles are actually quite large.[6] They are ashamed of their bodies and obsessed with working out with weights to develop muscular strength. They may avoid social contact because they believe other people are contemptuous of their bodies.

It is unclear why some people develop muscle dysmorphia. The condition may be related to obsessive-compulsive disorder, which is marked by recurring thoughts that people can't get out of their heads. The disorder may originate in childhood experiences that undermine self-esteem, such as taunting by peers, and it may be aggravated by media images that glorify bulging muscles and present them as a realistic goal. Still, many men are exposed to these experiences and images, and most do not develop muscle dysmorphia.

COSMETIC SURGERY

Some people with body dysmorphic disorder turn to cosmetic surgery to correct their supposed flaw in appearance. However, not everyone who turns to cosmetic surgery has this disorder. In fact, cosmetic surgery and makeovers of every kind have become commonplace in the last decade. The increase is most likely related to the ever-growing emphasis on appearance. Between 2000 and 2006 there was a 55 percent increase in the number of cosmetic procedures performed in the United States, with 11 million cosmetic surgery operations performed in 2006. Women have the majority of procedures, but rates are increasing in men. The most commonly performed surgical procedures were breast augmentation, rhinoplasty (nose reshaping), and liposuction. The most commonly performed nonsurgical procedures were Botox injections (for wrinkles), laser hair removal, skin resurfacing, and collagen injections.[23]

By definition, cosmetic surgery is elective; it is not done to treat a medical condition. As with any surgery or medical procedure, there are risks. A key risk is psychological: If a person is unhappy with her appearance because she has a distorted body image or is comparing herself to an unrealistic ideal, it is unlikely that a single operation is going to make her significantly happier. There are also physical risks, both at the time of surgery (for example, reactions to anesthesia, blood loss, infection) and later (for example, reactions to the silicone in breast implants).

Cosmetic surgery can also have psychological and physical benefits. Some people are happy with the results of cosmetic surgery. Some become more confident about their appearance and more successful socially or professionally. Surgeries such as otoplasty (cosmetic ear surgery) and rhinoplasty (nose reshaping) can change a physical characteristic that has caused a person emotional distress for years; breast reduction can enable a woman to feel less self-conscious about her appearance or engage in sports or activities that were previously uncomfortable.

BODY ART

Some people choose to use body art to express themselves and present a certain image. Like other forms of self-expression, body art is closely tied to an individual's sense of self. The tattoos, eyebrow rings, and nose piercing you see on campus may seem like a recent trend, but their roots go far back in history. Many cultures have used piercing or tattoos to mark tribal origin or status. Crusaders were tattooed with crosses so that they would be given a Christian burial. Ancient Egyptians used navel piercing as a sign of royalty.

In the United States, approximately one in four men and one in five women report having a tattoo. Of those, about one in five has considered removing the tattoo. The most common reasons given for wanting a tattoo removed are improved self-esteem, dislike for the design, and increased credibility.

Permanent tattooing involves making a puncture wound in the skin and injecting ink deep into the second layer of skin (called the dermis) to make the tattoo long-lasting. There is some pain, minor bleeding, and possible risk of infection. If a decision is made to remove the tattoo at a later date, it can be done with laser treatment, but the process is painful, time consuming, and expensive.[24]

Body piercing involves some of the same risks as tattooing. Certain body sites are more likely than others to result in problems. Piercing of the mouth and nose is often associated with infection, and tongue piercing can damage teeth. The longer a piercing is left in place, the more likely it is that

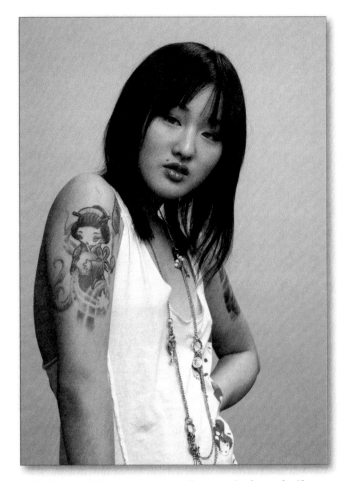

■ Tattoos and piercings are currently a popular form of self-expression. Over time, however, social norms around body art may shift, leaving some with regrets about these relatively permanent alterations.

scarring or a residual opening will occur should the jewelry be removed.

Tattoos and piercing should be approached with caution and considered permanent alterations of the body. If you decide to proceed with either, give yourself a waiting period to make sure that the location, design, and type of tattoo or piercing are what you really want. Consider how it will look 5, 10, or 20 years from now and how you might feel about it in a different phase of your life.

Exercise Disorders

Like eating disorders, exercise disorders are on the rise, and researchers are beginning to look into exercise patterns that may be abnormal. Such patterns may exist in conjunction with eating disorders or by themselves.[18]

FEMALE ATHLETE TRIAD

Female athletes are susceptible to a condition called the **female athlete triad,** a set of three interrelated

female athlete triad
Interrelated conditions of disordered eating, amenorrhea and osteoporosis.

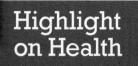

Highlight on Health

Ron: A Case of Muscle Dysmorphia and Activity Disorder

Ron had been concerned about his muscular development ever since he was a kid. At the age of 18, he still felt he wasn't big enough, even though he was bigger and stronger than the average man and quite athletic. Ron didn't socialize or go out much, mostly because he was usually at the gym working out. He avoided talking to people while he was there, because he was sure that they were all secretly laughing at how scrawny he was. Ron couldn't really enjoy a meal at a restaurant or a friend's house, either. He kept to a strict diet of high-protein foods and dietary supplements. Ron lifted weights in competition and was actually quite strong, but his muscles didn't look bulky enough to him. He thought about trying steroids to further increase his muscle size.

Not only was Ron obsessed with his muscular development; he was also using exercise to control his moods. He never really felt in control except when he was lifting weights. On a few occasions he injured himself by lifting too much weight, yet he couldn't rest long enough to heal properly. When he felt too sore to lift, he would run or do calisthenics. All the extra activity actually kept his muscles from bulking up further, but he saw the lack of new bulk as a sign that he wasn't working hard enough. Ron wasn't able to see how his pattern of exercise was hurting his health. It took the intervention of a personal trainer at the gym to help him start to understand that he needed to seek psychological help.

ACTIVITY DISORDER

People with **activity disorder** control their bodies or alter their moods by being overly involved in exercise or addicted to exercise. People who are addicted to exercise continue to exercise strenuously even when the activity causes such problems as illness, injury, or the breakdown of relationships. At the heart of activity disorder is the use of exercise to gain a sense of control and accomplishment, to maintain self-esteem, and to soothe emotions rather than to increase fitness, relaxation, or pleasure. The disorder is not about exercise itself but about meeting psychological needs through exercise. The hallmark of activity disorder is a pattern of exercise that becomes detrimental to health rather than beneficial (see the box "Ron: A Case of Muscle Dysmorphia and Activity Disorder").

> **activity disorder**
> Excessive or addictive exercising, undertaken to address psychological needs rather than to improve fitness.

The signs and symptoms of activity disorder often resemble those of anorexia and bulimia. Physical symptoms include fatigue, reduction in performance, decreased focus, increased compulsion to exercise, decreased heart rate response to exercise, and muscle degeneration. Cycles of repetitive overuse injuries are common.

Activity disorder is more common among men than among women, a difference that may be related to childhood experiences and cultural values. Males tend to be more active than females during childhood, and our culture supports male independence and physical achievement. The association between activity and achievement may influence active people with perfectionist tendencies to become addicted to exercise.

Treatment for activity disorder is similar to that for eating disorders, although most cases of pure activity disorder can be handled in an outpatient setting. Unfortunately, activity disorder often occurs in conjunction with an eating disorder; the combination can rapidly increase the physical problems of both disorders.

conditions: disordered eating patterns (often accompanied by excessive exercising), amenorrhea (cessation of menstruation), and premature osteoporosis (reduced bone density). The triad often begins when a female athlete engages in unhealthy eating patterns (restrictive or purging) and excessive exercise to lose weight or to attain a lean body appearance to fit a specific athletic image or improve performance. This then may lead to amenorrhea due to alterations in hormone levels (low estrogen and progesterone). Low estrogen leads to reduced calcium absorption and bone thinning.

This disorder overlaps with anorexia and bulimia, and risk factors are similar. Often, a first sign of a problem is a decrease in performance, a muscle injury, or an exercise-related stress fracture. Amenorrhea is another important sign. Female athletes need to understand the importance of good eating habits and moderation in exercise and recognize the patterns and dangers of eating disorders.

Awareness and Prevention: Promoting a Healthy Body Image

Promotion of healthy eating and a healthy body image involves many components and coordinated efforts.

COLLEGE INITIATIVES

Colleges have a role to play in ensuring that students learn how to transition successfully to new environments, new relationships, and different sociocultural pressures. These are skills that will translate well into future environments and relationships. Ideally, prevention efforts will include both individual measures and campuswide activities. Campus life typically affords many opportunities for people to recognize individuals who are at increased risk for disordered eating patterns and psychological distress. Residence advisors,

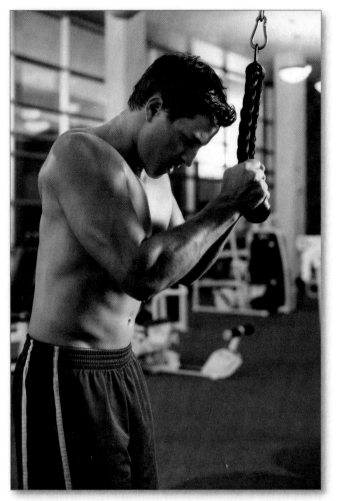

■ Like eating disorders, muscle dysmorphia involves a distorted body image and compulsive behaviors. People with this disorder exercise to feel in control and to manage uncomfortable emotions rather than to improve their fitness and health.

professors, coaches, trainers, and other college staff can be trained to watch for signs that students are having problems with the transition to college life. Health and counseling services can be visible and accessible so that students feel comfortable accessing help early if they are feeling distressed.

PUBLIC HEALTH APPROACHES

Public health approaches focus on raising awareness about eating disorders and changing widely accepted social norms. The "Love Your Body Day" campaign is one example of a public health approach aimed at promoting healthy body images. The idea of the campaign is to encourage acceptance

of physical differences, including different body shapes and sizes and the normal changes of healthy aging (see the box "Love Your Body Day").

Nationally, organizations and programs have been developed to promote healthy body image and lifestyle patterns for young people. For example, the Girl Scouts' "Free to Be Me" program emphasizes inner strength and healthy differences instead of outer appearances. It encourages girls to think about who they really are and what they like to do, to understand and resist peer pressure, to learn about eating disorders and substance abuse, and to celebrate their own diversity. The Boy Scouts' "Fit for Life" and "5-a-Day" badge programs, although not designed specifically to combat eating disorders, teach boys about the roles of healthy nutrition, fitness, and exercise.

Girls, Inc., is a nationwide educational and advocacy organization that encourages girls to be "strong, smart, and bold." This organization's programs focus on building girls' interest and skills in math, science, and technology; on developing media literacy, emotional literacy, strategies for self-defense, and leadership; and on helping girls participate in sports and take healthy risks in life. Dads and Daughters is an organization that recognizes the important role of parents in the lives of youth. Parents are powerful role models and can communicate a healthy body image, a healthy approach to weight management, and problem-solving skills. Parents can lead the way by emphasizing the importance of a balance between inner and outer beauty, healthy relationship patterns, and balanced achievements.

In addition to private efforts, the government sponsors a number of programs. The Office of Women's Health, operating under the U.S. Department of Health and Human Services, sponsors "Body Wise," an educational campaign aimed at increasing knowledge about eating disorders, promoting healthy eating, and reducing preoccupation with body weight and size. This office publishes information on boys and eating disorders as well.

In short, to counteract unhealthy attitudes, we can begin to resist current cultural messages and become active in changing them. The media and advertising industry spend millions of dollars every year finding out what consumers want and selling products. The industry conducts research on consumer attitudes, holds focus groups, monitors sales, and pays attention to consumer reactions. By supporting healthy body images and buying products that reflect diversity, we can move our society in the direction of realistic, accepting, and healthy attitudes toward the body.

Public Health in Action

Love Your Body Day

Since 1998, on a day in October, the National Organization for Women (NOW) has sponsored "Love Your Body Day." The day is promoted as a fun but serious way to help people "fight back" against Hollywood and the fashion, cosmetics, and diet industries. NOW encourages colleges and schools across the country to host events that draw attention to body image issues and that highlight the importance of diversity in body shape, size, and function.

Events have included picketing the headquarters of publications that promote offensive images of women and girls, creating T-shirts with slogans that will initiate discussions and questions (such as "This is what Barbie OUGHT to look like"), and hosting rallies and forums to discuss and highlight body image issues. Every year there is a Love Your Body poster contest; the winner receives a monetary prize, and the winning poster is distributed as the official poster for the upcoming year.

NOW provides other resources designed to help the public become active in confronting the media on the Love Your Body Web site. For example, it posts "Offensive Ads" and "Positive Ads" with explanations of why ads fall into different categories, thus enhancing media literacy skills. They also promote advocacy by asking visitors to nominate ads for posting. For further information and to find out when the next annual Love Your Body Day is scheduled, visit the Web site at www.loveyourbody.nowfoundation.org.

You Make the Call

Should the Fashion Industry Be Regulated?

- In August 2006 supermodel Luisel Ramos collapsed and died from heart failure after she left the runway during a fashion show in South America. At 22 years of age, she had a BMI of 14.5 and suffered from anorexia.

- In November of the same year, Ana Carolina Reston, an ultra-thin supermodel, died in Brazil from complications of anorexia. At the time of her death, she had a BMI of 13.4.

- In February 2007 model Eliana Ramos, the 18-year-old younger sister of Luisel, died at her grandparents' home, either from malnutrition or from a heart attack.

The deaths of these three supermodels within 6 months of each other spurred a crackdown on underweight models and highlighted efforts that were already taking place around the world. For example, in September 2006 the organizers of Spain's Madrid Fashion Week banned models with a BMI below 18, eliminating an estimated 30 percent of the models. In December 2006 the Italian National Fashion Chamber followed suit with a self-regulating code preventing models with a BMI below 18.5 from participating in Italian fashion shows.

In January 2007 the Academy for Eating Disorders issued guidelines designed to improve the health and safety of models and to reduce the impact of the media on people at risk for eating disorders. The academy recommended that a minimum age of 16 be established for models to reduce pressure on adolescent girls, that a minimum BMI of 18.5 be established for both men and women models older than 18, that a medical certificate be required for aspiring models to ensure that they are monitored for eating disorders, and that educational programs be provided for models and others in the fashion industry to raise awareness of the health risks associated with low body weight.

After the guidelines came out, the Council of Fashion Designers of America issued recommendations intended to raise awareness and promote a healthier work environment in the American fashion industry. It proposed that the industry be educated about early warning signs of eating disorders, that models with eating disorders be required to seek professional help, and that nutritious foods and snacks be provided at fashion shows. Compliance with these recommendations would be voluntary.

Those in favor of regulating the fashion industry argue that the pressures on young models to become super-thin are more than they can handle. Many of the models are very young and desperate for success, so they are particularly vulnerable. Often they travel around the world without supervision or healthy support systems. Increasingly, models are coming from developing countries, where they quickly become the primary breadwinners for their families, further increasing the pressure for success at any cost.

In response, members of the fashion industry assert that they are capable of monitoring and regulating themselves. They say they want healthy-looking models and deny that their employees are pressured to be thin. They also argue that BMI regulations discriminate against women who are naturally thin. They oppose regulations limiting models' weight or size.

Is the fashion industry responsible for encouraging eating disorders? Should there be regulations to protect vulnerable young women from becoming too thin? What do you think?

PROS

- Supermodels are dying of anorexia. Regulations would reduce the pressure on models to become super-thin.

- The fashion industry is an unhealthy business that needs regulation. The industry preys on vulnerable young women.

- The fashion industry exploits women; the least it can do is be proactive about protecting their health.

- Other industries and workplaces are regulated under the Occupational Safety and Health Administration to reduce the risk of health hazards on the job. There is no reason why the fashion industry should fall outside this standard.

CONS

- Fashion companies invest hundreds of thousands of dollars in their models; it doesn't make sense to think they would encourage their models to starve themselves to death.

- Models and supermodels enjoy success and admiration beyond the wildest dreams of most women. They choose the lifestyle that goes with success.

- The fashion industry is capable of monitoring itself; it does not need policing or bureaucratic regulations.

- It is discriminatory against naturally thin women to exclude models with a BMI below 18.5.

Sources: "For Some Fashion Models, Thin Is Definitely Not In," by Eve Bender, 2007, Psychiatric News, 42 (93), p. 10, retrieved October 14, 2007, from http://pn.psychiatryonline.org/cgi/content/full/42/3/10; "New Guidelines Hoped to Reduce Eating Disorders Among Fashion Models," 2007, Psychiatric News, 42 (3), p. 10, retrieved October 14, 2007, from http://pn.psychiatryonline.org/cgi/content/full/psychnews;42/3/10-a; "Extreme Diet Model Dies Six Months After Anorexic Sister," by Tom Hennigan, 2007, The Times, February 15, retrieved October 14, 2007, from www.timesonline.co.uk/tol/news/world/us_and_americas/article1386803.ece; "Everyone Knew She Was Ill," 2007, The Observer, January 14, retrieved October 14, 2007, from http://lifeandhealth.guardian.co.uk/fashion/story/0,1987945,00.html.

In Review

1. **What is body image, and how is it determined?** Body image is the mental representation a person has of his or her body. It includes perceptions, attitudes, thoughts, feelings, and judgments about one's body, and it is strongly influenced by culture. Via advertising, fashion, and language, our culture sends messages about appearance, beauty, and acceptable body size and shape, especially for women but increasingly for men.

2. **What is disordered eating, and what are eating disorders?** To meet society's standards, many people practice disordered eating behaviors like dieting or binging and purging on occasion, but some people develop full-blown eating disorders. These disorders are characterized by severe disturbances in eating behavior and by a distorted body image. They are serious, chronic illnesses and are classified as mental disorders. Related disorders are body dysmorphic disorder and activity disorder.

3. **Why do people develop eating disorders?** Aside from social pressures and cultural messages, which affect everyone, some people may be vulnerable to eating disorders because of a genetic predisposition, family factors, or other underlying emotional problems and characteristics, such as depression, anxiety, low self-esteem, a sense of powerlessness, perfectionism, and lack of other coping skills.

4. **What are the most common eating disorders?** Anorexia nervosa, characterized by self-starvation, is the most severe eating disorder. Bulimia nervosa, characterized by binging and purging, is more difficult to identify, because people with bulimia are of normal weight. Binge-eating disorder leads to obesity, but only a small percentage of obese people have this disorder. All eating disorders have serious health consequences.

5. **How are eating disorders treated?** Because they are mental disorders, treatment usually includes psychotherapy to address psychological issues, along with weight stabilization, behavior modification, nutritional rehabilitation and education, and, in some cases, medication. For anorexia, hospitalization may be required at first to prevent starvation. Treatment usually involves the whole family, and recovery can be lifelong. Communities have a role to play in promoting healthy body images for both women and men.

WWW For a detailed summary of this chapter and a comprehensive set of review questions, visit the Online Learning Center at **www.mhhe.com/teague2e**.

Web Resources

Body Positive: This educational organization teaches critical thinking about our culture's focus on thinness. Its resources include BodyTalk, a video on body acceptance for teen girls and boys, and links to other organizations that offer information on body image.
www.bodypositive.com

Girls, Inc.: Dedicated to inspiring all girls to be "strong, smart, and bold," Girls, Inc., offers educational programs throughout the United States, particularly to girls in high-risk, underserved areas. It teaches girls how to advocate for themselves and their communities and to promote positive change.
www.girlsinc.org

National Association for Self-Esteem: The aim of this organization is to improve self-esteem among Americans. Its Web site features a self-guided tour that lets you rate your self-esteem, as well as articles, a newsletter, FAQs, and links to other resources.
www.self-esteem-nase.org

National Eating Disorders Association: Promoting public understanding of eating disorders, this organization offers programs and services related to treatment and support of families affected by these disorders.
www.edap.org

TeensHealth: This site offers various topics of interest to teens, including body image and self-esteem, eating disorders, cutting, and emotional changes in adolesence.
www.kidshealth.org/teen

PART THREE

Your Health at Risk

Think It Over

- Do your social circles include both drinkers and nondrinkers?
- If all drugs were legal, would the "drug problem" be solved? If not, what problems would remain? What new problems might develop?
- What factors influence your decision to smoke or not smoke?

"We admitted we were powerless. . . ." So begins the first of the Alcoholics Anonymous famous 12 steps, the model for all the 12-step programs that followed. Virtually all the psychoactive drugs—including alcohol, tobacco, illicit drugs like marijuana and cocaine, and many prescription drugs—are capable of producing addiction and rendering individuals powerless over them. The chapters in Part 3 address how these substances work, the role they play in people's lives, and, most important, how you can make good decisions to avoid putting your health at risk from substance use, abuse, or dependence.

Chapter

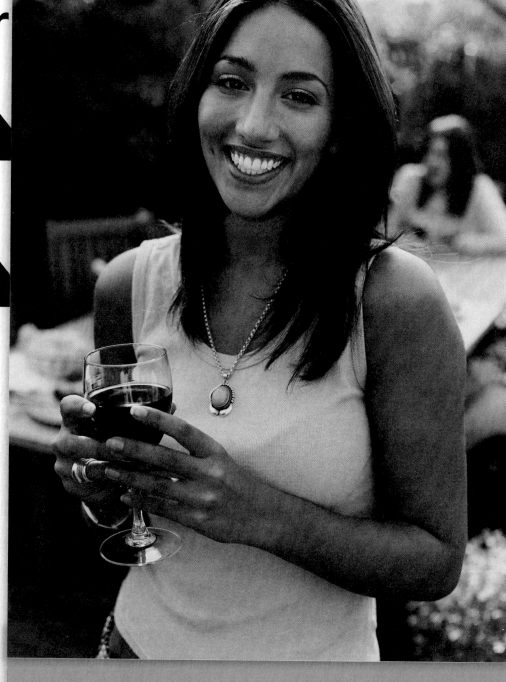

Alcohol
Responsible
Approaches
to Drinking

Ever Wonder...

- how "one drink" is defined?
- if drinking coffee or walking will help you sober up?
- if you have a problem with alcohol?

The alcohol culture permeates the environment on many college campuses, as seen in tailgate parties, bar crawls, twenty-one-shot birthday celebrations, and an endless variety of rituals marking the end of classes, the first snowfall, or spring break. For decades, college administrators ignored or condoned this culture. But recently, chilling statistics have brought alcohol-related problems to the forefront. High-risk alcohol drinking kills 1,700 students between the ages of 18 and 24 every year and causes injury to 599,000. Sexual assaults, physical violence, vandalism, and academic casualties are additional problems associated with the campus alcohol culture.[1]

Ambivalence toward college drinking reflects the ambivalence of the larger culture toward alcohol. We use alcohol to feel good, to celebrate, to toast one another and life, yet we also see the devastation that results when drinking gets out of control. Our society currently approves of the use of alcohol by adults, and alcohol advertising typically depicts drinkers as attractive, youthful members of a fun-loving circle of friends. We seldom if ever see images of drunks or alcoholics, nor do we see many images of drinkers vomiting, passing out, or being brought to hospital emergency rooms with alcohol poisoning.

Because alcohol is a **psychoactive drug**—it causes changes in brain chemistry and alters consciousness—it can have profound and wide-ranging effects on all aspects of our thinking, emotions, and behavior. It is in society's interest to regulate the use of such a powerful substance, but it is up to individuals to determine what role they want alcohol to play in their lives. In this chapter we explore the complexities of alcohol use as well as steps you can take to make sure your alcohol use, if any, is responsible.

psychoactive drug
A substance that causes changes in brain chemistry and alters consciousness.

Who Drinks? Patterns of Alcohol Use

More than 60 percent of American adults drink, at least occasionally. As many as 90 percent of American adults have had some experience with alcohol, and 60 percent of men and 30 percent of women have had a bad experience with alcohol, such as driving when intoxicated or missing work owing to a hangover.[2] **Intoxication** is an altered state of consciousness due to ingestion of alcohol or other substances.

About one-third of the adult U.S. population label themselves *abstainers.* They do not drink at all, or they do so less often than once a year. Of the two-thirds who do drink, 10 percent are considered *heavy drinkers,* and the remainder are *light drinkers* and *moderate drinkers.*[2,3] **Moderate drinking** is defined as two drinks a day for men and one drink a day for women; heavy drinking is defined as drinking more than this and light drinking as less.[4]

intoxication
Altered state of consciousness as a result of drinking alcohol or ingesting other substances.

moderate drinking
Two drinks a day for men; one drink a day for women.

"One drink" is defined by the National Institute on Alcohol Abuse and Alcoholism (NIAAA) as 0.5 ounce (or 15 grams) of alcohol, the amount contained in about 12 ounce of beer, 5 ounces of wine, a 1.5-ounce shot of 80-proof distilled liquor, or 1.5 ounces of liquor in a mixed drink (Figure 11.1). The term *proof* refers to the alcohol content of hard liquor, defined as twice the actual percentage of alcohol in the beverage; for example, 80-proof liquor is 40 percent alcohol by volume.

DRINKING PATTERNS ACROSS THE LIFESPAN

Drinking patterns for men and women in the United States, by age and ethnic group, are shown in Figures 11.2 and 11.3. As the figures indicate, the roots of drinking behavior are established by the adolescent years.

Consumption of alcoholic beverages is highest between the ages of 18 and 25 for Whites and then begins a steady descent. The peak period for heavy drinking among Hispanic and African American men occurs between the ages of 26 and 30, and the decline tends to be less marked than that for White men.[5] In general, people are more likely to

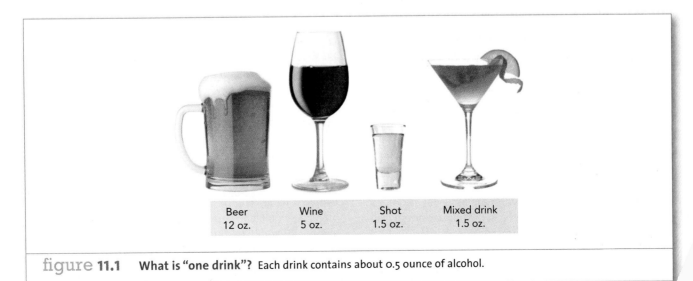

| Beer 12 oz. | Wine 5 oz. | Shot 1.5 oz. | Mixed drink 1.5 oz. |

figure **11.1** **What is "one drink"?** Each drink contains about 0.5 ounce of alcohol.

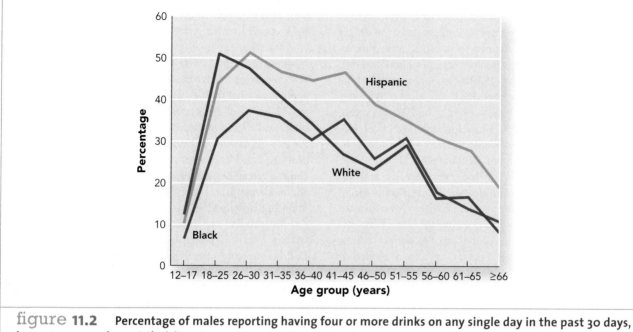

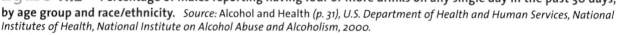

figure 11.2   Percentage of males reporting having four or more drinks on any single day in the past 30 days, by age group and race/ethnicity.   *Source: Alcohol and Health (p. 31), U.S. Department of Health and Human Services, National Institutes of Health, National Institute on Alcohol Abuse and Alcoholism, 2000.*

drink at certain stages in the lifespan, such as adolescence and early adulthood, the threshold of middle age, and following retirement.

Older adults drink significantly less than younger adults do. A high percentage of older adults, particularly older women, abstain from alcohol.[6] Alcoholism is five times more prevalent in older adult men than in older adult women, and it is more common among Whites than African Americans and Hispanic Americans.[7]

Women drink less than men do—60 percent of American women drink alcohol on a regular basis, and about 5 percent have two or more drinks daily—and start later.[8] However, it takes less time for women to develop a drinking problem than it does for men. Although the slope in drinking trajectories for men and women is different, recent research suggests that this gap is closing.

ETHNIC DIFFERENCES IN ALCOHOL USE

As shown in Figures 11.2 and 11.3, alcohol consumption is higher among Whites than among African Americans across most of the lifespan.[5] Alcohol consumption is high among Hispanic/Latino men, but it is very low among Hispanic/Latina women. Hispanic/Latina women are more likely to abstain from alcohol than are African American or White women. These differences may be the result of cultural norms and attitudes; in Hispanic culture, drinking tends to be encouraged for men but discouraged for women.[9]

Differences in alcohol consumption among ethnic groups are strongly influenced by sociocultural or environmental factors, including poverty, discrimination, feelings of powerlessness, immigration status, and degree of accul-

turation.[10] Economic factors, such as the heavy marketing of alcoholic beverages in minority neighborhoods, play a considerable role. For example, the number of liquor stores located in African American communities is proportionately much higher than the number in White communities.[5] Given these pressures, it is notable that alcohol consumption is generally lower among African Americans than among other groups.

Among Native Americans, alcoholism is recognized as the number one health problem.[5] The death rate from alcoholism for Native Americans is more than five times greater than that for other groups.[11] Of the 10 leading causes of death for Native Americans, 4 are alcohol related. Numerous factors contribute to these disparities, most notably sociocultural factors such as poverty and discrimination. Scientists have also suggested that genetic factors may contribute to patterns of alcohol use by Native Americans. In addition, the cultural belief that alcoholism is a spiritual disorder rather than a physical disease makes it less likely that Native Americans will seek treatment. Treatment programs that reflect tribal values may be more effective, such as those that incorporate traditional practices (sweat lodges, prayers, dances) into the therapeutic process.[11]

Among Asian Americans, alcohol consumption overall is lower than among White Americans. Many Asian Americans tend to drink very little or abstain because of a genetically based biological reaction to alcohol (see Chapter 2). Approximately half of all Asian Americans have a gene that impairs the metabolism of alcohol, causing a set of unpleasant reactions (facial flushing, sweating, nausea) referred to as the flushing effect.[8]

What Causes Problem Drinking?

Why do some people develop problems with alcohol while others do not? This question has no simple answers. Instead, a complex interaction of many factors—individual, psychological, and sociocultural—is at work.

GENETIC AND BIOLOGICAL FACTORS

As discussed in Chapter 2, some people may be genetically susceptible to the influences of alcohol. Family, twin, and adoption studies have shown a family pattern of alcohol dependence, with the risk of alcoholism three to four times greater in close relatives of an alcoholic than in the general population.[5] Inborn temperament may also play a role.

PSYCHOSOCIAL FACTORS

A family history of alcoholism as a risk factor for the development of alcoholism is well established.[12, 13] Family dysfunction in general, even without an alcoholic parent, increases the likelihood that children will grow up to have alcohol problems. Childhood traumas may predispose people to early alcohol use, which is associated with adult problem drinking.[5] Children in dysfunctional families are more likely to be exposed to high levels of stress and to experience negative emotions. Later, they may use drinking to soothe these negative feelings. Depression is associated with drinking at all stages of the lifespan for both men and women. Research suggests that family dysfunction is a stronger predictor of alcohol problems for women than it is for men.

Note that most children who grow up in dysfunctional family environments do not develop problems with alcohol. Two key protective factors are believed to prevent these problems: (1) parent-child connectedness and (2) school connectedness. High parent-child connectedness exists when children feel close to, loved by, or wanted by one or both parents. School connectedness occurs when students feel close to other students, feel that they are recognized as part of the school community, and believe they are treated fairly by teachers.[5] Individuals are further protected in adulthood by having work and marriage responsibilities and a supportive social network.

SOCIOCULTURAL OR ENVIRONMENTAL FACTORS

Because drinking occurs in a social and cultural context, sociocultural or environmental factors play an enormous role in how alcohol is used and misused. Some cultures have higher acceptance of alcohol use, more tolerant attitudes toward drinking and drunkenness, and/or higher levels of alcohol consumption than others do. Economic factors, such as the availability and cost of alcohol, and the ease of access, also play a role. Laws governing drinking age and the sale of alcoholic beverages affect who drinks. Stresses associated with minority status, including unemployment, discrimination, and poverty, are also associated with alcohol use.[14]

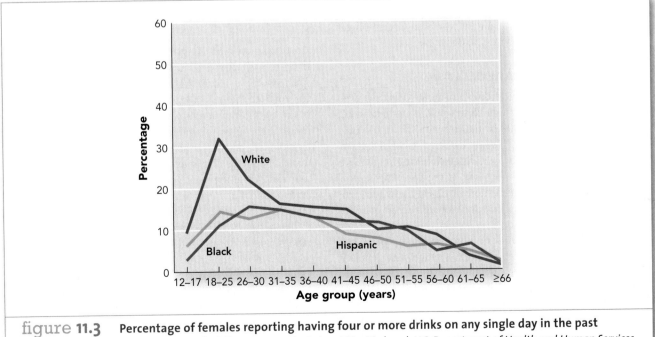

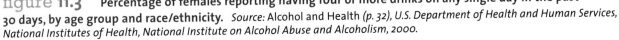

figure **11.3**   **Percentage of females reporting having four or more drinks on any single day in the past 30 days, by age group and race/ethnicity.** *Source: Alcohol and Health (p. 32), U.S. Department of Health and Human Services, National Institutes of Health, National Institute on Alcohol Abuse and Alcoholism, 2000.*

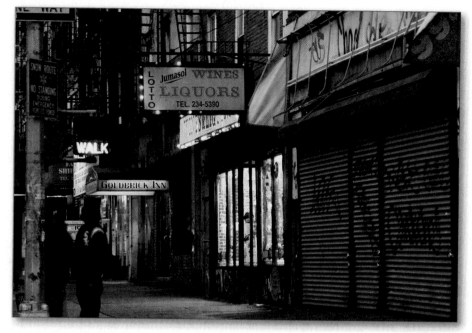

■ An oversupply of liquor stores in poor and minority neighborhoods plays a role in both the availability of alcohol and the social acceptability of alcohol use.

Drinking on the College Campus

If you take a walk on a college campus on a weekend morning, you may see broken liquor bottles, crushed beer cans, and fliers advertising specials at local bars littering the ground— the wreckage of the previous night's partying. Drinking rates at most colleges are very high; surveys indicate that up to 83 percent of college students drink alcoholic beverages.[15] Many students think of drinking as a recreational activity, part of having fun and letting off steam, but some engage in binge drinking, a particularly risky way to consume alcohol.

BINGE DRINKING

binge drinking
Consumption of five or more drinks in a row by a man or four or more drinks in a row by a woman.

The problem of binge drinking was brought to the public's attention in 2000 by the Harvard School of Public Health College Alcohol Study (CAS).[16] **Binge drinking** is defined in this study as the consumption of five or more drinks in a row for men and four or more drinks in a row for women at least once in the previous 2-week period.

Students who binged three or more times in the previous 2 weeks or more than once a week on average were labeled *frequent binge drinkers.* The study found that most college students—83 percent—drank alcohol. About half of all students were binge drinkers, and about one in five were frequent binge drinkers. A subsequent study found that rates of binge drinking were about the same or even higher in 2005 (see the box "College Students and Binge Drinking").[15]

Students at historically Black colleges and universities (HBCUs) have lower rates of binge drinking than students at other colleges. Family expectations, peer modeling, and religion and spirituality may account for some of the difference, but the most important factor may be community engagement. Research has shown that students engaged in civic duties on service-oriented campuses have lower rates of high-risk drinking. HBCUs have a stronger emphasis on character development, engaged learning, and service than many other colleges, perhaps leading students to be more focused on civic problem solving and leadership.[15]

Underage Drinking Very often, binge drinking does not begin in college. Many students binge drink in high school and come to college expecting to continue drinking heavily.[15, 18] This pattern suggests that colleges inherit the behavior of young people who binge drink. At the same time, college environments that promote drinking not only attract drinkers but also encourage drinking among people who were previously nondrinkers.

College students under the age of 21 consume 48 percent of all alcohol consumed by college students.[19] They drink less frequently than older students do, but they are more likely to binge drink during these episodes and to drink simply to get drunk.[20] They are also more likely to be injured or encounter trouble with law enforcement than are older students who binge drink.[21]

Consequences of Binge Drinking Binge drinking can have serious physical, academic, social, and legal consequences. (To evaluate the importance of such consequences for you, see the Add It Up feature for Chapter 11 at the end of the book.) Individuals who have been drinking heavily are more likely to be injured, to commit a crime or fall victim to violence, and to be involved with the law. Half to two-thirds of campus homicides and serious assaults are believed to involve drinking by the offender, the victim, or both.[3] One study found that 74 percent of perpetrators of sexual assaults on college campuses had been drinking.[1] Women who binge drink are nearly 150 percent more likely to be victims of date rape, sexual battering, and unplanned sexual activity than are women who do not drink alcohol.[22] (See the box "High-Risk College Drinking: A Snapshot of Consequences.")

Binge drinkers also cause problems for other students. About 9 out of 10 students reported experiencing at least one adverse consequence of another student's drinking during the school year.[23] These "secondhand effects" of binge drinking include serious arguments, physical assault, damaged property, interrupted sleep or studying, unwanted sexual advances, sexual assault, and having to take care of a drunk student.

Who's at Risk

College Students and Binge Drinking

- In 2005 83 percent of college students reported drinking alcohol. Nearly half qualified as binge drinkers, and 23 percent qualified as frequent binge drinkers.

- Men are more likely to binge drink than women. Male freshmen drink less than male upperclassmen, but female freshmen drink more than female upperclassmen.

- White college students are more likely to drink and binge drink than Hispanic, Asian American, or African American students. African American students are the least likely to binge drink.

- Members of fraternities have much higher rates of binge drinking than do non–fraternity members. Dormitory residents and students living off campus have about the same rates.

- Of college students who drink alcohol, about 25 percent began drinking in college, about 65 percent began drinking in high school, and about 8 percent began drinking in junior high. Students who began drinking in junior high consume more and drink more often than students who began drinking later.

- The highest prevalence of binge drinking occurs between ages 18 and 25. The peak rate of binge drinking occurs at age 21.

Sources: "Wasting the Best and the Brightest: Substance Abuse at America's Colleges and Universities," 2007, New York: National Center on Addiction and Substance Abuse at Columbia University; "A Matter of Degree: The National Effort to Reduce High-Risk Drinking Among College Students," American Medical Association, 2006, retrieved from www.ama-assn.org/ama/pub/category/3558.html.

Binge drinkers are more likely to meet the *Diagnostic and Statistical Manual of Mental Disorders* criteria for alcohol abuse and alcohol dependence 10 years after college and are less likely to work in prestigious occupations, compared with non–binge drinkers. Alcohol-related convictions for crimes like driving under the influence, vandalism, assaults, and providing alcohol to a minor may jeopardize ambitions in many careers, including accounting, architecture, engineering, medicine, law enforcement, and teaching. Many professional and graduate schools conduct background searches into criminal records as part of their admission procedures.

Why Do College Students Binge Drink? Students may drink to ease social inhibitions, fit in with peers, imitate role models, reduce stress, soothe negative emotions, or cope with academic pressure or for a variety of other reasons. The mistaken belief that alcohol increases sexual arousal and performance (heavy drinking actually suppresses sexual arousal) may also account for some binge drinking.[3] Young people who are inexperienced with alcohol may not realize how binge drinking will affect them, and they learn from these experiences.

Students who started drinking alcohol before age 16 are more likely to be binge drinkers, as are students with close friends or parents who binge drink. Binge drinking is also promoted by easy access to alcohol and cheap prices. Thus, social norms and the campus culture

contribute to patterns of drinking. Students are more likely to binge drink on campuses where heavy drinking is the norm and less likely to do so where drinking is discouraged.[24, 25]

Is the Definition of Binge Drinking Realistic? Some health experts disagree with the CAS definition of binge drinking (five or more drinks in a row for a man, four or more for a woman), pointing out that it does not take into consideration the size of the drink, the body weight of the drinker, the length of time during which the drinks are consumed, or other important factors. These experts believe the CAS definition is too broad and classifies a large number of

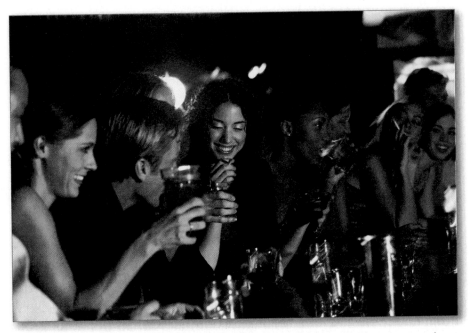

- Alcohol consumption among college students is influenced by the social norms around drinking on their campus. In some cases, there is a gap between student-perceived levels of alcohol consumption and actual consumption by most students.

Highlight on Health

High-Risk College Drinking: A Snapshot of Consequences

Death: Each year, 1,700 college students between the ages of 18 and 24 die from alcohol-related unintentional injuries, including motor vehicle crashes.

Injury: Each year, 599,000 students between the ages of 18 and 24 are unintentionally injured under the influence of alcohol.

Assault: Each year, more than 696,000 students between the ages of 18 and 24 are assaulted by another student who has been drinking.

Sexual assault: Each year, more than 70,000 students between the ages of 18 and 24 are victims of alcohol-related sexual assault or date rape.

Unsafe sex: In one year, 400,000 students between the ages of 18 and 24 had unprotected sex, and more than 100,000 students between the ages of 18 and 24 reported having been too intoxicated to know if they consented to having sex.

Academic problems: Each year, about 25 percent of college students report academic consequences of their drinking, including missing class, falling behind, doing poorly on exams or papers, and receiving lower grades .

Health problems/suicide attempts: More than 150,000 students develop an alcohol-related health problem every year, and between 1.2 and 1.5 percent of students indicate that they tried to commit suicide within the past year because of drinking or drug use.

Drunk driving: In one year, 2.1 million students between the ages of 18 and 24 drove under the influence of alcohol.

Vandalism: In one year, about 11 percent of college student drinkers reported that they damaged property while under the influence of alcohol.

Property damage: More than 25 percent of administrators from schools with relatively low drinking levels and over 50 percent from schools with high drinking levels say their campuses have a "moderate" or "major" problem with alcohol-related property damage.

Police involvement: Each year, about 5 percent of 4-year college students are involved with police or campus security as a result of their drinking, and an estimated 110,000 students between the ages of 18 and 24 are arrested for an alcohol-related violation, such as public drunkenness or driving under the influence.

Alcohol abuse and dependence: According to recent questionnaire-based self-reports about their drinking, 31 percent of college students met criteria for a diagnosis of alcohol abuse and 6 percent for a diagnosis of alcohol dependence in the previous 12 months.

Source: National Institute on Alcohol Abuse and Alcoholism, www.collegedrinkingprevention.gov.

people as binge drinkers who may not have a problem. They say that it is simply not true that half of all college students have problems with alcohol and that saying they do creates a credibility gap.[25–28]

Other terms, such as *heavy drinking* or *high-risk drinking,* may be preferable to describe the drinking currently labeled *binge drinking*. The Inter-Association Task Force on Alcohol and Other Substance Abuse Issues, a coalition of organizations that collaborate on substance-related issues in the higher education community, recommends that the term *binge drinking* be reserved for a prolonged period of intoxication (2 days or more). This definition would direct attention to the minority of students who have real problems with alcohol consumption.

The term *extreme drinking* is now being used to describe alcohol consumption that goes well beyond binge drinking, to double or triple the amounts in the CAS definition. In a survey of first-year students at 14 colleges, 20 percent of the men reported drinking 10 or more drinks on at least one day in the past 2 weeks, 10 percent of the women reported drinking 8 or more drinks on at least one day, 8 percent of the men reported drinking 15 or more drinks on at least one day, and about 2 percent of the women reported drinking 12 or more drinks on at least one day. Many colleges and universities are now targeting such extreme drinking on campus.

Addressing the Problem   The problem of excessive drinking by college students requires an integrated response at several levels. At the level of the individual student, the focus is on reducing the amount of drinking by students and identifying and helping high-risk students. One way high-risk students can be identified is through campus student health services, where brief screening interviews can be conducted during emergency room or routine health care visits and treatment services offered (see the section on brief interventions later in this chapter).

Screening tools can also be used to help students compare their drinking behaviors with those of other students. Many students have a misperception of the social norms around drinking on their campus, thinking more alcohol is being consumed than is the case. A screening tool that gives an accurate comparison of the student's alcohol intake with that of other students can be enlightening.[29, 30]

Other student-level measures include enforcing college alcohol policies consistently and punishing students who violate policies or break the law, mandating treatment for substance-related offenses, educating students to resist peer pressure, helping students cope with stress and time management issues, and targeting prevention messages to high-risk times and events, such as freshman year, athletic events, and spring break (see the box "Spring Break Safety Campaign").

Colleges can also implement strategies aimed more directly at changing the campus drinking culture. Some schools sponsor alcohol-free social and cultural events, while others have gone further by prohibiting alcohol at all college-sponsored events and maintaining alcohol-free residence halls and fraternity and sorority houses. Colleges have also focused on restricting alcohol advertising and promotion on campus, but this can be tricky because the alcohol industry provides significant financial support to athletic programs at many colleges.

Finally, colleges can work cooperatively with their communities to support such strategies as increased enforcement of drinking-age laws, provision of "safe rides" programs, and limits on the density of alcohol retailers near campus.

Effects of Alcohol on the Body

Alcohol is a very small molecule, and unlike food, which must be digested, it is quickly absorbed into the bloodstream through the walls of the stomach and the small intestine. Within minutes, alcohol is distributed to all the cells of the body, including the cells of the brain (Figure 11.4). In the brain, alcohol alters brain chemistry and changes neurotransmitter functions. It particularly affects the cerebellum—the center for balance and motor functions—and

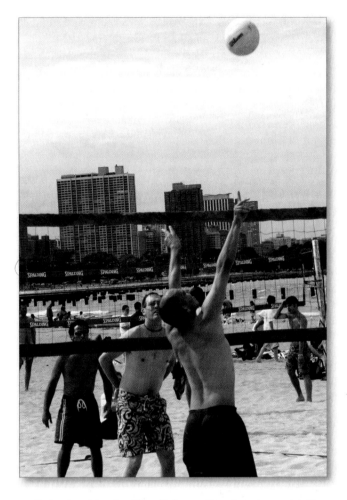

■ Spring break has traditionally been a time for extreme drinking accompanied by injury, property damage, and risky sexual encounters. Some colleges are establishing new, safer traditions.

Highlight on Health

Spring Break Safety Campaign

The ritual of spring break for college students is strongly associated with extreme drinking. Male college students at spring break destinations consume on average 18 drinks a day, and female college students consume 10 drinks a day. Seventy-five percent of males and 40 percent of females report being intoxicated at least once a day. More than 50 percent of males and 40 percent of females report drinking until becoming sick or passing out. One in five college women regretted sexual activity they engaged in during spring break, and 12 percent felt pressured to have sex. The risk of alcohol poisoning at beach destinations is much higher due to the combination of extreme drinking and dehydration from heat and humidity.

Colleges and universities have begun to respond to this problem by banning spring break promotions on college campuses, marketing community service spring break opportunities, and sponsoring spring break safety campaigns. The Boosting Alcohol Consciousness Concerning the Health of University Students (BACCHUS) Network Safe Spring Break program has received particular attention. It includes programming ideas for awareness tables and pledge signing, survival kits, speakers, health and fitness checkups, athletic events, impaired-driving awareness, sexual assault and predatory drug prevention, party planning, and many other activities. Model programs for making spring break safer are also provided on college campuses.

Sources: "Campus Programming for Spring Break," BACCHUS Network, retrieved May 14, 2008, from www.bacchusgamma.org/documents/ campusprogramming.pdf; "Wasting the Best and the Brightest: Substance Abuse at America's Colleges and Universities," March 2007, New York: National Center on Addiction and Substance Abuse at Columbia University; "Sex and Intoxication Among Women More Common on Spring Break According to AMA Poll," American Medical Association, March 8, 2006, retrieved May 14, 2008, from www.ama-assn.org/ama/pub/category/16083.html.

the prefrontal cortex—the center for executive functions, such as rational thinking and problem solving.

Alcohol is a **central nervous system depressant.** While alcohol levels in the blood and brain are rising, you experience feelings of relaxation and well-being, an expansive mood, and a lowering of social inhibitions. At higher levels, and especially when blood levels are falling, you are more likely to feel depressed and withdrawn and to experience impairments in thinking, balance, and motor coordination. As alcohol concentrations in the brain increase, more functions are depressed and greater impairment occurs. These effects last until all the alcohol is metabolized (broken down into energy and wastes) and excreted from the body.

central nervous system depressant
Chemical substance that slows down the activity of the brain and spinal cord.

ALCOHOL ABSORPTION

About 20–25 percent of the alcohol in a drink is absorbed into the bloodstream from the stomach, and 75–80 percent is absorbed through the upper part of the small intestine. A minimal amount of alcohol enters the bloodstream farther along the gastrointestinal tract. Many factors affect alcohol absorption:

- *Food in the stomach.* The type of food has not been shown to have a meaningful influence on alcohol absorption.

- *Gender.* Women absorb alcohol into the bloodstream more quickly than men do.

- *Age.* Older adults have a lower volume of water in the body; with less water to dilute alcohol, they are less tolerant of alcohol.

- *Drug interaction.* Interactions with many prescription and over-the-counter drugs can intensify a drinker's reaction to alcohol, leading to more rapid intoxication.

- *Cigarette smoke.* Nicotine extends the time alcohol stays in the stomach, increasing time for absorption into the bloodstream.

- *Mood and physical condition.* Fear and anger tend to speed up alcohol absorption. The stomach empties more rapidly than normal, allowing the alcohol to be absorbed more easily. People who are stressed, tired, or ill may also feel the effects sooner.

- *Alcohol concentration.* The more concentrated the drink, the more quickly the alcohol is absorbed. Hard liquor is absorbed faster than are beer and wine, which contain nonalcoholic substances that slow the absorption of alcohol.

- *Carbonation.* The carbon dioxide contained in champagne, cola, and ginger ale speeds the absorption of alcohol. Drinks that contain water, juice, or milk are absorbed more slowly.

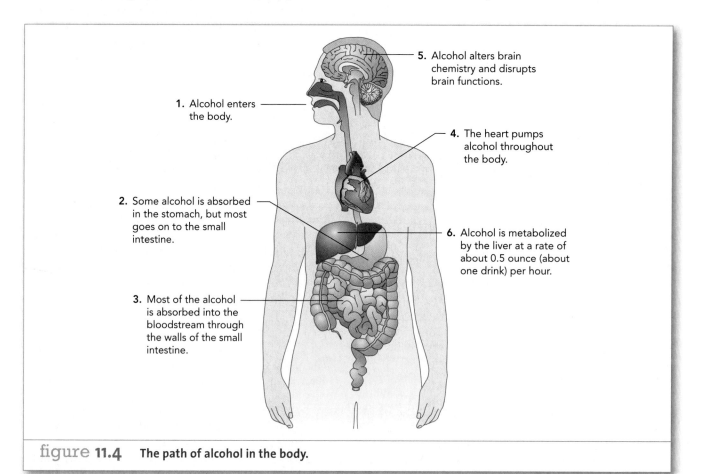

1. Alcohol enters the body.
2. Some alcohol is absorbed in the stomach, but most goes on to the small intestine.
3. Most of the alcohol is absorbed into the bloodstream through the walls of the small intestine.
4. The heart pumps alcohol throughout the body.
5. Alcohol alters brain chemistry and disrupts brain functions.
6. Alcohol is metabolized by the liver at a rate of about 0.5 ounce (about one drink) per hour.

figure **11.4**   **The path of alcohol in the body.**

■ *Tolerance.* The body adapts to a given alcohol level. Each time a person drinks to the point of impairment, the body attempts to minimize impairment by adapting to that level. More alcohol is needed to overcome the body's adaptation and achieve the desired effect.

Another factor that influences how alcohol affects a person is expectations. Studies using volunteers have found that people become more relaxed and talkative if they think they have been given alcoholic beverages, even when their drinks contained no alcohol.

ALCOHOL METABOLISM

A small amount of alcohol is metabolized in the stomach, but 90 percent is metabolized in the liver. Between 2 and 10 percent is not metabolized at all; instead it is excreted unchanged in the breath and urine and through the pores of the skin. This is why you can smell alcohol on the breath of someone who has been drinking.

In the liver, alcohol is converted to acetaldehyde, an organic chemical compound also known as *ethanol,* by the enzyme *alcohol dehydrogenase (ADH).* Acetaldehyde is then quickly converted to acetic acid (vinegar) by the enzyme *acetaldehyde dehydrogenase.* Acetic acid is eventually broken down into carbon dioxide and water.

The ability to metabolize alcohol is dependent on the amount and kind of ADH enzymes available in the liver. If more alcohol molecules arrive in the liver cells than the enzymes can process, the extra molecules circulate through the brain, liver, and other organs until enzymes are available to degrade them. Men make more ADH than women do, and alcoholics make less ADH than do nonalcoholics.

Blood Alcohol Concentration

blood alcohol concentration (BAC)
The amount of alcohol in grams in 100 milliliters of blood, expressed as a percentage.

Rates of alcohol absorption and metabolism affect how much alcohol is circulating in the blood at any given time. **Blood alcohol concentration (BAC)** is a measure of the amount of alcohol in grams in 100 milliliters of blood, expressed as a percentage. For example, for 100 milligrams of alcohol in 100 milliliters of blood, the BAC is .10 percent.

BAC provides a good estimate of the alcohol concentration in the brain, which is why it is used as a measure of intoxication by state motor vehicle laws. The alcohol concentration in the brain corresponds well with alcohol concentration in the breath, so breath samples are accurate indicators of BAC. For this reason, breath analyzers are legal in most states for identifying and prosecuting drunk drivers.[5]

BAC is influenced by the amount of alcohol consumed and the rate at which the alcohol is metabolized by the body. Because alcohol is soluble in water and somewhat less soluble in fat, it does not distribute to all body tissues equally.[5] The more body water a person has, the more the alcohol is diluted and the lower the person's BAC will be. The more body fat a person has, the less alcohol is absorbed by body tissue and the more there is to circulate in the bloodstream and reach the brain. Thus a 150-pound person with high body fat will have a higher BAC than will a 150-pound person with more lean body tissue who drinks the same amount. Body size alone influences BAC as well; a larger, heavier person has more body surface to diffuse the alcohol (as well as a higher body water content to dilute the alcohol).

Gender and Ethnic Differences in Alcohol Absorption and Metabolism Both of these factors—body size and body fat percentage—play a role in gender differences in the effects of alcohol. Women are generally more susceptible to alcohol's effects and have a higher BAC than men do after drinking the same amount. Women are generally smaller than men, and they have a higher body fat percentage.

Another factor is that women absorb more of the alcohol they drink because they metabolize alcohol less efficiently than men do. Women produce less of the alcohol-metabolizing enzyme ADH than men do; consequently, they absorb about 30 percent more alcohol into the bloodstream than men do, even if they consume the same number of drinks that the men consume. For example, if a 20-year-old, 200-pound man and a 20-year-old, 120-pound woman both have three beers in an hour, the man's BAC will be .06 percent at the end of the hour and the woman's will be .11 percent.

These differences make women more vulnerable to the health consequences of alcohol, including alcohol-related liver disease, heart disease, and brain damage.[8] The risk for cirrhosis starts at 2½ drinks to 4 drinks a day for a man, but for a woman this risk starts to increase at less than 2 drinks a day.[31] The rate of atrophy (wasting) of the brain is almost twice as great for women who are chronic drinkers as for men. Women are more susceptible to illness and die at higher rates than men do for every cause of death associated with alcohol. The relationship between alcohol intake and BAC for women and men is shown in Table 11.1.

Rates of alcohol metabolism are affected not just by gender but also by ethnicity. As mentioned earlier in this chapter and as discussed in Chapter 2, some ethnic groups have genetically based differences in the enzymes that metabolize alcohol, causing concentrations of alcetaldehyde to build up in the brain and body tissues. This buildup causes the unpleasant reaction referred to as flushing syndrome or flushing effect.

Drinking behavior also influences alcohol metabolism. Chronic drinkers metabolize alcohol more rapidly than nondrinkers do and may develop tolerance to alcohol, meaning they have to consume larger amounts to produce the same effects. Chronic users may have twice the tolerance for alcohol as the average person does.[1]

Rates of Alcohol Metabolism Alcohol is metabolized more slowly than it is absorbed. This means that the concentration of alcohol builds when additional drinks are consumed

Table 11.1 | Relationships Among Gender, Alcohol Consumption, and Blood Alcohol Concentration

Absolute Alcohol (ounces)	Beverage Intake in 1 Hour	Blood Alcohol Concentrations (g/100 ml)	
		Female (150 lb)	Male (150 lb)
½	1 drink*	0.030	0.025
1	2 drinks*	0.060	0.050
2	4 drinks*	0.120	0.100
3	6 drinks*	0.180	0.150
4	8 drinks*	0.240	0.200
5	10 drinks*	0.300	0.250

Source: Drugs, Society, and Human Behavior, 13th ed., by C.L. Hart, C. Ksir, and O. Ray, 2009, New York: The McGraw-Hill Companies.

*1 drink = 1 oz. spirits, 1 5-oz. glass of wine, or 1 12-oz. beer.

before previous drinks are metabolized. As a rule of thumb, people who have normal liver function metabolize about 0.5 ounce of alcohol (about one drink) per hour.[8] (Remember, rates of alcohol absorption and metabolism vary depending on gender, body weight, and numerous other factors.) For example, if you drink two drinks in 1 hour, you will still have 0.5 ounce of alcohol (one drink) in your system at the end of the hour.

Because of individual differences in sensitivity to alcohol, people experience impairment at different BAC levels. Some people experience nausea, headache, and impaired motor skills at very low BAC levels. The National Highway Traffic Safety Administration reports that driving function can be impaired by BAC levels as low as .02–.04 percent.[5]

The behavioral effects of alcohol, based on studies of moderate drinkers, are summarized in Table 11.2. As you can see, alertness, ability to think clearly, and reaction time are disrupted even at very low BAC levels. As BAC levels increase, thinking and motor skills become increasingly impaired. A person with a BAC of .08 percent is considered legally drunk in all states.

ACUTE ALCOHOL INTOXICATION

People who drink heavily in a relatively short time are vulnerable to **acute alcohol intoxication** (also called *acute alcohol shock* or *alcohol poisoning*), a potentially life-threatening BAC level. Acute alcohol intoxication can produce collapse of vital body functions, notably respiration and heart function, leading to coma and/or death (see the box "First Aid for Alcohol Poisoning").

acute alcohol intoxication
A life-threatening blood alcohol concentration.

Vomiting may occur during acute intoxication. If an unconscious drinker is lying in a position that allows the vomit to obstruct the airway passage, the person may die from asphyxiation. The vomiting reflex may be activated only if a BAC of .12 or higher is reached rapidly, however. Slow, steady drinking allows the vomiting reflex to be suppressed, and BAC can increase to dangerously high levels. At very high alcohol concentrations, .35 or greater, a person can become comatose, and death is possible.

BLACKOUTS

A **blackout** is a period of time during which a drinker is conscious but has impaired memory function; later, he or she has amnesia about events that occurred during this time. The blackout can be partial, or fragmentary (the person can recall events when reminded of them), or *en bloc* (the person has no memory of events). Whether a blackout is partial or en bloc depends on how much alcohol is consumed and how fast. The impairment is associated with changes in the hippocampus, a brain structure essential for memory and learning.[1] These changes may be temporary or permanent. Either way, a blackout is a warning sign that fundamental changes have occurred in the structure of the brain.[32, 33]

blackout
Period of time during which a drinker is conscious but has partial or complete amnesia for events.

Researchers once assumed that blackouts were an indicator of alcoholism. Today, alcohol-induced blackouts are recognized as a common experience among nonalcoholics who binge drink. Studies suggest that 25–50 percent of college students who drink alcohol have experienced a blackout. Women black out at half the consumption levels of alcohol reported by men; on average, women who reported blackouts consumed five drinks per occasion, whereas men consumed nine drinks per occasion.[1] Some people may be genetically predisposed to experience blackouts.

HANGOVERS

Less dangerous than blackouts but equally unpleasant, hangovers are a common reaction to alcohol toxicity. They are characterized by headache, stomach upset, thirst, and fatigue. Despite the consistency of these symptoms, the biological reasons behind them are not well understood. Health experts speculate that alcohol disrupts the body's water balance, causing excessive urination and thirst the next day. The stomach lining may be irritated by increased produc-

tion of hydrochloric acid, resulting in nausea. Alcohol also reduces the water content of brain cells. When the brain cells rehydrate and swell the next day, nerve pain occurs. Drinking more alcohol does not relieve these symptoms.[8] The only known remedy for a hangover is pain medication, rest, and time.

Table 11.2	Stages of Acute Alcoholic Influence/Intoxication	
Blood Alcohol Concentration (grams/100 ml)	**Stage of Alcoholic Influence**	**Clinical Signs/Symptoms**
0.01–0.05	Subclinical	Influence/effects usually not apparent or obvious Behavior nearly normal by ordinary observation Impairment detectable by special tests
0.03–0.12	Euphoria	Mild euphoria, sociability, talkativeness Increased self-confidence; decreased inhibitions Diminished attention, judgment, and control Some sensory-motor impairment Slowed information processing Loss of efficiency in critical performance tests
0.09–0.25	Excitement	Emotional instability; loss of critical judgment Impairment of perception, memory, and comprehension Decreased sensatory response; increased reaction time Reduced visual acuity and peripheral vision; slow glare recovery Sensory-motor incoordination; impaired balance; slurred speech; vomiting; drowsiness
0.18–0.30	Confusion	Disorientation, mental confusion; vertigo; dysphoria Exaggerated emotional states (fear, rage, grief, etc.) Disturbances of vision (diplopia, etc.) and of perception of color, form, motion, dimensions Increased pain threshold Increased muscular incoordination; staggering gait; ataxia Apathy, lethargy
0.25–0.40	Stupor	General inertia; approaching loss of motor functions Markedly decreased response to stimuli Marked muscular incoordination; inability to stand or walk Vomiting; incontinence of urine and feces Impaired consciousness; sleep or stupor
0.35–0.50	Coma	Complete unconsciousness; coma; anesthesia Depressed or abolished reflexes Subnormal temperature Impairment of circulation and respiration Possible death
Above 0.45	Death	Death from respiratory arrest

Source:

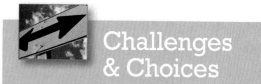

Challenges & Choices

First Aid for Alcohol Poisoning

People who have passed out from heavy drinking should be watched closely. All too often they are carried to bed and forgotten. For their safety, follow these measures:

- Know and recognize the symptoms of acute alcohol intoxication:
  — Lack of response when spoken to or shaken
  — Inability to wake up.
  — Inability to stand up without help.
  — Rapid or irregular pulse (100 beats per minute or more)
  — Rapid, irregular respiration or difficulty breathing (one breath every 3–4 seconds)
  — Cool, clammy, bluish skin
  — Bluish fingernails or lips
- Call 911. An intoxicated person who cannot be roused or wakened or has other symptoms listed above requires emergency medical treatment.
- Do not leave the person to "sleep it off." He or she may never awaken.
- Roll an unconscious drinker onto his or her side to minimize the chance of airway obstruction from vomit.
- If the person vomits, make certain his or her head is positioned lower than the rest of the body. You may need to reach into the person's mouth to clear the airway.
- Try to find out if the person has taken other drugs or medications that might interact with alcohol.
- Stay with the person until medical help arrives.

It's Not Just Personal ...
Drinking games, hazing rituals, and other excessive drinking practices contribute to cases of acute alcohol intoxication among college students. Every year, about 50 college students in the United States die from alcohol poisoning—about one person per weekend.

Health Risks of Alcohol Use

Excessive alcohol consumption causes more than 100,000 deaths each year in the United States. Alcohol is toxic and has an effect on virtually all body organs and systems as well as all aspects of a person's functioning.

MEDICAL PROBLEMS ASSOCIATED WITH ALCOHOL USE

The major organs and systems damaged by alcohol use are the cardiovascular system, the liver, the brain, the immune system, and the reproductive system (Figure 11.5). Alcohol use is associated with certain cancers, and when pregnant women drink, it can cause a set of fetal birth defects known as **fetal alcohol syndrome (FAS)** (discussed in Chapter 16). Children born with FAS have permanent physical and mental impairments.

fetal alcohol syndrome (FAS) Set of birth defects associated with use of alcohol during pregnancy.

Heart Disease and Stroke Chronic heavy drinking is a major cause of degenerative disease of the heart muscle, a condition called **cardiomyopathy,** and of heart arrhythmias (irregular heartbeat). Abnormal heart rhythm is one cause of sudden death in alcoholics, whether or not they already had heart disease. Heavy drinking also causes coronary heart disease (disease of the arteries serving the heart). Some studies have reported that binge drinkers have six times the risk for fatal attacks faced by moderate drinkers.[5]

cardiomyopathy Disease of the heart muscle.

In addition, long-term heavy drinking can elevate blood pressure and increase the severity of high blood pressure, which increases the risk for stroke (an interruption in the blood supply to the brain).

Liver Disease The liver is a vital organ with many metabolic, digestive, and regulatory functions, including filtering toxins and pathogens from the blood. Alcohol-related liver disease occurs in three phases. The first, called **fatty liver,** occurs when the liver is flooded with more alcohol than it can metabolize, causing it to swell with fat globules. This condition can literally develop overnight as a result of binge drinking. In men the alcohol capacity of the liver is about six drinks; in women it is three to four drinks. Drinking more than that at one sitting may cause fatty liver.

fatty liver Condition in which the liver swells with fat globules as a result of alcohol consumption.

Fatty liver is not a serious problem for most drinkers, because with abstinence (usually about 30 days or so), stored fatty acids are used as fuel energy and the condition is completely reversed. Serious health problems may develop, however, when stored fatty-acid molecules increase in size and their cell membranes rupture, causing liver cells to die.[8]

The second phase of liver disease is called **alcoholic hepatitis,** which includes both liver inflammation and liver function impairment. This condition typically occurs in parts of the liver where cells are dead or dying. Alcoholic hepatitis can occur in the absence of

alcoholic hepatitis Inflammation of the liver as a result of alcohol consumption.

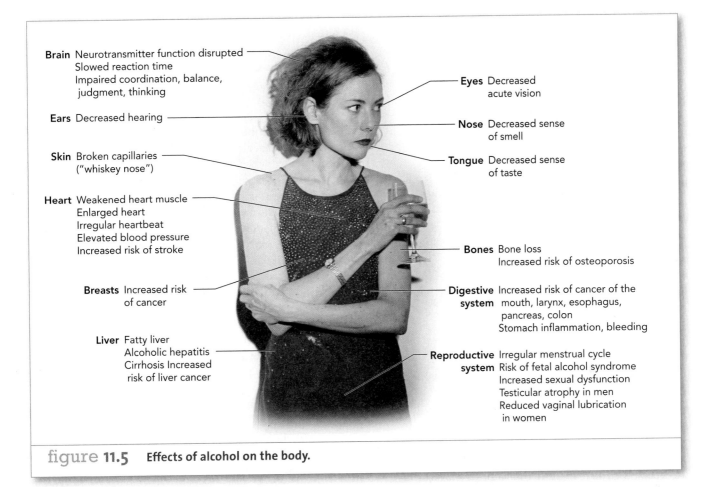

Brain Neurotransmitter function disrupted
Slowed reaction time
Impaired coordination, balance, judgment, thinking

Ears Decreased hearing

Skin Broken capillaries ("whiskey nose")

Heart Weakened heart muscle
Enlarged heart
Irregular heartbeat
Elevated blood pressure
Increased risk of stroke

Breasts Increased risk of cancer

Liver Fatty liver
Alcoholic hepatitis
Cirrhosis Increased risk of liver cancer

Eyes Decreased acute vision

Nose Decreased sense of smell

Tongue Decreased sense of taste

Bones Bone loss
Increased risk of osteoporosis

Digestive system Increased risk of cancer of the mouth, larynx, esophagus, pancreas, colon
Stomach inflammation, bleeding

Reproductive system Irregular menstrual cycle
Risk of fetal alcohol syndrome
Increased sexual dysfunction
Testicular atrophy in men
Reduced vaginal lubrication in women

figure **11.5**   **Effects of alcohol on the body.**

fatty liver, which suggests that direct toxic effects of alcohol may be the cause.[8]

The third phase of liver disease is **cirrhosis,** scarring of the liver tissue. Although other diseases can cause cirrhosis (such as viral hepatitis), between 40 and 90 percent of people with cirrhosis have a history of alcohol abuse.[3] The risk rises sharply with higher levels of consumption. It usually takes at least 10 years of steady, heavy drinking for cirrhosis to develop.[8]

cirrhosis
Scarring of the liver as a result of alcohol consumption.

As cirrhosis sets in, liver cells are replaced by fibrous tissue, called collagen, which changes the structure of the liver and decreases blood flow to the organ. Liver cells die and liver function is impaired, leading to fluid accumulation in the body, jaundice (yellowing of the skin), and an opportunity for infections or cancers to establish themselves. The prognosis for people with alcoholic hepatitis or cirrhosis is poor. The death rate exceeds 60 percent over a 4-year period, with most deaths occurring within the first year.[8]

Cancer   Alcohol is associated with several types of cancer, particularly cancers of the head and neck (mouth, pharynx, larynx, and esophagus), cancers of the digestive tract, and breast cancer.[5] Alcohol causes inflammation of the pancreas, but the link between this inflammation and pancreatic cancer remains unproven.

Substantial evidence from many countries suggests that the risk of breast cancer increases for women who consume more than three drinks per day compared with women who abstain.[5] The Nurses' Health Study found that women who consumed two drinks a day have a 10 percent higher risk of breast cancer than do women who consumed one drink per day.[1] Scientists theorize that alcohol increases a woman's exposure to estrogen and androgens, hormones that may increase cancer risk. The risk is more pronounced at heavy intake levels.

Brain Damage   Heavy alcohol consumption causes anatomical changes in the brain and directly damages brain cells. Alcohol can cause a loss of brain tissue, inflammation of the brain, and a widening of fissures in the cortex (covering) of the brain.[34] Heavy drinking, especially binge drinking, has been shown to disrupt short-term memory and the ability to analyze complex problems.[3]

In long-term alcohol abuse, loss of brain tissue is associated with a mental disorder called alcohol-induced persisting dementia, an overall decline in intellect. Some of this loss may be reversible if the person abstains from alcohol use for a few months, but after age 40, there is little improvement even with abstinence.[34]

Because the brain continues to grow and mature until the early 20s (see Chapter 3), there is concern that heavy alcohol use during the teen years can be harmful to the developing

MRI

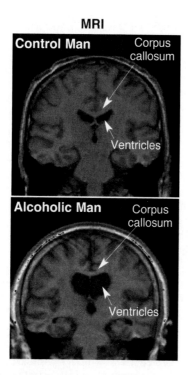

■ This magnetic resonance imaging (MRI) shows how chronic alcohol use can damage the frontal lobes of the brain, increase the size of the ventricles, and cause an overall reduction in brain size (shrinkage).

brain. Studies have revealed that the hippocampus (a center for learning and memory) is 10 percent smaller in teenagers who drink heavily than in those who don't.[34] Research has also found differences in the prefrontal cortex, the center for executive functions (rational thinking, planning). Teenagers who drink heavily score worse than nondrinkers do on tests, particularly tests involving verbal and nonverbal information recall, and they have an increased risk of school failure, social problems, depression, suicidal thoughts, and violence.[34, 35]

Body Weight and Nutrition   A regular beer has about 144 calories; a glass of wine, 100–105 calories; and a shot of gin or whiskey, 96 calories.[36] Mixers add more calories, as do *alcopops* or *malternatives*—sugary, fizzy, fruit-flavored drinks popular among younger drinkers (see the box "Malternatives: 'Starter' Beverages for Young Drinkers").

These calories are empty, providing almost no nutrients. It's easy to see that consuming alcohol can lead to weight gain; these calories have a tendency to be deposited in the abdomen, giving drinkers the characteristic "beer belly."

On the other hand, long-term heavy drinkers who substitute the calories in alcohol for those in food are at risk for weight loss and malnutrition. They are also vulnerable to mental disorders caused by vitamin deficiencies.

SOCIAL PROBLEMS ASSOCIATED WITH ALCOHOL USE

Alcohol reduces social inhibitions, and reduced inhibition may lead to high-risk sexual activity and a lowered likelihood of practicing safe sex (such as using a condom). One

study found that frequent binge drinkers were five times less likely to practice safe sex than were non–binge drinkers.[37] Heavy drinkers were more likely to have multiple sex partners and to engage in other high-risk sexual behaviors. These behaviors are associated with increased risk of sexually transmitted disease and unplanned pregnancy.[37]

Violence is another problem associated with alcohol use. The National Crime Victimization Survey (NCVS) has consistently found that alcohol is more likely than any other drug to be associated with violence. One study found that 15 percent of robberies, 28 percent of aggravated and simple assaults, and 37 percent of rapes and sexual assaults are committed by individuals who have been drinking. Alcohol is a factor in 67 percent of domestic violence cases and half of all homicides.[5] Women who binge drink or date men who binge drink are at increased risk for sexual exploitation (rape and other forms of nonconsensual sex).[38]

The relationship between alcohol and risk of injury has been established for a variety of circumstances, including automobile crashes, falls, and fires. Reduced cognitive function, impaired physical coordination, and increased risk-taking behavior (impulsivity) are the alcohol-related factors that lead to injury. Alcohol has also been shown to increase the risk of serious injury and decrease the probability of survival because it impairs heart and circulatory system function. The risk of injury increases steadily with the amount of alcohol consumed.[5]

Alcohol use is a factor in about one-third of suicides, and it is second only to depression as a predictor of suicide attempts by youth.[8] The relationship between alcohol and depression is very strong. Estimates are that 20–36 percent of people who commit suicide were drinking shortly before their suicide or had a history of alcohol abuse.[5] Alcohol-associated suicides tend to be impulsive rather than premeditated acts.

ANOTHER VIEW: HEALTH BENEFITS

The Health Professionals Study found that men and women who drink moderately on 5 to 7 days of the week have less risk of heart disease than do those who drink moderately on fewer days of the week.[39] Moderate drinkers also have less risk of heart disease than do either abstainers or heavy drinkers. The *Dietary Guidelines for Americans* notes that the lowest rates of death occur among people who consume one to two drinks a day.

Scientists speculate that moderate alcohol consumption increases high-density lipoproteins (HDL, also called "good cholesterol"), has an anticlotting effect on the blood, and reduces stress.[39] The beneficial effects of alcohol on HDL levels and blood clotting may be only temporary, lasting perhaps 24 hours, so that people who drink moderately every day maintain optimal protection against heart disease. It is apparently the pattern of drinking, not the type of alcoholic beverage, that confers benefits. People who drink wine, for example, tend to do so in small amounts every day rather than in large amounts. Binge drinking does not serve as a protective factor and can actually increase the risk for heart disease.[5] In women, the beneficial effects may be offset by an increased risk of breast cancer.

The *Dietary Guidelines for Americans* advises that moderate alcohol consumption—one drink a day for women and two drinks a day for men—can be beneficial for middle-aged and older adults, the age groups most susceptible to coronary heart disease. In younger adults, however, alcohol appears to have fewer, if any, health benefits, and it is associated with more deaths from injuries and accidents. Even light drinking can have adverse effects on certain people, such as individuals with liver disease or high blood pressure. It is not recommended that anyone begin drinking or drink more frequently because of anticipated health benefits.

Alcohol Misuse, Abuse, and Dependence

Between 20 and 25 percent of people who drink develop some alcohol-related problem(s) at some point.[6] About 4–5 percent develop alcohol dependence and are categorized as alcoholics.[40]

problem drinking
Pattern of alcohol use that impairs the drinker's life, causing difficulties for the drinker and for others.

Problem drinking is a pattern of alcohol use that impairs the drinker's life, causing personal difficulties and difficulties for other people. For college students, such difficulties might be missed classes or poor academic performance. **Alcohol abuse** is defined as the continued use of alcohol despite negative consequences. It is a pattern of drinking that leads to impairment in the person's ability to fulfill major obligations at home, work, or school or to legal or social problems.[13]

Alcohol dependence is considered a separate disorder; it is characterized by a strong craving for alcohol.[18] People who are dependent on alcohol use it compulsively, and most will eventually experience physiological changes in brain and body chemistry as a result of alcohol use. As described in Chapter 3, one indicator of dependence is the development of *tolerance*, reduced sensitivity to the effects of a drug so that larger and larger amounts are needed to produce the same effects.[6] Another indicator is experiencing *withdrawal*, a state of acute physical and psychological discomfort, when alcohol consumption stops abruptly.

Alcohol dependence is also known as **alcoholism,** defined as a

alcohol abuse
Pattern of alcohol use that leads to distress or impairment, increases the risk of health and/or social problems, and continues despite awareness of these effects.

alcohol dependence
Disorder characterized by a strong craving for alcohol, the development of tolerance for alcohol, and symptoms of withdrawal if alcohol consumption stops abruptly

alcoholism
A primary chronic disease characterized by excessive, compulsive drinking.

Consumer Clipboard

Malternatives: "Starter" Beverages for Young Drinkers

A new kind of beverage hit the shelves of convenience stores and liquor outlets in the mid-1990s—fruit-flavored alcoholic beverages with names like Skyblue, Smirnoff Ice, Tequiza, Snakebite, Moscow Mule, Hard Lemonade, and Wild Brew. Called "malternatives" or "alcopops," these drinks are malt based and contain 5 to 7 percent alcohol, about the same as beer.

Although alcohol manufacturers claim they market these beverages to 18- to 25-year-olds, the popularity of malternatives peaks between ages 13 and 16. Forty-one percent of teens say they have tried malternatives. Manufacturers use vibrant colors, rebellious or sexy names, and cartoon characters to target youth. Teens find malternatives appealing because they are more refreshing, taste less like alcohol, and are easy to get and cheap. (What they may not know is that malternatives are loaded with calories; most contain more calories than a Krispy Kreme donut.) Young people are much less likely to have experienced or under-

stand the potentially harmful effects of alcohol on the body, especially the maturing brain. As teens get older, they tend to switch to more mature types of alcoholic beverages.

Why should we be concerned about malternatives? Alcohol is the leading drug problem in the United States, killing six times as many teenagers as are killed by the use of illicit drugs. People who drink before age 15 are four times more likely to develop alcohol dependence than are those who wait until age 21. The U.S. Department of Justice estimates that underage drinking costs more than $53 billion every year by contributing to injuries, violence, rape, and other crime.

Health authorities are calling for tighter regulation of these "starter" alcoholic beverages. They want to make them less appealing to teenagers by revising names, packaging, and labeling so that they more closely resemble other alcoholic drinks. Labels would clearly and conspicuously identify them as alcoholic beverages and disclose their alcohol content. Consumer organizations have petitioned the Alcohol and Tobacco Tax and Trade Bureau to require "Alcohol Facts" labels on every alcoholic beverage container, including alcopops.

Source: "Alcohol Policies Project Issue: Alcopops," Center for Science in the Public Interest, retrieved April 20, 2008, from www.cspinet.org/booze/iss_alcopops.htm.

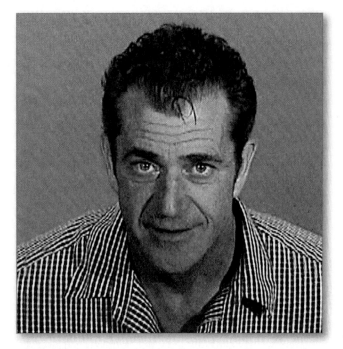

■ Alcohol abuse, alcohol dependence, or both? The Los Angeles County Sheriff's Department released this booking photo of actor Mel Gibson after he was charged with misdemeanor drunken driving in August 2006.

chronic disease with genetic, psychosocial, and environmental causes.[13] It is often progressive and fatal. The manifestations of alcoholism include lack of control over drinking, preoccupation with alcohol, use of alcohol despite adverse consequences, and distortions in thinking (most notably denial).

This definition is similar to that of problem drinking, but there is a difference in degree. Alcohol becomes a problem when individuals are impaired by their drinking, but drinkers become alcoholics when they become dependent on alcohol. Alcoholics spend time anticipating their next drink (craving), planning when and where to get it, and hiding their alcohol use from others.

Treatment Options

Treatment options for alcohol-related disorders include brief interventions, inpatient treatment programs, outpatient treatment programs, and self-help approaches.

BRIEF INTERVENTIONS FOR HIGH-RISK YOUNG ADULT DRINKERS

Early screening and intervention are critical for high-risk young adult drinkers. Almost half of those individuals who develop alcohol dependence have alcohol abuse problems before age 21. Many colleges and universities focus their high-risk programs on freshmen, athletes, and fraternity members. A growing body of research suggests that gay men, lesbians, and transgendered individuals should be included in the high-risk category.

General risk factors for alcohol problems include binge drinking in high school, family history of alcohol abuse, mental health problems, academic problems, legal infractions, and feeling overwhelmed by stress. Programs are also directed at high-risk times and events such as spring break, fraternity rushing, homecoming, and pre-graduation events for seniors.

The Alcohol Skills Training Program is a model brief intervention program adapted by many colleges and community-based organizations around the country. It is designed for college students and other young adults considered at risk for alcohol-related problems, such as poor class attendance and grades, accidents, sexual assault, and violence. It consists of a series of group sessions (usually six to eight) focusing on skills and knowledge development through lectures, discussion, and role plays. Students learn basic information about the physiology of alcohol addiction, drinking moderation skills, assertiveness skills, and relapse prevention strategies.

The Brief Alcohol Screening and Intervention for College Students (BASICS) program is another brief intervention model for college students who drink heavily and have experienced or are at risk for alcohol-related problems. BASICS is conducted in two 50-minute interviews and includes personalized feedback on the effects and consequences of alcohol use, strategies for reducing risks and making better decisions, and options that can help students make changes. Students who receive BASICS report fewer consequences and more rapid changes in their alcohol-related behavior and consequences than at-risk drinkers who do not receive the intervention.[41]

Motivational interviewing (MI) is a style of counseling frequently used in brief interventions. MI incorporates the stages of change model (see Chapter 1) and focuses on helping the student see the need for change. A typical strategy might be to question the student about his or her future plans and about how excessive drinking fits in with these plans. The intent is to create a discrepancy between what a person wants in life and his or her current state as a result of drinking.[41]

INPATIENT TREATMENT

When alcohol-related problems are severe, individuals benefit from placement in a residential facility specializing in alcohol recovery. The first stage of treatment is detoxification, the gradual withdrawal of alcohol from the body. Withdrawal symptoms include profuse sweating, rapid heart rate, elevated blood pressure, nausea, headache, difficulty sleeping, depression, and irritability.[40] People who have been heavy drinkers for a long time and/ or who have an underlying medical condition may experience more severe withdrawal symptoms, such as seizures and, rarely, a disturbance called **delirium tremens (DTs)**.[8] Symptoms of the DTs include delirium, disorientation, and hallucinations. An acute DT episode is a medical emergency requiring hospitalization.

delirium tremens (DTs)
Severe condition characterized by delirium, disorientation, and hallucinations, associated with withdrawal from alcohol.

The early phase of alcohol treatment may also include medications, such as anti-anxiety and antidepressant drugs, although such drugs are usually prescribed only when the person has an underlying medical or psychological disorder. Another drug that may be prescribed is disulfiram (Antabuse). This drug causes a person to become acutely nauseated if any alcohol is consumed, although it does not reduce alcohol cravings.[8] Researchers are exploring drugs that increase levels of the neurotransmitter serotonin as a way to reduce cravings and relapse.[3] Naltrexone, for example, is a drug that lessens alcohol craving by blocking opioid receptors in the brain.

Programs typically include education about alcohol and drugs, skills training, and group and individual counseling. Counseling is an important component in any kind of alcohol treatment. Family members are often encouraged to participate in the recovery process. This participation helps them better understand how they are personally affected and how they can help their loved one recover from alcoholism.

OUTPATIENT TREATMENT

Economic pressures have led to a reduction in the number of inpatient treatment days covered by health insurance companies, which in turn has led to greater use of outpatient programs. In these programs, patients participate in a treatment program during the day and return home in the evening. Treatment typically includes individual counseling, group counseling, and marital or family counseling. Research suggests that outpatient programs are as effective as, or more effective than, inpatient programs.[5]

SELF-HELP PROGRAMS

The best-known self-help program is Alcoholics Anonymous (AA). The goal of AA is total abstinence from alcohol. A basic premise of AA is that an alcoholic is biologically different from a nonalcoholic and consequently can never safely drink any alcohol at all. Although alcoholics are not to blame for their problem, they still must take responsibility for their behavior. In the 12-step path to recovery, members recognize that they are "powerless over alcohol" and have to seek help from a "higher power" (whatever the person considers to be a power greater than him- or herself, whether a divine being, nature, or even the AA community itself). Other key components of AA are group support and the use of sponsors—members who are paired with new members, who provide support if the tempta-

tion to relapse becomes overwhelming, and who help new members work their way through the steps.

Some people are uncomfortable with AA's focus on spirituality, and alternative programs have been developed that do not have this focus. One such group is Rational Recovery, which focuses on self rather than spirituality. Another objection to AA is its perceived masculine orientation, and alternative programs have been developed by and for women, such as Women for Sobriety. Although AA dominates self-help programs for alcoholism, it has not been shown to be more effective than some of these alternative programs.[5]

Self-help programs have also been developed for family members and friends of alcoholics. Al-Anon is a support program whereby individuals can explore how they may have enabled the alcoholic's behavior (for example, by covering up or rationalizing) and how they can change their behavior. Alateen is a support program for young people who have been affected by someone else's drinking. Adult Children of Alcoholics is a program that provides a supportive environment where people can confront the potentially lifelong emotional effects associated with growing up in an alcoholic household.

RELAPSE PREVENTION

Recovery from alcoholism is a lifelong process. The first two years after treatment are usually the hardest. The difficulty of recovery is thought to be due to the changes that alcohol has produced in the brain. The brain's circuitry has been reprogrammed such that pleasure has become associated primarily with alcohol. Craving can continue for years, even during sleep. MRI brain scans have shown that viewing

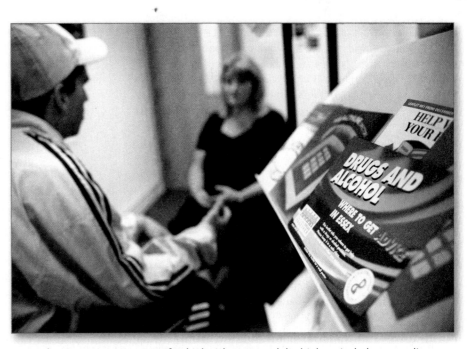

■ Brief intervention programs for high-risk young adult drinkers include counseling sessions that help individuals see the consequences of alcohol use and develop strategies for change.

a picture of an alcoholic drink activates a part of the frontal cortex in the brains of alcoholics but not in the brains of moderate drinkers. The mere thought of a drink can affect the brain of a recovering alcoholic.[42]

Relapse prevention focuses on social skills training (stress management, assertiveness, communication skills, self-control) and family and marital therapy. Despite a high relapse rate, those who participate in treatment programs do better than those who do not.

THE HARM REDUCTION APPROACH

Some health experts disagree with the disease model of alcoholism, in which it is viewed as a chronic disease that is either present or absent.[43] This view seems to rule out the possibility that there could be some middle ground or that some drinking by alcoholics might be acceptable. In contrast, the **harm reduction** approach focuses on reducing the harm associated with drinking, both to the individual and to society. An example of harm reduction is **controlled drinking,** which emphasizes moderation rather than abstinence.[44] Individuals are taught to practice responsible, controlled drinking through cognitive behavioral techniques, such as using a diary to chart drinking patterns, and consumption management techniques, such as limiting drinks to one per hour.

harm reduction
Approach to alcohol treatment that focuses on a broader range of drinking behaviors and treatments than those associated with abstinence programs.

controlled drinking
Approach to drinking that emphasizes moderation rather than abstinence.

Controlled drinking programs have long been promoted in Great Britain and Canada.[44] These programs are controversial precisely because they do not require abstinence. Some experts fear that making controlled drinking an option for alcoholism treatment will cause a stampede of patients away from abstinence programs, although research has not shown that this happens.[45] Most mental health experts agree that total abstinence is the most effective approach for recovery from alcoholism.[5] Controlled drinking is considered appropriate for early-stage problem drinkers.[46]

PUBLIC POLICIES AND LAWS AIMED AT HARM REDUCTION

A variety of public policies and laws are aimed at reducing the harm caused by alcohol consumption. These include the minimum drinking age, drunk driving laws, and various community ordinances.

Minimum Legal Drinking Age   Since 1984, all states have had laws prohibiting the purchase and public possession of alcohol by people under the age of 21. Despite inconsistent compliance with these laws, research suggests that they result in less underage drinking than occurred when the drinking age was 18.[47] Evidence also suggests that these laws result in less drinking after age 21.[5] Some people argue that the minimum drinking age laws are too restrictive and create

a mystique about alcohol that fosters irresponsible drinking, but research does not support this argument.

Drunk Driving Laws and Sobriety Checkpoints   Studies show that tough drinking laws are effective in preventing drunk driving,[44] despite problems with enforcement and detection of intoxicated drivers. Still, many people continue to drink and drive. Education and treatment programs used in conjunction with punishments, such as mandatory suspension of drivers' licenses for first-time offenders, have not proven to be effective in preventing driving under the influence.[5]

A practice that does substantially increase compliance with drunk driving laws is the use of sobriety checkpoints. Law enforcement agents check drivers for intoxication with alcohol sensors and breath analyzer tests. Alcohol sensors are noninvasive tests that can detect the presence of alcohol on the breath when held in the vicinity of a driver. Breath analyzer tests measure the amount of alcohol exhaled in the breath.

Laboratory tests, such as urinalysis and blood tests, are sometimes used to confirm BAC level. Many states now require people suspected of driving under the influence of alcohol or illicit drugs to undergo blood testing. Refusal to submit to either a breath analyzer test or urinalysis when requested by law enforcement can result in immediate revocation of the driver's license.

Server Liability Laws   Server liability laws make licensed establishments liable for injuries or property damage caused by an intoxicated or underage customer who is served by the establishment. These laws also apply to private individuals

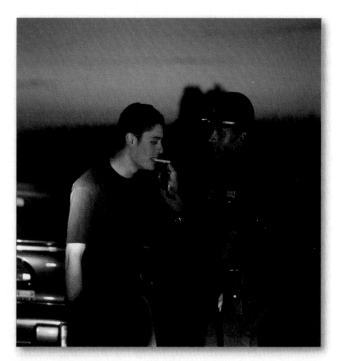

■ Breath analysis and sobriety checkpoints are public health measures designed to reduce the harm to self and others associated with alcohol use.

who serve alcohol at social functions. Under server liability laws, a third party who has been injured by a drunk driver can file a civil suit against the server for damages. The jury is still out on whether server liability laws are effective.[5] Few cases have been prosecuted, and few licensed establishments have been cited for serving alcohol to intoxicated patrons.[5]

Restrictions on Liquor Sales and Outlets Ease of access is a key factor in alcohol consumption. The more places there are to purchase alcohol within a certain geographical area, the higher the rates of alcohol consumption and alcohol-related harm.[5] Some communities have worked for a more even distribution of alcohol outlets throughout their area to curb this problem.

Studies show that alcohol is readily available to underage drinkers. Although parents and other adults are the most common source, underage drinkers also buy alcoholic beverages at convenience stores, liquor stores, and bars.[48] Recently, the Internet has become a source for underage purchase of alcoholic beverages, although regulations are being put in place to curb this practice.

Tax Increases Another way to control alcohol consumption is by increasing taxation. Research suggests that an increase in the price of alcohol is met by a corresponding decrease in consumption per capita. Higher prices appear to reduce consumption by underage and moderate drinkers but not by heavy drinkers. Raising prices too much might also create a black market for alcoholic beverages.[5, 47, 48]

Ignition Locks Some states are using interlock devices to crack down on drunk driving. The device acts like a breath analyzer. When the ignition key is turned on, a voice or tone prompts the driver to blow into the device within 10 seconds. The breath sample is analyzed, and if alcohol is present, the vehicle will not start. The device asks the driver for additional samples at any time the engine is on. If a sample is positive, the driver is instructed to pull over and shut off the engine. If the driver fails to comply after repeated warnings, the device will activate the horn and flash the vehicle lights. Records of violations are forwarded to law enforcement agencies.

As of 2007, 18 states had implemented mandatory interlock systems for drunk driving offenders, and Congress is considering a federal law that would require all states to use interlock systems for high-risk offenders. Parents are also installing interlock systems in vehicles operated by teenagers.

Community Ordinances Local communities have a variety of measures at their disposal for influencing alcohol consumption, including limiting drink specials at local bars, prohibiting out-of-sight sales (purchases made by one person for several others), and imposing a minimum drink price.[49] Communities can also enforce fines and revoke liquor licenses when bars serve underage drinkers. House parties can be controlled through public nuisance and noise

Public Health in Action

High-Tech Alcohol Monitors

Law enforcement agencies are using high-tech monitors to track alcohol consumption by people convicted of alcohol offenses, particularly chronic offenders. Test results are sent to the offender's probation officer on a daily or weekly basis. Recently developed devices include the following:

- *Visitel/Breath Alcohol Tester.* The offender is called at random times and asked to breathe into a breath alcohol tester. Test results, along with the offender's picture, are transmitted immediately to a monitoring center.

- *SleepTime Monitor.* This device tests the person's urine for ethyl glucuronide (EtG), a product of the metabolism of alcohol that stays in the urine for up to 5 days after alcohol consumption, long after alcohol itself has been eliminated from the body. The monitor samples urine while the person is sleeping and sends reports to law enforcement personnel. Extensive research has validated the accuracy of this test, but it has been criticized for being too sensitive to EtG to distinguish between alcohol consumption and exposure to alcohol in products like antiperspirant, aftershave, and hair spray.

- *Secure Continuous Remote Alcohol Monitor (SCRAM).* The offender wears two small black boxes strapped to both sides of the calf. The monitor takes hourly readings of the offender's perspiration for signs of alcohol use. A receiver is attached to the offender's home telephone or computer, and reports are sent to law enforcement personnel via telephone or computer. SCRAM devices received national attention in 2007 when actress Lindsay Lohan was ordered to wear one after being arrested for alcohol offenses.

- *Global Positioning System (GPS).* If an alcohol offender is under house arrest, his or her movement can be monitored on a daily basis using GPS. This approach is more commonly used for tracking sex offenders than alcohol offenders.

Sources: "Types of Monitoring," Lee's Home Confinement, Inc., retrieved May 14, 2008, from www.leeshomeconfinement.com/html/types_of_ monitoring.html; "Effectiveness of SCRAM Device Questioned," by D.S. Kabat, retrieved May 14, 2008, from http://alcoholism.about.com/od/ dui/a/kabat.htm.

laws. Research suggests that comprehensive community programs that unite city agencies and private citizens are effective in reducing drunk driving, related driving risks, and traffic deaths and injuries.[5] High-tech alcohol monitors are also used by communities as public health controls (see the box "High-Tech Alcohol Monitors").

Taking Action

Is alcohol a problem in your life? Do you wonder what you can do to reduce or prevent harm from alcohol-related activities? In this section we provide some suggestions for individual actions.

ARE YOU AT RISK?

Physicians sometimes use the CAGE questionnaire to identify individuals at risk for alcohol problems:

C: Have you ever tried to *cut down* on your drinking?

A: Have you ever been *annoyed* by criticism of your drinking?

G: Have you ever felt *guilty* about your drinking?

E: Have you ever had a morning "*eye-opener*"?

A yes answer to one or more of these question suggests that you may be at risk for alcohol dependence. To learn more about your risks, see the box "Assess Your Alcohol-Related Attitudes and Behavior."

DEVELOPING A BEHAVIOR CHANGE PLAN

If you decide you would like to change your behavior around alcohol, you can develop a behavior change plan to do so. First, keep track of when, how much, and with whom you drink for 2 weeks, and then analyze your record to discover your drinking patterns. Do you drink mostly on weekends, or do you drink every day? Do you drink mostly with certain people, or do you drink alone? Do you drink when you're under stress? Information like this can help you get a sense of the role alcohol plays in your life.

If you decide you want to change your drinking behavior, set goals for yourself. Goals should be specific, motivating, achievable, and rewarding. "I'm going to drink less" is too vague a goal. "I'm going to drink only once a week and have no more than four drinks" is a more specific, measurable goal.

Then develop specific strategies to attain your goals. For example, if you always have a drink when you get home from work or class and you want to eliminate that drink, don't keep alcohol in your house. If you drink in social situations or with certain people, learn to say no to some drinks. Tell people you feel better when you don't drink, and avoid people who can't accept that. Plan ahead what you will do when you're tempted to have a drink. Ask family and friends for their support. For more suggestions, see the box "Tips for Changing Your Alcohol-Related Behavior."

After a few weeks, evaluate the outcome of your behavior change plan. Did you achieve your goals? If not, what obsta-

Highlight on Health

Assess Your Alcohol-Related Attitudes and Behavior

Do you sometimes wonder if you have a problem with alcohol? This quick assessment will help you find out. Simply answer yes or no to the following questions:

1. Are you unable to stop drinking after a certain number of drinks?
2. Do you need a drink to get motivated?
3. Do you often forget what happened while you were partying (have blackouts)?
4. Do you drink or party alone?
5. Have others annoyed you by criticizing your alcohol use?
6. Have you been involved in fights with your friends or family while you were drunk or high?
7. Have you done or said anything while drinking that you later regretted?
8. Have you destroyed or damaged property while drinking?
9. Do you drive while high or drunk?
10. Have you been physically hurt while drinking?
11. Have you been in trouble with school authorities or campus police because of drinking?
12. Have you dropped or chosen friends based on their drinking habits?
13. Do you think you are a normal drinker despite friends' comments that you drink too much?
14. Have you ever missed classes because you were too hungover to get up on time?
15. Have you ever done poorly on an exam or assignment because of drinking?
16. Do you think about drinking or getting high a lot?
17. Do you feel guilty about your drinking?

If you answered yes to three or more questions, you may be consuming alcoholic beverages in a harmful manner. Consider contacting your student health clinic or counseling center for information or help.

Source: From "Alcohol Use and You: Decisions on Tap." Copyright © April 2008, American College Health Association. Reprinted by permission of American College Health Association, P.O. Box 28937, Baltimore, MD 21240-8937.

cles prevented you from succeeding? How can you overcome these obstacles? People who succeed at changing their behavior don't necessarily do so the first time they try. The key is to view each failure as an opportunity to learn more about yourself. Periodically assessing your progress allows you to devise alternative strategies for reaching your goals.

BE AN ADVOCATE

If you are interested in addressing irresponsible alcohol consumption, you can join an advocacy organization or concerned citizens group on your campus or in your community. Mothers Against Drunk Driving (MADD) is a nationwide advocacy organization with hundreds of local chapters throughout North America. It was founded to educate citizens about the effects of alcohol on driving and to influence legislation on drunk driving.

Students Against Destructive Decisions (SADD) initially focused on drunk driving by youth but has broadened its activities to include initiatives against underage drinking, illicit drug use, failure to use seat belts, and drugged driving. The central mission of SADD, however, remains a pact called "Contract for Life," an agreement parents and teenagers can make to provide safe transportation for one another, no questions asked, if any of them has become impaired by alcohol consumption.

Boost Alcohol Consciousness Concerning the Health of University Students (BACCHUS) is a nonprofit organization with hundreds of chapters across North America. It is run by student volunteers and promotes both abstinence and responsible drinking. Some BACCHUS chapters have joined with Greeks Advocating Mature Management of Alcohol (GAMMA) to provide a peer education network. This network program may be called BACCHUS or GAMMA on your college campus. The merging of BACCHUS and GAMMA has led to a broadening of approaches to health issues that affect college students.[1]

Many parents and students look into school alcohol policies as a factor in college selection. Some organizations publish rankings of the most notorious "party schools." Some colleges have signed on to national programs to combat binge drinking. These anti-alcohol actions have been fueled by the knowledge that a crackdown can play a key role in attracting applicants.

***

Whatever your attitudes toward alcohol, and whatever your alcohol-related behaviors have been thus far, remember that it is up to you to decide what role you want alcohol to play in your life. Many people do not drink at all, and many more drink only occasionally. Drinking is a serious problem for only about 5–10 percent of the population. You can make sure you are not among that group by making responsible decisions about alcohol use.

Challenges & Choices

Tips for Changing Your Alcohol-Related Behavior

- Stock your refrigerator with healthy beverages—juice, bottled water, milk, sports drinks, diet soda.
- If you want to have alcoholic beverages on hand, buy small quantities—one or two bottles of beer rather than a six-pack, for example.
- If you drink when you're upset, lonely, or stressed out, learn how to handle these feelings in a healthier way, such as exercising, meditating, or talking with a friend or counselor.
- If you drink when you're with other people, learn how to socialize without alcohol; try hiking or playing sports with friends, or attend alcohol-free events.
- If others are pressuring you to drink, learn how to say no.
- When you are drinking, keep your BAC low by drinking slowly, drinking water and nonalcoholic beverages along with alcoholic ones, eating food, and staying within your limits; avoid mixed or carbonated drinks.
- When you are the host, provide food and nonalcoholic beverages, and make sure no one who drives away from your house at the end of the party is drunk or impaired.

It's Not Just Personal . . .

Many people think that they can drink and still be capable of making rational decisions, that they can drive safely if they consume just a few drinks, that they can sober up quickly if they have to, and that drinking isn't dangerous. All are myths.

You Make the Call

Should Passive Alcohol Sensors Be Used by Law Enforcement?

The National Highway Safety and Traffic Administration estimates that about 40 percent of all traffic fatalities are alcohol related. One drunk driving death occurs every 30 minutes. To reduce alcohol-related crashes, law enforcement officials in many states now use passive alcohol sensors (PAS). PAS devices detect the presence of alcohol in the air surrounding the driver. They are often concealed in a flashlight or clipboard.

These devices are called passive because the driver being tested does not actually blow into the PAS. In fact, drivers are usually not aware that they are being tested for the presence of alcohol. The law enforcement officer holds the PAS 3 to 10 inches from the driver, and a light indicator displays an approximate level of alcohol in the air sample. The PAS reading is a simple pass or fail test; it does not measure BAC. If the driver fails, the officer may perform a breath analyzer test. Sensors have been used at sobriety checkpoints, during truck inspections, and during routine traffic stops.

A major legal issue is whether the use of PAS is a violation of an individual's rights under the Fourth Amendment, which provides protection from unreasonable search and seizure. Two exceptions to the Fourth Amendment may apply to this debate. One is the "plain view" doctrine—if something is in plain view, there cannot be a reasonable expectation of privacy. The argument is that a person's breath is openly displayed to the public. Law enforcement officers have long relied on sniffing the air for the presence of alcohol to determine whether the driver has been drinking. The other exception to the Fourth Amendment is the automobile exception doctrine, which holds that an individual should have less expectation of privacy in a vehicle than in his or her residence. In both cases, the law enforcement officer must be justified in making the stop. Sobriety checkpoints, truck stops, and stops for traffic violations have been found to meet this requirement.

Opponents of PAS object to their use as intrusive, sneaky, and a violation of civil rights. The American Civil Liberties Union (ACLU) has questioned their use because they allow law enforcement to check for alcohol without the knowledge or consent of the person being tested. According to the ACLU, such searches are conducted without probable cause.

Proponents point out that X-ray machines and dogs are used in airports to detect guns, explosives, drugs, and other dangerous or contraband items, often without probable cause. Drunk driving is a public health problem, and we should use advances in technology to protect the public. What do you think?

Pros

- PAS devices help officers identify a higher proportion of drivers who have been drinking, potentially reducing the number of injuries and deaths resulting from alcohol-related car crashes every year.

- Officers in routine traffic stops have only a short amount of time to evaluate drivers. The drivers' use of breath mints, cologne, and gum may interfere with the officer's ability to sniff alcohol. Car exhaust fumes can also interfere with this process. PAS devices provide a way around these problems.

- Arrests are not made on the basis of PAS results—a follow-up breath test is used to measure BAC—and PAS results cannot be used as evidence in court.

Cons

- Even if the use of PAS does not compromise an individual's civil liberties, it is intrusive and assumes guilt.

- PAS devices measure alcohol in the air and do not necessarily pinpoint its source. The alcohol officers detect could be on the breath of passengers rather than on the breath of the driver.

- PAS devices detect alcohol at very low levels. Alcohol from mouthwash or liquid cold medications can cause a person to fail a PAS test.

- Environmental conditions—wind, dampness, and extreme temperatures—interfere with PAS readings, leading to errors.

- PAS devices are costly and have not yet proven to be cost effective for detecting drunk driving.

Sources: "Combating Hardcore Drunk Driving: A Source Book of Promising Strategies, Laws, and Programs: Enforcement," National Commission Against Drunk Driving, 1997, www.ncadd.com; "A Survey of Strategies for Reducing Alcohol-Impaired Driving and Underage Drinking," by K. Orlansky, S. Richards, and K. Baker-Hernandez, 2001, Office of Legislative Oversight, www.montgomerycountymd.gov; "Passive Alcohol Sensors and the Fourth Amendment—The Impaired Driving Update," Spring 2001, www.ndaa.org; "Using a Passive Alcohol Sensor to Detect Legally Intoxicated Drivers," National Commission Against Drunk Driving, 1993, American Journal of Public Health, 83 (4), pp. 551–560; Dying to Drink, by H. Wechsler and B. Wuethrich, 2002, New York: Rodale Books.

In Review

1. **Why do people drink, and why do some people develop problems with alcohol?** People ingest psychoactive substances like alcohol for a wide range of reasons, from wanting to enhance positive feelings to wanting to numb negative feelings. A complex interplay of individual and environmental factors leads some people who drink to develop problems with alcohol, including alcohol dependence.

2. **Why is binge drinking on college campuses a problem?** Binge drinking, defined as five or more drinks in a row for men and four or more drinks in a row for women, can have serious social, academic, and legal consequences. Binge drinkers are more likely to be alcohol dependent 10 years after college. Some experts believe the term *binge drinking* should be reserved for prolonged periods of intoxication of 2 days or more.

3. **What are the effects of alcohol on the body?** Alcohol is a central nervous system depressant, lowering inhibitions and depressing breathing and heart rates. In the brain, it causes changes in thinking, balance, and more coordination. People who drink heavily in a short period of time are at risk for alcohol poisoning.

4. **What are the health risks of alcohol consumption?** Over the long term, alcohol consumption can cause cardiovascular disease, liver disease, cancer, brain damage, and unhealthy changes in body weight and food absorption. Alcohol use is also associated with high-risk sexual activity, violence, injury, and suicide.

5. **What are alcohol abuse and alcohol dependence, and how are they treated?** Alcohol abuse is defined as the continued use of alcohol despite negative consequences. Alcohol dependence, or alcoholism, is the compulsive use of alcohol, usually accompanied by the development of tolerance and withdrawal symptoms when alcohol is not present in the body. Treatment options include brief interventions for young adults, inpatient and outpatient programs, and self-help programs like Alcoholics Anonymous. The harm reduction approach focuses on reducing the harm associated with drinking both to the drinker and to society.

6. **How can you know if you have a problem with alcohol?** You can use the CAGE questionnaire or other, more extensive assessments to get an idea of whether you are at risk for alcohol problems. If you have alcoholism in your family health history, you may want to take extra precautions.

WWW For detailed summary of this chapter and a comprehensive set of review questions, visit the Online Learning Center at **www.mhhe.com/teague2e**.

Web Resources

Alcoholics Anonymous (AA) World Services: This organization provides information on Alcoholics Anonymous, including the philosophy of its 12-step program. It features a preventive approach to alcohol abuse.
www.alcoholics-anonymous.org

BACCHUS and GAMMA Peer Education Network: Made up of college and university students, this organization promotes peer education programs designed to prevent alcohol abuse.
www.bacchusgamma.org

The College Alcohol Study, Harvard School of Public Health: To learn more about studies of binge drinking on college campuses, visit this site.
www.hsph.harvard.edu/cas

National Council on Alcoholism and Drug Dependence (NCADD): Besides offering counseling referrals, this council is a valuable resource for various types of information on alcoholism.
www.ncadd.org

National Institute on Alcohol Abuse and Alcoholism (NIAAA): Visit this organization's Web site for authoritative information on alcohol abuse and alcoholism. NIAAA is dedicated to public education on these topics and offers various helpful publications.
www.niaaa.nih.gov

Substance Abuse and Mental Health Services Administration: The U.S. Department of Health and Human Services sponsors this site, which features a wide range of resources on substance abuse and closely related issues, such as mental health, homelessness, and AIDS/HIV.
www.samhsa.gov

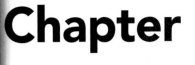

Chapter 12

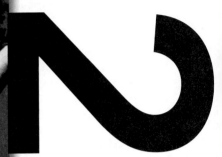

Drugs Use, Abuse, and Control

Ever Wonder...

- how addictive drugs change the brain?

- why some people can't seem to stop using drugs?

- how to know if someone is starting to have a problem with drugs?

WWW

Your Health Today

www.mhhe.com/teague2e

Go to the Online Learning Center for *Your Health Today* for interactive activities, quizzes, flashcards, Web links, and more resources related to this chapter.

Like alcohol, drugs have a pervasive presence in American life. We use them for headaches, insomnia, anxiety, stress—and some of us use them for fun. In 2006 an estimated 20.4 million Americans aged 12 or older were current users of illicit (illegal) drugs, representing 8.3 percent of the population (Table 12.1).[1] Although these numbers seem large, it's worth noting the other side of the picture, namely, that 91.7 percent of the population age 12 or over—more than 200 million people—do not use illicit drugs.

Drugs are used by different people for different reasons. Many people take drugs as a recreational activity—to alter their state of consciousness, to relax and feel more sociable, to experience euphoria, to get high. Some people take drugs to rebel—to experiment, take risks, seek new and exciting sensations. Others take drugs to conform—to fit in with a peer group or to avoid having to say no. For some people, drug use is a way to cope with stress, pain, or adversity, whether the adversity comes in the form of an unexpected life event, such as loss of a job, or in the form of oppressive social conditions experienced daily, such as poverty and discrimination. And for some people, drug use is a way of life, a behavior they can no longer control.

Who Uses? Patterns of Illicit Drug Use

Rates of illicit drug use vary by age, gender, race and ethnicity, education, employment status, and geographical region (see the box "Rates of Illicit Drug Use"). Among Americans aged 12 or older, more than 45 percent report having used an illicit drug in their lifetime (see Table 12.1). The most commonly used drug is marijuana, with nearly 15 million current users among Americans aged 12 or older.[1] An estimated 7 million Americans use prescription-type drugs nonmedically, including pain relievers, tranquilizers, stimulants, and sedatives (Figure 12.1).[1]

Among young adults aged 18–25, the most commonly used drugs are marijuana, prescription-type drugs, cocaine, and hallucinogens. The use of marijuana declined from 2002 to 2006, but nonmedical use of prescription-type drugs increased. According to a 2007 survey, the percentage of college students who abuse prescription drugs increased dramatically over the 12-year period from 1993 to 2005:[2]

Table 12.1	Illicit Drug Use in Lifetime, Past Year and Past Month Among Persons Aged 12 or Older: Percentages, 2006		
	Time Period		
Drug	**Lifetime**	**Past Year**	**Past Month (Current)**
Any illicit drug	45.4	14.5	8.3
Marijuana and hashish	39.8	10.3	6.0
Cocaine	14.3	2.5	1.0
Crack	3.5	0.6	0.3
Heroin	1.5	0.2	0.1
Hallucinogens	14.3	1.6	0.4
LSD	9.5	0.3	0.1
PCP	2.7	0.1	0.0
Ecstasy	5.0	0.9	0.2
Inhalants	9.3	0.9	0.3
Nonmedical use of any prescription drug	20.3	6.6	2.8
Pain relievers	13.6	5.1	2.1
OxyContin	1.7	0.5	0.1
Tranquilizers	8.7	2.1	0.7
Stimulants	8.2	1.4	0.5
Sedatives	3.6	0.4	0.2

Source: Results from the 2006 National Survey on Drug Use and Health: National Findings, Substance Abuse and Mental Health Services Administration, 2007, Rockville, MD: Office of Applied Studies.

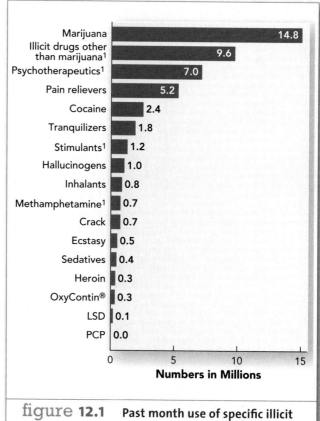

figure 12.1 **Past month use of specific illicit drugs among persons aged 12 or older: 2006**
Source: Results from the 2006 National Survey on Drug Use and Health: National Findings, Substance Abuse and Mental Health Services Administration, 2007, Rockville, MD: Office of Applied Studies.

Who's at Risk

Rates of Illicit Drug Use

- **Age.** The highest rates of illicit drug use occur among young adults aged 18–20 (Figure 12.2), with these rates remaining stable from 2002 to 2006. Among teenagers, rates decreased during this period, from 11.6 to 9.8 percent. Among those aged 50–54, rates of illicit drug use nearly doubled between 2002 and 2006, from 3.4 percent to 6.0 percent, perhaps reflecting the aging of the baby boomers, whose lifetime use of illicit drugs is higher than that of older cohorts.

- **Gender.** Males are more likely to use drugs than females, at rates of 10.5 percent versus 6.2 percent among persons aged 12 or older. The rate of marijuana use is about twice as high among males as females (8.1 percent versus 4.1 percent), but rates are similar for stimulants, Ecstasy, sedatives, OxyContin, LSD, and PCP. Rates for all of these drugs are less than 1 percent.

- **Race/ethnicity.** Rates are highest among American Indian/Alaskan Natives (13.7 percent) and lowest among Asian Americans (3.6 percent), with rates for Blacks (9.8 percent), persons reporting two or more races (8.9 percent), Whites (8.5 percent), Native Hawaiians or Other Pacific Islanders (7.5 percent), and Hispanics (6.9 percent) falling in between.

- **Education.** Rates are lower among college graduates than among those with some college education, high school graduates, and those who did not graduate from high school. However, adults who had graduated from college were more likely than adults who had not completed high school to have tried illicit drugs in their lifetime.

- **Employment.** Rates are higher for adults who are unemployed than for those who are employed either full-time or part-time. However, 75 percent of drug users are employed. Of the 17.9 million adults aged 18 or older who used illicit drugs in 2006, 13.4 million were employed.

- **Geographical Region.** Among persons aged 12 or older, rates are highest in the West (9.5 percent) compared with the Northeast (8.9 percent,) the Midwest (7.9 percent), and the South (7.4 percent). For methamphetamine use, however, rates are higher in the West and the South than in the Northeast or Midwest.

Source: Results from the 2006 National Survey on Drug Use and Health: National Findings, Substance Abuse and Mental Health Services Administration, 2007, Rockville, MD: Office of Applied Studies.

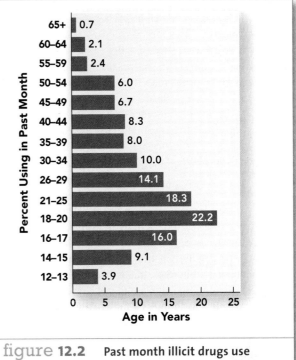

figure **12.2**   **Past month illicit drugs use among persons aged 12 or older: 2006**
Source: Results from the 2006 National Survey on Drug Use and Health: National Findings, Substance Abuse and Mental Health Services Administration, 2007, Rockville, MD: Office of Applied Studies.

- Pain relievers (for example, OxyContin, Vicodin, Percocet): Use increased by 343 percent

- Stimulants (for example, Ritalin, Adderall): Use increased by 93 percent

- Tranquilizers (for example, Xanax, Valium): Use increased by 450 percent

- Sedatives (for example, Nembutal, Seconal): Use increased by 225 percent

Nonmedical use of prescription-type drugs is also the most common form of drug use among young teens aged 12–13.[1] More than half of those who used prescription drugs nonmedically report that they obtained the drug from a friend or relative for free.[1]

What Is a Drug?

A **drug** is a substance other than food that affects the structure or the function of the body through its chemical action. Alcohol, caffeine, aspirin, and nicotine are all drugs, as are amphetamines, cocaine, hallucinogens, sedatives, and inhalants. The drugs discussed here are *psychoactive drugs*—substances that cause changes in brain

drug
Substance other than food that affects the structure or function of the body through its chemical action.

chemistry and alter consciousness, perception, mood, and thought. This state is known as *intoxication.*

Psychoactive drugs are used for both medical and non-medical (recreational) purposes. For example, Ritalin, a central nervous system (CNS) stimulant with effects similar to amphetamine, is prescribed to treat hyperactivity in children—a medical use. Cocaine, another CNS stimulant, is used recreationally to cause a burst of pleasurable sensations and to increase energy and endurance—a nonmedical use. When a medical drug is used for nonmedical (recreational) purposes, or when a drug has no medical uses, it is referred to as a **drug of abuse.**

drug of abuse
Medical drug used for nonmedical (recreational) purposes or a drug that has no medical uses.

All drugs have the potential to be toxic, that is, poisonous, dangerous, or deadly. Central nervous system depressants, such as alcohol, barbiturates, tranquilizers, and opium-derived drugs such as morphine and heroin can cause death if used in sufficient amounts to suppress vital functions like respiration. At the other extreme, CNS stimulants such as cocaine can cause sudden death by speeding up heart rate, elevating blood pressure, and accelerating other body functions to the point that systems are overwhelmed and collapse. The American Psychiatric Association (APA) uses the term **substance** to refer to a drug of abuse, a medication, or a toxin.[3] In this chapter we use the terms *drug* and *substance* interchangeably.

substance
Drug of abuse, a medication, or a toxin; the term is used interchangeably with *drug.*

TYPES OF DRUGS

Drugs are classified in several different ways. A basic distinction is often made between legal drugs and illicit (illegal) drugs. *Legal drugs* include medications prescribed by physicians, over-the-counter (OTC) medications, and herbal remedies. Drugs developed for medical purposes, whether OTC or prescription, are referred to as **pharmaceutical drugs.**

pharmaceutical drugs
Drugs developed for medical purposes, whether over-the-counter or prescription.

OTC medications can be purchased easily by consumers without a prescription. They include common remedies for headache, pain, colds, coughs, allergies, stomach upset, and other mild symptoms and complaints. Herbal

---

Consumer Clipboard

Taking a Smart Approach to Self-Medication

More than 700 products sold over the counter today include ingredients or dosage strengths that were available only by prescription just 30 years ago. With this wide range of products to choose from, self-medication has become common. Helpful as these products may be, they need to be approached with caution and common sense. When choosing to use over-the-counter drugs, keep these points in mind:

■ Read the label each time you purchase an OTC medication. The format for OTC drug labels is set by the FDA and includes ingredients, uses, warnings, directions, and additional information, including a phone number to call for questions or comments.

■ Do not exceed the recommended dose or take the medication for a longer period of time than recommended. If your condition does not improve, you need to see a physician.

■ Be alert for possible interactions with other drugs you may be taking. Here are a few cautions:

– Avoid alcohol if you're taking antihistamines, cough or cold products that contain dextromethorphan, or drugs used to treat sleeplessness.

– Don't use drugs for sleeplessness if you're taking prescription sedatives or tranquilizers.

– If you're taking a prescription blood thinner, or if you have diabetes or gout, check with your physician before taking any product that contains aspirin.

– Unless your physician has instructed you to do so, don't use a nasal decongestant if you're taking a prescription drug for high blood pressure or depression, or if you have thyroid disease, diabetes, or prostate problems.

■ Dietary supplements are not regulated by the FDA, so the ingredient amounts listed on the label are not always accurate. In addition, the manufacturer's claims about the safety and effectiveness of their products are not always backed up by solid research.

■ If possible, select a medication with a single ingredient targeted at your symptoms rather than a combination of ingredients. You may not have all the symptoms treated by the multiple ingredients and may expose yourself to side effects unnecessarily.

■ Choose a generic product over a brand-name product to save money. The active ingredients are the same.

■ If the product has an expiration date, it refers to how long the drug will be active in an unopened package. Once the package is opened, the drug will probably be good for about a year.

Source: Data from "Over-the-Counter Medicines: What's Right for You?" 2005, U.S. Food and Drug Administration, www.fda.gov.

remedies are usually botanical in origin; there are more than 700 substances in this group. At this time, the federal government's Food and Drug Administration (FDA) does not regulate herbal remedies before they are brought to market the way it regulates the development and approval of pharmaceutical drugs. The FDA does have the power to remove an herbal remedy from the market if it has proven harmful. This was the case with the dietary supplement ephedra, a stimulant used for weight loss and body building, which the FDA banned after it was linked with more than 100 deaths from heart attack and stroke (see the box "Taking a Smart Approach to Self-Medication").

Prescription drugs can be ordered only by a licensed medical doctor (MD). They must undergo a rigorous testing and approval process by the FDA. Today the pharmaceutical industry is one of the largest and most profitable industries in the United States, with sales well over $100 billion a year. Despite these astronomical sales, however, more than half of all prescriptions are filled with only 200 drugs.

Illicit drugs are generally viewed as harmful, and it is illegal to possess, manufacture, sell, or use them. Many drugs that are available by prescription are legal when obtained through a physician but illicit when manufactured or sold outside of the regulated medical system. Tobacco and alcohol are illegal drugs in the hands of minors, but they are usually not considered illicit because of their widespread availability to adults.

illicit drugs
Drugs that are unlawful to possess, manufacture, sell, or use.

In an effort to reduce the use of illegal drugs and the nonmedical use of certain prescription drugs, Congress passed the Comprehensive Drug Abuse Prevention and Control Act, usually referred to as the Controlled Substance Act, in 1970. This act categorized drugs into five groups according to their addictive quality and medical uses. Table 12.2 summarizes the controlled substance schedules and gives examples for each group.

DRUG MISUSE AND ABUSE

The term **drug misuse** generally refers to the use of prescription drugs for purposes other than those for which they were prescribed or in greater amounts than prescribed. The term can also refer to the use of nonprescription drugs or chemicals such as glues, paints, or solvents for any purpose other than that intended by the manufacturer.

The term **drug abuse** generally means the use of a substance in amounts, situations, or a manner such that it causes problems, or greatly increases the risk of problems, for the user or for others. The APA's *Diagnostic and Statistical Manual of Mental Disorders* (*DSM-IV-TR*) defines *substance abuse* as a maladaptive pattern of use leading to impairment or distress that continues despite serious negative consequences, such as losing a job or getting in fights.

drug misuse
Use of prescription drugs for purposes other than those for which they were prescribed or in greater amounts than prescribed, or the use of nonprescription drugs or chemicals for purposes other than those intended by the manufacturer.

drug abuse
Use of a substance in amounts, situations, or a manner such that it causes problems, or greatly increases the risk of problems, for the user or for others.

Table 12.2	Summary of Controlled Substance Schedules	
Schedule	**Criteria**	**Examples**
Schedule I	a. High potential for abuse b. No currently acceptable medical use in treatment in the United States c. Lack of accepted safety for use under medical supervision	Heroin Marijuana LSD
Schedule II	a. High potential for abuse b. Currently accepted medical use c. Abuse may lead to severe psychological or physical dependence	Morphine Cocaine Methamphetamines
Schedule III	a. Potential for abuse less than I and II b. Currently accepted medical use c. Abuse may lead to moderate physical dependence or high psychological dependence	Anabolic steroids Most barbiturates Dronabinol
Schedule IV	a. Low potential for abuse relative to III b. Currently accepted medical use c. Abuse may lead to limited physical or psychological dependence relative to III	Alprazolam (Xanax) Barbital Chloral hydrate Fenfluramine
Schedule V	a. Low potential for abuse relative to IV b. Currently accepted medical use c. Abuse may lead to limited physical or psychological dependence	Mixtures having small amounts of codeine or opium relative to IV

Source: Drugs, Society, and Human Behavior (13th ed.), by C.L. Hart, C. Ksir, and O. Ray, 2009, New York: The McGraw-Hill Companies.

Drug abuse is not the same as drug dependence; a person can abuse a drug—for example, by binge drinking—without being dependent on it. We discuss drug dependence later in the chapter.

Effects of Drugs on the Body

All psychoactive drugs have an effect on the brain, and they reach the brain by way of the bloodstream. Like alcohol, some psychoactive drugs are consumed by mouth, but other routes of administration are used as well.

ROUTES OF ADMINISTRATION

Psychoactive drugs can be taken by several methods: orally (by mouth), injection, inhalation, application to the skin, or application to the mucous membranes. The speed and efficiency with which the drug acts are strongly influenced by the route of administration (Figure 12.3; Table 12.3).

Oral   Most drugs are taken orally. Although this is the simplest way for a person to take a drug, it is the most complicated way for the drug to enter the bloodstream. A drug

in the digestive tract must be able to withstand the actions of stomach acid and digestive enzymes and not be deactivated by food before it is absorbed. Drugs taken orally are absorbed into the bloodstream in the small intestine.

Injection   The injection route involves using a hypodermic syringe to deliver the drug directly into the bloodstream (intravenous injection), to deposit it in a muscle mass (intramuscular injection), or to deposit it under the upper layer of skin (subcutaneous injection). With an intravenous (IV) injection ("mainlining"), the drug enters the bloodstream directly; onset of action is more rapid than with oral administration or other means of injection.

Inhalation   The inhalation route is used for smoking tobacco, marijuana, and crack cocaine and for "huffing" gasoline, paints, and other inhalants. An inhaled drug enters the bloodstream quickly because capillary walls are very accessible in the lungs.

Application to Mucous Membranes   Application of a drug to the mucous membranes results in rapid absorption, because the mucous membranes are moist and have a rich blood supply. People who snort cocaine absorb the

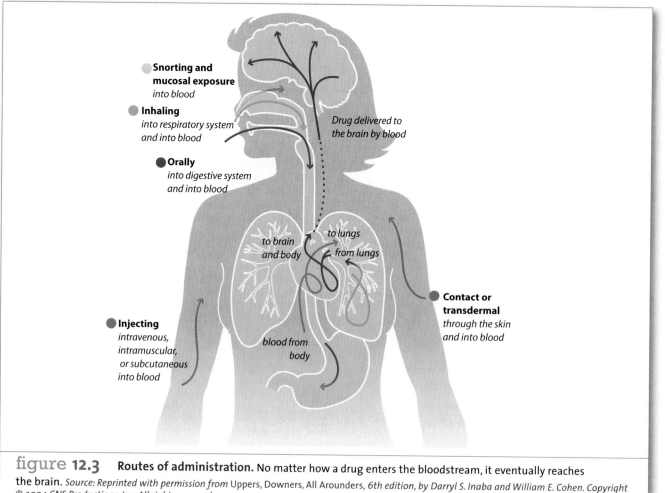

figure 12.3   **Routes of administration.** No matter how a drug enters the bloodstream, it eventually reaches the brain. *Source: Reprinted with permission from Uppers, Downers, All Arounders, 6th edition, by Darryl S. Inaba and William E. Cohen. Copyright © 2004 CNS Productions, Inc. All rights reserved.*

Table 12.3 | Routes of Administration

Route	Time to Reach Brain	Drug Example	Potential Adverse Effects

Inhalation
  Smoking
  Huffing
	7–10 seconds	Marijuana
		Crack cocaine
		Tobacco
		Inhalants
			Irritation of lungs

Injection
  Intravenous
  Intramuscular
  Subcutaneous
	
	15–30 seconds
	3–5 minutes
	5–7 minutes
		Heroin
		Cocaine
		Methamphetamine
			Danger of overdose
			Collapsed veins
			Infection at injection site
			Blood infection
			Transmission of HIV, hepatitis C, and other pathogens

Mucous membranes Snorting	3–15 minutes	Cocaine Methamphetamine Heroin	Irritation or destruction of tissue Difficulty controlling dose
Oral ingestion Eating, drinking	20–30 minutes	Alcohol Pills	Vomiting

Skin contact
  Dermal
  Transdermal
	1–7 days	Oils, ointments
		Nicotine patch
			Irritation of skin

drug quickly into the bloodstream through the mucous membranes of the nose. People who chew tobacco absorb nicotine through the mucous membranes lining the mouth. Rectal and vaginal suppositories are also absorbed quickly, although these methods are less commonly used.

Application to the Skin Application to the skin is a less common method of drug administration. Most drugs are not well absorbed through the skin. *Dermal absorption* occurs when an oil or ointment is rubbed on the skin, producing a topical, or local, effect. *Transdermal absorption* occurs when a longer lasting application produces a systemic effect, such as when a patch delivers estrogen or nicotine. The advantage of the transdermal route is that it affords slow, steady absorption over many hours, producing stable levels of the drug in the blood.

FACTORS INFLUENCING THE EFFECTS OF DRUGS

The effect a drug has on a person depends on a number of variables, including the characteristics of the drug, the characteristics of the person, and the characteristics of the situation.

The first of these categories includes the chemical properties of the drug and its actions. Depending on the drug's chemical composition, it may speed up body processes or slow them down, produce a mild high or acute anxiety, or cause disorientation or hallucinations. These effects also depend on how much of the drug is taken, how often it is taken, and how recently it was taken.

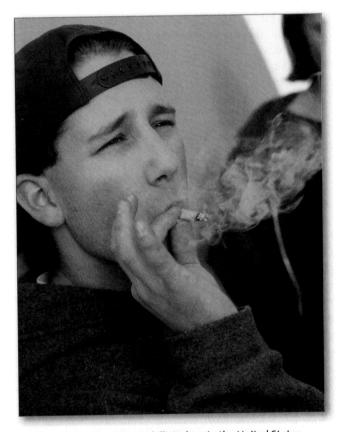

■ The most commonly used illicit drug in the United States is marijuana. Nearly 15 million Americans are current users.

Characteristics of the person include age, gender, body weight and mass, physical condition, mood, experience with the drug, and expectations. Generally speaking, the same amount of a drug has less effect on a 180-pound man than on a 120-pound woman. If a person has taken other drugs, the interactions of the chemicals can influence outcomes, as when one CNS depressant intensifies the effect of another.

The effects of drugs are also influenced by the characteristics of the situation or the environment. Taking a drug at home while relaxing with a group of friends may produce a different experience than will taking the same drug at a crowded, noisy bar or club, surrounded by strangers.

DRUG DEPENDENCE

As we saw in the case of alcohol, continued use of a drug can lead to *dependence* (or *addiction*), a condition characterized by a strong craving for a drug and by compulsive use of the drug despite serious negative consequences. Dependence usually means that physiological changes have taken place in brain and body chemistry as a result of using the drug. As described in Chapter 3, the main two indicators of physiological dependence are the development of *tolerance,* reduced sensitivity to the effects of the drug, and *withdrawal,* the experience of uncomfortable feelings when drug use stops.

Withdrawal symptoms are different for different drugs. For example, withdrawal from amphetamines is marked by intense feelings of fatigue and depression, increased appetite and weight gain, and sometimes suicidal thinking. Withdrawal from heroin causes nausea, vomiting, sweating, diarrhea, yawning, and insomnia. To assess whether you are at risk for developing dependence on a drug, see the Add It Up feature for Chapter 12 at the end of the book.

EFFECTS OF DRUGS ON THE BRAIN

What accounts for the phenomenon of drug dependence? Scientists studying the effects of drugs on the brain have found that many addictive drugs, including cocaine, marijuana, opioids, alcohol, and nicotine, act on neurons in three brain structures—the ventral tegmental area (VTA) in the midbrain, the nucleus accumbens, and the prefrontal cortex.[4] Neurons in these three structures form a pathway referred to as the **pleasure and reward circuit** (Figure 12.4).

pleasure and reward circuit
Pathway in the brain involving three structures—the ventral tegmental area, the nucleus accumbens, and the prefrontal cortex—associated with drug dependence.

Under normal circumstances, this network of neurons is responsible for the feelings of satisfaction and pleasure when a physical, emotional, or survival need is met (for example, hunger, thirst, bonding, sexual desire). When it is activated, the circuit powerfully reinforces the behavior that satisfied the need (for example, eating), sending the message to "do it again." Neurons in the VTA increase production of dopamine, a neurotransmitter associated with feelings of pleasure. The VTA neurons pass messages to clusters of neurons in the nucleus accumbens, where the release of dopamine produces intense pleasure, and to the prefrontal cortex, where thinking, motivation, and behavior are affected.

Addictive psychoactive drugs activate this same pathway, causing an enormous surge in levels of dopamine and the associated feelings of pleasure. The nucleus accumbens sends the message to repeat the behavior that produced these feelings, and using the drug begins to take on as much importance as normal survival behaviors. Because the drug produces such huge surges of dopamine, the brain responds by reducing normal dopamine production. Eventually the person is unable to experience any pleasure, even from the drug, due to the disrupted dopamine system. Parts of the brain involved in rational thought and judgment are also disrupted, leading to loss of control and powerlessness over drug use. The very parts of the brain needed to make good life decisions are "hijacked" by addiction. Nonaddictive drugs do not cause these changes.

All or nearly all addictive drugs, whether "uppers" or "downers," operate via the pleasure and reward circuit, but some also operate via additional mechanisms. An example is the opioids (opium and its derivatives, morphine, codeine, and heroin). The brain has neurons with receptors for **endorphins,** its own "natural opiates"—brain chemicals that block pain when the body undergoes stress, such as during extreme exercise or childbirth. The structure of drugs in the opium family is similar to the structure of endorphins, so opioids readily bind to endorphin receptors, reducing pain

endorphins
Natural chemicals in the brain that block pain during stressful or painful experiences.

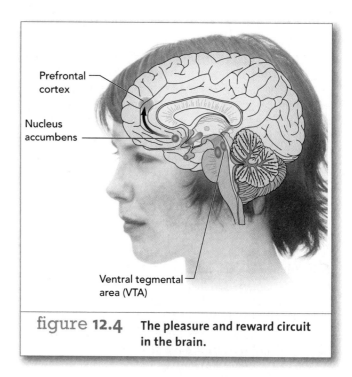

Prefrontal cortex

Nucleus accumbens

Ventral tegmental area (VTA)

figure **12.4**   **The pleasure and reward circuit in the brain.**

and increasing pleasure. These effects occur in addition to the dopamine-related changes in the pleasure and reward circuit.

Individuals trying to recover from addiction are disadvantaged by their altered brain chemistry, drug-related memories, and impaired impulse control. Recovery is not simply a matter of will power, nor does it involve abstinence from substances alone. Rather, multiple areas of the person's life have to be addressed—emotional, psychological, social, occupational, and so on. As a chronic, recurring disease, addiction typically involves repeated relapses and treatments before the person achieves recovery and return to a healthy life.

Drugs of Abuse

Drugs of abuse are usually classified as stimulants, depressants, opioids, hallucinogens, inhalants, and cannabinoids (Figure 12.5). For an overview of commonly abused drugs, their trade and street names, their intoxication effects, and their potential health consequences, see Table 12.4.

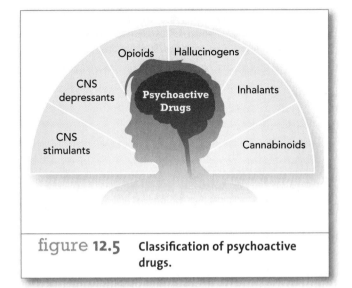

figure 12.5   **Classification of psychoactive drugs.**

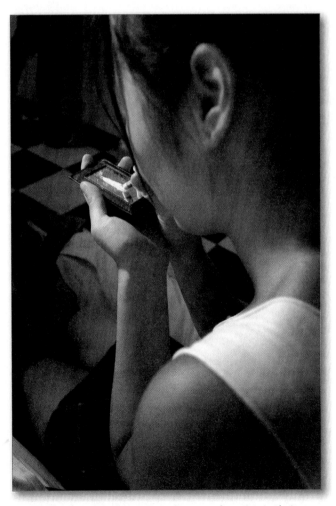

■ About 14 percent of Americans have used cocaine in their lifetime, but only 1 percent are current users.

CENTRAL NERVOUS SYSTEM STIMULANTS

Drugs that speed up activity in the brain and sympathetic nervous system are known as **stimulants.** Their effects are similar to the response evoked during the fight-or-flight reaction (see Chapter 5). Heart rate accelerates, breathing deepens, muscle tension increases, the senses are heightened, and attention and alertness increase. These drugs can keep people going, mentally and physically, when they would otherwise be fatigued. The drugs may stimulate movement, fidgeting, and talking, and they may produce intense feelings of euphoria and create a sense of energy and well-being (see the box "Signs of Drug Use: CNS Stimulants on p. 243").

stimulants
Drugs that speed up activity in the brain and the sympathetic nervous system.

Cocaine   A powerful CNS stimulant, cocaine heightens alertness, inhibits appetite and the need for sleep, and provides intense feelings of pleasure. Pure cocaine was first extracted from the leaves of the coca plant in the mid-19th century; it was introduced as a remedy for a number of ailments and used medically as an anesthetic.[5] Cocaine has high potential for abuse.

The most common form of pure cocaine is cocaine hydrochloride powder, made from coca paste. It can be snorted or mixed with water and injected intravenously. Snorting produces a relatively quick effect that lasts from 15 to 30 minutes; IV injection produces a rapid, powerful, and brief effect.

Two other methods of use are freebasing and smoking crack cocaine. Freebasing involves heating cocaine hydrochloride with a volatile solvent such as ether or ammonia and smoking it. This practice is dangerous because the solvent can ignite and burn the user. Crack is a form of cocaine that appeared in the mid-1980s and led to an epidemic of cocaine use in the United States. When crack is smoked in a pipe, its effects are extremely rapid and intense. This method

Table 12.4 | Commonly Abused Drugs

Category & Name	Trade Names/Street Names	Intoxication Effects	Potential Health Consequences
CNS Stimulants		**Increased heart rate, blood pressure; metabolism; feelings of exhilaration, increased mental alertness**	**Rapid or irregular heart rate, reduced appetite, weight loss, heart failure**
Cocaine	*Cocaine hydrochloride/*Coke, blow, crack, snow, toot, rock, bump, C, candy, Charlie, flake	Also: Increased body temperature	Also: Chest pain, respiratory failure, strokes, seizures, headaches, malnutrition
Amphetamine	*Biphetamine, Dexedrine/*Bennies, uppers, black beauties, speed, crosses, hearts, truck drivers	Also: Rapid breathing, hallucinations	Also: Tremor, irritability, anxiety, impulsivity, aggressiveness, restlessness, panic, paranoia
Methamphetamine	Desoxyn/Meth, speed, crank, crystal, chalk, glass, ice	Also: Aggression, violence, psychotic behavior	Also: Memory loss, cardiac and neurological damage
MDMA	Ecstasy, X, XTC, Adam, Eve, clarity, peace, STP	Mild hallucinogenic effects, increased tactile sensitivity, empathic feelings	Impaired memory and learning, hyperthermia, renal failure
CNS Depressants		**Reduced pain and anxiety, feeling of well-being, lowered inhibitions, slowed pulse and breathing, lowered blood pressure**	**Fatigue; confusion; impaired memory, judgment, coordination; respiratory depression and arrest**
Barbiturates (sedatives)	*Amytal, Nembutal, Seconal, Phenobarbital/*Barbs, reds, red birds, yellows, yellow jackets	Also: Sedation, drowsiness	Also: Depression, fever, irritability, poor judgment, dizziness, slurred speech
Benzodiazepines (tranquilizers)	*Ativan, Librium, Valium, Xanax/* Candy, downers, sleeping pills, tranks	Also: Sedation, drowsiness	Also: Dizziness
Flunitrazepam	*Rohypnal/*Roofies, R2, forget-me pill, Mexican Valium, rope, rophies		Memory loss for time under the drug's effects, visual and gastrointestinal disturbances, urine retention
GHB	*Gamma-hydroxybutyrate/*G, Georgia home boy, grievous bodily harm, liquid ecstasy		Drowsiness, nausea, vomiting, headache, loss of consciousness, loss of reflexes, seizures, coma, death
Opioids (Narcotics)		**Pain relief, euphoria, drowsiness**	**Nausea, constipation, confusion, sedation, respiratory depression and arrest, unconsciousness, coma, death**
Morphine	*Roxanol, Duramorph/*M, Miss Emma, monkey, white stuff		
Heroin	*Diacetyl-morphine/*H, junk, smack, brown sugar, skag, skunk, white horse	Also: Staggering gait	
Synthetic opioids	*OxyContin, Vicodin, Percodan, Percocet, Demerol, Darvan/* Oxy 80s, oxycotton, oxycet, hillbilly heroin, percs, demmies		
Hallucinogens		**Altered states of perception and feeling, nausea**	**Persisting perception disorder (flashbacks)**
LSD	*Lysergic acid diethylamide/*Acid, blotter, boomers, microdot, yellow sunshines	Also: Increased body temperature, heart rate, blood pressure; loss of appetite; sleeplessnesss; tremors	Also: Persisting mental disorders
PCP	*Phencyclidine/*Angel dust, boat, love boat, hog, peace pill	Also: Increased heart rate and blood pressure; impaired motor function; panic, aggression, violence	Also: Memory loss, numbness, nausea, vomiting, loss of appetite, depression
Inhalants	*Solvents, gases, nitrites/*Laughing gas, poppers, snappers	Stimulation; loss of inhibition, headache, nausea, vomiting, slurred speech, loss of motor coordination	Unconsciousness, cramps, weight loss, muscle weakness, depression, memory impairment, damage to cardiovascular and nervous systems, sudden death
Cannabinoids		Euphoria, slowed thinking and reaction time, confusion, impaired balance and coordination	Cough, frequent respiratory infections, impaired memory and learning, increased heart rate, anxiety, panic attacks
Marijuana	Pot, grass, weed, dope, ganja, Mary Jane, reefer, sensamilla, herb		Also: Chronic bronchitis
Hashish	Hash, hemp, boom, gangster		

Source: "Commonly Abused Drugs," National Institute on Drug Abuse, retrieved May 17, 2008, from www.nida.nih.gov/DrugPages/DrugsofAbuse.html.

of use also produces the highest rate of dependence. Cocaine mixed with heroin produces a drug called a "speedball."

Cocaine is still used as a local anesthetic, often for surgeries in the areas of the nose and throat. Most uses, however, are recreational. Like other CNS stimulants, cocaine causes acceleration of the heart rate, elevation of blood pressure, dilation of the pupils, and an increase in alertness, muscle tension, and motor activity. It produces feelings of euphoria, often accompanied by talkativeness, sociability, and a sense of grandiosity. These effects appear almost immediately after a single dose and usually last for 15 minutes to an hour. When the effects wear off, the user typically wants to repeat the experience. Dependence can occur after only a few uses. Withdrawal after prolonged use is characterized by a depressed mood, fatigue, sleep disturbances, unpleasant dreams, and increased appetite.

At higher doses, cocaine use can lead to cardiac arrhythmias, respiratory distress, bizarre or violent behavior, psychosis, convulsions, seizures, coma, and even death. Regular snorting can irritate the nasal passage and result in a chronic runny nose. Some users may become malnourished because the drug suppresses appetite.

Amphetamines For centuries practitioners of Chinese medicine have made a medicinal tea from herbs called Ma-huang. In the 1920s a chemist working for the Eli Lilly Company identified the active ingredient in Ma-huang as the compound ephedrine. The actions of this compound include opening the nasal and bronchial passages, allowing people to breathe more easily. The drug quickly became an important treatment for asthma, allergies, and stuffy noses. Researchers worked to develop synthetic forms of this botanical product, and a few years later, amphetamine was synthesized. Nasal amphetamine inhalers quickly grew in popularity; consumers found that they not only cleared the bronchioles but also produced elation.

In the 1930s amphetamines were put to additional uses: helping patients with narcolepsy stay awake, suppressing appetite in people who wanted to lose weight, and treating depression. In the 1940s soldiers fighting in World War II took amphetamines to stay alert and combat drowsiness. By the 1960s amphetamines were so widely available that they were quickly swept up into the drug culture of that period.

Amphetamines are no longer recommended for depression or weight control. Particularly in the case of depression, a host of newer, more effective drugs is available. Amphetamines are still used to treat *attention deficit/hyperactivity disorder (ADHD)* in children and adults. Although they are stimulants, they have a paradoxical effect in individuals with ADHD, helping them gain control of their behavior. More than 1 million children in the United States now take Ritalin and other amphetamines to control hyperactivity.

Concerns about the use of amphetamines involve their effects on the heart, lungs, and many other organs. At low levels they may cause loss of appetite, rapid breathing, high blood pressure, and dilated pupils. Decision making can be impaired even at moderate dosage levels. At higher levels, amphetamines can cause paranoia, panic, fever, sweating,

Highlight on Health

Signs of Drug Use: CNS Stimulants

Cocaine

- Excessive activity, excess energy, talkativeness, pressured speech, lack of focus
- Irritability, argumentativeness
- Lack of interest in food or sleep
- Runny nose, chronic sinus or nasal problems
- Dilated pupils
- Dry mouth

Methamphetamine

- Excessive activity, excess energy, talkativeness
- Irritability, argumentativeness
- Lack of interest in food or sleep
- Overconfidence, grandiosity, paranoia
- Decayed teeth ("meth mouth")
- Acne, oily skin

MDMA (Ecstasy)

- Clenched teeth and jaw (use of pacifiers), twitching eyelids
- Dilated pupils
- Reduced inhibitions, excess energy
- High body temperature, sweating, chills

headaches, blurred vision, dizziness, and sometimes aggressiveness and violence. Very high doses may cause flushing, rapid or irregular heartbeat, tremors, and even collapse. Deaths due to heart failure and burst blood vessels in the brain have also been reported. Withdrawal symptoms after continued amphetamine use include a drop in energy, feelings of helplessness, and thoughts of suicide. The person may "crash" into depression or sleep for 24 hours. Some symptoms can continue for days or weeks.

Methamphetamine ("speed") has a chemical structure similar to that of amphetamine and produces similar but more intense effects. It is usually snorted. A very pure form of methamphetamine, called "ice" or "crystal meth," can be smoked, producing an intense rush of pleasure lasting a few minutes.

Methamphetamine is more addictive and dangerous than most other forms of amphetamine because it contains so many toxic chemicals. Small doses can have powerful effects for hours, including heightened concentration, increased alertness, high energy, wakefulness, and loss of appetite. Aside from addiction and brain damage, health effects of

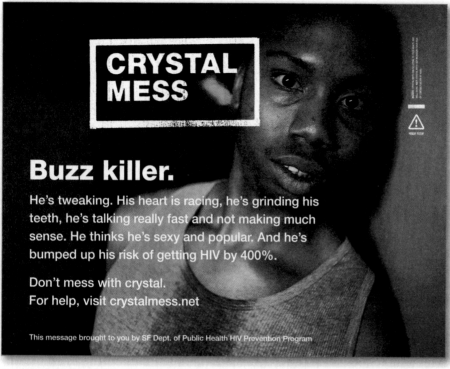

CRYSTAL MESS

Buzz killer.

He's tweaking. His heart is racing, he's grinding his teeth, he's talking really fast and not making much sense. He thinks he's sexy and popular. And he's bumped up his risk of getting HIV by 400%.

Don't mess with crystal.
For help, visit crystalmess.net

This message brought to you by SF Dept. of Public Health HIV Prevention Program

■ In 2004, the San Francisco Department of Public Health's HIV Prevention Program launched its confrontational "crystal mess" campaign, with ads posted in subways stations and bus shelters and on outdoor billboards. The campaign was aimed particularly at the city's gay population, which had experienced a dramatic increase in rates of HIV infection in the previous few years.

meth use include severe weight loss, cardiovascular damage, increased risk of heart attack and stroke, extensive tooth decay and tooth loss ("meth mouth"), and oily skin and acne. Users are also at risk for paranoia and violent behavior.

Rates of meth use have soared in the past decade, in part due to its easy manufacture in makeshift labs from relatively inexpensive and commonly available drugs and chemicals.[6] One such drug is pseudoephedrine, a nasal decongestant used in some cold and allergy medications. In 2005 Congress passed the Combat Methamphetamine Epidemic Act requiring that over-the-counter drugs like pseudoephedrine be sold from behind the counter and subjected to additional regulations. Some law enforcement agencies consider meth the number-one drug problem in the United States.

MDMA Also known as Ecstasy, MDMA has chemical similarities to both stimulants (such as methamphetamine) and hallucinogens (such as mescaline).[7] Thus it produces both types of effects. MDMA appears to elevate levels of the neurotransmitter serotonin, the body's primary regulator of mood, perhaps in a manner similar to the action of antidepressants. Users experience increased energy, feelings of euphoria, and a heightened sense of empathy with and closeness to those around them. Some users report enhanced hearing, vision, and sense of touch, but only a few report actual visual hallucinations.

In addition to the drug's euphoric effects, MDMA can cause increased heart rate, elevated body temperature (sometimes to dangerous levels), profuse sweating, dry mouth, muscle tension, blurred vision, and involuntary teeth clench-

ing. Serious risks include dehydration, hypertension, and heart or kidney failure. MDMA use can lead to psychological problems, such as depression, anxiety, confusion, paranoia, and sleep disturbances. Findings from several studies show that long-term users of MDMA can suffer cognitive defects, including problems with memory. However, more research on the long-term effects of this drug is needed.

Caffeine The mild stimulant caffeine is probably the most popular psychoactive drug. Common sources of caffeine include coffee, tea, soft drinks, headache and pain remedies like Excedrin, stay-awake products like No-Doz, and weight loss aids. Chocolate contains caffeine but at much lower levels than these sources.

At low doses caffeine increases alertness; at higher doses it can cause restlessness, nervousness, excitement, frequent urination, and gastrointestinal distress. At very high levels of consumption (1 gram a day, or 8–10 cups of coffee), symptoms of intoxication can include muscle twitching,

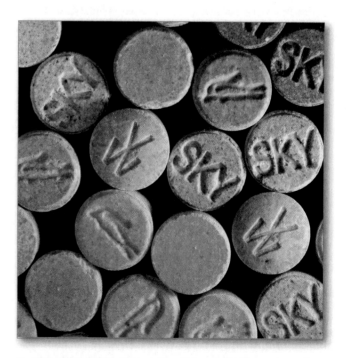

■ MDMA (Ecstasy) is frequently adulterated with a variety of other drugs and toxic substances. At some clubs, raves, and other dance events, pills can be screened by volunteers from DanceSafe, a harm reduction organization with services aimed at "non-addicted, recreational drug users."

irregular heartbeat, insomnia, flushed face, excessive sweating, rambling thoughts or speech, or excessive pacing or movement. People can develop tolerance to caffeine and experience withdrawal symptoms (usually irritability, headache, and fatigue) when cutting back on or eliminating it.

CENTRAL NERVOUS SYSTEM DEPRESSANTS

Central nervous system **depressants** slow down activity in the brain and sympathetic nervous system (see the box "Signs of Drug Use: CNS Depressants"). This category of drugs includes sedatives (for example, barbiturates), hypnotics (sleeping medications), and most anti-anxiety drugs. They can be deadly if misused, especially when mixed with one another or with alcohol (another CNS depressant). CNS depressants carry a high risk for dependence.

depressants
Drugs that slow down activity in the brain and sympathetic nervous system.

Highlight on Health

Signs of Drug Use: CNS Depressants

Barbiturates, benzodiazepines
- Reduced anxiety, euphoria
- Relaxation, drowsiness, sedation

Flunitrazepam (Rohypnol)
- Relaxation, sedation, lowered inhibitions, incapacitation
- Disrupted memory, amnesia

Barbiturates and Hypnotics Barbiturates ("downers") are powerful sedatives that produce pleasant feelings of relaxation when first ingested, usually followed by lethargy, drowsiness, and sleep. Users experience impairments in judgment, decision making, and problem solving, as well as slow, slurred speech and lack of coordination. Dependence is common among middle-aged and older adults who use barbiturates as sleep aids. Withdrawal is difficult, and symptoms, including insomnia, anxiety, tremors, and nausea, can last for weeks; they can be mitigated by gradually tapering off the drug.

Hypnotics are prescribed for people with insomnia and other sleep disorders. People working on the night shift or traveling through multiple time zones may use them to get to sleep quickly and at odd hours. Hypnotics are also used to control epilepsy and to calm people before surgery or dental procedures.

Anti-Anxiety Drugs The most widely prescribed CNS depressants fall into the group of anti-anxiety drugs known as the *benzodiazepines;* examples are Xanax, Valium, and Ativan. Also known as *tranquilizers*, the benzodiazepines are used to control panic attacks and anxiety disorders. Users are at risk for dependence and for increasing dose levels as they become tolerant.

rebound effect
Phenomenon that occurs when a person stops using a drug and experiences symptoms that are worse than those experienced before taking the drug.

Another concern is the **rebound effect,** which occurs when a person stops using a drug and experiences symptoms that are worse than those experienced before taking the drug. The rebound effect can make it difficult to stop taking a particular medication.

Rohypnol A relatively new CNS depressant is flunitrazepam (Rophynol); it started appearing in the United States in the 1990s. This powerful sedative has depressive effects and causes confusion, loss of memory, and sometimes loss of consciousness. It is especially dangerous when mixed with alcohol. Rohypnol is known as a "date rape drug" because men have slipped it into women's drinks in order to sexually assault them later. As of this time the drug's manufacturer has changed the formulation of this drug so that it will not remain colorless when dissolving in a drink.

GHB Another so-called date rape drug is gamma hydroxybutyrate (GHB). This CNS depressant produces feelings of pleasure along with sedation and is a drug of choice among young people at bars, clubs, and parties. It can be produced in several forms, including a clear, tasteless, odorless liquid and a powder that readily dissolves in liquid. Like Rohypnol, it has been slipped into the drinks of women who later did not remember being sexually assaulted. It usually takes effect within 15 to 30 minutes and lasts from 3 to 6 hours. Besides sedation and amnesia, GHB can cause nausea, hallucinations, respiratory distress, slowed heart rate, loss of consciousness, and coma. Users are at risk for dependence with sustained use.

GHB, Rohypnol, and MDMA are sometimes referred to as *club drugs* because of their widespread use at clubs and parties. Their use is particularly dangerous because of the unpredictable setting in which they are usually taken. When GHB and Rohypnol are consumed with alcohol, the combined sedative effects can lead to life-threatening conditions. Additionally, all of these drugs are typically produced in basement labs, so dose and purity are uncertain.

OPIOIDS

Natural and synthetic derivatives of opium, a product harvested from a gummy substance in the seed pod of the opium poppy, are known as **opioids.** Opium originated in the Middle East and has a long history of medical use for pain relief and treatment of diarrhea and dehydration. Currently, opioids are prescribed as

opioids
Natural and synthetic derivatives of opium.

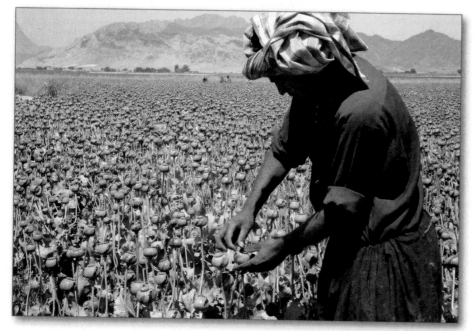

■ Opium poppies are an important cash crop for subsistence farmers in developing countries around the world. Although there are legal medical uses for opium, virtually all of Afghanistan's opium poppy harvest is sold on the international market as heroin.

pain relievers, anesthetics, antidiarrheal agents, and cough suppressants.

Drugs in this category include morphine, heroin, codeine, and oxycodone. Also known as *narcotics,* opioids are commonly misused and abused. They produce a pleasant, drowsy state in which cares are forgotten, the senses are dulled, and pain is reduced. They act by altering the neurotransmitters that control movement, moods, and a number of body functions, including body temperature regulation, digestion, and breathing.

With low doses, opioid users experience euphoria, followed by drowsiness, constriction of the pupils, slurred speech, and impaired attention and memory (see the box "Signs of Drug Use: Opioids"). With higher doses, users can experience depressed respiration, loss of consciousness, coma, and death. When first used, opioids often cause nausea, vomiting, and a negative mood rather than euphoria. Chronic users usually experience dry mouth, constipation, and vision problems.

Opioids can be smoked, snorted, injected, or taken orally. They have a high potential for dependence. Withdrawal symptoms include anxiety, restlessness, craving, irritability, nausea, muscle aches, negative mood, runny nose, insomnia, and diarrhea.

Morphine The primary active chemical in opium, morphine is a powerful pain reliever. Its first widespread use, facilitated by the development of the hypodermic syringe in the 1850s, was during the Civil War. So many soldiers became addicted that after the war, morphine addiction was called "the soldier's disease."[8] Because of the high risk of dependence, physicians prescribing morphine today do so conservatively.

Heroin Heroin is three times more potent than morphine. It was developed in the late 19th century as a supposedly nonaddictive substitute for codeine (another derivative of morphine, useful for suppressing coughs). Just as Civil War veterans suffered from morphine addiction, many soldiers came home from the war in Vietnam addicted to heroin.

Whereas morphine has medical uses, heroin is almost exclusively a drug of abuse. Its use is associated with unemployment, divorce, and drug-related crimes. Users are at risk for such diseases as hepatitis, tuberculosis, and HIV infection from contaminated needles. Heroin dependence is also associated with a high rate of death, primarily from overdoses, accidents, injuries, AIDS, and incidents involving violence.[9] Babies born to women who used heroin during pregnancy are often drug dependent at birth. When heroin addicts are seen scratching their bodies in a frantic way, it usually indicates the drug was mixed with additives or contaminants prior to sale and is causing an allergic reaction.

Synthetic Opioids Some of the most widely prescribed drugs in the United States are synthetic opioids, made from oxycodone hydrochloride. Brand names include OxyContin, Vicodin, Demerol, Percocet, and Percodan.

Highlight on Health

Signs of Drug Use: Opioids

Heroin
- Drowsiness, nodding out, drooping eyelids
- Slurred speech, slowed movement, impaired coordination, insensitivity to pain, confusion
- Pinpoint pupils
- Dry, itchy skin, scratching

Oxycodone
- Excess energy, talkativeness at first, then relaxation and drowsiness
- Slightly slurred speech, impaired coordination
- Constricted pupils

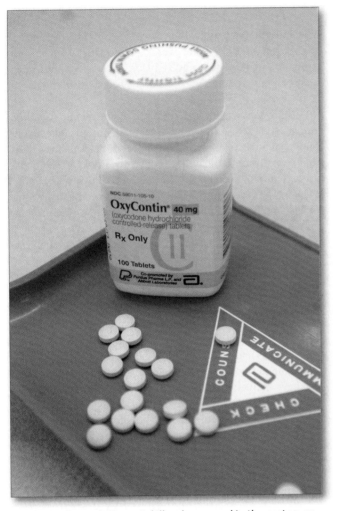

■ Abuse of prescription painkillers has soared in the past 10–15 years, especially among teenagers and young adults. Overdoses from these central nervous system depressants now kill more people than overdoses from either heroin or cocaine.

Some people who start using these drugs for pain become addicted and misuse or abuse them.

OxyContin, for example, provides long-lasting, timed-release relief for moderate to severe chronic pain when taken in tablet form. If the tablets are chewed, crushed and snorted, or dissolved in water and injected, they provide an immediate, intense rush similar to that of heroin. One group particularly susceptible to opioid misuse is medical personnel with access to controlled substances.

hallucinogens
Drugs that alter perceptions and thinking, intensifying and distorting visual and auditory perceptions and producing hallucinations; also called *psychedelics*.

HALLUCINOGENS

LSD, psilocybin, and mescaline are a few of the so-called **hallucinogens** (also called *psychedelics*). They differ chemically, but their effects are similar: They alter perceptions and thinking in characteristic ways. They produce intensification and distortion of visual and auditory perceptions as well as hallucinations (see the box "Signs of Drug Use: Hallucinogens and Inhalants").

Some hallucinogens are synthetic (for example, LSD), and others are derived from plants (for example, mescaline, from peyote, and psilocybin, from psilocybin mushrooms). They are Schedule I drugs with no current medical uses.[10]

LSD Lysergic acid diethylamide (LSD) is a synthetic hallucinogen that alters perceptual processes, producing visual distoßrtions and fantastic imagery. Use of LSD peaked in the late 1960s and then declined, as reports circulated of "bad trips," prolonged psychotic reactions, "flashbacks," self-injurious behavior, and possible chromosomal damage.

LSD is one of the most potent psychoactive drugs known. It is odorless, colorless, and tasteless, and a dose as small as a single grain of salt (about .01 mg) can produce mild effects. At higher doses (.05 mg to .10 mg), hallucinogenic effects are produced. Most users take LSD orally; absorption is rapid. Effects last for several hours and vary depending on the user's mood and expectations, the setting, and the dose and potency of the drug. It usually takes hours or days to recover from an LSD trip. Although LSD is thought to stimulate serotonin receptors in the brain, its exact neural pathway is not completely understood.

Besides visual distortion, LSD can produce auditory changes, a distorted sense of time, changes in the perception of one's own body, and *synesthesia*, a "mixing of senses," in which sounds may appear as visual images or a visual image changes in rhythm to music. Feelings of euphoria may alternate with waves of anxiety. In a bad trip, the user may experience acute anxiety or panic.

Tolerance to the effects of LSD develops quickly for some users, and they must increase their intake of LSD to get the same effects. Repeated daily doses become ineffective in 3 to 4 days. LSD does not produce compulsive drug-seeking behaviors, and physiological withdrawal symptoms do not occur when use is stopped.

Phencyclidine (PCP) First developed in the 1950s as an anesthetic, PCP was found to produce such serious side effects—agitation, delusions, irrational behavior—that its use was discontinued. Since the 1960s it has been manufactured illegally and sold on the street, often under the name "angel dust." It has fewer hallucinogenic effects than LSD and more disturbances in body perception. A drug with similar effects is ketamine.

PCP is a white crystalline powder that is readily soluble in water or alcohol. It can be smoked, snorted, or injected intravenously. At low doses it produces euphoria, dizziness, nausea, slurred speech, rapid heartbeat, high blood pressure, numbness, and slowed reaction time. At higher doses it causes disorganized thinking and feelings of unreality, and at very high doses it can cause amnesia, seizures, and coma. A person who has taken PCP is anesthetized enough to undergo surgery. The drug is particularly associated with aggressive behavior, probably as a result of impaired judgment and disorganized thinking. Combined with insensitivity to pain, these effects can produce dangerous or deadly results. PCP is involved in about 3 percent of drug-related emergency room visits and about 3 percent of drug-related deaths.[11]

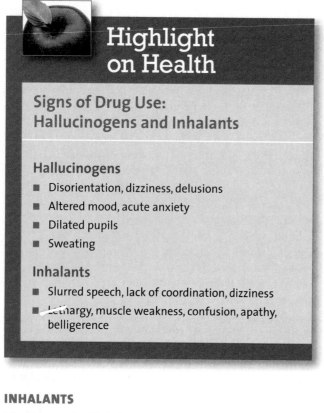

Highlight on Health

Signs of Drug Use: Hallucinogens and Inhalants

Hallucinogens

- Disorientation, dizziness, delusions
- Altered mood, acute anxiety
- Dilated pupils
- Sweating

Inhalants

- Slurred speech, lack of coordination, dizziness
- Lethargy, muscle weakness, confusion, apathy, belligerence

INHALANTS

The drugs called **inhalants** are breathable chemical vapors that alter consciousness, typically producing a state of intoxication that resembles drunkenness. The vapors come from substances like paint thinners, gasoline, glue, and spray can propellant. The active ingredients in these products are chemicals like toluene, benzene, acetone, and tetrachlorethylene—all dangerously powerful toxins and carcinogens.[12]

inhalants
Breathable chemical vapors that alter consciousness, producing a state resembling drunkenness.

Vapors can be inhaled using different methods. A user can inhale the fumes from a rag that has been soaked in the substance and placed over the mouth and nose ("huffing") or breathe into a bag containing the substance ("bagging"). Users also inhale fumes directly from containers and even spray aerosols into the nose and mouth. Vapors reach the lungs and enter the bloodstream very quickly.

At low doses inhalants cause light-headedness, dizziness, blurred vision, slurred speech, lack of coordination, and feelings of euphoria. At higher doses they can cause lethargy, muscle weakness, and stupor. An overdose of an inhalant can result in a loss of consciousness, coma, or death. Inhalants can also cause behavioral and psychological changes, including belligerence, confusion, apathy, and impaired social and occupational functioning. Perhaps the most significant negative effect for chronic users is widespread and long-lasting brain damage.

Initial use of inhalants often starts early, with 16.1 percent of 8th graders having tried some type of an inhalant. Over 72 percent of those using inhalants for the first time during 2005 were under the age of 18.[12]

MARIJUANA

The most widely used illicit drug in the United States is marijuana. In 2006 there were an estimated 14.8 million users among Americans aged 12 or older, and over 15 percent of young people aged 12 to 17 had used marijuana at least once.[1]

Marijuana is derived from the hemp plant, *Cannabis sativa*. The leaves of the plant are usually dried and smoked, but they can also be mixed in tea or food. Hashish is a resin that seeps from the leaves; it is usually smoked. The active ingredient in marijuana is delta-9-tetrahydrocannabinol (THC). The potency of the drug is determined by the amount of THC in the plant, which in turn is affected by the growing conditions. Since the 1960s, the amount of THC in marijuana sold on the street has increased from 1–5 percent to as much as 10–15 percent.

Marijuana use produces mild euphoria, sedation, lethargy, short-term memory impairment, distorted sensory perceptions, a distorted sense of time, impaired motor coordination, and an increase in heart rate (see the box "Signs of Drug Use: Marijuana"). Effects typically begin within a few minutes and last from 3 to 4 hours. Sometimes the drug causes anxiety or a negative mood. At high doses marijuana can have hallucinogenic effects, accompanied by acute anxiety and paranoid thinking. Chronic, heavy users of marijuana may develop tolerance to its effects and experience some withdrawal symptoms if they stop using it, but most dependence seems to be psychological.

Researchers have found that THC has a variety of effects on the brain. One effect is the suppression of activity in the information processing system of the hippocampus, perhaps accounting for some impairments in problem solving and decision making associated with being high on marijuana. Marijuana smoke has negative effects on the respiratory system; it contains more carcinogens than tobacco smoke and is highly irritating to the lining of the bronchioles and lungs.

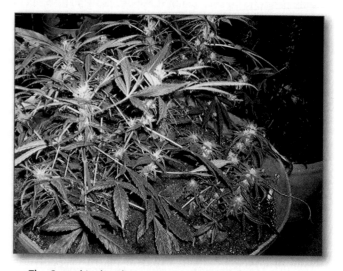

■ The *Cannabis* plant has a variety of uses, including fiber (hemp), food, mediations, and psychedelic effects. From its probable origin in China or central Asia, the plant spread to India, ancient Rome, Africa, Europe, and the Americas.

Highlight on Health

Signs of Drug Use: Marijuana

- Talkativeness, loud laughter, then drowsiness
- Increased appetite
- Bloodshot eyes, dilated pupils
- Forgetfulness, distractibility
- Distorted sense of time

In addition to coughs and chest colds, users may experience more frequent episodes of acute bronchitis and may be more likely to develop chronic bronchitis.[13]

Many people claim that marijuana does have medical uses, especially as a treatment for glaucoma, for the pain and nausea associated with cancer and chemotherapy, and for the weight loss associated with AIDS. Research suggests that smoking marijuana is no more effective than taking THC in pill form for these purposes, but the use of marijuana for medical reasons has become a matter of political debate. Proponents of its use assert that it makes life livable for many people with painful and debilitating medical conditions and that there is no reason not to legalize it. Opponents argue that legalizing marijuana would imply approval of its use for recreational purposes and open the floodgates to abuse of all drugs.

Like alcohol, marijuana affects the skills required to drive a car safely, including concentration, attention, coordination, reaction time, and the ability to judge distance. Because it also impairs judgment, people who are high may not realize their driving skills are impaired. It also appears that marijuana use during pregnancy affects both the likelihood of miscarriage and the health of the fetus.[13] Babies born to mothers who use marijuana may be smaller and more likely to develop health problems once they are born. During infancy and early childhood, these children may have more behavioral problems and cognitive deficits, and in school, they have more difficulty with tasks requiring memory, attention, and decision making.[14]

Approaches to the Drug Problem

Drug abuse and dependence have negative consequences affecting individuals, communities, and society. In addition to the human costs, illicit drug use causes considerable economic damage. An estimated $180 billion is drained from the U.S. economy by drug use annually, largely in lost productivity due to drug-related illness and death and in health care costs.[15] In 2005 1.4 million drug-related hospital emergency room visits were reported in the United States.[16] About 27 percent of these visits were related to the use of alcohol in combination with other drugs, most commonly, cocaine, marijuana, and heroin.

Other economic costs of illicit drug use include social welfare costs, workplace accidents, property damage, incarceration of otherwise productive individuals, goods and services lost to crime, work hours missed by victims of drug-related crime, costs of law enforcement, and costs of the criminal justice system. A large part of these costs—about $40 billion annually—is incurred by the war on drugs, especially the operation of the prison system.

Government approaches to the drug problem have traditionally fallen into two broad categories: supply reduction and demand reduction. A newer approach to the drug problem is harm reduction, an approach used in alcohol treatment programs as well.

SUPPLY REDUCTION STRATEGIES

Strategies to reduce the supply of drugs are aimed at controlling the quantity of illicit substances that enter or are produced in the United States. An example is *interdiction,* the interception of drugs before they enter the country, as when customs officials use dogs to sniff out drugs at airports or when the Coast Guard boards ships to search for drugs as they enter U.S. waters.

The U.S. government also puts pressure on governments in other countries to suppress the production and exportation of drugs. Unfortunately, the plants that yield drugs are important and profitable cash crops for peasant farmers in many countries, and the drug smuggling business is controlled by criminal interests that are often beyond the control of the government. Efforts to reduce the drug supply at the international level have led to human rights abuses, an expansion of oppressive regimes, and increased corruption among police, government, and military personnel.

The government also attempts to prevent domestic production of drugs by raiding suspected underground drug labs or stamping out enterprises that grow marijuana on a large scale. Another domestic supply-side strategy is to obstruct the distribution of drugs, such as when a massive police presence is used in an area where drugs are sold or when legal means are used to disrupt money laundering and other practices that underlie the financial structures of the drug business. Federal statutes now authorize the seizure of any property used in connection with the sale or possession of illegal drugs, including cars, boats, planes, and homes.

DEMAND REDUCTION STRATEGIES

Demand-side strategies include penalizing users through incarceration; preventing drug use, primarily through education; and treating individuals once they have become dependent on drugs.

Incarceration for Drug-Related Crimes Penalizing users means enforcing the laws against drug possession, arresting offenders, and putting people in prison. The assumptions behind this approach are that incarceration will reduce drug-related crime by getting users off the streets and that the threat of punishment will deter others from using drugs. Most states mandate harsh prison terms for the possession or sale of relatively small quantities of drugs, regardless of whether the person is a first-time or repeat offender. As a result, U.S. prisons are crowded with people convicted of drug-related crimes; in fact, more than half of the people in U.S. prisons are serving time for such offenses. The United States imprisons a larger percentage of its population than does any other nation. Elsewhere, low-level crimes like drug possession do not draw a prison sentence.

Since prisoners are a captive audience, it would make sense to provide treatment while they are in jail, but only a small percentage of prisoners who need drug treatment receive it. Instead, prison time serves mainly to disrupt people's lives and turn young people who may have been experimenting with drugs into criminals. Incarceration does little to address the larger problem of drug use in our society.

Prevention Strategies   A second demand-side strategy is prevention through education. Prevention strategies focus on reducing the demand for drugs by increasing an individual's ability to decline drug use when confronted with an opportunity to experiment. Programs involve primary, secondary, or tertiary prevention, depending on their targeted audience. *Primary, or universal, prevention programs* are designed to reach the entire population without regard to individual risk factors. Public service commercials on television asking us

Public Health in Action

Combating Teen Prescription Drug Abuse

> *"Don't look at me, man. Ain't my problem. I didn't do it."*

A drug dealer stands by a public phone complaining that he's losing his customers—they're now getting their drugs from their parents' medicine cabinets. This ad, called "Drug Dealer Testimonial," aired during Super Bowl XLII on February 3, 2008. It was the first ad in a media campaign launched by the federal government's Office of National Drug Control Policy (ONDCP) to educate parents about prescription and over-the-counter drug abuse by teenagers. A second TV ad, called "All My Pills," featured a teenage boy showing off his stash of pills to the camera and bragging that he got them for free at home.

Although teen drug use is down overall, more teens abuse prescription drugs than any illicit drug except marijuana. In 2006 more than 2.1 million teenagers abused prescription drugs; the most commonly abused are painkillers (for example, OxyContin, Vicodin), depressants (for example, sleeping pills, anti-anxiety drugs), and stimulants (for example, Ritalin). Teens are also abusing over-the-counter drugs like cough and cold medications that contain the cough suppressant dextromethorphan, such as NyQuil and Robitussin.

Research suggests that teenagers believe that taking prescription medications is safer than using street drugs, not realizing the risks of addiction and overdose, especially if the medications are combined with alcohol or other drugs. Between 1999 and 2004, fatal overdoses from prescription drugs increased by 84 percent, and between 1995 and 2005, admissions to treatment programs for prescrip-

tion drug abuse increased by 300 percent. Many parents are not aware of these dangers either, nor do they realize how much influence they have with their teenagers.

The media campaign was developed in collaboration with the Partnership for a Drug-Free America at a cost of about $30 million in advertising. Designed to reach more than 90 percent of parents a dozen times, the campaign includes two TV ads, an Open Letter to Parents printed in 43 national and regional newspapers, print ads in national magazines, online ads directing parents to the campaign's Web site, information sheets on prescription drugs placed in pharmacies nationwide, a tool kit to help community groups implement local prescription drug abuse prevention efforts, and a report entitled *Prescription for Danger: A Report on Prescription and Over-the-Counter Drug Abuse Among the Nation's Teens.* For more information on the campaign and to view the ads, visit www.theantidrug.com.

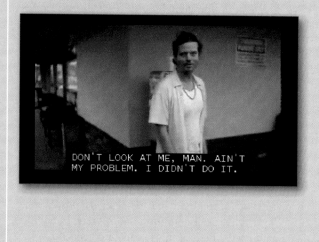

DON'T LOOK AT ME, MAN. AIN'T MY PROBLEM. I DIDN'T DO IT.

Sources: "ONDCP Launches First Major Initiative to Combat Teen Prescription Drug Abuse," Office of National Drug Control Policy, 2008, retrieved April 20, 2008, from www.mediacampaign.org/newsroom/press08/012408.html; Prescription for Danger: A Report on Prescription and Over-the-Counter Drug Abuse Among the Nation's Teens, Office of National Drug Control Policy, 2008, retrieved April 20, 2008, from http://theantidrug.com/pdf/prescription_report.pdf.

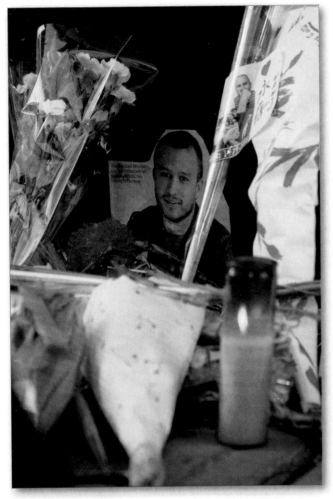

■ Actor Heath Ledger was only 27 when he died from the combined effects of prescription painkillers, sleeping pills, and anti-anxiety medications. His death was ruled accidental.

to imagine a world without cigarettes or billboards referring to crystal meth as "crystal mess" are examples of primary prevention strategies (see the box "Combating Teen Prescription Drug Abuse").

Secondary, or selective, strategies focus on those subgroups that are at greatest risk for use or abuse, with the aim of increasing protective factors and decreasing potential risk factors. An example is a class that teaches problem-solving skills to adolescents.

Tertiary, or indicated, strategies target at-risk individuals rather than groups, again focusing on protective factors such as academic, interpersonal, social, or job skills. An example is a program that tutors individual students in ways to manage emotions and maintain self-esteem without drugs.

A prevention strategy used in the workplace is drug testing, usually random urine screening. The goal of drug testing is not to catch drug users and fire them but to create an environment in which it is clear that drug use is not condoned. Companies also want to limit their liability by reducing the likelihood that an employee will make a mistake that causes someone harm. Federal law requires that people in jobs involving transportation, such as air traffic controllers, train engineers, and

truck drivers, undergo regular testing to ensure public safety. U.S. military personnel also undergo regular drug testing. Although some see the practice as an infringement of privacy rights, so far it has withstood judicial challenges.

On college campuses, a number of steps can be taken to prevent drug use and to reduce harm to those students who do use (see the box "Do you Know Someone With a Drug Problem?"). A comprehensive approach, known as *environmental management*, can be implemented to modify an environment that often benignly accepts or overlooks drug use and experimentation during college. The most effective approaches seem to have a number of common factors:[2]

■ Sending clear messages that drug use is not acceptable.

■ Changing the climate of drug tolerance on campus, if it exists.

■ Engaging parents.

■ Identifying and intervening with at-risk students.

■ Providing alternative activities.

■ Involving students in the planning of prevention programs.

For those individuals who will experiment regardless of changes made on campus, harm reduction strategies are important. Implementing such strategies should not be seen as "giving permission" to students to use; rather, it reduces the likelihood that they will harm themselves or others. The following are some harm reduction strategies that have been implemented on college campuses:

■ Providing containers in college buildings for the safe disposal of needles and syringes.

■ Providing condoms so that students will not transmit infectious diseases if drug use leads to sexual activity.

■ Making naloxone (Narcan) available in case of opioid overdose. Naloxone is an opiate antagonist that can counteract life-threatening depression of the respiratory system.

Drug Treatment Programs The third type of demand-side strategy is helping people to stop using drugs after they have started, that is, providing treatment. Evidence indicates that treatment is a more effective strategy for reducing drug use than locking up dealers or cutting off supplies at our borders.[17, 18] As with alcohol, treatment is available in a variety of formats, ranging from hospital-based inpatient programs to self-help/mutual-help groups such as Narcotics Anonymous (NA).

In 2006 approximately 23.6 million people in the United States—9.6 percent of the population aged 12 or older—needed treatment for an illicit drug or alcohol abuse problem, but only 4 million received treatment.[1] More than half received treatment in a self-help group, and most of the remainder received treatment at a specialty substance abuse facility. Overall treatment effectiveness (defined as being drug-free 1 year after finishing a program) ranges from 25 percent to 50 percent.

Most experts agree that treatment is a long-term process, often marked by relapses and requiring multiple treatment episodes. The first step is acknowledging that there is a problem and getting into a program. No single treatment is appropriate for everyone; matching services to individual needs is important.

Treatment is more successful when the program lasts at least 3 months, includes individual counseling, and addresses all aspects of the client's life, including medical treatment, family therapy, living skills, and occupational skills. In counseling, clients work to increase motivation, build relapse prevention skills, improve problem-solving and interpersonal skills, and develop life-enhancing behaviors. Participating in self-help support programs during and following treatment often helps maintain abstinence.

HARM REDUCTION STRATEGIES

As described in Chapter 11, harm reduction strategies are based on the idea that attempting to completely eliminate substance use is futile and that efforts should be focused on helping addicts reduce the harm associated with their substance use.[19-21]

Advocates of the harm reduction approach assert that drug users are in need of treatment rather than punishment. Examples of harm reduction strategies are needle exchange programs, in which addicts are provided with sterile needles in exchange for their used ones, and drug substitute programs, in which individuals are maintained on addictive but less debilitating drugs, such as methadone for heroin addicts.

Other harm reduction strategies include controlled availability (certain drugs are available through a government monopoly), medicalization (drugs are available by prescription but only to individuals who are already addicted to them), and decriminalization (the penalty for possession of certain drugs is reduced or eliminated if the quantity held is below a certain limit).

Proponents of harm reduction strategies claim that they represent a more realistic approach to the drug problem and would allow resources to be directed away from punishment, which is ineffective, and toward treatment, which is effective. Opponents of harm reduction strategies argue that they are thinly disguised forms of drug legalization and that any softening of a zero tolerance position would result in an epidemic of drug use. Although effective harm reduction programs are in place in England and Canada, harm reduction is rejected as an official policy by the U.S. government.

***

Challenges & Choices

Do You Know Someone With a Drug Problem?

College students turn to illicit drugs for a variety of reasons. They may want to experiment, relax, reduce stress, stay up late to study, or even self-medicate psychiatric problems. Some are continuing a pattern of drug use they began in high school, while others are experimenting with their new-found freedom away from home. Many young adults do not realize how easy it is to become dependent on a drug, whether physiologically or psychologically.

Most colleges identify alcohol abuse as their most pressing substance-related issue and focus their attention on alcohol-related programs. Very few schools report having programs specifically aimed at early identification of drug-related problems. Without formal programs, it is important that students take a role in the early identification of such problems in their friends, roommates, and fellow students. The following behaviors may indicate that someone is having a problem with drugs:

- A noticeable change in behavior, such as withdrawal or agitation.
- A change in sleep habits, needing either more or less.
- Nodding out during conversations or in class on a regular basis.

- Lack of interest in activities that used to be a source of enjoyment.
- An increase in physical complaints or pain.
- Preoccupation with a drug; activities scheduled around drug use.
- An increase in money borrowing.

If you notice these behaviors in a friend, you may want to express your concerns—keeping silent does nothing to help your friend acknowledge and address the problem. Be prepared to offer suggestions about where he or she might go to get help, such as the college counseling center, and also be prepared to be rebuffed in case your friend is in denial. The best thing you can do is continue to be supportive of your friend and look out for his or her best interest.

It's Not Just Personal . . .

According to the Monitoring the Future research project, conducted for the past 30-plus years by the University of Michigan, five classes of illicit drugs—marijuana, amphetamines, cocaine, LSD, and inhalants—have had an impact on young people in their late teens and early 20s. Use of LSD has fallen precipitously in all age groups, but the abuse of prescription drugs has risen. Rates of use of narcotics other than heroin (pain relievers) are about 9 percent among college students. For tranquilizers, rates are about 6–7 percent, and for sedatives (barbiturates), about 4 percent.

Source: Monitoring the Future: National Survey Results on Drug Use, 1975–2006: Volume II, College Students and Adults Ages 19–45 *(NIH Publication No. 07-6206), by L.D. Johnson, P.M. O'Malley, J.G. Bachman, and J.E. Schulenberg, 2007, Bethesda, MD: National Institute on Drug Abuse.*

The use of drugs in our society is widespread. If you have not already had a personal encounter with recreational drugs, you are likely to have one at some point in your life. As with other aspects of health-related behavior, making responsible decisions about drug use depends on information, self-knowledge, and behavioral strategies and skills. Use the material in this chapter as the basis for making the right decision for yourself.

You Make the Call

Is Law Enforcement the Best Way to Fight the War on Drugs?

Imagine that your child is about to start attending a high school where drug use has been increasing and a star athlete recently overdosed on cocaine. You and other parents meet with teachers, school and district administrators, and local and state government officials to discuss solutions to the growing drug problem. To your surprise, the range of opinions is broad and the debate is heated. Some people want to build up the police force, use drug-sniffing dogs to patrol the school, and impose mandatory drug testing for school athletes. Others want to implement drug awareness and education programs and set up more after-school clubs and activities. At the end of the evening, the advocates of increased law enforcement have prevailed.

A local debate such as this mirrors the national debate over solutions to the drug problem. The ratio of government spending on prevention, education, and treatment to spending on law enforcement (including spending on military interdiction by the Department of Defense, court costs incurred by the Justice Department, and maintenance of the prison system by the Bureau of Prisons) is roughly 30:70, despite abundant evidence that law enforcement is not solving the problem. Although billions of dollars are spent every year on the war on drugs, illicit substances are readily available in high schools, on college campuses, and in communities across the country.

Proponents of the law enforcement approach point out that possession of drugs, even in small quantities, is illegal and that to have an orderly and safe society the law must be upheld. Arresting individuals who use drugs and sentencing them to jail discourages dealers and sellers and serves as a deterrent to those considering drug use. Because adolescents often have poor judgment, lack impulse control, and take risks without thinking about consequences, efforts to get through to them have to be tough and harsh.

Opponents of this approach point out that research supports prevention and treatment as far more effective responses to the drug problem than enforcement. They argue that drugs will always be available and that families, schools, and communities need to help young people acquire problem-solving and decision-making skills. Relying on the police and drug testing can lead to civil rights abuses and violations of privacy rights. In the war on drugs, one side lines up with a "law and order" approach, and the other emphasizes prevention and treatment. What do you think?

PROS

- Criminal activity calls for criminal punishment.
- Drug dealers and sellers need to be driven from the community.
- Harsh punishments deter young people from trying drugs.
- Public safety and security are of the highest importance and override concerns about civil liberties abuses.

CONS

- Most young people are experimenting with drugs; they are not criminals. Arrests and jail time can permanently derail the lives of promising young citizens.
- Imprisonment and long sentences have not been shown to reduce the number of subsequent drug arrests; the deterrent argument is faulty.
- We always need to be vigilant about our civil liberties, especially when the public is vulnerable to fears about safety and security.
- Drug users are in need of treatment and rehabilitation, not punishment and incarceration.

In Review

1. **Why do people use drugs, and what are current patterns of drug use?** As with alcohol, people use drugs to feel better, often as a recreational activity; however, some people become addicted and lose control of their drug use. The most commonly used illicit drug is marijuana, but the nonmedical use of prescription-type drugs has increased dramatically in recent years.

2. **How do drugs affect the body?** As psychoactive substances, drugs affect the brain and central nervous system (CNS). Effects vary depending on the chemical properties of the drug, the characteristics of the person, and the environment. Drug dependence occurs when the drug causes changes in the brain, particularly the brain structures that make up the pleasure and reward circuit and those parts of the brain involved in rational thought and judgment.

3. **What are the different categories of drugs?** Drugs are classified as CNS stimulants (for example, cocaine, methamphetamine), CNS depressants (barbiturates, benzodiazepines), opioids (heroin, oxycodone), hallucinogens (LSD), inhalants (paint thinner, glue), and cannabinoids (marijuana).

4. **What are the main approaches to the drug problem?** The main approaches are supply reduction strategies (for example, interdiction), demand reduction strategies (incarceration, prevention through education, treatment), and harm reduction strategies (needle exchange programs). Because colleges are often focused more on alcohol-related problems than on drug-related problems, students may have to be more proactive in identifying and helping friends who are developing a drug problem.

 For a detailed summary of this chapter and a comprehensive set of review questions, visit the Online Learning Center at **www.mhhe.com/teague2e.**

Web Resources

ClubDrugs.Org: This Web site offers information on club drugs such as Ecstasy, GHB, and LSD, including trends and statistics for these and other drugs of abuse. www.clubdrugs.org

Higher Education Center for Alcohol and Other Drug Abuse and Violence Prevention: This government organization looks at problems of drug abuse and violence in context, emphasizing the importance of managing the environment, using educational campaigns, and promoting early intervention treatment and recovery strategies. www.edc.org/hec

Narcotics Anonymous (NA): NA resources include drug information, help lines, contact information, news features, publications, and links. www.na.org

National Clearinghouse for Alcohol and Drug Information: This site features a RADAR network—Regional Alcohol and Drug Awareness Resource—consisting of more than 700 active centers for substance abuse prevention and treatment. www.health.org

National Institute on Drug Abuse: This government site features in-depth information on various drugs of abuse, offering research reports and drug information along with many other helpful resources. www.nida.nih.gov

Substance Abuse and Mental Health Services Administration (SAMHSA): SAMHSA offers information and resources on mental health, drug abuse prevention and treatment, and workplace issues. www.samhsa.gov

U.S. Drug Enforcement Administration: Drugs of Abuse: This comprehensive resource includes fact sheets on drugs of abuse and briefs and background information on topics such as drug trafficking and abuse, law enforcement, and drug policy. www.dea.gov

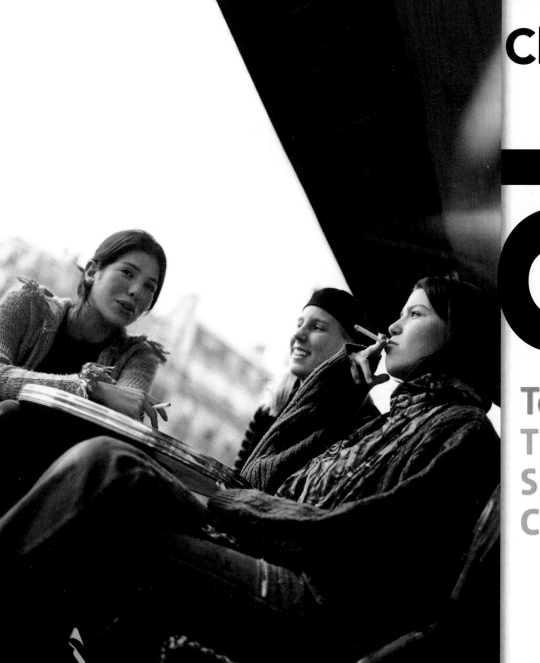

Tobacco
The
Smoking
Challenge

Ever Wonder...

- if flavored cigarettes or little cigars are safer than regular cigarettes?

- if secondhand smoke is really that bad for you?

- if you gain weight when you quit smoking?

WWW

Your Health Today

www.mhhe.com/teague2e

Go to the Online Learning Center for *Your Health Today* for interactive activities, quizzes, flashcards, Web links, and more resources related to this chapter.

College students have been smoking more in recent years. When students are asked why they smoke, the most common reasons given are to relax or reduce stress, to fit in or relieve social pressure, to control weight, and to satisfy nicotine craving (for those who are addicted). Male students who smoke are generally perceived by both genders in a positive light—as cool or manly. In contrast, female smokers are perceived by both genders in a more negative light—as trashy or unfeminine. The aggressive marketing of tobacco products to college students fuels their smoking habits.[1]

Tobacco use is the leading preventable cause of death in the United States, implicated in a host of diseases and debilitating conditions. The health hazards of tobacco use are well known, yet one in five Americans smokes, and nearly 4,000 young people under the age of 18 start smoking every day.[2] If you are one of the 80 percent of Americans who *don't* smoke, this chapter offers information about how you can protect yourself and others from the dangers of tobacco use. If you are one of the 20 percent of Americans who *do* smoke, this chapter will give you some ideas about how you can quit.

Who Smokes? Patterns of Tobacco Use

About 20.8 percent of the adult population of the United States 18 years old or over are smokers—about one in five Americans (Table 13.1). The percentage of Americans who smoke is down from a high of nearly 42 percent in 1965. In that year, more than half of all men smoked (51.2 percent), and a third of all women smoked (33.7 percent).[3] The decline since then has occurred largely as a result of public health campaigns about the hazards of smoking, beginning with the 1964 surgeon general's *Report on Smoking and Health.*

Although the prevalence of smoking in the United States continues to decline, the rate of decline has slowed since 1990. Rates of smoking vary across states, with the highest rates in Kentucky, Alaska, West Virginia, Tennessee, and Indiana and the lowest rates in Utah, California, Massachusetts, New Jersey, and Connecticut.[3]

More than 20 percent of Americans are former smokers, and about 60 percent have never smoked.[2] By far the most popular tobacco product is cigarettes, followed by cigars and smokeless tobacco (chewing tobacco). Sixteen percent of men and 4 percent of women smoke cigars, and 9 percent of men and 1 percent of women use smokeless tobacco.[3]

GENDER AND AGE GROUP DIFFERENCES

Smoking is more prevalent among men than women (see the box "Tobacco Use"). Rates of smoking are higher among young people than among older people. Most smokers get hooked in adolescence—more than 90 percent of smokers begin smoking before the age of 21.[2] Many young smokers think they can easily quit at any time, but adolescents who smoke regularly have just as hard a time quitting as older smokers do.

Currently, college students are more likely than the general population to smoke. Overall, however, cigarette

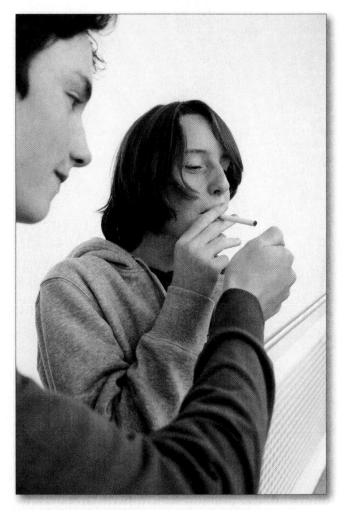

■ The vast majority of smokers start when they are teenagers. Many young smokers don't realize they are addicted to nicotine until they try to quit.

Table 13.1	Cigarette Smoking by Persons 18 Years of Age or Over, United States, Selected Years 1965–2006					
	Percentage of Persons Who Are Current Cigarette Smokers					
	1965	**1985**	**1995**	**2000**	**2002**	**2006**
All persons	41.9	29.9	24.6	23.1	22.4	20.8
Male	51.2	32.2	26.5	25.2	24.8	23.6
Female	33.7	27.9	22.7	21.1	20.1	18.1

Source: Health, United States, 2007, *National Center for Health Statistics, 2007, Hyattsville, MD: Author.*

Who's at Risk

Tobacco Use

- Rates of smoking are higher among men (23.6 percent) than women (18.1 percent). Women smoke less than men in all ethnic groups.

- Smoking is more prevalent among the White population (23.9 percent) than among African Americans (22 percent), Hispanics (18 percent), or Asian Americans and Pacific Islanders (17 percent). The highest smoking rate occurs among American Indians and Alaskan Natives (34 percent).

- Smoking is more common among young adults (25 percent) than among middle-aged adults (22 percent) or older adults (9 percent).

- Currently, 26 percent of high school seniors, 22 percent of 10th graders, and 12 percent of 8th and 9th graders smoke.

- The rate of current smoking by college students decreased from 30.6 percent in 1993 to 23.8 percent in 2005. College men and women have almost equivalent smoking rates (23.7 percent versus 23.8 percent), but college women are slightly more likely to smoke daily. Rates of heavy smoking (more than 10 cigarettes a day) are 7.1 percent for college women and 6.0 percent for college men.

- Current smoking is more common among White college students (30.4 percent) than among Hispanic (25.4 percent), Asian (22.4 percent), or Black (13.7 percent) students.

- Smoking rates are lower at historically Black colleges and universities (22 percent) than at other colleges and universities (40 percent).

- About half of college smokers are social smokers, defined as smoking regularly but not daily and primarily in social situations. Health experts are not sure whether these smokers will stop smoking, continue smoking at a low level, or become heavy smokers.

- Individuals above the poverty line are less likely to smoke (22.2 percent) than are those below the poverty line (32.9 percent).

- One out of every two long-term smokers will die from their tobacco habit. More than 400,000 Americans die each year from smoking-related causes.

- Exposure to environmental tobacco smoke (ETS) causes about 3,000 lung cancer deaths each year. Nonsmokers exposed to ETS have a 20–30 percent increased risk for lung cancer and a 25–30 percent increased risk for heart disease.

- Children exposed to ETS are at increased risk for respiratory disorders and sudden death infant syndrome.

Sources: "Wasting the Best and the Brightest: Substance Abuse at America's Colleges and Universities," 2007, New York: National Center on Addiction and Substance Abuse at Columbia University; The Guide to Community Preventive Services, by S. Zaza, P.A. Briss, and K.W. Harris (Eds.), 2005, New York: Oxford University Press; Ending the Tobacco Problem: A Blueprint for the Nation, Report Brief, Institute of Medicine, 2007, Washington, DC: National Academies Press; Health, United States, 2007, National Center for Health Statistics, 2007, Hyattsville, MD: Author.

smoking is negatively correlated with educational attainment. Adults with less than a high school education are three times as likely as those who graduate from college to smoke.[3]

Other psychosocial factors that increase the likelihood that a person will smoke include having a parent or sibling who smokes, associating with peers who smoke, being from a lower socioeconomic status family, doing poorly in school, and having positive attitudes about tobacco.

SMOKING AND ETHNICITY

Smoking is more prevalent among the White population than among African Americans, Hispanics, and Asian Americans and Pacific Islanders.[7] The highest rates of smoking occur among American Indians and Alaska Natives.[4, 5]

Smoking rates can vary tremendously among groups within broad ethnic categories. For example, despite low rates of smoking overall among Asian Americans and Pacific Islanders, rates are very high among some of the 50 distinct ethnic groups that fall under this umbrella label. Among Tongan American men, the smoking rate is 65 percent; among

Cambodian American men, 71 percent; and among Laotian American men, 72 percent.[4] Clearly, behaviors like smoking are influenced by sociocultural factors, including acculturation and access to health information and health care.

Tobacco Products

Tobacco is a broad-leafed plant that grows in tropical and temperate climates. Tobacco leaves are harvested, dried, and processed in different ways for the variety of tobacco products—rolled into cigars, shredded for cigarettes, ground into a fine powder for inhalation as snuff, or ground into a chewable form and used as smokeless tobacco.

SUBSTANCES IN TOBACCO

When tobacco leaves are burned, more than 4,800 distinct substances are produced. So far, nearly 70 of these substances have been identified as carcinogenic (cancer causing), and many more are harmful in other ways. The most harmful substances are tar, carbon monoxide, and nicotine.

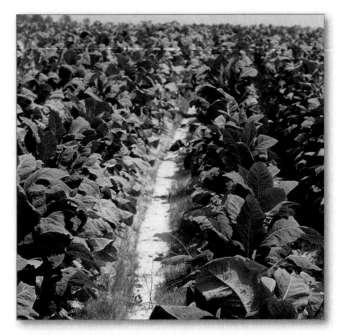

■ Tobacco use originated in the Americas, where it was used ceremonially and medicinally by native populations. By 1600, it was being exported to Europe and Asia. Today, tobacco is still an important crop in Virginia, Kentucky, North and South Carolina, and other southeastern states.

Tar   Tar is a thick, sticky residue that consists of hundreds of different chemical compounds and contains many of the carcinogenic substances in tobacco smoke. Tar coats the smoker's lungs and creates an environment conducive to the growth of cancerous cells. Tar is responsible for many of the changes in the respiratory system that cause the hacking "smoker's cough."

tar
Thick, sticky residue formed when tobacco leaves burn, containing hundreds of chemical compounds and carcinogenic substances.

Carbon Monoxide   One of the most hazardous gaseous compounds in burning tobacco is carbon monoxide, the same toxic gas emitted from the exhaust pipe of a car. Carbon monoxide interferes with the ability of red blood cells to carry oxygen, so that vital body organs, such as the heart, are deprived of oxygen. Many of the other gases produced when tobacco burns are carcinogens, irritants, and toxic chemicals that damage the lungs. For example, tobacco smoke contains nitrous oxide and hydrogen cyanide,[6] two gases that cause lung cancer; toluene, an industrial solvent; and acetone (nail polish remover).

Nicotine   **Nicotine** is the primary addictive ingredient in tobacco. It is carried into the body in the form of thousands of droplets suspended in solid particles of partially burned tobacco. These droplets are so tiny that they penetrate the alveoli (small air sacs in the lungs) and enter the bloodstream, reaching body cells within seconds.

Nicotine is both a poison (it is used as a pesticide) and a powerful psychoactive drug. The first time it is used, it usually produces dizziness, light-headedness, and nausea, signs of mild nicotine poisoning. These effects diminish as tolerance grows. Nicotine causes a cascade of stimulant effects throughout the body by triggering the release of adrenaline, which increases arousal, alertness, and concentration. Nicotine also stimulates the release of endorphins, the body's "natural opiates" that block pain and produce mild sensations of pleasure. (We discuss the effects of nicotine in greater detail later in the chapter.)

nicotine
Primary addictive ingredient in tobacco; a poison and a psychoactive drug.

CIGARETTES

Cigarettes account for nearly 95 percent of the tobacco market in the United States.[3] Nicotine from a cigarette reaches peak concentration in the blood in about 10 minutes and is reduced by half within about 20 minutes, as the drug is distributed to body tissues. Rapid absorption and distribution of nicotine enable the smoker to control the peaks and valleys of nicotine absorption and effect. This process of control—absorption, distribution, elimination—makes cigarettes an effective drug-delivery system for nicotine.[7]

Hookahs, or water pipes, have recently become popular among college students and other young adults as a supposedly safe alternative to cigarettes. Groups of smokers pass the

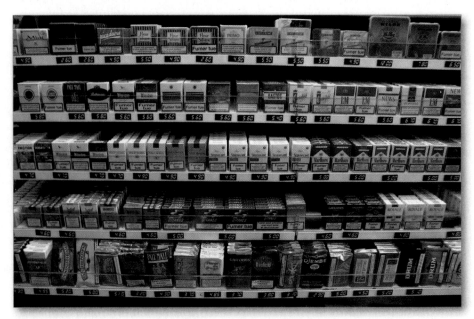

■ Tobacco is processed and packaged into a huge array of products, mostly cigarettes. Besides the common brands, this tobacco shop sells hand rolling tobacco, mini cigars, flavored cigarettes, and French short filter cigarettes.

Consumer Clipboard

Hookah Smoking: An Unsafe Alternative

Hookahs (water pipes) have been used in North Africa, the Middle East, and Central and South Asia for hundreds of years, primarily as a social activity. Although the tobacco mixture smoked in a hookah does not look, smell, taste, or burn like a cigarette, it is not safer to smoke than cigarettes. The World Health Organization warns that hookah use exposes the user to more smoke over a longer period of time than cigarettes, and the CDC reports that hookah use poses a serious potential health hazard to smokers and others exposed to the smoke:

- Hookah tobacco and smoke contain numerous toxins known to cause lung cancer, heart disease, and other diseases.
- Even after passing through water, hookah smoke contains high levels of toxic compounds, including nicotine, carbon monoxide, heavy metals, and cancer-causing chemicals.
- The mode of smoking (frequency of puffing, depth of inhalation, and length of time in the smoking session) may lead to higher absorption of toxic chemicals. A typical 1-hour session involves inhaling 100 to 200 times the volume of smoke inhaled from one cigarette.
- Exposure to smoke and tobacco juice increases the risk for oral cancers.
- Sharing a hookah pipe can expose users to orally transmitted viruses like herpes and hepatitis.
- Secondhand smoke from hookahs poses a serious risk to nonsmokers.

Studies are currently under way to determine whether hookah smoking leads to the same levels of addiction as smoking cigarettes and to further investigate the health effects of hookah use.

Sources: "Fact Sheet: Hookahs," Centers for Disease Control and Prevention, 2007, retrieved April 27, 2008, from www.cdc.gov/tobacco/data_statistics/Factsheets/hookahs.htm; "Waterpipe Tobacco Smoking: Health Effects, Research Needs, and Recommended Actions by Regulators," WHO Study Group on Tobacco Regulation, 2005, retrieved April 27, 2008, from www.who.int/tobacco/global_interaction/tobreg/Waterpipe%20recommendation_Final.pdf.

mouthpiece around, inhaling *shisah,* a mixture of tobacco, molasses, and fruit flavors. The aromatic flavors of hookah tobacco and the smooth smoke produced by the water pipe, which is less irritating to the throat than cigarette smoke, have driven the perception that hookah use is safe. The World Health Organization and the CDC warn that hookah use can pose even greater dangers than cigarette smoking (see the box "Hookah Smoking: An Unsafe Alternative").[8]

Flavored cigarettes are another relatively recent offering of the tobacco industry. Critics claim that tobacco manufacturers are targeting young people with cigarettes flavored with such ingredients as cocoa, sugar, licorice, pineapple, coconut, and lime and bearing names like Kauai Kolada, Caribbean Chill, Midnight Berry, and Winter Warm Toffee. One survey found that 20 percent of smokers aged 17 to 19 smoke flavored cigarettes, compared with 6 percent of smokers over age 25. Several states have sued tobacco companies for violating the ban on marketing cigarettes to children and are considering a ban on the sale of flavored cigarettes.[9]

Clove Cigarettes   Clove cigarettes, which consist of about 60 percent tobacco and 40 percent cloves (an aromatic spice), are also promoted as safer cigarettes. However, they actually contain higher levels of tar and carbon monoxide than regular cigarettes. The active ingredient in cloves causes a numbing effect that allows smokers to inhale the smoke more deeply and to hold the smoke in their lungs for a longer time, giving the smoke more time to do damage.[9]

Herbal Cigarettes   Herbal cigarettes contain herbs such as ginseng rather than tobacco. They come in flavors like cherry and mint and are packaged to look like candy cigarettes. Since they contain no tobacco or nicotine, they are billed as healthier alternatives to tobacco or as aids to quitting.[9] They are not subject to FDA regulation or to the laws that prevent sale to minors.

Despite their popularity, herbal cigarettes are harmful to health. Like tobacco, herbs produce an assortment of dangerous chemicals when they burn. Smoking herbal cigarettes also ingrains the behaviors associated with smoking tobacco cigarettes and may make it more likely that a young person will move on to cigarettes.

Bidis   Bidis are cigarettes made in India from unprocessed, sun-dried tobacco. They are smaller than cigarettes, contain less tobacco, and come in flavors like chocolate and strawberry. No chemicals or additives are used in their manufacture.[11] They are less expensive than cigarettes and can be sold to minors in some states.

Because they contain only natural ingredients, their manufacturers claim they are safer than regular cigarettes. Health experts disagree and call them "cigarettes with training wheels."[12] The unprocessed tobacco in bidis actually produces smoke three times higher in nicotine, three times higher in carbon monoxide, and four times higher in tar than that in cigarettes. Because the tobacco is wrapped in a nonporous leaf rather than cigarette paper, bidis do not burn well, forcing smokers to inhale more deeply to keep the cigarette lit. Studies from India suggest that bidis pose a greater risk for cancers of the oral cavity, throat, lung, esophagus, stomach, and liver, as well as for coronary artery disease, than regular cigarettes do.[10, 12]

Most bidi smokers are Latino and African American teens and adults in their 20s.[12] About 6 percent of college students use bidis.[13] Bidis account for less than 1 percent of all cigarette sales in the United States, but health experts are concerned about their appeal to youth and their marketing on the Internet. At the request of the U.S. government, some importers are voluntarily putting health warning labels on bidis.

CIGARS

Cigars have more tobacco and nicotine per unit than cigarettes do, take longer to smoke, and generate more smoke and more harmful combustion products than cigarettes. The tobacco mix used in cigars has a different pH (relative acidity) than the tobacco mix used in cigarettes, making it easier for cigar smoke to be absorbed through the mucous membranes of the oral cavity than is the case with cigarettes. Nicotine absorbed via this route takes longer to reach the brain than nicotine absorbed in the lungs and has a less intense but longer lasting effect.

Cigar smokers typically do not inhale; those who do are usually former cigarette smokers. Cigar smokers who do not inhale have lower mortality rates than cigar smokers who do.[14] Inhalation substantially increases the cigar smoker's exposure to carcinogenic chemicals and increases the risk for lung cancer and chronic respiratory disease.[15]

Whether or not smoke is inhaled, cigar smoking exposes the oral mucosa to large amounts of carcinogenic chemicals; consequently, cigar smokers have a higher risk than cigarette smokers for oral cancers. When compared with people who don't smoke at all, cigar smokers have 8 times the risk for oral cancers, 7 times the risk for throat cancer, 4.5 times the risk for obstructive lung disease, and twice the risk for lung cancer.[15]

Black and Mild is a brand of "little cigars" or cigarillos that are popular among teens and young adults, particularly

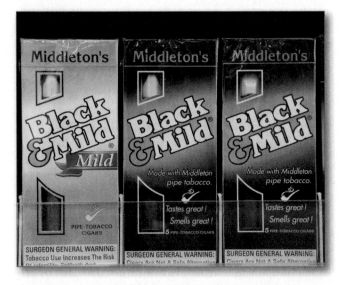

■ Black and Milds are little cigars filled with pipe tobacco. In 2007, John Middleton's, the manufacturer of Black and Milds, was bought by tobacco giant Philip Morris.

young African Americans. Black and Milds are long and thin like a cigarette but wrapped in tobacco leaf rather than paper, like a cigar. The difference in wrapping means they are not subject to certain cigarette regulations and taxes. They come in flavors like apple, cream, and wine, and many varieties have a plastic tip. Black and Mild little cigars contain more tobacco and more nicotine than cigarettes and are addictive if inhaled. Use of Black and Mild cigars is much higher among African Americans (54 percent) than in any other ethnic group.

PIPES

Pipe smoke has more toxins than cigarette smoke does and is more irritating to the respiratory system. Pipe smokers who do not inhale are at less risk for lung cancer and heart disease than cigarette smokers are. Like cigar smokers, however, pipe smokers who are former cigarette smokers tend to inhale and consequently are exposed to more toxins than they were when they smoked cigarettes. Pipe smokers are just as likely as cigarette smokers to develop cancer of the mouth, larynx, throat, and esophagus.[16]

SMOKELESS TOBACCO

There are two types of smokeless tobacco, snuff and chewing tobacco. *Snuff* is a powdered form of tobacco that can be inhaled through the nose or placed between the bottom teeth and lower lip. *Chewing tobacco* is used by lodging a cud or pinch of smokeless tobacco between the cheek and gum. It is available as loose leaf or as a plug (a compressed, flavored bar of processed tobacco). Smokeless tobacco is sometimes called *spit tobacco* because users spit out the tobacco juices and saliva that accumulate in the mouth.

Because users do not inhale toxic gases, manufacturers of smokeless tobacco have promoted their product as a safe alternative to cigarettes. This is not the case. Tobacco does not have to burn to cause health hazards. Spit tobacco contains at least 28 carcinogens, and use of spit tobacco is believed to cause about 10–15 percent of oral cancers, leading to about 6,000 deaths each year. When spit tobacco is kept in contact with the oral mucosa, it can cause *dysplasia,* an abnormal change in cells, and *oral lesions,* whitish patches on the tongue or mouth that may become cancerous. Spit tobacco also causes gum disease, tooth decay and discoloration, and bad breath.[17–20] The amount of nicotine absorbed from smokeless tobacco is two to three times greater than that delivered by cigarettes.

Snus is a smokeless tobacco that is being marketed as a safer alternative to cigarettes. It is made from tobacco mixed with water, salt, sodium carbonate, and aroma and is often packaged in small bags resembling teabags. It is produced and sold mainly in Sweden and Norway but is being test-marketed in other countries, including the United States. Snus contains more nicotine than cigarettes but lower levels of other dangerous compounds, and since it isn't burned, there is no secondhand smoke. Users have lower rates of certain cancers, but snus may cause oral lesions, hypertension, and complications of pregnancy.[19]

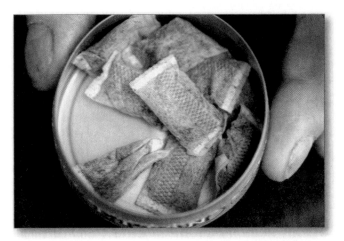

■ Snus is a form of smokeless tobacco produced in Sweden and Norway, where it is marketed as a safe way to enjoy tobacco. Users place one of the small prepackaged bags under the upper lip and leave it there for an extended period of time.

Why Do People Smoke?

Tobacco use and its relationship to health are complex issues that involve nicotine addiction, behavioral dependence, and aggressive marketing by tobacco companies, among other factors.

NICOTINE ADDICTION

Nicotine is a highly addictive psychoactive drug—some health experts believe it is the most addictive of all the psychoactive drugs—and tobacco products are very efficient delivery devices for this drug. Once in the brain, nicotine follows the same pleasure and reward pathway—involving the ventral tegmental area (VTA), the nucleus accumbens, and the prefrontal cortex—as other psychoactive drugs follow (see Chapter 12 and Figure 12.4). Increases in release of the neurotransmitter dopamine produce feelings of pleasure and a desire to repeat the experience. As noted earlier, nicotine also affects alertness, energy, and mood by increasing levels of endorphins and other neurotransmitters, including serotonin and norepinephrine.

With continued smoking, neurons in the VTA become more sensitive and responsive to nicotine, causing *addiction,* or dependence on a steady supply of the drug; *tolerance,* or reduced responsiveness to its effects; and *withdrawal* symptoms if it is not present. Nicotine withdrawal symptoms include irritability, anxiety, depressed mood, difficulty concentrating, restlessness, decreased heart rate, increased appetite, and increased craving for nicotine.

More than two-thirds of cigarette smokers who attempt to quit relapse within 2 days, unable to tolerate the period when withdrawal symptoms are at their peak. It takes about 2 weeks for a person's brain chemistry to return to normal. Withdrawal symptoms decrease and become more subtle with prolonged abstinence, but some smokers continue to experience intermittent cravings for years. Smoking tobacco may cause permanent changes in the nervous system, which may explain why some people who haven't smoked in years can become addicted again after smoking a single cigarette.[33–35]

Tobacco manufacturers long argued that nicotine use is a habit and not an addiction, but in 1988 the surgeon general issued a report stating that nicotine meets all the criteria for classification as an addictive drug. According to this report, cigarettes and other forms of tobacco are addictive, nicotine is the drug in tobacco that causes this addiction, and pharmacological and behavioral processes that determine tobacco addiction are similar to those that determine addiction to other drugs such as cocaine and heroin.[21]

BEHAVIORAL DEPENDENCE

People who smoke are not just physiologically dependent on a substance; they also become psychologically dependent on the habit of smoking. Through repeated paired associations, the effects of nicotine on the brain are linked to places, people, and events. Individuals may associate smoking with drinking a cup of coffee in the morning, drinking alcohol in the evening, or other daily activities, and these sensory or environmental stimuli may trigger the urge for a cigarette. Tobacco companies design their advertising to take advantage of these associations.

Many smokers have a harder time imagining their future life without cigarettes than they do dealing with the physiological symptoms of withdrawal. Simply holding a cigarette may have a tranquilizing effect on some smokers. Some ex-smokers remain vulnerable to sensory and environmental stimuli—smelling tobacco smoke, seeing a cigarette ad, and so on—for years after quitting.[7] Stress is a common cause of relapse.

WEIGHT CONTROL

Nicotine suppresses appetite and slightly increases basal metabolic rate (rate of metabolic activity at rest). People who start smoking often lose weight, and continuing smokers gain weight less rapidly than nonsmokers. Weight control is one of the major reasons young women give for smoking, and weight gain can be a deterrent to quitting.[22]

When individuals stop smoking, their appetite returns, along with craving for sweet foods, which nicotine also suppresses. In addition, many people eat more while they are quitting just to have something in their mouths. Gaining 7 to 10 pounds is typical before the body adjusts to the absence of nicotine.[23] Once a person has successfully quit, this weight can be lost through exercise and sensible eating.

TOBACCO MARKETING AND ADVERTISING

Every day, the tobacco industry loses 4,600 smokers, either to quitting or to death.[21] These users have to be replaced if tobacco companies are to stay in business. Because most smokers get hooked in adolescence, children and teenagers are prime targets of tobacco advertising. Tobacco advertising aimed at children associates smoking with cartoon characters, and advertising aimed at teenagers associates smoking with alcohol, sex, and independence. Judging by the number of people who take up tobacco use every year, tobacco advertising and marketing are extremely effective. Although the industry continues to claim that it does not market its products to children, research suggests otherwise.[21, 24]

Effects of Tobacco Use on Health

By the 18th century, scientists suspected that tobacco smoke caused cancer. By the mid-20th century, research showed that it was also a causal factor in heart disease, respiratory diseases, and numerous other debilitating conditions. Today, overwhelming evidence confirms that smoking is the single greatest preventable cause of illness and premature death in North America.[21]

SHORT-TERM EFFECTS

Smoking affects virtually every system in the body (Figure 13.1). When a smoker lights up, nicotine reaches the brain within 7 to 10 seconds, producing both sedating and stimulating effects. Adrenaline causes heart rate to increase by 10 to 20 beats per minute, blood pressure to rise by 5 to 10 points,[25] and body temperature in the fingertips to decrease by a few degrees.

The tar and toxins in tobacco smoke damage cilia, the hairlike structures in the bronchial passages that prevent toxins and debris from reaching delicate lung tissue. Researchers believe that chemicals in tar, such as benzopyrene, switch on a gene in lung cells that causes cell mutations that can lead to cancerous growth.[26] These chemicals may also damage a gene with a role in killing cancer cells.

Carbon monoxide in tobacco smoke affects the way smokers process the air they breathe. Normally, oxygen is carried through the bloodstream by hemoglobin, a protein in red blood cells. When carbon monoxide is present, it binds with hemoglobin and prevents red blood cells from carrying a full load of oxygen. Since there is only so much hemoglobin in the body at any given time, oxygen delivery to the cells is impaired. Smokers' bodies try to compensate by creating more red blood cells, but such compensation is insufficient. Heavy smokers quickly become winded during physical activity because the cardiovascular system cannot effectively deliver oxygen to muscle cells.[7]

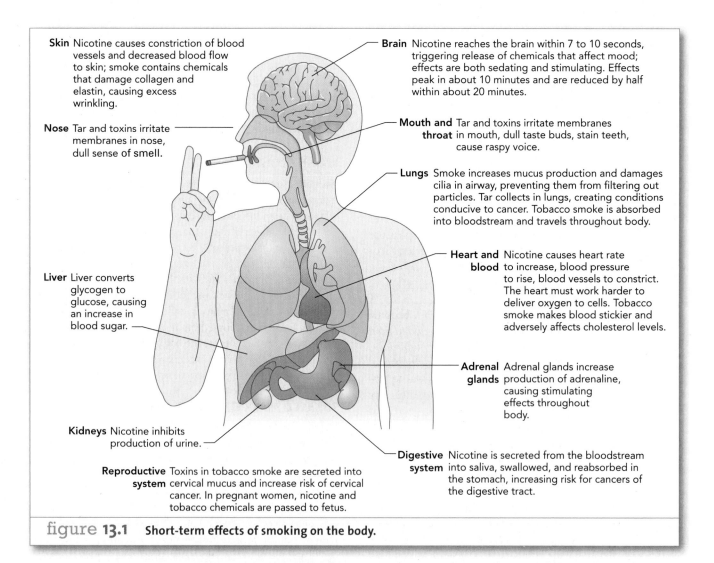

Skin Nicotine causes constriction of blood vessels and decreased blood flow to skin; smoke contains chemicals that damage collagen and elastin, causing excess wrinkling.

Nose Tar and toxins irritate membranes in nose, dull sense of smell.

Liver Liver converts glycogen to glucose, causing an increase in blood sugar.

Kidneys Nicotine inhibits production of urine.

Reproductive system Toxins in tobacco smoke are secreted into cervical mucus and increase risk of cervical cancer. In pregnant women, nicotine and tobacco chemicals are passed to fetus.

Brain Nicotine reaches the brain within 7 to 10 seconds, triggering release of chemicals that affect mood; effects are both sedating and stimulating. Effects peak in about 10 minutes and are reduced by half within about 20 minutes.

Mouth and throat Tar and toxins irritate membranes in mouth, dull taste buds, stain teeth, cause raspy voice.

Lungs Smoke increases mucus production and damages cilia in airway, preventing them from filtering out particles. Tar collects in lungs, creating conditions conducive to cancer. Tobacco smoke is absorbed into bloodstream and travels throughout body.

Heart and blood Nicotine causes heart rate to increase, blood pressure to rise, blood vessels to constrict. The heart must work harder to deliver oxygen to cells. Tobacco smoke makes blood stickier and adversely affects cholesterol levels.

Adrenal glands Adrenal glands increase production of adrenaline, causing stimulating effects throughout body.

Digestive system Nicotine is secreted from the bloodstream into saliva, swallowed, and reabsorbed in the stomach, increasing risk for cancers of the digestive tract.

figure **13.1**   **Short-term effects of smoking on the body.**

LONG-TERM EFFECTS

Smoking accounts for 15 percent of all adult deaths in a given year—more than AIDS, car crashes, alcohol, homicides, illegal drugs, suicides, fires, poor diet, and physical inactivity combined.[27] The greatest health concerns associated with smoking are heart disease, cancer, and chronic lower respiratory diseases.

Cardiovascular Disease The increased heart rate, increased tension in the heart muscle, and constricted blood vessels caused by nicotine lead to hypertension (high blood pressure), which is both a disease in itself and a risk factor for other forms of heart disease, including coronary artery disease, heart attack, stroke, and peripheral vascular disease. Nicotine also makes blood platelets stickier, increasing the tendency of blood clots to form. It raises blood levels of low-density lipoproteins ("bad cholesterol") and decreases levels of high-density lipoproteins ("good cholesterol").[25] People who smoke more than one pack of cigarettes per day have three times the risk for heart disease and congestive heart failure as nonsmokers.[25]

Cancer Smoking is implicated in about 30 percent of all cancer deaths. It is the cause of 87 percent of deaths from lung cancer, and it is associated with cancers of the pancreas, kidney, bladder, breast, and cervix. Smoking and using smokeless tobacco play a major role in cancers of the mouth, throat, and esophagus. Among men, oral cancers are the seventh most frequently occurring cancer. Oral cancers caused by smokeless tobacco tend to occur early in adulthood. The use of alcohol in combination with tobacco increases the risk of oral cancers.[26]

Smoking also increases the cancer-causing potential of occupational and environmental pollutants, such as asbestos and radon. The lung cancer risk associated with exposure to radon, for example, is 6 to 11 times higher in smokers than nonsmokers.[28]

The association between smoking and cancer varies greatly according to the number of cigarettes smoked per day, the degree of inhalation, the age at smoking initiation, and, if the person no longer smokes, the number of years since he or she quit.[23] The likelihood of dying from lung cancer increases with the number of cigarettes smoked, deeper inhalation, and earlier initiation age.

Chronic Obstructive Pulmonary Disease Smoking is a key factor in causing the diseases encompassed by the catgegory *chronic obstructive pulmonary disease* (COPD, also called chronic lower respiratory disease). These are emphysema, chronic bronchitis, and asthma. **Emphysema** is an abnormal condition of the lungs in which the alveoli (air sacs) become enlarged and their walls lose their elasticity. Late in the disease, it becomes increasingly difficult to breathe. Although there may

emphysema
Abnormal condition of the lungs characterized by decreased respiratory function and increased shortness of breath.

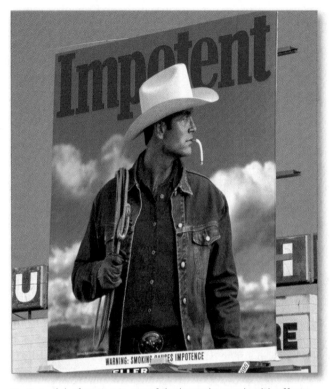

■ Sexual dysfunction is one of the lesser known health effects of tobacco use for both men and women. This billboard is part of an antismoking campaign warning that "smoking causes impotence."

be a hereditary component, people with emphysema almost always have a history of smoking. Bronchitis is irritation and inflammation of the bronchi, the airway passages leading to the lungs. **Chronic bronchitis** is characterized by mucus secretion, cough, and increasing difficulty in breathing. **Asthma** is a respiratory disorder characterized by recurrent episodes of difficulty in breathing, wheezing, coughing, and thick mucus production. Almost as many people die from COPD today as from lung cancer.[21] Thousands more people live with COPD complications and discomfort that seriously compromise their quality of life.

chronic bronchitis
Respiratory disorder characterized by mucus secretion, cough, and increasing difficulty in breathing.

asthma
Respiratory disorder characterized by recurrent episodes of difficulty in breathing, wheezing, coughing, and thick mucus production.

Other Health Effects of Tobacco Use Tobacco is associated with a variety of other health conditions, including changes in the skin (wrinkling), increased risk during surgery, infertility and sexual dysfunction, periodontal disease, duodenal ulcers, osteoporosis, and cataracts. Smoking also reduces the effectiveness of some medications, particularly anti-anxiety drugs and penicillin.

Athletes who smoke have to work harder than nonsmokers in the same physical activity. Respiration is immediately affected by smoking because of the increased presence of carbon monoxide in the blood and decreased oxygen absorption. Nicotine constricts bronchial tubes, and lung function is compromised further by phlegm production. The smoker has less oxygen available for exercise as well as for recovery.

SPECIAL HEALTH RISKS FOR WOMEN

Increased smoking among women since the 1970s has led to an increase in rates of lung cancer, heart disease, and respiratory disease in women; deaths from lung cancer in women, for example, have increased by 400 percent. Women are also more vulnerable to the addictive properties of nicotine.[29, 30]

In addition, smoking is associated with fertility problems in women, menstrual disorders, early menopause, and problems in pregnancy. Women who smoke during pregnancy are at increased risk for miscarriage, stillbirths, preterm delivery, low birth weight in their infants, and perinatal death (infant death a few months before or after birth). Research indicates that infants are at higher risk for sudden infant death syndrome (SIDS) if their mothers smoked during pregnancy. Their risk continues to be higher after birth if they are exposed to environmental tobacco smoke.[31]

SPECIAL HEALTH RISKS FOR MEN

The overall drop in smoking rates for men in the past three decades has led to a reduction of lung cancer deaths in men, but the greater use by men of other forms of tobacco—cigars, pipes, and smokeless tobacco—places them at higher risk for cancers of the mouth, throat, esophagus, and stomach. Like women, men who smoke experience problems with sexual function and fertility. Smoking adversely affects blood flow to the erectile tissue, leading to a higher incidence of erectile dysfunction (impotence); it also alters sperm shape, reduces sperm motility, and decreases the overall number of viable sperm.[32]

SPECIAL HEALTH RISKS FOR ETHNIC MINORITY GROUPS

Mortality rates from several diseases associated with tobacco use, including cardiovascular disease, cancer, and SIDS, are higher for ethnic minority groups than for Whites.[5] For example, African American men and women are more likely to die from lung cancer, heart disease, and stroke than are members of other ethnic groups, despite lower rates of tobacco use. Reductions in smoking among African Americans since the mid-1980s have led to a decline in lung cancer for African American men and a leveling off in African American women.

Reduced smoking rates have also led to a decrease in lung cancer deaths in Hispanic men.[4]

Dependence on tobacco and desire to quit appear to be prevalent across all ethnic groups, but groups vary in rates of smoking, smoking patterns, quitting behavior, and awareness of the health effects of smoking. Health experts stress the need to deliver effective and appropriate tobacco intervention programs to various ethnic groups.

BENEFITS OF QUITTING

Smokers greatly reduce their risk of many health problems when they quit. Health benefits begin immediately and become more significant the longer the individual stays smoke free. Respiratory symptoms associated with COPD, such as smoker's cough and excess mucus production, decrease quickly after quitting. Infection rates for bronchitis and pneumonia drop significantly, and recovery from illnesses like colds and flu is more rapid. Taste and smell return and circulation improves, raising body temperature in the hands and feet and improving brain, heart, and lung function.

Within 1 year, the risk of heart attack and coronary artery disease is reduced by half, and within 5 years, risk approaches that of nonsmokers, as does the risk of stroke.[27] Within 10 years, the risk of lung cancer is cut by 23–50 percent (see the box "When You Quit Smoking: Health Benefits Timeline").

Quitting also increases longevity. Individuals who quit before the age of 50 cut their risk of dying within the next 15 years in half. Men who quit between ages 35 and 39 add an average of 5 years to their lifespan, and women add 3 years. Even quitting after the age of 70 substantially lowers the risk of dying and improves the quality of life.

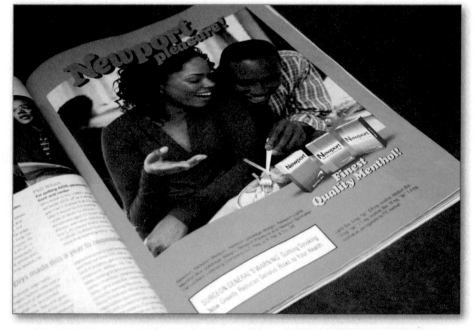

■ African Americans have higher mortality rates from smoking-related illnesses despite lower rates of smoking. Tobacco manufacturers deny that they promote certain products and brands to minority populations and other segments of the general population.

Highlight on Health

When You Quit Smoking: Health Benefits Timeline

Immediately	You stop polluting the air with secondhand smoke; the air around you is no longer dangerous to children and adults.
20 minutes	Blood pressure decreases; pulse rate decreases; temperature of hands and feet increases.
12 hours	Carbon monoxide level in blood drops; oxygen level in the blood increases to normal.
24 hours	Chance of heart attack decreases.
48 hours	Nerve endings start to regrow; exercise gets easier; senses of smell and taste improve.
72 hours	Bronchial tubes relax, making breathing easier; lung capacity increases.
2–12 weeks	Circulation improves; lung functioning increases up to 30 percent.
1–9 months	Fewer coughs, colds, and flu episodes; fatigue and shortness of breath decrease; lung function continues to improve.
1 year	Risk of smoking-related heart attack is cut by half.
5 years	Risk of dying from heart disease and stroke approaches that of a nonsmoker; risk of oral and esophageal cancers is cut by half.
10 years	Risk of dying from lung cancer is cut by half.
10–15 years	Life expectancy reaches that of a person who never smoked.

Source: Health Canada: On the Road to Quitting, © 2008 Health Canada. Reproduced with the permission of the Minister of Public Works and Government Services Canada, 2008.

EFFECTS OF ENVIRONMENTAL TOBACCO SMOKE

You don't have to be a smoker to experience adverse health effects from tobacco smoke. Abundant evidence shows that inhaling the smoke from other people's tobacco products—called **environmental tobacco smoke (ETS),** secondhand smoke, or passive smoking—has serious health consequences. Even 30 minutes of daily secondhand smoke exposure causes heart damage similar to that experienced by a habitual smoker. People who are exposed daily to secondhand smoke have a 30 percent higher rate of death and disease than nonsmokers. In 1993 the Environmental Protection Agency designated ETS a Class A carcinogen—an agent known to cause cancer in humans—and in 2000 the U.S. Department of Health and Human Services added it to their list of known human carcinogens. In 2006, the U.S. surgeon general stated that there is *no* safe level of exposure to secondhand smoke (see the box "Health Effects of Secondhand Smoke").

The effects of ETS vary depending on whether the smoke is coming from the burning end of a cigarette or cigar or the burning tobacco in a pipe (*sidestream smoke*)

environmental tobacco smoke (ETS) Smoke from other people's tobacco products; also called *secondhand smoke* or *passive smoking.*

or has been inhaled and exhaled by the smoker (*mainstream smoke*). Sidestream smoke contains more tar, nicotine, carbon monoxide, and other toxic and carcinogenic compounds than mainstream smoke does.[33] About 85 percent of ETS is sidestream smoke, and 15 percent is mainstream smoke.

Scientists estimate that for every pack of cigarettes smoked by a smoker, the nonsmoker sharing a common air supply will have involuntarily inhaled the equivalent of three to five cigarettes. Scientific evidence supports a significant relationship between long-term exposure to ETS and both heart disease and lung cancer. ETS may also increase the risk of breast cancer, especially if exposure to the smoke occurs during a period when the breasts are growing rapidly, such as puberty or first pregnancy.[33]

ETS can also cause allergic reactions, with symptoms such as eye irritation, headache, cough, nasal congestion, and asthma. About 15 percent of ETS allergies are severe enough to cause disability and qualify people with allergies for occupational disability insurance.[33] This is one reason that employers have implemented smoke-free workplaces.

Because of their smaller body size, infants and children are especially vulnerable to the effects of ETS. Children exposed to ETS experience 10 percent more colds, flu, and other acute respiratory infections than do those not exposed.

Highlight on Health

Health Effects of Secondhand Smoke

The 1986 surgeon general's report entitled *The Health Consequences of Involuntary Smoking* concluded that environmental tobacco smoke was a cause of disease in nonsmokers. Since the publication of this report, the evidence of the harm caused by ETS has become even stronger. In 2006 an updated version of this publication reported four key findings:

- Secondhand smoke exposure causes heart disease and lung cancer in adults and sudden infant death syndrome and respiratory problems in children. Secondhand smoke is responsible for 50,000 deaths annually.

- There is *no* risk-free level of secondhand smoke exposure, with even brief exposure adversely affecting the cardiovascular and respiratory systems. Secondhand smoke can have immediate adverse health effects on blood and blood vessels and quickly irritates the lungs. People with heart disease or respiratory disorders are at especially high risk for adverse effects.

- Only smoke-free environments effectively protect nonsmokers from secondhand smoke exposure in indoor spaces. Although separating smokers and nonsmokers within the same air space confinement reduces adverse effects, it does not eliminate the risks, nor do sophisticated ventilation systems completely eliminate secondhand smoke from indoor areas.

- While great strides have been made in recent years in reducing nonsmoking Americans' secondhand smoke exposure, an estimated 126 million Americans continue to be exposed to secondhand smoke in their homes and workplaces.

As of 2006, 13 states had passed laws prohibiting smoking in restaurants and most bars. Cities have also become proactive in banning smoking in public places and prohibiting smoking near building entrances. The tobacco industry has successfully lobbied state governments to pass preemption laws, which prevent local governments from passing laws more restrictive than those at the state level. Many states have now moved to override such preemptive loopholes.

Sources: "The Health Effects of Secondhand Smoke," remarks by the U.S. surgeon general, 2006, Washington, DC: U.S. Department of Health and Human Services, retrieved from www.surgeongeneral.gov/news/speeches/06272006a.html; "New Dangers of Secondhand Smoke," by A. Park, 2007, Time, June 28, retrieved May 16, 2008, from www.time.com/time/health/article/0,8599.1638535.00.html?cnn=yes.

ETS aggravates asthma symptoms and increases the risk of SIDS.[35]

Some states, including California, Arkansas, and Louisiana, have moved to ban smoking in cars when children under the age of 6 are present. The rationale is twofold: first, secondhand smoke is especially hazardous to young children, and second, children are incapable of making a decision about whether to be in a smoke-filled car and so deserve protection. The American Medical Association supports such legislation.

Quitting and Treatment Options

Once a person becomes an established smoker, quitting is exceptionally difficult. Nearly four of every five smokers want to quit smoking. Many daily smokers believe they will not be smoking in 5 years, but 75 percent are still smoking 5 to 6 years later. Only about 7 percent of smokers who quit are successfully abstaining a year later. Even among smokers who have lost a lung or undergone major heart surgery, only about 50 percent stop smoking for more than a few weeks.[5, 23, 35]

The good news is that smokers who quit for a year have an 85 percent chance of maintaining their abstinence. Those who make it to 5 years have a 97 percent chance of continued success. Most people don't succeed the first time they try to quit—in fact, the average number of attempts required for successful smoking cessation is seven—but many succeed on subsequent attempts.[23]

TREATMENT PROGRAMS TO QUIT SMOKING

Treatment programs can be quite effective; 20–40 percent of smokers who enter good treatment programs are able to quit smoking for at least a year.[33] Some programs are provided by hospitals. At the Mayo Hospital Nicotine Dependence Center, for example, smokers participate in an intensive residential smoking cessation program that includes daily group and individual therapy, stress reduction techniques, nutrition information, exercise, and a 12-step program similar to Alcoholics Anonymous.

Many programs encourage smokers to limit or eliminate their consumption of alcohol while they are quitting, because alcohol interacts with nicotine in complex ways and can make quitting more difficult. Dieting is not recommended while trying to quit, despite the potential for weight gain. Research suggests that individuals who diet while also trying to stop smoking are vulnerable to relapse. A more effective strategy is to tolerate the weight gain for the time being and address it after successfully quitting. Combining exercise with smoking cessation appears to be the most effective approach to managing the potential for weight gain. Another element is social support and encouragement from important people in the smoker's life.

MEDICATIONS TO QUIT SMOKING

In **nicotine replacement therapy (NRT),** a controlled amount of nicotine is administered, which gradually reduces daily nicotine use with minimal withdrawal symptoms. The transdermal patch and nicotine gum are the most common delivery systems, but also available are a nicotine inhaler, a nicotine spray, a nicotine lozenge, and a nicotine hand gel. The gel, sold under the name Nicogel, is marketed as a product for tobacco users who find themselves in situations where they can't smoke. A quick-evaporating hand gel made from tobacco extracts, Nicogel can reduce nicotine cravings for up to 4 hours.

nicotine replacement therapy (NRT)
Treatment for nicotine addiction in which a controlled amount of nicotine is administered to gradually reduce daily nicotine use with minimal withdrawal symptoms.

Although nicotine is addictive no matter how it is administered, NRT products contain none of the carcinogens or toxic gases found in cigarette smoke, so they are a safer form of nicotine delivery.[34] Using one or more of the NRT products doubles a person's chances of success in quitting. NRT is beneficial when used as part of a comprehensive physician-promoted cessation program. It can help control withdrawal symptoms and craving while the individual is learning new behavioral patterns.[35, 36]

Other smoking cessation aids work not by replacing nicotine but by acting on the neurotransmitter receptors in the brain that are affected by nicotine. Bupropion is a prescription smoking cessation drug that acts in this way. It was approved in 2001 by the FDA and is marketed under the trade name Zyban. Bupropion is also prescribed as an antidepressant under the name Wellbutrin; Zyban and Wellbutrin should not be taken together.

Varenicline (marketed in the United States as Chantix) is another smoking cessation drug that acts on neurotransmitter receptors. It was approved by the FDA in 2006. Clinical studies have found that more than one in five people using varenicline quit smoking for at least 1 year, a significant improvement over other smoking cessation drugs.

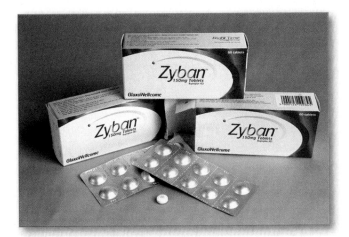

■ Zyban and Chantix belong to a newer category of smoking cessation aids that work by acting on neurotransmitter receptors in the brain rather than replacing nicotine. Smokers are sometimes advised to continue smoking or to use a nicotine replacement product for the first few days of using these products to ease nicotine withdrawal symptoms.

NicVax is an experimental nicotine vaccine that blocks the pleasurable effects of smoking. It works by eliciting the production of antibodies that bind with nicotine molecules in the bloodstream, preventing them from entering nicotine receptors in the brain. NicVax has not been approved by the FDA, but early studies have been encouraging.

QUITTING ON YOUR OWN: DEVELOPING A BEHAVIOR CHANGE PLAN

Despite the hardships of withdrawal and the challenges of behavior change, quitting smoking is worth it, and the majority of people who quit do so on their own.

One approach is to develop a behavior change plan similar to the one we described for cutting back on alcohol consumption in Chapter 11. A first step is determining your readiness to quit. As discussed in Chapter 1, trying to change a behavior when you are not ready to change is pointless and counterproductive. It will only lead to failure and discouragement. Refer to the box "Assesssing Your Stage of Change" in Chapter 1 (p. 12) for a quick evaluation of your own stage of change in regard to quitting smoking. If you are in the contemplation or action stage, you can develop a behavior change plan by following the steps described next.

Record and Analyze Your Smoking Patterns First, keep track of your smoking for 2 weeks, noting when, where, and with whom you smoke. Note the triggers or cues for smoking and your thoughts and feelings at the time. Then analyze your record to get a sense of your smoking patterns. Do you always smoke in certain situations or at certain times? The Add It Up activity for Chapter 13 at the end of the book can help you analyze your smoking patterns and identify your reasons for smoking.

Establish Goals Set a specific date to quit. Choose a time when you will be relatively stress free—not during exams, for example—so that you will have the needed energy, attention, and focus. Experts recommend aiming for some time within 2 weeks of when you begin to plan. Plan to quit completely on that date; tapering off rarely works because it only prolongs withdrawal.

Prepare to Quit Your most important asset in quitting is your firm commitment to do so. At the same time, you can take specific, concrete steps to increase your chances of success. Consider these questions:

■ Why do you want to quit? Make a list of your reasons and post them on your refrigerator or in another prominent place in your home. Examples are better health, cleaner clothes, more spending money, and a sense of achievement.

■ If you tried to quit in the past, what helped and what didn't? Learn from your mistakes. Don't be discouraged—as noted earlier, many people try several times before they finally succeed in quitting.

■ What situations are going to be the most difficult? How can you plan ahead to handle them? To the extent you can, reorganize your life to avoid situations in which you were accustomed to smoking and to include situations that are smoke free.

- What pleasures do you get from smoking? How can you get those pleasures from life-enhancing activities instead of smoking?

- Who can help you? Tell your family and friends you are planning to quit and ask for their support. Find out if your state has a telephone quitline. See the box "Preparing to Quit Smoking" for more tips.

Implement Your Plan Make sure you no longer have any tobacco products when your quit day arrives. Be prepared to experience symptoms of withdrawal and have a plan for handling them, even if it's just "toughing it out." Exercise will help ease cravings for nicotine and elevate your mood, so make sure you exercise daily. About one in five smokers may experience mild depression after quitting. Exercise will also improve sleep and help you limit weight gain. Drink plenty of fluids; they help flush nicotine from your body. Don't drink as much caffeine as you are used to, though; the effects of caffeine become more pronounced when you stop smoking and can lead to nervousness or jitters.

Prevent Relapse Symptoms of nicotine withdrawal last from 2 to 3 weeks, although the most acute symptoms may last only a few days. See Table 13.2 for a summary of symptoms, their causes, and suggested relief strategies.

Abstinence becomes easier with time, although it can still be difficult. Most relapses occur within the first 3 months.[23] There are two main lines of defense for maintaining prolonged abstinence. First, avoid high-risk situations. Relapse episodes are much more likely to occur if you are near someone else who smokes or you are in a smoky environment. Seek out smoke-free restaurants and bars and make your home smoke free.[37, 38]

Second, develop coping mechanisms. Relapses are prompted by stress, anger, frustration and depression.[39] Make sure you have strategies to deal with these feelings, whether relaxation techniques, exercise, social support, or cognitive techniques. Examples of cognitive techniques are reminding yourself of why you quit, thinking about the people you know who have quit, adjusting your self-image so that you think of yourself as an ex-smoker or a nonsmoker rather than a smoker, reminding yourself that withdrawal symptoms mean your body is flushing out toxic nicotine residue, and congratulating yourself every time you beat an urge to smoke. Remember, you are overcoming an addiction to an extremely harmful and addictive drug; your discomfort and effort will be repaid with better health and longer life.

Confronting the Tobacco Challenge

The cost of tobacco use to individuals and society is enormous. An estimated 440,000 Americans die every year from smoking-related causes. The financial losses from tobacco smoke amount to billions of dollars in lost work productiv-

Challenges & Choices

Preparing to Quit Smoking

When you have decided to quit and set a quit date, you can make adjustments in your environment and lifestyle that will improve your chances of success. Here are some tips:

- Make your home a smoke-free zone. If feasible, ask your friends not to smoke around you.

- Throw away all your cigarettes and ashtrays.

- Get your clothes cleaned so that they don't smell of cigarette smoke. Air out your car and house.

- Make an appointment with your dentist to get your teeth cleaned.

- If you want to use nicotine replacement therapy, consult with your physician about what product may work best for you.

- Stock up on low-calorie munchies to help you handle cravings with minimal weight gain.

- Make sure your social support system is established. Let your family and friends know your quit date.

- Try to make your last few days of smoking inconvenient, such as smoking only outdoors when it is very cold.

- Write a good-bye letter to cigarettes as a symbolic way of letting go.

It's Not Just Personal . . .

The decision to quit smoking is a personal one. Yet experts say that "going public" with this decision is usually best. You'll need the support of those closest to you—family and friends—to help you create an environment for success and to keep you going when you want to give up.

Sources: Dying to Quit: Why We Smoke and How to Stop, by J. Brigham, 1998, Washington, DC: National Academies Press; Treating Tobacco Use and Dependence: Clinical Practice Guideline, by M.C. Fiore, W.C. Bailey, S.S. Cohen, et al., 2000, Rockville, MD: U.S. Department of Health and Human Services, Public Health Service.

ity ($92 million), health care expenditures ($89 billion), and Social Security survivor insurance (between $0.6 and $3 billion) each year.[40] Given this devastation, why are the manufacture and sale of tobacco products legal in this country?

The answer to this question is complex. Tobacco has been part of the agricultural economy of the country since colonial times, and today it is a multibillion-dollar industry with tremendous lobbying power and a huge impact on the nation's economic health. Many state economies depend on tobacco, and elected representatives from those states make sure tobacco interests are protected at the federal level. Because smoking is viewed as a personal decision, there are many constraints on the government's ability to protect citizens and consumers from the hazards of tobacco use. Still, significant inroads have been made in confronting the challenge posed by tobacco, and the tobacco industry is facing tremendous pressure on many fronts.

THE NONSMOKERS' RIGHTS MOVEMENT AND LEGISLATIVE BATTLES

Beginning in the 1970s, a nonsmokers' rights movement took shape as a result of growing public awareness and outrage at the damage inflicted by tobacco. Smoking came to be seen as both a public health problem and a problematic behavior.[41]

By 2003, thousands of local laws and ordinances were in place across the country, creating smoke-free workplaces, restaurants, bars, and public places. Some tobacco control laws have also been passed at the state level. In 1975 Minnesota became the first state to enact a clean indoor air act requiring nonsmoking areas in public places. California has had a ban on smoking in workplaces since 1994 and on smoking in bars since 1998. The federal government also has tobacco control measures in place, such as the ban on smoking on domestic airline flights.

LAWSUITS AND COURT SETTLEMENTS

In the 1990s tobacco companies began to face class action suits, cases representing claims of injury by hundreds or thousands of smokers. In addition, states began suing tobacco companies for losses incurred by state health insurance funds used to pay for tobacco-related diseases.

These pressures led to the 1998 Master Settlement Agreement (MSA), in which the tobacco industry agreed to pay $206 billion to 46 states over a 25-year period in exchange for protection from future lawsuits by the states and other public entities. Other provisions of the MSA included a ban on billboard advertising and restrictions on advertising aimed at children. The settlement money from the MSA was to be used by the states primarily to fund tobacco education and prevention programs.

Some of the money went to the American Legacy Foundation's "Truth" campaign, a nationwide effort to tell the truth about tobacco products to youth. Studies indicate that this campaign was successful in deterring children and teenagers from taking up smoking.[42] Still, the campaign's annual spending pales in comparison with the billions spent by tobacco companies on advertising and promoting tobacco products. Furthermore, money from the settlement may dry up as a result of loopholes in the agreement.[43] For more on

Table 13.2 | What to Expect When You Quit

Symptom	Reason	Duration	Relief
Irritability	Body craves nicotine.	2–4 weeks	Take walks, hot baths; use relaxation techniques.
Fatigue	Nicotine is a stimulant.	2–4 weeks	Take naps; don't push yourself.
Insomnia	Nicotine affects brain waves.	2–4 weeks	Avoid caffeine after 6:00 p.m.; use relaxation techniques.
Coughing, dry throat, nasal drip	Body is getting rid of excess mucus.	A few days	Drink fluids; try cough drops.
Dizziness	Brain is getting more oxygen.	1–2 days	Be cautious moving; change positions slowly.
Poor concentration	Nicotine is a stimulant, boosts concentration.	1–2 weeks	Get enough sleep; exercise; eat well.
Tightness in chest	Muscles are tense from nicotine craving or sore from coughing.	A few days	Use relaxation techniques, especially deep breathing; take hot baths.
Constipation, gas, stomach pain	Intestinal movement decreases for brief time.	1–2 weeks	Drink fluids; add fiber to diet (fruits, vegetables, whole grains).
Hunger	Nicotine craving can feel like hunger.	Up to several weeks	Drink water or low-calorie drinks; have low-calorie snacks on hand.
Headaches	Brain is getting more oxygen.	1–2 weeks	Drink water; use relaxation techniques.
Craving for a cigarette	Withdrawal from nicotine.	Most acute first few days; can recur for months	Wait it out; distract yourself; exercise; use relaxation techniques.

Source: www.quitnet.com.

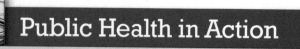

Public Health in Action

Ending the Tobacco Problem

Although smoking rates have declined significantly since 1960, the rates have stabilized at about 20 percent for adults. Aggressive measures will be needed to further reduce smoking rates and the impact of tobacco use on morbidity and mortality. In 2007 the American Legacy Foundation and the Institute of Medicine released a joint report, *Ending the Tobacco Problem: A Blueprint for the Nation,* outlining several important public health targets:

■ *Helping smokers quit.* Telephone help lines have been effective in increasing smoking abstinence by as much as 30–50 percent. The U.S. Department of Health and Human Services provides a national quitline network that supports states in establishing and maintaining quitlines. Insurance companies, managed care, and employee benefit plans should cover reimbursement for effective cessation programs as a lifetime benefit.

■ *Encouraging community action.* Comprehensive state programs are essential for reducing smoking rates. State tobacco control programs, the CDC, philanthropic foundations, and voluntary organizations should actively support community coalitions advocating smoke-free environments. States and cities should enact complete bans on smoking in all nonresidential indoor locations, including workplaces, malls, restaurants, and bars. Parents should maintain smoke-free homes and smoke-free vehicles. Owners of multi-apartment buildings and condominium developers should include and enforce nonsmoking clauses in their leases and sales agreements.

■ *Increasing tobacco excise taxes.* Variations in state tobacco excise taxes encourage tobacco smuggling across states and tax evasion. States with excise taxes below the level applied by the top one-fifth of states should significantly increase their excise taxes to prevent smuggling. The federal excise tax should be significantly increased. One-third of the revenue from the federal excise tax should be set aside to support comprehensive state smoking cessation programs.

■ *Supporting stronger federal regulation.* The FDA should have broad regulatory authority over the manufacture, distribution, marketing, and use of tobacco products. Manufacturers should be required to list the quantities of all chemicals in their tobacco products and product smoke. Tobacco manufacturers should be banned from targeting their products to youth for any purpose, including surveys of youth opinions, attitudes, and behaviors. Health warnings on tobacco products should be strengthened and placed under the FDA's regulation.

Source: Ending the Tobacco Problem: A Blueprint for the Nation, *eds. Richard J. Bonnie, Kathleen Stratton, and Robert B. Wallace, Institute of Medicine, 2007, Washington, DC: National Academies Press.*

the American Legacy Foundation's efforts, see the box "Ending the Tobacco Problem."

REGULATION AND TAXATION: HARM REDUCTION STRATEGIES

The U.S. government doesn't prohibit tobacco use by adults or force individuals to stop smoking, but it does take actions aimed at reducing the harm associated with the use of tobacco products by those who continue to smoke. A *harm reduction approach* to tobacco use focuses on reducing a smoker's exposure to nicotine, tar, and carbon monoxide. One way to achieve this is by limiting access to tobacco products, such as by increasing the price through taxes. Another way, one promoted by tobacco companies, is the use of "light" cigarettes. The latter approach has proved to be just another way to dupe consumers.

Limiting Access to Tobacco Access to tobacco can be limited by increasing cost, reducing physical availability, and regulating tobacco marketing campaigns. When taxes on tobacco products are increased, raising their price, sales and use decline. Cigarette tax increases have been particularly effective in discouraging people from starting smoking.[44]

Physical availability of tobacco products is reduced when the laws restricting sales to minors are enforced. States are required to conduct random, unannounced inspections of places where tobacco is sold, and reports detailing results of these inspections must be submitted to the federal government each year. Physical availability is also reduced when smoking is prohibited in workplaces and public spaces.

Restrictions on tobacco advertising may affect access to tobacco as well.[45] Tobacco companies argue that their advertising efforts are aimed solely at creating brand loyalty, not at attracting new smokers. Antitobacco activists draw from extensive research to refute this claim. Tobacco marketing campaigns appear to be specifically directed at children, women, and minorities. Children as young as age 6 have reported familiarity with cigarette ads using cartoon characters.[45]

The Scam of "Light" Cigarettes "Light" cigarettes with lower levels of tar and nicotine have been promoted by the tobacco industry as safer than regular cigarettes. This marketing campaign has been successful: Lower tar cigarettes have become the best-selling cigarettes in North America.[46]

Lower tar cigarettes are not safer than regular cigarettes. Smokers who switch to these cigarettes compensate

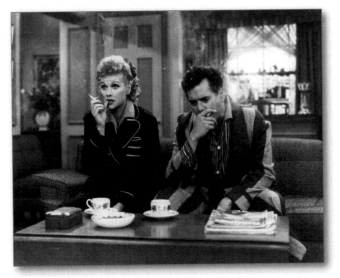

■ Fifty years ago, the cultural climate included acceptance and normalization of smoking in virtually all settings. Lucille Ball and Desi Arnaz were just two of the many TV actors and celebrities who modeled smoking for the public.

for reduced yields of tobacco and nicotine by taking more puffs per cigarette, inhaling more deeply, and smoking more cigarettes per day.[47] Large studies of mortality risks have found no evidence that lower tar cigarettes reduce health risks.[48] Public health experts strongly argue that the tobacco industry should not be allowed to market cigarettes using the terms *mild, light,* or *ultra-light,* and the World Health Organization Framework Convention on Tobacco Control specifically outlaws these terms. The truth is that there is no such thing as a safe cigarette.

EDUCATION AND PREVENTION: CHANGING THE CULTURAL CLIMATE

In the 1950s, cigarette smoking was an accepted part of everyday life. People smoked in restaurants, movie theaters, concert halls, college classrooms, offices, and airplanes. On television, quiz show panelists, newshour anchormen, and sitcom characters smoked on the air. In movies, smoking was associated with the elegant, sophisticated lifestyle of characters played by actors such as Katharine Hepburn and Humphrey Bogart.

Those days are gone, along with the social norms that made smoking a socially acceptable behavior. Awareness of the health hazards of smoking and ETS, greater skepticism toward tobacco advertising and promotion, and increased willingness on the part of nonsmokers to assert their rights have all contributed to changes in the cultural climate surrounding tobacco use.

Clearly, however, there is more to do. Movies still depict attractive characters smoking, cigarette ads still lead young people to associate smoking with fun and relaxation, and teenagers still try cigarettes every day. Antismoking campaigns that focus on the risks of smoking fail to counter the positive images that are conveyed by movies, media,

and advertising and that motivate young people to take up smoking.[36] Research indicates that perception of risk is not a deterrent when teenagers are thinking about experimenting with tobacco.

One recommendation by health experts is that antismoking campaigns use some of the same strategies that have worked for the tobacco companies.[48] For example, they should target specific market segments, focusing on young people and their attitudes, values, and lifestyles. Messages should be delivered repeatedly over long periods of time in a multitude of formats, and they should be varied to appeal to the age and ethnic/cultural identity of the intended audience. As many forms of media as possible should be used, including public service announcements, paid advertising during prime time, and celebrity endorsement and support.

Community interventions are also recommended, working through schools, local government, civic organizations, and health agencies. Many colleges and universities are now smoke-free environments, as are many fast-food restaurant chains and a majority of the country's shopping malls. All of these efforts have the potential to create a fundamental change in social norms and in public attitudes toward tobacco use. Such a change, in turn, has the potential to close the pipeline of new smokers and motivate current smokers to quit.

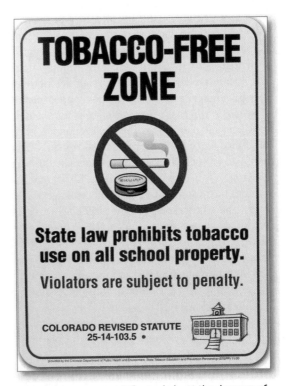

■ As people become more informed about the dangers of smoking and of secondhand smoke, smoke-free environments proliferate and are more accepted. The cultural climate is changing, but more needs to be done, especially to help adolescents keep from getting hooked.

You Make the Call

Smoking Restrictions in Public Places

There is no longer any doubt that environmental tobacco smoke (ETS) significantly increases the risk of smoking-related diseases in individuals who do not smoke. For example, the rate of lung cancer among spouses of smokers is higher than among spouses of nonsmokers, and rates of respiratory infections in children are higher in families with smokers than in families without smokers. In such cases, smoking or not smoking is a personal issue with ethical dimensions.

ETS becomes a public policy issue when smoking affects people in public accommodations, where access is open to everyone. There are two types of public accommodations: those operated by the government on behalf of taxpayers and those operated by private business owners on their own behalf. Most people agree that facilities operated with taxpayer support, such as public universities, courthouses, and libraries, have the right to ban smoking, since most taxpayers—75–80 percent of the population—are nonsmokers. (Some people do argue that public facilities should take into consideration the rights of smokers as well, since they are also taxpayers.)

More controversial are efforts to ban smoking in facilities operated by private owners, such as restaurants, bars, movie theaters, and stores. Technically, any place that allows a person to walk in off the street can be defined as a public accommodation, and many cities include such small businesses in their laws and ordinances restricting smoking. In some local jurisdictions, nonsmoking restrictions are extended to outdoor areas like beaches, parks, pedestrian malls, and areas within a certain distance—for example, 50 feet—of doors and entries to buildings. Proponents of smoking restrictions argue that government has not only the right but the duty to protect the public from known health hazards. They cite rates of disease and death from ETS and point out that even brief exposure causes respiratory irritation. People who work in bars and restaurants are particularly at risk from ETS when patrons are allowed to smoke. Proponents argue that the right of nonsmokers to breathe clean air supersedes the rights of smokers to light up.

Opponents of smoking restrictions argue that the government does not have the right to intrude on small businesses. They view such restrictions as an oppressive crusade by nonsmokers to impose their tastes and preferences on smokers, and they suggest government controls may next extend into private residences. They point out that businesses like bars and restaurants depend on customer satisfaction, and when smoking is prohibited, revenues may go down. Evidence to date has not been conclusive on this possible effect.

Laws are changing, but restrictions on smoking in public places are still controversial. What do you think?

PROS

- Since the 1986 surgeon general's report, ETS has been identified as a cause of cancer, including lung cancer, in healthy nonsmokers and has been associated with an increased frequency of respiratory infections in the children of smokers.

- Even brief exposure to ETS can cause headaches, coughing, dizziness, nausea, and irritation to the eyes, nose, and throat.

- Nonsmoking employees and patrons are exposed to ETS when patrons are allowed to smoke.

- Loss of revenue by restaurants and bars that adopt smoke-free accommodations has not been proven by objective studies.

- Any greater revenue taken in by bars and restaurants that allow smoking is offset by higher costs in other areas—maintenance expenses (cleaning of carpets, drapes, clothes), insurance premiums (fire, health, worker compensation), and labor costs (absenteeism, productivity).

- The right to smoke should not interfere with the nonsmoker's right to breathe smoke-free air.

CONS

- Restaurant owners are entrepreneurs and have the right to operate their businesses without undue local government interference.

- Bans on smoking may reduce revenue at restaurants and bars and put them out of business.

- Many restaurants and bars have implemented self-imposed bans; government action is not needed.

- If people don't like smoke, they can go to another restaurant.

- If local government can control the actions of private citizens in restaurants, what is to stop it from extending its reach into private residences?

Sources: "Reducing Tobacco Use: A Report of the Surgeon General," U.S. Department of Health and Human Services, 2000, Atlanta, GA: Centers for Disease Control and Prevention; "Smoke-free Laws Do Not Harm Profits," by N. Simpson, 2005, Tobacco Control, 14 (4), pp. 75–76.

In Review

1. **Who smokes, and why is it a problem?** About 20 percent of the U.S. adult population are smokers, with higher rates of smoking among men than women and among college students than the general population. Tobacco use is the leading preventable cause of death in the United States.

2. **What are the main tobacco products?** Cigarettes are by far the most commonly used tobacco products, trailed by cigars, pipes, and smokeless (chewing) tobacco. Most newer products (for example, flavored cigarettes, tobacco for water pipes, little cigars, snus) are marketed as safer alternatives, but nearly all contain nicotine and, when burned, produce thousands of toxic substances.

3. **Why do people smoke?** Nicotine is one of the most highly addictive psychoactive drugs, and quitting is exceptionally difficult. Most users start in adolescence and become both physiologically and psychologically (behaviorally) dependent. The tobacco industry targets young people and minorities and advertises smoking as glamorous and rebellious.

4. **How does tobacco use affect your health?** In the short term, smoking produces both sedating and stimulating effects; it increases heart rate and blood pressure, damages cilia in the lungs, and impairs oxygen delivery to cells. In the long term, it causes cardiovascular disease, cancer, chronic obstructive pulmonary disease, and numerous other effects in virtually every body system. Environmental tobacco smoke, or secondhand smoke, causes health problems in nonsmokers comparable with those caused in smokers. There is no safe level of exposure to secondhand smoke.

5. **How can you quit?** Treatment programs are available, but most people who quit do so on their own; a structured behavior change plan can help. Smoking cessation products can help, too. They work either by replacing nicotine or by acting on neurotransmitter receptors in the brain. Despite pressure from the tobacco industry, the antismoking movement is gaining ground, supported by court decisions and government actions.

WWW For a detailed summary of this chapter and a comprehensive set of review questions, visit the Online Learning Center at **www.mhhe.com/teague2e**.

Web Resources

Action on Smoking and Health (ASH): This site covers a wide range of information on smoking, including nonsmokers' rights, guidelines on quitting smoking, smoking risks, and statistics on smoking.
www.ash.org

American Lung Association: See the Quit Smoking feature of the association's Web site for news articles, resources for support, information on legislation, and fact sheets.
www.lungusa.org

Americans for Nonsmokers' Rights: This organization offers information on environmental smoke; how to protect yourself from smoke at home, at work, and in the community; legal issues related to smoking; and special concerns for youth.
www.no-smoke.org

The BACCHUS Network: This site provides information aimed at helping people quit smoking. It includes a clock showing the benefits of smoking cessation over time.
www.bacchusnetwork.org.

CDC's Tobacco Information and Prevention Sources (TIPS): Everything from the surgeon general's reports to Celebrities Against Smoking and community action programs can be found here.
www.cdc.gov/tobacco

Center for Tobacco Cessation: Look for the Resources section of this site for a varied list of links offering information on smoking cessation, including special groups such as women and young girls, useful information for smokers, and vital information on nicotine addiction.
www.ctcinfo.org

Smokefree.Gov: The online guide to quitting smoking offered at this site includes practical steps for preparing to quit, quitting, and "staying quit." You can also instant-message an expert or get telephone support.
www.smokefree.gov

PART FOUR

Your Relationships and Sexuality

People are social beings; we spend our lives, from birth to death, embedded in relationships with others. Healthy relationships—with friends, intimate partners, and family members—support and enhance our well-being and life satisfaction. What constitutes a healthy relationship? What role does our sexuality play in our partnerships? How can we ensure healthy families? These are some of the questions addressed by the chapters in Part 4.

Think It Over

- Are family ties, friendships, or intimate relationships most important to you at this time in your life?
- What does being sexually responsible mean to you?
- What factors influence your opinions about reproductive choices?

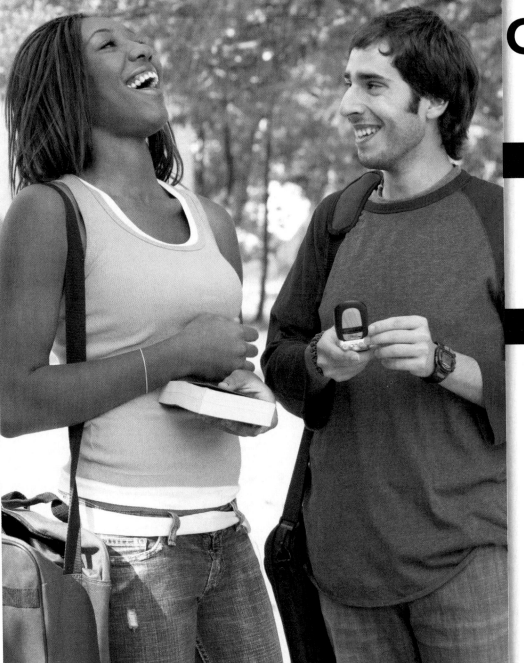

14

Relationships
Connection
and
Communication

Ever Wonder...

- if your primary relationship is a healthy one?

- how you can get better at resolving conflict in your relationships?

- why so many marriages end in divorce?

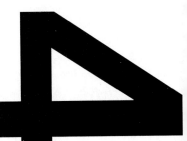

Your Health Today

www.mhhe.com/teague2e

Go to the Online Learning Center for *Your Health Today* for interactive activities, quizzes, flashcards, Web links, and more resources related to this chapter.

Relationships are at the heart of human experience. We are born into a family; grow up in a community; have class-mates, teammates, and colleagues; find a partner from among our acquaintances and friends; and establish our own family. Yet for all their importance in our lives, relationships are fraught with difficulties and challenges. About half of all marriages in the United States end in divorce, and many children grow up in a single-parent or blended family of one kind or another. Many people also live alone in the United States, either by choice or by chance.

We sometimes take relationships for granted, but they deserve as much attention and effort as other aspects of our lives. They are a vital part of wellness. People with a strong social support system have better mental and physical health, are more capable of dealing with stress and adverse life events, and may even live longer than those without such support (see the box "Relationships and Health").[1] Social isolation contributes to depression and feelings of helpless-ness and hopelessness; being isolated undermines a person's self-esteem and sense of purpose in life.

Healthy Relationships

Three kinds of important relationships are the one you have with yourself, the ones you have with friends, and the ones you have with intimate partners. In each, certain qualities serve to enhance the relationship's positive effects.

A HEALTHY SENSE OF SELF

All your relationships begin with who you are as an indi-vidual. A healthy sense of self, reasonably high self-esteem, a capacity for empathy, and the ability both to be alone and to be with others are examples of such individual attributes. Many people develop these assets growing up in their fami-lies, but if you experience deficits in childhood, you can still make up for them later in life.

In Chapter 3 we discussed the characteristics of men-tally healthy people. They include optimism, resilience, a sense of self-efficacy, and emotional intelligence. We also discussed ways of enhancing your mental health, such as cultivating a supportive social network, developing good communication skills, and maintaining a healthy lifestyle. The attributes and skills that enhance the mental health of individuals are also the building blocks of healthy relationships.

FRIENDSHIPS AND OTHER KINDS OF RELATIONSHIPS

Friendship is a reciprocal relationship based on mutual liking and caring, respect and trust, interest and compan-ionship. We often share a big part of our personal history with our friends. Compared with romantic partnerships, friendships are usually more stable and longer lasting; in fact, some last a lifetime. Many people have hundreds of

Who's at Risk

Relationships and Health

- People with lower levels of social involvement are one and a half times more likely than people with stronger support systems to have a first heart attack, and they are more likely to be readmitted to the hospital after discharge.

- Better relationship quality has been shown to have a positive effect on health promotion behav-iors in long-term marriages.

- Married men—regardless of race, age, income, or education—have been found to be healthier than men who are single, divorced, or widowed.

- Men who have secure marriages and who con-tinue to be sexually active tend to live longer, heal faster, and get sick less often.

- Married women in satisfying relationships have a health advantage when compared to mar-ried women with low levels of satisfaction and women who are unmarried. The advantage includes having lower blood pressure, lower cholesterol levels, and lower levels of depression, anxiety, and anger.

acquaintances but only three to seven people they would really call friends.

A recent survey found that despite experiencing very high levels of stress, 97 percent of Americans report hav-ing people in their lives that they trust and can turn to when they need support. More than one-third of respondents said they had up to five people, more than half said they had more than five people, and only 3 percent reported having no one. Women (58 percent) were more likely than men (48 percent) to have more than five people. Men are more likely to turn to their spouse or partner for emotional sup-port, and women are more likely to turn to other family members.[2] Another study found that, in 2004, 15 percent of respondents said they were close friends with a mem-ber of another race, up from the percentage in 1985, and that the least socially isolated people were White and well educated.[3]

Along with family ties and involvement in social activi-ties, friendships offer a psychological and emotional buffer against stress, anxiety, and depression. They help protect you against illness, and they help you cope with problems if you do become ill. Friendships and other kinds of social support increase your sense of belonging, purpose, and self-worth.[1] For tips on cultivating friendships, see the box "Expanding Your Circle of Friends."

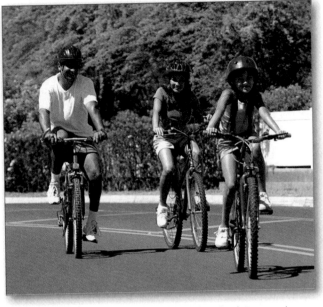

■ A healthy sense of self begins in childhood, when parents can let their children know they are valued by spending time with them. People carry their early sense of self into all their adult relationships.

Strengths of Successful Partnerships

An intimate relationship with a partner has many similarities with friendships, but it has other qualities as well. Compared with friendships, partnerships are more exclusive, involve deeper levels of connection and caring, and have a sexual component. The divorce rate tells us that many intimate partnerships are not successful. What makes them succeed? The following are some characteristics of successful partnerships:

■ The more mature and independent individuals are, the more likely they are to establish intimacy in their relationship. Independence and maturity often increase with age; in fact, the best predictor of a successful marriage is the age of the partners.

■ The partners have both self-esteem and mutual respect.

■ The partners understand the importance of good communication and are willing to work at their communication skills. They know that listening to the other's feelings and trying to see things from the other's perspective are key in communication, even if they do not ultimately agree.

■ The partners have a good sexual relationship, one that includes the open expression of affection and respect for the other's needs and boundaries.

■ The partners enjoy spending time together in leisure activities, but they also value the time they spend alone pursuing their own interests.

■ The partners are able to acknowledge their strengths and failings and take responsibility for both.

■ The partners are assertive about what they want and need in the relationship and flexible about accommodating the other's wants and needs. They can maintain a sense of self in the face of pressure to agree or conform.

Challenges & Choices

Expanding Your Circle of Friends

Some people prefer a small circle of friends, and others enjoy having a large and diverse social support system. If you want to expand your circle of friends, here are some tips:

■ *Get out with your pet.* Take your dog to a beach or dog park. Conversation happens naturally between pet owners.

■ *Work out.* Join a class at the gym or community center, get a group of people to take yoga at lunchtime, or start a walk group.

■ *Do lunch.* Invite someone to join you for lunch, or for breakfast or dinner.

■ *Volunteer.* Many organizations need volunteers, including museums, concert halls, churches, hospitals, community centers, and campus programs. Common interests are a positive basis for relationships.

■ *Join an organization in support of an issue or a cause you believe in.* People working toward common goals often form strong bonds, whether it's cleaning up the environment, working in a political campaign, or rescuing abandoned animals.

■ *Join a hobby group.* Find a group with similar interests, such as gardening, hiking, cycling, books, crafts, or singing.

■ *Go back to school.* Take a college course or adult education class in something you've been meaning to pursue but never had time for before, such as painting, interior design, or auto mechanics.

It's Not Just Personal . . .

According to the U.S. Bureau of Labor Statistics, about 60.8 million Americans, or 26.2 percent of the population over 16 years of age, volunteered through or for an organization between September 2006 and September 2007. About 23 percent of all men and 29 percent of all women do some kind of volunteer work.

Source: "Social Support: A Buffer Against Life's Ills," Mayo Clinic, 2005, www.mayoclinic.com.

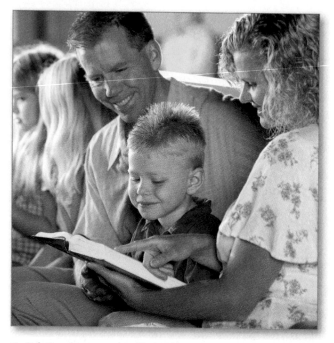

■ Relationships are more likely to be strong and lasting when partners share important values, including spiritual values.

■ The partners know that disagreement is normal in relationships and that when conflict is handled constructively, it can strengthen the relationship.[4]

■ The partners are friends as well as lovers, able to focus unselfish caring on each other.

■ The couple has good relationships with family and friends, including in-laws, members of their extended family, and other couples.

■ The partners have shared spiritual values.

Developing and maintaining a successful intimate relationship takes time and effort, but it is a challenge worth pursuing (see the box "Healthy Vs. Unhealthy Relationships").

Love and Intimacy

How do we go about finding the right person for a successful partnership, and what is involved when we fall in love? Is it all about magic and chemistry, or is there something more deliberate and purposeful about it?

ATTRACTION

People appear to use a systematic screening process when deciding whether someone could be a potential partner. According to one scholar, love is not blind, and we do not fall in love accidentally.[5] Some of the conscious and unconscious factors that affect this process include proximity, physical attractiveness, similarity, and perhaps even a bit of biological instinct.

Proximity is an often overlooked but significant factor in how we find our romantic partners.[6, 7] Simply being physically close to people makes it more likely that we will establish a relationship with them. Sometimes attraction is a function of familiarity, and proximity determines how often we are exposed to another person.

Of the people in proximity to us, we are most interested in those we find physically attractive. Only if we find a person attractive are we willing to consider his or her other traits. In general, people who are perceived as attractive in our society have an advantage. They are evaluated more positively by parents, teachers, and potential employers; make more money; and report having better sex with more attractive partners.

We are also drawn to people who are similar to ourselves, usually in characteristics such as age; physical traits such as height, weight, and attractiveness; educational attainment; family, ethnic, and cultural background; religion; political views; and values, beliefs, and interests. We are attracted to people who agree with us, validate our opinions, and share our attitudes. Even though opposites may initially attract, partners who are like each other tend to have more successful relationships. The more differences partners have, the more important communication skills become.

Some theorists propose that our attractions to potential mates have a biological, evolutionary basis. They suggest that on some level, women seek mates who have or can obtain necessary resources and can provide a safe and comfortable home for them and their children. They are less interested in a man's physical attractiveness and more interested in his social and economic status, his ambition and power, and his character and intelligence.[5] Women are willing to marry less attractive older men if the men earn more money and have more education than the women do.

Men, according to this view, seek mates who can give them strong and healthy children, and consequently they pursue women who are physically attractive (which can be an

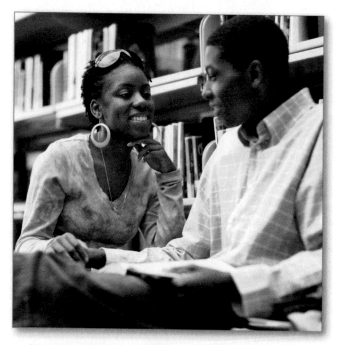

■ Attraction includes a mysterious "chemistry" but is also based on more mundane factors like proximity and similarity.

Highlight on Health

Healthy Vs. Unhealthy Relationships

Being in a HEALTHY RELATIONSHIP means . . .	If you are in an UNHEALTHY RELATIONSHIP . . .
Loving and taking care of yourself, before and while in a relationship.	You care for and focus on the other person only and neglect yourself, or you focus only on yourself and neglect the other person.
Respecting individuality, embracing differences, and allowing each person to "be themselves."	You feel pressure to change to meet the other person's standards, you are afraid to disagree, and your ideas are criticized. Or you pressure the other person to meet your standards and criticize his or her ideas.
Doing things with friends and family and having activities independent of each other.	One of you has to justify what you do, where you go, and who you see.
Discussing things, allowing for differences of opinion, and compromising equally.	One of you makes all the decisions and controls everything without listening to the other's input.
Expressing and listening to each other's feelings, needs, and desires.	One of you feels unheard and is unable to communicate what you want.
Trusting and being honest with yourself and each other.	You lie to each other and find yourself making excuses for the other person.
Respecting each other's need for privacy.	You don't have any personal space and have to share everything with the other person.
Sharing sexual histories and sexual health status with a partner.	Your partner keeps his or her sexual history a secret or hides a sexually transmitted infection from you, or you do not disclose your history to your partner.
Practicing safer sex methods.	You feel scared about asking your partner to use protection, or he or she has refused your requests for safer sex. Or you refuse to use safer sex methods after your partner has requested, or you make your partner feel scared.
Respecting sexual boundaries and being able to say no to sex.	Your partner has forced you to have sex, or you have had sex when you don't really want to. Or you have forced or coerced your partner to have sex.
Resolving conflicts in a rational, peaceful, and mutually agreed-upon way.	One or both of you yells and hits, shoves, or throws things at the other in an argument.
Having room for positive growth and learning more about each other as you develop and mature.	You feel stifled, trapped, and stagnant. You are unable to escape the pressures of the relationship.

Source: Adapted from "Healthy vs. Unhealthy Relationships," Copyright © Advocates for Youth. Reprinted with permission.

indicator of good health). Men are willing to marry women who are younger than them, who have less education, who are not likely to hold a steady job, and who are likely to earn less money than they do, all because such women are thought (on some level) to be better procreators. This evolutionary view has incited controversy and debate, with opponents insisting such differences in attraction are the result of socialization and learning.

THE PROCESS OF FINDING A PARTNER: DATING AND MORE

How do people actually find a suitable mate? A generation or two ago, dating fulfilled this function. Although many people still date, others prefer a different approach. Accord-

ing to a survey of more than 1,000 college women, the newer trends of "hanging out" and "hooking up" are popular alternatives to traditional dating.[8] Singles might hang out with a group of 5 or 10 friends rather than pairing off with a partner and doing only couples' activities. Hooking up (sex without commitment) was reported to be widespread on many campuses and had many levels, from kissing, to oral sex, to intercourse. The survey found it was rare for college men to ask women out on dates or to acknowledge they had become a couple. Still, the study reported that marriage remains a major life goal for the majority of college women; most would like to meet a spouse while at college.

Both in and out of college, many people prefer a more flexible approach to finding a life partner than traditional dating. For example, women often take the lead in asking men out and play a more assertive role in the development of the relationship. Many people place personal ads in newspapers, search for partners on the Internet, or use dating services to find a suitable mate. Others participate in "speed dating" events, in which they spend a designated period of time talking with each of several other participants over the course of the evening, often over dinner.

It makes sense to cast a wide net in the search for a partner. Even participating in such activities as social groups, volunteering, sports, and church may not bring you in contact with a broad range of people. Furthermore, most people lead busy lives, and these approaches to dating enhance your ability to be selective. For example, Internet dating services provide detailed personal profiles of potential partners so that you can eliminate those who will not be a good match for you. Aside from dating and matchmaking sites, social networking sites like MySpace and Facebook now account for a large proportion of the time people spend connecting with others. MySpace has over 85 million users and continues to grow at an exponential pace. Still, if you decide to pursue a relationship with someone you meet over the Internet, be cautious. For some guidelines, see the box "Tips for Internet Dating."

No matter how you approach the process of finding a suitable partner, it should be a time for fun and mutual enjoyment and a way to get to know another person. The following are some suggestions for making this experience rewarding:

- Take things slowly. Reveal information about yourself gradually; otherwise, it can be overwhelming to the other person.
- Do not feel the need to become physically involved right away; becoming friends first is better for a relationship.
- Get to know the person's friends and family members if you can. You can learn a great deal about someone from the other people in his or her life. Also notice how the person treats other people. Look for someone who is respectful to everyone.
- Keep in mind that the traits you dislike in the beginning will probably bother you even more as time goes by.
- Be honest about who you are.

WHAT IS LOVE?

Of all the people we are attracted to and all the potential mates we screen, what makes us fall in love with one or two or a few in a lifetime? Some theorists propose that we fall in love with people who are similar to us in important ways (*similarity theory*). Couples with more similarities seem to have not only greater marital harmony but also higher fertility rates. Other theorists suggest that falling in love and choosing a partner are based on the exchange of "commodities" like love, status, property, and services (*social exchange theory*). According to this view, we are looking for someone who fills not just our emotional needs but also our needs for security, money, goods, and more.

Consumer Clipboard

Tips for Internet Dating

Know how to guard your safety, privacy, and emotional energy when dating through the Internet. Here are some tips:

- Allow for the "cyber exaggeration" factor. Most people lie a little about their age, looks, job, salary, or marital status. Some people lie a lot.
- Use your instincts. If you feel uncomfortable, discontinue the conversation and do not meet the person. Advise the dating service or bulletin board if you feel your experience with the person was threatening or dangerous.
- If you decide to meet someone in person, choose a public place and make it a coffee date. A person who insists on meeting for dinner or at a bar might be overeager or need to drink to feel comfortable.
- Tell a friend you are meeting someone you met on the Internet and say where and when. Print the profile of the person you are meeting and give it to your friend. Ask your friend to call you on your cell phone during the meeting to check in with you.

- Be aware that communication on the Internet can become intimate quickly and you may find yourself writing things you would never say to someone in person at an early stage of a relationship. When meeting in person, do not skip the usual steps in getting to know someone. Act in a manner appropriate to meeting a person for the first time, regardless of previous conversations or perceived closeness.
- Schedule a half-hour meeting at most. If it's not working out, be ready with a simple statement, such as "I've really appreciated meeting you, but I think I'm looking for a different match and I don't want to take more of your time. Thank you and good luck." Don't invent ridiculous excuses. Be polite and decisive.
- Limit your search to people who live within 30 or 40 miles of you. Otherwise, you may end up having a long-distance relationship, or the relationship will suffer from time and distance strains.
- Don't get discouraged. Ask your friends for their support and encouragement in your search.

The Course of Love The beginning stages of falling in love can feel like a roller-coaster ride, taking the lovers from the heights of euphoria to the depths of despair. They may actually become "love sick" and find themselves unable to eat, sleep, or think of anything but the object of their desire. These early stages of a love relationship are typically romantic, idealistic, and passionate. The lovers are absorbed in each other and want to spend all their time together, sometimes to the exclusion of other people and everyday responsibilities.

Researchers think this experience of love involves increased levels of the neurotransmitter dopamine in the brain.[6] As we have seen in the context of psychoactive drugs (Chapter 12), dopamine is associated with the experience of pleasure. Love also causes arousal of the sympathetic nervous system, as evidenced by such physiological signs as increased heart rate, respiration, and perspiration.

These responses gradually decrease as the relationship develops and progresses. Intense passion may subside as lovers become habituated to each other. In some cases, passion continues at a more bearable level and intimacy deepens; the relationship becomes more fulfilling and comes to include affection, empathy, tolerance, caring, and attachment. The partners are able to become involved in the world again, while maintaining their connection with each other. In other cases, the lessening of passion signals the ending of the relationship; the lovers drift apart, seeking newer, more satisfying partnerships.

Sternberg's Love Triangle Psychologist Robert Sternberg has proposed a view of love that can give us insight into its various aspects. In this view, love has three dimensions: intimacy, passion, and commitment. **Intimacy** is the emotional component of love and includes feelings of closeness, warmth, openness, and affection. **Passion** is the sexual component of love; it includes attraction, romance, excitement, and physical intensity. **Commitment** is the decision aspect of a relationship, the pledge that you will stay with your partner through good times and bad, despite the possibility of disappointment and disillusionment.[9]

According to Sternberg, passion peaks relatively quickly in a relationship and then decreases to a stable level as a result of habituation. After a relationship breaks up, a person's capacity for passion may go underground for a while, as he or she overcomes feelings of loss. Intimacy tends to peak more slowly than passion and then levels out at a relatively low level of manifest intimacy, as interpersonal bonding continues to grow. Changes in circumstances can activate latent intimacy,

intimacy
Emotional component of love, including feelings of closeness, warmth, openness, and affection.

passion
Sexual component of love, including attraction, romance, excitement, and physical intensity.

commitment
The decision aspect of a relationship, the pledge to stay with a partner through good times and bad.

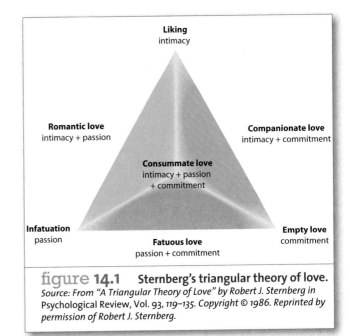

figure 14.1 Sternberg's triangular theory of love.
Source: From "A Triangular Theory of Love" by Robert J. Sternberg in Psychological Review, Vol. 93, 119–135. Copyright © 1986. Reprinted by permission of Robert J. Sternberg.

causing the manifest level to return to or exceed its earlier peak. Commitment builds slowly at first, then speeds up and gradually levels off. When relationships fail, commitment decreases back the baseline level.

Different combinations of these three components, represented metaphorically as a triangle, produce different kinds of love (Figure 14.1). When there is only intimacy, the relationship is likely to be a friendship. Passion alone is infatuation, the high-intensity early stage of a love relationship. Commitment alone is characteristic of a dutiful, obligatory relationship, one that many people would consider empty. When there is both intimacy and passion, the relationship is a romantic one; commitment may develop in time. When there is passion and commitment, the relationship has probably developed rapidly, without the partners getting to know each other very well; when passion fades, there may not be much substance to this type of relationship. When there is intimacy and commitment but no passion, the relationship may have evolved into more of a long-term friendship; Sternberg calls this relationship *companionate love*. Finally, when all three components are present, the couple has *consummate love*.[9] This type of relationship is what we all dream of, but it's difficult to find and even harder to sustain. To evaluate your relationship, see the Add It Up feature for Chapter 14 at the end of the book.

Some researchers have found that life satisfaction is more strongly predicted by companionate love (high levels of commitment and intimacy, low level of passion) than by passionate love (high level of passion).[10] Companionate love is more characteristic of couples who have been married for years. Passionate love includes more intense emotions, both positive and negative. However love is conceptualized, it is something that enhances happiness and satisfaction in life.

Communication

We establish, maintain, and nourish our relationships—or, alternatively, damage and destroy them—through communication. Clear, positive communication is a key to successful intimate relationships. This doesn't mean you should "tell all" at the beginning of a relationship or deliver the "brutal truth" in the middle of a heated argument. It does mean that you are honest and open and communicate in a caring, respectful way. It also means learning to listen when your partner has the floor.

NONVERBAL BEHAVIOR AND METAMESSAGES

A good deal of communication takes place as **nonverbal communication,** through facial expressions, eye contact, gestures, body position and movement, and spatial behavior (how far apart people sit or stand). People tend to monitor their verbal behavior—what they say—much more carefully than their nonverbal behavior, yet nonverbal communication may convey their real message. Researchers studying nonverbal communication in married couples have found correlations between the quality of a relationship and nonverbal behavior. Couples with less disagreement in their relationship sit closer to each other, touch each other more during discussion, make eye contact more frequently, and display more open body postures than do couples with more disagreement.

Nonverbal behavior is part of the **metamessage,** the unspoken message you send or get when you are communicating. The metamessage encompasses all the conscious and unconscious aspects of a message, including the way something is said, who says it, when and where it is said, or even that it is said at all. It includes the meaning and intent behind a message.

Often, the metamessage is what triggers an emotional response rather than just the words someone says. When you find yourself in an escalating argument, stop and "metacommunicate," or talk about the way you are talking. What you are perceiving as condescending or insulting, for example, may not be meant that way; if you seek clarification, you may discover this. On the other hand, a gut reaction can be an accurate reading of intent, and metacommunicating is a way to explore feelings and meanings that may be hidden or unconscious.

BUILDING COMMUNICATION SKILLS

People who are good communicators have many personal attributes that contribute to their success, such as empathy, interest in others, a sense of humor, and a history of positive interactions with others. There are also some specific skills

nonverbal communication
Communication that takes place without words, mainly through body language.

metamessage
The unspoken message in a communication; the meaning behind the message, conveyed by nonverbal behavior and by situational factors such as how, when, and where the message is delivered

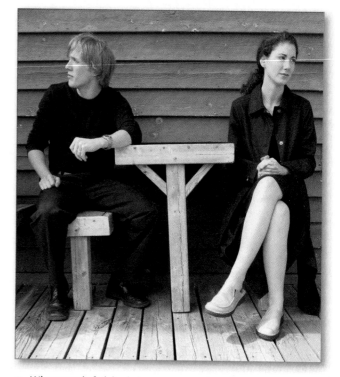
■ When words fail, body language speaks volumes.

that people can learn and practice in order to be better communicators, both when they speak and when they listen.

One aspect of being an effective communicator when you speak is knowing what you want to say. Examine your own feelings, motives, and intentions before you speak. When you do speak, use "I" statements to state what you feel or want in a clear, direct way without blaming or accusing the other person. Using "I" statements helps you take responsibility for your own emotions and reactions rather than trying to place responsibility on someone else. For example, it is more productive to say, "I feel . . . when you . . ." than to say, "You make me feel . . ." Saying what you would like to have happen is also more productive than complaining about what isn't happening. Other keys to positive, effective communication are avoiding generalizations, making specific requests, and remaining calm. If you feel yourself starting to get angry, take a time-out and come back to the conversation after you cool off.

When you are the listener, do just that—listen. Don't interrupt, give advice, explain, judge, analyze, defend yourself, or offer solutions. Give the other person the time and space to say fully what is on his or her mind, just as you would like when you are speaking. Show with your body language that you are paying attention and are present. If you don't understand something, seek clarification at an appropriate point. Attentive listening shows that you respect the other person and care about him or her. It is the cornerstone of good communication.

If you and your partner are experiencing conflict, good communication skills can help you resolve it constructively. Conflict is a normal part of healthy relationships. Often, it is a sign that partners are maintaining their right to be different people and to have different points of view; it can also indicate that the relationship is changing or growing. See the box "A Caring Approach to Conflict Resolution" for some insights on how partners in successful relationships approach conflict.

When you are trying to resolve a conflict with your partner, keep the topic narrow. Try not to generalize to other topics, incidents, or issues. You might want to set a specific time and place to have your conversation, making sure it's quiet and private. You might also want to set a time limit on your discussion. Avoid being either passive or aggressive; **assertiveness** means speaking up for yourself without violating someone else's rights. Don't exaggerate or use sarcasm, and don't be afraid to admit you are wrong or sorry. Be prepared to negotiate and compromise, but don't give up something that is really important to you (for example, time to keep up your other friendships). If you feel that demands are being made on you that you cannot or do not want to meet, this may not be the right relationship for you. Communicating clearly about that is important, too.

assertiveness
The ability to stand up for oneself without violating other people's rights.

GENDER DIFFERENCES IN COMMUNICATION STYLES

Like other aspects of behavior, patterns of communication are learned and therefore subject to social and cultural influences, including gender expectations. According to linguistics scholar Deborah Tannen, gender differences in communication patterns have a significant impact on relationships. Tannen suggests that men are more likely to use communication to compete and women are more likely to use communication to connect. Men want to establish their dominance, competence, and knowledge in a conversation, and women are interested in finding commonalities, sharing experiences, and giving and receiving support.[11]

Consider this example: A woman comes home from work and tells her partner about an upsetting incident that occurred that day. He responds by giving her advice on what she should have done and said. A few days later, she tells him about another, similar incident at work. He responds by saying, "I already told you how to handle this situation." The woman feels unsupported and disappointed by this response, and her partner doesn't understand why. In this example, the woman wants to talk about the incident and have her partner show his understanding and caring by listening to her. The man wants to fix the problem; he shows his understanding and caring by giving her advice.

Although these patterns are broad and general, they are sometimes at the root of misunderstandings between men and women. If you find yourself experiencing confusion or conflict in your communications with the other sex, consider whether gender differences may be involved. Neither style is right or wrong, better or worse—they are just different.

Highlight on Health

A Caring Approach to Conflict Resolution

Research indicates that all couples fight and that most fights are never resolved. The difference between unhappy and happy couples is *how* they fight. Although effective listening contributes to the overall health of a relationship, it appears that being a good listener requires too much of partners when the argument gets heated. Instead, partners in successful marriages seem to be able to moderate their responses during conflict to avoid inflicting permanent damage on the relationship. Here are some characteristics of this approach to conflict:

■ Gentleness and compassion are key ingredients in successful relationships. Partners who couch their criticisms and complaints in a gentle, soothing, and even humorous approach are more likely to have a happy relationship than those who are belligerent.

■ Anger itself is not destructive in a relationship, but criticism, defensiveness, contempt, and stonewalling are counterproductive and damaging during conflict. They can lead to escalation, withdrawal, and distancing, all of which are associated with lower relationship satisfaction.

■ When the focus is more on having a good discussion than on finding a solution to a problem, the outcome is more satisfactory. Discussion and problem solving can be treated as two separate parts of conflict resolution.

■ Couples who report being happy have come to terms with their irresolvable differences and have learned to work around them while continuing to love each other. They don't let the differences poison the wonderful things in their relationship.

Sources: "Predicting Marital Happiness and Stability From Newlywed Interactions," by J. Gottman et al., 1998, Journal of Marriage and Family, 60, pp. 5–22 © 1998 by the National Council on Family Relations, reprinted by permission of Blackwell Publishing; "Married With Problems? Therapy May Not Help," by Susan Gilbert, April 19, 2005, New York Times.

Sex and Gender

Most adult partnerships and intimate relationships include a sexual component. Sexuality encompasses not just sexual behavior but also a broad set of values, beliefs, attitudes, and social behaviors. As discussed in Chapters 15 and 16, it includes biological, psychological, sociological, and cultural dimensions. In this section, we consider just two such dimensions—gender roles and sexual orientation.

Gender Roles

Although they are often used interchangeably, the terms *sex* and *gender* have different meanings. **Sex** refers to a person's biological status as male or female; it is usually established at birth by the appearance of the external genitals. A person with female genitals usually has XX chromosomes, and a person with male genitals usually has XY chromosomes.

Sex is not always clear-cut, however. As discussed in Chapter 2, chromosomes are sometimes added, lost, or rearranged during the production of sperm and ova, causing such conditions as Klinefelter syndrome (XXY) and Turner syndrome (XO). Sometimes, as a result of genetic factors or prenatal hormonal influences, a baby is born with ambiguous genitals—a condition referred to as **intersex.** In such cases, parents and physicians may be faced with the difficult task of deciding which sex to "assign" the child to. Other times, a person experiences a sense of inappropriateness about his or her sex and identifies psychologically or emotionally with the other sex.

sex
A person's biological status as a male or a female, usually established at birth by the appearance of the external genitals.

intersex
Condition in which the genitals are ambiguous at birth as a result of genetic factors or prenatal hormonal influences.

gender
Masculine or feminine behaviors and characteristics considered appropriate for a male or a female in a particular culture.

gender role
Set of behaviors and activities a person engages in to conform to society's expectations of his or her sex.

Gender refers to the behaviors and characteristics considered appropriate for a male or a female in a particular culture. "Masculine" and "feminine" traits are learned largely via the process of socialization during childhood. **Gender role** is the set of behaviors and activities a person engages in to conform to society's expectations. In our culture, for example, the traditional male gender role has been that of breadwinner and provider, and the traditional female gender role has been homemaker, wife, and mother. Gender role stereotypes suggest that a masculine man is competitive, aggressive, ambitious, power-oriented, and logical and that a feminine woman is cooperative, passive, nurturing, supportive, and emotional.

Today, we commonly assume that both genders are capable and can be successful in a variety of roles at home and at work. However, gender roles and gender stereotypes are learned in childhood and become part of who we are. They are ingrained and hard to change, even when we are aware of them. For example, both men and women have been shown to play the stereotyped role assigned to their gender in order to appear romantically attractive to the other sex, and both men and women may be initially attracted to romantic partners because they fit the gender role stereotype.[12]

After the initial attraction phase of a relationship, however, many partners are irritated by the stereotypical traits they originally found exciting or endearing, such as talkativeness in a woman or reticence in a man. In long-term relationships, both sexes value traits such as honesty, empathy,

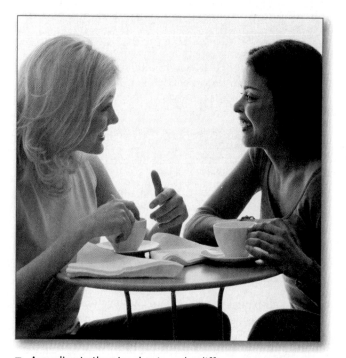

■ According to theories about gender differences in communication style, women are interested in sharing, finding similarities, and giving and receiving support when they interact with others.

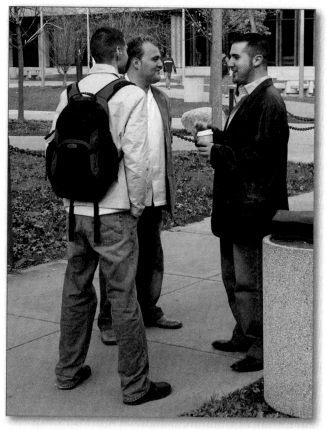

■ Men supposedly establish dominance in their interactions with others by showing off their knowledge and competence.

responsibility, open-mindedness, and humor, and both tend to prefer a partner who integrates so-called masculine and feminine traits. The term *androgynous* is applied to a person who displays characteristics or performs tasks traditionally associated with the other sex; sometimes it is also applied to a person who does not display overt characteristics of either sex.

SEXUAL ORIENTATION

Sexual orientation refers to a person's emotional, romantic, and sexual attraction to a member of the same sex, the other sex, or both. It exists along a continuum that ranges from exclusive heterosexuality through bisexuality to exclusive homosexuality. Although the role of genes in sexual orientation is not clearly understood (see Chapter 2), sexual orientation is known to be influenced by a complex interaction of biological, psychological, and societal factors, and these factors may be different for different people.

sexual orientation
A person's emotional, romantic, and sexual attraction to a member of the same sex, the other sex, or both.

Sexual orientation involves a person's sense of identity. Most experts believe that it is not a choice and does not change (perhaps more so for men than for women). It is not the result of how a person was raised or of experiences the person had as a child. A person's sexual orientation may or may not be evidenced in his or her appearance or behavior, and the person may choose not to act on his or her sexual orientation. For example, a bisexual may have a committed relationship with a person of one sex and therefore decide not to act on an attraction to the other sex. Some people who are homosexual or bisexual may choose to hide their sexual orientation or live as heterosexuals to avoid prejudice or, if their sexual orientation is incompatible with their personal beliefs, to avoid their own internal dilemmas.

Heterosexuality is defined as emotional and sexual attraction to members of the other sex. Heterosexuals are often referred to as *straight*. Throughout the world, laws related to marriage, child rearing, health benefits, financial matters, sexual behavior, and inheritance generally support heterosexual relationships. **Homosexuality** is defined as emotional and sexual attraction to members of the same sex. In today's usage, homosexual men are typically referred to as *gay*, and homosexual women are referred to either as gay or as *lesbians*.

heterosexuality
Emotional and sexual attraction to members of the other sex.

homosexuality
Emotional and sexual attraction to members of the same sex.

Homosexuality occurs in all cultures, but researchers have generally had difficulty determining exactly what proportions of the population are straight and gay. Sex researcher Alfred Kinsey estimated that about 4 percent of American males and 2 percent of American females were exclusively homosexual.[13, 14] The popular media tend to place the combined figure for gay men and lesbians at about 10 percent of the population.

Emotional and sexual attraction to both sexes is referred to as **bisexuality.** Bisexuals may date members of both sexes, or they may have a relationship with a member of one sex for a period of time and then a relationship with a member of the other sex for a period of time. After having relationships with members of both sexes, a bisexual may move toward a more exclusive orientation, either heterosexual or homosexual.

Individuals who experience discomfort or a sense of inappropriateness about their sex (called *gender dysphoria*) and who identify strongly with the other sex are referred to as cross-gender identified, transsexual, or **transgender.** The term *transgender* can describe anyone whose **gender identity** differs from the sex of

bisexuality
Emotional and sexual attraction to members of both sexes.

transgender
Having a sense of identity as a male or female that conflicts with one's biological sex; transgendered individuals experience a sense of inappropriateness about their sex and identify strongly with the other sex.

gender identity
Internal sense of being male or female.

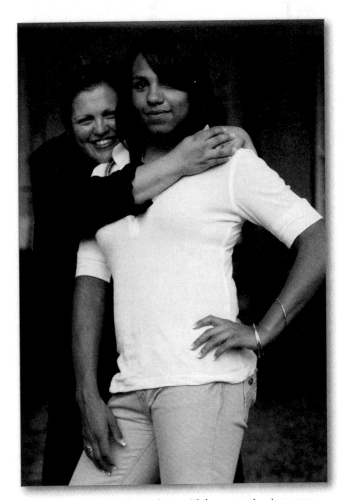

■ Rochelle Evans, 15, shown here with her mom, is a transgender teen living in Texas. She started high school as Rodney Evans and fought a public battle to be allowed to wear women's clothes to school.

their birth. The *Diagnostic and Statistical Manual of Mental Disorders* includes gender identity disorder as a diagnostic category.

Many transgender individuals dress in the clothes of the other sex (*cross-dressing*) and live in society as the other sex. Some undergo surgery and hormone treatments to experience a more complete transformation into the other sex, and others do not. Transgender individuals have typically experienced gender dysphoria since earliest childhood, but there is controversy about using the gender identity disorder diagnosis with children.[15] Most children who do not fit the cultural stereotype of masculinity or femininity do not grow up to be transgender. According to the National Center for Transgender Equality, fewer than 1 percent of the population in the United States (between 750,000 and 3,000,000 people) are transgender.

Whether straight, gay, bisexual, or transgender, human beings seek the same things in relationships, whether conceptualized as intimacy, passion, and commitment or some other combination of qualities and experiences. We all want to be affirmed, to be wanted, to love someone and be loved in return, to belong. These (and many others) are basic human needs and desires that are fulfilled only in relationships with other human beings.

Committed Relationships and Lifestyle Choices

In this section we consider marriage, one of the most important social and legal institutions in societies throughout the world, along with other relationship and lifestyle choices that many people make today.

MARRIAGE

Marriage is not only the legal union of two people but also a contract between the couple and the state. In the United States, each state specifies the rights and responsibilities of the partners in a marriage. Although marriage has traditionally meant the union of a man and a woman, many same-sex couples are interested in marriage, and some states now issue marriage licenses to same-sex couples.

Although the percentage of Americans who marry and live together as married couples continues to decline, marriage still appears to be the most popular living arrangement. The decline in the number of married people may be accounted for by the increase in cohabiting couples, a decrease in the number of people getting married for a second time, and the choice made by many individuals to postpone marriage until they are older (Table 14.1).

It appears, however, that the marriage rate is now higher among people with a college education than among their non-college-educated peers and that their divorce rate has been dropping. It also appears that there has been a movement toward modifying gender roles and toward more equitable relationships, at least among individuals with a college education. Marriage rates among those who are not college educated have continued to decline. This trend has public health implications, because marriage is associated with better health outcomes and greater longevity.[16]

Marriage is an opportunity to develop a physically and emotionally intimate and supportive relationship with another person. Marriage partners typically merge their social networks and their financial resources as well as their lives. Most married couples expect to become parents and view raising children as a purpose of the marriage.

Marriage confers benefits in many domains. Partnerships and family relationships provide emotional connection for individuals and stability for society. Married people live longer than single or divorced people, partly because they lead a healthier lifestyle. Married people report greater happiness than do single, widowed, or cohabiting people. Married couples have sex more frequently and consider their sexual relationship more satisfying emotionally and physically than do single people. Married people are more successful in their careers, earn more, and have more wealth. Children brought up by married couples tend to be more academically successful and emotionally stable.

What makes a marriage successful? One predictor of a successful marriage is positive reasons for getting married. Positive motivations include companionship, love and intimacy, supportive partnership, sexual compatibility, and interest in sharing parenthood. Poorer reasons for getting married, those associated with less chance of having a successful marriage, include premarital pregnancy, rebellion against parents, seeking independence, seeking economic security, family or social pressure, and rebounding from another relationship.

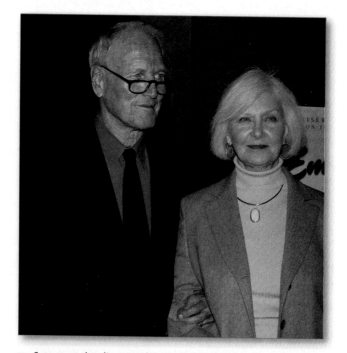

■ Some couples discover the secrets to a long and happy marriage. Paul Newman and Joanne Woodward celebrated their 50th wedding anniversary in January 2008.

Table 14.1	Percentage of All Persons Aged 15 or Older Who Were Married, by Sex and Race, 1960–2005, United States					
	Males			**Females**		
Year	**Total***	**Black**	**White**	**Total***	**Black**	**White**
1960	69.3	60.9	70.2	65.9	59.8	66.6
1970	66.7	56.9	68.0	61.9	54.1	62.8
1980	63.2	48.8	65.0	58.9	44.6	60.7
1990	60.7	45.1	62.8	56.9	40.2	59.1
2000	57.9	42.8	60.0	54.7	36.2	57.4
2005**	55.0	37.9	57.5	51.5	30.2	54.6

* Includes races other than Black and White.

** In 2003 the U.S. Census Bureau expanded its racial categories to permit respondents to identify themselves as belonging to more than one race. This means that racial data computations beginning in 2004 may not be strictly comparable with those of prior years.

Source: America's Families and Living Arrangements: March 2000 *and earlier reports, U.S. Bureau of the Census, Current Population Reports, Series P20-506; data calculated from Current Population Surveys, March 2005 Supplement.*

Love alone is not enough to make a marriage successful. Research has found that the best predictors of a happy marriage are realistic attitudes about the relationship and the challenges of marriage; satisfaction with the personality of the partner; enjoyment of communicating with the partner; ability to resolve conflicts together; agreement on religious and ethical values; egalitarian roles; and a balance of individual and joint leisure activities. The characteristics associated with successful and unsuccessful marriages are typically present in a couple's relationship before they are married.[17]

Infidelity mars some marriages, though it does not necessarily end them. Men are twice as likely as women to have a sexual affair during marriage, but women are more likely to have an affair to end a bad marriage.[18] Men are more threatened if their partner has a sexual affair than if she falls in love with someone else, whereas women are more distressed if their partner falls in love with someone else (see the box "The Numbers on Cheating").

GAY AND LESBIAN PARTNERSHIPS

Like heterosexual couples, same-sex couples desire intimacy, companionship, passion, and commitment in their relationships. Because they often have to struggle with "coming out" and issues with their families, gay men and lesbians frequently have communication skills and strengths that are valuable in relationships. These qualities include flexible role relationships, the ability to adapt to a partner, the ability to negotiate and share decision-making power, and effective parenting skills among those who choose to become parents.[19, 20] Unfortunately, gay men and lesbians often have to deal with discrimination and **homophobia** (irrational fear of homosexuality

homophobia
Irrational fear of homosexuality and homosexuals.

and homosexuals). Same-sex relationships do not receive the same level of societal support and acceptance as heterosexual relationships.

Researchers looking at relationship satisfaction among comparable samples of gay, lesbian, and heterosexual couples found that all three groups reported similar levels of relationship quality and satisfaction.[21] The options of domestic partnership, civil union, and marriage have become available for same-sex partners in some states. The issue of gay marriage has become a hot political topic in the United States in recent

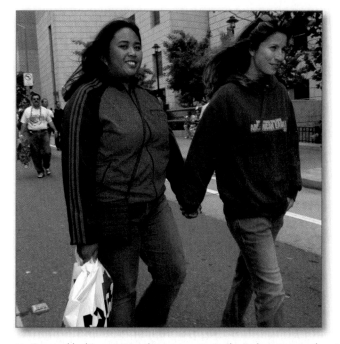

■ Gay and lesbian partnerships are very similar to heterosexual partnerships, but same-sex couples often have to deal with bias and discrimination.

Highlight on Health

The Numbers on Cheating

Percentage of adults in monogamous relationships
who say they have had an affair 20

Percentage of married men who say they have had
an affair.. 22

Percentage of married women who say they have
had an affair 13

Percentage of adults who think that sexual
intercourse or oral sex is cheating 100

Percentage of adults who think that romantically
kissing someone is cheating 83

Percentage of adults who think that virtual affairs
are cheating.. 65

Percentage of men who engage in online sex or
sex webcamming.. 15

Percentage of women who engage in online sex or
sex webcamming...7

Men's top reasons for cheating:

    Want more sex 44

    Want more sexual variety 40

    Want more satisfying sex 38

Women's top reasons for cheating:

    Want emotional attention 40

    Want reassurance of desirability 33

    Have fallen in love with someone else 20

Percentage of cheaters who say they do not
regret their infidelity.. 66

Percentage of cheaters who say the affair left them
with lingering feelings of

    Sadness.. 75

    Guilt 49

    Stress.. 32

Percentage of relationships that broke up
immediately after affair 19

Percentage of relationships that broke up
eventually due to continued feelings of
betrayal 22

Percentage of men in committed relationships
of 30 years or more who say they have been
faithful throughout the entire relationship 67

Percentage of women in committed relationships
of 30 years or more who say they have been
faithful throughout the entire relationship.............. 80

Sources: "Cheating Hearts: Who's Doing It and Why," retrieved May 19, 2008, from www.msnbc.msn.com/id/17951664; "American Sexual Behavior: Trends, Socio-Demographic Differences, and Risk Behavior," GSS Topical Report No. 25, by Tom W. Smith, 2006, National Opinion Research Center, University of Chicago.

years, with one side asserting that marriage must be defined as a union between a man and a woman and the other side arguing that denying marriage to gay people is a violation of their civil rights.[22] For a discussion of the debate surrounding the issue of same-sex marriage, see You Make the Call at the end of the chapter.

COHABITATION

The U.S. government defines **cohabitation** as two people of the opposite sex living together as unmarried partners.

cohabitation
Living arrangement in which two people of the opposite sex live together as unmarried partners.

Since the 1960s, cohabitation has become one of the most rapidly growing social phenomena in the history of our society. The rate of cohabitation has increased tenfold since the 1960s, when about half a million people were living together. In 2005 approximately 4.8 million couples, or 9.6 million men and women, were identified as cohabiting (Table 14.2). About a quarter of unmarried

women between the ages of 25 and 39 are currently living with a partner.

Cohabitation seems to have become an accepted part of the process of finding a mate. Most couples today believe it is a good idea to live together in order to decide if they should get married, and more than 50 percent do live together before getting married. Yet an estimated 40 percent of these arrangements do not result in marriage.[16]

Currently, cohabitation is more common among individuals of lower socioeconomic levels. Recent data show that among women between 19 and 44 years of age, 60 percent of high school dropouts have cohabited, whereas 37 percent of college graduates have done so. Cohabitation is also more common among individuals who have been divorced or have experienced the divorce of their parents. Individuals who are less religious than their peers, have been fatherless, or grew up in families with serious marital conflict are also more likely to cohabit.[16]

Some studies have shown that cohabitation actually decreases the likelihood of success in marriage and increases the likelihood of divorce. Such findings are controversial,

Table 14.2	Number of Cohabiting, Unmarried, Adult Couples of the Opposite Sex, by Year, United States
Year	**Number of Couples (millions)**
1960	0.439
1970	0.523
1980	1.589
1990	2.856
2000	4.736
2005	4.855

Sources: "America's Families and Living Arrangements: March 2000," Current Population Reports, Series P20-537, 2001, Washington, DC: U.S. Bureau of the Census; Current Population Survey, 2005 Annual Social and Economic Supplement, U.S. Bureau of the Census, Population Division, retrieved from www.census.gov/population/socdemo/hh-fam/cps2005.

however, because of the difficulty in determining whether this effect results from the characteristics of those who choose to cohabit before marriage or from the experience of living together before marriage.[16, 23]

DIVORCE

For a large percentage of couples, the demands of marriage prove too difficult, and the couple choose to divorce. The current divorce rate is nearly twice what it was in 1960, although it has declined since reaching its highest point in the 1980s. The lifetime probability of a couple in their first marriage experiencing divorce is between 40 and 50 percent.[16] Some observers suggest that approximately 60 percent of second marriages end in divorce. However, the length of first and second marriages appears to be about the same, with the median length of first marriages about 7.8 years for males and 7.9 years for females and the median length of second marriages about 7.3 years for males and 6.8 years for females.

Most people who divorce in the United States are younger than 45 years old. Couples who marry when they are 20 or younger are more likely to split up than couples who are older when they marry. Overall, people with lower incomes and less education tend to have higher rates of divorce. Two-thirds of all divorces are initiated by women, probably because it gives them a better chance of retaining custody of their children in most states. Women may also be less satisfied with their marriages than men.

Why do so many couples divorce in our society? Many couples simply cannot handle the challenges of married life. They may not have the problem-solving skills, or they may not be sufficiently committed to the relationship. Many people enter marriage with unrealistic expectations, and some people choose an unsuitable mate.

Although divorce may seem to be a single event in a person's life, the termination of a marriage is almost always a traumatic process lasting months or years. Divorce is a leading cause of poverty, leaving many children in impoverished homes headed by a single parent, often the parent with the lower income. The number of single-mother families in the United States rose from 3 million in 1970 to 10 million in 2003, and the number of single-father families rose from under half a million to 2 million in the same period. In all, there were 12 million single-parent families in 2003.[24] Most single-parent families cannot maintain the same lifestyle that they had before the divorce.

Divorce also appears to damage physical health. Gastrointestinal and respiratory problems increase after divorce, as does the incidence of hypertension. Divorce is one of the most stressful life events a person can experience. It is especially hard on children, leading to different kinds of problems for children of different ages (see the box "Children and Divorce"). Counseling can help both children and adults deal with the stress of divorce and adjust to a new life. Children are best served by continuing to have contact with both parents as long as the adults can get along.

BLENDED FAMILIES

Many divorced people eventually remarry, and **blended families,** in which one or both partners bring children from a previous marriage, are becoming a common form of family.

Just as it takes time for a family to reorganize and stabilize itself after a divorce, it also takes time for a blended family to achieve some measure of cohesion after parents remarry. It can take 2 years or more for stepparents and stepchildren to build relationships. Adults should allow time for trust and attachment to develop before they take on a parenting role with their stepchildren. When children regularly see their noncustodial parent, they are better able to adjust to their new family. Children also adjust better if the parents in the blended family have a low-intensity relationship and if the relationships between ex-spouses are civil.

blended families
Families in which one or both partners bring a child or children from a previous marriage.

SINGLEHOOD

Although marriage continues to be a popular institution, a growing number of people in our society are unmarried. In 2003 25 percent of women and 32 percent of men over the age of 15 had never been married. For the age group 30 to 34, 33 percent of men and 23 percent of women had never been married.[24] The biggest change in the profile of U.S. families between 1970 and 2003 was the increase in the percentage of households that were one-person households, from 17 percent to 26 percent. In other words, one in four Americans lived alone in 2003.

Part of the reason for this shift is that young people have been staying single longer and getting married later.

Public Health in Action

Children and Divorce

Divorce in the United States has become fairly common, with almost half of all first marriages ending in divorce and one-third ending within the first 10 years. Many of these divorcing couples have children; more than half of all children will experience divorce at least once.

The many stressors associated with divorce can have an impact on children's health and increase their risk for a number of physical and mental-health-related problems. When a divorce involves a lot of conflict, children can become depressed and anxious, have academic problems, and have difficulty with friendships and peer relationships. Research suggests that about a third of children are subjected to high-conflict divorces and are at risk for such problems. When parents can maintain a relatively conflict-free relationship after the divorce, children generally do well.

Several programs have been developed to help children negotiate their parents' divorce process successfully. An example is the Children in Divorce Intervention Program, a school-based intervention designed to help prevent long-term emotional problems in school-age children who are adjusting to divorce. Meeting with children for 15 sessions, trained group leaders work to build a supportive group environment that promotes understanding of divorce, encourages expression of feelings, and enhances self-esteem. One evaluation found that positive outcomes for children in the program included reduced anxiety and blaming, an increased ability to problem solve, and an understanding that they could not fix problems that were beyond their control. The program has won several awards for its work.

Parents who are divorcing can help their children by following a few guidelines:

- Both parents should tell the children about the divorce together.

- The children's welfare should be given higher priority than the parents' desire to argue, be right, or have the last word.

- Questions should be answered honestly and children reassured that they are not responsible for what has occurred.

- Children should also be reassured that they will be cared for and that both parents will continue to have an active role in their lives.

- Parents should avoid arguing in front of the children, creating loyalty binds, or allowing a situation to develop in which children feel they need to choose between parents.

Between 1970 and 2003, age at first marriage in the United States rose from 20.8 to 26.6 for women and from 23.2 to 28.6 for men.[24]

As the age of first marriage rises, the number of single people in the population increases. Many of these young adults are delaying marriage to pursue educational and career goals, but an increasing number of people view singlehood as a legitimate, healthy, and satisfying alternative to marriage. Some people, including some highly educated professionals and career-oriented individuals, prefer to remain unmarried. In singlehood they find the freedom to pursue their own interests, spend their money as they wish, invest time in their careers, develop a broad network of friends, have a variety of sexual relationships, and enjoy opportunities for solitude. For them, being single is a positive choice.

The ranks of the single also include those who are involuntarily single. These include people who are divorced, separated, and widowed; they may or may not be satisfied with their unmarried state. People who enjoy being single are socially and psychologically independent, are able to handle loneliness, are able to make it on their own financially, and are proactive about creating an interesting life.

KEEPING YOUR RELATIONSHIPS STRONG AND VITAL

A characteristic of relationships—both partnerships and families—is that they change over time. Many researchers and clinicians have studied how individuals deal with roles and developmental tasks within a relationship or family unit as they move through the life cycle. No matter what specific challenges come up, three basic qualities seem to make partnerships and families strong: cohesion, flexibility, and communication.[25]

Cohesion is the dynamic balance between separateness and togetherness in both couple and family relationships. Relationships are strongest when there is a balance between intimacy and autonomy. There are times when partners and family members spend more time together and other times when they spend more time apart, but they come back to a comfortably cohesive point. *Flexibility* is the dynamic balance between stability and change. Again, relationships are strongest when there is a balance. Too much stability can cause rigidity; too much change can cause chaos. Communication is the tool that partners and families use to adjust levels of cohesion or flexibility when change is needed. It is important that communication with a partner includes expressions of appreciation, healthy complaining, and the recognition of both partners' levels of sensitivity.[4]

When relationship problems persist for 2 or 3 months and the partners are not able to resolve them, the couple should probably seek help. Couples who receive help with difficulties before they become too severe have a better chance of overcoming the problems and developing a stronger relationship than do those who delay. Marriage and family therapists are specifically trained to help couples and families with relationship problems. Look for a therapist who is licensed by your state or who is a certified member of the American Association for Marriage and Family Therapists. Your physician or clergyperson may be able to recommend a qualified professional. A couples therapist can help you develop the strengths and resources you need to nourish and enhance this vital part of your life.

You Make the Call

Should Same-Sex Marriage Be Legal?

Although marriage has traditionally been defined as a religious and legal commitment between a man and a woman, many committed same-sex partners are challenging this definition and demanding the right to marry. In a few states, they have won some rights. In Vermont and Connecticut, same-sex civil unions offer couples many of the rights of marriage, and Hawaii's Reciprocal Beneficiaries law offers some marriagelike benefits. Maine and New Jersey offer domestic partnerships, with a range of rights and benefits. In Massachusetts and California, same-sex couples are entitled to full marriage rights as a result of supreme court rulings in those states. Changes in state laws and court rulings are ongoing.

Other states have passed "defense of marriage" acts, stating that marriage is a union between one man and one woman. They have done so because the "full faith and credit" clause of the U.S. Constitution requires that any law passed in one state be honored in all other states. To further circumvent this clause, President Clinton signed the Defense of Marriage Act in 1996, making the same claim law at the federal level. The passage of these laws creates a conflict with laws allowing same-sex unions. The debate continues.

What is at stake in this issue? Proponents of same-sex marriage point out that the 14th Amendment to the U.S. Constitution prohibits the states from denying any citizen the equal protection of the laws, and many state constitutions protect equal rights for all. Proponents claim that same-sex couples are being discriminated against and denied equal rights by not being allowed to marry. Marriage gives heterosexual couples hundreds of legal, economic, and social benefits and rights, in areas such as child custody, joint ownership of property, taxation, health insurance, Social Security and pensions, medical decision making, inheritance, legal protection, and many others. Proponents argue that gay people are unfairly denied access to the same benefits that are available to heterosexual people.

Opponents of same-sex marriage argue that the Bible condemns homosexuality and that virtually all major religions consider gay relationships sinful or immoral. They further argue that a nation's laws should reflect the moral values on which it is founded and that many U.S. laws have their origin in religious teachings, such as the injunction against murder. Because laws imply moral approval of a behavior and shape the attitudes of society, legalizing same-sex unions condones behavior that the majority of people find unacceptable. Some but not all opponents with a religious orientation also argue that the purpose of marriage is procreation and because same-sex couples do not produce children, they are not entitled to be married.

Supporters of same-sex marriage respond to the religious argument by citing the U.S. Constitution. The First Amendment prohibits the establishment of a state religion, which is the basis for the separation of church and state in the United States. Laws based on religious views are not constitutional, nor is discrimination against an individual or a group on the basis of religious views. Even if certain churches do not want to perform same-sex marriages, marriage as a secular institution should be available to all.

Another argument against legalizing same-sex marriage is that doing so threatens the sanctity of marriage, one of society's most revered institutions. Marriage is the basis of the family, and one of the family's most important functions is raising and socializing children. Marriage is already in a precarious state in the United States, and legalizing gay marriage would further weaken it and cause it to lose respect, according to this view. Some opponents argue that if marriage is opened up to same-sex couples, it would lead down the "slippery slope" to marriage between multiple persons, marriage between friends for tax purposes, or even marriage to an animal. We need a firm definition of marriage to discourage such an explosion of possibilities, in the opinion of these opponents.

Continued . . .

Continued . . .

Supporters of same-sex marriage respond that society is changing and that sometimes the law has to take the lead in securing social justice for all. They point out that civil rights laws had to be passed to back up principles on which the United States was founded, such as that all people have equal rights. They note that interracial marriage was illegal in the United States until the Supreme Court ruled otherwise in 1967. Prohibiting marriage between same-sex partners is a form of minority discrimination, as it would be if African American or Hispanic partners were not allowed to marry. Like interracial marriage, gay marriage is an idea whose time has come.

Proponents also say that allowing gay people to marry would only strengthen the institution of marriage, creating more families and environments for child rearing and promoting family values. They note that no research has ever shown that being raised by same-sex parents results in psychological or emotional harm or causes children to become gay or lesbian. They assert that the institution of marriage is far less threatened by gay marriage than by the social forces that have been eroding it for the past 50 years.

Some opponents say that same-sex partners who want to publicly declare their commitment to each other should be satisfied with the options of civil union or domestic partnership where available, leaving the institution of marriage to heterosexual couples. Proponents respond that these are second-class options, analogous to the "separate but equal" schools and facilities provided for African Americans until they were declared unconstitutional by the Supreme Court in 1954.

Should marriage be an option for everyone, or should it be limited to heterosexual couples? What do you think?

PROS

- All citizens are entitled to equal rights and equal protection under the law. When same-sex partners are prohibited from marrying, they are denied access to the many rights and benefits available to their fellow citizens who are heterosexual and thus allowed to marry. Prohibiting same-sex marriage is a form of discrimination.

- Prohibiting gay marriage on religious grounds is unconstitutional, as is discrimination based on religious views.

- Society is changing, and sometimes law and society have to lead the way in areas of social justice, setting a standard that encourages people to reconsider their prejudices. This was the case with many civil rights laws. Gay marriage is an idea whose time has come.

- Gay people form the same kind of loving, committed relationships as heterosexual people and have the same right to formalize their relationships in the eyes of society and the law.

- Gay marriage increases the number of committed relationships and families in society and promotes family values.

- Domestic partnerships and civil unions provide couples some rights at the state level, but many of the rights and benefits of marriage are conferred at the federal level, as, for example, in tax laws. Thus, these options are not the same as marriage.

CONS

- Virtually all major religions consider homosexuality sinful or immoral; this value should be reflected in the nation's laws. Legalizing gay marriage would condone behavior that the majority of people consider immoral or unacceptable.

- Legalizing gay marriage weakens the institution of marriage and threatens its sanctity. Opening up marriage to same-sex partners would lead to new definitions of marriage and family, contributing to a further devaluation of marriage and a decline in family values.

- The purpose of marriage is procreation. Since same-sex couples do not procreate, they do not need the protection or validation of marriage.

- Marriage is one of the most important traditional social institutions, and in nearly all societies it is considered to be a union between one man and one woman.

In Review

1. **Why are relationships important for health?** People are social beings and need connections with others to live fully functioning lives. People with strong social support networks tend to enjoy better health than do those with fewer connections, although the mechanisms behind this difference are not fully known.

2. **What kinds of relationships are important?** Two important kinds of relationships are friendships and intimate partnerships. Friendships are reciprocal relationships based on mutual liking; intimate partnerships have additional qualities, usually including exclusivity, commitment, and sexuality. Healthy relationships allow people to be themselves and to grow.

3. **How do intimate relationships form and develop?** People are often attracted to others who are similar to them in significant ways. The more differences there are, the more important are good communication skills. Sternberg conceptualizes love as composed of intimacy, passion, and commitment, with different kinds of love formed by different combinations of these three elements.

4. **What is the role of communication in relationships?** Clear, positive communication is the key to successful intimate relationships. Empathy and the ability to listen are important communication skills, as are using "I" statements, practicing assertiveness, and developing conflict resolution strategies.

5. **What are gender roles and sexual orientation?** Gender roles are the sets of behaviors individuals engage in, whether "masculine" or "feminine," to conform to society's expectations based on their biological sex. Sexual orientation is a person's emotional, romantic, and sexual attraction to someone of the same or other sex or both.

6. **What living arrangements and lifestyle choices are common in our society?** Marriage is the most common and popular living arrangement; it has traditionally been defined as a union between a man and a woman, but same-sex couples are increasingly seeking the social, economic, and psychological benefits of marriage. Cohabitation (defined by the government as two people of the opposite sex living together) is a living arrangement that has become phenomenally popular in the past 40 to 50 years. Singlehood is another increasingly popular choice.

7. **What makes a relationship and a family strong?** A balance of cohesion and flexibility, facilitated by communication, appears to make relationships and families strong and resilient.

 For a detailed summary of this chapter and a comprehensive set of review questions, visit the Online Learning Center at **www.mhhe.com/teague2e**.

Web Resources

American Association for Marriage and Family Therapy: At this Web site, you can view FAQs about marriage and family therapy, read updates on family problems, locate a family therapist in your area, and find listings of resources.
www.aamft.org

American Psychological Association Help Center: The Families and Relationships section of this site features a wide variety of information, such as communication tips, psychological tasks for a good marriage, stepfamily issues, and social life problems.
www.apahelpcenter.org

Family Pride Coalition: This organization promotes equality for lesbian, gay, bisexual, and transgendered parents and their children.
www.familypride.org

National Council on Family Relations: This professional organization offers information on families and family relationships. Go to its Families section for family tips, expert information on family life, and links to other resources on family issues.
www.ncfr.org

Parents Without Partners: This international organization addresses the special issues of rearing children alone for adults who are divorced, widowed, or never married.
www.parentswithoutpartners.org

Prepare-Enrich / Life Innovations: This site offers a stronger-marriage inventory, a quiz for couples, information on finding a marriage counselor, and other resources for couples.
www.prepare-enrich.com

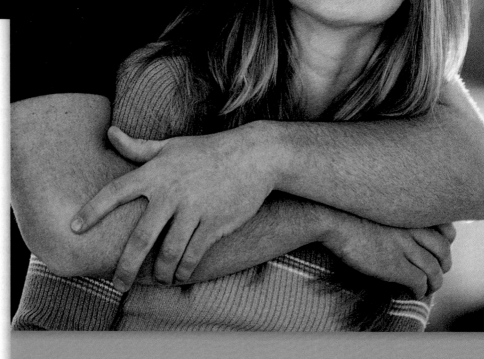

Chapter

15

Sexual Health Biology, Society, and Culture

Ever Wonder...

- if you are "normal"?
- how Viagra works?
- how to talk with a prospective partner about your sexual history?

Like health in general, sexual health is not limited to the absence of symptoms of disease. It includes healthy sexual functioning across the lifespan, satisfying intimate relationships based on mutual respect and trust, and the ability and resources to procreate if so desired. It involves acceptance of one's own sexual feelings and tolerance for those of others. It also includes knowledge about sexuality and access to the information needed to make responsible decisions about your sexual health.

Studies show that an active sex life is good for your health. It reduces the risk of heart disease, decreases risk of depression, provides temporary relief from chronic pain, boosts the immune system, and lowers the risk of death.[1] But sexuality is a complex human behavior, and it can be associated with negative experiences, such as worries and anxieties, relationship discord, health issues, and social problems. This chapter addresses some of these complexities and helps you build a foundation for lifelong sexual health.

Biology, Culture, and Sexual Pleasure

Although sexual anatomy and physiology are similar in all human beings, sexual behavior and expression vary tremendously across societies, cultures, and eras. There are even differences in what is considered sexually pleasurable, a phenomenon that highlights the role of the brain in sexuality. **Sexual pleasure** has been defined as positively valued feelings induced by sexual stimuli.[2]

sexual pleasure
Positively valued feelings induced by sexual stimuli.

Sensory signals arriving in the brain are not inherently pleasurable; rather, the brain interprets them as pleasurable. This interpretation and evaluation of stimuli by the brain as sexually pleasurable is influenced by everything the individual has learned about sex in his or her society and culture, including expectations, attitudes, and values. Thus the experience of sexual pleasure is profoundly affected by context and culture.

American culture projects mixed attitudes about sex and sexual pleasure. Our Puritan forebears believed that the sole purpose of sexuality was procreation and that sexual expression for any other purpose was sinful. Partly as a result of these attitudes, sexuality was shrouded in mystery and silence for generations, and this Puritan legacy continues to influence our cultural character today.

On the other hand, the 20th century, especially the second half of the 20th century, was characterized by a drive for greater openness and freedom of expression, including sexual expression. The "sexual revolution" of the 1960s and 1970s made sexuality something to be talked about, studied, and celebrated.

Sexual attitudes in U.S. society are marked by an ongoing tension between the two poles of sexual restrictiveness and sexual freedom. As with all issues, attitudes toward sex shift over time. The sexual revolution gave way to a more conservative climate in the 1980s and 1990s. Prevailing

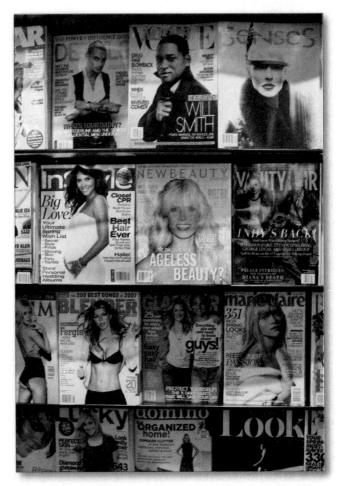

■ What we find sexually exciting, attractive, and acceptable is largely determined by the messages we get from our culture.

attitudes toward sex and sexual pleasure in the early 21st century will be determined, in part, by college students and other young adults (see the box "Sexual Behavior").

Sexual Anatomy and Functioning

Although sexuality serves many purposes in human experience, the biological purpose of sexuality is reproduction. In this section we explore some of the biological aspects of sexuality.

SEXUAL ANATOMY

The male and female sex organs arise from the same undifferentiated tissue during the prenatal period, becoming male or female under the influence of hormones (discussed later in this section). In this sense, the sexual organs of males and females are very similar, and their purpose and functions are complementary. The female sex organs are responsible for the production of ova and, if pregnancy occurs, the development of the fetus. The male sex organs are responsible for producing sperm and delivering them into the female reproductive system to fertilize the ovum.

Who's at Risk

Sexual Behavior

The National Youth Risk Behavior Survey tracks trends in health risk behaviors that contribute to the leading causes of death, disability, and social problems among youth and adults in the United States. The survey is conducted every 2 years among students in grades 9 through 12 in public and private schools in the United States. These are selected behaviors from 2005, the latest year for which data are available:

All Respondents

47% Ever had sexual intercourse.

14% Had sexual intercourse with four or more people.

34% Are currently sexually active (intercourse during the last 3 months).

63% Used a condom during last sexual intercourse.

18% Used birth control pills before last sexual intercourse.

43% Currently use alcohol.

74% Used alcohol in lifetime.

23% Drank alcohol or used drugs before last sexual intercourse (among students who are currently sexually active).

88% Were ever taught in school about AIDS or HIV infection.

Males

48% Ever had sexual intercourse.

17% Had sexual intercourse with four or more people.

33% Are currently sexually active (intercourse during the last 3 months).

30% Did not use a condom during last sexual intercourse.

44% Currently use alcohol.

74% Used alcohol in lifetime.

28% Drank alcohol or used drugs before last sexual intercourse (among students who are currently sexually active).

Females

45% Ever had sexual intercourse.

12% Had sexual intercourse with four or more people.

35% Are currently sexually active (intercourse during the last 3 months).

44% Used a condom during last sexual intercourse.

43% Currently use alcohol.

75% Used alcohol in lifetime.

19% Drank alcohol or used drugs before last sexual intercourse (among students who are currently active).

Blacks

68% Ever had sexual intercourse.

28% Had sexual intercourse with four or more people.

17% Had first sexual intercourse before age 13.

47% Are currently sexually active (intercourse during the last 3 months).

31% Did not use a condom during last sexual intercourse.

Hispanics

51% Ever had sexual intercourse.

16% Had sexual intercourse with four or more people.

7% Had sexual intercourse before age 13.

35% Are currently sexually active (intercourse during the last 3 months).

42% Did not use a condom during last sexual intercourse.

Whites

43% Ever had sexual intercourse.

11% Had sexual intercourse with four or more people.

5% Had first sexual intercourse before age 13.

32% Are currently sexually active (intercourse during the last 3 months).

37% Did not use a condom during last sexual intercourse.

Sources: "YRBSS: Youth Risk Behavior Surveillance System," Centers for Disease Control and Prevention, retrieved May 4, 2008, from www.cdc.gov/ healthyyouth/yrbs.

Female Sex Organs and Reproductive Anatomy In both sexes, there are external and internal sex organs. The external genitalia of the female are called the vulva and include the mons pubis, the labia majora and labia minora, the clitoris, and the vaginal and urethral openings (Figure 15.1). The mons pubis is a mound or layer of fatty tissue that pads and protects the pubic bone. The labia majora (major lips) and labia minora (minor lips) are folds of tissue that wrap around the entrance to the vagina. Pubic hair typically covers the mons pubis and the outer surface of the labia majora. The inner surfaces of the labia majora are smooth and contain several oil and sweat glands. The labia minora form a protective hood, or prepuce, over the clitoris. The clitoris is a highly sensitive, cylindrical body about 3 centimeters in length that fills with blood during sexual excitement. Consisting of a glans, corpus, and crura, the clitoris is located at the top of the vulva between the lips of the labia minora.

The urethral opening, the passageway for urine from the urinary bladder, is located immediately below the clitoris. The hymen is a thin membranous fold, highly variable in appearance, which may partially cover the opening of the vagina. The hymen has no known biological function and is frequently absent. The perineum is the area between the bottom of the vulva and the anus. It contains many nerve endings. The anus is the lower opening of the digestive tract.

The internal sex organs of the female include the vagina, cervix, uterus, fallopian tubes, and ovaries. The vagina is a hollow, muscular tube extending from the external vaginal opening to the cervix. It serves as both the organ for heterosexual intercourse and the birth canal. In most women, it is 3 to 4 inches long. The walls of the vagina are soft and flexible and have several layers. The existence of an area called the G-spot on the lower front wall of the vagina is a subject of debate; if it is present, it may feel like an elevated bump.

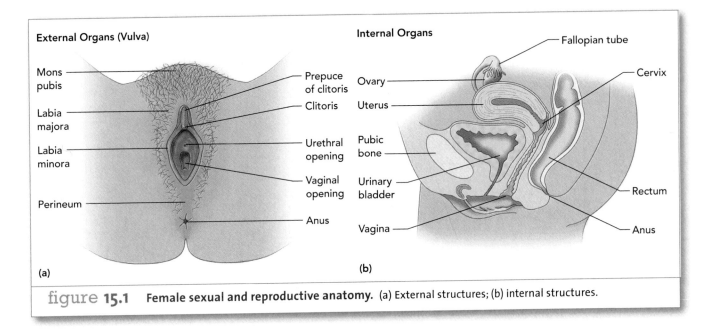

External Organs (Vulva)

Mons pubis
Labia majora
Labia minora
Perineum

Prepuce of clitoris
Clitoris
Urethral opening
Vaginal opening
Anus

(a)

Internal Organs

Ovary
Uterus
Pubic bone
Urinary bladder
Vagina

Fallopian tube
Cervix
Rectum
Anus

(b)

figure 15.1 **Female sexual and reproductive anatomy.** (a) External structures; (b) internal structures.

Located on either side of the vagina under the labia are the crura, extensions of the clitoris.

The cervix is the lower part of the uterus; it extends into the vagina and contains the opening to the uterus. The cervix produces a mucus that changes with different stages of the menstrual cycle. The uterus is the organ in which a fertilized egg develops into an embryo and then a fetus. Approximately the size of a pear (3 inches long), the uterus is made up of several layers of muscle and tissue. The endometrium is the layer that is shed during menstruation.

The ovaries are the female reproductive glands that store and release the ova (eggs) every month, usually one at a time—the process of ovulation. They also produce the female sex hormones estrogen and progesterone. The ovaries are about 1½ inches long and are located on either side of the uterus. Extending from the upper sides of the uterus are the fallopian tubes (or oviducts), the passageways through which ova move from the ovaries into the uterus. They are about 4 inches long. Their openings are lined with fimbria, appendages with beating cilia that sweep the surface of the ovaries during ovulation and guide the ovum down into the tubes.

The mammary glands, or breasts, are also part of female sexual and reproductive anatomy. They consist of 15 to 25 lobes that are padded by connective tissue and fat. Within the lobes are glands that produce milk when the woman is lactating following the birth of a baby. At the center of each breast is a nipple, surrounded by a ring of darker colored skin called the areola. The nipple becomes erect when stimulated by cold, touch, or sexual stimuli.

Male Sex Organs and Reproductive Anatomy The external genitalia of the male include the penis and the scrotum, which contains the testes (Figure 15.2). The penis, when erect, is designed to deliver sperm into the female reproductive tract. The shaft of the penis is formed of three columns of sponge-like erectile tissue that fill with blood during sexual excitement. The glans, or head of the penis, is an expansion of the corpus spongiosum (one of the three columns of erectile tissue in the penis shaft). The glans contains a higher concentration of nerve endings than the shaft and is highly sensitive.

The corona is a crownlike structure that protrudes slightly and forms a border between the glans and the shaft; it is also highly sensitive. The frenulum is a fold of skin extending from the corona to the foreskin. The foreskin, or prepuce, covers the glans, more or less completely. **Circumcision** involves removing this skin and leaving the head of the penis permanently exposed. The urethral opening, through which both urine and semen pass (at different times), is located at the tip of the penis in the glans. The urethra runs the length of the penis from the urinary bladder to the exterior of the body.

circumcision
Removal of the foreskin of the penis; a procedure often routinely performed on newborn male infants in the United States.

The scrotum, a thin sac composed of skin and muscle fibers, contains the testes. The scrotum is separated from the body to keep the testes at the lower temperature that is needed for sperm production. The area between the scrotum and the anus is the perineum; as in females, it contains many nerve endings. The anus is the lower opening of the digestive tract.

The male internal reproductive organs include the testes; a series of ducts that transport sperm (the epididymis, vas deferens, ejaculatory ducts, and urethra); and a set of glands that produce semen and other fluids (the seminal vesicles, prostate gland, and Cowper's glands). The two testes, located in the scrotum, are the male reproductive glands; they produce both sperm and male sex hormones such as testosterone. Once sperm are produced in the testes, they enter the epididymis, a highly coiled duct lying on

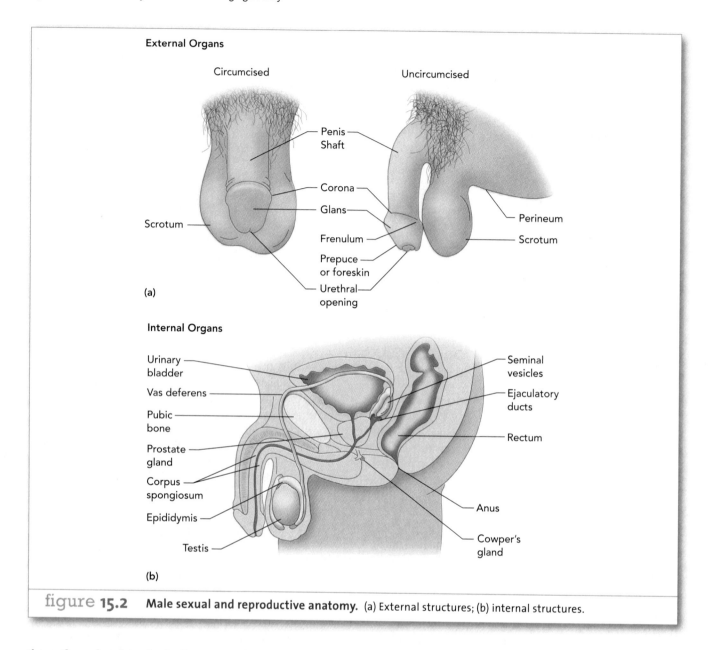

External Organs

Circumcised

Uncircumcised

Penis
Shaft

Corona

Glans

Perineum

Scrotum

Frenulum

Scrotum

Prepuce
or foreskin

Urethral
opening

(a)

Internal Organs

Urinary
bladder

Seminal
vesicles

Vas deferens

Ejaculatory
ducts

Pubic
bone

Prostate
gland

Rectum

Corpus
spongiosum

Epididymis

Anus

Testis

Cowper's
gland

(b)

figure **15.2** **Male sexual and reproductive anatomy.** (a) External structures; (b) internal structures.

the surface of each testis. As they move along the length of the epididymis (which, if uncoiled, would measure about 20 feet in length), immature sperm mature and develop the ability to swim.

When the male ejaculates, sperm are propelled from the epididymis into the vas deferens, another duct, which joins with ducts from the seminal vesicles to form the short ejaculatory ducts. The two seminal vesicles, located at the back of the bladder, produce about 60 percent of the volume of semen, the milky fluid that carries sperm and contains nutrients to fuel them. The sperm and semen travel through the ejaculatory ducts to the prostate gland, a doughnut-shaped structure that encircles the urethra and contributes the remaining volume of semen. The semen is then ejaculated through the urethra. The two Cowper's glands, located below the prostate gland, produce a clear mucus that is secreted into the urethra just before ejaculation. The volume of semen in one ejacula-

tion is about 2 to 5 milliliters, containing between 100 and 600 million sperm.

SEXUAL RESPONSE

In order for reproduction to occur, ova and sperm have to be brought into close association with each other. The psychological and motivational mechanism for this is the human sexual response, which includes sex drive, sexual arousal, and orgasm.

Sex Drive Sex drive—sexual desire, or libido—is defined as a biological urge for sexual activity. The principal hormone responsible for the sex drive in both males and females is testosterone, produced by the testes in males and by the adrenal

sex drive
Biological urge for sexual activity; also called sexual desire or libido.

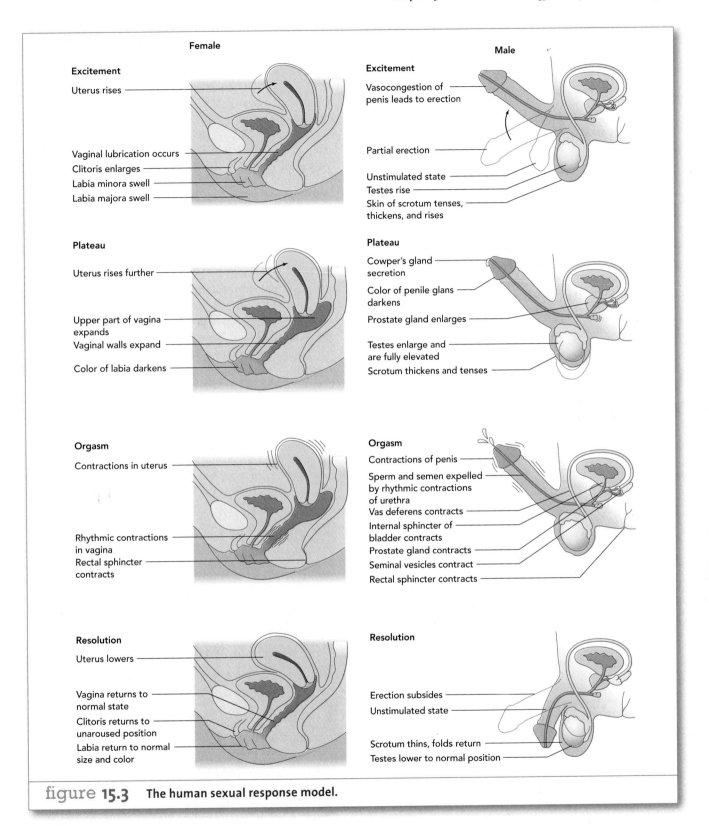

figure **15.3**   **The human sexual response model.**

stimulation of the clitoris with fingers or a vibrator can help women reach orgasm.

When a woman is unable to reach orgasm, it is usually due to inhibition or lack of needed stimulation. Some women may be tempted to fake orgasm, perhaps out of fear of being perceived as sexually deficient, but doing so can undermine a relationship. A satisfying relationship includes having honest discussions about what helps both partners respond orgasmically (see the box "Discussing a Sexual Problem With Your Partner").

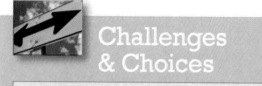

Challenges & Choices

Discussing a Sexual Problem With Your Partner

Conversations about sex are part of virtually all successful intimate relationships. Sexual desires are personal, and partners can't read each other's minds. At some point you may need to speak up about a sexual problem. Here are some guidelines:

- Be assertive about your needs, but be tactful and considerate. Sex is a sensitive topic for most people.
- Admit frustration but avoid anger. Anger is a roadblock to effective communication.
- Avoid blame. Take responsibility for whatever part of the problem you may have control over.
- Avoid words like *should, ought,* and *must.* They sound like demands and imply that there is some standard your partner has to meet. Improving a sexual relationship means working together for your mutual pleasure and satisfaction.
- If your partner approaches you with a problem, try not to be defensive. When people want to solve sexual problems, it means they care about the relationship.

It's Not Just Personal . . .

If you and your partner are having a sexual problem, keep in mind that this is more common than you might think. For example, 8% of women say that they rarely achieve orgasm. For men, premature ejaculation is common, with 28% reporting that they experience this problem often.

Source: Sexuality Information and Education Council of the United States, www.siecus.org.

SEXUAL DEVELOPMENT AND HEALTH ACROSS THE LIFESPAN

androgens
Male sex hormones, secreted primarily by the testes.

estrogens
Female sex hormones; secreted by the ovaries.

progestins
Female sex hormones; secreted by the ovaries.

The biology of sexual and reproductive development is directed by hormones, beginning in the womb. Male sex hormones, called **androgens**, are secreted primarily by the testes, and female sex hormones, called **estrogens** and **progestins**, are secreted by the ovaries. The adrenal glands also secrete androgens in both males and females. The pituitary gland and the hypothalamus in the brain both have roles in regulating levels and functions of the sex hormones.

Prenatal Development During prenatal development, the presence of a Y chromosome causes the reproductive glands to develop into testes; the testes produce testosterone, which causes the undifferentiated reproductive structures to become male sex organs. If there is no Y chromosome, the glands develop into ovaries and the reproductive structures become female sex organs. At birth, the appearance of the external sex organs signals the biological sex of the baby to the world.

Puberty Hormones come into play again at puberty, when the secondary sex characteristics appear and the reproductive system matures. There is a growth spurt in both sexes (about 2 years earlier in girls than in boys), the sex organs become larger, and pubic and underarm hair appears. In boys, the voice deepens, facial hair begins to grow, and the onset of **ejaculation** occurs. Boys begin to experience **nocturnal emissions** (orgasm and ejaculation during sleep), and the testes start to produce sperm. In girls, breasts develop, body fat increases, and **menarche**, the onset of menstruation, occurs.

ejaculation
Emission of semen during orgasm.

nocturnal emission
Orgasm and ejaculation during sleep.

menarche
Onset of menstruation.

Menstruation Every month between the ages of about 12 and about 50, except during pregnancy, women experience monthly menstrual periods. During the first half of the cycle, the lining of the uterus thickens with blood vessels in prepa-

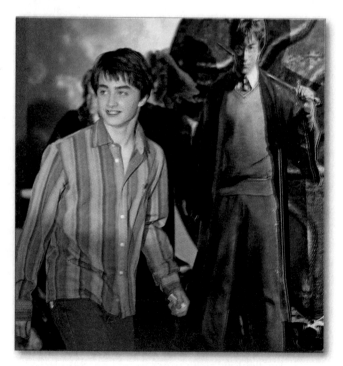

■ Movie viewers watched Daniel Radcliffe transition from a prepubescent boy to a young man as he played the lead role in the Harry Potter movie series. Radcliffe was 15 when *Harry Potter and the Prisoner of Azkaban* was released in 2004, two years older than his character.

ration for the possibility of pregnancy, and an ovum matures in one of the ovaries. About halfway through the cycle, the ovum is released (ovulation) and is carried into the uterus. If sperm are present, the ovum may be fertilized and begin to develop into an embryo. If sperm are not present, the uterine lining is shed, causing **menses**, and the cycle begins again.

menses
Flow of menstrual blood; the menstrual period.

Some girls and women experience uncomfortable physical symptoms during their periods, such as cramps and backache, and some experience physical and emotional symptoms before their periods, such as headache, irritability, and mood swings, referred to as premenstrual tension or premenstrual syndrome (PMS). If symptoms are severe and interfere with usual work, family, or social activities, the woman may be diagnosed with premenstrual dysphoric disorder (PMDD). The exact causes of PMS and PMDD are not known, but lifestyle changes, such as exercising, eating well, and avoiding alcohol, may help relieve symptoms. A physician may prescribe medications for more severe symptoms.

Menopause   In middle age, hormonal changes cause a gradual reduction in ovarian functioning that culminates in **menopause**, the cessation of menstruation. Although the average age at menopause in the United States is 52, a small percentage of women experience premature menopause before age 40.[7]

menopause
Cessation of menstruation.

During the time leading up to menopause, a period of 3 to 7 years called *perimenopause,* many women experience symptoms caused by hormonal fluctuations, such as hot flashes, night sweats, irritability, and insomnia. A decrease in estrogen production can cause less visible symptoms as well, such as a reduction in bone density and changes in blood levels of cholesterol. These changes contribute to women's increased risk of osteoporosis and heart disease later in life.

Loss of estrogen also causes changes in the genitals, which can lead to changes in sexual functioning. These changes may be minimal for some women but dramatic for others. The vaginal walls become thinner and lubrication may decrease, making intercourse less comfortable. Vaginal lubrication during the excitement phase may take from 1 to 5 minutes to occur, whereas in a young woman it takes only 15 to 20 seconds. It may take longer to reach orgasm, and orgasm may be less intense. In some women, sex drive may decrease. Because sexuality has so many emotional, psychological, and interpersonal dimensions, however, the physical changes associated with menopause do not necessarily have a major impact on a woman's sex life.

Hormone replacement therapy (HRT) has been a popular treatment for the symptoms of menopause and perimenopause. At first, estrogen was used alone, but evidence surfaced that estrogen replacement therapy increased the risk of endometrial cancer. Then estrogen and progesterone were used together in HRT, not only to treat the symptoms of menopause but also to lower the risk of heart disease and osteoporosis in menopausal women.

In 1991 the National Institutes of Health began a research project called the Women's Health Initiative Study to provide definitive conclusions on the relationship between HRT and osteoporosis, breast cancer, heart disease, stroke, blood clots, and colon cancer. Results were due in 2005, but in 2002, the portion of the study involving women taking a combination of estrogen and progestin was abruptly stopped when researchers concluded that the risks of HRT far outweighed the benefits.[8] The risk of breast cancer rose more quickly for women on HRT after 4 years, and the risk of heart disease and blood clots increased each year for women on HRT.

Based on results from the Women's Health Initiative Study, doctors generally advise women to avoid HRT if at all possible. New drugs called selective estrogen receptor modulators may allow women to take advantage of estrogen's benefits without incurring its risks. Uncomfortable symptoms of perimenopause and menopause can be improved in many cases by lifestyle changes like increased physical activity, stress management, and weight loss. Women who elect to use HRT are advised to take the lowest effective dose for the shortest possible time.[8] The U.S. Preventive Services Task Force and the American Heart Association currently recommend that HRT not be used to protect against heart disease.

Viropause   Men do not experience a dramatic change in reproductive capacity in midlife as women do; the testes continue to produce sperm throughout life. Some researchers believe, however, that middle-aged men experience a 5- to 12-year period during which their testosterone levels

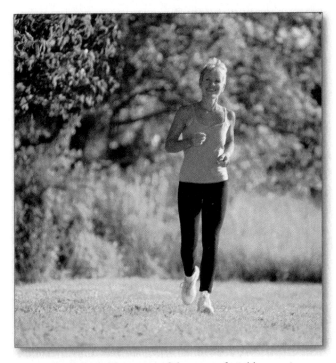

■ Exercise helps relieve many of the uncomfortable symptoms of menopause.

fluctuate.[9] The term **viropause** (pronounced VEER-o-pause) has been coined to refer to changes in virility or sexual desire in middle-aged men, analogous to menopause in women. The condition is also referred to as androgen decline in aging males. Common symptoms include irritability, sluggishness, mild to moderate mood swings, and a sense of declining vitality. A sudden loss of self-respect may reduce testosterone levels, which can in turn reduce a man's sex drive.[9]

viropause
Changes in virility or sexual desire in middle-aged men.

As testosterone levels decline in later life, men experience some changes in sexual functioning. It may take up to several minutes to achieve an erection during stimulation, whereas in younger men it takes from 3 to 5 seconds. It may also take longer to reach orgasm, and orgasm may be less intense. The refractory period usually becomes longer as men get older.

Men aged 50 and older who are bothered by symptoms of viropause should consult their family physician.

The doctor will measure blood levels of total testosterone in the morning when these levels are the highest. Testosterone levels above 400 nanograms per deciliter (ng/dl) are considered normal, and levels between 200 and 400 ng/dl are borderline. If testosterone is deficient, treatments are available to increase levels.[10] For both men and women, biological changes in the sexual response phases have only a marginal effect on sexual interest and activity. There does tend to be a slow, steady decline in sexual activity over the course of life, caused by lower levels of sex hormones and physiological changes. The more sexually active a person is, the less effect these biological changes have.

Varieties of Sexual Behavior and Expression

What is "normal" sexual behavior? By now it should be clear that what is defined as normal depends on social and cultural

Highlight on Health

Sexuality and Disability

A wide range of disabling conditions can affect a person's sexuality, from Down syndrome to spinal cord injury. Although individuals with disabilities may experience limitations on their sexuality or may have to develop new or alternative forms of sexual activity, most people with disabilities can have a rewarding sex life. Information and education can help individuals with disabilities, as can counseling that focuses on building self-esteem; overcoming shame, guilt, fear, anger, and unrealistic expectations; and developing a holistic approach to sexuality that includes all activities that offer pleasure and intimacy. Information and education are also important for members of the general public, who too often fail to acknowledge the full humanity of individuals with disabilities, including their sexuality.

For people with physical limitations, a major challenge can be finding a sexual partner. Individuals may not want to risk rejection and may hide their feelings behind a mask of anger or indifference. Potential partners may need to be open-minded, patient, persistent, and willing to experiment to find out what works.

Depending on the type of condition or injury, different forms of sexual expression may be possible. A person with a spinal cord injury may or may not be able to have an orgasm, but he or she may be able to have intercourse, may experience sensuous feelings in other parts of the body, and may be able to have a child. As in any relationship, the key is discovering who the other person is and nurturing emotional as well as sexual intimacy. When a partner in an established relationship is facing a disability, the couple

may want to seek information and counseling on how the disability will affect their sexual functioning.

Changes in sexual functioning and desire can also be caused by chronic diseases, such as diabetes, arthritis, and cardiovascular disease, as well as by the medications used to treat them. Diabetes can cause nerve damage and circulatory problems that affect erectile functioning in men; arthritis causes pain that can make sexual activity uncomfortable; cardiovascular disease can lead to depression or to fear that sexual activity will cause another heart attack or stroke. Individuals and couples may have to make significant adjustments in their forms of sexual expression to accommodate such disabling conditions.

Individuals with mental or developmental disabilities also face challenges in sexual expression. Depending on the degree of disability, some such individuals may be unable to learn the basics of reproduction or how to behave appropriately in public, while others are able to marry and raise children. Sex education is important for all people with developmental disabilities, especially adolescents. Children and young teens need to know about puberty and the hormonal and physical changes they will experience, and they especially need to know that these changes are normal. Both boys and girls need to learn about masturbation and that, if done, it should be done in private.

For more severely disabled people, education may be limited to teaching them not to undress or touch their genitals in public. For those with milder disabilities, learning about companionship, safe sex practices, and sexual relationships is appropriate. In general, the best approach is to tailor sex education to the needs of the individual.

Sources: Human Sexuality, 6th ed., by B. Strong, W. Yarber, B. Sayad, and C. DeVault, 2008, New York: McGraw-Hill; The Sexual Male: Problems and Solutions, by R. Milsten and J. Slowinski, 1999, New York: W.W. Norton and Company.

context. For example, individuals with a disability will have special issues related to having a sexual life (see the box "Sexuality and Disability"). Rather than thinking in terms of normalcy, social scientists think in terms of behavior that is typical and behavior that is less typical.

TYPICAL AND COMMON FORMS OF SEXUAL EXPRESSION

Typical forms of sexual behavior and expression in U.S. society include celibacy, kissing, erotic touch, self-stimulation, oral-genital stimulation, and intercourse.

Celibacy   Continuous abstention from sexual activities with others is called **celibacy**. People may be completely celibate (do not engage in masturbation) or partially celibate (engage in masturbation). Moral and religious beliefs lead some people to choose celibacy. Lack of a suitable sexual partner or sexual relationship may be another reason for celibacy.[6]

Some people use the term *abstinence* interchangeably with *celibacy*, but **abstinence** usually means abstention only from sexual intercourse. As such, abstinence is promoted as a way to avoid sexually transmitted diseases and unintended pregnancy. It is discussed further later in this chapter and in Chapter 16.

celibacy
Continuous abstention from sexual activities with others.

abstinence
Abstention from sexual intercourse, usually as a way to avoid conception or STDs.

Kissing   Kissing is usually the first sexual experience with another person. The act of kissing stimulates all of the body senses simultaneously. The lips physically respond to a kiss by swelling, darkening in color, and congesting with blood. These physical changes make nerve endings in the lips more sensitive, heightening the pleasurable sensation.

Erotic Touch   Touch is a sensual form of communication that can elicit feelings of tenderness and affection as well as sexual feelings. It is an important part of **foreplay**, touching that increases sexual arousal and precedes sexual intercourse. Some areas of the body are more sensitive to touch than others. Skin in the nonspecific erogenous zones of the body (the inner thighs, armpits, shoulders, feet, ears, and sides of the back and neck) contains more nerve endings than do many other areas; these areas are capable of being aroused by touch. Skin in the specific erogenous zones (penis, clitoris, vulva, perineum, lips, breasts, and buttocks) has an even higher density of nerve endings, and nerve endings are closer to the skin surface.[6] These erogenous zones are more sensitive to sexual arousal by touch. The landscape of erotic touch includes holding hands, stroking, caressing, squeezing, tickling, scratching, and massaging.

foreplay
Touching that increases sexual arousal before sexual intercourse.

Self-Stimulation   The two most common self-stimulation sexual activities, called **autoerotic behaviors**, are sexual

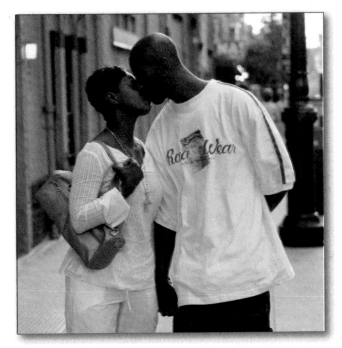

■ The lips are a highly sensitive part of the body, making kissing an intimate act.

fantasies and masturbation. Sexual fantasies are mental images, scenarios, and daydreams imagined to initiate sexual arousal. They range from simple images to complicated erotic stories.[11] One study found that college men fantasize or think about sex about seven times a day, compared to four to five times a day for college women. Men are more likely to focus on their partner's physical characteristics, while women focus more on their partner's emotional and personal characteristics.[11]

autoerotic behaviors
Self-stimulating sexual activities, primarily sexual fantasies and masturbation.

The fact that the body can become aroused when a person thinks about sex highlights the fact that the brain is a major player in sexual functioning. Many people feel guilty about sexual fantasies,[6] but fantasies are actually effective and harmless ways of exploring sexual fulfillment. People often fantasize about situations and behaviors they would never choose to experience in real life.

Masturbation is self-stimulation of the genitals for sexual pleasure. It is usually done manually or with a vibrator or other sex toy. The stigma attached to masturbation is left over from a previous era, when it was considered sinful and dangerous to one's health, probably because its purpose was pleasure rather than procreation. Today, masturbation is better understood and more widely accepted as a natural and healthy sexual behavior. Masturbation is a part of sex therapy programs designed to help people overcome sexual problems, and mutual masturbation is promoted as a way to practice safer sex. Still, about half of all men and women feel guilty about masturbating.[12]

masturbation
Self-stimulation of the genitals for sexual pleasure.

Oral-Genital Stimulation **Cunnilingus** is the oral stimulation of the female genitals with the tongue and lips; it includes licking, kissing, and gently sucking the clitoris, labia, or vaginal area. **Fellatio** is the oral stimulation of the male genitals with the tongue, lips, and mouth. Oral stimulation can be part of foreplay, or it can be a sexual activity leading to orgasm. Some people find oral-genital stimulation very pleasurable; others refrain because of religious or moral beliefs. Oral sex is not an entirely safe form of sex, because infections can be transmitted via the mouth. Using some form of protection during oral sex is recommended, as discussed later in this chapter.

cunnilingus
Oral stimulation of the female genitals with the tongue and lips.

fellatio
Oral stimulation of the male genitals with the tongue, lips, and mouth.

Anal Intercourse A small percentage of heterosexual couples and a larger percentage of gay male couples practice anal intercourse, the penetration of the rectum with the penis. The anal area has a high density of nerve endings and is sensitive to stimulation. Because the skin and tissue of the anus and rectum are delicate and can be easily torn, anal intercourse is one of the riskiest sexual behaviors for the transmission of infections. Condom use is strongly recommended during anal intercourse.

Sexual Intercourse Sexual intercourse, also known as coitus or making love, is by far the most common form of adult sexual expression. It is a source of sexual pleasure for most couples. In sexual intercourse, a man typically inserts his erect penis into a woman's vagina and thrusts with his hips and pelvis until he ejaculates. A woman who is aroused responds with matching hip and pelvic thrusts, but she may or may not reach orgasm solely from penetration and thrusting, as mentioned earlier.

Sexual intercourse can be performed in a variety of positions. The most common is the so-called missionary position, in which the man lies on top of the woman. In this position, the penis can penetrate deeply into the vagina. When the woman lies on top of the man, penetration may not be as deep, but the woman has more control, an important psychological factor for some women. When the woman sits or kneels on top of the man, penetration is deeper and the woman can increase clitoral stimulation by rocking back and forth.[6]

In the rear-entry position, the woman lies face down and the man lies on top of her, or both lie on their sides. Although penetration is not as deep in this position, there is more opportunity for clitoral stimulation by either the woman or the man. Side-by-side positions may be popular for sexual partners with significant weight differences, pregnant women, partners with chronic pain disorders like arthritis, and partners who do not enjoy deep thrusting.[6]

ATYPICAL SEXUAL BEHAVIORS AND PARAPHILIAS

Some sexual practices are much less common statistically in our society than those already described. If they are practiced between consenting adults and no physical or psychological harm is done to anyone, they are simply considered atypical. Examples are sex games in which partners enact sexual fantasies, use sex toys (vibrators, dildos), or engage in phone sex (talk about sex, describe erotic scenarios). Another kind of sex game is bondage and discipline, in which restriction of movement (using handcuffs or ropes, for example) or sensory deprivation (using blindfolds or masks) is employed for sexual enjoyment. Most sex games are safe and harmless, but partners need to openly discuss and agree beforehand on what they are comfortable doing.

Atypical sexual practices that do not meet the criteria described above (being consensual and causing no harm) are called paraphilias; they are classified as mental disorders, and many are illegal. According to the American Psychiatric Association's *Diagnostic and Statistical Manual of Mental Disorders (DSM-IV-TR)*, a **paraphilia** is a mental disorder characterized by recurrent, intense sexual urges, fantasies, or behaviors generally involving (1) nonhuman objects, (2) the suffering and humiliation of oneself or one's sexual partner, or (3) children or other nonconsenting adults.[13] The urges occur over a period of at least 6 months and cause significant distress or impairment.

paraphilia
Mental disorder characterized by recurrent, intense sexual urges, fantasies, or behaviors generally involving (1) nonhuman objects, (2) the suffering and humiliation of oneself or one's sexual partner, or (3) children or other nonconsenting adults.

Examples of paraphilias are exhibitionism (exposing one's genitals to strangers), voyeurism (observing others' sexual activity without their knowledge), and pedophilia (sexual attraction to and activity with children). A person with a paraphilia usually seeks treatment only when compelled to do so by the law. Treatment focuses initially on reducing the danger to the patient and potential victims and then on strategies to suppress the behavior. Relapse prevention is essential since these behaviors are usually long-standing.[6]

Sexual Dysfunctions

At some point in their lives, many people experience some kind of **sexual dysfunction**—a disturbance in sexual drive, performance, or satisfaction. Up to 50 percent of couples report having experienced sexual dissatisfaction or dysfunction.[14] Sexual difficulties may occur at any point in the sexual response, although lack of sexual desire is cited as the most frequent problem in marriage and long-term relationships.[15] Fortunately, most forms of sexual dysfunction are treatable.

sexual dysfunction
Disturbance in sexual drive, performance, or satisfaction.

FEMALE SEXUAL DYSFUNCTIONS

Common sexual dysfunctions in women include pain during intercourse, sexual desire disorder, female sexual arousal disorder, and orgasmic dysfunction.

Pain During Intercourse Some women experience pain during intercourse as a result of **vaginismus**, intense involuntary contractions of the outer third of the muscles of the vagina that tighten the vaginal opening when penetration is attempted. The muscle spasm may range from mild, causing discomfort during intercourse, to severe, preventing intercourse altogether. Vaginismus may be caused by the physiological effects of a medical condition, such as a pelvic or vaginal infection, by psychological factors, such as fear of intercourse, or by lack of vaginal lubrication. A physician may recommend **Kegel exercises**, the alternating contraction and relaxation of pelvic floor muscles, to relieve vaginismus. Referral to psychotherapy or sex therapy may be needed if the condition persists.

vaginismus
Intense involuntary contractions of the outer third of the muscles of the vagina that prevent penetration or make it uncomfortable.

Kegel exercises
Alternating contraction and relaxation of pelvic floor muscles, performed to help relieve vaginismus, among other effects.

Sexual Desire Disorder Sexual desire disorder is characterized by lack of sexual fantasies and desire for sexual activity. Because individuals have different normal levels of sexual desire, a problem is considered to exist only if a person is dissatisfied with her own or her partner's level of sexual desire. Low sexual desire can have physical causes, such as medications and drugs, hormonal changes, alcohol, nicotine, recreational drugs, some antidepressants, birth control pills, and medical problems such as chronic pain.[16] Low sexual desire can also be caused by psychological, emotional, and relationship problems.[20]

Female Sexual Arousal Disorder This disorder is characterized by an inability to attain or maintain the lubrication-swelling response of sexual arousal to the completion

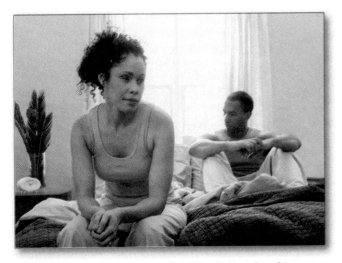

■ Sexuality has physical, psychological, emotional, and interpersonal dimensions. Although sexual problems can have medical or physical causes, they often occur because of relationship problems.

of sexual activity. The symptoms do not occur because of insufficient or misplaced sexual stimulation. Like sexual desire disorder, this disorder is considered a problem only if the individual experiencing it considers it a problem.

Orgasmic Dysfunction Orgasmic dysfunction is defined as the persistent inability to have an orgasm following normal sexual arousal. Between 25 and 35 percent of women report having had difficulty with orgasm on one or more occasions, and 10–15 percent of women report that they have never had an orgasm.[17] Some women can achieve orgasm through masturbation or oral sex but not with penile penetration. Although orgasm is not necessary for conception or enjoyment of sex, difficulty achieving orgasm can become a frustrating experience.

Orgasmic dysfunction may be influenced by psychological and emotional factors, by lack of knowledge and experience, or by the person's beliefs and attitudes about sex.[18] Certain medications, including some antidepressants, also reduce the ability to reach orgasm. Orgasmic dysfunction may be more common in younger women; as they gain experience, learn more about their bodies, and are exposed to a wider variety of stimulation, they may be less likely to have difficulties reaching orgasm. Therapy for orgasmic dysfunction focuses on encouraging women to experiment with their own bodies to discover what stimulates them to orgasm. They are then encouraged to transfer this learning to their sexual relationships.

Treatment of Female Sexual Dysfunctions Much of what is known about the neurophysiology of sexual arousal, desire, and orgasm has come from research on men and has been applied to women.[19] But women's sexuality is different from men's and much more complex than previously thought. Currently, there is a new interest in female sexuality on the part of scientists, sex therapists, and pharmaceutical companies, partly as a result of the success of Viagra in relieving men's sexual problems.

One approach to treatment of sexual problems in women is testosterone replacement therapy. As noted earlier, testosterone is responsible for sex drive in both men and women. Women typically experience a 15 percent drop in testosterone levels during their 30s and 40s.[7] Women with deficient testosterone levels may experience decreased sexual arousal, less sexual fantasizing, and less sensitivity to the stimulation of their nipples, vagina, or clitoris.

Sensibly prescribed, medically necessary testosterone can increase a woman's sex drive without serious side effects. Benefits of testosterone treatments have included increased feelings of vitality and sexual desire, but possible side effects include increased risk of heart disease and liver damage.[7]

Viagra has been tried in women to treat low sexual desire, but results have been disappointing. Viagra has the same effect on the clitoris that it has on the penis, allowing tissue to swell with blood during sexual arousal. Although the ability to become aroused may be enhanced, the desire to have sex may not. A few studies suggest that Viagra combined with a low doses of testosterone replacement may have good results.[7] Despite setbacks, the drug market for treating female sexual dysfunction is likely to grow.

MALE SEXUAL DYSFUNCTIONS

Male sexual dysfunctions include pain during intercourse, sexual desire disorder, erectile dysfunction, and ejaculation dysfunction.

Pain During Intercourse

Pain during intercourse or after intercourse is rarely cited as a sexual dysfunction in men, but it can reduce sexual pleasure and satisfaction. Penile pain usually results from infections from sexually transmitted diseases. Herpes can cause painful lesions on the penis, and gonorrhea and chlamydia cause a penile discharge and pain with urination or ejaculation for most men. Peyronie's disease, an abnormal curvature of the penis, can also make intercourse painful. Infections of the prostate and epididymis also cause pain and should be treated.

Sexual Desire Disorder

Like women, men sometimes experience reduced interest in sex. Sexual desire disorders are frequently caused by emotional problems, including relationship difficulties, depression, guilt over infidelity, worry, stress, and overwork. Reduced sexual desire also can have some physical causes, such as changes in testosterone level. Some health conditions can reduce the production of testosterone by the testes. One out of every four men over 30 years of age has low testosterone levels, and 1 out of every 20 has clinical symptoms associated with deficient levels.

Erectile Dysfunction

As noted earlier, erection occurs when arterioles supplying blood to the penis relax, allowing the spongy chambers of the penis to fill with blood. In men with **erectile dysfunction (ED)**, smooth-muscle cells constrict the local arteries and reduce blood flow to a trickle, preventing a buildup of blood. The penis remains flaccid if the smooth-muscle cells are contracted.

erectile dysfunction (ED) Condition in which the penis does not become erect before sex or stay erect during sex.

The causes of erectile dysfunction (formerly called impotence) can be psychological or physical or both. The best way to determine the cause is to observe overnight erection patterns. Starting in early childhood, males experience erections during normal sleep. If the cause of ED is emotional, erections will continue to occur during sleep. Less than 20 percent of ED cases have emotional causes.[6, 21] Examples of such causes are anxiety about sexual performance and problems in the relationship with the partner.

Some of the physical causes of ED are low testosterone levels, medications (some antidepressants, blood pressure medications), drugs (alcohol, tobacco), injury, vascular disease, blood flow problems in the genitals, and nerve damage, such as from diabetes, injury, or prostate surgery (see the box "Sex and Alcohol").

Long-term excessive pressure from riding a bicycle also may cause erectile dysfunction. Blood vessels that supply the penis are located in the area between the base of the scrotum and the anus, and excessive pressure in this area can reduce blood flow to the penis. Numbness in the penis and scrotum is a warning sign of excessive pressure. If you experience this problem, try adjusting the bicycle seat so your legs don't extend as far while pedaling, or buy a wider bicycle seat. Personnel in most bicycle shops can help you adjust your seat properly.[14]

Ejaculation Dysfunction

Premature ejaculation, defined as ejaculation less than 2 minutes after the beginning of intercourse, is probably the most common type of ejaculation dysfunction.[21] (Men typically average 2 to 7 minutes before ejaculation.) About one-third of sexually active men experience premature ejaculation; gay men have lower rates of premature ejaculation.[21] Like ED, premature ejaculation often results from anxiety about sexual performance or unreasonable expectations. For example, a man might be worried about maintaining an erection and rush to a climax.[14]

An effective technique for preventing premature ejaculation is to stop before orgasm, slow down, and then start again. The stop-start method trains the body to lengthen the duration of the sexual arousal state and can increase enjoyment. Numbing creams can work but may inhibit arousal;

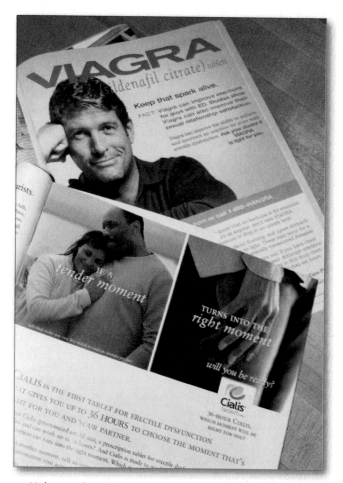

■ Male sexual problems have become a public topic as a result of the development of a new class of drugs that treat erectile dysfunction. Viagra is the most frequently prescribed drug in the United States.

Challenges & Choices

Sex and Alcohol

Have you ever . . .

- Had regrets about sex the next day?
- Suspected that you might be pregnant because of unprotected sex?
- Had sex with someone you would not choose to have a relationship with?
- Been unable to remember the events from a previous night?
- Wondered whether you were victimized by a date rape drug?
- Been unable to perform sexually?

All of these concerns are much more likely to be on your mind if you consume excessive amounts of alcohol. Alcohol lowers sexual inhibitions and impairs judgment, decision making, effective listening, rational thinking, and the ability to assess risky behaviors and potentially dangerous situations. Alcohol consumption also reduces erectile response in men and vaginal lubrication in women. Heavy consumption of alcohol is even riskier, making it more difficult to maintain control. Psychoactive drugs like marijuana and Ecstasy also increase your risk of engaging in behavior you might regret later.

The physical consequences of sexual activity under the influence of alcohol are well known: increased risk for STDs, sexual assaults, and unwanted pregnancy. The emotional consequences are too often overlooked. Honesty, respect, trust, and communication are likely to be compromised

under the influence of too much alcohol. Crossing sexual boundaries, acting against personal values, and rushing into sexual intimacy can cause awkwardness in an otherwise promising relationship.

To make sure you don't jeopardize your sexual health through alcohol consumption, you can take two simple precautions: first, know your alcohol limit and don't exceed it, and second, enlist a buddy when you go to a bar or party and look out for each other. Also, take time to clarify your values, attitudes, and standards about your own sexuality. Is your behavior consistent with your values? Are you influenced by media images and peer pressure, or are your decisions about sexual activity intentional and voluntary?

When you are going to be in a potentially sexual situation, consider these questions ahead of time: (1) Will I be sexually active and, if so, to what degree? (2) How does being sexually active fit with my personal values and beliefs? (3) If I choose to be sexually active, how can I ensure my physical and emotional safety? Along with all the sexual information and freedom available to people in our society comes the responsibility to make informed, healthy choices.

It's Not Just Personal . . .

Researchers have recently become concerned that extreme drinking is being glamorized by videos and photos of 21st birthday binges posted at YouTube and MySpace. In a study of more than 2,500 college students, 34 percent of the men and 24 percent of the women reported consuming 21 or more drinks to celebrate their 21st birthday. Such extreme drinking puts people at risk not only for unprotected sexual activity and sexual assault but also for alcohol poisoning, respiratory shutdown, and death.

Source: "Drinking to Extremes to Celebrate 21," New York Times, April 8, 2008.

they can also produce numbing in a female partner unless a condom is used.[6]

Treatment of Male Sexual Dysfunction Treatment of sexual dysfunction in men often relies on testosterone. Men with a low testosterone level may benefit from testosterone replacement therapy. It can be injected, administered through a patch, or applied to the skin as an ointment. It is not prescribed for men with normal testosterone levels because it can increase blood pressure, affect blood cholesterol levels, and possibly increase risk for prostate cancer.[14]

Treatments for erectile problems include drugs taken orally and by injection, mechanical devices (penile implants), and surgery to repair arteries supplying blood to the penis. Today, Viagra (sildenafil) is the treatment of choice for ED. Viagra was introduced in 1998 and has become the most frequently prescribed drug in the United States. Taken an hour before sex, Viagra works by increasing the concentration of the chemical that allows smooth-muscle cells in the erectile tissue to stay relaxed so that the spongy chambers of

the penis can remain filled with blood. Its effects last about 4 hours. Studies suggest that about 80 percent of men with varying degrees of ED have benefited from Viagra.[14]

Common side effects of Viagra include flushing, indigestion, nasal congestion, nausea, and headaches. Overuse can cause a dangerous condition called priapism, a state of continuous erection that can permanently damage the penis. Use of Viagra is dangerous for men with preexisting health conditions such as heart disease, high blood pressure, and diabetes, and fatalities have been reported in connection with its use.

Viagra is just one of several drugs now on the market for erectile problems. Levitra (Vardenafil) and Cialis (Tadolifil) are chemically similar to Viagra but more potent and efficient. Levitra takes about 16 minutes to work and may last 2 hours longer than Viagra. Cialis also takes about 16 minutes to work but may last up to 36 hours. Both have side effects similar to those of Viagra.

Drug approaches to sexual dysfunctions do not take into account the importance of relationships. They may offer a temporary confidence-builder, but they do not provide a long-term solution to issues that may lie behind sexual problems. Correcting unhealthy lifestyles, working on relationships, and cultivating a more realistic expectation of aging can improve mid- and late-life sexuality. Exercise, good nutrition, and emotional intimacy with one's partner are as important as Viagra.

Misuse of ED Drugs by Young Men   The misuse of Viagra and other ED drugs on college campuses has recently come to the attention of health experts. Viagra has been tagged the "thrill pill" on many campuses, where young men are taking it as a party drug at clubs, raves, and private parties. They mistakenly believe they will quickly and easily attain an erection that will allow them to have sex for hours. Erection drugs do not work unless nitric oxide is present in the penis, and nitric oxide is produced only in response to physical and mental stimulation. Any effect these drugs seem to have is more likely a placebo effect in healthy young men.

More important, the combination of ED drugs with alcohol or illicit drugs such as cocaine, amphetamines, or Ecstasy can be life-threatening. Even more dangerous is combining them with amyl nitrate ("poppers"). The combination of ED drugs with any stimulant drug dilates blood vessels, which can result in a sudden drop in blood pressure.[22]

Protecting Your Sexual Health

One of the biggest threats to your sexual health is infection with a sexually transmitted disease (STD). These infections range from annoyances like pubic lice to life-threatening diseases like AIDS. We discuss STDs in detail in Chapter 20; here, we discuss **safer sex** practices, which prevent the exchange of body fluids during sex. Two safer sex practices are using condoms and having sex that does not involve genital contact or penetration. A third practice is abstinence, considered the only way to completely guarantee protection against STDs. (These practices are also discussed in Chapter 16 as ways to prevent conception.) Another key to safeguarding your sexual health is communicating about sex.

safer sex
Sexual activities that do not include exchange of body fluids during sex.

USING CONDOMS

The **condom** (or *male condom*) is a thin sheath, usually made of latex, that fits over the erect penis during sexual intercourse. It provides a barrier against penile, vaginal, or anal discharges and genital lesions or sores. Although condoms do not provide complete protection against all STDs, they greatly reduce the risk of infection when used correctly (see Figure 16.2 in the next

condoms
Thin sheaths, usually made of latex, that fit over the erect penis during sexual intercourse to prevent conception and protect against STDs.

chapter). Latex condoms should not be used with any oil-based lubricants (such as Vaseline or hand lotion) because such products cause latex to deteriorate. Plastic (polyurethane) condoms are also available and can be used by people who are allergic to latex. They are thinner, stronger, and less constricting than latex, and they are not eroded by oil-based lubricants. However, they are more expensive than latex condoms and have not been tested as fully for effectiveness.

Protection against STDs is also offered by the **female condom**, a soft pouch of thin polyurethane that is inserted into the vagina before intercourse. The female condom has a soft flexible ring at both ends. The ring at the closed end is fitted against the cervix, and the ring at the open end remains outside the body (see Figure 16.3 in the next chapter). Both male and female condoms can be purchased at drugstores and grocery stores. The female condom covers more of the genital area, so it may provide more protection against an STD lesion or sore than the male condom does.

female condom
Soft pouch of thin polyurethane that is inserted into the vagina before intercourse to prevent conception and protect against STDs.

Condoms and **dental dams** (a small latex square placed over the vulva) should be used during oral sex because bacteria and viruses can be transmitted in semen and vaginal fluids. Plastic wrap placed over the vulva, or a piece of latex cut from a latex glove, is an alternative to a dental dam. Protection is especially important if there are any cuts or sores in the mouth; even bleeding gums can increase the risk of getting an infection.

dental dam
Small latex square placed over the vulva during oral sex.

Sexual activities that do not involve genital or skin contact are safer than those that do. Many people find enjoyment in such activities as hugging, massage, and erotic touching, stroking, and caressing with the clothes on.

PRACTICING ABSTINENCE

People practice abstinence for a variety of reasons. Some are abstinent for moral or religious reasons; they believe that sexual activity should be reserved for marriage. Abstinence is often promoted as a positive choice for young people; when this is the case, however, individuals should be provided with information and education about both contraception and STDs (see the box "Abstinence-Only Sex Education"). Some unmarried couples choose to be abstinent until they are married, and some married couples use periodic abstinence as a contraceptive method. As noted earlier, abstinence is the only way that people can be completely certain they are not at risk for STDs and unintended pregnancy.

COMMUNICATING ABOUT SEX

Conversations about sexual topics are important to your health, your partner's health, and the success of your relationship. If you are about to begin a sexual relationship, take

Public Health in Action

Abstinence-Only Sex Education

Abstinence-only sex education programs became more common in the United States after the federal government began directing funds toward them in 1996. In that year, under a provision of a welfare reform law (referred to as Title V), Congress established a program of special grants to states that implemented abstinence-only-until-marriage sex education programs. Between 1996 and 2007, Congress directed more than $1.4 billion toward such programs, in both federal and state matching funds.

Abstinence-only sex education programs teach that social, psychological, and health benefits are attained through sexual abstinence, that mutually faithful monogamous relationships in the context of marriage are the expected standard of sexual activity, and that sexual activity outside of marriage is likely to have harmful psychological and physical effects. The programs are not allowed to discuss safer sex approaches or contraceptive methods, including condoms, except to emphasize their failure rates.

For the first 5 years, all states except California participated in the program. Since then, many states have declined further funding, after evaluations failed to demonstrate the effectiveness of their programs. In 2000 the Bush administration established another program, Community-Based Abstinence Education (CBAE), that bypassed state governments and offered grants directly to community and faith-based organizations that provide abstinence-only education programs. The goal of CBAE is to persuade unmarried people to refrain from any activity that might be construed as sexually stimulating and to adhere to this standard at any age. In 2006 CBAE granted $115 million to organizations that agreed to carry out this mission.

Abstinence-only sex education programs have been criticized on many counts: They fail to address the needs of young people who are sexually active; they fail to provide young people with the information they need to protect themselves from pregnancy and STDs, including HIV; and they have not been shown to delay initiation of sexual activity. Evaluations of abstinence-only programs found little evidence that they have any long-term impact on attitudes, intentions, or sexual behaviors. Many young people become sexually active while they are participating in the programs but have no information about contraception or STDs.

Furthermore, abstinence-only programs are out of step with sexual behavior patterns in the United States. For example, the average age at first intercourse is 17 for females and 16 for males, almost a decade before the average age of first marriage. According to the National Survey of Family Growth, 53 percent of females and 49 percent of males aged 15 to 19 said they had had vaginal intercourse, and about half of respondents said they had had oral sex. One study found that most teenagers who pledged to remain virgins until marriage broke their pledges and were less likely to use safer sex practices or seek testing for STDs than teens who did not make such pledges. It could be that breaking a virginity pledge causes guilty feelings that lead to denial of sexual feelings and lack of responsible behavior around sexual activity. Organizations that have issued formal statements criticizing abstinence-only programs include the American Medical Association, the American Psychological Association, the American College Health Association, and the American Public Health Association.

The alternative to abstinence-only sex education is comprehensive sex education, which includes information on contraception and STDs. Proponents of comprehensive sex education point to the example of European models. In Sweden and the Netherlands, for example, it is accepted that older teenagers will be sexually active. Rather than exerting societal pressure for abstinence, these countries promote a cultural norm that sexual activity takes place only in the context of long-term committed relationships, married or unmarried. Teenagers in these countries have longer lasting relationships as well as lower rates of STDs and unintended pregnancies than their counterparts in the United States.

In 2007 a bill called the Responsible Education About Life Act was introduced in the U.S. Senate. This bill would provide for the funding of comprehensive sex education programs that include science-based, medically accurate, and age-appropriate public health information about both abstinence and contraception. These programs would also teach sexual decision-making skills, provide information about the effects of alcohol and drugs, and encourage family communication about sex. An abstinence-only message can still be the centerpiece of sex education in such programs, but they also provide much-needed information on safe sex practices and technologies that protect young people's health and futures.

Sources: "Legislating Against Sexual Arousal: The Growing Divide Between Federal Policy and Teenage Sexual Behavior," by C. Dailard, 2006, Guttmacher Policy Review, Vol. 9 (3), retrieved April 30, 2008, from www.guttmacher.org/pubs/gpr/09/3/gpr090312.html; "Responsible Education for Life (REAL) Act," Advocates for Youth, retrieved April 30, 2008, from www.advocatesforyouth.org/real.htm; "A Brief History of Abstinence-Only-Until-Marriage Education," Sexuality Information and Education Council of the United States, 2005, retrieved May 20, 2008, from www.nomoremoney.org/history.

the time to tell your partner your sexual health history and find out about his or hers. Here are some questions to guide your conversation:

- Are you having sex with anyone else? Are you willing to be monogamous with me?

- Have you ever had an STD? If so, how long ago, and what treatment did you get? Do you now have a clean bill of health?

- How many sexual partners have you had? As far as you know, did any of them ever have an STD?

- Do you know how to tell if you have an STD? Do you have any STD symptoms, such as sores, warts, pain, or discharge?

- Are you willing to use condoms every time we have sex?

If you are not satisfied with the answers you get, take care of yourself by insisting on further conversations and behavioral changes before you begin a sexual relationship.

Sex and Culture: Issues for the 21st Century

Woody Allen's 1973 movie *Sleeper* may have captured some of the sexual realities of our current cultural scene. In this movie, set in the future, all of a person's sexual needs can be taken care of by a sophisticated mechanical masturbator called an "orgasmatron." People no longer have to deal with the difficulties of relationships to get sexual satisfaction.

Like the orgasmatron, the Internet offers people immediate, anonymous, and solitary sex without the complexities of relationships. The same can be said for pornography and prostitution, two other commonplace features of contemporary culture. In this section, we take a brief look at some of these complex issues.

CYBERSEX

If you are looking for sex on the Internet—**cybersex**—you can easily find pornography, sexually explicit Web sites, erotic chat rooms, interactive games, and sex toys for sale. Some Web sites offer instant partners for mutual sexual fantasies, and some provide live video of performers who can respond to suggestions made by the viewer.

People access this explicit but virtual sex for many reasons—to obtain sexual gratification, to search for romance, to relieve boredom, to satisfy their curiosity. Issues arise

over whether the availability of cybersex has harmful consequences, for adults, for children, for society (see the box "Are You at Risk for Sex Addiction?"). An exploration of the issues associated with cybersex is provided in You Make the Call at the end of the chapter.

cybersex
Sexual material and activity available on the Internet, including pornography, sexual chatting, and interactive sex with a virtual partner.

PORNOGRAPHY

The definition of **pornography** has been a matter of debate for generations, but it is widely held to include materials created, distributed, or sold for the sole purpose of sexual arousal. Pornography has long been part of human culture, but every society and era has its own versions. An issue for our time is whether pornography promotes violence against women and sexual abuse of children. Some social scientists have suggested that exposure to depictions of sexual violence and exploitation can increase criminal behavior, especially on the part of men with psychological problems or other vulnerabilities. Some feminists have argued that pornography contributes to the sexual subordination of women and ongoing social inequalities for women.[23] The distribution of child pornography on the Internet has vastly increased its availability and emboldened its practitioners. For reasons such as these, some people want government to do more to suppress X-rated materials and punish those who promote them.

pornography
Materials created, distributed, or sold for the sole purpose of sexual arousal.

Defenders of pornography respond that the use of explicit sexual materials by adults is protected by the right to

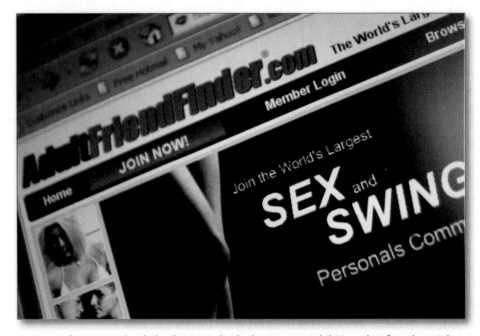

Sex on the Internet has helped some individuals overcome inhibitions, but for others, it has meant time lost to isolation, fantasy, and even sex addiction.

free speech. They argue that pornography—both "hard core" and "soft core" (erotic material aimed more at couples)—provides harmless pleasure and has educational and therapeutic benefits. They also point out that research has yet to establish a relationship between pornography and sexual violence.[23] With the Internet becoming ever more pervasive in our society, the debate is likely to continue.

PROSTITUTION

Like pornography, **prostitution**—the exchange of sex for money—has been around since the beginning of recorded history and probably before. An issue in our era is the spread of HIV infection and AIDS by prostitutes throughout the world. Commercial sex is associated with very high rates of HIV infection worldwide. In some developing countries, prostitu-

prostitution
Exchange of sex for money; prostitutes are sometimes called sex workers.

tion is forced on young girls and adolescents, and condom use by men is rare. In some places, these "sex workers" are organizing to protect their health and human rights.[24]

In the United States, many prostitutes use injection drugs, one of the principal sources of HIV infection, or have customers who use them. In some parts of the country, up to 50 percent of the prostitutes are estimated to be infected with HIV.[14] Some public health experts have argued that prostitution should be decriminalized so that prostitutes can be licensed and required to have regular health exams. They point to the counties in Nevada where prostitution is legal and prostitutes are required by law to use condoms and be tested monthly for HIV. No legal working prostitute in these counties is HIV-positive. Decriminalizing prostitution on a national level is unlikely at this time, however; at most, it will remain a major cultural issue in the 21st century.[25]

Consumer Clipboard

Are You at Risk for Sex Addiction?

Do you spend more time on sexual activities than you intend to? Do you continue engaging in them despite negative consequences (risking your relationships, your job, your health, your legal status)? Are you obsessed or preoccupied with these activities when you should be focusing on other aspects of your life? If you answered yes to these three questions, you may be at risk for sex addiction, which is defined as compulsive, out-of-control sexual behavior that results in severe negative consequences.

Whether through cybersex, phone sex lines, porn magazines, or porn videos, sex addicts lose time every day to the isolating activities of fantasy and masturbation. The Internet is a particularly seductive medium; research indicates that cybersex addicts spend at least 11–12 hours per week and often two to three times that amount of time on Internet sex. These are hours that the person is not spending on real-life activities, including time spent developing intimate relationships with real partners.

Even if the individual is interacting with another person in a chat room, such interactions usually lack the honesty, trust, respect, and dignity that characterize healthy relationships.

In some cases, cybersex addiction is a continuation of compulsive sexual behaviors that began in adolescence, such as phone sex, voyeurism, and viewing pornography. Some experts worry that cybersex will promote more extreme forms of real-life sexual behavior in the adult years. Studies have found that 70 percent of sex addicts suffer from depression and 83 percent have concurrent addictions such as eating disorders, compulsive gambling, and alcoholism. One study found that the vast majority of sex addicts grew up in abusive family environments.

If you think you might be at risk for sex addiction, talk to a mental health professional at your campus counseling center. Sex addiction can cause serious physical, emotional, spiritual, family, financial, and legal problems, but treatment is available. You can also learn more about sex addiction at the Sexual Recovery Institute (www.sexualrecovery.com).

Sources: "Frequently Asked Questions About Sexual Addiction," Sexual Recovery Institute, retrieved May 4, 2008, from www.sexualrecovery.com/resources/articles/faq.php; "Cybersex Use and Abuse: Implications for Health Education," by D.D. Rimington and J. Gast, 2007, American Journal of Health Education, 38 (1), pp. 34–39.

You Make the Call

Cybersex: Harmless Fun or Moral Black Hole?

Cybersex, cyber porn, virtual sex—whatever you call it, it's available on the Internet. A major objection to the widespread availability of this material is that children can easily access it. Although owners of adult Web sites say they are not interested in attracting children, there is no foolproof way to prevent sexually curious children from gaining access to many of these sites. Some children use their parents' credit cards to pay for access and simply click on the "I am over 18" button. Other children come across the sites by accident when researching innocent topics.

In 1995 Congress passed the Communications Decency Act (CDA), imposing fines and possible prison sentences on anyone who knowingly made sexually explicit material on the Internet available to children. The Supreme Court struck down the CDA in 1997 as a violation of the right to free speech guaranteed by the First Amendment. In 1998, President Clinton signed the 1998 Child Online Protection Act, but this act has also been challenged under the First Amendment.

Another objection is that the Internet has vastly expanded the range over which pornographic material, including child pornography, can be distributed. It has emboldened pedophiles and enhanced their ability to pursue their activities, and it has led people to explore a world of atypical sexual behaviors and sexual subcultures in ways that were not feasible in the past.

Opponents also question the effect of cybersex on mental health; they argue that engaging in sex with virtual partners impairs real relationships and robs people of the ability to experience sexual pleasure through interpersonal connections and intimacy. Laboratory studies have found that men are less enthusiastic about the attractiveness of their real-life partners after viewing attractive women in pornographic videos. Some people become addicted to Internet sex and devote large portions of their lives and financial resources to it, at the expense of their relationships, families, and jobs. Finally, opponents argue that the proliferation of sexual material on the Internet represents a degradation of society's morals and standards of decency.

Defenders of cybersex point out that it is intended for adults, who have the right to choose what they want to view on the Internet. Parents are responsible for keeping their children from accessing explicit sexual materials. Censoring or suppressing this material would be a violation of First Amendment rights, as the courts have already ruled. Defenders also argue that all forms of sexual expression are natural and that it is puritanical to condemn the behaviors depicted in pornography as immoral or abnormal. Defenders argue in addition that the kind of sexually explicit material available on the Internet can be used to educate and treat people with sexual dysfunctions by exposing them to a broad range of sexual activity without negative judgments.

Some people see cybersex as harmless entertainment that provides a needed outlet for responsible adults. Others view it as a threat to the moral development of children and the moral fiber of society. What do you think?

PROS

- Cybersex is a healthy outlet for sexual expression that fulfills sexual fantasies and needs for both men and women.
- Cybersex is not harmful. A 1970 review of scientific evidence by the Commission on Obscenity and Pornography concluded that pornography is not harmful. Cybersex would fall into the same category.
- Cybersex is an educational tool that can be used to teach sexual anatomy and functioning to people as they become sexually mature. It reinforces acceptance of a wide range of behaviors and enhances people's ability to enjoy their full sexuality.
- Cybersex is a useful therapeutic treatment for some sexual problems and dysfunctions, especially for sexually inhibited individuals.
- Adults have the right to view sexually explicit materials if they wish. Cybersex is protected by the First Amendment right to free speech.
- There is no practical way to regulate and police sexual material on the Internet.
- Children are much more likely to be exposed to sexual images and references in movies, television shows, and song lyrics than on the Internet.

CONS

- Like pornography, cybersex objectifies and exploits women. Much of the sexually explicit material on the Internet depicts women in dehumanizing ways.
- Cybersex endangers children by facilitating the widespread distribution of child pornography and promoting pedophilia.
- The findings of the 1970 review of obscenity and pornography are not relevant today. Sexually explicit material today is much more violent and exploitative than in 1970.
- Pornography is illegal for children under age 18, but the Internet does not have any effective ways to block children from accessing sexually explicit sites. Operators of adult sites know they are going to break the law.
- Cybersex has a negative effect on people's real lives and relationships.
- Cybersex is degrading and has an emotionally and morally damaging effect on people.

Sources: Pornography: The Production and Consumption of Inequality, *by G. Dines, R. Jensen, and A. Russo, 1998, New York: Routledge;* Growing Up Digital: The Rise of the Net Generation, *by D. Tapscott, 1998, New York: McGraw-Hill;* Tangled in the Web: Understanding Cybersex From Fantasy to Addiction, *by K.S. Young, 2001, Austin, TX: 1st Book Library;* The Psychology of the Internet, *by P. Wallace, 1999, New York: Columbia University Press.*

In Review

1. **What sexuality related attitudes and behaviors are prevalent in our society?**
American attitudes are marked by tension between the poles of sexual restraint and sexual permissiveness. Most Americans are engaged in committed, monogamous relationships, and marital infidelity is relatively uncommon. Statistically speaking, men have about 13 years of premarital sexual activity and women have about 10 years.

2. **What are the basics of sexual anatomy and functioning?** Both men and women have external and internal sexual organs, designed for the biological purpose of reproduction. Sex drive, sexual arousal, and sexual response also work to facilitate reproduction. The human sexual response model conceptualizes sexual response as occurring in four phases. Sexual development and change begin prenatally and extend across the lifespan, driven by hormones.

3. **What are the varieties of sexual behavior and expression?** Typical and common forms of sexual behavior include celibacy, kissing, erotic touch, self-stimulation (fantasy and masturbation), oral-genital stimulation, and intercourse. Atypical behaviors include both consensual sex games and nonconsensual sexual activities considered paraphilias. Sexual dysfunctions are common in both women and men and include, in women, vaginismus, low sexual desire and arousal, and orgasmic dysfunction and, in men, pain during intercourse, low sexual desire and arousal, erectile dysfunction, and ejaculation dysfunction. Treatments are available for all sexual dysfunctions.

4. **What are the best ways to protect your sexual health?** Using condoms, practicing abstinence, avoiding alcohol in sexual situations, and practicing good communication skills are the best ways to protect your sexual health.

5. **What societal issues arise in connection with sexuality?** Current issues include sex on the Internet, including pornography and child pornography; sex addiction; and prostitution, with its associated dangers of HIV infection.

For a detailed summary of this chapter and a comprehensive set of review questions, visit the Online Learning Center at **www.mhhe.com/teague2e**.

Web Resources

Go Ask Alice: This Columbia University site features questions and answers of interest to young adults. The section on sexuality addresses a wide range of topics—from kissing to achieving orgasm. The sexual health section offers information on issues such as reproduction, contraception, and STDs.
www.goaskalice.columbia.edu

National Men's Health Network: In addition to offering basic information related to men's health, this site includes a resource center with links to articles, books, government sites, health organizations, and other health resources of special interest to men.
www.menshealthnetwork.org

National Sexuality Resource Center: This organization addresses issues in contemporary sexuality. Its sexual literacy campaign is designed to counteract negative messages about sexuality and promote healthy attitudes toward sexuality.
http://nsrc.sfsu.edu

National Women's Health Network: Organized to promote women's involvement in the health care system, this group offers news updates, fact sheets, and health information packets. It encourages critical analysis of health issues related specifically to women.
www.womenshealthnetwork.org

Planned Parenthood: The Sexual Health section of this Web site offers a guide to sexuality for young women and another for young men. It also features topics such as safer sex, condom use, and STDs, with questions and answers on a variety of sexuality issues.
www.plannedparenthood.org

Sexuality Information and Education Council of the United States: This organization's Web site includes FAQs, information updates, fact sheets on sexuality at different life stages, gay and lesbian issues, and approaches to sex education.
www.siecus.org

Chapter

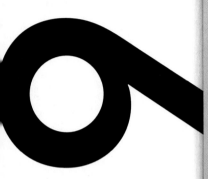

Reproductive Choices
Contraception, Pregnancy, and Childbirth

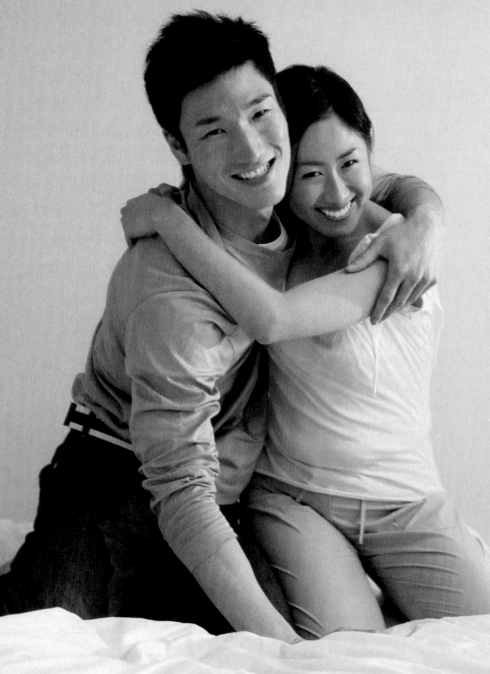

Your Health Today

www.mhhe.com/teague2e

Go to the Online Learning Center for *Your Health Today* for interactive activities, quizzes, flashcards, Web links, and more resources related to this chapter.

Ever Wonder...

- what the best form of contraception is?

- what your chances of getting pregnant are if you are sexually active and don't use any form of contraception?

- how much it costs to raise a child?

Are you ready to be a parent? If your answer is no, many safe and effective methods of contraception are available that you and your partner can use to avoid an unintended pregnancy. If your answer is yes, a wealth of knowledge is available that you can use to increase the likelihood that your pregnancy is a positive experience and that your baby is healthy. If you want to have children some time in the future, planning for it now—by using contraception and choosing healthy lifestyle behaviors—can give you peace of mind and the knowledge that you are doing everything you can to protect the health of your future family. This chapter builds on the topics discussed in Chapters 14 and 15—relationships and sexual health—to discuss reproductive choices and issues in creating a family.

Choosing a Contraceptive Method

Choosing and using a contraceptive method that is right for you is important for one very significant reason: It lowers your risk of unintended pregnancy. About half of all pregnancies in the United States are unintended, and many are unwanted, either because the couple doesn't want a child at this time or because they don't want a child at all. Unintended pregnancies occur among women of all ages and ethnic groups, but rates are highest among low-income, minority (Black, American Indian, Alaska Native, and Hispanic) women in the 18- to 24-year-old age group. Unintended pregnancies nearly always cause stress and life disruption and are associated with poorer health outcomes (see the box "Teen Pregnancies"). Compared with women having planned pregnancies, women with unintended pregnancies are less likely to receive adequate **prenatal care**, are more likely to drink alcohol and smoke, and are more likely to have babies with **low birth weight** (less than 5.5 pounds).[1]

prenatal care
Regular medical care during pregnancy, designed to promote the health of the mother and the fetus.

low birth weight
Birth weight of less than 5.5 pounds, often as a result of preterm delivery.

Advances in reproductive technology have led to the development of many acceptable and reliable contraceptive methods. In this section we take a look at several of these methods.

ABSTINENCE

The only guaranteed method of preventing pregnancy and sexually transmitted diseases (STDs) is *abstinence*. As noted in Chapter 15, abstinence is usually defined as abstention from sexual intercourse; that is, there is no penile penetration of the vagina. In heterosexual couples who have vaginal intercourse and use no contraceptive method, 85 percent of the women will become pregnant in one year.[2]

Abstinence is free, is available to all, and can be started at any time. The downside of abstinence as a contraceptive method is that it requires control and commitment—that is, the ability or the determination not to change one's mind in the heat of the moment. Recent years have seen a decline in the rates of teen pregnancy, and some of this decline is attributed to increased rates of abstinence among teenagers, especially those in the 15- to 17-year-old age group. The primary determinant, however, appears to be increasing use of contraceptives.[3]

HORMONAL CONTRACEPTIVE METHODS

Hormonal methods come in a variety of forms—pills, injections, patches, and vaginal rings—and work by preventing ovulation. They also alter cervical mucus, making it harder for sperm to reach ova, and they affect the uterine lining so that a fertilized egg is less likely to be implanted. They are prescribed or administered by a physician. The advantages of hormonal methods include their effectiveness, their ease of use, their limited side effects, and the fact that they do not permanently affect fertility. They do not require any action at the time of intercourse. In addition, they offer some general health benefits. They reduce menstrual cramping and blood loss, premenstrual symptoms, ovarian cysts, endometriosis, and the risk of endometrial and ovarian cancer. In addition, they can improve acne.

A major disadvantage associated with hormonal contraceptives is that they offer no protection against STDs. In some women, they can cause some minor side effects, including symptoms of early pregnancy (nausea, bloating, weight gain, and breast tenderness), mood changes, and headaches. Serious side effects are rare and more common in women who are older and who smoke (Figure 16.1). Hormonal contraceptives require a visit to a health provider to determine which method is best for you and to ensure you do not have a contraindication for use.

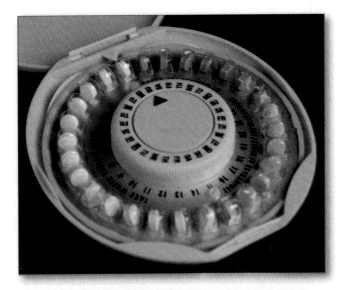

■ The development of "the pill" and its approval by the FDA in 1960 ushered in an era of more relaxed sexual attitudes and behaviors—the so-called sexual revolution. Today, birth control pills remain the most popular form of contraception among unmarried women.

Birth control pills (*oral contraceptives*) are the most popular reversible form of contraception. They usually contain a combination of estrogen and progesterone. A pack of birth control pills typically contains a month's worth of pills. Most packs contain 21 active, hormone-containing pills and 7 placebo pills (for a 28-day cycle); others are sold as 21-pill packs and call for a 7-day break between packs. Another formulation has 84 active pills and 7 placebo pills, resulting in just four periods a year. Some formulations contain only progesterone; they are slightly less effective but can be used by women who can't take estrogen (for example, because they are breastfeeding or have a family history of blood clots).

The *transdermal patch* works by slowly releasing estrogen and progesterone into the bloodstream through the skin. A woman places a new patch on her skin every week for 3 weeks; during the 4th week, she does not use a patch and has a light period. Because the patch is changed once a week, it can be useful for women who have a hard time remembering to take a daily pill. Potential side effects are similar to those of the pill, except that the patch results in higher levels of estrogen in the blood (about 60 percent higher than a typical birth control pill) and has been associated with about twice the risk of blood clots as pills.[4]

The *vaginal contraceptive ring* is a soft, flexible plastic ring that is placed in the vagina and slowly releases estrogen and progesterone. It is left in place for 21 days and then removed. After 7 days, a new ring is inserted. Women and their partners report that they rarely feel the ring during intercourse. The advantage of the ring is the monthly application; side effects are similar to those of birth control pills.

The *injectable contraceptive* currently available in the United States is Depo-Provera. A progesterone-only injection, it is administered as a shot in a health care provider's office every 3 months. It is highly effective and requires little action

Who's at Risk

Teen Pregnancies

When teenagers get pregnant and give birth, their future prospects decline, as do those of their children. Compared with non-teenage mothers, teen mothers are less likely to finish high school or attend college, less likely to marry or stay married, and more likely to require public assistance. They are less likely to receive prenatal care and more likely to smoke, factors associated with poor birth outcomes.

About one-third of girls in the United States get pregnant before age 20. More than 80 percent of these pregnancies are unintended. In 2006 more than 435,000 infants were born to mothers aged 15–19 years, a birth rate of 41.9 live births per 1,000 females in this age group. Although pregnancy and birth rates among girls aged 15–19 years have declined 34 percent since 1991, birth rates increased for the first time in 2006.

Major disparities exist in pregnancy and birth rates. In 2005 Washington, D.C., had the highest teen birth rate, followed by Texas and New Mexico. New Hampshire had the lowest teen birth rate. The highest birth rate in 15- to 19-year-olds was among Latinas; the rate was 83 live births per 1,000 females, twice the overall rate. Among non-Hispanic Black females in this age group, the rate was 63.7; among American Indian or Alaska Native females, 54.7; and among non-Hispanic White females, 26.6.

International comparisons show that the behavior of American teenagers is similar to that of teens in other developed countries in terms of when they start having sex and how often they have it. However, teen pregnancy and birth rates in the United States are the second highest of any of these countries. Compared with the teens of other developed countries, American teens are less likely to use contraception or to consistently use more effective methods of contraception. Data show that 77 percent of the decline in teen pregnancy rates among U.S. teens aged 15–17 years is due to increased use of contraception and 23 percent is due to reduced sexual activity.

Health organizations are working to promote healthy decision-making among teenagers, such as reducing numbers of partners, delaying initiation of sex, and increasing contraception and condom use. More work is needed, however, to identify interventions that speak to the social, cultural, and environmental influences on teen pregnancy. The National Campaign to Prevent Teen Pregnancy has these suggestions:

- Involve parents and encourage them to teach their children and adolescents about sex, love, relationships, and expected behavior.
- Stop fighting about "abstinence versus contraception"—more of both are needed.
- Intensify efforts in communities with especially high rates of teen pregnancy, particularly Latinas and African American girls.
- Make the connection between pregnancy and poverty.
- Increase the focus on boys in teen pregnancy prevention.
- Target younger teens.
- Recognize the challenge and opportunity represented by ever-advancing technology and take advantage of the media to prevent teen pregnancy.

Sources: "Adolescent Reproductive Health: Teen Pregnancy," Centers for Disease Control and Prevention, retrieved May 3, 2008, from www.cdc.gov/ reproductivehealth/AdolescentReproHealth/index.htm; "Why It Matters?" The National Campaign to Prevent Teen Pregnancy, retrieved May 3, 2008, from www.thenationalcampaign.org/default.aspx; "Teen Pregnancy in America," by S. Brown, in United Health Foundation, America's Health, retrieved May 3, 2008, from www.unitedhealthfoundation.org/download/ahrcomments/TeenPreg-2005.pdf.

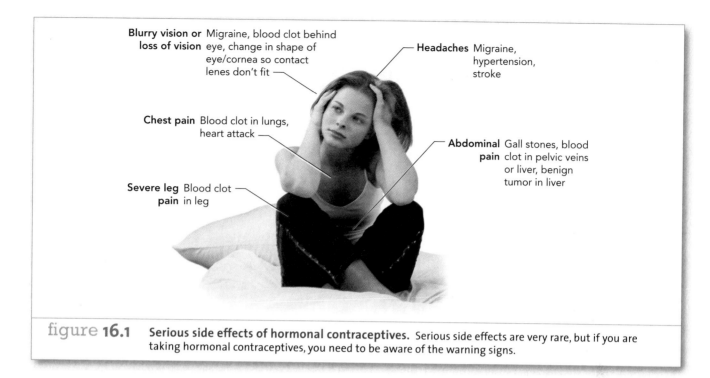

Blurry vision or loss of vision Migraine, blood clot behind eye, change in shape of eye/cornea so contact lenes don't fit

Headaches Migraine, hypertension, stroke

Chest pain Blood clot in lungs, heart attack

Abdominal pain Gall stones, blood clot in pelvic veins or liver, benign tumor in liver

Severe leg pain Blood clot in leg

figure **16.1**   **Serious side effects of hormonal contraceptives.** Serious side effects are very rare, but if you are taking hormonal contraceptives, you need to be aware of the warning signs.

on the part of a woman except regular visits to the provider. Depo-Provera can cause menstrual changes with irregular bleeding early on and amenorrhea (no periods) in 50 percent of women after 1 year. Most women consider this an advantage. Disadvantages specific to Depo-Provera include weight gain (about 5.4 pounds on average in the first year) and decreased bone density with prolonged use (longer than 2 years).

A *contraceptive implant* is a small, flexible plastic rod that contains progesterone. It is inserted under the skin on the inner side of the upper arm and slowly releases hormones. The only implant currently available in the United States is Implanon. Once inserted, it can be left in place for 3 years, thus eliminating user error. It may be less effective for women with a body mass greater than 30 percent of ideal.

BARRIER METHODS

---

barrier methods
Contraceptive methods based on physically separating sperm from the female reproductive tract.

spermicide
Chemical agent that kills sperm.

Contraceptive methods known as **barrier methods** physically separate the sperm from the female reproductive tract. These methods include the male condom, the female condom, the diaphragm, Lea's shield, the cervical cap, and the contraceptive sponge. To increase their effectiveness, the diaphragm and cervical cap should be used with **spermicide,** chemical agents that kill sperm. Spermicide usually comes in a foam or jelly and can be purchased at a grocery store or drugstore at a cost of $10–$15 per tube.

The chance of becoming pregnant while using a barrier method is low if the method is used consistently and correctly. Correct use of a barrier method means that the

barrier is used 100 percent of the time in which there is contact between the penis and the vagina and that spermicide is correctly applied with the diaphragm and the cervical cap. Unfortunately, this is often not the case. The typical pregnancy rates are 15 percent with the male condom and 16 percent with the diaphragm. With correct use during every act of intercourse, however, the pregnancy rates drop to 2 percent for condoms and 6 percent for diaphragms.

Condoms—Male and Female   The only form of contraception proven to decrease the risk of contracting an STD is the male condom. As described in Chapter 15, the *male condom* is a thin sheath, usually made of latex, that is rolled down over

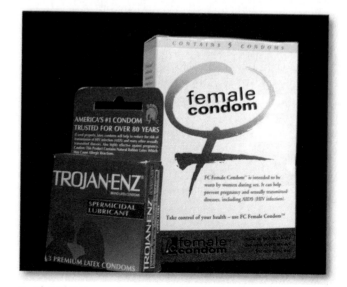

■ The advantages of condoms are that they are portable, available over the counter, and inexpensive. Male condoms provide some protection against STDs, including HIV.

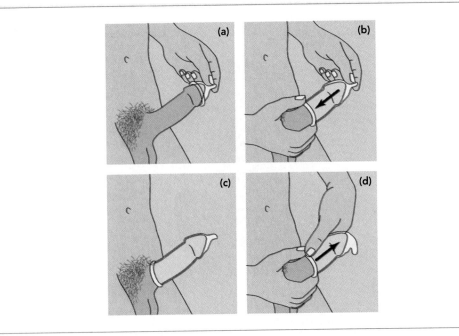

figure **16.2**   **Use of the male condom.** (a) Place the rolled condom over the head of the erect penis. Hold the top one-half inch of the condom with one hand, and squeeze the air out to allow space for semen. (b) With the other hand, unroll the condom downward, smoothing out any air bubbles. (c) Continue unrolling the condom down to the base of the penis. (d) After ejaculation, hold the condom around the base of the penis until the penis has been withdrawn completely to avoid any leakage of semen.

Challenges & Choices

Buying and Using Condoms

The advantages of condoms are that they are available over the counter, relatively low in cost, fairly convenient to use, effective in protecting against STDs, and moderately effective in protecting against unintended pregnancy. Here are some tips to ensure the lowest risk of an unwanted outcome:

■ Buy latex condoms if you are not allergic to them. Latex is the best material for preventing the spread of STDs.

■ Check the expiration date before buying or using condoms. Outdated condoms are more likely to break during use.

■ Condoms are available with or without spermicide. The most commonly used spermicide is nonoxynol-9. Because of recent evidence that this product can cause skin irritation, it is currently recommended that condoms without spermicide be purchased.

■ Don't remove the condom from its wrapper until you are ready to use it.

■ Don't leave condoms in the glove compartment of your car. Temperature extremes weaken the condom and make it more likely to break. Don't store them in your wallet either.

■ Use only water-based lubricants. Oil-based products quickly cause latex to deteriorate, leading it to leak or break.

■ If you are buying a female condom, check the expiration date and make sure it includes directions. Practice inserting the condom before you actually use it. During use, make sure the man's penis is inserted inside the condom.

■ Correct use of condoms means not only that they are placed on the penis correctly before intercourse and removed correctly afterward (see Figure 16.2) but also that they are used for every occasion of sexual intercourse and do not leak or break. Most failures occur because of incorrect or inconsistent use.

It's Not Just Personal . . .

In many developing nations, such as Ivory Coast, Togo, and Ghana in West Africa, condoms are widely used for contraception because of their availability and their low cost in comparison with oral contraceptives. Even when not used specifically to prevent the spread of HIV/AIDS and other STDs, condoms have this added benefit in countries where such diseases are often present at epidemic levels.

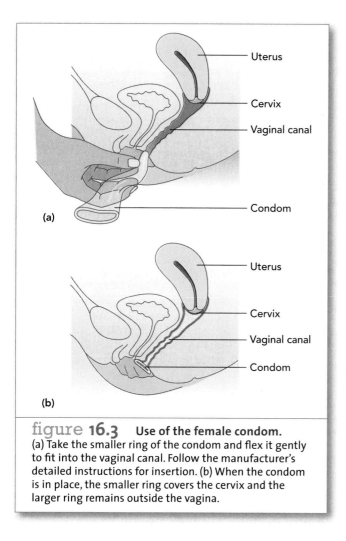

figure **16.3** **Use of the female condom.**
(a) Take the smaller ring of the condom and flex it gently to fit into the vaginal canal. Follow the manufacturer's detailed instructions for insertion. (b) When the condom is in place, the smaller ring covers the cervix and the larger ring remains outside the vagina.

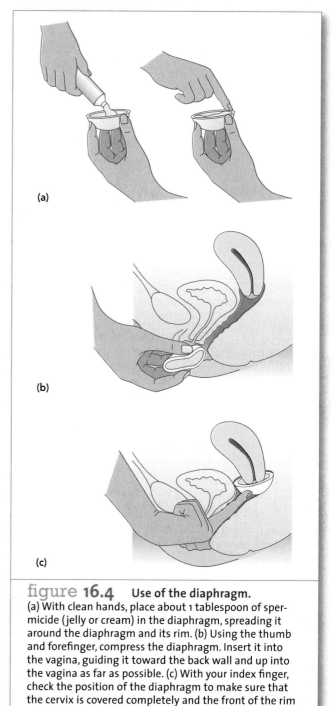

figure **16.4** **Use of the diaphragm.**
(a) With clean hands, place about 1 tablespoon of spermicide (jelly or cream) in the diaphragm, spreading it around the diaphragm and its rim. (b) Using the thumb and forefinger, compress the diaphragm. Insert it into the vagina, guiding it toward the back wall and up into the vagina as far as possible. (c) With your index finger, check the position of the diaphragm to make sure that the cervix is covered completely and the front of the rim is behind the pubic bone.

the erect penis before any contact occurs between the penis and the woman's genitals. The correct application of a condom is illustrated in Figure 16.2. Male condoms come with or without spermicide. There is no evidence that spermicide is necessary to reduce the risk of pregnancy, and spermicide can cause irritation for some users. Condoms can be purchased over the counter in grocery stores and drugstores (see the box "Buying and Using Condoms"). They cost between 27 cents and 1 dollar each, but they are often given out free at clinics.

Also as described in Chapter 15, the *female condom* is a pouch of thin polyurethane that is inserted into the vagina before intercourse (Figure 16.3). Like male condoms, female condoms can be purchased at grocery stores or drugstores for about $2.

Female Barrier Methods The vaginal **diaphragm** is a circular rubber dome that is inserted in the vagina before intercourse; correct placement is shown in Figure 16.4. It fits between the pubic bone and the back of the vagina and covers the cervix. Spermicidal jelly or foam is placed in the dome, or cup, of the diaphragm before it is inserted; thus the spermicide

diaphragm
Circular rubber dome that is inserted in the vagina before intercourse to prevent conception.

covers the cervix, where it provides the best protection. Spermicide must be reapplied into the vagina if a second act of sex occurs. The diaphragm is removed 6 to 12 hours after sex (see the box "Toxic Shock Syndrome" on the next page).

A woman has to be fitted with the correctly sized diaphragm by a health care provider and shown how to insert and remove it. The cost of this method includes the physician visit (between $50 and $150), the diaphragm (usually $30–$50), and spermicide. A diaphragm can be used for 2 years with correct care.[2]

Lea's shield is an oval device made of silicone rubber that is quite similar to a diaphragm. One size fits all, but it is available only by prescription. Lea's shield is used with spermicide and is reusable. It should be left in place for 6 to 24 hours after intercourse. The cost is similar to that of a diaphragm.

Lea's shield
Oval, silicone rubber device that is inserted in the vagina before intercourse to prevent conception.

cervical cap
Small, cuplike rubber device that covers only the cervix and is inserted in the vagina before intercourse to prevent conception.

contraceptive sponge
Small polyurethane foam device presaturated with spermicide that is inserted in the vagina before intercourse to prevent pregnancy.

The **cervical cap** is a small, cuplike device that covers the cervix and prevents sperm from entering the uterus. As with a diaphragm, the cervical cap requires a fitting by a health care provider; it is replaced annually. Currently the FemCap is the only available model. It is made of non-allergenic silicone and comes in three sizes. A small amount of spermicide is placed in a groove on the vaginal side of the cap prior to insertion (Figure 16.5). It should be left in place for 6 to 48 hours after intercourse. The cost includes the provider visit, the cervical cap itself (approximately $70), and spermicide.[5]

The Today **contraceptive sponge** is a small, polyurethane foam device that is presaturated with 1 gram of the spermicide nonoxynol-9. The sponge is moistened with water and inserted into the vagina. It fits snugly over the cervix, becomes immediately effective, and remains effective for 24 hours (see Figure 16.6). It should be left in place for at least 6 hours after intercourse and should then be removed. The sponge is available over the counter without prescription; one size fits all. The sponge should not be used during menstruation or if the user or her partner is allergic

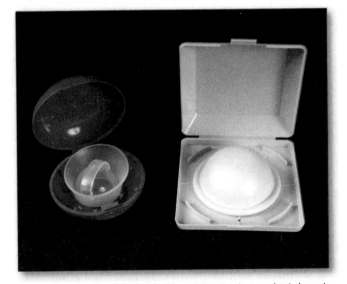

■ The FemCap cervical cap (left) and the diaphragm (right) work by creating a physical barrier at the cervical opening, preventing sperm from entering the uterus. Both are used with spermicidal cream or jelly.

to sulfa medicines or polyurethane. It may be less effective in women who have had a pregnancy. The cost is approximately $2.50 per sponge.[2]

THE IUD

The **intrauterine device (IUD)** has a complex history in the United States. Because of a design flaw, IUDs in the 1960s and 1970s were associated with a high rate of pelvic inflammatory disease, an infection of the ovaries and fallopian tubes. The design of IUDs has

intrauterine device (IUD)
Small T-shaped device that when inserted in the uterus prevents contraception.

Highlight on Health

Toxic Shock Syndrome

Toxic shock syndrome is a very rare, potentially life-threatening infection usually caused by the bacterium *Staphylococcus aureus* (it can also occur in association with *Streptococcal* infection). In the 1980s, there was a sudden increase in the number of cases of toxic shock syndrome affecting young women who were using superabsorbent tampons. It is not clear why these particular tampons caused the disease; they may have been left in place for a long time and allowed bacteria to grow in the vagina.

Toxic shock syndrome also has been associated with the use of contraceptive sponges and diaphragms. The risk is very low, but to reduce risk further, women should change tampons frequently (at least every 4 to 8 hours) and should not leave female barrier methods of contracep-

tion in place beyond the recommended time. Symptoms of toxic shock include

■ A sudden high fever.

■ Vomiting or diarrhea.

■ A rash that looks like a sunburn and eventually leads to peeling of the skin on the hands and feet.

■ Muscle aches.

■ Headache.

■ Seizure and confusion.

The sudden onset of these symptoms should be evaluated immediately. If you are using a tampon or female barrier method of contraception, remove it and tell the health care provider what you were using. Toxic shock syndrome is usually treated in a hospital with intravenous antibiotics.

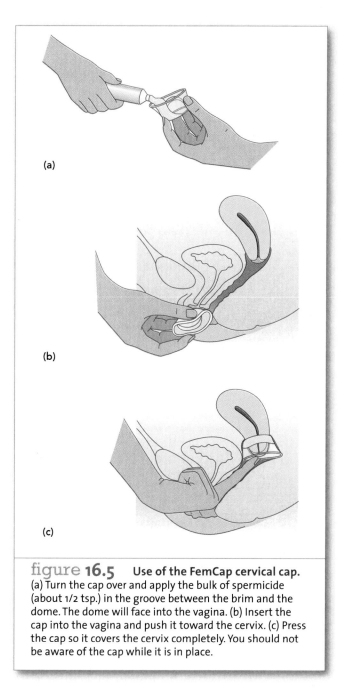

figure **16.5**   **Use of the FemCap cervical cap.**
(a) Turn the cap over and apply the bulk of spermicide (about 1/2 tsp.) in the groove between the brim and the dome. The dome will face into the vagina. (b) Insert the cap into the vagina and push it toward the cervix. (c) Press the cap so it covers the cervix completely. You should not be aware of the cap while it is in place.

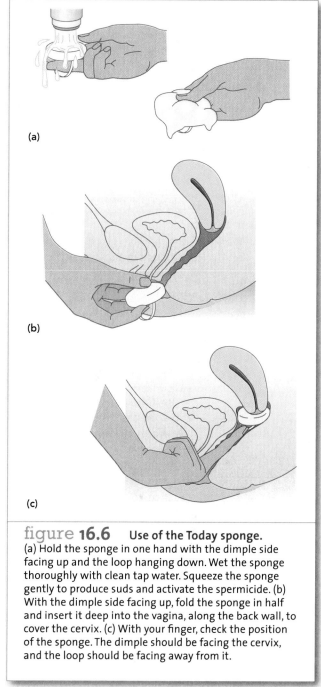

figure **16.6**   **Use of the Today sponge.**
(a) Hold the sponge in one hand with the dimple side facing up and the loop hanging down. Wet the sponge thoroughly with clean tap water. Squeeze the sponge gently to produce suds and activate the spermicide. (b) With the dimple side facing up, fold the sponge in half and insert it deep into the vagina, along the back wall, to cover the cervix. (c) With your finger, check the position of the sponge. The dimple should be facing the cervix, and the loop should be facing away from it.

been made safer, and they are currently regaining popularity. Two types are used, the copper IUD and the progesterone IUD. Both are small, T-shaped devices that a health care provider inserts through the cervix into the uterus. A correctly placed IUD is shown in Figure 16.7.

The IUD is believed to work by altering the uterine and cervical fluids to reduce the chance that sperm will move up into the fallopian tubes where they can fertilize an ovum. In addition, some women using the progesterone-containing IUD do not ovulate.

IUDs are highly effective and require little maintenance after they are in place, but several problems are associated with their use. Women can experience irregular bleeding. Because the IUD can move or fall out of the uterus, the woman must

learn how to check to make sure the device is still properly located each month. Currently, the role that IUDs play in the spread of STDs and pelvic inflammatory disease is unclear. Any woman at risk for STDs should use condoms.

The cost of an intrauterine device is about $200 to $300, including the physician fee and the cost of the device. The copper IUD can remain in place for up to 10 years; the progesterone IUD can remain in place for 5 years.

THE FERTILITY AWARENESS METHOD

Women can usually become pregnant in a window of time around ovulation (release of an ovum). The **fertility**

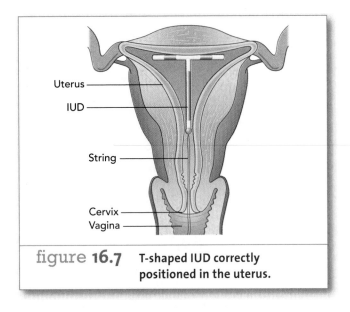

figure 16.7 T-shaped IUD correctly positioned in the uterus.

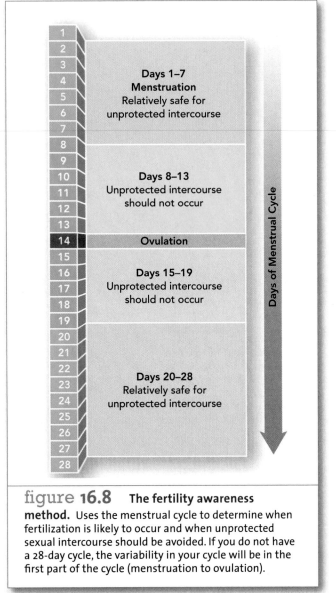

figure 16.8 **The fertility awareness method.** Uses the menstrual cycle to determine when fertilization is likely to occur and when unprotected sexual intercourse should be avoided. If you do not have a 28-day cycle, the variability in your cycle will be in the first part of the cycle (menstruation to ovulation).

awareness method of birth control, sometimes called the *rhythm method,* is based on abstaining from sex during the time that conception might take place. Ovulation usually occurs 14 days *before* the menstrual period begins (Figure 16.8). For a woman with a 28-day cycle, ovulation usually occurs on day 14. However, for a woman with a shorter or longer cycle, the time difference is in the first part of the cycle (from menstruation to ovulation), not in the second part of the cycle (from ovulation to menstruation). For example, if a woman has a 21-day cycle, ovulation will usually occur on day 7. If a woman has a 32-day cycle, ovulation will usually occur on day 18.

> **fertility awareness method**
> Contraceptive method based on abstinence during the window of time around ovulation when a woman is most likely to conceive.

The ovum is most likely to become fertilized within 24 hours after release from the ovary if it is to happen at all; however, the ovum can remain viable for 4 days. Sperm can survive up to 7 days in cervical mucus. Thus any sperm deposited in the vagina after day 8 of the menstrual cycle could still be around on day 14, when the woman ovulates (in a 28-day cycle). To avoid pregnancy, the couple would need to avoid intercourse or use another method of contraception between day 8 and day 19.

The fertility awareness method requires that the woman have a regular cycle (same number of days every month), because abstinence or barrier methods must be used for 7 days before ovulation. Although both regular and irregular cycles are normal, the fertility awareness method is appropriate only for women with a regular cycle.

Ovulation is accompanied by certain signs that a woman can recognize in order to learn her own patterns. Couples also use these signs to pinpoint the time of ovulation when they are trying to conceive. One sign is that cervical mucus becomes thinner and stretchier, resembling egg white, and increases in quantity before ovulation, so the vagina feels wetter. Another sign is that, because of hormone activity, basal body temperature rises by about half a degree when ovulation occurs and remains higher until the end of the cycle. A woman can take her temperature each morning with a basal temperature thermometer to see when this increase occurs.

Some couples who use the fertility awareness method rely on **withdrawal** when they have intercourse during the fertile period; that is, the man removes his penis from the woman's vagina before he ejaculates. With perfect use, withdrawal may be an effective form of contraception; however, for typical users, this is not an effective or reliable way to prevent conception, for several reasons. One is that sperm are frequently released before ejaculation; another is that sperm ejaculated near the entrance

> **withdrawal**
> An ineffective contraceptive method in which the man removes his penis from the vagina before ejaculating.

to the vagina can sometimes find their way inside; a third is that the man may not be able to withdraw quickly enough.

EMERGENCY CONTRACEPTION

Also referred to as the *morning-after pill, post-sex contraception*, or *back-up birth control*, **emergency contraception**

emergency contraception (EC)
Pill containing hormones that can be taken within 48 to 72 hours of unprotected sex to prevent pregnancy.

(**EC**) can prevent pregnancy after unprotected vaginal intercourse. It is most effective if taken within 48 to 72 hours and must be taken within 5 days of unprotected intercourse. EC reduces the chance of pregnancy by preventing ovulation and fertilization. It may reduce the likelihood of implantation, but this is not proven. EC will not cause the termination of an existing pregnancy and thus is not an *abortogenic* (abortion-causing) agent.

Emergency contraception is useful when another method fails, such as when a condom breaks or a diaphragm or cervical cap slips out of position. It is also useful in cases of forced sex, including rape and incest. Plan B is an emergency contraceptive now available over the counter for women aged 18 or older. It consists of two pills, containing progesterone only, that can be taken at the same time or 12 hours apart. Other progesterone-only formulations or estrogen-progesterone combinations are available by prescription. Plan B ranges in cost from $10 to $45.

STERILIZATION

Sterilization is a surgical procedure that permanently prevents any future pregnancies. It is the most commonly chosen form of contraception and is especially popular with married couples who do not want to have any more children.

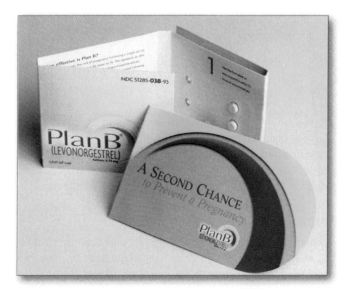

■ Emergency contraception can be taken to prevent pregnancy after unprotected sex or used as a backup when another form of contraception fails, as when a condom breaks.

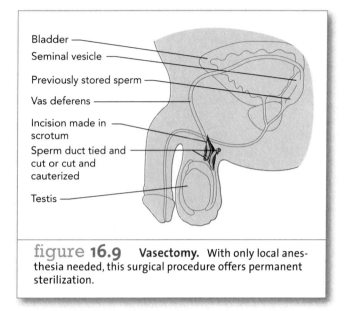

Bladder
Seminal vesicle
Previously stored sperm
Vas deferens
Incision made in scrotum
Sperm duct tied and cut or cut and cauterized
Testis

figure 16.9 **Vasectomy.** With only local anesthesia needed, this surgical procedure offers permanent sterilization.

Besides condoms, sterilization is currently the only form of contraception available to men.

The male sterilization procedure is **vasectomy.** In this procedure, a health care professional makes a small incision or puncture in the scrotum, then ties off and severs the vas deferens, the duct that carries sperm from the testes to the seminal vesicle, where sperm would mix with semen (Figure 16.9). This is done on both sides of the scrotum because each testicle has a vas deferens.

sterilization
Surgical procedure that permanently prevents any future pregnancies.

Vasectomy is usually a relatively quick procedure performed with a local anesthetic. Most men return to their usual activities within 2 to 3 days. Vasectomy does not interfere with sexual function or alter the level of male hormones. Semen is still produced and does not change in appearance. The cost of a vasectomy can range from $350 to $755, and the sterilization effect lasts for life.

vasectomy
Male sterilization procedure, involving tying off and severing the vas deferens to prevent sperm from reaching the semen.

The most common female sterilization procedure is **tubal ligation.** In this procedure, a physician makes an incision in the abdo-

tubal ligation
Female sterilization procedure involving severing and tying off or sealing the fallopian tubes to prevent ova from reaching the uterus.

men, then severs and ties or seals the fallopian tubes, the ducts through which ova pass from the ovaries to the uterus (Figure 16.10). The procedure can be done via a surgical method called *laparoscopy*. A laparoscope, a tube that the surgeon can look through with a tiny light on the end, is inserted through a small incision, and the surgical instruments are inserted through another small incision. Recovery usually takes somewhat longer than recovery from a vasectomy.

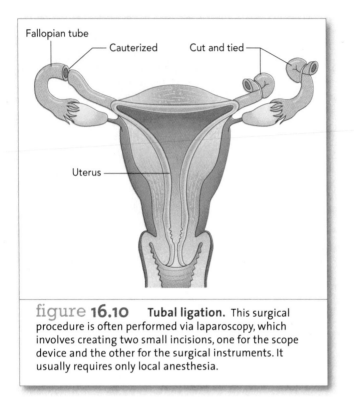

figure 16.10 **Tubal ligation.** This surgical procedure is often performed via laparoscopy, which involves creating two small incisions, one for the scope device and the other for the surgical instruments. It usually requires only local anesthesia.

Tubal ligation does not alter a woman's menstrual cycle or hormone levels. The ovaries continue to function, but ova are prevented from traveling through the fallopian tubes to the uterus and thus cannot be fertilized. A tubal ligation costs between $1,200 and $2,500 and lasts for life.[2] Although in rare cases pregnancy does occur after a vasectomy or tubal ligation, these procedures should be considered permanent.

Another option for permanent sterilization in women, called Essure, was approved by the FDA in 2003. It involves the placement of a micro-rod in each of the fallopian tubes. Tissue begins to develop around the micro-rods, and after 3 months this tissue barrier prevents sperm from reaching the egg.

WHICH CONTRACEPTIVE METHOD IS RIGHT FOR YOU?

Given all the options available for contraception and the number of variables that have to be taken into account in choosing a method—effectiveness, cost, convenience, permanence, safety, protection against STDs, and consistency with personal values—deciding which method is the best one for you can be difficult. (For an overview of methods, see Table 16.1.) Here are some questions to consider:

■ Is your main concern preventing pregnancy? Or do you also need to worry about sexually transmitted diseases? If you are concerned about STDs, you need to use condoms. If you are in a mutually faithful, monogamous relationship and neither you nor your partner has an STD, then a barrier method may not be necessary. You may want to consider birth control pills, an injectable contraceptive, or an IUD.

■ Are you planning to have children with this partner at some time in the future? If so, are you comfortable with a form of contraception that may be slightly less reliable but that has other advantages? The male and female condoms, the diaphragm, Lea's shield, the cervical cap, and the contraceptive sponge are all safe, nonpermanent methods.

■ Do you already have children and know that you do not want any more? Surgical sterilization is a highly effective method with no hassles after the initial procedure.

■ How much can you afford to pay for contraception? There are several factors to consider here. For example, how often do you need contraception? If you have sex daily, the cost of buying condoms for every time can quickly add up, whereas the one-time cost of an IUD or sterilization may be less. If you have sex once a month or less, the opposite may be true. If you need to use two forms of contraception, one to prevent STDs and one to decrease your chances of pregnancy, again, the costs can add up. Don't forget to take into account the cost if you or your partner gets pregnant with the form of contraception you select. It might be the cost of having an abortion, or it might be the cost of raising a child.

■ Are you worried about the safety and health consequences of contraception? These are important concerns, but people are often surprised to learn how safe all the contraceptive options available today have become. To put the risks in perspective, consider that the risk of being killed in a car crash in a given year is 1 in 5,900; the risk of dying from a pregnancy carried past 20 weeks is 1 in 10,000; and the risk of dying from the use of birth control pills in a nonsmoking woman aged 15 to 44 years is 1 in 66,700.[2]

■ Is your choice influenced by your religious, spiritual, or ethical beliefs? Some people are not comfortable with any method that interferes with natural processes. Abstinence, periodic abstinence, or the fertility awareness method may be the right choice.

Unintended Pregnancy

If you or your partner becomes pregnant unexpectedly, you have to make a monumental decision in a very short period of time. Your options are to (1) carry the pregnancy to term and raise the child, (2) carry the pregnancy to term and place the child in an adoptive family, or (3) terminate the pregnancy.

SIGNS OF PREGNANCY

Some signs of pregnancy are common early on, even before a missed period, as a result of hormonal changes. They can include breast tenderness and swelling, fatigue, nausea and vomiting, and light-headedness or mood swings. Some women have light vaginal bleeding or spotting 10 to 14 days after conception—about the time of a normal period but

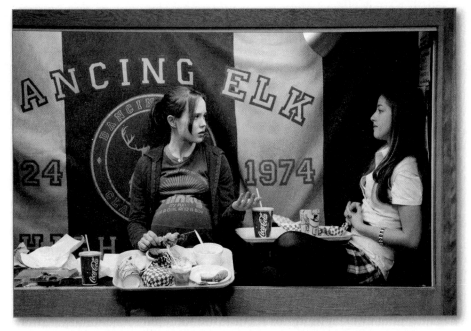

In the 2007 movie *Juno*, Ellen Page plays 16-year-old who considers abortion but opts for adoption as the solution to her unintended pregnancy. The movie underplays the hardship experienced by many teenagers who find themselves in this situation.

shorter in duration. If you experience any of these symptoms after unprotected sex or a missed period, you may want to take a pregnancy test.

A rare complication of early pregnancy is **ectopic pregnancy**, a potentially life-threatening condition. The fertilized egg implants or attaches outside of the uterus, usually in the fallopian tube. Signs of ectopic pregnancy are severe lower abdominal pain or cramping on one or both sides, vaginal spotting or bleeding with abdominal pain, or light-headedness, dizziness, or fainting (a possible sign of internal bleeding). If you experience any of these signs, contact your physician or go to the emergency room immediately.

ectopic pregnancy
A pregnancy in which a fertilized egg implants or attaches outside of the uterus, usually in a fallopian tube.

DECIDING TO BECOME A PARENT

Are you ready to become a parent? Here are some questions to consider:

■ What are your long-term educational, career, and life plans? How would having a child at this time fit in with those plans?

■ What is the status of your relationship with your partner? Is he or she someone you want to commit to and share parenthood with? If you are the mother, the greater part of the pregnancy experience will fall on you, but parenting will involve making decisions with your partner about child rearing (see the box "The Role of Fathers"). Do you have similar goals for a child? Can you communicate well with each other?

■ Do you feel emotionally mature enough to take on the responsibility of raising a child? Parenthood can be demanding, bewildering, and frustrating, and it requires patience, sacrifice, and the ability to put aside your own needs to meet the needs of another person.

■ What are your financial resources at this point? Having a child is expensive. In 2006 the total cost of having a child and raising the child through age 18 was estimated at between \$190,000 and \$381,000.[6] If you are the father, even if you do not want to be emotionally or physically involved, you will probably be legally required to remain financially involved.

■ How large is your social support system? Do you have family members and friends who will help you? Does your community have resources and support services? Social support has been found to be one of the most important factors in helping couples make a successful adjustment to parenthood.

■ What is your health status and age? Do you smoke, drink, or use recreational drugs? Do you have an STD or other medical condition that needs to be treated? Are you under 18 or over 35? Babies born to teenagers and women over 35 have a higher incidence of health problems.

ADOPTION

Adoption can be a positive solution for an unintended pregnancy if you and your partner are not able or willing to become parents at this time in your lives. All forms of adoption require that both biological parents relinquish their parental rights.

In an *open adoption*, the biological parents help to choose the adoptive parents and can maintain a relationship with them and the child. The degree of involvement can range from the exchange of information through a third party to a close and continuous relationship among all parties throughout the child's life. This choice can make it easier for parents to give up a baby, and it allows the child to know his or her biological parents, siblings, and relatives. Many adoption agencies offer this option.

In a *closed adoption*, the more traditional form of adoption, the biological parents do not help choose the adoptive parents, and the adoption records are sealed. This type of adoption provides more privacy and confidentiality than open adoption does. In some states, the child may access the sealed records at the age of 18, and many states are in

Table 16.1   Overview of Contraceptive Methods

Method of Birth Control	Failure Rate (%)		Advantages	Disadvantages	Cost	STD Protection	Rate of User Continuation (%)
	Perfect Use	Actual Use					
No method	85	85		No protection against pregnancy	*	None	?
Abstinence	0	?	Available to all	Requires control; interrupts sexual expression Must agree on definition	None	++	?
Oral contraceptives (birth control pills)	0.3	8	Easy to use Does not interrupt intercourse Safe for most women Noncontraceptive benefits	Possible side effects/rare serious health problems Must be taken daily Prescription required	$$	None	68
Transdermal patch (Ortho Evra Patch)	0.3	8	Easy-to-use weekly application Does not interrupt intercourse Safe for most women Noncontraceptive benefits	Possible side effects/rare serious health problems Greater risk of blood clots than with oral contraceptives or other hormonal methods Prescription required	$$	None	68
Vaginal contraceptive ring (NuvaRing)	0.3	8	Easy-to-use monthly application Does not interrupt intercourse Safe for most women Noncontraceptive benefits	Possible side effects/rare serious health problems Prescription required	$$	None	68
Injection (Depo-Provera)	0.3	3	Very effective Contains no estrogen Requires action only every 3 months	Possible side effects/rare serious health problems Visit to provider every 3 months Weight gain May decrease bone density over time	$$	None	56
Emergency contraception			Reduces risk of pregnancy in case of rape, unprotected sex, or failure of barrier Available over the counter for those aged 18 or older	Must be used within 5 days of unprotected intercourse Nausea/vomiting May alter menstrual cycle Not intended for regular use	$**	None	Not intended for ongoing use
Spermicides	18	29	Available over the counter Increase effectiveness of barriers Female involvement only	May cause allergic reaction Must be inserted with every act of intercourse May increase transmission of HIV	$	None	42
Male condom	2	15	Accessible, inexpensive, easily carried, over the counter Male involvement Reduces risk of STD transmission	Requires interruption of intercourse Male involvement Possible embarrassment Possible breakage	$	+/++	53
Female condom	5	21	No male involvement Can insert up to 8 hours before intercourse Accessible, easily carried, over the counter	Difficult for some women to insert Not as readily available More expensive	$$	+	49

Method of Birth Control	Failure Rate (%)		Advantages	Disadvantages	Cost	STD Pro-tection	Rate of User Continuation (%)
	Perfect Use	Actual Use					
Diaphragm	6	16	May reduce risk of some STDs May be inserted prior to onset of sexual activity	Requires provider appointment/prescription May cause allergic reaction Rarely, may be associated with toxic shock syndrome Must be used with every act of intercourse	$$	+	57
Cervical cap (FemCap) w/o prior pregnancy	4	14	May reduce risk of some STDs May be inserted prior to onset of sexual activity	Requires provider appointment/prescription May cause allergic reaction Rarely, may be associated with toxic shock syndrome Must be used with every act of intercourse	$$	+	57
Sponge w/o prior pregnancy	9	16	Over the counter Immediately effective upon insertion	May cause allergic reaction Rarely, may be associated with toxic shock syndrome Must be used with every act of intercourse	$	+	57
Fertility awareness	3–5	25	Requires knowledge of fertility cycle Male actively involved No serious side effects	Requires knowledge of fertility cycle Male actively involved Variations in cycle may make difficult for some women	None	None	51
IUD (ParaGard Copper)	0.6	0.8	Always in place Effective for 10 years Very effective but reversible	May have pain/heavy menstrual flow Initial expense is high Requires provider visit Possible complications	$$$	None	80
IUD (Mirena)	0.2	0.2	Always in place Effective for 5 years Very effective but reversible Decreased menstrual flow	Initial expense high Requires provider visit Possible complications	$$$	None	80
Sterilization (female)	0.5	0.5	Permanent and highly effective No further action needed No significant long-term side effects	Permanent; difficult to reverse Requires surgery/anesthesia Initial expense is high Risk of ectopic pregnancy if failure	$$$	None	Permanent
Sterilization (male)	0.1	0.15	Permanent and highly effective No further action needed No significant long-term side effects Male involvement	Permanent; difficult to reverse Initial expense is high Requires local anesthesia and minor surgery	$$$	None	Permanent

Cost: none; $ (low), $$ (low/moderate), $$$ (high).

Sexually transmitted disease (STD) protection: none; + (low—may offer some protection); ++ (high).

* "No method" has no initial cost but carries with it a high risk of pregnancy and associated costs.

** Emergency contraception is inexpensive for single use but expensive for regular use.

Source: Adapted from Contraceptive Technology, *19th rev. ed., by R.A. Hatcher, J. Trussell, F. Stewart, et al., 2007, New York: Ardent Media.*

Public Health in Action

The Role of Fathers

With dual-career households, increased rates of divorce, and high rates of childbirth outside of marriage, the role of fathers is changing. In some ways, fathers are more involved than they used to be. They are more likely to drop off children at school or daycare, stay home with a sick child, and go to school meetings than were fathers in the past. For most children, a father's active role promotes physical, economic, and educational well-being.

Unfortunately, 36 percent of children in the United States are in a living situation that does not include their biological father. These children, on average, are more likely than children living with both parents to be poor, to be less educated, to use drugs, to be victims of child abuse, to engage in criminal behavior, and to have more health, emotional, and psychological problems. A Gallup Poll reported that 79 percent of Americans feel "the most significant family or social problem facing America is the physical absence of the father from the home."

All heterosexually active men should take responsibility for the role they play in contraception. They should talk to their partners about birth control options *prior* to the initiation of sexual intercourse. Many men assume the woman is taking charge of the situation, only to find out later that she was not. A single act of intercourse that results in the conception of a child can link the lives of a man and a woman together for life.

During pregnancy, men can play an important role, attending prenatal visits and childbirth classes and discussing issues like parenting styles and financial planning. Many men attend their partner's childbirth and provide emotional and physical support (for example, walking with their partner while she is in labor, encouraging her during contractions). After delivery, men can help their partner recover from the experience of birth. Many employers now offer paternity leave so that fathers can spend time at home and be involved in newborn care and emotional bonding.

As children grow, the role of fathers becomes even more important. On the occasion of Father's Day 2005, the U.S. surgeon general offered a set of tips to fathers and fathers-to-be for keeping their children healthy and safe. Among the guidelines for fathers are these:

- Teach healthy habits for life, such as 60 minutes or more of physical activity every day; limited television, video, and computer time; and avoidance of alcohol, tobacco, and drugs.

- Practice injury prevention and safety, such as by having your child wear appropriate protective gear when bicycling, playing contact sports, using in-line skates, or riding a skateboard.

- Teach and practice healthy eating, and share meals as a family. Offer children nutritious foods and let them decide how much to eat.

- Practice positive parenting: Show affection for your child, recognize his or her accomplishments, encourage your child to express his or her feelings, teach family rules, and set limits.

- Maximize school success by meeting with teachers and being involved in school activities.

- Prevent violence by teaching peaceful resolution to conflict and building positive relationships. Encourage respect for others and set an example with your words and actions. Limit your child's exposure to violence in the media.

- Make sure your child has a primary health care provider, such as a pediatrician or family practitioner, who knows your child before your child has an illness, an injury, or a developmental delay that requires medical attention.

Sources: "Fatherhood Facts," National Fatherhood Initiative, retrieved May 3, 2008, from www.fatherhood.org/fatherfacts/; "U.S. Surgeon General Gives Tips to Fathers and Fathers-to-Be: Father's Day Tips for a Healthy Childhood," U.S. Department of Health and Human Services, retrieved May 3, 2008, from www.surgeongeneral.gov/pressreleases/sg06172005.html.

the process of passing legislation that would open previously sealed records, even for adoptions that occurred decades ago. This change could affect many men and women who thought their adoption decisions would remain confidential forever. One of the reasons for the proposed change is the realization that knowledge about one's biological parents can be important for both psychological and health reasons.

International adoptions have become increasingly common, with children being adopted from countries around the world. For many couples, the decision to adopt a child from another country is based on a desire to help a child who is already alive and in need of care. A major legislative change now allows children in international adoptions to automatically be granted U.S. citizenship at the time of their adoption.

ELECTIVE ABORTION

Terminating the pregnancy through **elective abortion** is the third option for a woman with an unintended pregnancy. (This type of abortion is called *elective* to distinguish it from

elective abortion
Voluntary termination of a pregnancy.

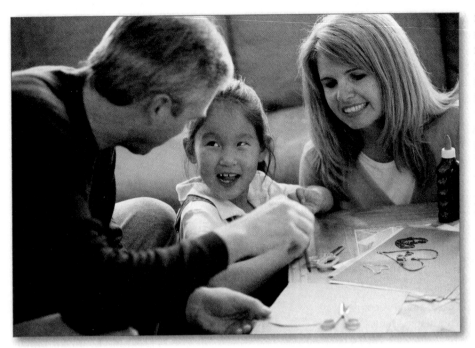

■ Adoption offers the possibility of parenting to people who are not able to conceive a child or who choose not to. It is also one of three possible choices for women who experience an unintended pregnancy.

relief after the abortion. However, about 20 percent of women experience mild, transient depressive symptoms that pass quickly after an abortion. These are similar to symptoms experienced by 70 percent of women after childbirth. The risk of emotional problems after an abortion is increased if depression is present before an unplanned pregnancy or if the abortion is performed due to fetal abnormalities in a desired pregnancy. Even if women do not regret the decision to terminate a pregnancy, they may still experience feelings of regret and sadness. Expressing such feelings may help the recovery process.[8]

If you are pregnant and considering abortion, seek health care counseling to discuss all your options, the risks associated with the procedure, and the technique to be used. The most common technique currently in use is surgical abortion, but the use of medical abortion is increasing.

spontaneous abortion, or miscarriage.) Since 1973 elective abortion has been legal in the United States. In the case of *Roe v. Wade*, the U.S. Supreme Court ruled that the decision to terminate a pregnancy must be left up to the woman, with some restrictions applying as the pregnancy advances through three *trimesters* (divisions of the pregnancy into parts, each about three months long).

Since the passage of *Roe v. Wade*, many attempts have been made at state and national levels to limit access to legal abortion. The debate over abortion between pro-life and pro-choice activists is one of the most highly charged political issues of our time. In 2007 the U.S. Supreme Court upheld the Partial Birth Abortion Ban Act of 2003, the first federal legislature to criminalize a form of abortion. "Partial birth" refers to a rarely performed procedure that aborts a fetus in the third trimester, virtually always for medical reasons. The vast majority of abortions—88 percent—are performed during the first 12 weeks of pregnancy.

International studies show that the legality of abortion does not influence abortion rates. Women around the world seek abortion regardless of the legality of the procedure. In fact, the lowest rates of abortion occur in countries where abortion is legal (Western Europe), and the highest rates of abortion occur in countries where abortion is illegal (Latin America). When abortion is illegal, it is more likely to be unsafe and to be associated with a higher rate of maternal death.[7]

Unintended pregnancy raises complex emotions. The majority of women who have an abortion report a feeling of

spontaneous abortion Involuntary termination of a pregnancy, or miscarriage.

Surgical Abortion In **surgical abortion,** the embryo or fetus and other contents of the uterus are removed through a surgical procedure. (Between 2 and 8 weeks of gestation, the term *embryo* is used; after the 8th week, the term *fetus* is used.) The most common method of surgical abortion performed between the 6th and 12th weeks is vacuum aspiration; it is used for about 90 percent of all abortions performed in the United States. A physician performs this procedure in a clinical setting, such as a medical office or hospital. The cervix is numbed with a local anesthetic and opened with an instrument called a dilator. After the cervix has been opened, a catheter, a tubelike instrument, is inserted into the uterus. The catheter is attached to a suction machine, and the contents of the uterus are removed.

surgical abortion Surgical removal of the contents of the uterus to terminate a pregnancy.

The procedure takes about 10 minutes and requires a few hours' recovery before the woman can return home. A follow-up appointment is needed about 2 weeks after the procedure to ensure that the body is healing. When performed in a legal and safe setting, elective abortion does not increase the risk of infertility or of complications in future pregnancies.

For later stage pregnancies, usually when the mother's life is at risk, a procedure called dilatation and extraction ("partial birth abortion") is sometimes used. Fetal death is caused by a fetal injection; then the cervix is dilated and the contents of the uterus removed by a combination of suction, curette, and forceps.[8]

Medical Abortion   An alternative to surgical abortion is **medical abortion**, in which a pharmaceutical agent is used to induce an abortion. Medical abortions can be performed very early in pregnancy (less than 7 weeks of gestation) or in late pregnancy (after 15 weeks). Between these gestational ages, the surgical techniques are recommended.

medical abortion
Use of a pharmaceutical agent to terminate a pregnancy.

The drug mifepristone (RU486) is used during the first 7 weeks of gestation (or 9 weeks of pregnancy, dated from the first day of the last menstrual period). It is taken in a pill and followed 2 or 3 days later by another drug, misoprostol, which induces contractions. Most women have cramping and bleeding and abort the pregnancy within 2 weeks, although in some cases abortion may occur in a few hours or days. The success rate is nearly 90 percent, and serious complications are rare. After 15 weeks of gestation, different medications are used to induce labor. If abortion does not occur with medication, a surgical abortion is recommended, because the drugs can harm the developing fetus.[8]

Infertility: Causes and Treatment Options

About 7 percent of married couples experience **infertility**,[9] the inability to become pregnant after not using any form of contraception during sexual intercourse for 12 months. The longer childbearing is delayed, the higher the chances that conception will be difficult and that pregnancy will be complicated.

infertility
Inability to become pregnant after not using any form of contraception during sexual intercourse for 12 months.

In about one-third of cases, infertility stems from male factors, such as low sperm count or lack of sperm motility. In another one-third of cases, infertility results from blockage in the woman's fallopian tubes, often scarring that has occurred as a result of pelvic inflammatory disease or another complication of an STD. Blockage can also be caused by an unsterile abortion or by endometriosis, a condition in which uterine tissue grows outside the uterus. In the remaining one-third of cases, the problem is lack of ovulation, abnormalities in the cervical mucus or in anatomy, or unknown causes.

Treatment options for infertility are increasingly being used by couples experiencing difficulty conceiving and by single and lesbian women. The decision to use reproductive techniques can be difficult. The evaluation and treatment often involve detailed questions about sexual activity. Treatment options can be expensive and may not be covered by insurance. In addition, procedures involving the use of hormones to stimulate egg production increase the risk of having multiple births (twins, triplets, quadruplets).

Treatments include surgery to open blocked fallopian tubes or correct anatomical problems, fertility (hormonal) drugs to promote ovulation and regulate hormones, and more advanced reproductive techniques. Intrauterine (artificial) insemination is a process whereby sperm are collected and placed directly into a woman's uterus by syringe. This procedure can be helpful if a man has a low sperm count or low sperm mobility. Donor sperm can be used if a man has a genetic abnormality or in the case of a single woman or a lesbian woman.

In vitro fertilization is a technique by which hormones are used to stimulate egg production in the ovaries, multiple eggs are collected through a surgical procedure, the eggs are fertilized in the clinic, and the fertilized eggs are transferred to the woman's uterus. Other techniques used include gamete intrafallopian transfer or zygote intrafallopian transfer. Both techniques involve induction of multiple eggs with hormones, surgical collection, and manual reintroduction into the fallopian tubes.

Pregnancy and Prenatal Care

Many women do not realize they are pregnant until they are beyond the crucial early phase of development. During this time they may have inadvertently caused harm to their developing child by drinking, smoking, taking medications or recreational drugs, or being exposed to hazardous substances. Research is now indicating that events and conditions during pregnancy can not only cause **congenital abnormalities** (birth defects) but also influence the individual's development throughout life, affecting cognitive development in childhood and health risks, including mental health risks, in adulthood. The best approach to ensuring good health is to give every child the best possible start in life.

congenital abnormalities
Birth defects.

PREGNANCY PLANNING

When is the best time to have a child? Although this is a highly personal decision influenced by many factors—educational and career plans, relationship status, health issues, and others—evidence indicates that the least health risk occurs when women have pregnancies between the ages of 18 and 35. Before age 18, a woman's body is still growing and developing. The additional demands of pregnancy and nursing can impair her health, and the baby is more likely to be born early and have a low birth weight.

After age 35, a woman is more likely to have difficulty getting pregnant, because fertility declines as a woman gets older. Women over 35 are also more likely to have medical problems during pregnancy, including miscarriage, and to have a baby who is born prematurely, has low birth weight, or has a genetic abnormality like Down syndrome.

Male fertility also declines with age. After age 35, men are twice as likely to be infertile as men in their early 20s.

Men over age 40 have an increased risk of fathering a child with autism, schizophrenia, or Down syndrome.[10]

PREPREGNANCY COUNSELING

Couples who practice family planning can take advantage of **prepregnancy counseling,** which typically includes an evaluation of current health status, health behaviors, and family health history. A woman who smokes, uses drugs, or drinks alcohol will be encouraged to quit *before* trying to become pregnant, as will her partner. Existing health conditions will be treated and medications adjusted to the safest options for pregnancy. This can be especially important if a woman is taking medications for high blood pressure or seizure disorder or if she is taking some psychiatric medications. If obesity is an issue, a woman may be counseled about a weight management program. If a couple appear to be at increased risk for a genetic disease on the basis of their ethnic background or family history, they may be referred at this point for genetic counseling and testing.

prepregnancy counseling Counseling before conception that may include an evaluation of current health behaviors and health status, recommendations for improving health, and treatment of any existing conditions that might increase risk.

NUTRITION AND EXERCISE

Because so many women become pregnant unintentionally, every sexually active woman who might become pregnant should be aware of the importance of healthy lifestyle factors. A balanced, nutritious diet before and during pregnancy helps ensure that both you and your child get required nutrients. Total calorie intake needs increase by about 300 calories a day during the second and third trimesters, equivalent to an extra apple and glass of milk each day. The goal for weight gain during pregnancy is 20 to 30 pounds, most of it during the second half of pregnancy.[11]

A baby needs calcium for its growing bones, and this is linked to the mother's calcium intake. A pregnant teenager needs to consume more calcium than an older woman does because she needs more calcium for her own bones. Getting folic acid in food or in a folate supplement is also recommended to reduce the risk of neural tube defects (problems in the development of the brain and spinal cord). Women should increase their folic acid intake during the 3 months *before* getting pregnant so that they have a high level of folic acid in their bodies at the time of conception. The 2005 *Dietary Guidelines for Americans* recommends that all women of childbearing age who may become pregnant consume at least 400 micrograms of folic acid a day and that pregnant women consume 600 micrograms a day.[12] You can reach this intake by eating several servings of dark green, leafy vegetables a day, by taking vitamin supplements, or by eating grain products and cereals fortified with folic acid.

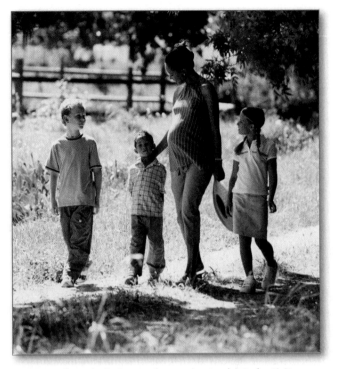

■ Prenatal care includes regular, moderate physical activity, especially cardiorespiratory endurance exercise like walking and swimming.

Foodborne infections can have more serious effects in pregnant women than in the general population, and the FDA advises pregnant women to avoid unpasteurized foods, soft cheese (for instance, Brie, Camembert, and feta), and raw or smoked seafood. Pregnant women, women who might become pregnant, nursing mothers, and young children are advised to monitor their fish and shellfish intake because of contamination with mercury.[13] For guidelines on safe fish consumption, see Chapter 7.

Regular exercise during pregnancy is recommended to help maintain muscle strength, circulation, and general well-being. Women can usually maintain their prepregnancy level of activity. In the second and third trimesters, women should be cautious about exercise that might cause injury or trauma, such as team sports, and favor safer forms of exercise like walking and swimming.

MATERNAL IMMUNIZATIONS

Women should be up to date on routine vaccinations *before* pregnancy. Especially important are vaccination for rubella (German measles) and hepatitis B. Rubella can cause spontaneous abortion or serious birth defects, including deafness and blindness. Hepatitis B is a highly infectious disease that causes liver damage and can be transmitted from mother to child during pregnancy and delivery (called **vertical transmission**). Pregnant women are also

vertical transmission Transmission of an infection or disease from mother to child during pregnancy and delivery.

at high risk of complications from influenza and should get a flu shot during the flu season.

MEDICATIONS AND DRUGS

The uterus is a highly protected place, but most substances that the mother ingests or that otherwise enter her bloodstream eventually reach the fetus. These include prescription medications as well as other drugs and toxic substances. Some substances, called **teratogens,** can cause physical damage or defects in the fetus, especially if they are present during the first trimester, when rapid development of body organs is occurring.

teratogens
Substances that can cause physical damage or defects in the fetus, especially if they are present during the first trimester, when rapid development of body organs is occurring.

Tobacco and alcohol are the drugs most commonly used during pregnancy, with 22 percent of pregnant women using tobacco and 20 percent using alcohol. Women report lower rates of illegal drug use with pregnancy, with 7 percent using marijuana and 2 percent using cocaine, heroin, or methamphetamine. Almost 50 percent of women stop using these drugs once they learn they are pregnant.[14]

If you have a condition for which you take prescription medication, such as diabetes, epilepsy, high blood pressure, acne, or asthma, consult with your physician to make sure the medication does not cause harm to a fetus. You may need to change medications or consider making lifestyle changes to maintain your health during pregnancy while also protecting the health of your fetus. If you suffer from depression or anxiety, your symptoms may worsen during pregnancy and the **postpartum period** (the 3-month period following childbirth) as a result of hormonal and emotional fluctuations. Your physician may be able to help you find natural ways to deal with these changes or recommend starting or continuing medication.

postpartum period
Three-month period following childbirth.

Tobacco Use During Pregnancy   Risk of spontaneous abortion, low birth weight, early separation of the placenta from the uterine wall, and infant death increases with the use of tobacco during pregnancy. If you smoke, try to quit before you get pregnant or abstain during pregnancy and after the baby is born. Avoid places where you and your child will be exposed to environmental tobacco smoke. Babies living in homes where adults smoke have a higher incidence of respiratory infections and **sudden infant death syndrome (SIDS).**

sudden infant death syndrome (SIDS)
Unexpected death of a healthy baby during sleep.

Alcohol and Pregnancy   Consuming 3 or more ounces of alcohol daily (about six drinks) during pregnancy is associated with **fetal alcohol syndrome (FAS).** This condition is characterized by abnormal facial appearance, slow growth, mental retardation, and social, emotional, and behavior problems in the child. A safe level of alcohol consumption during pregnancy has not been established, and even occasional binge drinking may carry significant risk. If you are pregnant or may become pregnant, avoid drinking alcohol.

fetal alcohol syndrome (FAS)
Combination of birth defects caused by prenatal exposure to alcohol, characterized by abnormal facial appearance, slow growth, mental retardation, and social, emotional, and behavior problems.

Illicit Drugs and Pregnancy
Illicit drugs have a variety of effects on a fetus, depending on the chemical action of the drug. Cocaine causes blood vessels to constrict in the placenta and fetus, increasing the risk of early separation of the placenta from the uterine wall, low birth weight, and possible birth defects. Heroin can cause retarded growth or fetal death as well as behavior problems in a child exposed to it in the womb. A baby whose mother used heroin during pregnancy is born addicted and experi-

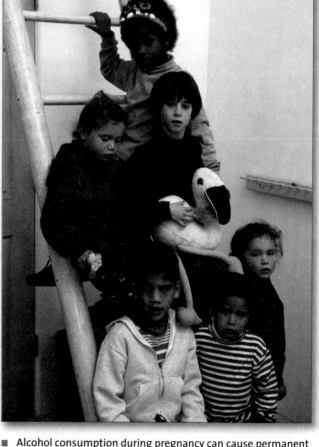

■ Alcohol consumption during pregnancy can cause permanent damage to the fetus, with physical, learning, and behavioral effects. These children with fetal alcohol syndrome exhibit some of the facial characteristics associated with FAS, including a short nose, low nasal bridge, and thin upper lip.

Consumer Clipboard

Choosing a Health Care Provider for Labor and Delivery

When you are thinking about prenatal care and delivery, you have a number of options. Factors influencing your choice include your personal preferences, your medical and health history, and the likelihood of complications during your pregnancy. Here is a general description of the kinds of providers who may be available.

Midwives can be certified nurse-midwives or licensed midwives. A certified nurse-midwife has graduated from a school of nursing, passed a nursing certification exam, and received additional training in midwifery. A licensed midwife has completed a training program in midwifery similar to that of a certified nurse-midwife but may or may not have a prior background in nursing. Licensing laws for midwives vary from state to state. Depending on the state, midwives may be allowed to deliver babies at home, in birthing centers, or in hospitals.

Midwives usually take patients who are at low risk for medical or pregnancy complications. If complications develop during prenatal care or delivery, a midwife will refer the case to a family physician or an obstetrician. Midwives tend to view pregnancy and birth as a family event. They are usually trained in support techniques (such as breathing and relaxation techniques) so the woman can

have a delivery without anesthetic medications, and they usually stay with the woman throughout labor.

Family physicians have completed 4 years of medical school and 3 years in a residency training program. Some family physicians provide pregnancy-related care only for low-risk pregnancies; others receive extra training so they can manage complicated pregnancies and perform caesarean sections if necessary. Family physicians may deliver babies in birthing centers or hospitals but rarely perform home births. Like midwives, many family physicians view pregnancy and birth as a family event, and some use the same kind of support techniques.

Obstetricians have completed 4 years of medical school and an additional 4 years in a residency training program in obstetrics and gynecology. They are trained to handle all kinds of pregnancies, from low risk to high risk. Obstetricians tend to spend limited time at the bedside of a laboring patient; instead, they monitor labor for signs of problems and are present for delivery. Obstetricians usually have a medical orientation to labor management and delivery.

Perinatologists are obstetricians with additional training in the management of high-risk pregnancy. These specialists consult with and accept referrals from obstetricians. They are usually found at major medical centers. Most women see a perinatologist only if serious complications arise in the pregnancy.

---

ences withdrawal symptoms, which can include seizures, irritability, vomiting, and diarrhea. Illicit drugs are also dangerous because they are often contaminated with other agents, such as glass, poisons, and other drugs.

REGULAR HEALTH CARE PROVIDER VISITS

Every pregnant woman should visit her health care provider once a month until the 30th week, once every 2 weeks from the 31st to the 36th week, and once a week from the 37th to the 40th week for *prenatal care* (see the box "Choosing a Health Care Provider for Labor and Delivery"). Week of pregnancy is calculated from the date of the last menstrual period, which is 2 weeks before ovulation and conception occurred. A full-term baby has a gestational period of 38 weeks and is considered to have reached its due date 40 weeks after the woman's last menstrual period.

After the first visit, the health care provider uses the subsequent visits to monitor the fetus for normal growth and development and the woman for complications of pregnancy.

Complications of Pregnancy   Although it is shocking to hear that a woman has died in childbirth in the 21st century, such deaths do occur. Mortality is higher in ethnic and

racial minority groups, pointing to the role of socioeconomic factors, such as lack of prenatal care, lack of access to health information, and dietary differences.

Early complications of pregnancy include the diagnosis of STDs. All women are screened during early pregnancy for gonorrhea, chlamydia, syphilis, hepatitis B, and HIV. Gonorrhea, chlamydia, and syphilis are treated with antibiotics. The viral infections cannot be cured, but the risk of passing these infections to the infant can be reduced through antiviral medications.

Miscarriage is another early complication. Approximately 15–50 percent of all pregnancies end in miscarriage. Most occur during the first trimester (before 12 weeks of gestation). Early symptoms of a miscarriage are vaginal spotting and menstrual cramping. If pain becomes intense, it may be a sign of an ectopic pregnancy.

Pregnancy predisposes some women to develop diabetes, called *gestational diabetes*. Most women are screened between 24 and 28 weeks, since the condition occurs midway through pregnancy. Women with gestational diabetes are advised to exercise, control their diet, and monitor glucose levels, but some women need to start taking insulin.

Toward the end of pregnancy, the risk for several conditions increases. An especially dangerous condition is

preeclampsia
Dangerous condition that can occur during pregnancy, characterized by high blood pressure, fluid retention, possible kidney and liver damage, and potential fetal death.

eclampsia
Potentially life-threatening disease that can develop during pregnancy, marked by seizures and coma.

preeclampsia, characterized by high blood pressure, fluid retention, possible kidney and liver damage, and potential fetal death. Signs include facial swelling, headaches, blurred vision, nausea, and vomiting. If not treated, the condition can progress to **eclampsia**, a potentially life-threatening disease marked by seizures and coma.

Preterm or early labor is another complication of pregnancy. If a woman experiences contractions, cramping, pelvic pressure, or vaginal bleeding before 37 weeks, she should be evaluated to prevent preterm labor.

Complications of Pregnancy for the Child   Approximately 1.2 percent of all pregnancies end in infant death. Half of these deaths occur before the fetus is born, and 80 percent occur before the 28th week of pregnancy (**stillbirth**). After birth, the leading causes of infant death are preterm birth, low birth weight, and SIDS. Before 1980, an infant born early and weighing less than 750 grams (about 1.65 pounds) would not have survived. Now it is standard practice to treat any infant weighing at least 500 grams (about 1.1 pounds).[15]

stillbirth
Infant death before or at the time of expected birth.

Rates of both low birth weight and infant mortality are significantly higher for African Americans in the United States than for members of other groups. Reducing such disparities through improved access to health information and prenatal care is a national health goal.

DIAGNOSING PROBLEMS IN A FETUS

About 5 percent of babies born in the United States have a birth defect.[9] Several tests have been developed to detect abnormalities in a fetus before birth. The most frequently performed tests are alpha-fetoprotein (AFP) measurement, ultrasound, and chromosomal analysis through chorionic villus sampling or amniocentesis.

Alpha-Fetoprotein Triple Screen Measurement   Alpha-fetoprotein (AFP) is a protein produced by the infant and released into the amniotic fluid. It then crosses into the mother's blood, where it can be measured along with other hormone levels and compared with normal ranges. Abnormally high levels have been associated with problems in brain and spinal cord development, and abnormally low levels have been associated with chromosomal abnormalities in the fetus, especially Down syndrome. AFP testing is often done as part of triple screening or quadruple screening (screening for certain hormone levels) at 16 to 18 weeks of pregnancy.

alpha-fetoprotein (AFP)
Protein produced by the infant and released into the amniotic fluid; AFP measurement is used to screen for some fetal abnormalities.

ultrasound
Technique for producing a visual image of the fetus using high-frequency sound waves.

Ultrasound   Ultrasound is the use of high-frequency sound waves to produce a visual image of the fetus in the womb. It is commonly used to determine the size and gestational age of the fetus, its location in the uterus, and any major anatomical abnormalities. It can also reveal the sex of the fetus.

Chromosomal Analysis Many chromosomal abnormalities are fatal and cause spontaneous abortion, but some are not fatal. Chromosomal abnormalities cause from 20 to 25 percent of all birth defects. The most common is Down syndrome (see Chapter 2 for more on this syndrome). Chromosomal abnormalities occur with greater frequency as maternal age increases. For example, the risk of Down syndrome in a 20-year-

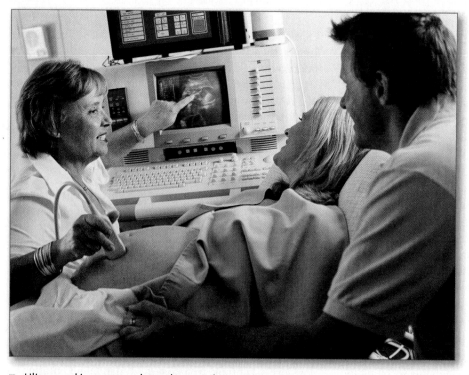

■ Ultrasound is a commonly used prenatal screening tool that can reveal the sex of the fetus, along with other information. Sonograms give expectant parents their first view of their child.

chorionic villus sampling (CVS)
Technique for testing fetal cells for chromosomal abnormalities by removing cells from the chorionic villus, part of the placenta in the uterus.

amniocentesis
Technique for testing fetal cells for chromosomal abnormalities by removing a sample of amniotic fluid from the amniotic sac.

old woman is 1 in 1,400, but the risk in a 40-year-old woman is 1 in 100.[15] The most common reasons for chromosomal testing are advanced maternal age (35 years or older) and an abnormal triple screen finding.

In both **chorionic villus sampling (CVS)** and **amniocentesis,** a needle is passed through the abdomen of a pregnant woman into the uterus. (CVS can also be done by passing a thin catheter through the vagina and cervix.) In CVS, a sample is taken from the chorionic villus, part of the placenta (fetal support system) in the uterus. In amniocentesis, a sample of amniotic fluid, the fluid that fills the pouch enclosing the fetus in the uterus, is taken. In both cases, fetal cells from the samples are subjected to chromosomal analysis. CVS can be performed between weeks 10 and 12, and amniocentesis can be performed between weeks 14 and 18. If a chromosomal problem is detected, the parents are faced with the difficult choice of continuing or terminating the pregnancy.

FETAL DEVELOPMENT

Within 30 minutes of fertilization in the fallopian tube, the single-celled fertilized ovum, called a *zygote,* starts to divide. By the end of 5 days, the cluster of cells has made its way down the tube into the uterus. By the end of a week, it attaches to the uterus and starts to send small rootlike attachments into the uterine wall to draw nourishment. By the end of the 2nd week, it is fully embedded in the lining of the uterus.

The period from week 2 to week 8, called the embryonic period, is a time of rapid growth and differentiation. By 4 weeks, the cluster of cells has divided into cells of different types, forming an embryo, a **placenta,** and an **amniotic sac.** By 8 weeks, all body systems and organs are present in rudimentary form, and some, including the heart, brain, liver, and sex organs, have started to function.

placenta
Structure that develops in the uterus during pregnancy and links the circulatory system of the fetus with that of the mother.

amniotic sac
Membrane that surrounds the fetus in the uterus and contains amniotic fluid.

The period from the end of the 8th week after conception to birth is called the fetal period. By 12 weeks, bones have formed and blood cells are beginning to be produced in the bone marrow. By 16 weeks, the sex of the fetus can be readily determined, and the mother can feel fetal movements. By 24 weeks, the fetus makes sucking movements with its mouth. It typically weighs about 640 grams and is starting to assume a fetal position because of space restrictions in the uterus. If a fetus is born between about 24 and 25 weeks of gestation, it can survive with aggressive medical intervention.

By week 26, the eyes are open, and by week 30, a layer of fat is forming under the skin. At 36 weeks, the fetus weighs about 2,500 grams and has an excellent chance of survival. The lungs are usually mature at this point. As noted earlier, a baby is considered to be full term at 38 weeks of gestation, 40 weeks after the mother's last menstrual period. Full-term babies usually weigh about 7½ pounds and are about 20 inches long. An overview of fetal development is shown in Figure 16.11.

Childbirth

By the 9th month, the pregnant woman is usually uncomfortably large and eager to have the baby, despite any apprehension she may harbor about the process of giving birth.

LABOR AND DELIVERY

Labor begins when hormonal changes in both the fetus and the mother cause strong uterine contractions to begin. The pattern of labor and delivery can be different for every woman, but often it begins with irregular uterine contractions.

labor
Physiological process by which the mother's body expels the baby during birth.

When labor begins in earnest, the contractions will become regularly spaced and begin to get stronger and more painful. The contractions cause the cervix to gradually pull back and open (dilate), and they put pressure on the fetus, forcing it down into the mother's pelvis. This first stage of labor can last from a few to many hours.

When the cervix is completely open, the second stage of labor begins. The baby slowly moves into the birth canal, which stretches open to allow passage. The soft bones of the baby's head move together and overlap as it squeezes through the pelvis. When the top of the head appears at the opening of the birth canal, the baby is said to be *crowning.* After the head emerges, the rest of the body usually slips out easily.

The third stage of labor is the delivery of the placenta, which usually takes another 10 to 30 minutes. An overview of the process of labor and delivery is shown in Figure 16.12.

Many techniques have been developed to help women with the discomfort of the labor and delivery process. Childbirth preparation classes help women and their partners learn breathing and relaxation techniques to use during contractions. Several medication options are available in hospitals to further help with the discomfort.

Occasionally the birthing process does not go smoothly. Sometimes the infant is too big to pass through the mother's pelvis or is in the wrong position, either sideways, buttocks first, or face first. Occasionally, the placenta covers the cervix so the baby cannot move into the birth canal. And sometimes the infant just does not tolerate the stress of the process well.

Time	Changes/milestones
8 weeks (end of embryonic period)	*By week 8, pregnancy is detectable by physical examination.* Head is nearly as large as body. First brain waves can be detected. Limbs are present. Ossification (bone growth) begins. Cardiovascular system is fully functional. All body systems are present in at least basic form. Crown-to-rump length: 30 mm (1.2 inches) Weight: 2 grams (0.06 ounces)
9–12 weeks (3rd month)	*By week 10, fetus responds to stimulation.* Head is still large, but body is lengthening. Brain is enlarging. Spinal cord shows definition. Facial features begin to appear. Internal organs are developing. Blood cells are first formed in bone marrow. Skin is apparent. Limbs are well molded. Sex can be recognized from genitals. Crown-to-rump length: 90 mm
13–16 weeks (4th month)	*By week 14, skeleton is visible on X-ray.* Cerebellum becomes prominent. Sensory organs are defined. Blinking of eyes and sucking motions of lips occur. Face has human appearance. Head and body come into greater balance. Most bones are distinct. Crown-to-rump length: 140 mm
17–20 weeks (5th month)	*By week 17, mother can feel movement of fetus.* Fatty secretions (vernix caseosa) cover body. Lanugo (silky hair) covers skin. Fetal position is assumed. Limbs are reaching final proportions. Mother feels "quickening" (movement of fetus). Crown-to-rump length: 190 mm
21–30 weeks (6th and 7th months)	*By weeks 25–27, survival outside the womb is possible.* Substantial weight gain occurs. Myelination (formation of sheath around nerve fibers) of spinal cord begins. Eyes are open. Bones of distal limbs ossify. Skin is wrinkled and red. Fingernails and toenails are present. Tooth enamel is forming. Body is lean and well proportioned. Blood cells are formed in bone marrow only. In males, testes reach scrotum at 7th month. Crown-to-rump length: 280 mm
30–40 weeks (8th and 9th months)	*Between weeks 32 and 34, survival outside the womb is probable.* Skin is whitish pink. Fat is present in subcutaneous tissue. Crown-to-rump length: 360–400 mm Weight: 2.7–4.1 kg (6–10 pounds)

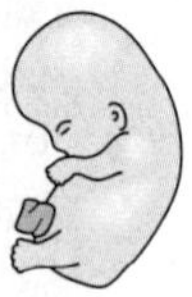

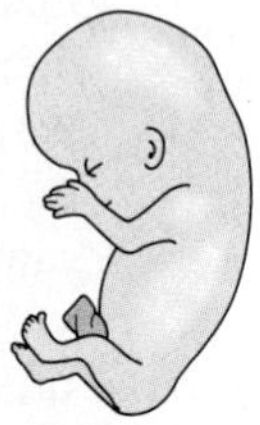

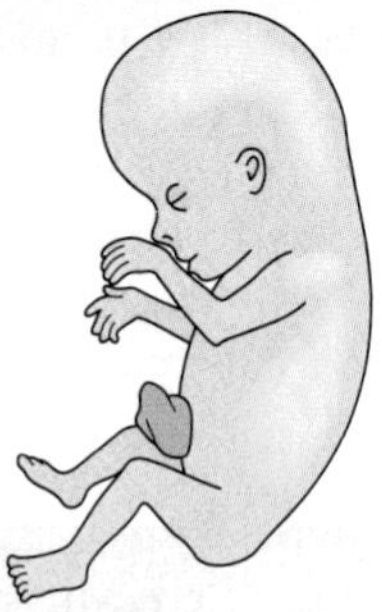

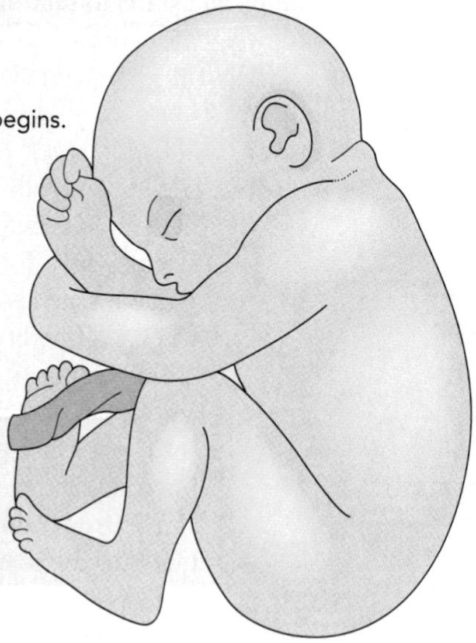

figure **16.11** **Fetal development.**
Sources: Data from Human Anatomy and Physiology, 6th ed., by E.N. Marieb, 2004, San Francisco: Benjamin-Cummings; Understanding Children and Adolescents, 4th ed., by J.A. Schickedanz et al., 2001, Boston: Allyn & Bacon.

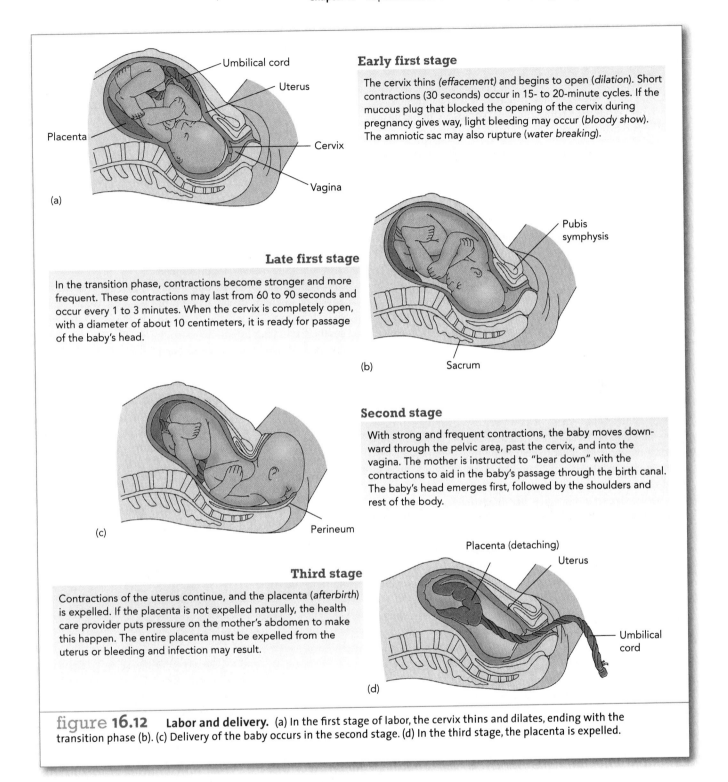

Early first stage

The cervix thins (*effacement*) and begins to open (*dilation*). Short contractions (30 seconds) occur in 15- to 20-minute cycles. If the mucous plug that blocked the opening of the cervix during pregnancy gives way, light bleeding may occur (*bloody show*). The amniotic sac may also rupture (*water breaking*).

Late first stage

In the transition phase, contractions become stronger and more frequent. These contractions may last from 60 to 90 seconds and occur every 1 to 3 minutes. When the cervix is completely open, with a diameter of about 10 centimeters, it is ready for passage of the baby's head.

Second stage

With strong and frequent contractions, the baby moves downward through the pelvic area, past the cervix, and into the vagina. The mother is instructed to "bear down" with the contractions to aid in the baby's passage through the birth canal. The baby's head emerges first, followed by the shoulders and rest of the body.

Third stage

Contractions of the uterus continue, and the placenta (*afterbirth*) is expelled. If the placenta is not expelled naturally, the health care provider puts pressure on the mother's abdomen to make this happen. The entire placenta must be expelled from the uterus or bleeding and infection may result.

figure **16.12**   **Labor and delivery.** (a) In the first stage of labor, the cervix thins and dilates, ending with the transition phase (b). (c) Delivery of the baby occurs in the second stage. (d) In the third stage, the placenta is expelled.

In these situations, the health care provider usually recommends **cesarean section (C-section),** the surgical delivery of the infant through the abdominal wall. Although most women are not enthusiastic about this option, it has saved many infants' and mothers' lives. Most hospitals now allow a woman to have her support person with her during the surgery. She can be awake and see her infant as it is born.

cesarean section (C-section)
Surgical delivery of the infant through the abdominal wall.

NEWBORN SCREENING

Babies are evaluated at birth to determine whether they require any medical attention or will need developmental support later. The Apgar scale is used as a quick measure of the baby's physical condition: a score of 0 to 2 is given for heart rate, respiratory effort, muscle tone, reflex irritability, and color. The scores are added for a total score of 0 to 10. The baby's neurological condition may also be assessed, and various screening tests may be given, such as tests for hearing and for phenylketonuria (see Chapter 2). Most babies are pronounced healthy and taken home within 24 to 48 hours of birth.

THE POSTPARTUM PERIOD

Many expectant parents spend the 9 months of pregnancy focusing on the upcoming birth and thinking about the baby's sex, possible names, *circumcision* (whether or not to remove the foreskin of the penis), and breast-feeding versus bottle feeding. They may have spent little time thinking about exactly what it is like to be responsible for a baby. The first few weeks or months of parenthood are a period of profound adjustment, as parents learn how to care for their newborn (or **neonate**) and the newborn takes his or her place in the family. A few issues that deserve attention are growth and nutrition, illness and vaccinations, and attachment.

neonate
Newborn.

Growth and Nutrition Babies have very high calorie requirements. One reason for this is their rapid rate of growth—they triple their birth weight by their first birthday—and another reason is the great relative mass of the infant's organs, especially the brain and liver, compared with muscle. Organs have much higher metabolic and energy requirements than muscle does.

Most organizations agree that breastfeeding is the best way to feed babies. Breast milk is perfectly suited to babies' nutritional needs and digestion; it also contains antibodies that reduce the risk of infections, allergies, asthma, and SIDS. For mothers, breastfeeding enhances bonding with the baby, contributes to weight loss after pregnancy, and may decrease the risk of ovarian cancer and breast cancer after menopause.

Breastfeeding can be more convenient and less expensive than bottle-feeding. New mothers who have difficulty with breastfeeding can get advice and support from a lactation consultant, their health care provider, or support groups like LaLeche League. When a woman is breastfeeding, she may not get her menstrual period for up to 6 months after giving birth; however, ovulation can still occur, so breastfeeding is not a reliable form of birth control.

Because of illness, breast infection, or other reasons, about 10 percent of women are unable to breastfeed, and they bottle-feed their infants instead. Bottle-feeding provides adequate nutrition and enables parents to know how much food the baby is consuming. It also allows the mother more freedom and gives other family members the opportunity to feed and bond with the baby.

Illness and Vaccinations Childbirth and the neonatal period are times of increased risk of infection for an infant. Starting at 2 months, children receive vaccinations against several childhood diseases that, in the past, caused serious illness and death. They include diphtheria, pertussis (whooping cough), tetanus, measles, rubella (German measles), mumps, and polio, among others. The vaccinations are inexpensive and safe, especially when compared with the physical, emotional, and social costs of childhood diseases.

Most states require that children be vaccinated before they are allowed to start public school. The National Immunization Survey reports that current childhood vaccination levels are at their highest ever, with 90 percent of children receiving the primary recommended vaccines. However, rates vary among racial and ethnic groups; again, reducing such disparities is a goal of national health policies.

Adjustment and Attachment Although babies are tiny, they quickly become the center of attention in the household. They spend their time in recurring states of crying, alertness, drowsiness, and sleep. Parents spend much of their time feeding their newborn (at first, every 2 hours or so), changing diapers, and trying to soothe the crying infant. The strong emotional bond between parents and infant known as **attachment** develops during this period, and the infant begins to have feelings of trust and confidence as a result of a comforting, satisfying relationship with parental figures. This sense of trust is crucial for future interpersonal relationships and social and emotional development. Thus a healthy infancy lays the foundation for a healthy life.

attachment
Deep emotional bond that develops between an infant and its primary caregivers.

About 13 percent of women experience depression in the first year after giving birth, referred to as *postpartum depression.* Rapid hormone changes after delivery, broken sleep patterns, self-doubt about one's ability to provide for an infant, a sense of loss of control, and changes in one's

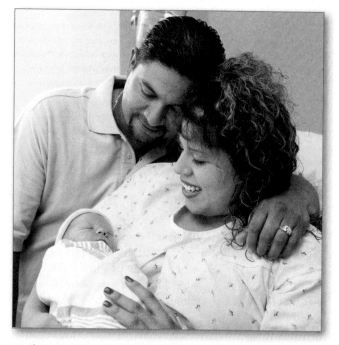

■ The arrival of a newborn signals not just the beginning of a new life but a radical change in how the family will function.

support system can all contribute to feelings of sadness, restlessness, loss of interest, guilt, difficulty focusing, and withdrawal. Postpartum depression can have significant effects on a woman's relationships with her partner and baby. Effective treatments exist for depression, and women and their partners should be aware of the signs and symptoms of the condition.

You Make the Call

Egg and Sperm Donation: A Booming Business

Imagine this scenario: You are in your senior year of college, the bills are adding up, and you are starting to realize how big those student loans really are. You're also thinking how nice it would be to take a week off and go on vacation—if only you had some extra cash. You open the campus newspaper and see an ad that reads, "Egg donors needed: $10,000." Is this the answer to all your problems?

The fertility industry has become just that—an industry that addresses people's fertility needs by creating babies. Egg donors (and sperm donors, too) are often recruited on college campuses. College students are among the most coveted donors because they are typically young, healthy, and smart. They usually are also financially limited and thus become an appealing target. But a number of issues arise in association with this practice.

One issue is health risk and safety. A woman who agrees to donate eggs first undergoes personal and family health screening. She is then given a series of hormonal medications, often by injection, to induce the formation of multiple eggs at one time in her ovaries. She then goes to a health care facility to have the eggs collected. During the procedure, for which the woman is sedated, a needle is inserted through the vagina, bladder, or abdominal wall and guided by ultrasound to the ovaries, where the eggs are removed. Potential risks from the medications include nausea, diarrhea, abdominal bloating, shortness of breath, sleeplessness, moodiness, and rarely, ovarian hyperstimulation (a condition in which too many eggs are produced). It is not known how or whether egg donation affects a young woman's own future fertility, but over a woman's reproductive lifespan, she produces many more eggs than she will use for her own pregnancies.

For sperm donations, the man also undergoes personal and family health screening. He has to refrain from intercourse or ejaculation for a few days prior to the donation and then has to ejaculate into a cup. Men produce millions of sperm, so donation does not limit a man's future fertility. The smaller time investment and the lower risk for men translate into less compensation for sperm donation—usually about $150.

Compensation for egg and sperm donations raises another issue. Many countries have banned payments to egg donors, arguing that a child is not a commodity to be bought and sold. When compensation is high, it can induce financially strapped individuals to take actions they might otherwise find morally or ethically repugnant or later think of as coerced.

Perhaps most important, this practice raises questions that must be answered by each prospective donor: What does your DNA mean to you? Is it just a set of genes and chromosomes that you can separate from yourself and your family? Or is a child created with your DNA somehow connected to you? Most egg and sperm donors sign a legal agreement relinquishing all parental rights, and most arrangements are anonymous. It is unlikely that a donor could ever track down his or her genetic offspring in the future or that the offspring could locate his or her genetic donor. The personal, biological, and ethical implications of these situations are yet to be fully explored.

This rapidly growing area of reproductive technology has been portrayed both as a boon to infertile couples and as a seriously questionable practice. What do you think?

PROS

- Reproductive technology allows many couples and individuals access to pregnancy and childbearing that they would otherwise not have had. It allows them to achieve their dream of parenthood. Often the child is biologically related to one of the parenting adults.

- Men produce millions of sperm, and donation does not limit a man's fertility.

- Women produce more eggs than they use for their own pregnancies and thus can perform a service for an infertile couple without risking their own future childbearing.

- Financial compensation for time spent and medical risks is appropriate.

CONS

- Paying women and men for egg or sperm amounts to buying and selling children.

- Women or men in financial need may be exploited by couples or fertility clinics with the means to pay them.

- A child may suffer psychological harm when told of the donated egg or sperm.

- Donors may struggle with their role (or lack thereof) in the life of a child genetically related to them.

- Egg and sperm donations result in the birth of children who may be related to each other and not know it. As adults, such individuals may meet and become romantically involved, creating the potential for relationships that could be genetically problematic.

In Review

1. **What are the commonly available contraceptive methods?** The most reliable method is abstinence. Other methods include hormonal methods (birth control pills, the transdermal patch, the contraceptive ring, the injectable contraceptive, and the contraceptive implant), barrier methods (male and female condoms, the diaphragm, Lea's shield, the cervical cap, and the contraceptive sponge), the IUD, the fertility awareness method, emergency contraception, and male and female sterilization. Methods vary in their effectiveness, cost, convenience, permanence, safety, protection against STDs, and consistency with personal values.

2. **What are a person's options in the event of unintended pregnancy?** The three options are having and keeping the baby, placing the baby for adoption, and having an abortion. The vast majority of abortions, nearly 90 percent, are performed during the first 12 weeks of pregnancy. Abortion can be performed surgically or medically (with drugs).

3. **What happens when a couple cannot conceive?** Treatments are increasingly available for infertility and include surgery, fertility drugs, intrauterine fertilization, in vitro fertilization, and other advanced technologies.

4. **What are the basics of prenatal care?** Prepregnancy care can include genetic counseling and vaccinations against common infectious diseases, especially rubella and hepatitis B. Once a woman is pregnant, prenatal care includes good nutrition and exercise, avoidance of substances that could harm the fetus, and regularly scheduled health care visits. Problems in the fetus can be diagnosed prenatally by advanced technologies.

5. **What happens during prenatal development?** The fertilized egg (zygote) implants in the uterine wall and begins a period of repid growth and differentiation. During the first trimester, all the body systems form and start functioning (for example, the heart starts beating), the limbs are molded, and the sex of the fetus can be recognized. During the second trimester, the fetus continues to develop, and the proportion of the body to head becomes more balanced. The third trimester is a period of rapid weight gain. At birth, the typical baby weighs about 7 1/2 pounds and is about 20 inches long.

6. **What happens during labor and delivery?** During the first stage of labor, strong uterine contractions cause the cervix to shorten and open and push the baby down into the mother's pelvis. During the second stage of labor, the baby moves into the birth canal and emerges from the mother's body, usually head first. During the third stage of labor, the placenta is delivered.

7. **What concerns arise during the postpartum period?** Breastfeeding is considered the best way to feed a baby, but bottle-feeding is an acceptable alternative. Newborns are especially vulnerable to infections; they start receiving routine vaccinations at about 2 months. The newborn period is one of profound adjustment for all family members.

www For a detailed summary of this chapter and a comprehensive set of review questions, visit the Online Learning Center at **www.mhhe.com/teague2e.**

Web Resources

American Society for Reproductive Medicine: Offering publications on sexual and reproductive health, this organization also provides fact sheets, FAQs, and information booklets.
www.asrm.org

Guttmacher Institute: This organization publishes journals and special reports related to sexual and reproductive health. Online articles address topics such as abortion, pregnancy and childbirth, contraception, and STDs.
www.guttmacher.org

Managing Contraception: This site offers a Q&A page with helpful information about sexual and reproductive health issues. It also features links related to abortion, contraception, counseling, and emergency contraception.
www.managingcontraception.com

NARAL Pro-Choice America: This pro-choice organization works for better access to effective contraceptive options and to reproductive and other health care services.
www.naral.org

National Adoption Clearinghouse: This organization offers information on adoption, adoption counseling, birth family search, and more, including referrals and links.
www.adoption.org

National Right to Life Committee: This group works for legislative reform related to abortion and promotes alternatives to abortion. Its Web site features fact sheets and links to other resources.
www.nrlc.org

Planned Parenthood Federation of America: This organization provides health information on birth control, emergency contraception, abortion, adoption, and pregnancy. Its resources include fact sheets, reports, and links.
www.plannedparenthood.org

PART FIVE

Protecting Your Health

Even with healthy lifestyles, people get sick. They catch colds, come down with the flu, and are sometimes exposed to foodborne illness or sexually transmitted diseases. Many people discover they've developed heart disease, and others receive a diagnosis of cancer. The American health care system provides a multitude of ways to meet these challenges, and complementary and alternative medicine offers additional options. Most important, there are many steps you can take to improve your chances of avoiding these conditions. The chapters in Part 5 show you how.

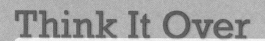

Think It Over

- Given the prevalence of sexually transmitted diseases, do you take the risks seriously enough on every sexual occasion?

- Do you have a history of cardiovascular disease or cancer in your family? If so, do you take extra lifestyle precautions?

- Will complementary and alternative medicine ever gain the same degree of acceptance in the United States as conventional medicine?

Infectious Diseases
Prevention and Management

Ever Wonder...

- if there's any risk in getting a tattoo or piercing?

- if you should buy antibacterial soaps and cleaning products?

- if people are more likely to get sick after they've traveled somewhere by airplane?

WWW

Your Health Today

www.mhhe.com/teague2e

Go to the Online Learning Center for *Your Health Today* for interactive activities, quizzes, flashcards, Web links, and more resources related to this chapter.

The moment you enter the world, your body is colonized by millions of bacteria. Your whole life is shared with other organisms, some helpful and some harmful. The strongest influence on human evolution has been the microscopic world. Microorganisms have affected where, how, with whom, and how long we live. They have determined the outcomes of wars and attempts at colonization, and they have shaped the way populations have moved around the globe.

Prior to 1900 infectious diseases were the leading cause of death in the United States, with 30 percent of all deaths occurring among young children. Public health measures, vaccinations, and antibiotics are responsible for the reduction in the death rate from infectious diseases in the United States to about 2 percent by the end of the 20th century. Perhaps the greatest reductions in infectious diseases have come from improved sanitation and hygiene practices, especially clean water supplies. In recent years, however, death rates from infectious diseases have started to creep up again, as a result of new diseases such as AIDS and the reemergence of existing diseases once thought vanquished. This chapter provides an overview of infectious diseases, including sexually transmitted diseases, and offers guidelines for protecting yourself from infections.

The Process of Infection

Microorganisms, the tiniest living organisms on earth, do what all living organisms do: eat, reproduce, and die. An **infection** occurs when part of a microorganism's life cycle involves you. An infection is considered an illness or disease if it interferes with your usual lifestyle or shortens your life.

infection
Disease or condition caused by a microorganism.

Infections can result in different outcomes. Some infections cause a sudden illness with a high risk of death, such as infection with the Ebola virus. Some infections stimulate your body's immune response, causing the death of the microorganism, as occurs with the common cold virus. Still other infections may persist without signs of illness for years and yet be passed on to other people, as is the case with the human immunodeficiency virus (HIV). Finally, some infections are walled off by the immune system, as in the case of tuberculosis, and held at bay for as long as the immune system is healthy.

The process of infection often follows a typical course, with the length of each stage depending on the pathogen (Figure 17.1). Some infections will have a latent phase, when the infectious organism is dormant or walled off in the body prior to causing symptoms. Latent infections may activate at a later point. Other infections are incompletely cleared by the body and continue at a low level indefinitely.

THE CHAIN OF INFECTION

The **chain of infection** is the process by which an infectious agent, or **pathogen,** passes from one organism to another. Pathogens often live in large communities, called *reservoirs,* in soil or water or within organisms. Many pathogens cannot survive in the environment and require a living *host.* To cause infection, pathogens must have a *portal of exit* from the reservoir or host and a *portal of entry* into a new host (Figure 17.2).

A pathogen can exit a host in respiratory secretions (coughing, sneezing); via feces, genital secretions, blood or blood products, or skin; or through an insect or animal bite. The pathogen enters the new host in similar ways: through skin-to-skin contact, genital-to-genital contact, inhalation of respiratory droplets, exposure to blood products, or insect or animal bites. If the transfer from host to host or reservoir to host is carried out by an insect or animal, that organism is said to be a **vector.**

chain of infection
Process by which an infectious agent passes from one organism to another.

pathogen
Infectious agent capable of causing disease.

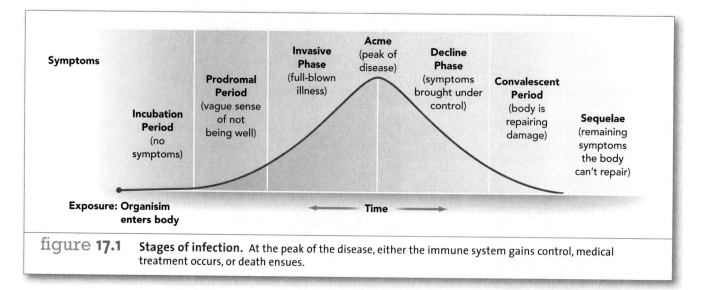

Symptoms

Incubation Period (no symptoms)

Prodromal Period (vague sense of not being well)

Invasive Phase (full-blown illness)

Acme (peak of disease)

Decline Phase (symptoms brought under control)

Convalescent Period (body is repairing damage)

Sequelae (remaining symptoms the body can't repair)

Exposure: Organisim enters body

Time

figure **17.1**   **Stages of infection.** At the peak of the disease, either the immune system gains control, medical treatment occurs, or death ensues.

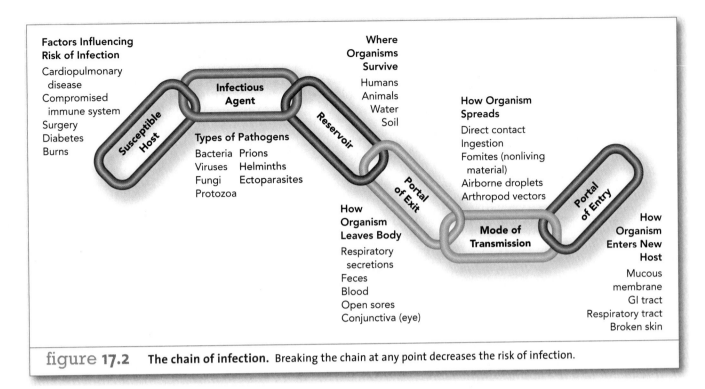

figure **17.2**   **The chain of infection.** Breaking the chain at any point decreases the risk of infection.

vector
Animal or insect that transmits a pathogen from a reservoir or an infected host to a new host.

Breaking or altering the chain of infection at any point can either increase or decrease the risk of infection. For example, chlorinating drinking water reduces the number of pathogens and the size of reservoirs for waterborne infections; using condoms disrupts both the portal of exit and the portal of entry for infectious agents that may be present in semen or vaginal secretions; controlling mosquito populations eradicates vectors and disrupts a pathogen's mode of transmission.

The extent or spread of an infection depends on several factors, including the **virulence** (speed and intensity) of the pathogen, the mode of transmission (how an infection spreads from person to person), the ease of transmission, the duration of infectivity (how long a person with infection can spread it to other people), and the number of people an infected person has contact with while he or she is infectious. If an infected person does not transmit the infection to anyone else, that person's disease dies out. If the person transmits it to at least one other person, the infection continues. If the infection is transmitted to many people, an **epidemic** may occur.

virulence
Speed and intensity with which a pathogen is likely to cause an infection.

epidemic
Widespread outbreak of a disease that affects many people.

PATHOGENS

Millions of different pathogens cause human infections, but they fall into several broad categories (Figure 17.3).

Viruses   Viruses represent some of the smallest pathogens. They are also among the most numerous; it is estimated that there are more different types of viruses than all other creatures combined.

Viruses consist of a genome (a genetic package of either DNA or RNA), a capsid (protein coat), and in some cases an outer covering or envelope. They are unable to reproduce on their own; they can replicate only inside another organism's cells. Viruses do not survive long outside of humans or other hosts. A virus infects a host cell by binding to its receptors and injecting its genetic material into the cell. Once inside, the virus can have a number of different effects. It can make many copies of itself, burst the cell, and release the copies to infect more cells. It can persist within the cell, slowly continuing to cause damage or becoming inactive and reactivating at a later time. Some viruses integrate themselves into a cell's DNA and alter the growth pattern of the cells. This process can lead to the development of a tumor or cancer.[1]

Bacteria   Bacteria are single-celled organisms that can be found in almost all environments. They are classified based on shape (spherical, rodlike, spiral), the presence or absence of a cell wall, and growth requirements. Speed of replication varies from 20 minutes to 2 weeks. Some bacteria can enter a dormant or spore state in which they can survive for years.

Many bacteria inhabit a person harmlessly or helpfully and are considered part of the person's **normal flora.** Sometimes, bacteria that are normal in one body location are pathogens in another location, as

normal flora
Bacteria that live in or on a host at a particular location without causing harm and sometimes benefiting the host.

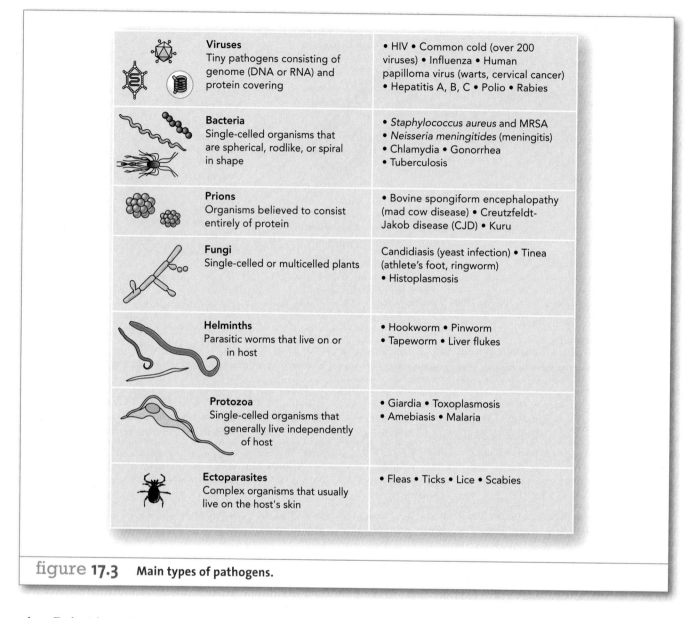

Viruses
Tiny pathogens consisting of genome (DNA or RNA) and protein covering

- HIV • Common cold (over 200 viruses) • Influenza • Human papilloma virus (warts, cervical cancer) • Hepatitis A, B, C • Polio • Rabies

Bacteria
Single-celled organisms that are spherical, rodlike, or spiral in shape

- *Staphylococcus aureus* and MRSA • *Neisseria meningitides* (meningitis) • Chlamydia • Gonorrhea • Tuberculosis

Prions
Organisms believed to consist entirely of protein

- Bovine spongiform encephalopathy (mad cow disease) • Creutzfeldt-Jakob disease (CJD) • Kuru

Fungi
Single-celled or multicelled plants

- Candidiasis (yeast infection) • Tinea (athlete's foot, ringworm) • Histoplasmosis

Helminths
Parasitic worms that live on or in host

- Hookworm • Pinworm • Tapeworm • Liver flukes

Protozoa
Single-celled organisms that generally live independently of host

- Giardia • Toxoplasmosis • Amebiasis • Malaria

Ectoparasites
Complex organisms that usually live on the host's skin

- Fleas • Ticks • Lice • Scabies

figure **17.3**   **Main types of pathogens.**

when *Escherichia coli,* a bacterium that inhabits the large intestine and aids in digestion, enters the bladder, where it causes a bladder or urinary tract infection.

Prions   Prions, the least understood infectious agents, are known to be responsible for the neurodegenerative disease bovine spongiform encephalopathy (BSE), or mad cow disease. The term *prion* was coined as a shortened form of *proteinaceous infectious particle.* Prions are believed to be made entirely of protein. They are found in brain tissue and appear to alter the function or shape of other proteins when they infect a cell, initiating a degeneration of brain function. Prions appear to spread by the ingestion of infected brain or nerve tissue.[1]

Fungi   A fungus is a single-celled or multicelled plant. Several kinds of fungi, including yeasts and molds, cause infection in human beings. Fungi reproduce by budding or by making spores; many fungal infections result from exposure to spores in the environment, such as in the soil or on tile floors. Except for tinea (ringworm) in children, fungal infections rarely spread from person to person.

Dermatophytes are a group of fungi that commonly infect the skin, hair, or nails; they are responsible for tinea, athlete's foot, and nail fungus. The yeast *Candida* may be part of a person's normal flora but can overgrow and cause a yeast infection in the vagina or mouth. All of the fungi can become serious infections in a person with a compromised immune system (for example, someone with HIV infection or AIDS, someone undergoing chemotherapy for cancer, or someone taking immunosuppressant drugs following an organ transplant).[1]

Helminths   Helminths, protozoa, and ectoparasites are broadly grouped in the category *parasites*—organisms that live on or in a host and get food at the expense of the host. Helminths, or parasitic worms, include roundworms, flukes, and tapeworms. They are large compared with other infectious agents, ranging in length from 1 centimeter to 10 meters.

People usually become infected with parasites by accidentally ingesting worm eggs in food or water or by having the skin invaded by worm larvae. Worldwide, parasitic worms cause a huge disease burden. For example, hookworm, which attaches to the human intestine and causes blood loss, is a leading cause of anemia and malnutrition in developing countries.[1, 2]

Protozoa   Protozoa are single-celled organisms; most can live independently of host organisms. Protozoal infection is a leading cause of disease and death in Africa, Asia, and Central and South America. Infection may be transmitted by contaminated water, feces, or food, as is the case in protozoal infections such as giardia, toxoplasmosis, and amebiasis; by air, as is the case in *Pneumocystis carinii* pneumonia; or by a vector, such as the mosquito in the case of malaria.[1, 2]

Ectoparasites   Ectoparasites are complex organisms that usually live on or in the skin, where they feed on the host's tissue or blood. They cause local irritation and are frequently vectors for serious infectious diseases. Examples are fleas, ticks, lice, mosquitoes, and scabies.[1, 2]

The Body's Defenses

A single square inch of skin on your arm is home to thousands of bacteria. A sneeze projects hundreds of thousands of viral particles into the air. Bacteria can double in number every 20 minutes, and a virus can replicate thousands of times within a single human cell. Although you are substantially larger than microorganisms, you feel the power of their numbers each time you catch a cold. Considering these facts, our ability to overcome invasion and survive infectious diseases is remarkable.

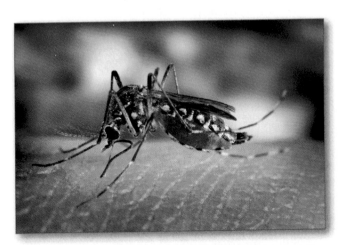

■ Skin is an excellent physical barrier, but the female mosquito is able to penetrate it with her proboscis. Mosquitoes serve as vectors for several diseases caused by bloodborne pathogens, including encephalitis, West Nile virus, and malaria.

EXTERNAL BARRIERS

The skin is the first line of defense against infection. Most organisms cannot get through skin unless it is damaged, such as by a cut, burn, or infection, or if passage is aided by an insect bite or needle stick. Most portals of entry into the body, such as the mouth, lungs, nasal passages, and vagina, are lined with mucous membranes. Although these linings are delicate, mucus traps many organisms and prevents them from entering the body. Nasal passages and ear canals have hair that helps trap particles. The lungs are protected by the cough reflex and by cilia, tiny hairlike structures that rhythmically push foreign particles up and out. Damage to these physical barriers increases risk of infection. For example, tobacco, alcohol, and some illnesses can decrease the effectiveness of the cough reflex and the clearing of mucus from the body; burns and cuts compromise the integrity of the skin and allow entry by infectious agents.

If pathogens get past these barriers, they often encounter chemical defenses. Saliva contains special proteins that break down bacteria, and stomach acids make it difficult for most organisms to survive. The small intestine contains bile and enzymes that break down pathogens. The vagina normally has a slightly acidic environment, which favors the growth of normal flora and discourages the growth of other bacteria. The body protects pores and hair follicles in the skin by excreting fatty acids and lysozyme, an enzyme that breaks down bacteria and reduces the likelihood of infection. Some medications reduce the effectiveness of chemical barriers, as when medications for acid reflux decrease stomach acidity or antibiotics kill normal flora in the vagina and create conditions conducive to a yeast infection. The physical and chemical barriers to infection are illustrated in Figure 17.4.

THE IMMUNE SYSTEM

The **immune system** is a complex set of cells, chemicals, and processes that protects the body against pathogens when they succeed in entering the body. The immune system is organized to fulfill three functions: recognize foreign particles or infectious organisms, attack and destroy these agents, and communicate with other parts of the immune system about when to begin and end an attack.

The immune system has two subdivisions: the innate immune system and the acquired immune system. These two overlap in many of their functions, and both operate largely through the action of white blood cells, but there are some key differences. The **innate immune system** is a rapid response designed to catch and dispose of foreign

immune system
Complex set of cells, chemicals, and processes that protects the body against pathogens when they succeed in entering the body.

innate immune system
Part of the immune system designed to rapidly dispose of pathogens in a nonspecific manner.

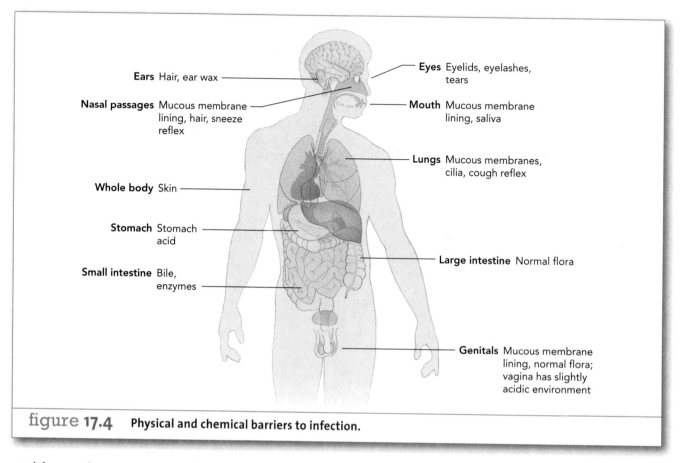

Ears　Hair, ear wax

Nasal passages　Mucous membrane lining, hair, sneeze reflex

Whole body　Skin

Stomach　Stomach acid

Small intestine　Bile, enzymes

Eyes　Eyelids, eyelashes, tears

Mouth　Mucous membrane lining, saliva

Lungs　Mucous membranes, cilia, cough reflex

Large intestine　Normal flora

Genitals　Mucous membrane lining, normal flora; vagina has slightly acidic environment

figure 17.4　**Physical and chemical barriers to infection.**

particles or pathogens in a nonspecific manner. The **acquired immune system** is a highly specialized response that recognizes specific targets.

The Innate Immune System

The body's initial reaction to tissue damage, whether it is due to trauma or infection, is an **acute inflammatory response**, a series of changes that increase the flow of blood and its cellular contents to the site. A complicated series of molecular and cellular events occurs when the innate immune system is activated. Signs of the inflammatory response are redness, warmth, pain, and swelling.

The cells of the innate immune system are neutrophils, macrophages, and natural killer cells. Neutrophils and macrophages are white blood cells that travel in the bloodstream to areas of infection or tissue damage. These phagocytes ("cell eaters") digest damaged cells, foreign particles, and bacteria. Natural killer cells are white blood cells that recognize and destroy virus-infected cells or cells that have become cancerous.

The Acquired Immune System　Your acquired (or adaptive) immunity develops as you are exposed to potential infections, infections, and vaccinations. Each time the cells of the acquired immune system are exposed to a pathogen, they form a kind of memory of it and can mount a rapid response the next time they encounter it.

The defining white blood cells of the acquired immune system are **lymphocytes,** which circulate in the bloodstream and lymphatic system. The lymphatic system is a network of vessels and organs throughout the body that serves to move fluid from body tissues and clear infection. It includes the lymph nodes, spleen, and thymus.

If the lymphocytes encounter an **antigen** (a marker on the surface of a foreign substance), they rapidly duplicate and "turn on" their specific function. The two main types of lymphocytes are *T cells* and *B cells*. T cells monitor events that may be occurring inside the body's cells. If a cell is infected, molecules on its surface are altered that indicate it is now "nonself." *Helper T cells* "read" this message and trigger the production of killer T cells and B cells; helper T cells also enhance the activity of the cells of the innate immune system and of B cells once they are activated. *Killer T cells* attack and kill foreign cells and body cells that have been infected by a virus or have become cancerous. *Suppressor T cells* slow down and halt the immune response when the threat has been handled.

acquired immune system
Part of the immune system that recognizes specific targets.

acute inflammatory response
Series of cellular changes that bring blood to the site of an injury or infection.

lymphocytes
White blood cells that circulate in the bloodstream and lymphatic system.

antigen
Marker on the surface of a foreign substance that identifies it to immune cells as "nonself."

B cells monitor the blood and tissue fluids. When they encounter a specific antigen, they mature to become cells that produce **antibodies**—proteins that circulate in the blood and bind to specific antigens, triggering events that destroy them. Antibodies may neutralize the pathogen just because they are bound to the antigen; they may signal other cells to destroy the organism that has the antigen on its outside; or they may activate parts of the innate immune system, which destroy the pathogen.

antibodies
Proteins that bind to specific antigens and trigger events that destroy them.

Immunization   Once a person has survived infection by a pathogen, he or she often acquires **immunity** to future infection by the same pathogen. The reason for this is that some B and T cells become *memory cells* when exposed to an infectious agent; if they encounter the same antigen in the future, they can respond rapidly, destroying the invader before it can cause illness. Immunization is based on this principle: The immune system is exposed to part of an infectious agent so that an immune response is triggered. On subsequent exposures, the immune system mounts a rapid response, preventing disease.

immunity
Reduced susceptibility to a disease based on the ability of the immune system to remember, recognize, and mount a rapid defense against a pathogen it has previously encountered.

vaccines
Preparations of weakened or killed microorganisms or parts of microorganisms that are administered to confer immunity to various diseases.

The concept of immunization was first introduced in 1796 by English physician Edward Jenner. Jenner realized that people who had been infected with cowpox, a disease that causes mild illness in humans, seldom became ill or died when exposed to smallpox, a related but often fatal disease. Jenner's observation led to the development of **vaccines,** preparations of weakened or killed microorganisms or parts of microorganisms that are administered to confer immunity to various diseases. Since 1900, vaccines have been developed for many infectious diseases, and significant reductions in death rates from these diseases have occurred (see the box "Vaccination: Not Just for Kids").[3]

Vaccination serves two functions. The first is to protect an individual, frequently but not always a child, by stimulating an immune response. The second is to protect society. Widespread vaccination shrinks the reservoir of infectious agents, protecting the community through "herd" immunity. For example, widespread use of the smallpox vaccine has led to the elimination of naturally occurring smallpox worldwide. All future generations benefit from the earlier smallpox vaccination campaigns and no longer require vaccination themselves. Deaths from vaccine-preventable diseases are at an all-time low, but high vaccination levels are necessary to maintain this effect.[4]

RISK FACTORS FOR INFECTION

Your risk for infections depends on numerous factors, some within your control and others beyond your individual control.

Controllable Risk Factors   You can reduce your risk of infection by adopting behaviors that support and improve the health of your immune system. One such behavior is eating a balanced diet; poor nutrition is associated with a higher risk of infectious disease. Other behaviors that support a healthy immune system are exercising, getting enough sleep, and managing stress. Vaccination, when available, can boost your immune system and facilitate a quicker response to pathogens. Good hygiene practices like hand washing reduce the risk of many infections, and protecting your skin from damage keeps many pathogens out of your body. Avoiding tobacco and environmental tobacco smoke improves your defenses against respiratory illness.

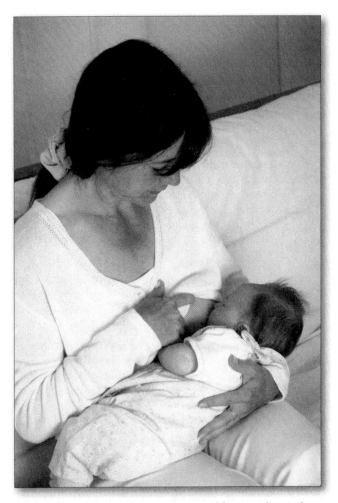

■ Antibodies for some diseases are passed from mothers to babies in breast milk. Breastfeeding has been shown to reduce the incidence of infections, allergies, and diarrhea in infants and even to promote good health later in the child's life.

Public Health in Action

Vaccination: Not Just for Kids

As a child, you almost certainly received a series of routine vaccinations. As an adult, you need vaccinations, too. It's especially important for college students to be up to date on their vaccinations because of crowded living quarters and close social interactions. Check this list to see if your vaccinations are current:

- **Varicella (chickenpox) vaccine.** Many adults have immunity to chickenpox from a childhood exposure. If you are not sure whether you had chickenpox, you can have a blood test to assess your immunity. If you did not receive two doses of the varicella vaccine as a child and do not have signs of immunity, you should receive one dose now and a second dose in 8 weeks. Pregnant women should wait until after they deliver to be immunized.

- **Human papillomavirus (HPV) vaccine.** HPV causes genital warts and cervical cancer. The vaccine is recommended for all girls and women aged 9 to 26 years—ideally, prior to the onset of sexual activity. However, women with a history of HPV infection, abnormal Pap tests, or genital warts may still benefit from vaccination, since the vaccine protects against multiple strains of HPV. The vaccination is a three-shot series—one now, the second in 2 months, and the third in 6 months.

- **Tetanus, diphtheria, and acellular pertussis (Tdap) vaccine.** This vaccine boosts immunity against three diseases; most adults received a similar series in childhood. The current recommendation is that adults receive a booster of tetanus, diphtheria (Td) vaccine every 10 years. However, immunity to all three infections decreases with age, and recently pertussis was added to this combination vaccine. A single dose of Tdap should replace the Td for all adults under 65 years of age.

- **Influenza vaccine.** Vaccination against influenza is recommended for anyone with an increased risk of complications or anyone living with someone at increased risk. People at high risk include children aged 6 months to 5 years, pregnant women, people aged 50 or older, and people with chronic health conditions (including asthma, heart disease, lung disease, and compromised immune function). The vaccine is available as a shot or nasal spray and becomes available each fall for that year.

- **Hepatitis A vaccine.** Hepatitis A vaccination is recommended for certain persons who have liver disease or are receiving clotting factors; men who have sex with men; people who use intravenous drugs; and people who plan to travel where hepatitis is common, such as Mexico, Central America, or South America. The vaccine is a two-shot series, one now, the second in 8 weeks.

- **Hepatitis B vaccine.** Hepatitis B vaccination is recommended for all sexually active persons not in a long-term, mutually monogamous relationship; men who have sex with men; and injection drug users. It is also recommended for persons with chronic liver disease, kidney disease, HIV infection, or other sexually transmitted diseases, and for those who work in health care or other settings where they could be exposed to blood products. The vaccination is a three-shot series, administered now, in 2 months, and in 6 months.

- **Mumps, measles, and rubella (MMR) vaccine.** Many adults received one or two doses of this vaccine in childhood. If you didn't, you should receive this vaccination to boost your immunity against these three diseases. The second dose is especially important for international travelers, health care workers, and college students. Many colleges and universities are moving toward requiring two doses of this vaccine. Pregnant women should wait until after they deliver to receive this vaccine.

- **Meningococcal vaccine.** The vaccine protects against a dangerous form of meningitis and is recommended for first-year college students living in the dormitories, military recruits, people in other close living situations, and travelers to areas where infection is common. The vaccine is a single dose, although revaccination in 3 to 5 years may be indicated if risk of disease remains high.

- **Pneumococcal vaccine.** A single dose of the pneumococcal vaccine is recommended routinely for all adults 65 years of age or older and for younger adults if they have risk factors for pneumonia, such as HIV, compromised immune function, diabetes, heart disease, chronic lung disease, alcoholism, liver disease, kidney disease, or sickle cell disease.

- **Herpes zoster (shingles) vaccine.** Herpes zoster is a reactivation of the varicella (chickenpox) virus; it increases in frequency with age or in times of stress. A single dose of the zoster vaccine is recommended for all people aged 60 years or older as a way to reduce episodes.

- **Other vaccinations.** Other vaccines may be recommended for you (for example, for rabies, yellow fever, and typhoid fever) if you were not immunized in childhood, if you plan to travel to other countries, or if you have other risks based on your occupation or exposures. Visit the Centers for Disease Control and Prevention (CDC) Web site for travel recommendations and vaccine recommendations.

Sources: "Recommended Adult Immunization Schedule, United States, October 2007–September 2008," U.S. Department of Health and Human Services, October 19, 2007, MMWR QuickGuide, retrieved May 28, 2008, from www.cdc.gov/MMWR/PDF/wk/mm5641-Immunization.pdf; data from Global Alliance for Vaccines and Immunization, retrieved from www.gavialliance.org; "Malaria: Eliminating an Old Adversary," retrieved from www.gatesfoundation.org/ GlobalHealth/Pri_Diseases/Malaria/.

Uncontrollable Risk Factors Age plays a role in vulnerability to infection, with higher risks at both ends of the lifespan. Newborns and young children are at increased risk because they have not been exposed to many infections; pregnancy and breast feeding confer **passive immunity**—a mother's antibodies can pass to the fetus or child to provide temporary immune protection. Older people are at increased risk due to a gradual decline in the immune system that can occur with aging. Other factors that increase vulnerability include undergoing surgery, having a chronic disease such as diabetes, and being bedbound.

passive immunity
Temporary immunity provided by antibodies from an external source—such as passed from mother to child in breast milk.

Genetic predisposition may play a role in susceptibility to infectious disease. It is unclear why certain people develop an overwhelming, life-threatening illness when exposed to a pathogen while others develop only a mild fever. Certain sociocultural factors are associated with higher risk for infectious disease; in many situations, these are not controllable risk factors. Overcrowded living environments (including dormitories, fraternities, and sororities) increase the risk for any infectious disease that is spread from person to person, such as influenza, meningitis, and tuberculosis. Poverty is associated with increased risk for many illnesses, probably owing to poor nutrition, stress, and lack of access to health care, among other factors.

DISRUPTION OF IMMUNITY

Because the immune system is so complex, it is occasionally subject to malfunctions. Two such disruptions are autoimmune diseases and allergies.

Autoimmune Diseases Sometimes, a part of the body is similar enough to an antigen on a foreign agent that the immune system mistakenly identifies it as "nonself." Other times, the immune control system fails to turn off an immune response once an infection is over. In both cases, a process of self-destruction can ensue, causing damage to body cells and tissues. Autoimmune diseases vary in their effects, depending on which part of the body is seen as foreign. In rheumatoid arthritis, the immune system can cause destruction of joints, kidneys, and other internal organs. In psoriasis, the immune system causes severe rashes and damage to internal organs. Other autoimmune diseases include multiple sclerosis, scleroderma, and lupus erythematosis. Genetics is known to play a role in some autoimmune diseases.[1] For unknown reasons, autoimmune diseases are more common in women than in men.

Allergies Allergic reactions occur when the immune process identifies a harmless foreign substance as an infectious agent and mounts a full-blown immune response. Allergic responses to substances like pollen or animal dander, for example, may include a runny nose, watery eyes, nasal congestion, and an itchy throat. Asthma, a condition character-

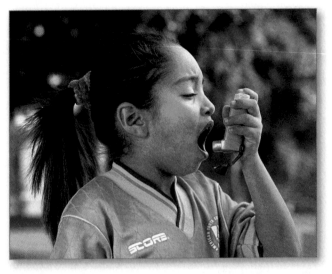

■ The incidence of asthma has increased dramatically in recent years, particularly among ethnic minorities, low-income populations, and children living in inner cities.

ized by wheezing and shortness of breath, is caused by inflammation of the bronchial tubes and spasm of the muscles around the airways in response to an allergen or other trigger (see the box "Asthma: a Treatable Condition").

Anaphylactic shock is a life-threatening systemic allergic response. Medications containing antihistamine can help relieve mild allergy symptoms; powerful drugs called steroids are sometimes used to decrease an immune response that has become chronic. Epinephrine (adrenaline) is used in an emergency situation to reduce the swelling associated with anaphylactic shock.

anaphylactic shock
Hypersensitive reaction in which an antigen causes an immediate and severe reaction that can include itching, rash, swelling, shock, and respiratory distress.

Immunity and Stress As described in Chapter 5, stress can have a significant impact on the immune system. Short-term stress can actually enhance immune system functioning by activating the body's responses to stressors like puncture wounds, scrapes, and animal bites. Chronic, long-term stress, however, suppresses immune system functioning; the longer lasting the stress, the greater the negative effect on immune system functioning. Although the relationship between stress and immune system change has been verified by more than 300 studies conducted over the past 30 years, it is not clear that stress "causes" illness. Further research is needed to determine the exact nature of the relationship.[5]

Changing Patterns in Infectious Disease

In 1969 the surgeon general of the United States reportedly declared before Congress that it was time to close the book on infectious diseases. Dramatic declines in the death rate from infectious diseases during the 20th century inspired

Highlight on Health

Asthma: A Treatable Condition

Asthma is a chronic lung condition that affects the airways, or bronchial tubes (the tubes that carry air in and out of the lungs). In asthma, inflammation makes the smooth muscle that lines the airways very sensitive. The muscles go into spasm in response to irritants in the air, making the airways even narrower and reducing the amount of air that can move in and out. Symptoms range from mild to life threatening and include wheezing, coughing, shortness of breath, chest tightness, and difficulty breathing.

Rates of asthma have been increasing over the past 50 years, especially among children and in racial and ethnic minorities. About 20 million Americans have asthma, nearly 9 million of them children. What causes the disorder is unclear, but it does run in families and is more common in people with allergies. Exposure to cigarette smoke and other irritants early in life and some infections may play a role.

An asthma attack—a sudden worsening of symptoms—can be set off by a range of triggers, including exer-cise, cold air, pet dander, foods, air pollution, tobacco smoke, and viral infections. Although asthma cannot be cured, it can be controlled. Some medications work over the long term to reduce inflammation; others provide quick relief by relaxing the muscles causing the spasm. The National Heart, Blood, and Lung Institute offers the following recommendations:

- If you think you might have asthma, see your physician to get tested. Medications can significantly improve the quality of your life.

- Identify your irritants and learn to avoid them.

- Respond quickly at the onset of an attack to treat it effectively, and seek medical care if your medications are not controlling symptoms.

- If your asthma is exacerbated by exercise, ask your physician how to use your medications so that you can lead an active life.

- Get annual flu shots. People with asthma are at increased risk of complications if they get a respiratory infection.

Source: "What Is Asthma?" National Heart, Lung, and Blood Institute, retrieved November 30, 2007, from www.nhlbi.nih.gov/health/dci/Diseases/Asthma/Asthma_WhatIs.html.

this bold statement (Figure 17.5). Within a little more than 10 years, however, the first cases of what would soon be identified as human immunodeficiency virus (HIV) infection were causing perplexity and alarm in hospitals in several U.S. cities. Since then, the appearance of other new infections, changes in patterns of infection, and the development of antibiotic resistance in many strains of bacteria have demonstrated that infectious diseases remain an important health concern.

TECHNOLOGY-RELATED CHANGES THAT AFFECT DISEASE TRANSMISSION

Technological advances that have increased the ease with which infectious organisms can get from one person to another include blood banks and centralized food production.

Blood Products and Organ Transplants Each year, approximately 11 to 12 million units of blood are transfused and 27,000 organs are transplanted in the United States. These lifesaving treatments serve as a potential vector for transmitting infectious diseases from donor to recipient. Confirmed transmission of viruses (HIV; hepatitis A, B, and C; West Nile virus; rabies), bacteria (syphilis), and parasites (malaria) has occurred.[6–9]

Blood banks in the United States and Canada screen donors through questionnaires prior to donation and test blood for numerous infectious diseases. People are restricted from donating if they have lived or traveled in areas at high risk for malaria or mad cow disease. Blood banks in the United States and Canada have never been safer. Due to the screening programs in place, the risk of infection from HIV, hepatitis B, and hepatitis C is exceedingly low.[7, 8] New infections continue to arise, however, and screening requirements are constantly being reviewed and updated. For instance, in 2007, the Red Cross began screening all blood for evidence of Chagas, a bloodborne parasitic infection affecting an estimated 11 million people in Latin America.[10]

Food Production and Distribution For the most part, the days of backyard gardens, local butchers, and corner groceries are gone. Much of our food is grown in one part of the country or in a foreign country, shipped to a central processing plant, packaged, and then distributed to locations from coast to coast. This widespread distribution of food lowers some costs and makes production more convenient, but it may decrease nutrient value and increase the risk that contaminated food will cause infectious disease in many people.

More than 250 organisms are associated with food-related illnesses. They include viruses, bacteria, prions, and parasites. As described in Chapter 2, a national network of public health officials monitors reported cases of foodborne illness in the United States and investigates unusual increases in cases involving particular strains of pathogens. For example, in October 2006, an outbreak of salmonella poisoning with cases in 47 states was traced to a single peanut butter

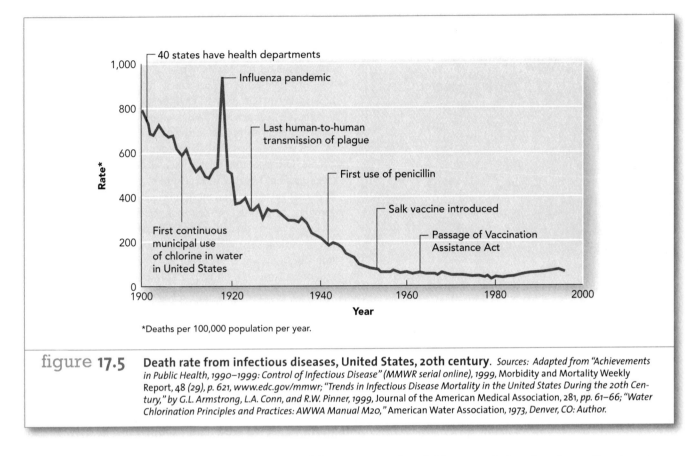

figure 17.5 **Death rate from infectious diseases, United States, 20th century.** *Sources: Adapted from "Achievements in Public Health, 1990–1999: Control of Infectious Disease" (MMWR serial online), 1999,* Morbidity and Mortality Weekly Report, *48 (29), p. 621, www.edc.gov/mmwr; "Trends in Infectious Disease Mortality in the United States During the 20th Century," by G.L. Armstrong, L.A. Conn, and R.W. Pinner, 1999,* Journal of the American Medical Association, *281, pp. 61–66; "Water Chlorination Principles and Practices: AWWA Manual M20," American Water Association, 1973, Denver, CO: Author.*

processing plant in Georgia.[11] For guidelines on avoiding foodborne illness, see the tips provided in Chapter 7.[12]

BEHAVIOR-RELATED CHANGES THAT AFFECT DISEASE TRANSMISSION

Disease transmission has also been affected by changes in behavior, including travel, sexual behavior, drug use, and tattooing and piercing.

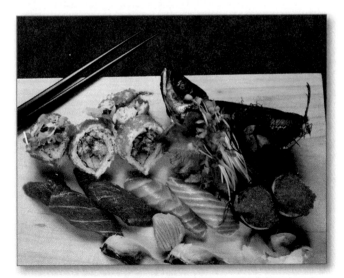

■ Although many sushi bars offer freshly caught fish, some also serve fish that was caught in distant locations, processed at a central distribution plant, and shipped nationwide. By the time the sushi reaches the table, there have been many opportunities for contamination.

Travel and Disease Before the advent of modern transportation systems—for example, when it took weeks to cross the ocean on a ship—a passenger who became sick en route could be quarantined (separated from others to prevent transmission of disease). Nowadays, people can travel immense distances in hours, carrying incubating pathogens with them. University students and staff are particularly vulnerable to disease transmission because higher education is an international endeavor, with academics traveling around the world in pursuit of their interests.

The severe acute respiratory syndrome (SARS) outbreak in 2003 is an excellent example of how travel affects the spread of disease and how community efforts can control it. In March 2003 the World Health Organization activated a Global Outbreak Alert concerning an atypical pneumonia that was believed to have originated in southern China at the end of 2002. By February 2003 it had spread to Hong Kong, Vietnam, Singapore, Germany, and Canada. By the time the disease was contained in July 2003, there had been 8,098 probable cases and 774 deaths in 26 countries.

SARS is caused by a previously unknown corona virus and is spread directly from person to person by coughing, sneezing, and skin contact. Air travel was identified as a key reason for its rapid spread. With no vaccine or treatment, isolation and quarantine of potentially infected people was the key to stopping the spread of infection. The disease has an incubation period of 2 to 10 days, and transmission appears to occur only while people have symptoms.

During the outbreak, airlines and travelers were alerted to the early symptoms, which include fever, cough, and

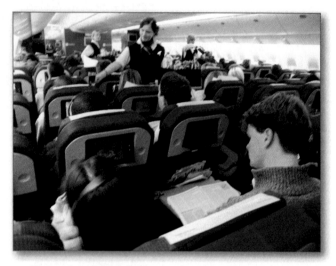

■ Air travelers are vulnerable to infectious diseases because of close proximity with other passengers who may be ill.

body aches; these symptoms can progress fairly rapidly to a severe form of pneumonia. Travelers boarding planes that were departing from cities with SARS cases were screened for symptoms and prevented from travel if symptomatic. If a traveler became ill in flight, health officials boarded the plane upon arrival to examine and possibly quarantine the individual. Travelers were advised to avoid cities with SARS cases, and many locales suffered financially until the advisory ended. Countries around the world remain on alert for a recurrence. International surveillance and preparedness have significantly improved as a result of this experience. Such awareness is important, because new diseases—such as avian flu—will continue to arise and spread.[13]

Sexual Behavior and Disease Sexual behavior also affects the transmission of disease. A variety of factors make a difference in how likely it is that a person will be exposed to a sexually transmitted disease (STD). These factors can be categorized as partner variables, susceptible person variables, and sex act variables.

Partner variables that increase the risk of being exposed to an STD include the total number of sex partners a person has, how frequently he or she acquires new sex partners, and the number of concurrent sexual partners. Certain types of partners are associated with an increased risk of infection; the highest risks are associated with commercial sex workers (people who are paid to have sex) and unknown partners (for example, people picked up at bars or bath houses).[14]

Variables associated with increased susceptibility to infection if exposed to an STD include gender, age at first intercourse, and the general health of the susceptible person. Women are at greater risk than men due to anatomy (the larger mucosal surface of the vagina and the cervix in comparison to the penis). Young women are at particular risk because the cervix is more susceptible to infection in the first few years after the start of menstruation. The overall health of a person is important because it affects the strength of the immune response and the integrity of the mucosal surfaces. For instance, a person with one sexually transmitted infection may be more likely to contract a second infection, as discussed later in this chapter.

The sexual acts performed by a couple also affect how likely it is for an STD to be passed from one person to another. Nonpenetrative sex (fondling, mutual masturbation) has the lowest risk, followed in increasing order of risk by oral sex, penile-vaginal intercourse, and penile-anal intercourse. Other factors further increase or decrease the risk of transmission. The risk of exposure increases with the number of sexual acts. The amount of lubrication, either natural from foreplay or applied, affects risk, because abrasions to the mucosa make it easier for the STD to be transmitted. Forced sex or violent sex increases the risk of abrasions and of STD transmission. When used correctly, condoms decrease the risk of transmission of many STDs, but they are not 100 percent effective, and there are currently no data showing that they reduce the risk of transmission of the human papillomavirus, which causes genital warts and cervical cancer.[14, 15]

Highlight on Health

The ABCDs of STD Prevention

You can significantly reduce your risk of contracting an STD by taking charge of your behaviors. Here are some tips in an easy-to-remember ABCD format:

■ **A**bstinence is the only 100 percent sure way to avoid contracting an STD. Delaying the onset of sexual activity until you are ready for a long-term committed relationship will reduce your risk, as will abstaining from sex between long-term relationships. Periodic abstinence also means you will probably have fewer sexual partners, which reduces risk further.

■ **B**e faithful: Maintain a mutually monogamous relationship with a noninfected partner. In addition to agreeing to be mutually monogamous, you and your partner will have to have a conversation about your sexual histories. Some tips on how to have this conversation are included in Chapter 15.

■ **C**ondoms, if used consistently and correctly, can reduce transmission of some—but not all—STDs. Directions for using male and female condoms are included in Chapter 16.

■ **D**etection is critical, because some STDs have no symptoms. If you are at risk, see your health care provider to be tested for STDs.

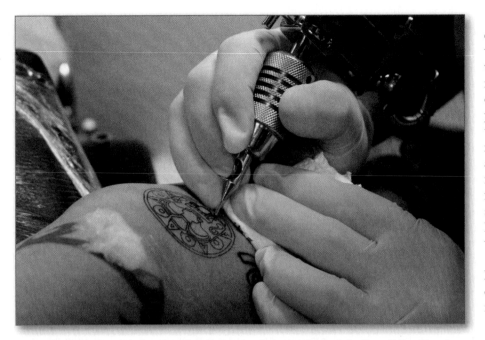

■ Anything that causes a break in the skin carries the potential for infection. Tattooists who don't follow infection control measures like wearing gloves, changing gloves between clients, and disinfecting their equipment can place their clients at risk for diseases like MRSA and hepatitis C.

The most effective ways to prevent the transmission of STDs are to abstain from intimate sexual activities and to be in a mutually monogamous, long-term relationship with an uninfected partner (see the box "The ABCDs of STD Prevention").

Illicit Drug Use: The Case of Hepatitis C When users of illicit drugs share needles and syringes, some blood from the first user is injected into the bloodstream of the next user, creating an effective means of transmitting bloodborne infections. Several viral infections, specifically HIV, hepatitis B, and hepatitis C, are easily transmitted through shared needles. We discuss HIV and hepatitis B later in the chapter; here, we consider hepatitis C.

All hepatitis viruses cause inflammation of the liver, with symptoms such as fatigue, weakness, loss of appetite, and jaundice (a yellow discoloring of the skin and eyes). The hepatitis C virus was discovered in 1989. Before 1990 approximately 10 percent of blood transfusion recipients developed hepatitis, nearly always from hepatitis C. After blood banks started screening for hepatitis C, transfusion-related infection dropped.

Hepatitis C is not a highly infectious virus and requires introduction directly into the bloodstream for transmission. Risk factors include intravenous drug use or sharing of other drug paraphernalia that may have infected blood on it; receipt of blood or blood products prior to 1990; sex with a person infected with hepatitis C; or sharing personal items, such as a razor or toothbrush, with a person who has hepatitis C. Sexual transmission is rare, but hepatitis C can be transmitted through contaminated tattoo or body piercing equipment.

An estimated 4.1 million Americans are infected with hepatitis C, the majority of whom have no symptoms. The incubation period for the infection is about 4 to 6 weeks, but only about 20 percent of infected people will develop symptoms. The virus causes a chronic, low-level infection in 55–85 percent of people, and after about 20 years, one in five infected people will develop liver failure, scarring of the liver (cirrhosis), or liver cancer. Hepatitis C is the leading reason for the need for liver transplants.[16]

Individuals reduce their risk for hepatitis C by not using injection drugs and by maintaining mutually monogamous sexual relationships with noninfected partners. Those who do use drugs should reduce risk by not sharing needles or syringes or, at the very least, cleaning them with bleach after every use. People with hepatitis C can reduce the risk of disease progression by avoiding alcohol, limiting the use of medications that affect the liver (such as acetaminophen), and getting vaccinated for hepatitis A and B. Community programs have helped reduce risk by linking drug users with treatment programs and by encouraging safe injection programs for addicts until they are able to receive treatment. Community programs can also raise awareness about this asymptomatic disease and encourage testing of persons at risk.

Tattoos and Body Piercing As described in Chapter 10, tattoos and piercings are popular these days as body ornamentation and alteration. However, they do carry a risk of infection, because the insertion of needles breaks down the body's protective skin barrier and also because equipment and dyes can be contaminated with bloodborne pathogens. Recently, cases of methicillin-resistant *Staphylococcus aureus* (MRSA) have been associated with tattooing. This form of bacterial infection can spread quickly and be difficult to treat. To reduce risk, carefully consider your decisions to obtain a tattoo or piercing, and make sure you obtain services from a licensed provider who follows infection control practices.[17] Licensing and regulating authorities for tattooing and piercing vary from state to state.

ANTIBIOTIC RESISTANCE

In 1928 British bacteriologist Alexander Fleming observed that a common mold, *Penicillium*, prevented the growth of bacteria. When penicillin, the first **antibiotic,** was isolated from this mold, it was declared a miracle drug. It was widely

antibiotic
Drug that works by killing or preventing the growth of bacteria.

used during World War II and saved the lives of many wounded soldiers. By the 1950s, however, the bacterium *Staphylococcus aureus* was already showing signs of resistance to penicillin. A new antibiotic, methicillin, was introduced in 1960 and proved effective, but resistance began developing by 1961. Since then, hundreds of new antibiotics have been developed.[18]

The 21st century may mark the beginning of a postantibiotic era as **antibiotic resistance** grows (as well as antiviral and antifungal resistance). Sharp increases in antibiotic resistance have been noted, whether infections are acquired in hospitals, nursing homes, or the community. Some bacteria are becoming resistant to all known antibiotics.[18, 19] Two factors are believed to account for bacterial resistance: the frequency with which resistant genes arise naturally among bacteria through mutation and the extent of antibiotic use.

antibiotic resistance
Lessened sensitivity to the effects of an antibiotic.

Resistant genes arise naturally because bacteria reproduce quickly, and mutations in their DNA occur frequently. The appearance of resistant genes in bacteria through mutation is amplified when a population of bacteria is exposed to an antibiotic. The most sensitive bacteria die quickly, while those with some resistance survive. Once the nonresistant bacteria are out of the way, the resistant bacteria have more space and food, and they quickly produce more resistant bacteria. Thus frequent and widespread antibiotic use is accompanied by increased antibiotic resistance.

Another way that resistance is promoted is through the action of antibiotics on the bacteria that are part of the normal flora. Antibiotics are nonspecific, so they kill helpful bacteria as well as pathogens and increase antibiotic resistance in helpful bacteria as well as in pathogens. Such resistance can be passed on to pathogens during a subsequent infection (see the box "Reducing Antibiotic Resistance").

VACCINATION CONTROVERSIES

Many of today's parents and health care providers have never seen a case of measles, mumps, polio, diphtheria, or rubella. Vaccine-preventable childhood diseases that devastated previous generations are at an all-time low. However, as the diseases become less common, people begin to question the necessity and safety of the vaccines themselves. In response, public health officials point out that although cases of these diseases may be infrequent, the viruses and bacteria that cause them still exist. As rates of vaccination drop, the likelihood of a disease recurrence increases. For example,

Consumer Clipboard

Reducing Antibiotic Resistance

Have you ever asked your physician for antibiotics when you had a stuffy nose, a sore throat, muscle aches, and fever—symptoms of the common cold or flu? Even though antibiotics are not effective against viral infections, physicians sometimes prescribe them when they are uncertain about a diagnosis, when they don't have time to explain the difference between bacterial and viral infections, or when patients pressure them for a prescription. Estimates are that antibiotics are not needed and do not alter the course of an illness in up to 50 percent of cases in which they are prescribed.

This is just one example of the type of antibiotic misuse that is promoting antibiotic resistance. As a consumer of health care and other products, you play an active role in reducing the risk of antibiotic resistance. Here are some guidelines:

■ Don't take antibiotics unnecessarily. Talk with your health care provider about why an antibiotic may or may not be helpful. If your illness is viral, an antibiotic won't help.

■ Take antibiotics as prescribed. If you do need an antibi-

otic, complete the full course even if you feel better, and don't skip doses. When you don't take the full course, a few resistant bacteria can survive and grow. This is the mechanism by which antibiotic resistance increases.

■ Avoid antibacterial products in daily personal use. There is no evidence that products containing antibiotics offer any benefit over routine hygiene measures. To reduce the risk of spreading infection, wash your hands frequently with soap and water for a full 20 seconds. When water is not available, use an alcohol-based hand sanitizer.

■ Clean and disinfect with detergent-based cleaners and dilute bleach solutions. Antibacterial cleaning products offer no additional benefit.

■ Purchase foods that have been grown with minimal use of antibiotics. Approximately 70 percent of the antibiotics produced in the United States are used on livestock. Low doses of antibiotics are often mixed with animal feed to reduce illness and promote growth; however, such nonspecific use promotes resistance. Many European countries have banned this practice, and in the United States, measures are being supported that would reduce the nonspecific use of antibiotics in livestock feed.

Sources: "Antibiotic/Antimicrobial Resistance," Centers for Disease Control and Prevention, retrieved January 7, 2008, from www.cdc.gov/drugresistance; "Antimicrobial Resistance Interagency Task Force 2006 Annual Report," Centers for Disease Control and Prevention, 2007, retrieved January 7, 2008, from www.cdc.gov/drugresistance/actionplan/2006report/index.htm.

if someone traveling to a part of the world where a disease still occurs brings the pathogen back to the local community, the disease could spread quickly if local vaccination rates are low.

Some people oppose vaccination because they believe the risks associated with the vaccines themselves are too great. Some minor, temporary side effects do occur after vaccination, such as local reactions, fever, discomfort, irritability, and, more rarely, allergic reactions. However, serious reactions to currently recommended vaccinations are very rare. The risk of the vaccine must be weighed against the risk of the disease. For example, the risk of developing encephalitis (brain inflammation) after a dose of the MMR (measles-mumps-rubella) vaccine is less than 1 in 1 million, whereas the risk of developing encephalitis from measles is 1 in 1,000 and the risk of death is 2 in 1,000.[20]

Some people have postulated links between the MMR vaccine and autism, a developmental disorder that begins in childhood. However, to date, no scientific studies have found any link between the two.[21] As new vaccines are developed and introduced, they are constantly monitored in efforts to improve vaccine safety. The CDC and the Food and Drug Administration jointly run the Vaccine Adverse Events Reporting System, which collects and analyzes information on possible adverse events that occur after vaccinations.

Infectious Diseases Worldwide and on Campus

Of the hundreds or thousands of infectious diseases that occur in the world, a handful, relatively speaking, are responsible for most cases of illness and death.

GLOBAL INFECTIOUS DISEASES

From an infectious disease perspective, the world has become a small community. Diseases do not respect borders or boundaries. New diseases arise, such as SARS, and other diseases reemerge as public health concerns, such as tuberculosis. In this section we consider the four leading causes of global infectious disease mortality (Table 17.1).

Pneumonia Pneumonia—infection of the lungs or lower respiratory tract—is the leading cause of infectious disease and death. Young children and older adults are at greatest risk for pneumonia; besides age, factors that increase risk include exposure to environmental pollutants and use of tobacco, alcohol, or drugs, all of which reduce the lungs' ability to clear infection. Close living situations, such as college dormitories or military barracks, can also increase risk.

Pneumonia can be viral or bacterial (it can also be caused by other organisms). The pathogens are usually inhaled in infected air droplets, transmitted from an infected person who is coughing or sneezing nearby. Symptoms of pneumonia include fever, cough, chest pain, shortness of breath, and

Table 17.1	Top 10 Infectious Diseases: Global Mortality	
Condition	**Frequency (× 1,000)**
Pneumonia	4,400
Diarrhea	3,100
Tuberculosis	3,100
Malaria	2,100
AIDS	1,500
Hepatitis B	1,100
Measles	1,000
Neonatal tetanus	460
Pertussis	350
Worms	135

Source: Johns Hopkins Infectious Diseases, http://hopkins-id.edu.

chills. Viral pneumonia tends to come on more gradually and is often milder than bacterial pneumonia, but both types can be serious and deadly.

Vaccines are available to reduce the risk of contracting pneumonia, and some antiviral and antibacterial medications can shorten the course of the illness. Prevention strategies include avoiding tobacco smoke and crowded living conditions, practicing good hygiene, and following vaccination recommendations. Antibiotic resistance is a growing problem in treating pneumonia. Up to 40 percent of the *Streptococcus* bacterium that causes pneumonia is resistant to penicillin, and approximately 96 percent of influenza A, one of the viruses that causes pneumonia, is resistant to two of the four antiviral drugs used for treatment.[18, 20] (See the box "An Influenza Pandemic: Could It Happen Again?")

Diarrhea In the developing world, severe diarrhea kills 2 to 3 million children each year. As with most infectious diseases, the young are at greatest risk. Severe diarrhea leads to dehydration and electrolyte imbalances, and repeated episodes lead to malnutrition and growth delay. Multiple organisms cause diarrhea, including viruses and bacteria; rotavirus is responsible for 25 percent of diarrhea deaths worldwide. Diarrhea illnesses are spread through contaminated food and water. In the developed world, sanitation and clean water have substantially reduced the risk and severity of diarrhea illness.

Treatment usually consists of supportive care with fluid and electrolyte replacement. In the developing world, access to oral rehydration solutions (clean water, salt, and sugar) can be life saving. Prevention depends on effective sanitation systems and access to clean water and food. In addition, a vaccine against rotavirus has been recommended for all infants starting at age 2 months.[22]

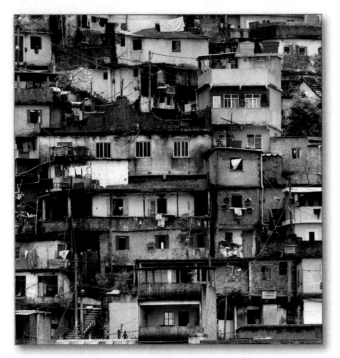

■ Crowded living conditions, poor sanitation, and poverty create perfect conditions for the transmission of infectious diseases, including tuberculosis. These hillside structures in Rio de Janeiro are home to thousands of impoverished people squatting on public land.

Tuberculosis   Worldwide, *Mycobacterium tuberculosis* (TB) is the most common infectious disease, with approximately 30 percent of the world population infected.[23] Each year, nearly 9 million people develop TB, and about 1.6 million die. The disease is caused by a mycobacterium, a subset of bacteria, and is spread primarily through aerosolized droplets coughed out of the lungs of an infected person and breathed in by another person. Once the mycobacterium is inhaled, a healthy immune system creates a wall around it and prevents it from growing or spreading. In this **latent infection,** the bacterium is in the body but not causing any signs of disease or infection.

latent infection
Infection that is not currently active but could reactivate at a later time.

About 5–10 percent of infected people develop the active disease at some point in their lives, meaning that the bacterium is no longer controlled and can replicate, spread, and be transmitted to other people. Symptoms of active tuberculosis include cough, fatigue, weight loss, night sweats, fever, and coughing up blood. The active disease is more likely to develop if the immune system is impaired, as in HIV infection.

Tuberculosis has reemerged as a major health problem because of the rapid spread of HIV. People with HIV/ AIDS are at increased risk of developing and dying from active tuberculosis. TB is now the leading cause of death among people with HIV.[24] Changes in population patterns have also influenced the spread of TB. Poverty and crowded living situations enhance the spread of disease. Close living quarters vastly multiply the number of people who can become infected by a single person with active tuberculosis. In the United States, the people at highest risk for tuberculosis are recent immigrants (particularly from Asia, Africa, Mexico, and South and Central America), homeless people, prison populations, and people infected with HIV.

Active tuberculosis is treated with a combination of three or four anti-tuberculosis drugs taken for 6 to 9 months (making it a difficult treatment to complete). Multi-drug-resistant TB (MDR-TB) has become a major public health concern in recent years; it has been identified around the world. It is resistant to the standard medications and must be treated with second-line medications, which are more expensive, take longer to work, and have more side effects. An even more resistant strain, called extensively drug-resistant tuberculosis (XDR-TB), has recently developed in 41 countries. In these cases, treatment options are very limited, and more than 50 percent of people will die within 5 years.[23, 25]

International public health efforts are essential for the control of TB. Screening of people at risk for tuberculosis, access to appropriate medications, and tracking systems to ensure successful completion of treatment are essential. Researchers are trying to develop simpler treatments, and new vaccines are being studied that will reduce the risk of infection and progression to active disease.

Malaria   Malaria is a mosquito-borne disease caused by four species of the *Plasmodium* parasite. Approximately 350 to 500 million people are infected annually, with over 1 million deaths, mostly among young children. Currently, about 60 percent of malaria cases and 80 percent of malaria deaths occur in sub-Saharan Africa.[26]

Malaria symptoms, which include high fever, chills, sweats, headache, nausea, vomiting, and body aches, develop 7 to 30 days after a bite from an infected Anopheles mosquito. Symptoms are often cyclic, recurring every few days. Severe malaria can lead to confusion, seizures, coma, heart failure, kidney failure, and death. Treatment varies depending on the species of *Plasmodium* and medication-resistant patterns in the country where it occurs.

Prevention strategies include eliminating mosquito breeding grounds (for example, standing water), applying insecticides, using screens and mosquito netting, and staying inside during peak mosquito hours (dawn and dusk). Travelers to areas where there is a risk for malaria usually take antimalarial medication before, during, and after their trip.

Malaria used to be endemic in parts of the southeastern United States, but the CDC, working with local health agencies, undertook a program that targeted mosquito breeding grounds and included other anti-mosquito measures. In 1946, when the program began, there were 15,000 cases of malaria in these areas; by 1951 there were none. Vigilant monitoring remains essential, since the Anopheles mosquito is still

Highlight on Health

An Influenza Pandemic: Could It Happen Again?

In 1918–1919, the infamous "Spanish flu" swept the globe, causing an estimated 50 million deaths. The world saw two more influenza pandemics—worldwide epidemics—in the 20th century: the "Asian flu" of 1957 and the "Hong Kong flu" of 1968. In each of these pandemics, serious illness and death were not limited to high-risk groups, such as older adults or infants; in 1918–1919, death rates were highest among healthy young adults. Today, people are asking if an influenza pandemic could happen again.

Two types of influenza virus, influenza A and influenza B, cause "flu" in humans. Influenza A is further divided into subtypes based on antigens on the surface of the virus, called H and N; subtypes are named according to these antigens, such as "H1N1." Like other viruses, the influenza virus is subject to frequent minor genetic changes as well as infrequent, abrupt, major genetic change. When a slight change occurs, many people will have partial immunity from previous infection with a similar strain or vaccination. When a substantial change occurs, however, most people will have little or no immunity to the new strain.

An additional concern is that, although only three influenza A subtypes commonly infect humans (H1N1, H1N2, and H3N2), many others infect birds, pigs, horses, dogs, and other animals. Recently, outbreaks of avian (bird) influenza subtype H5N1 occurred in several Asian countries among domesticated birds, and some humans also were infected, most from direct contact with poultry but a few

apparently from contact with an infected person. Because people have little or no immunity to the H5N1 virus, the risk of serious complications is high; in some areas nearly 50 percent of humans infected with H5N1 have died.

The fear is that the H5N1 virus could "jump" to humans—that is, that it could change such that it could easily infect people and spread by person-to-person contact (via droplets carried in coughs or sneezes). Such a shift could result in another influenza pandemic. Vaccination would not be effective in such a scenario. Each year a new flu shot is developed in an attempt to respond to newer viral strains, but a major genetic shift is difficult to predict. Treatment of avian flu is also problematic, although some of the current antiviral medications are believed to be effective.

History suggests that it is only a matter of time before another influenza pandemic occurs. The virus would spread quickly around the world through international travel, leaving little time for preparation. A vaccine would not be available in the early stages. When vaccines and antiviral medications became available, there would not be enough for everyone, and decisions would have to be made about access. In some places quarantines might be imposed. All of these problems highlight the difficult issues involved in balancing the rights of individuals with society's role in serving the greater good.

While the public discussion continues, remember to practice basic good health habits: Avoid people who are sick, stay home when you are sick, wash your hands often, and take good care of your immune system. For more information on protecting yourself from influenza, visit the CDC Web site at www.cdc.gov/flu.

---

present in many Southern states and periodically causes small outbreaks of malaria.[27]

INFECTIOUS DISEASES ON CAMPUS

Infectious diseases also cause illness on college campuses (Table 17.2). College students consistently list colds, flu, sore throat, and sinus infection among the top 10 impediments to academic performance.[28]

Pertussis (Whooping Cough)   *Whooping cough* is the common name for an infection of the respiratory tract caused by the pertussis bacterium. It is highly contagious, transmitted by inhaling respiratory droplets from an infected person's cough or sneeze. Initial infection may seem similar to a common cold, with nasal congestion, runny nose, mild fever, and a dry cough, but after 1 to 2 weeks, the coughing occurs in spells lasting a few minutes and ending in a "whooping" sound as the person gasps for air. Almost all infants and nearly half of older babies with pertussis require hospitalization. The illness is milder in older children, adolescents, and young adults, but the cough can be disruptive and persist for months.

Most infants and young children are vaccinated against pertussis, but immunity begins to wear off after 5 to 10 years,

leaving adolescents and young adults susceptible to infection. Studies on college campuses show that among students with a prolonged cough, approximately 30 percent may have pertussis. Pertussis is treated with antibiotics if diagnosed early. Antibiotics may also be given to household members or roommates to decrease the spread of disease. Reported cases of pertussis have increased 20-fold in the past 30 years. It is now recommended that all adolescents and adults receive a booster vaccination to enhance their immunity against this infection.[29]

Mumps   Mumps is a viral illness characterized by fever, headache, and swollen salivary and parotid glands. The parotid glands are located on either cheek just in front of the ears and above the jaw line; swelling causes a classic "chipmunk" appearance. Serious complications of mumps are rare, but they include inflammation of the brain, testicles, ovaries, or breast. Long-term complications can include deafness, sterility, and even death. Transmission is by respiratory secretions from an infected person. There is no antiviral medication for treatment.

Widespread transmission of mumps on campuses is due to group living environments, social interaction, and local and interstate travel. Although they are rare, campus outbreaks

Table 17.2 | Infectious Diseases on Campus

Illness	Cause (Pathogen)	Incubation	Symptoms	Home Treatment	When to Seek Medical Care	Prevention
Common cold	Over 200 different viruses including rhinovirus, adenovirus, coronavirus	1–4 days	Runny nose (often clear initially, then turning thicker, darker), nasal congestion, mild cough, sore throat, low-grade fever (< 101° F), sneezing.	Usually resolves on its own; fluids, rest, over-the-counter decongestant, antihistamines, cough suppressant, antipyretic/analgesic; avoid alcohol and tobacco.	Inability to swallow, worsening symptoms after 3rd day, difficulty breathing, stiff neck.	Hand washing, avoid sharing personal items, balanced nutrition, exercise, adequate sleep.
Influenza ("the flu")	Influenza A or B virus	1–5 days	Sudden-onset fever (usually > 101° F), headache, tiredness (can be extreme), body aches, cough, sore throat, runny or stuffy nose.	Usually resolves on its own; as for common cold; in addition, antiviral medications can be used by prescription.	Immediately if in group with high risk for complications such as pregnant women, those with chronic lung or heart disease, those with asthma. Otherwise, difficulty breathing, severe headache or stiff neck, confusion, fever lasting more than 3 days, new pain localizing to one area (ear, chest, sinuses).	Annual flu shot in October or November, frequent hand washing; avoid close contact with sick people.
Strep throat	*Streptococcus* bacteria	2–5 days	Sudden-onset sore throat and fever (often > 101° F); may have mild headache, stomachache, nausea; back of throat red and white pus on tonsils, sore lymph nodes in neck; absence of cough, stuffy nose, or other cold symptoms (as most common cause of sore throat is common cold).	Salt water gargles, analgesics, antipyretics, throat lozenges.	Strep throat is treated with antibiotics to reduce duration of symptoms and reduce risk of complications. If symptoms are consistent with strep, a health provider visit is appropriate.	Same as common cold.
Acute sinus infection	Virus: most common cause; same as common cold Bacteria: *Streptococcus, Haemophilus influenza*; less common, often as complication of common cold or allergies	Varies	Pain or pressure in the face, stuffy or runny nose, upper teeth pain, fever; may have headache, bad breath, yellow or green nasal discharge.	Same as for common cold: decongestants or antihistamines; nasal irrigation; most sinus infections resolve on their own with opening and drainage of the sinuses.	Fever > 101° F after 3 days, no improvement in facial pain or pressure after 2 days of home treatment with decongestant, cold symptoms continue beyond 10 days or worsen after 7 days.	Same as common cold. Early treatment of nasal congestion with decongestant or antihistamine.

Illness	Cause (Pathogen)	Incubation	Symptoms	Home Treatment	When to Seek Medical Care	Prevention
Mononucleosis ("mono")	Epstein-Barr virus (EBV)	4–6 weeks	High fever (> 101° F), severe sore throat, swollen glands, weakness and fatigue; loss of appetite; nausea, and vomiting can occur.	Usually resolves on its own; rest, fluids; avoid contact sports until symptoms resolve due to risk of spleen rupture.	Fever > 101°F after 3 days, unable to maintain fluids; low energy, body aches, swollen glands lasting longer than 7–10 days; severe pain in belly can indicate spleen rupture and is a medical emergency.	Do not kiss or share utensils or foods with someone who has mono; EBV is spread from saliva.
Bronchitis or cough	Virus: same as common cold Bacteria: rare Other lung irritants: tobacco smoke	Varies	Initial dry, hacking cough; after a few days, may be productive of mucus; may have associated low fever and fatigue; often develops 3–4 days into a cold; may last 2–3 weeks.	Rest, fluids, cough drops, and avoidance of lung irritants such as tobacco; over-the-counter cold medications may help.	If you feel short of breath, have history of asthma or chronic lung disease, or develop signs of pneumonia: high fever, shaking chills, shortness of breath; also, if symptoms last more than 4 weeks.	Avoid tobacco smoke; get annual flu shot; good hand washing.
Meningitis	Virus: fairly common, usually not serious Bacteria: less common, must be treated immediately to avoid brain damage and death	Varies	Stiff and painful neck, fever, headache, vomiting, difficulty staying awake, confusion, seizures.	Home treatment is not appropriate if signs of meningitis are present until a health care provider determines if symptoms are due to a virus or bacteria; if viral cause, home treatment to relieve fever and pain symptoms is appropriate.	Immediately if signs of meningitis are present.	Viral: Immunization against some of the pathogens reduces risk; these include measles, mumps, rubella; chicken pox; *Neisseria meningitides* (meningococcal vaccine). Bacterial: Antibiotics when you have come in close contact with someone who is infected; insect repellent; special immunizations for certain areas of the world.
Cellulitis	Bacteria: most common are *Streptococcus* and *Staphylococcus aureus*	Varies	Infected area will be warm, red, swollen, and painful; if infection spreads, may have associated fever, chills, swollen glands.	Warm compresses; keep area clean and dry; topical antibiotics if small area of skin involved.	Cellulitis is usually treated with antibiotics; any symptoms of cellulitis should be evaluated by a health care provider.	Healthy skin protects you from infection; keep cuts, burns, and insect bites clean and dry; treat chronic skin conditions such as eczema, ulcers, psoriasis; avoid intravenous drug use; avoid piercing and tattoos.

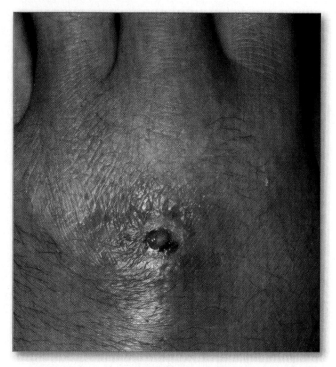

■ A skin infection caused by MRSA is easy to get and hard to treat.

can be highly disruptive (see You Make the Call at the end of this chapter). Campus outbreaks underscore the importance of being up to date on all recommended vaccinations.[30, 31]

***Staphylococcus aureus* Skin Infections** *Staphylococcus aureus* (often called "Staph"), a common bacterium carried on the skin or in the noses of healthy people, is one of the most common causes of skin infection. Usually these infections are mild, taking the form of a pimple or small boil. Many infections can be treated by keeping the area clean and dry. Sometimes these infections can spread, creating a large abscess (pocket of infection), which can require incision, drainage, and treatment with antibiotics. Less often, Staph can cause infection of the blood or pneumonia. These cases usually require hospitalization and intravenous antibiotic treatment.

Some strains of Staph are becoming increasingly resistant to antibiotics. Methicillin-resistant *Staphylococcus aureus* (MRSA), mentioned earlier in the context of tattooing and piercing, causes a hard-to-treat skin infection that can be transmitted through skin-to-skin contact and that is becoming more common among college students. At present, other classes of antibiotics can be used to treat MRSA.

Good hygiene practices can reduce the risk of MRSA infection. Keep your hands clean by washing frequently with soap and water, or use an alcohol-based hand sanitizer. Shower after exercising, and avoid sharing personal items such as towels, razors, clothing, and uniforms. Keep cuts and scrapes clean and covered until healed. If you have been diagnosed with an MRSA infection, avoid skin-to-skin contact (including contact sports) until the area has healed.[32]

Urinary Tract Infections Urinary tract infections (UTIs) are believed to be the most common bacterial infection.

They are more common in women than in men. One in three women will have a UTI by age 24, and more than 50 percent of women will have at least one UTI in their lifetime. Most UTIs involve the lower urinary tract or the bladder. Less frequently, they involve the upper urinary tract or the kidneys. The vast majority of UTIs are caused by the bacterium *E. coli*, although they can be caused by other bacteria.

Symptoms include pain or burning with urination, pain in the lower abdomen, urgency and frequency of urination, and, if the kidneys become involved, pain in the back and fever. Recent sexual activity and history of UTI are risk factors for infection. If a woman is at risk for STDs or has vaginal symptoms, such as discharge or irritation, she should be tested to rule out STDs. Treatment includes fluids and antibiotics, although *E. coli* is becoming increasingly resistant to commonly used antibiotics.[33]

Sexually Transmitted Diseases

Sexually transmitted diseases (STDs) are infections that are spread from one person to another predominantly through sexual contact. Some health experts prefer the term *sexually transmitted infection* (*STI*), because often there are no symptoms, and by definition, a disease is an infection that causes symptoms. However, the CDC continues to use the term *sexually transmitted disease,* and this text follows their usage.

The primary pathogens responsible for STDs are viruses and bacteria. We begin this section with HIV infection, one of the most serious threats to public health worldwide, and then we discuss the other STDs by type of pathogen.

HIV/AIDS

Acquired immunodeficiency syndrome (AIDS) is caused by the human immunodeficiency virus (HIV). Since the first case was diagnosed in 1981, more than 20 million people have died from HIV/AIDS. The pandemic is considered the most serious infectious disease challenge in public health today. At the end of 2007, an estimated 33.2 million people worldwide were infected, two-thirds of them in sub-Saharan Africa and another 20 percent in Asia (Figure 17.6). In 2007 2.5 million new infections and 2.1 million deaths occurred (three-quarters of the deaths were in sub-Saharan Africa). Furthermore, in sub-Saharan Africa, an estimated 11.4 million children have been orphaned by AIDS.[34]

Currently, there appear to be two patterns of infection. In sub-Saharan Africa, the epidemic is in the general population, with women representing 61 percent of the people living with HIV, and transmission is predominantly via heterosexual contact. In other parts of the world, HIV remains concentrated in populations of increased risk, such as men who have sex with men, injection drug users, and sex workers and their sexual partners.[34]

An estimated 1.3 million people are living with HIV in North America. New technology reveals the rate of new HIV infection in the United States is higher than previously believed. Results indicate an estimated 56,300 new HIV

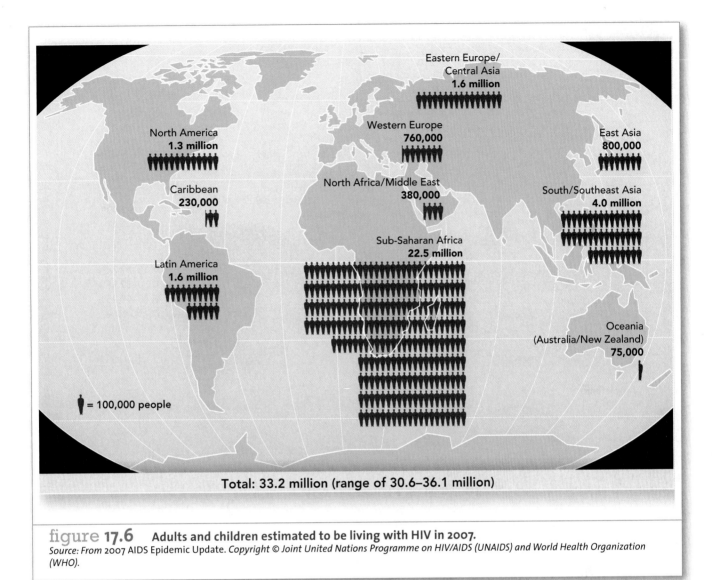

North America
1.3 million

Caribbean
230,000

Latin America
1.6 million

Eastern Europe/
Central Asia
1.6 million

Western Europe
760,000

North Africa/Middle East
380,000

Sub-Saharan Africa
22.5 million

East Asia
800,000

South/Southeast Asia
4.0 million

Oceania
(Australia/New Zealand)
75,000

= 100,000 people

Total: 33.2 million (range of 30.6–36.1 million)

figure **17.6**   **Adults and children estimated to be living with HIV in 2007.**
Source: From 2007 AIDS Epidemic Update. Copyright © Joint United Nations Programme on HIV/AIDS (UNAIDS) and World Health Organization (WHO).

infections occurred in 2006 (40 percent higher than previous estimates of 40,000 new infections per year).[35] In the United States, sexual contact is involved in about 85 percent of newly diagnosed HIV infections (men who have sex with men account for more than half of all infections), and intravenous drug use is involved in about 18 percent. Racial and ethnic minority populations continue to be affected disproportionately (see the box "Disproportionate Risk for HIV Infection").

HIV most likely originated from a similar virus, the simian immunodeficiency virus found in chimpanzees in Africa. It is believed to have jumped from animal host to human host approximately 50 to 75 years ago. The virus may have entered a human being from the bite of an infected chimpanzee or during the slaughtering of a chimpanzee. Once in a human host, the simian immunodeficiency virus evolved through mutation into human immunodeficiency virus.[36] There are two main strains of the virus: HIV-1 is the predominant strain in North America and most of the rest of the world; HIV-2 is found primarily in Africa.

Course of the Disease   HIV targets the cells of the immune system, especially macrophages and CD4 cells (a subcategory of helper T cells). Once inside these host cells, the virus uses the cell's DNA to replicate itself and disable the host cell. During the initial infection with HIV, known as *primary infection,* the virus replicates rapidly. Within 4 to 11 days of exposure, several million viral copies may circulate in the bloodstream. The immune system mounts a rapid response in an attempt to control and remove the virus, but HIV is able to mutate quickly and avoid complete eradication.

Between 40 and 90 percent of people infected with HIV experience an acute infection phase approximately 4 to 6 weeks after exposure with symptoms such as fever, weight loss, fatigue, sore throat, lymph node swelling, night sweats, muscle aches, rash, and diarrhea. The symptoms may last for a few weeks and are easily mistaken for other infections, such as influenza, mononucleosis, or herpes.[37]

After the early phase, the immune system and the virus come to a balance with the establishment of a *viral load set point,* a level of virus that continues to circulate in the blood

Who's at Risk

Disproportionate Risk for HIV Infection

Certain groups are at disproportionate risk for HIV infection. Here is a profile of new HIV cases in the United States.

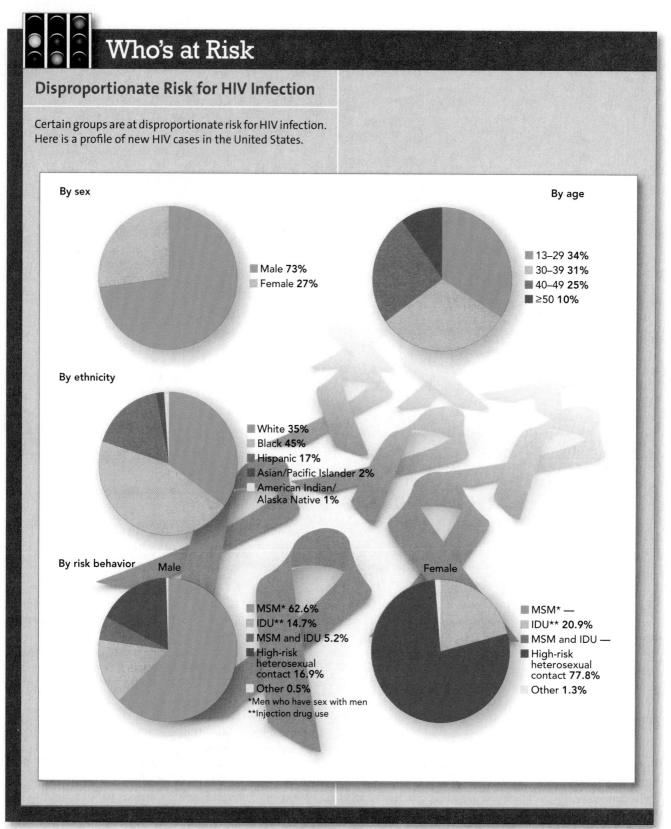

By sex

- Male **73%**
- Female **27%**

By age

- 13–29 **34%**
- 30–39 **31%**
- 40–49 **25%**
- ≥50 **10%**

By ethnicity

- White **35%**
- Black **45%**
- Hispanic **17%**
- Asian/Pacific Islander **2%**
- American Indian/ Alaska Native **1%**

By risk behavior

Male

- MSM* **62.6%**
- IDU** **14.7%**
- MSM and IDU **5.2%**
- High-risk heterosexual contact **16.9%**
- Other **0.5%**

*Men who have sex with men
**Injection drug use

Female

- MSM* —
- IDU** **20.9%**
- MSM and IDU —
- High-risk heterosexual contact **77.8%**
- Other **1.3%**

Sources: "A Glance at the HIV/AIDS Epidemic," Centers for Disease Control and Prevention, retrieved May 19, 2008, from www.cdc.gov/hiv/resources/ factsheets/PDF/At-A-Glance.pdf; "Update to Racial/Ethnic Disparities in Diagnoses of HIV/AIDS—33 States, 2001–2005," Centers for Disease Control and Prevention, retrieved May 19, 2008, from www.cdc.gov/hiv/resources/reports/mmwr/mm5609a1.htm. Estimation of HIV incidence in the United States by H.F. Hall, et al., 2008, Journal of the American Medical Association, 300 (5): 520–529.

and body fluids. During this phase, a person is asymptomatic and may remain so for 2 to 20 years. The virus continues to replicate, and the immune system continues to control it without completely removing it.

Eventually the immune system is weakened significantly and can no longer function fully, signaling the onset of AIDS. Symptoms of AIDS include rapid weight loss, cough, night sweats, diarrhea, rashes or skin blemishes, and memory loss. These symptoms are due to **opportunistic infections**—infections that occur when the immune system is no longer able to fight them off. Common opportunistic infections include *Pneumocystis carinii* pneumonia, Kaposi's sarcoma (a rare cancer), and tuberculosis.

opportunistic infections
Infections that occur when the immune system is weakened. These infections do not usually occur in a person with a healthy immune system.

A note of caution: The symptoms associated with acute HIV infection and AIDS are also associated with many other illnesses. A person experiencing such symptoms should not automatically assume they are signs of HIV infection or AIDS. However, if the person is at risk, he or she should get tested for HIV infection.

Methods of Transmission HIV cannot survive long outside of a human host, and thus transmission requires intimate contact. The virus can be found in varying concentrations in an infected person's blood, saliva, semen, genital secretions, and breast milk. It usually enters a new host either at a mucosal surface or by direct inoculation into the blood. HIV is not transmitted through casual contact, such as by shaking hands, hugging, or a casual kiss, nor is it spread by day-to-day contact in the workplace, school, or home setting. Although HIV has been found in saliva and tears, it is present in very low quantities. It has not been found in sweat. Contact with saliva, tears, or sweat has not been shown to result in transmission of HIV.

Risk of HIV transmission is influenced by factors associated with the host (the already infected person), the recipient (the currently uninfected person), and the type of interaction that occurs between the host and recipient (behaviors). An important host factor is the level of virus circulating in the blood. High levels of circulating virus, such as during the initial infection stage, increase the risk of transmission. In addition, some people may have a higher viral load set point during the equilibrium period. Antiviral treatment (discussed in a later section) lowers the level of circulating virus and may reduce the risk of transmission.

Sexual Contact The primary exposure risk for 85 percent of cases of HIV infection in the United States and for 82 percent of cases in Canada is sexual contact.[34] HIV can enter the body through the mucosa or lining of the vagina, penis, rectum, or mouth. If the mucosa is cut, torn, or irritated (as can happen with intercourse or if there is another STD), the risk increases. The sexual behaviors associated with transmission are receptive anal sex, insertive anal sex, penile-vaginal sex, and oral sex.

Although discussing HIV status with a potential sexual partner may be awkward, its importance cannot be overemphasized. As noted, the time of highest circulating virus is shortly after initial infection; the person may not have any symptoms and may not know he or she is infected. In fact, 25 percent of HIV-positive people in the United States do not know they are infected. Unless you have a conversation about whether your potential partner has been tested for HIV, what risky behaviors he or she has engaged in, and what other sexual partners he or she has been involved with, you do not know what your risk is in starting a sexual relationship.[38]

Injection Drug Use Injection drug use is reported as the method of HIV transmission by 20 percent of people with AIDS in Canada and 18 percent of people with AIDS in the United States. Another 4 percent and 5 percent, respectively, report both injection drug use and being a man who has sex with other men as combined risk factors. Individuals can reduce their risk of HIV infection by avoiding injection drug use. People who are already using drugs can reduce their risk by using sterile needles and not sharing needles with others. Communities can play a role in decreasing the spread of HIV by implementing needle exchange programs and ensuring adequate access to drug treatment programs.

Contact With Infected Blood or Body Fluids HIV can be transmitted by direct contact with the blood or body fluids of an infected person. The risk of transmission again varies depending upon how much virus is in the body fluid, how much fluid gets onto another person, and where the fluid contacts the other person. A small amount of infected blood on the intact skin of another person carries essentially no risk. A larger amount of blood on cut or broken skin or mucosal membranes has a greater risk. The accidental injection of infected blood through a needle stick has an even greater risk.

universal precautions
A set of precautions designed to prevent transmission of bloodborne infections. Blood and certain body fluids of *all* patients are considered potentially infectious for HIV and hepatitis B and C. Protective barriers, such as gloves, aprons, and protective eyewear, are used in health settings.

These types of exposure are most likely to occur in health care settings, and to reduce the risk of transmission of HIV, hepatitis B and C, and other bloodborne infections, the **universal precautions** approach has been instituted in these settings.

Universal precautions include the use of gloves, gown, mask, and other protective wear (such as eyewear or face shields) in settings where someone is likely to be exposed to the blood or infected body fluids of another person. These precautions should be taken with every patient.[39]

Perinatal Transmission Perinatal, or vertical, transmission—the transmission of HIV from an infected mother to her child—can occur during pregnancy, during delivery (when the fetus is exposed to the mother's blood in the birth canal), or after delivery (if the baby is exposed to the mother's breast milk). The risk of transmission from mother to child can be reduced through the use of antiretroviral medications during pregnancy and around the time of delivery. Infected mothers also reduce the risk to their babies by electing not to breastfeed.

In the United States and Canada, women are routinely offered HIV testing as part of prenatal care. If she tests positive, a woman is offered preventive therapy with antiretroviral medications to reduce her child's risk. In untreated women with HIV, approximately 30 percent of infants are infected; in treated women, less than 2 percent are infected.

HIV Testing   The earlier HIV infection is recognized, the sooner treatment can begin, the longer a person is likely to remain symptom free, and the fewer people he or she is likely to expose to the virus. The only way to confirm HIV infection is by laboratory testing. In the United States, an estimated 75 percent of infected people know their HIV status. In sub-Saharan Africa, only 12 percent of men and 10 percent of women know their status.[34]

To increase the number of HIV cases that are diagnosed early, the CDC recommends that everyone between the ages of 13 and 64 be tested for HIV infection at least once during routine medical care. Testing is strongly recommended for anyone who has engaged in any of the following behaviors or has a partner who has done so:

- Injected drugs, including steroids
- Had unprotected vaginal, anal, or oral sex with men who have had sex with men
- Had multiple partners or anonymous partners or has exchanged sex for drugs or money
- Been diagnosed with an STD

Anyone who continues to engage in these risk behaviors should be tested at least annually. All pregnant women should be screened for HIV.[38]

Most HIV tests are designed to detect antibodies to HIV circulating in the bloodstream. After an HIV exposure, it can take 2 to 8 weeks for a sufficient quantity of antibodies to be produced for an HIV test to detect them. This time is referred to as a "window period"—a time when the HIV test may result in a false negative. If the test is done within the first 3 months after a potential exposure, the test should be repeated 3 months later.

Several HIV screening tests are available. The standard test is an enzyme immune assay (EIA) that screens a person's blood for antibodies to HIV. Newer EIA tests use oral fluid or urine instead of blood. It takes several days to get results from most EIA tests, but rapid tests are also available, and some can produce results in 20 minutes. If the result of any of these screening tests is positive, a confirmatory test called a Western blot is performed. The Western blot also detects antibodies to HIV but can distinguish false positives

from actual infection. If the Western blot confirms that there are circulating antibodies to HIV, the person is said to be HIV-positive. It is also possible to test for recent HIV infection by looking for the actual virus through a viral load test. This test is used if HIV infection is suspected based on acute symptoms, but it is not used routinely because of its greater cost.[40]

A home test called the Home Access HIV-1 Test System was licensed and approved by the FDA in 1997. The kit and others like it can be purchased at a pharmacy or drugstore. The consumer collects a small amount of blood from a finger prick, places the blood on a card, mails the card to a registered laboratory, and telephones for results using an identification number. All people with a positive result are referred to a health clinic because the positive result must be confirmed by the Western blot test. Consumers are warned to use only FDA-approved test kits, since others may not be as accurate.[41]

Management of HIV/AIDS   The development of new medications and improved understanding of the HIV disease process have contributed to prolonged survival by some people infected with HIV. However, the benefits of medical treatment have been slow to reach people in low- and middle-income populations around the world. In these areas, only an estimated 28 percent of infected people receive treatment.[42]

Antiretroviral Agents   The most important medications in HIV treatment are antiviral drugs—or, more accurately, antiretroviral drugs, since HIV is a type of virus called a retrovirus. Antiretroviral medications do not cure the infection, but they slow the rate at which the virus replicates and destroys the immune system, thus prolonging life and improving the quality of life for people who are HIV-positive. Four different categories of drugs are used against HIV, each functioning in a different way to stop replication of HIV. Drugs within each category have slight differences in side effects, frequency of use, cost, and number of pills taken a day. These factors can be extremely important when a medication must be taken for years.

Drug Cocktails   HIV has an uncanny ability to develop drug resistance. On average, 10 billion viral particles are produced every day in an infected person, offering many opportunities for mutation and the development of resistance. If a single antiretroviral medication is used, resistant strains develop fairly quickly. To combat resistance, scientists have developed complicated drug combinations, called **drug cocktails,** that usually include a medication from two to four of the drug categories. A viral strain is less likely to develop several mutations allowing it to evade the combination of drugs than to develop one or a few mutations allowing it to evade a single drug. However, the complexity, cost, and risk of side effects for the person taking the drugs are all increased.

drug cocktails
Complicated drug combinations used to overcome drug resistance in different strains of HIV.

New Prevention Possibilities Since the identification of the virus, researchers have been attempting to develop a safe, effective, and inexpensive HIV vaccine, but the challenge is enormous. To develop a vaccine, scientists must be able to identify a part of the virus that could produce protective immunity if injected into a host. However, the immune system does not seem to be able to clear HIV and produce immunity; instead, the virus produces lifelong infection. Furthermore, the virus is a moving target; it mutates frequently and develops new strains rapidly. That said, more than 30 vaccine trials are under way around the world. Unfortunately, vaccine trials experienced a setback in 2007, when a vaccine appeared to increase risk of HIV infection among study participants.[43, 44]

Another avenue being pursued is the development of a **microbicide,** a compound or chemical in the form of a cream, gel, or suppository that would kill microorganisms and that could be applied topically to the vagina or rectum before intercourse, reducing the risk of STD transmission. Many such products are currently under study. Microbicides would offer an alternative to condoms and could be especially important to women. Condom use requires the cooperation of a woman's partner; microbicides can be used without the consent or cooperation of a partner and so could empower women and reduce their risk of infection.[45]

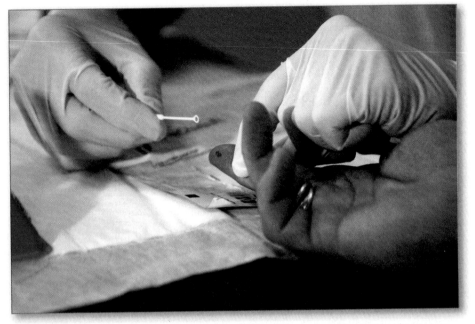

■ The CDC recommends voluntary testing for HIV for all persons aged 13 to 64 at least once during routine medical care. HIV testing is done via a blood test that detects antibodies in the bloodstream. Sexually active individuals should undergo screening for all STDs on a regular basis.

microbicide
Compound or chemical in the form of a cream, gel, or suppository that would kill microorganisms and that could be applied topically to the vagina or rectum before intercourse, reducing the risk of STD transmission.

BACTERIAL STDS

Bacterial STDs are curable infections if identified early. Undiagnosed, they can cause serious consequences, including pelvic inflammatory disease, reduced fertility, ectopic pregnancy, and increased risk for HIV transmission. Chlamydia, gonorrhea, pelvic inflammatory disease, syphilis, and bacterial vaginosis are the most common bacterial STDs.

Chlamydia The most commonly reported bacterial STD is chlamydia infection; it is caused by the bacterium *Chlamydia trachomatis*. Rates of infection are increasing in the United States, with an estimated 1.0 million cases diagnosed annually. A random study of women and men aged 18 to 26 in the general population revealed that 4.1 percent had chlamydia infection. Young women are at greatest risk for chlamydia, with rates three times that of young men. Seven percent of women aged 15 to 24 visiting family planning clinics are infected. Approximately half of all reported chlamydia cases occur in 15- to 19-year-olds, and another third occur in 20- to 24-year-olds. Although all racial and ethnic groups are affected, Black women have rates eight times higher than White women.[46, 47, 48]

Chlamydia can be transmitted via vaginal, anal, or oral sex. Most people with chlamydia are not aware they are infected, since 75 percent of women and 50 percent of men have no symptoms. If symptoms do develop, they occur about 1 to 3 weeks after exposure. For women, symptoms could include a mild burning sensation with urination and a slight increase in vaginal discharge. Infected men may have a watery penile discharge, a burning sensation with urination, or pain and swelling in the scrotum.

Untreated infection can persist for months or years and can lead to pelvic inflammatory disease in women (discussed later in this section). There is also an association between chlamydia infection and increased risk of HIV acquisition and transmission for both men and women. Chlamydia can be effectively treated with antibiotics; however, a person can be reinfected if re-exposed. If there has been scarring of the fallopian tubes or other parts of the female reproductive system from pelvic inflammatory disease, that damage cannot be reversed.

A screening test for chlamydia can be performed on urine or on a specimen collected from the penis, cervix, or throat. All sexually active women under age 26 should be screened regularly for chlamydia, as should women who are at increased risk because they have a new sexual partner or multiple sexual partners or are infected with another STD. There is debate about the cost effectiveness of screening all sexually active men under age 26. Men should be tested if they have symptoms or have a new sexual partner or if their sexual partner has been diagnosed with chlamydia. They also should be aware that rates of chlamydia infection are increasing among men and that they can be infected yet have no symptoms.

Gonorrhea   The second most commonly reported bacterial STD is gonorrhea; it is caused by the bacterium *Neisseria gonorrheae.* A random study of women and men aged 18 to 26 indicated that .4 percent had gonorrhea infection. As with chlamydia, the highest rates occur in young women. Rates of gonorrheal infection are increasing, with an estimated 358,000 cases diagnosed annually.

Gonorrhea can be transmitted via vaginal, anal, or oral sex. Symptoms, if they develop, will usually develop 2 to 5 days after exposure. Most women will not develop symptoms, which would include a mild burning sensation with urination, increased vaginal discharge, or vaginal bleeding. The majority of men infected with gonorrhea eventually develop a penile discharge. Infection can also occur in the rectum or the throat in people who engage in anal or oral sex. Because men often (but not always) have symptoms, they usually notice the infection early and get treatment.

Gonorrhea tests can be performed on samples taken from the throat, penis, anus, or vagina or on a urine sample. Regular screening is recommended for women at high risk of infection—those who are under 25 and have had two or more sex partners in the past year, who exchange sex for money or drugs, or who have a history of repeated episodes of gonorrhea. It is less clear if asymptomatic men should be screened, because most men eventually develop symptoms.

Gonorrhea is treated with antibiotics, but drug resistance is a growing problem. In 2007 the CDC issued new treatment guidelines for gonorrhea, recommending that fluoroquinolones, the leading class of antibiotics previously used in treating gonorrhea, no longer be used because of widespread resistance. Now, cephalosporins are the only class of antibiotics available to treat gonorrhea infection.[46]

Pelvic Inflammatory Disease   Pelvic inflammatory disease (PID) is an infection of the uterus, fallopian tubes, and/or ovaries. The infection occurs when bacteria from the vagina or cervix spread upward into the uterus and fallopian tubes. The bacteria involved are usually from STDs, such as chlamydia or gonorrhea, but they can be bacteria that are normally found in the vagina.

Symptoms of PID include fever, abdominal pain, pelvic pain, and vaginal bleeding or discharge. A woman experiencing any of these symptoms should see her health care provider. If PID is suspected, a combination of antibiotics is prescribed to cover gonorrhea, chlamydia, and vaginal bacteria. If symptoms are severe, hospitalization may be required. About 18 percent of women with PID develop chronic abdominal or pelvic pain that lasts more than 6 months.

PID can cause severe consequences and can be life threatening if untreated. Most of the long-term problems arise from scarring in the fallopian tubes, which increases the risk of ectopic pregnancy (a pregnancy that implants outside of the uterus) and infertility. Women with a history of PID have a 7- to 10-fold increased risk of ectopic pregnancy, and about 20 percent of women with PID will experience infertility. Regular screening for asymptomatic chlamydia infection in sexually active women under age 25 has been shown to reduce the risk of PID by detecting infection early.[49]

Syphilis   Rates of syphilis, a disease caused by infection with the bacterium *Treponema pallidum,* decreased throughout the 20th century but began to increase in 2001. Since then, rates among men who have sex with men have increased rapidly, such that rates among men are now six times those among women (they were nearly equal 10 years ago). Although rates in women are lower than they are in men, they are increasing. In particular, rates among Black women have increased.[46]

Untreated syphilis progresses through several stages. In the first stage, called *primary syphilis,* a moist, painless sore called a *chancre* appears 10 days to 3 months after sexual contact with an infected person. The chancre is usually in the genital area, mouth, or anus and heals on its own within a few weeks. The primary stage can go unnoticed because the sore is painless. The second stage, *secondary syphilis,* occurs 3 to 6 weeks after the appearance of the chancre and is characterized by a skin rash that often involves the palms of the hands and soles of the feet. The rash can be accompanied by fever, fatigue, sore throat, joint pain, and a headache. Secondary syphilis also resolves without treatment, but it can recur over several years.

Many people then enter a period in which the syphilis is latent or inactive; the infected person is no longer contagious and may show no signs of disease. However, about a third of secondary syphilis cases progress to a final stage, called *tertiary syphilis,* many years after the initial infection. In this stage, the disease causes deterioration of the brain, arteries, bones, heart, and other organs, leading to dementia, ataxia (lack of coordination), and severe pain. Death can result from nervous system deterioration or heart failure. The treatment for syphilis in all stages is penicillin. However, in the late stages, organ damage cannot be reversed.

A pregnant woman with active syphilis can transmit infection to her fetus, causing serious mental and physical problems. Infection with syphilis also increases the risk of transmitting and acquiring HIV infection. The usual screening test for syphilis is a blood test.[50] Screening is recommended for all pregnant women at their initial prenatal care visit and for persons at increased risk for syphilis infection. This includes men who have sex with men, commercial sex workers, and anyone who tests positive for another STD, exchanges sex for drugs, or has sex with partners who have syphilis.

Bacterial Vaginosis   Bacterial vaginosis (BV) is an alteration of the normal vaginal flora; Lactobacillis, the usually predominant bacteria, is replaced with different bacteria, causing a vaginal discharge and unpleasant odor. It is not clear why women develop bacterial vaginosis. Although it is not considered an STD, women who have never had sex rarely experience the condition. Treatment of male partners does not alter the rate of recurrence for women.

BV is diagnosed by an evaluation of the vaginal flora under a microscope. Treatment is recommended not just because the symptoms are unpleasant but also because BV has been associated with increased risk of PID, complications in pregnancy, and transmission of HIV. The condition is treated with the antibiotic metronidazole, which can be taken orally or vaginally.[14]

VIRAL STDS

Viral STDs cannot be cured, making prevention even more important than in cases of bacterial STDs. Vaccination is an option for some of the viral STDs, and symptoms can be treated. Here we discuss human papillomavirus, herpes virus, and hepatitis A and B.

Human Papillomavirus   Human papillomavirus (HPV) is the most common STD in the United States. There are more than 100 types of HPV. Some types are associated with genital warts, others with cancers of the cervix, vulva, penis, anus, and other areas. Strains associated with cancer are called high-risk strains; of these, two strains (HPV 16, 18) are associated with 70 percent of cervical cancer. Strains associated with genital warts are called low-risk strains; of these, two strains (HPV 6, 11) are most commonly associated with genital warts.

Estimates are that 15 percent of the general population is currently infected with HPV, but rates are higher in certain populations. Studies have found HPV in 46 percent of women on college campuses and in more than 50 percent of men who have sex with men. HPV is transmitted by skin-to-skin contact, usually through penetrative vaginal or anal sex.

Most HPV infections are transient and asymptomatic, and the majority of people do not know they are infected. However, weeks to months after an exposure to a low-risk strain of HPV, both men and women can develop genital warts—flat or raised, small or large, pinkish lesions—on the penis, scrotum, vagina, anus, or skin around the genital area. Warts are diagnosed by their appearance. Most will resolve on their own, or they can be treated with medication. However, treatment is primarily for cosmetic purposes and may not alter the risk of transmitting the virus to another person.

Most women with HPV are diagnosed through screening with the Papanicolaou smear (Pap test). The Pap test was implemented as a way to detect cervical cancer or precancerous lesions. After infection with HPV, the cells of the cervix undergo specific changes that can be identified under a microscope. If mild abnormalities in the cervical cells are noted, HPV testing can be performed to determine if a high-risk (cancer-causing) strain of HPV is present. Among women with HPV infection of the cervix, 90 percent spontaneously clear the infection within 2 years. However, 10 percent of women have persistent infection and are at high risk for cervical cancer. Pap testing is recommended for all sexually active women.[51]

Men and women who have receptive anal intercourse are at high risk for anal HPV infection and anal cancer. A test called an anal pap can be used to collect a sample of cells from the rectum to be evaluated for precancerous changes. Currently, anal pap or HPV testing is not recommended as a routine screening for men, but men at high risk should discuss this test with their health care provider.[51] Consistent and correct use of condoms may reduce the risk of transmission of HPV but may not provide full protection, since HPV can infect skin not covered by the condom.

A vaccine for HPV (Gardasil) was approved by the FDA in 2006, and additional vaccines are in development. Gardasil protects against four HPV strains (HPV 6, 11, 16, and 18). As noted, two of these strains—16 and 18—cause 70 percent of cervical cancer, and two others—6 and 11—cause 90 percent of genital warts. The vaccine is approved for girls and women aged 9 to 26; ideally, it is administered before the onset of sexual activity. At present, the vaccine is not approved for males, but studies are under way to determine its safety and possible benefits.[51] A second vaccine, Cervarix, with FDA approval pending in the United States, protects against HPV strains 16 and 18.

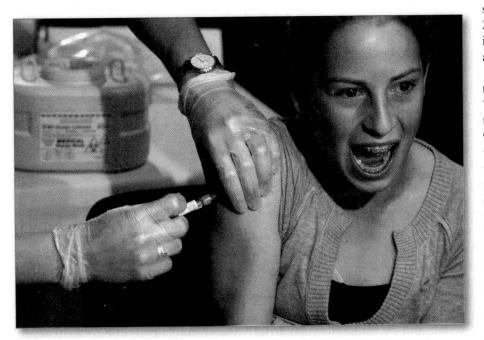

■ Fourteen-year-old Sophie Weisz was one of the first people to receive the HPV vaccine when the campaign was launched in August 2006.

Genital Herpes   Genital herpes is caused by the herpes simplex virus

(HSV), which has two strains, called HSV-1 and HSV-2. Both strains can infect the mouth, genitals, or skin. HSV-1 is often associated with lesions in and around the mouth (cold sores). This type of herpes is frequently acquired in childhood from nonsexual transmission, although up to 30 percent of genital herpes has been associated with HSV-1. The type more frequently associated with genital herpes is HSV-2.[14]

The first sign of herpes simplex infection, usually 2 to 7 days after exposure, is the appearance of small, painful ulcers or sores at the site where the person first contacted HSV, in or around the genitals or mouth. The initial illness can be quite severe, with fever and swelling of the lymph nodes. This acute stage may last from 7 to 10 days. The virus then becomes latent, remaining in the body and reactivating periodically with painful sores at the site of initial contact. The virus is shed or released even without evidence of a sore or an ulcer; an infected person can spread the infection to another even if there is no visible lesion.

Because there is no cure for HSV infection, prevention is particularly important. Condoms partially protect people against infection with HSV, but they are not 100 percent effective. Condoms must be used at all times and not just when a lesion is present. Several different vaccines for HSV are currently under study. Antiviral medications are available that shorten the course of outbreaks and reduce their frequency. These medications may also reduce the risk of transmission to sexual partners.

Herpes can be transmitted to a newborn during delivery. The risk is greatest if a woman contracts a new herpes infection near the end of pregnancy. All pregnant women should be screened for symptoms of genital herpes during labor. If symptoms are present, women should be offered delivery by cesarean section. Some women with herpes take antiviral medications to reduce the risk of an outbreak at delivery.[14]

Hepatitis   Hepatitis (inflammation of the liver) can be caused by several viruses, but the most common ones are hepatitis A, B, and C. We discussed hepatitis C earlier in the context of injection drug use, the most common route of acquiring the infection. There is debate over whether hepatitis C can be transmitted sexually. It does appear that sexual transmission can occur, but the virus is not efficient at getting from one person to another via this route.

Hepatitis A and B are both easily transmitted through sexual acts. Hepatitis A is transmitted through fecal-oral contact and can be spread through contact with contaminated food or water. The people at greatest risk for sexual transmission of hepatitis A are those who have oral-anal contact or penile-anal intercourse. About 4 weeks after exposure to the virus, hepatitis A causes a self-limited inflammation of the liver; symptoms include nausea, vomiting, abdominal pain, and jaundice. The diagnosis is confirmed by a blood test for the virus. A safe and effective vaccine is available for hepatitis A and is recommended for men who have sex with men, illicit drug users, people with chronic liver disease, and the general population in areas that have high rates of hepatitis A or before travel to such areas.[14]

Most hepatitis B infections in the United States are sexually transmitted, although the infection can also be spread by exposure to infected blood. Worldwide, hepatitis B is a major cause of liver disease, liver failure, and liver cancer; unlike hepatitis A, it can cause chronic liver disease. The chance of developing chronic disease varies by age at the time of infection, with risk decreasing with age at exposure. Chronic infection carries an increased risk of liver failure and liver cancer.

A safe and effective vaccine for hepatitis B is available, and universal vaccination of all children is recommended. Adolescents and adults who were not vaccinated in childhood and are sexually active should be vaccinated; some colleges encourage hepatitis B vaccinations for all entering students. Because of the risk of transmission by blood, hepatitis B vaccinations are currently required for all health care workers. In addition, all pregnant women are screened to determine whether their infants are at high risk of infection during delivery. High-risk infants can be vaccinated immediately after birth to further decrease risk of infection.[14]

OTHER STDS

Several other nonbacterial, nonviral infections are transmitted sexually or involve the genital area. Most are treatable infections. They include trichomoniasis, candidiasis, and pubic lice and scabies.

Trichomoniasis   Trichomoniasis is caused by the protozoa *Trichomonas vaginalis* and is transmitted from person to person by sexual activity. Men infected with "trich" may have pain with urination or a watery discharge from the penis, but they usually have no symptoms. Infected women may experience vaginal soreness and itchiness, a frothy yellow-green vaginal discharge, and a musty, fishy vaginal odor. The diagnosis is confirmed by examination of the vaginal discharge under a microscope. Like bacterial vaginosis, trichomoniasis is treated with the antibiotic metronidazole. Sexual partners of the infected person need to be contacted and treated to prevent the further spread and recurrence of the infection.[14]

Candidiasis   Candidiasis is usually caused by the yeast *Candida albicans;* symptoms of yeast infection include vaginal discharge, itching, soreness, and burning with urination. About 75 percent of women have an episode of candidiasis during their lifetime. Yeast infections are not usually acquired through sexual intercourse, but they can be mistaken for an STD because the symptoms are similar. *C. albicans* can be a normal part of the vaginal flora and may overgrow in response to changes in the vaginal environment, such as when a woman takes antibiotics or if she has diabetes.

Candidiasis is treated by antifungal medications that can be taken orally as a pill or applied to the vagina with a tablet or as a cream. Several antifungal creams, such as miconazole or clotrimazole, are available over the counter. If a woman is unsure of the diagnosis, has recurrences, or is at risk for STDs, she should have the diagnosis confirmed by a health care provider before she treats herself.[14]

Pubic Lice and Scabies   Pubic lice and scabies are ectoparasites that can be sexually transmitted. Pubic lice (or "crabs") infect the skin in the pubic region and cause intense itching. Scabies can infect the skin on any part of the body and, again, cause intense itching. In adults, both pubic lice and scabies are most often sexually transmitted, but in children, scabies is usually acquired through nonsexual contact. Both infections are treated with a medicated cream or shampoo called permethrin or lindane. Bedding and clothing must be decontaminated to prevent reinfection, either by machine washing and drying or by enclosure in a plastic bag for at least 72 hours.[14]

Prevention and Treatment of Infectious Diseases

There are many steps that you as an individual can take to protect yourself from infectious diseases and prevent their spread. Here are a few:

- Support your immune system by eating a balanced diet, getting enough exercise and sleep, managing stress, not smoking, and adopting other practices that are part of a healthy lifestyle.

- Follow government recommendations for vaccinations for both adults and children. If you are in a high-risk group, get a flu shot when it is offered in the fall.

- If you have been exposed to an infectious disease, minimize the chances that you will pass it on to someone else. For example, if you have a cold or the flu, follow good hygiene practices such as washing your hands frequently; stay home from work; and avoid crowded public places. If you have been exposed to an STD, take appropriate action (see the box "Tips for Telling a Partner You Have an STD").

- Minimize your use of antibiotics. Don't buy antibacterial soaps, try to avoid meat or poultry from animals that have been fed antibiotics, and don't take antibiotics for viral infections. When prescribed antibiotics for a bacterial infection, take them as directed and complete the full course of treatment.

- Practice the ABCDs of STD prevention. If you have been exposed to an STD, see your physician for testing and treatment, and tell any sexual partners that they have been exposed so that they can be treated too.

- If you are planning a trip to a new part of the country or a new country, learn what infectious diseases are common in that location and how you can decrease your risk of infection while visiting or living there.

- Reduce the likelihood that new diseases will take hold in your community, such as by getting rid of any standing water in your yard where mosquitoes could breed.

Infectious diseases will always be part of human existence. We may discover treatments for some diseases, but new organisms are continually evolving, independently and in response to human behaviors and activities. By being vigilant, we can reduce their negative impact on our lives.

Challenges & Choices

Tips for Telling a Partner You Have an STD

Telling a partner you have an STD is not easy. Being candid and honest at the outset of the relationship is highly recommended. Here are some tips:

- If you are currently undergoing treatment for the STD, tell your partner; do not have sex until treatment is complete.

- Be open about how you contracted the STD and share the information you have about the disease. Do not share any medication you are taking. Most antibiotics are effective only if you take the entire course prescribed for you.

- Encourage your partner to be tested if it is possible that he or she has become infected. This might happen if you realize you have an STD after you and your partner begin a sexual relationship. Symptoms of some STDs don't appear for some time; other STDs don't have any visible symptoms at all.

- If your partner resists getting tested, emphasize that consequences can be very serious if an STD is left untreated.

- You can be reinfected with an STD after you have been treated if your partner isn't treated as well. Some STDs are passed back and forth between partners several times, sometimes becoming more resistant to treatment. Make sure you are both free of infection before you start or resume sexual activity.

It's Not Just Personal . . .

According to the CDC National Prevention Information Network (www.cdcnpin.org), the United States has the highest rates of STDs in the industrialized world. In fact, those rates are 50 to 100 times higher than those of other industrialized countries. An estimated 15.3 million new cases of STDs are reported each year in the United States.

Source: Sex Q & A, by A. Hooper, 2001, New York: DK Publishing.

You Make the Call

Should Colleges Tighten Vaccination Requirements?

In November 2007 a student at the University of Southern Maine was diagnosed with mumps. Although mumps is usually mild, it occasionally has serious complications, and it is extremely contagious. At the time, USM students were required by state law to show proof that they had received one dose of measles-mumps-rubella (MMR) vaccine. Following the diagnosis, the requirement was changed to two doses of MMR vaccine. Students who could not show such proof or who did not comply with the requirement were not allowed on campus. The student with mumps was sent home for 9 days to reduce the risk of a widespread outbreak.

This case exemplifies the ethical dilemma frequently faced by society, in which individual freedom is pitted against the collective welfare of the community, or the "common good." College campuses are uniquely vulnerable to these issues. Colleges and universities are small communities of people living in close contact with each other, whether in dormitories, off-campus housing, classrooms, or shared eating facilities. In addition, students, faculty, and staff frequently travel around the world for recreation, academic research, and family opportunities. As such, they have an increased likelihood of exposure to infectious disease. Returning students, faculty, and staff can bring infections back to campus, where they may spread rapidly.

The University of Southern Maine implemented a relatively mild requirement—a second immunization. Some health experts have proposed stricter requirements in such situations, including the following:

- *Immunizations for a range of diseases could be required prior to entry onto campus.* Currently most colleges require one or two doses of MMR and recommend but do not require immunization for such diseases as meningococcal infection, varicella (chickenpox), pertussis (whooping cough), and other childhood and adult infectious diseases. To increase herd immunity and reduce the risk of outbreaks, colleges could require immunization for all these diseases.

- *Travel to high-risk areas by students, faculty, and staff could be restricted.* Currently the CDC and the World Health Organization offer travel warnings, precautions, and news of outbreaks in the states and around the world; occasionally they recommend that travelers avoid certain areas or countries if an outbreak risk is high. Colleges could similarly limit or restrict travel.

- *Travelers returning from certain parts of the world could be prevented from entering campus for a certain period of time.* The CDC recommends that travelers returning from countries with outbreaks of new and emerging diseases monitor themselves for symptoms for 10 days prior to returning home or stay at home for 10 days after returning. Colleges could enforce this restriction on campus.

- *Individuals with infectious diseases could be quarantined.* This course of action has been proposed in the event of a pandemic flu outbreak. Colleges could house students, faculty, or staff in separate facilities for the duration of their illness so that the disease could be contained.

Each of these proposals has its advantages and its drawbacks. Some people think colleges and universities should tighten their restrictions to protect the community and promote the common good. Others see such restrictions as violations of personal freedom, if not civil rights. What do you think?

PROS

- Required vaccination reduces the risk of disease for the entire college community. When vaccination levels are high overall, even the few who aren't vaccinated are protected by herd immunity, because widespread vaccination shrinks the reservoir of infectious agents.

- College campuses are unique, tightly linked communities with a high risk of contagion should an infectious agent be introduced.

- Colleges have a responsibility to protect students and other community members from unnecessary risk. Requiring vaccination and taking other restrictive measures helps ensure health and safety for everyone.

CONS

- Individuals should have freedom of choice about health risks and what they do with their bodies. They should not have to take personal risks, such as those associated with vaccination, for the good of the community.

- Travel advisories by the CDC and the World Health Organization are usually issued as recommendations. Colleges do not have the right to enforce a different standard.

- Isolation and quarantine are difficult to enforce, and the threat of such treatment may discourage people from seeking appropriate medical care. Thus, these measures could actually increase the risk of infectious disease outbreaks.

Source: "Mumps Confirmed on USM Campus," News Releases 2007–2008, University of Southern Maine, November 29, 2007.

In Review

1. **What causes infection, and how does the body protect itself from infectious diseases?** Several different types of pathogens cause infection and illness in humans, categorized as viruses, bacteria, prions, fungi, helminths, protozoa, and ectoparasites. Infection occurs when one of these microorganisms gains entry to the body and reproduces, causing symptoms of illness. The body has external barriers to keep pathogens out and a complex immune system to destroy them when they get in.

2. **What changing patterns in infectious diseases are occurring?** Technological advances, like blood banks, organ transplants, and centralized food distribution, have created new opportunities for widespread disease transmission, as have global travel, changes in sexual behavior, injection drug use, and tattooing and piercing. Overuse of antibiotics has led to the appearance of resistant strains of many bacteria.

3. **What are the most common infectious diseases?** Currently the top four infectious diseases worldwide are pneumonia, diarrhea, tuberculosis, and malaria. On college campuses in the United States, the top four are pertussis (whooping cough), mumps, *Staphylococcus aureus* skin infections, and urinary tract infections.

4. **What are the most serious and most common sexually transmitted diseases?** HIV/AIDS is the most serious STD because it is fatal, although it is now possible, with medications, to live with HIV infection as a chronic condition for many years. The virus attacks and eventually overwhelms the immune system, leaving the body vulnerable to opportunistic infections like tuberculosis. The bacterial STDs, which include chlamydia, gonorrhea, pelvic inflammatory disease, syphilis, and bacterial vaginosis, can be treated with antibiotics. The viral STDs, which include human papillomavirus, genital herpes, and hepatitis A and B, can be controlled but not cured. Other STDs include trichomoniasis, candidiasis, and pubic lice and scabies.

5. **How can infectious diseases be prevented?** The best defense is being in good health, so a healthy lifestyle is important. Getting all recommended vaccinations also helps, as do avoiding exposure, practicing safer sex, and minimizing unnecessary use of antibiotics.

www For a detailed summary of this chapter and a comprehensive set of review questions, visit the Online Learning Center at **www.mhhe.com/teague2e**.

Web Resources

CDC National Center for Infectious Diseases Traveler's Health: This comprehensive Web site offers information on safe food and water, tips on traveling with children, travelers with special needs, illness and injury abroad, cruises, and air travel. Its Travel Notices section is updated regularly for health warnings and precautions.
www.cdc.gov/travel

CDC National Prevention Information Network: This site focuses on prevention of HIV/AIDS, STDs, and tuberculosis. Its many resources include information about HIV testing and statistics, organizations, and infectious diseases in the news.
www.cdcnpin.org

HIV InSite: Gateway to AIDS Knowledge: This organization looks at AIDS from a global perspective, offering research and news information about advances in knowledge about this disease, treatment approaches, and trends in the spread of the disease.
http://hivinsite.ucsf.edu

National Foundation for Infectious Diseases: Publications offered by NFID include immunization guides, clinical updates, reports on special populations, and a newsletter. Its online fact sheets cover topics such as adult immunizations, foodborne diseases, herpes, and measles in adults.
www.nfid.org

National Institute of Allergy and Infectious Diseases: This organization provides publications on AIDS, allergies, asthma, hepatitis, Lyme disease, SARS, and West Nile virus. It also features links to information on clinical trials.
www.niaid.nih.gov

World Health Organization: Infectious Diseases: This site offers a comprehensive list of health topics that provide in-depth information on infectious diseases, including STDs. It also features links to other resources, such as journals and reports.
www.who.int/health-topics/idindex.htm

Chapter

18

Cardiovascular Disease Risks, Prevention, and Treatment

Ever Wonder...

- what heart disease is?

- if young people ever have heart disease?

- how to know if someone is having a heart attack—and what to do?

WWW

Your Health Today

www.mhhe.com/teague2e

Go to the Online Learning Center for *Your Health Today* for interactive activities, quizzes, flashcards, Web links, and more resources related to this chapter.

Not long ago, people believed that heart attacks and strokes were like bolts out of the blue—they happened without warning. Today we know that heart attacks and strokes are the result of disease processes that begin much earlier, often in childhood. Behavior patterns that contribute to risk for **cardiovascular disease (CVD)** include tobacco use, physical inactivity, and poor diet. Early detection and treatment of precursors to CVD, such as high blood pressure, diabetes, and elevated cholesterol levels, can help young people reduce the risk of developing this disease. This chapter presents an overview of CVD, along with guidelines for living a heart-healthy life.

cardiovascular disease (CVD)
Any disease involving the heart and/or blood vessels.

The Cardiovascular System

cardiovascular system
The heart and blood vessels that circulate blood throughout the body.

The **cardiovascular system** consists of a network of blood vessels (arteries, veins, and capillaries) and a pump (the heart) that circulate blood throughout the body. The heart is a fist-sized muscle with four chambers, the right and left atria and the right and left ventricles, separated from one another by valves.

The right side of the heart is involved in **pulmonary circulation**—pumping oxygen-poor blood to the lungs and oxygen-rich blood back to the heart. The left side of the heart is involved in **systemic circulation**—pumping oxygen-rich blood to the rest of the body and returning oxygen-poor blood to the heart (Figure 18.1).

In pulmonary circulation, oxygen-poor (or deoxygenated) blood returning from the body to the heart enters the right atrium via large veins called the inferior and superior **vena cava**. After the right atrium fills, it contracts and moves the blood into the right ventricle. The right ventricle fills and contracts, moving the blood into the lungs via the right and left pulmonary arteries. The pulmonary artery branches into a network of smaller arteries and arterioles that eventually become the pulmonary capillaries. Capillaries are the smallest blood vessels; some capillary

pulmonary circulation
Pumping of oxygen-poor blood to the lungs and oxygen-rich blood back to the heart by the right side of the heart.

systemic circulation
Pumping of oxygen-rich blood to the body and oxygen-poor blood back to the heart by the left side of the heart.

vena cava
Largest veins in the body; they carry oxygen-poor blood from the body back to the heart.

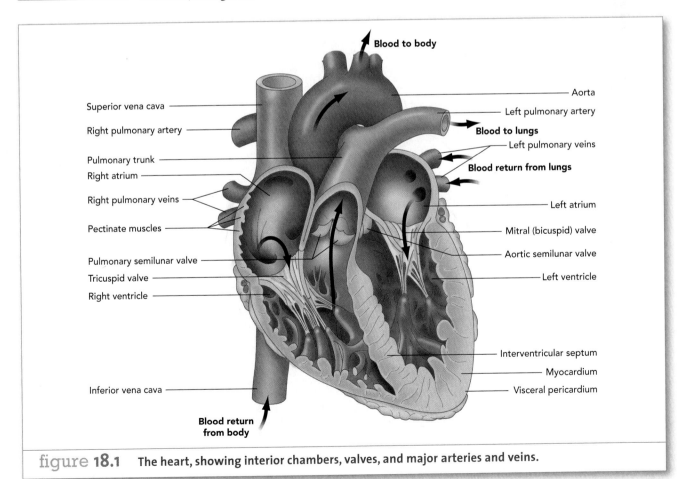

figure **18.1**   **The heart, showing interior chambers, valves, and major arteries and veins.**

walls are only one cell thick, readily allowing the exchange of gases and molecules. In the interweaving network of capillaries, the red blood cells in the blood pick up oxygen and discard carbon dioxide, a waste product from the cells. The capillaries then unite and form venules, and venules join to become pulmonary veins. The pulmonary veins return oxygen-rich blood from the lungs to the left atrium of the heart.

In systemic circulation, the left atrium fills and contracts to move oxygen-rich blood into the left ventricle. The left ventricle fills, contracts, and moves oxygen-rich blood into the body via the **aorta,** the largest artery in the body. The aorta branches into smaller and smaller arteries, and eventually, oxygen-rich, nutrient-rich blood enters the capillaries located throughout the body. At these sites, red blood cells release oxygen and nutrients to the tissues and pick up carbon dioxide to be carried back to the lungs. The capillaries unite to form veins and eventually connect to the inferior and superior **vena cava,** which returns the oxygen-poor blood to the heart. The cycle then repeats.

aorta
Largest artery in the body; it leaves the heart and branches into smaller arteries, arterioles, and capillaries carrying oxygen-rich blood to body tissues.

vena cava
Largest veins in the body; they carry oxygen-poor blood from the body back to the heart.

Like other muscles of the body, the heart needs oxygen and nutrients provided by blood; the blood being pumped through the heart does not provide nourishment for the heart muscle itself. Two medium-sized arteries, called **coronary arteries,** supply blood to the heart muscle. The main vessels are the right coronary artery and the left coronary artery, each distributing blood to different parts of the heart (Figure 18.2). The distribution of blood flow is important, because when a blood vessel is narrowed, the section of muscle that it supplies does not get enough blood.

coronary arteries
Medium-sized arteries that supply blood to the heart muscle.

The four chambers of the heart contract to pump blood in a coordinated fashion. The contraction occurs in response to an electrical signal that starts in a group of cells called the **sinus node** or **sinoatrial (SA) node** in the right atrium. The signal spreads through a defined course leading first to contraction of the right and left atria, then to contraction of the right and left ventricles. The contraction and relaxation of the ventricles is what we feel and hear as the heartbeat. The contraction phase is called *systole* and the relaxation phase is called *diastole*.

sinus node or **sinoatrial (SA) node**
Group of cells in the right atrium where the electrical signal is generated that establishes the heartbeat.

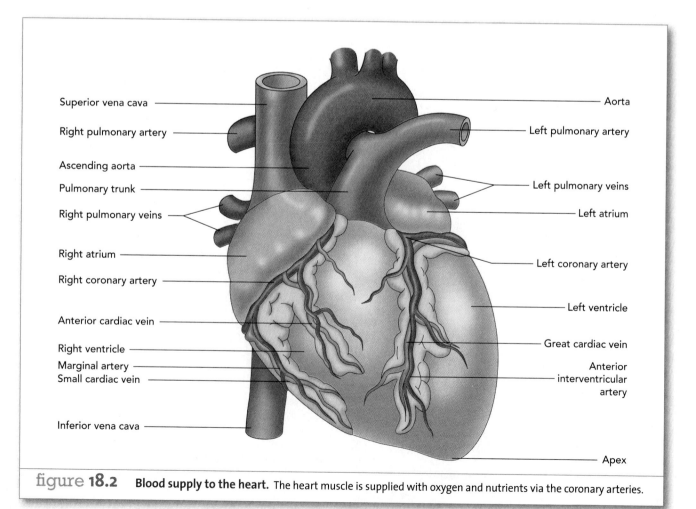

Superior vena cava

Right pulmonary artery

Ascending aorta

Pulmonary trunk

Right pulmonary veins

Right atrium

Right coronary artery

Anterior cardiac vein

Right ventricle

Marginal artery

Small cardiac vein

Inferior vena cava

Aorta

Left pulmonary artery

Left pulmonary veins

Left atrium

Left coronary artery

Left ventricle

Great cardiac vein

Anterior interventricular artery

Apex

figure **18.2**   **Blood supply to the heart.** The heart muscle is supplied with oxygen and nutrients via the coronary arteries.

Cardiovascular Disease

The leading cause of death in the United States, cardiovascular disease (CVD) accounts for 36.3 percent of all deaths. Approximately 1.4 million Americans die each year from various forms of this disease. Since 1900 CVD has been the leading cause of death in the United States, except for 1918, when infectious disease was the leading cause. Some good news can be seen in the fact that the death rate from CVD for men has decreased over the past 30 years (Figure 18.3). The drop in the death rate is believed to be the result of lifestyle changes, improved recognition and treatment of risk factors, and improved treatment of disease. The drop in death rate has not been seen for women, and some reasons for this are discussed later in the chapter.[1]

Cardiovascular disease is a general term that includes heart attack, stroke, peripheral artery disease, congestive heart failure, and other conditions (Figure 18.4). The disease process underlying many forms of CVD is atherosclerosis (hardening of the arteries), which causes damage to the blood vessels.

ATHEROSCLEROSIS

A progressive process that takes years to develop and starts at a young age, **atherosclerosis** is a thickening or hardening of the arteries due to the buildup of fats, cholesterol, cellular waste products, calcium, and other substances in artery walls. Autopsies of people aged 15 to 35 who died from unrelated trauma show that some young people already have the beginnings of significant atherosclerosis.[2]

atherosclerosis
Thickening or hardening of the arteries due to the buildup of lipid (fat) deposits.

Healthy arteries are strong and flexible. Arteries can harden and become stiff in response to too much pressure, a process generally referred to as *arteriosclerosis*. Atherosclerosis is a common form of arteriosclerosis, and the terms are often used interchangeably. Atherosclerosis starts with damage to the inner lining and the formation of a **fatty streak** in an artery. Fatty streaks consist of an accumulation of lipoproteins within the walls. A **lipoprotein** is a combination of proteins, phospholipids (fat molecules with phosphate groups chemically attached), and **cholesterol** (a waxy, fatlike substance that is essential in small amounts for certain body functions). Lipoproteins can be thought of as packages that carry cholesterol and fats through the bloodstream.

An artery wall has several layers, including an inside lining consisting of a single layer of endothelial cells and a layer behind this consisting of smooth muscle cells. When the inner lining of the wall is damaged (by tobacco smoke, high blood pressure, or infection, for example), creating a *lesion,* lipoproteins from the blood can accumulate within the wall. Here, they can undergo chemical changes that trigger an inflammatory response, attracting white blood cells.

Once at the site, white blood cells take up the altered lipoproteins. Some white blood cells leave the site, cleaning lipids from the artery wall, but if blood lipoprotein levels are high, more lipoproteins continue to accumulate. Many of the white blood cells die within the lesion, forming a core of lipid-rich material—a fatty streak.

The process may stop at this point, leaving a dynamic lesion that can still undergo repair, or may develop further, with increased involvement of the artery's smooth muscle

fatty streak
Accumulation of lipoproteins within the walls of an artery.

lipoprotein
Package of proteins, phospholipids (fat molecules with phosphate groups chemically attached), and cholesterol that transports lipids in the blood.

cholesterol
Type of fat that is essential in small amounts for certain body functions.

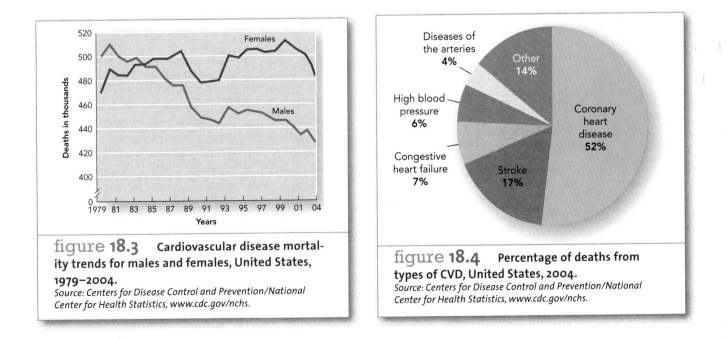

figure 18.3 **Cardiovascular disease mortality trends for males and females, United States, 1979–2004.**
Source: Centers for Disease Control and Prevention/National Center for Health Statistics, www.cdc.gov/nchs.

figure 18.4 **Percentage of deaths from types of CVD, United States, 2004.**
Source: Centers for Disease Control and Prevention/National Center for Health Statistics, www.cdc.gov/nchs.

cells. Together with the white blood cells, smooth muscle cells release collagen and other proteins to form a **plaque,** an accumulation of debris that undergoes continuing damage, bleeding, and calcification. Plaques cause the artery wall to enlarge and bulge into the *lumen,* the channel through which the blood flows, slowing blood flow and reducing the amount of blood that can reach the tissue supplied by the artery. Plaques can also break off and completely block the artery, preventing any blood from flowing through (Figure 18.5).

plaque
Accumulation of debris in an artery wall, consisting of lipoproteins, white blood cells, collagen, and other substances.

Heart attacks, strokes, and peripheral vascular disease are all consequences of the narrowing of arteries caused by atherosclerosis. A diagnosis of one of these diseases suggests risk for the others. Atherosclerosis may also weaken an artery wall, causing a stretching of the artery known as an **aneurysm.** Aneurysms can rupture, tear, and bleed, causing sudden death.

aneurysm
Weak or stretched spot in an artery wall that can tear or rupture, causing sudden death.

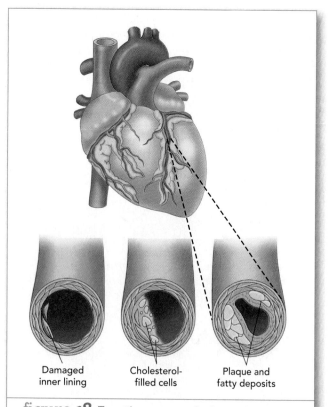

Damaged   Cholesterol-   Plaque and
inner lining   filled cells   fatty deposits

figure 18.5   The process of atherosclerosis.
The process begins with damage to the lining of an artery and progresses to narrowing or blockage of the artery by fatty deposits and plaques.

CORONARY HEART DISEASE

When atherosclerosis involves a coronary artery, the result is **coronary heart disease (CHD)** and, often, a heart attack. Coronary heart disease (also called coronary artery disease) is the leading form of CVD. An estimated 16 million Americans are living with CHD. Those who survive a heart attack are often left with damaged hearts and significantly altered lives.

coronary heart disease (CHD)
Atherosclerosis of the coronary arteries.

Heart Attack and Angina   When a coronary artery becomes narrowed or blocked, the heart muscle does not get enough oxygen-rich blood, a condition called **ischemia.** If the artery is completely blocked, the person has a heart attack, or **myocardial infarction (MI).** The blockage may be caused by an atherosclerotic plaque that has broken loose or a blood clot (a *thrombus*) that has formed in a narrowed or damaged artery. The latter condition is called a **coronary thrombosis** and may cause sudden death. During a heart attack, the area of muscle supplied by the blocked coronary artery is completely deprived of oxygen. If blood flow is not quickly restored, that part of the heart muscle will die.

ischemia
Insufficient supply of oxygen and nutrients to tissue, caused by narrowed or blocked arteries.

myocardial infarction (MI)
Lack of blood to the heart muscle with resulting death of heart tissue; often called a heart attack.

coronary thrombosis
Blockage of a coronary artery by a blood clot that may cause sudden death.

The severity of a heart attack is determined by the location and duration of the blockage. If the blockage occurs close to the aorta where the coronary arteries are just starting to branch, a large area of heart muscle is deprived of oxygen. If the blockage is farther out in a smaller coronary artery, the area of muscle supplied is smaller. The duration of the blockage is usually determined by the time between onset of symptoms and initiation of medical or surgical treatment to reopen the artery. Duration is directly dependent on how quickly a person recognizes the symptoms of a myocardial infarction and gets help.

A heart attack may occur when extra work is demanded of the heart, such as during exercise or emotional stress, or it may occur during light activity or even rest. A classic symptom of a heart attack is chest pain, often described as a sensation of pressure, fullness, or squeezing in the midportion of the chest. The pain can radiate to the jaw, shoulders, arms, or back (see the box "Signs of a Heart Attack"). For an unfortunate 20 percent of people who have a heart attack, sudden death may be the only sign of coronary artery disease. Not all symptoms occur in all cases. Approximately 37 percent of women and 27 percent of men in large studies did not have chest pain or discomfort with their heart attack. The sex difference may be explained partially by the fact that women are, on average, 10 years older than men when they have a first heart attack, and absence of chest pain is more common with heart attack at older ages. At present, the American Heart Association does not list different symptoms of presentation for men and women.[1, 3]

angina
Intermittent pain, pressure, heaviness, or tightness in the center of the chest caused by a narrowed coronary artery.

When coronary arteries are narrowed but not completely blocked, the person may experience **angina**—pain, pressure, heaviness, or tightness in the center of the chest that may radiate to the neck, arms, or shoulders. Half of all heart attacks are preceded by angina. The difference between a heart attack and angina is that the pain of angina resolves, whereas the pain of a heart attack continues. Angina can be controlled with medical treatment. However, if angina is becoming more frequent or starting to occur with less exercise or at rest, it may mean that coronary artery disease is progressing, increasing the risk for a heart attack.

Many physical conditions can cause pain in the chest, including irritated esophagus, arthritis of the neck or ribs, gas in the colon, stomach ulcers, and gallbladder disease. Chest pain can also be caused by weight lifting or other heavy lifting or vigorous activity. If you are used to chest pain from any of these causes, you may be inclined to ignore angina or chest pain from a heart attack. Don't let complaisance or confusion delay your efforts to seek help if you experience the signs of a heart attack.

Arrhythmias The pumping of the heart is usually a well-coordinated event, controlled by an electrical signal emanating from the sinus node in the right atrium, as described earlier. The sinus node establishes a rate of 60 to 100 beats per minute for a normal adult heart. The rate increases in response to increased demand on the heart, such as during exercise, and slows in response to reduced demand, such as during relaxation or sleep. If the signal is disrupted, it can cause an **arrhythmia,** or disorganized beating of the heart. The disorganized beating is usually not as effective at pumping blood.

arrhythmia
Irregular or disorganized heartbeat.

An arrhythmia is any type of irregular heartbeat. It may be an occasional skipped beat, a rapid or slow rate, or an irregular pattern. Not all arrhythmias are serious or cause for concern. In fact, most people have occasional irregular heartbeats every day; some people do not even notice them. However, arrhythmia may cause noticeable symptoms, including palpitations, a sensation of fluttering in the chest, chest pain, light-headedness, shortness of breath, and fatigue.

Arrhythmias occur for a variety of reasons. The sinus node may be damaged and not produce a regular signal, or the normal electrical conduction course may be damaged, preventing the signal from traveling from the atria to the ventricles. Such damage can be the result of coronary artery disease; structural abnormalities of the heart (such

as valve abnormalities or congenital heart disease); chemical imbalances; or the use of caffeine, alcohol, tobacco, cocaine, or medications, including some over-the-counter cold medications.

Sudden Cardiac Death **Ventricular fibrillation** is a particular type of arrhythmia in which the ventricles contract rapidly and erratically, causing the heart to quiver or "tremor" rather than beat. Blood cannot be pumped by the heart when the ventricles fibrillate. The result is **sudden cardiac death**—an abrupt loss of

ventricular fibrillation
Type of arrhythmia in which the ventricles contract rapidly and erratically, causing the heart to quiver or "tremor" rather than beat.

Highlight on Health

Signs of a Heart Attack

Recognizing the signs of a heart attack and getting treatment quickly are critical to survival. Although symptoms may vary, the following signs may indicate that a heart attack is occurring:

- *Chest discomfort.* Most heart attacks involve discomfort in the center of the chest that lasts more than a few minutes, or that goes away and comes back. It can feel like uncomfortable pressure, squeezing, fullness, or pain.
- *Discomfort in other areas of the upper body.* Symptoms can include pain or discomfort in one or both arms, the back, neck, jaw, or stomach.
- *Shortness of breath.* May occur with or without chest discomfort.
- *Other signs.* These may include breaking out in a cold sweat, nausea, or light-headedness.

Note: For both men and women, chest pain or discomfort is the most common symptom of heart attack. However, women are more likely than men to experience middle or upper back pain, neck pain, jaw pain, shortness of breath, nausea or vomiting, weakness or fatigue, insomnia, or loss of appetite as their presenting symptoms. Women are less likely than men to believe they are having a heart attack and more likely to delay seeking treatment.

If you or someone you are with experiences one or more of these signs, seek emergency medical treatment by calling 911 immediately.

Sources: American Heart Association, www.americanheart.org; "Symptom Presentation in Women with Acute Coronary Syndromes: Myth vs. Reality," by J.G. Canto, R.J. Goldberg, M.M. Hand, et al., 2007, Archives of Internal Medicine, 167 (22), pp. 2405–2413.

Consumer Clipboard

Does Your Home Need an Automated External Defibrillator?

As you walk through airports or other public areas, you have probably noticed the increasing visibility of automated external defibrillators (AEDs). The proliferation of AEDs is due to the growing recognition that defibrillation (an external shock of the heart) after sudden cardiac arrest can save a life—if it is administered in time. The U.S. Food and Drug Administration has decided that AEDs are safe enough for the general public to operate and has approved over-the-counter sales of AEDs for use in the home. An AED currently costs between $1,500 and $3,000. They are easy to transport, are easy to use, and are becoming less expensive. Some health experts think that home AEDs will soon become as common as home fire extinguishers.

It is true that cardiac arrest often occurs in the home, and the use of home AEDs may reduce the time between cardiac arrest and defibrillation. So far, however, there is no evidence that this is what happens. When deciding whether to purchase a home AED, consider these questions:

■ What are the cardiac risk factors of your family members or housemates? How likely is it that someone who lives with you will experience sudden cardiac arrest?

■ How likely is it that a guest in your home will experience sudden cardiac arrest?

■ Do you live alone? If so, a home AED may be of little use to you, since someone else is needed to operate it.

If you decide to get an AED, it is important to learn how to use it and maintain it properly. Enroll yourself and family members or housemates in a CPR course that includes instruction on the use of AEDs, even if your home AED comes with an instructional video. Practice using it, and store it in an easily accessible location. Make sure everyone knows where it is, and also make sure everyone knows they still need to call emergency medical services (911).

Source: "An Overview of Automated External Defibrillators," by L.A. Lewis, 2007, American Journal of Clinical Medicine, 4 (1).

---

sudden cardiac death
Abrupt loss of heart function caused by an irregular or ineffective heartbeat.

---

heart function. An estimated 7,000 to 14,000 infants and children die each year from sudden cardiac death, and sudden cardiac death is the leading cause of death in high school and college athletes, with an estimated incidence at 1 in 200,000 athletes (see Chapter 2 for a discussion of the genetic contributing factors). Vigorous exercise can be a trigger for lethal arrhythmia when an underlying heart abnormality is present. Under age 35, sudden cardiac death is usually due to congenital cardiac abnormalities. Over age 35, the cause is usually coronary artery disease.

Ventricular fibrillation can be reversed with an electrical shock from a defibrillator, which can restart the heart's normal rhythm (see the box "Does Your Home Need an Automated External Defibrillator?"). Every minute counts, however: The chances of survival are reduced by 8–10 percent for every minute following cardiac arrest. About 310,000 Americans die each year from sudden cardiac death in emergency rooms or prior to reaching the hospital. Response to sudden cardiac death provides an example of how communities must work together to improve health (see the box "The Chain of Survival" on p. 384).

STROKE

When blood flow to the brain or part of the brain is blocked, the result is a **stroke,** or **cerebrovascular accident (CVA).** Stroke is the third-leading cause of death in the United States, after heart disease and cancer, and is a leading cause of severe, long-term disability.

Ischemic strokes are 87 percent of all strokes and occur when an artery in the brain becomes blocked, in the same way that a heart attack occurs when a coronary artery is blocked, and prevents the brain from receiving blood flow (Figure 18.6). The blockage can be due to a **thrombus** (a blood clot that develops in a narrowed artery) or an **embolism** (a clot that develops elsewhere, often in the heart, travels to the brain, and lodges in an artery).

Hemorrhagic strokes are 13 percent of strokes and occur when a brain artery ruptures, bleeds into the surrounding area, and compresses brain tissue. There are two types of hemorrhagic stroke. *Intracerebral hemorrhagic* strokes account for 10 percent and occur when the ruptured artery is within brain tissue. *Subarachnoid hemorrhagic* strokes account for 3 percent and occur when the ruptured artery is on the brain's surface and blood accumulates between the brain and the skull. Hemorrhagic strokes may be due to a head injury or a ruptured aneurysm.[1]

---

stroke, or cerebrovascular accident (CVA)
Lack of blood flow to the brain with resulting death of brain tissue.

ischemic strokes
Strokes caused by blockage in a blood vessel in the brain.

thrombus
Blood clot that forms in a narrowed or damaged artery.

embolism
Blood clot that travels from elsewhere in the body.

hemorrhagic strokes
Strokes caused by rupture of a blood vessel in the brain, with bleeding into brain tissue.

As with the heart, different arteries supply different areas of the brain. Strokes may have a variety of symptoms, depending on the area of the brain involved. However, symptoms usually involve the sudden onset of neurological problems, such as headaches, numbness, weakness, or speech problems (see the box "Signs of a Stroke").

A small percentage of people have **transient ischemic attacks (TIAs)** before having a stroke. Sometimes called "ministrokes," TIAs are periods of ischemia that produce the same symptoms as a stroke, but in this case the symptoms resolve within 24 hours with little or no tissue death. A TIA should be viewed as a warning sign of stroke. After a TIA, 3–17 percent of people will have a stroke within the next 90 days. Early recognition and rapid treatment are as important for TIA and stroke as they are for heart disease. Treatment can improve survival and reduce complications but must be given quickly (treatment is discussed further later in the chapter).

transient ischemic attacks (TIA)
Periods of ischemia that temporarily produce the same symptoms as a stroke.

blood pressure
Force exerted by the blood against artery walls.

hypertension
Blood pressure that is forceful enough to damage artery walls.

HYPERTENSION

Blood pressure is the pressure exerted by blood against the walls of arteries, and high blood pressure, or **hypertension,** occurs when the pressure is great

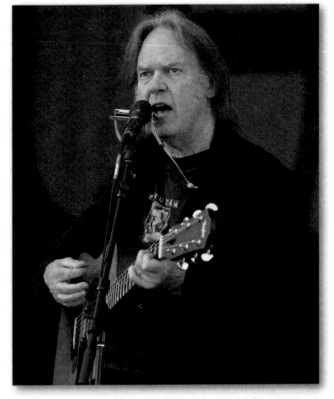

In April 2005, Neil Young underwent treatment for a brain aneurysm, a bulge in a blood vessel that can burst and cause a hemorrhagic stroke. The 59-year-old singer sought treatment after he experienced symptoms that included blurred vision. .

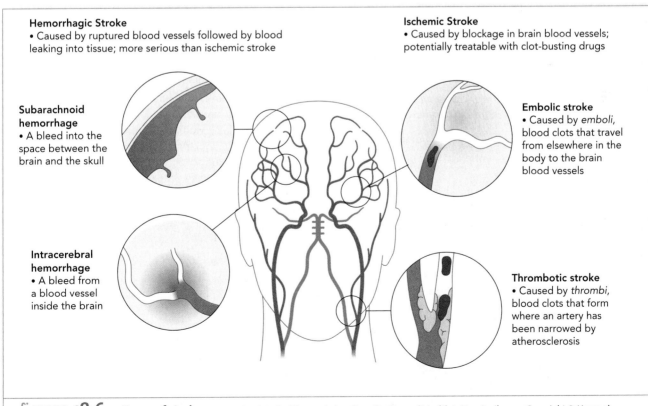

Hemorrhagic Stroke
• Caused by ruptured blood vessels followed by blood leaking into tissue; more serious than ischemic stroke

Ischemic Stroke
• Caused by blockage in brain blood vessels; potentially treatable with clot-busting drugs

Subarachnoid hemorrhage
• A bleed into the space between the brain and the skull

Embolic stroke
• Caused by *emboli*, blood clots that travel from elsewhere in the body to the brain blood vessels

Intracerebral hemorrhage
• A bleed from a blood vessel inside the brain

Thrombotic stroke
• Caused by *thrombi*, blood clots that form where an artery has been narrowed by atherosclerosis

figure **18.6**   **Types of stroke.** *Source: Reprinted with permission from the* Harvard Health Letter, *April 2000. Copyright © Harvard University and Harriet Greenfield. For more information, visit: www.health.harvard.edu. Harvard Health Publications does not endorse any products or medical procedures.*

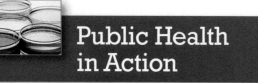

Public Health in Action

The Chain of Survival

Sudden cardiac arrest is a leading cause of death in the United States and Canada. Survival depends on a quick, well-organized community response. Resuscitation is most successful when a collapsed victim receives cardiopulmonary resuscitation (CPR) and defibrillation within 5 minutes of collapse. Initiation of the American Red Cross Chain of Survival is critical and involves four steps:

- Step 1: Early activation of emergency medical services (call 911 or other local emergency number).

- Step 2: Early cardiopulmonary resuscitation (CPR).

- Step 3: Early defibrillation.

- Step 4: Early advanced cardiac life support (transfer to a hospital).

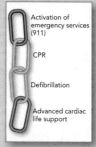

Each step depends on individuals and factors in the surrounding environment. Early activation of emergency medical services requires a bystander to recognize that an athlete, colleague, friend, family member, or stranger may be having sudden cardiac arrest. Sudden collapse and loss of consciousness should prompt an immediate call for help.

Early cardiopulmonary resuscitation depends on a trained and willing public. When performed immediately after collapse, CPR can double or triple the chance for survival. New CPR guidelines, discussed in Chapter 22, make it easier for bystanders to perform it.

Early defibrillation requires quick access to defibrillators. In recognition of the fact that the time between a first call to emergency medical services and the arrival of medics is often greater than 5 minutes, automated external defibrillators (AEDs) are now recommended in many public locations. They are frequently found in airports, health clubs, shopping malls, and sports events. Many schools are starting to incorporate AEDs in their emergency planning. Early defibrillation depends on bystanders being trained to use AEDs.

Early advanced cardiac life support depends on the arrival of medics to assist with resuscitation, stabilization, and transfer to a hospital where definitive treatment can begin. This requires community investment and support of the emergency medical services infrastructure.

Source: "American Heart Association Guidelines for Cardiopulmonary Resuscitation and Emergency Cardiovascular Care," 2005, Circulation, 112: pp. IV-12–IV-18.

enough to damage artery walls. Untreated high blood pressure can weaken and scar the arteries and makes the heart work harder, weakening it as well. Hypertension can cause heart attacks, strokes, kidney disease, peripheral artery disease, and blindness.[1, 4]

Blood pressure is determined by two forces—the pressure produced by the heart as it pumps the blood and the resistance of the arteries as they contain blood flow. When arteries are hardened by atherosclerosis, they are more resistant. Blood pressure is measured in millimeters of mercury and stated in two numbers, such as 120/80. The upper number represents **systolic pressure,** the pressure produced when the heart contracts; the lower number represents **diastolic pressure,** the pressure in the arteries when the heart is relaxed, between contractions. There is no definite line dividing normal blood pressure from high blood pressure, but categories have been established as guidelines on the basis of increased risk for CVD; see Table 18.1.

systolic pressure
Pressure in the arteries when the heart contracts, represented by the upper number in a blood pressure measurement.

diastolic pressure
Pressure in the arteries when the heart relaxes between contractions, represented by the lower number in a blood pressure measurement.

Prehypertension is a category of blood pressure measurement higher than recommended but not meeting criteria for hypertension; the category has been identified to target people at high risk of developing hypertension. An estimated 37 percent of the U.S. population aged 20 and older have prehypertension. Blood pressure in this range should prompt aggressive lifestyle change and increased monitoring to reduce future risk.

Hypertension is often referred to as the "silent killer," because it usually causes no symptoms. More than 73 million people in the United States (nearly one in three adults) and more than 1 billion people worldwide are estimated to have high blood pressure. Although people are becoming more aware of this condition, 28 percent of people with high blood pressure do not know they have it. Of those who know they have the condition, only 61 percent are receiving treatment, and of those, only 35 percent are adequately treated.

Table 18.1	Blood Pressure Guidelines	
Category	**Systolic**	**Diastolic**
Normal	Less than 120 *and*	Less than 80
Prehypertension	120–139 *or*	80–89
Hypertension		
Stage 1	140–159 *or*	90–99
Stage 2	160 and above *or*	100 and above

Source: "The Seventh Report of the Joint National Committee on Prevention, Detection, Evaluation and Treatment of High Blood Pressure" (NIH Publication No. 03–5233), 2003, Bethesda, MD: National Heart, Lung, and Blood Institute, National Institutes of Health.

Highlight on Health

Signs of a Stroke

Neurological problems that have a sudden onset and are unremitting, especially if they involve only one side of the body, may be signs that a stroke is occurring or has occurred. Although some of the following symptoms may occur with other illnesses, such as migraine headache, the more symptoms there are, and the more severe they are, the more likely they are to be the result of a stroke.

- Sudden numbness or weakness of the face, arm, or leg, especially on one side of the body.
- Sudden confusion, trouble speaking or understanding.
- Sudden trouble seeing in one or both eyes.
- Sudden trouble walking, dizziness, loss of balance or coordination.
- Sudden, severe headache with no known cause.

    If you or someone you are with experiences one or more of these symptoms, seek emergency medical treatment by calling 911 immediately. Remember the acronym FAST:

- **F**acial numbness or weakness
- **A**rm numbness or weakness
- **S**lurred speech
- **T**ime to call 911

Source: Adapted from American Stroke Association, www.stroke.org.

Thus there is room for significant improvement by individuals and communities.[1,4]

In approximately 95 percent of cases, the cause of hypertension is unknown. In Western societies, aging seems to be a factor, but this is not the case in other cultures. Genetics plays a role in some cases. Racial differences exist, with Blacks having the highest rates. Other factors that contribute to elevated blood pressure include high salt consumption, use of alcohol, low potassium levels, physical inactivity, and obesity. Less frequently, medical conditions can cause hypertension. Women can develop hypertension during pregnancy or while taking oral contraceptive pills; even children and adolescents occasionally develop hypertension, often as a result of underlying medical conditions or congenital problems.

CONGESTIVE HEART FAILURE

When the heart is not pumping the blood as well as it should, a condition known as **congestive heart failure** occurs. It can develop after a heart attack or as a result of hyperten-

sion, heart valve abnormality, or disease of the heart muscle. When the heart cannot keep up its regular pumping force or rate, blood backs up into the lungs, and fluid from the backed-up blood in the pulmonary veins leaks into the lungs. A person with congestive heart failure experiences difficulty breathing, shortness of breath, and coughing, especially when lying down. Blood returning to the heart from the body also gets backed up, causing fluid to leak into the ankles and legs and causing swelling of the lower legs. When blood fails to reach the brain efficiently, fatigue and confusion can result.

congestive heart failure
Condition in which the heart is not pumping the blood as well as it should, allowing blood and fluids to back up in the lungs.

Approximately 5.3 million Americans live with congestive heart failure.[1] Symptoms can be treated with medications that help draw off extra fluid, decrease blood pressure, and improve the heart's ability to pump. Other factors that contribute to the development of congestive heart failure include cigarette smoking, high cholesterol, and diabetes. Lifestyle changes such as weight loss, exercise, and smoking cessation can reduce symptoms and the risk of disease progression. In some instances, surgery can be done to repair a heart valve or the damage incurred by coronary heart disease. In extreme cases, the only recourse may be a heart transplant.

OTHER CARDIOVASCULAR DISEASES

Other conditions can affect the structure of the heart and blood vessels and their ability to function. Some of these conditions are congenital (present from birth), and others occur as progressive diseases.

Heart Valve Disorders   Four valves in the heart keep blood flowing in the correct direction through the heart (see Figure 18.1). A normally functioning valve opens easily to allow blood to flow forward and closes tightly to prevent blood from flowing backward. Sometimes a valve does not open well, preventing the smooth flow of blood, and sometimes a valve does not close tightly, allowing blood to leak backward. These problems can be caused by congenital abnormalities, rheumatic heart disease, or an aging-related degeneration process. When valves are not functioning normally, the flow of blood is altered and the risks of blood clots and infection increase. Often, the person experiences no symptoms; if symptoms do occur, they can include shortness of breath, dizziness, fatigue, and chest pain.

The most common heart valve defect is **mitral valve prolapse** (the mitral valve separates the left atrium from the left ventricle). In this condition, the mitral valve billows backward and the edges do not fully close when the left ventricle contracts to move blood into the aorta, allowing blood to leak backward into the

mitral valve prolapse
Heart valve disorder in which the mitral valve, which separates the left ventricle from the left atrium, does not close fully, allowing blood to leak backward into the atrium.

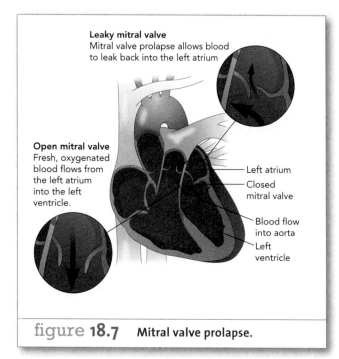

Leaky mitral valve
Mitral valve prolapse allows blood to leak back into the left atrium

Open mitral valve
Fresh, oxygenated blood flows from the left atrium into the left ventricle.

Left atrium
Closed mitral valve
Blood flow into aorta
Left ventricle

figure **18.7**   **Mitral valve prolapse.**

atrium (Figure 18.7). Mitral valve prolapse is common, affecting 5–10 percent of the population. It can occur at any age and affects both men and women; it is often detected when a physician hears a "click" or "murmur" in the heartbeat. With certain types of mitral valve prolapse, individuals should take antibiotics before dental surgery and other procedures to reduce the risk of infection from bacteria introduced into the bloodstream by the procedure.

Rheumatic Heart Disease   A common cause of heart valve disorders and other heart damage is **rheumatic fever,** leading to **rheumatic heart disease**. In this disease, the heart is scarred following an infection with a strain of streptococcus bacteria (Group A streptoccocus, usually as strep throat). Symptoms of rheumatic fever include fever, joint pain, fatigue, and rash; when the heart is affected, there can be congestive heart failure, valve dysfunction, or arrhythmia. Acute rheumatic fever can occur 2 to 3 weeks after a strep throat infection (although almost one in three people did not have a sore throat) and last weeks to months. Heart damage can occur over years. The condition is prevented by treating strep throat infections with antibiotics. Rheumatic fever often occurs in children, and worldwide it is a major cause of heart disorders. The incidence of rheumatic heart disease has declined significantly in developed countries, partly as a result of aggressive diagnosis and treatment of strep throat.

rheumatic fever
Acute disease that can occur as a complication of an untreated strep throat infection.

rheumatic heart disease
Disease in which the heart is scarred following strep throat infection and rheumatic fever.

Congenital Heart Disease   A variety of structural defects that are present at birth can involve the heart valves, major arteries and veins in or near the heart, or the heart muscle.

An abnormality can cause the blood to slow down, flow in the wrong direction, or not move from one chamber to the next. More than 35 types of heart defects have been described. One of the more common defects is a **septal defect,** in which an extra hole in the heart allows blood to flow from one atrium to the other or from one ventricle to the other. When a septal defect is present, poorly oxygenated blood from the body mixes with oxygenated blood from the lungs, resulting in lower oxygen supply to the body.

septal defect
Congenital heart defect in which an extra hole allows blood to flow from one atrium to the other or from one ventricle to the other.

Approximately 36,000 babies are identified at birth with congenital heart defects each year in the United States.[5] Other congenital or genetic diseases may go undetected until an older age. Undetected congenital cardiac abnormalities are the leading cause of death in competitive athletes. Conditions such as hypertrophic cardiomyopathy, abnormal coronary arteries, and underlying electrical conduction abnormalities are present in approximately 0.3 percent of the athletic population.[6] Indications and recommendations for pre-participation screening of athletes are discussed at the end of the chapter in You Make the Call.

Peripheral Vascular Disease   The result of atherosclerosis in the arteries of the arms or legs (more commonly, the legs), **peripheral vascular disease (PVD)** causes pain, aches, or cramping in the muscles supplied by a narrowed blood vessel. Although it is usually not fatal, PVD causes a significant amount of disability, limiting the activity level of many older people because of pain with walking. If circulation is severely limited by the ischemia, the affected leg or arm may have to be amputated.

peripheral vascular disease (PVD)
Atherosclerosis in the blood vessels of the arms or legs.

Eight million people live with PVD (12–20 percent of older adults). It is a clue to advanced atherosclerosis and indicates the need for lifestyle change or medical treatment in order to reduce the risk of heart attack or stroke. High levels of daily physical activity are associated with better survival and lower risk of death. Anyone who experiences unexplained pain in the legs or arms, especially if it is associated with exercise, should see a health care provider.[1]

Cardiomyopathy   Deaths from **cardiomyopathy**—disease of the heart muscle—account for 1 percent of heart disease deaths in the United States, with the highest rates occurring among men and Blacks. The most common form of cardiomyopathy is *dilated cardiomyopathy,* an enlargement of the heart in response to weakening of the muscle. The cause is often unknown, although a virus is suspected in some cases. Other factors that can weaken the heart muscle are toxins (alcohol, tobacco, heavy metals, and some medications), drugs, pregnancy, hypertension, and coronary artery disease.

cardiomyopathy
Disease of the heart muscle.

Another form is **hypertrophic cardiomyopathy,** an abnormal thickening of one part of the heart, frequently the left ventricle. The thickened wall makes the heart abnormally stiff, so the heart doesn't fill well. Although most people with hypertrophic cardiomyopathy have no symptoms, the condition can cause heart failure, arrhythmia, and sudden death. In fact, 36 percent of cases of sudden death in young competitive athletes are due to hypertrophic cardiomyopathy. The cause of the condition is unknown in about 50 percent of cases, but in the rest, there is a genetic link.

hypertrophic cardiomyopathy Abnormal thickening of one part of the heart, frequently the left ventricle.

Risk Factors for CVD

A rapid increase in cardiovascular disease occurred in the United States in the 1930s, and by the late 1940s, CVD had become the leading cause of death. In an effort to understand this pattern, the U.S. Public Health Service joined with a group of researchers to look at differences between people who developed CVD and those who did not. This was the origin of the Framingham Heart Study, which began in 1948 and continues to this day.

The town of Framingham, Massachusetts, was chosen as the site of the study; 2,336 men and 2,873 women signed up to be studied longitudinally (followed over time). In the years since then, more participants have been added, including members of Framingham's minority communities. Every 2 to 4 years, participants in the study undergo extensive testing to evaluate their behaviors and health status. More than 50 years of study and the participation of more than 10,000 men and women have allowed researchers to identify multiple factors that alter the risk of cardiovascular disease.[7]

As discussed in Chapter 2, cardiovascular disease is a multifactorial disease, the result of genetic, environmental, and lifestyle factors interacting over time. Some factors are controllable, while others are not. Worldwide, nine risk factors account for more than 90 percent of the risk for initial heart attack: cigarette smoking, abnormal lipid levels, hypertension, diabetes, abdominal obesity, lack of physical activity, low daily fruit and vegetable intake, excessive alcohol intake, and psychosocial stress. This holds true for men and women and for different ethnic groups.[8]

MAJOR CONTROLLABLE RISK FACTORS IN CVD

Controllable risk factors are factors associated with CVD that can be altered through individual behavior or community intervention. The American Heart Association lists six major controllable risk factors: tobacco use, hypertension, unhealthy blood cholesterol levels, physical inactivity, overweight, and diabetes. Ninety percent of persons with heart disease will have at least one of these risk factors.[1]

Tobacco Use and CVD Risk Tobacco use is the leading risk factor for all forms of CVD. Cigarette smokers develop coronary artery disease at two to four times the rate of nonsmokers and have twice the risk of sudden cardiac death as nonsmokers. Cigar and pipe smoking are also associated with an increased risk of coronary artery disease and perhaps an increased risk of stroke, although not as great an increase as with cigarettes.

Tobacco smoke functions in a variety of ways to increase risk. Components of tobacco smoke damage the inner lining of blood vessels, speeding up the development of atherosclerosis. Toxins in tobacco smoke can stimulate the formation of blood clots in the coronary arteries and trigger spasms that close off the vessels. Smoking raises blood levels of LDL cholesterol ("bad" cholesterol) and decreases blood levels of HDL cholesterol ("good" cholesterol). Exposure to environmental tobacco smoke (secondhand smoke) is also a risk factor for CVD; risk appears to be proportional to the amount of daily exposure. The risk for CVD decreases within a few years of quitting smoking. For more on tobacco use and strategies for quitting, see Chapter 13.[1, 9]

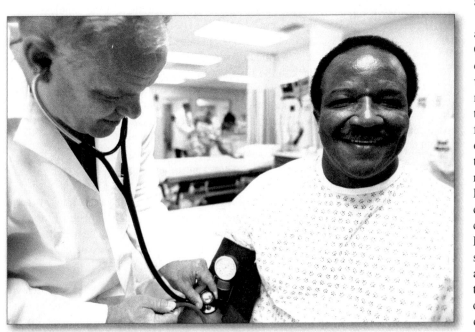

■ African Americans have higher rates of hypertension than the rest of the population, probably due to a combination of genetic, sociocultural, and behavioral factors. Regular screening can help keep blood pressure under control.

Hypertension and CVD Risk Hypertension increases the risk for heart attack, stroke, congestive heart failure, and kidney disease; the higher the blood pressure, the greater the risk. Hypertension makes the heart work harder to circulate the blood. The increased work may cause the heart to enlarge, which may lead to congestive heart failure. Hypertension can also cause damage to the lining of arteries, promoting atherosclerosis and causing blood vessel walls to weaken.

There are significant differences in the prevalence of high blood pressure across different minority populations. In Blacks, hypertension is not only more common; it also appears to follow a different course than it does in other groups. It develops earlier, is more severe, and is associated with more complications, such as heart attacks, stroke, and kidney failure. Blacks tend to excrete sodium (salt) at a slower rate than Whites do, possibly making them more sensitive to dietary salt. This difference may contribute to the higher rate of stroke among Blacks. To date, there has not been a clear genetic explanation for the ethnic differences. Socioeconomic and behavioral factors may be involved as well, as discussed later in the chapter.[10]

Unhealthy Cholesterol Levels and CVD Risk Cholesterol is a waxy, fat-like substance essential to the body; it is used in cell membranes, in some hormones, in brain and nerve tissue, and in bile acids that help digest fats. The amount of cholesterol in your body is affected by what you eat and by how fast your body makes and gets rid of cholesterol (see Chapter 7). Because it is fat-like, cholesterol cannot circulate in the blood in a free-floating state; instead, it is combined with proteins and other molecules in packages called *lipoproteins*.

Lipoproteins are spherical and smaller than red blood cells; they are categorized into five main classes according to density, with each class playing a different role in the body. The categories that have received the most study are total cholesterol and the LDL and HDL subcategories. Levels of total cholesterol are directly related to frequency of coronary heart disease; that is, as cholesterol levels rise, so does the incidence of heart disease (Table 18.2). An estimated 48 percent of the adult U.S. population has total cholesterol greater than 200 mg/dl, and 17 percent have a level greater than 240 mg/dl.[1]

low-density lipoproteins (LDLs) "Bad" cholesterol; lipoproteins that accumulate in plaque and contribute to atherosclerosis.

Low-density lipoproteins (LDLs)—"bad" cholesterol—are clearly associated with atherosclerosis. The higher the level of LDLs, the higher the risk of atherosclerosis. Lowering LDL cholesterol through dietary change, exercise, and medication reduces risk. Goals for LDL levels (in mg/dl) are influenced by the number of other risk factors for coronary artery disease a person has (for example, tobacco use, hypertension, older age):[11, 12]

- No risk factors or one other risk factor: < 160
- Two risk factors: < 130
- Already have heart disease or diabetes: < 100
- Very high risk (for example, recent heart attack): < 70

High-density lipoproteins (HDLs)—"good" cholesterol—consist mainly of protein and are the smallest of the lipoprotein particles. HDLs help clear cholesterol from cells and atherosclerotic deposits and transport it back to the liver for recycling. Thus they decrease blood levels of cholesterol and reverse the development of deposits and plaque. High HDL levels provide protection from CVD.

HDL levels are determined mainly by genetics, but they are influenced by exercise, alcohol, and estrogen. They are higher among Blacks and among women, especially before menopause, and they change little with age. The protective effect of HDL is quite significant: A 1 percent decrease in HDL level is associated with a 3–4 percent increase in heart disease.[11]

high-density lipoproteins (HDLs) "Good" cholesterol; lipoproteins that help clear cholesterol from cells and atherosclerotic deposits and transport it back to the liver for recycling.

Physical Inactivity and CVD Risk A sedentary lifestyle is another major risk factor for CVD, and regular physical activity reduces the risk of CVD and many cardiovascular risk factors, including high blood pressure, diabetes, and obesity. Physical activity conditions the heart, reduces high blood pressure, improves HDL cholesterol levels, helps maintain a healthy weight, and helps control diabetes.

Table 18.2	Cholesterol Guidelines
Total cholesterol (mg/dl)	
Less than 200	Desirable
200–239	Borderline high
240 or greater	High
LDL cholesterol (mg/dl)	
Less than 100*	Optimal
100–129	Near or above optimal
130–159	Borderline high
160–189	High
190 or greater	Very high
HDL cholesterol (mg/dl)	
Less than 40	Low (undesirable)
60 or greater	High (desirable)
Triglycerides (mg/dl)	
Less than 150	Normal
150–199	Borderline high
200–499	High
500 or greater	Very high

*Achieving a goal of less than 70 is an option if there is a high risk for heart disease.

Source: "Executive Summary of the Third Report of the National Cholesterol Education Program Expert Panel on Detection, Evaluation, and Treatment of High Blood Cholesterol in Adults," 2001, by Journal of the American Medical Association, *285 (19), pp. 2486–2497.*

Unfortunately, the majority of adults in the United States are not active at levels that can promote health. Only 46.7 percent of women and 49.7 percent of men report achieving the goal of 30 minutes of moderate-intensity exercise most days of the week or 20 minutes of vigorous exercise on three or more days a week. Disparities exist by racial/ethnic group, with 49 percent of White women, 40.5 percent of Hispanic women, and 36.1 percent of Black women meeting the goal, and 52 percent of White men, 41.9 percent of Hispanic men, and 45.3 percent of Black men meeting the goal. One in four adults reports no leisure-time physical activity at all.[13] Exercise is especially important for children, because it is associated with lower blood pressure and weight control and because active children tend to become active adults.

Obesity and CVD Risk Overweight and obesity are associated with increased risk for CVD and greater seriousness of the disease. Excess weight puts a strain on the heart and contributes to other risk factors such as hypertension, high LDL levels, and diabetes. The association among all these risk factors is found across ethnic groups, including Mexican Americans, non-Hispanic Blacks, and non-Hispanic Whites.

As discussed in Chapter 9, body fat distribution plays a role in CVD risk. Waist-to-hip ratio may play a greater role than absolute body mass index. People with central fat distribution—those who are apple-shaped, as suggested by an abdominal circumference of greater than 40 inches for men and greater than 35 inches for women—have a higher risk for diabetes, high blood pressure, and CVD. Weight loss of 10–15 percent for an overweight individual, if maintained, is associated with an improved cardiovascular risk profile. Diet and exercise are recommended ways to reduce overweight and obesity.[1, 8]

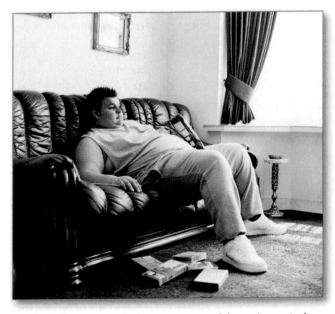

■ Physical inactivity and obesity are two of the major controllable risk factors for cardiovascular disease.

Diabetes and CVD Risk **Diabetes** is a metabolic disorder in which the production or use of insulin is disrupted, as described in Chapter 9. Elevated levels of glucose circulating in the bloodstream cause changes throughout the body, including damage to artery walls, changes in some blood components, and damage to peripheral nerves and organs. People with diabetes are two to four times more likely than people without diabetes to develop cardiovascular disease. Their arteries are particularly susceptible to atherosclerosis, and it occurs at an earlier age and is more extensive. The incidence of Type-2 diabetes has doubled in the past 30 years and is expected to double again by 2050. Currently, 7.3 percent of the U.S. adult population has been diagnosed with diabetes. An estimated 2.8 percent of adults have diabetes that has not been diagnosed.[1]

diabetes
Metabolic disorder in which the production or use of insulin is disrupted, so that body cells cannot take up glucose and use it for energy, and high levels of glucose circulate in the blood.

Another concern for people with diabetes is that their symptoms of heart attack may be different from the norm. They are more likely to have a "silent" heart attack. Their only symptoms may be nausea, vomiting, sweating, or dizziness, any of which could be easily mistaken for another illness. Control of diabetes reduces risk, and it is especially important for people with diabetes to control other risk factors.[1]

CONTRIBUTING RISK FACTORS IN CVD

Besides the six major controllable risk factors for CVD, other risk factors that can be controlled have been identified. These factors contribute to risk, but their role is either slightly less than that of the major risk factors or has not been as clearly delineated yet.

High Triglyceride Levels **Triglycerides** are another form in which fat exists in the body. Body triglycerides are derived from fats eaten or produced by the body from other energy sources, such as excess carbohydrates. High blood levels of triglycerides are a risk factor for CVD, although they are not linked to CVD as strongly as are cholesterol levels. A triglyceride level of less than 150 is desirable (see Table 18.2). High triglyceride levels are associated with excess body fat, diets high in saturated fat and cholesterol, alcohol use, and some medical conditions, such as poorly controlled diabetes. The main treatment for high triglycerides is lifestyle modification, but medications can also be used.

triglycerides
Blood fats similar to cholesterol.

High Alcohol Intake The relationship between alcohol and CVD is complicated because different levels of alcohol consumption have different effects. Heavy drinking, defined as more than three drinks per day, can damage the heart, increasing the risk of cardiomyopathy, some arrhythmias, and neurological complications. Light to moderate alcohol intake, defined as fewer than two drinks per day, appears

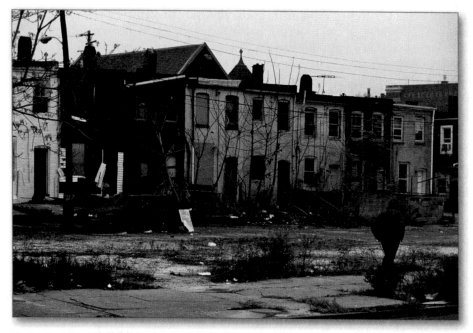

■ Low socioeconomic status is associated with greater risk for cardiovascular disease. Contributing factors may be the stress of poverty and discrimination and lack of access to health information and health care services.

to have a protective effect against heart disease and stroke, increasing HDL levels.

The benefit associated with light to moderate alcohol use is seen regardless of the beverage, which suggests that the protective factor is alcohol itself, rather than another substance in some beverages, such as the tannins in red wine. The disadvantages of alcohol consumption are that it may contribute to weight gain, higher blood pressure, and elevated triglycerides, as well as alcoholism in vulnerable individuals. The possible cardiovascular benefits have to be weighed against the disadvantages and potential harm associated with drinking.[1]

Psychosocial Factors Five psychosocial factors have been studied that appear to play a role in the development and outcomes of CVD: personality, chronic stress, socioeconomic status, depression, and social support.

As described in Chapter 5, traits and behavior patterns associated with the so-called Type A personality—specifically, anger and hostility—have been shown to contribute to CVD risk. These feelings cause the release of stress hormones. When anger, hostility, and stress in general are persistent and pervasive, the continuous circulation of stress hormones in the blood increases blood pressure and heart rate and triggers the release of cholesterol and triglycerides into the blood. All these changes may promote the development of atherosclerosis and, for those with atherosclerosis, increase vulnerability to heart attack or stroke.[14, 15]

People with low socioeconomic status and low levels of educational attainment have a greater risk for heart attack, stroke, congestive heart failure, and hypertension. Income inequality in a country—the gap between the rich and the poor—is directly related to national rates of death from CVD, coronary artery disease, and stroke. Numerous factors may help explain the link between poverty and poor health. For example, poverty limits people's ability to obtain the basic requisites for health, such as food and shelter, as well as their ability to participate in society, which creates psychological stress. Poverty also limits access to health-related information, health care, medications, behavior change options, and physical activity. In addition, racism, prejudice, and discrimination can act as psychosocial stressors and lead to increased risk of CVD.[1, 8, 16]

Depression has a bidirectional relationship with CVD; that is, depression increases risk of CVD, and CVD increases risk of depression. Depression can play a role in all stages in the development of CVD. People who are depressed have a more difficult time choosing healthy lifestyle options, making lifestyle changes, initiating access to health care, and adhering to medication regimens. Early diagnosis and treatment of depression may help reduce risk of CVD in vulnerable individuals.[1, 8, 14]

People who lack social support or live in social isolation are at increased risk for many health conditions, including CVD. Strong social networks have been shown to decrease the risk of CVD, and social support, altruism, faith, and optimism are all associated with a reduced risk of CVD. Thus, it appears that the strength of a person's relationships and the nature of his or her basic attitudes toward life play important roles in maintaining health and protecting against disease, as discussed in Chapter 4.[17]

POSSIBLE RISK FACTORS IN CVD

Factors that contribute to CVD are not fully understood, and some people with heart disease have none of the risk factors discussed so far. Researchers are constantly trying to identify additional risk factors; in this section we consider a few promising areas of ongoing research.

Vitamin D Deficiency An estimated 30–50 percent of middle-aged and older adults have low levels of vitamin D intake. Vitamin D has long been known to play an important role in calcium absorption and bone health; however, it is becoming increasingly clear that low levels of vitamin D may increase risk of CVD. Vitamin D is believed to affect blood clotting, inflammation, and the cells in the walls of arteries. At present, there are not enough data to recommend routine screening of vitamin D blood levels, nor are there data to show that treatment of vitamin D deficiency reduces risk of CVD. However, this may become an important risk factor in the future, given that vitamin D deficiency is so common and is relatively easy to treat with sunshine or vitamin supplementation.[18]

Lipoprotein(a) A subgroup of LDL cholesterol, **lipoprotein(a)** is similar to LDL but has an additional protein

___

lipoprotein(a)
Subgroup of LDL cholesterol that is thought to increase blood clotting.

___

attached. This particular subtype of LDL may increase blood clotting and atherosclerosis. Higher levels of lipoprotein(a) are associated with an increased risk of coronary artery disease. Screening for lipoprotein(a) is possible but not currently recommended. The question of whether screening specifically for lipoprotein(a) further identifies people at risk for CVD beyond what can be learned from screening for LDLs has not been answered definitively. In addition, there are currently no treatments that specifically target lipoprotein(a). Steps that decrease LDL levels, such as dietary modifications and medications, also decrease levels of lipoprotein(a).[19]

Homocysteine High blood levels of **homocysteine,** an amino acid, have been associated with increased risks of

___

homocysteine
Amino acid that circulates in the blood and may damage the lining of blood vessels.

___

CVD. Homocysteine may damage the lining of blood vessels, leading to inflammation and atherosclerosis. Both genetics and diet appear to play a role in setting homocysteine levels. Meats are high in methionine, which the body converts into homocysteine. Blood levels of homocysteine are higher in people with diets high in animal protein and low in vitamin B_6, vitamin B_{12}, and folic acid (commonly found in fruits, vegetables, and enriched grains).

At this time, there is no recommendation for measuring homocysteine levels in the general population, nor is there evidence to show that reducing homocysteine levels can

___

metabolic syndrome
Condition characterized by a combination of obesity, especially central obesity; elevated blood pressure; dyslipidemia (high triglycerides and low HDL cholesterol); and glucose intolerance, a pre-diabetes condition.

___

reduce risk of CVD. For now, testing remains controversial. However, individuals can reduce their blood level of homocysteine by eating a diet rich in fruits, vegetables, and grains, especially grains fortified with folic acid.

Metabolic Syndrome A condition associated with a significantly increased risk of CVD and the development of Type-2 diabetes, **metabolic syndrome** is characterized by a combination of risk factors. Although several criteria have been identified, the condition is commonly diagnosed when three of the following five risk factors are present:

- Fasting glucose level ≥ 100

- HDL cholesterol < 40 in men or < 50 in women

- Triglycerides ≥ 150

- Waist circumference ≥ 102 cm for men or ≥ 88 cm for women

- Systolic blood pressure ≥ 130 and diastolic blood pressure ≥ 85

An estimated 47 million adult Americans meet the criteria for diagnosis, but prevalence varies by ethnic and racial group. For example, prevalence is 21.6 percent in Blacks, 31.9 percent in Mexican Americans, and 23.8 percent in Whites.[1] The causes are believed to be a combination of genetics and central obesity. Recommendations for metabolic syndrome include increasing physical activity, losing weight, and making dietary changes.

Inflammatory Response and C-Reactive Protein
Inflammation is well established as a factor in all stages of atherosclerosis. Several blood test markers can be used to

identify and measure an ongoing inflammatory response, and elevated levels of **C-reactive protein,** fibrinogen, and white blood cell count have been associated with an increased risk of CVD. High levels of C-reactive protein are associated with increased risk for coronary

___

C-reactive protein
Blood marker for inflammation that may indicate an increased risk for coronary heart disease.

___

heart disease in both men and women and have also been associated with more rapid progression of CVD.

Routine screening of all populations for C-reactive protein is not recommended at this time. Such screening may be helpful for people at moderate risk for CVD due to other risk factors. Aspirin and statin medications, which are used to lower LDL cholesterol levels, have been shown to reduce C-reactive protein levels, but, again, it remains unclear whether these drugs should be used for elevated C-reactive protein independent of other risk factors.[20, 21]

Infectious Agents Hard as it may be to believe, increasing evidence suggests that infections play a role in CVD. Infections appear to promote atherosclerosis and may cause atherosclerotic plaques to break free and block arteries. *Chlamydia pneumoniae*, a strain of *Chlamydia* that causes lung infections (not the strain that causes the sexually transmitted disease), was the first organism to be shown to have a potential role. The organism was found in 59 percent of arteries containing atherosclerotic plaques and only 3 percent of arteries without atherosclerotic plaques. Other studies have shown an association between heart attack and stroke in the month of a respiratory infection and pneumonia. Risk appears to be greatest in the few days to a week after infection. Lung infections may stress the heart by causing an increase in oxygen demand.

There still is no conclusive evidence to support the use of antibiotics to reduce risk of infection-associated CVD. However, two vaccines can significantly reduce the risk of influenza and pneumococcal pneumonia (the most common form of bacterial pneumonia). The influenza vaccine is routinely recommended annually for all adults aged 50 or older or at any age if a person has a medical indication such as heart disease or lung disease. The pneumococcal vaccine is recommended once at age 65 or earlier if a medical indication is present.[22–25]

Fetal Origins Research has shown a relationship between birth weight and risk of CVD, with lower birth weight associated with higher risk. This represents what is called a *programming phenomenon*. Tissues (in this case the heart muscle and blood vessels) may be damaged during a sensitive stage of fetal development in a way that programs them to develop problems later in life. Changes may occur due to undernutrition. Poor fetal growth has been associated with increased risk of other common adult health problems as well, such as hypertension, stroke, diabetes, and obesity.[26, 27] Such findings further demonstrate the importance of providing healthy conditions for prenatal development.

NONCONTROLLABLE RISK FACTORS IN CVD

Age, gender, ethnicity and race, family history, and postmenopausal status are the noncontrollable risk factors for cardiovascular disease (see the box "Risk for CVD by Age, Gender, Race/Ethnicity, and Geographical Location"). Individuals with noncontrollable risk factors, especially, should choose healthy behaviors that do not promote CVD.

Age and CVD Risk Age is probably the most important noncontrollable risk factor. The Framingham Study confirmed a progressive increase in CVD risk with each additional year of life, probably reflecting the progressive nature of atherosclerosis. There is a significant rise in deaths due to heart disease and stroke after age 65. Heart disease and stroke are responsible for 40 percent of deaths in people aged 65 to 74 and for 60 percent of deaths in people over age 85. Age alone does not cause CVD, however; there is great variation in CVD among older people of the same age.[28]

Gender and CVD Risk Although heart disease is often thought of as a man's disease, CVD is the leading cause of death for both men and women. There are some differences between the sexes, however. A 40-year-old man without evidence of heart disease has a 1 in 2 chance of developing CVD in his lifetime, whereas a 40-year-old woman has a 1 in 3 chance. Women tend to develop heart disease about 10 years later than men, perhaps because of the protective effect of estrogen before menopause. After age 50 (the average age of menopause), the difference in risk between men and women starts to decrease.

The death rates for CVD are higher in women, both Black women and White women; this is true of heart attack, stroke, hypertension, and congestive heart failure. One reason for this is that women tend to be older and frailer when they develop heart disease and so are less likely to survive. Another reason is that women are more likely to have either no symptoms before a heart attack or symptoms that make the diagnosis of heart disease more confusing, such as stomach complaints. One study showed that women delay seeking treatment as much as 3.5 hours longer than men do. Because

treatment is more effective the sooner it is started, this delay means that more damage occurs. A third reason is that health care providers may also delay treatment because they do not recognize the symptoms or are less likely to think about heart disease in women.[1]

Genetics and Family History and CVD Risk Individuals who have a relative with a history of CVD have a higher risk of CVD themselves. The risk for heart attack appears to be greatest if a male relative had a heart attack before age 55 or a female relative had a heart attack before age 65. The risk for stroke is increased if a relative has had a stroke, regardless of age. High rates of CVD in a family may be related to genetics or lifestyle patterns or both. A large part of the family risk is due to other risk factors such as hypertension, elevated lipids, and diabetes. As mentioned previously, a history in the family of sudden cardiac death at a young age is

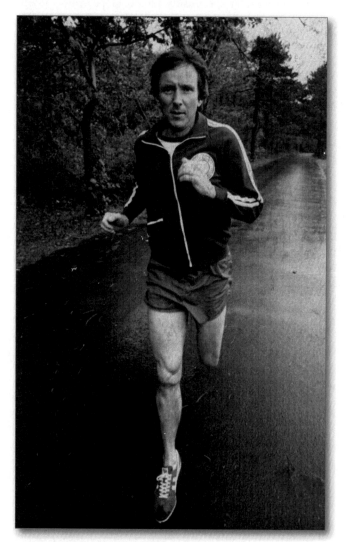

■ After his father died of a heart attack at age 43, Jim Fixx took up running and published the best-selling book *The Complete Book of Running*. When he died suddenly of a heart attack, the running world was stunned. An autopsy revealed that his coronary arteries were almost completely blocked by atherosclerotic plaque. His death at 52 suggests that his condition had a strong genetic component.

Who's at Risk

Risk for CVD by Age, Gender, Race/Ethnicity, and Geographical Location

Noncontrollable risk factors for CVD include age, gender, and race/ethnicity, among others. Risk for CVD also varies by the state in which a person lives. Why do you think geographical location makes a difference in risk for CVD?

Prevalence of CVD in Adults Aged 20 and Older by Age and Gender

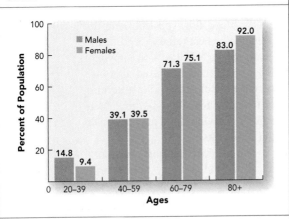

Source: Reprinted with the permission from Heart Disease and Stroke Statistics—2008 Update. *Copyright © 2008 American Heart Association, Inc.*

Prevalence of Hypertension in Adults by Age, Gender, and Race/Ethnicity

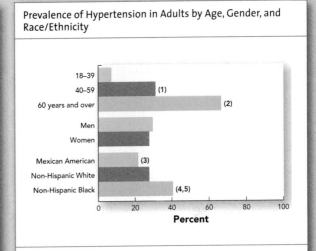

Source: Data from National Center for Health Statistics, National Health and Nutrition Examination Survey, 1999–2004.

Prevalence of Heart Attack or Coronary Artery Disease Among Adults Aged 18 and Older, by U.S. State

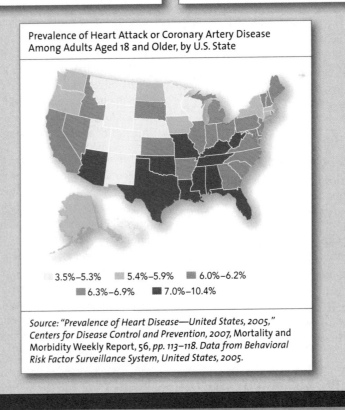

3.5%–5.3% 5.4%–5.9% 6.0%–6.2%
6.3%–6.9% 7.0%–10.4%

Source: "Prevalence of Heart Disease—United States, 2005," Centers for Disease Control and Prevention, 2007, Mortality and Morbidity Weekly Report, 56, pp. 113–118. Data from Behavioral Risk Factor Surveillance System, United States, 2005.

important, since it may signify a genetic risk for cardiomyopathy or another congenital cardiac disease.[6, 8]

Ethnicity and Race and CVD Risk Minority and low-income populations in the United States carry a disproportionate burden of CVD. Blacks have a higher risk of CVD and stroke than do Whites, as well as higher rates of hypertension, obesity, and diabetes. Mexican Americans, American Indians, and Native Hawaiians also have a higher risk of CVD than do Whites, along with higher rates of obesity and diabetes.

Recent improvements in cardiovascular health have not been shared evenly by all racial or ethnic groups. Although the death rate from heart attack has declined across all groups, it has declined less among minority groups and women. Several pathways may lead to these health disparities, including differences in such risk factors as hypertension, genetics, stress, and psychosocial factors.[29]

Postmenopausal Status and CVD Risk The hormone estrogen has long been thought to protect premenopausal women from CVD. When levels of estrogen fall during menopause, levels of HDL also decline, and body fat distribution shifts to a more central distribution pattern, similar to the male pattern.

For many years, medical practitioners prescribed hormone replacement therapy (HRT) for postmenopausal women to relieve the symptoms of menopause, lower the risk of osteoporosis (bone thinning), and reduce the risk of CVD. The belief in the benefits of estrogen was so strong that at one point, nearly one in three postmenopausal women was on HRT. As described in Chapter 15, research has now shown that HRT actually increases rather than decreases the risk of heart attack and stroke. HRT is still prescribed as a treatment for the symptoms of menopause and prevention of osteoporosis, but these benefits must now be weighed against an individual woman's risk for CVD.[30]

Testing and Treatment

People with no symptoms of CVD are usually not tested for evidence of disease; instead the focus is on screening for risk factors (hypertension, cholesterol levels, family health history, and so on). An exception is people in certain occupations, such as airline pilots or truck drivers, whose sudden incapacity would place other people at risk. Such individuals may be tested for asymptomatic CVD as part of an employment physical examination. People may also be screened for signs of CVD before surgery, and the American College of Sports Medicine recommends that an exercise stress test be performed on men older than age 40 and women older than age 50 if they are sedentary and about to begin an exercise program.

TESTING AND TREATMENT FOR HEART DISEASE

For people with a family history of sudden death or symptoms suggestive of CVD, such as shortness of breath, dizziness, or exertional chest pain, physical examination and diagnostic tests can determine the presence of disease and the extent of the problem. If disease is present, a variety of steps can be taken, from lifestyle changes, to medication, to surgery.

Diagnostic Testing for Heart Disease Several tests are available to evaluate heart function and determine if underlying disease is present. An **electrocardiogram** (ECG or EKG), a record of the electrical activity of the heart as it beats, can detect abnormal rhythms, inadequate blood flow (possibly due to ischemia or heart attack), and heart enlargement. A *Holter* or *event monitor* is an ECG that is worn at home during normal activity for a period of time (such as 24 hours) to detect abnormal rhythms that may be causing symptoms.

An **echocardiogram** (or echo), an ultrasound test that uses sound waves to visualize the heart structure and motion, can detect structural abnormalities (changes in the underlying structure of the valves, arteries, or heart chambers), thickness of the muscle walls, and how well the heart pumps. An **exercise stress test** evaluates how well the heart functions with exercise.

Blood tests can be performed to detect certain proteins in the blood that are released by a damaged heart muscle. A variety of other procedures allows visualization of the heart, heart valves, and any blocked or narrowed coronary arteries; they include **coronary angiogram** (injection of a dye with multiple X-rays), computerized tomography (CT) scans, and magnetic resonance imaging (MRI).

Medical Management of Heart Disease Multiple categories of medications can be used in the treatment of heart disease, depending on the underlying problem. There are medications that help control heart rhythm (anti-arrhythmics), dilate the coronary arteries and reduce angina (anti-anginals), decrease blood clotting (anti-coagulants), and dissolve blood clots during a heart attack (thrombolytics).

When a heart attack occurs, emergency treatment is critical. The effectiveness of treatment depends on the time elapsed from first symptoms until the reestablishment of blood flow to the heart muscle. Thrombolytics are most effective when given within the first hour after a heart attack. Other medications are used to control risk factors and reduce the chance of developing heart disease or a recurrence of heart disease. These include anti-hypertensives, cholesterol-lowering medications, and antiplatelet medications.

Surgical Management of Heart Disease Every day thousands of people have heart surgery; there are many dif-

electrocardiogram
Record of the heart's electrical activity as it beats.

echocardiogram
Diagnostic test for a heart attack in which sound waves are used to visualize heart valves, heart wall movement, and overall heart function.

exercise stress test
Procedure that evaluates how well the heart functions with exercise.

coronary angiogram
Diagnostic test for a heart attack in which a dye is injected into a fine catheter that is passed into the heart and X-rays are taken as the dye moves through the heart, showing any blocked or narrowed coronary arteries.

ferent types of surgery, depending on the underlying problem. For structural abnormalities, surgeons can repair or replace heart valves, close septal defects (holes) that allow blood to flow abnormally, reposition arteries and veins that are attached incorrectly, and repair aneurysms in the aorta. If the problem is related to abnormal electrical conduction through the heart, a cardiologist can destroy a small amount of heart tissue in an area that is disturbing the flow of electricity or can implant a defibrillator into the chest that will automatically shock the heart if a life-threatening arrhythmia develops. Also, often as a last resort, a surgeon can replace a damaged heart completely with a heart from a donor.

angioplasty
Procedure to reopen a blocked coronary artery, in which a balloon catheter (a thin plastic tube) is threaded into the narrowed area and inflated to stretch the vessel open again.

coronary artery bypass grafting
Surgical procedure in which a healthy blood vessel is taken from another part of the body and grafted to the coronary arteries to allow a bypass of blood flow around a narrowed vessel.

If the underlying abnormality is related to coronary artery disease, a few surgical options exist. One is **angioplasty**, in which a balloon catheter (a thin plastic tube) is threaded into a blocked or narrowed artery and inflated to stretch the vessel open again. A *coronary stent,* a springy framework that supports the vessel walls and keeps the vessel open, is often permanently placed in the artery to prevent it from closing again. Another surgical option is **coronary artery bypass grafting,** usually just called *bypass.* A healthy blood vessel is taken from another part of the body, usually the leg, and grafted to the coronary arteries to allow a bypass of blood flow around a narrowed vessel.

TESTING AND TREATMENT FOR STROKE

Before the 1990s, little could be done to alter the natural course of a stroke. Today we know that the same thrombolytic (clot-dissolving) medications used in heart attacks can decrease the damage incurred by a stroke. As with heart attacks, the clot-dissolving medications work best when given soon after the onset of symptoms; in fact, they can be administered only within the first 3 hours of the onset of symptoms. Thus, it is critical that a person experiencing symptoms of a stroke receive medical care immediately.

Diagnostic Testing for Stroke   At the hospital, a CT scan or an MRI can be used to generate images of the brain and blood flow and to determine whether a stroke has occurred. These tests can also show whether a stroke has been caused by a blockage or by a hemorrhage. Further testing may be done to find the source of the blockage. The carotid arteries, the large arteries on the sides of the neck that supply blood to the brain, are examined to see if they are blocked with atherosclerotic plaques. If so, part of the plaque may have broken off and become the source of an embolism blocking a blood vessel in the brain.

Management of Stroke   If a stroke is found to be thrombotic (caused by a blockage) and there is no evidence

of bleeding in the brain, thrombolytic medications can be administered to dissolve the clot and restore blood flow to the brain. Thrombolytic medications must not be given if the stroke is hemorrhagic, because they can cause increased bleeding. Aspirin and other anticlotting medications can be used after a thrombotic stroke to reduce the risk of another stroke. Control of blood pressure and other risk factors is important for all people who have a stroke, whether thrombotic or hemorrhagic.

Rehabilitation is a component of treatment for stroke. If an area of the brain is damaged or destroyed, the functions that were controlled by that part of the brain will be impaired. Rehabilitation consists of physical therapy (to strengthen muscles and coordination), speech therapy (to improve communication and eating), and occupational therapy (to improve activities of daily living and job retraining if appropriate). Progress and return of functions vary by individual. Some people recover fully within a few days to weeks, while others are left with long-term impairment.

Protecting Yourself from CVD

As scientists learn more about the progressive nature of cardiovascular disease, the significance of early prevention becomes clearer. Adopting healthy lifestyle habits now, regardless of your age or current health status, is the best way to reduce your risk of developing CVD in the future.

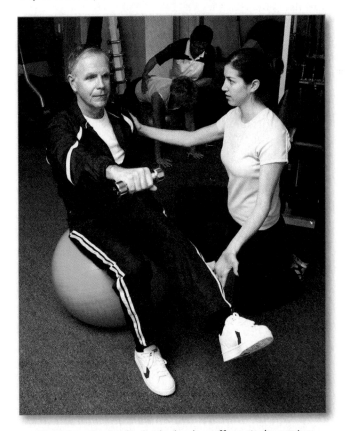

■ About two-thirds of individuals who suffer a stroke survive and require rehabilitation. When a stroke has caused muscle weakness or paralysis, therapy focuses on regaining use of impaired limbs, improving coordination and balance, and developing strategies for bypassing deficits.

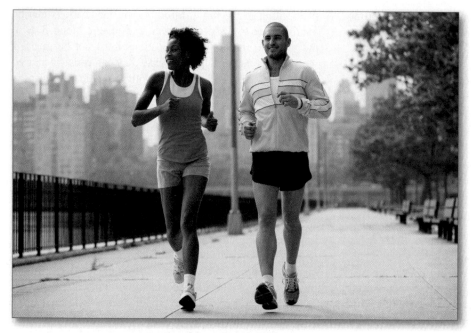

■ Cardiorespiratory endurance exercise is one of the best antidotes to heart disease. The current recommendation for most adults is 30 minutes of moderate-intensity physical activity on most days of the week or 20 minutes of vigorous activity on three days of the week.

EATING FOR HEART HEALTH

Diet and nutrition have been extensively studied and found to alter risk for heart disease and stroke. Diet also plays a role in controlling the major risk factors such as diabetes, hypertension, and obesity. A diet that supports cardiovascular health emphasizes fruits, vegetables, whole grains, low-fat dairy products, fish, and lean meat and poultry. The American Heart Association Dietary Guidelines are summarized in the box "Choosing a Heart-Healthy Diet."

Micronutrients appear to play a role in cardiovascular health. Many micronutrients, especially antioxidants, are more plentiful in a plant-based diet than in a diet based on foods from animal sources. Foods high in important antioxidants are brightly colored fruits and vegetables and nuts and seeds (see Chapter 7). Experts recommend that micronutrients be consumed in foods rather than in supplements.

One supplement that may be beneficial for some people with CVD is coenzyme Q_{10} (CoQ_{10}), an enzyme used by cells in energy production that may have a special role in the health of heart muscle. Levels of CoQ_{10} are lower in some people with heart disease, and levels may decrease progressively with the severity of the disease. Supplementation may improve symptoms and survival rates for people with some forms of heart disease, although there is no general recommendation at this time.[31]

Other specific foods have been shown to alter cholesterol levels. Soy products and legumes, such as lentils and chickpeas, have both been shown to decrease LDL. Garlic appears to have a similar effect on total cholesterol, although fresh garlic (one to two cloves per day) is recommended over synthesized garlic capsules. Foods rich in fiber also help reduce cholesterol levels; they include fruits, vegetables, oats, and barley.

EXERCISING REGULARLY

Exercise has an effect on many CVD risk factors. It has a direct conditioning effect on the heart, improving the health of the heart muscle and enhancing its ability to pump blood efficiently. Exercise helps in weight loss and weight-maintenance programs by increasing energy output. It also has more subtle effects, such as improving HDL levels and increasing the number of insulin receptors, which enhances the ability of people with diabetes to use insulin. Even low-intensity activities, such as walking, gardening, or climbing stairs, can be helpful. See Chapter 8 for more information on exercising for health and fitness.

AVOIDING TOBACCO USE

Smoking is the leading preventable cause of CVD. It poses both an immediate hazard for heart attack and a long-term hazard for atherosclerosis. Because nicotine is so addictive, the best prevention is never to start smoking. If you do smoke, quitting now can significantly reduce your risk of developing CVD. See Chapter 13 for more information on tobacco use and strategies for quitting.

CONTROLLING BLOOD PRESSURE

Regular screening for hypertension is recommended for individuals over age 18.[1] For anyone in the prehypertension or hypertension category, lifestyle changes are recommended, including weight reduction, dietary changes, low salt intake, physical activity, and moderate alcohol intake.[4] If lifestyle changes alone do not reduce blood pressure, medications are recommended. Hypertension can be controlled in most cases, but sometimes it takes lifestyle change plus two or more medications.

The DASH diet was developed to reduce elevated blood pressure (see Chapter 7). The *2005 Dietary Guidelines for Americans* recommends a limit of 1,500 mg of sodium per day for individuals with hypertension, middle-aged and older adults, and Blacks.

MANAGING CHOLESTEROL LEVELS

The National Cholesterol Education Program recommends that all adults over age 20 have their cholesterol checked at least once every 5 years. If you find that your LDL cholesterol levels, in combination with other risk factors, put you at risk for CVD, your physician will work with you to develop an LDL goal and a plan for reaching it. Exercising, maintaining a healthy weight, and dietary changes, including reducing total and saturated fat intake and increasing dietary fiber, are first-line actions.

However, as with high blood pressure, these changes may not be enough for some people and medication may be required. Some cholesterol-lowering drugs decrease cholesterol absorption from the diet; others decrease cholesterol synthesis by the liver. Taking medication to control cholesterol levels is complicated and should always be done under the guidance of a health care provider.[11, 12, 32]

USING ASPIRIN THERAPY

Nearly 36 percent of American adults—more than 50 million people—take aspirin regularly to reduce their risk of CVD. Aspirin inhibits the clotting function of platelets and thus reduces the risk of blood clots. However, aspirin also increases the risk of bleeding, and the higher the aspirin dose, the greater the risk of bleeding.

Aspirin is generally recommended for anyone who has a history of heart attack, unstable angina, ischemic stroke, or transient ischemic attack if the person has no contraindications (such as allergy to aspirin or a history of bleeding ulcer). In others, both men and women, benefits have to be weighed against risks, and decisions should be made in collaboration with a physician.[33]

CONTROLLING DIABETES

People with diabetes must control their blood glucose levels to reduce their risk of cardiovascular complications. For Type-1 diabetes, in which the pancreas produces no insulin, treatment requires lifelong self-administered insulin injections to maintain blood glucose levels as close to normal as possible. For Type-2 diabetes, in which body cells no longer respond well to insulin, exercise and weight loss are often enough to correct the condition without medication. When needed, pills can be taken to help improve the cellular response to insulin, or insulin injections may be given. People with diabetes also have to control their other CVD risk factors, such as high cholesterol levels, high triglyceride levels, and high blood pressure, all of which are more likely to occur in association with this disorder.[1]

MANAGING STRESS AND IMPROVING MENTAL HEALTH

Stress, anger, hostility, and depression can all contribute to CVD. If you frequently feel overwhelmed by negative feelings and moods, try some of the stress management and relaxation techniques described in Chapters 3, 4, and 5. You may want to increase your social support system by expanding your connections to family, friends, community, or church. You may want to simplify your schedule and slow down. Meditating can lower blood pressure and blood cholesterol levels, thereby slowing the process of atherosclerosis. Biofeedback may help reduce blood pressure. Hypnosis may be useful to help control hypertension and other chronic health problems. Whatever approach you choose to manage stress and enhance your mental health, try to incorporate a daily practice into your life.

Challenges & Choices

Choosing a Heart-Healthy Diet

The American Heart Association encourages all Americans, young and old, to adopt a heart-healthy diet. AHA guidelines include the following recommendations:

- Balance your calories in to calories out. Don't eat more calories than you use each day. Aim for at least 30 minutes of moderate physical exercise on most days of the week.

- Eat a variety of nutritious foods from all the food groups. Eat plenty of nutrient-rich foods such as fruits, vegetables, and whole-grain products. These are high in vitamins, minerals, and fiber and are low in calories.

- Aim to eat fish twice a week; omega-3 fatty acids may reduce risk of CVD.

- Eat less of the foods that are low in nutrients and high in calories:
  - Choose lean meats and poultry without skin, and prepare them without added saturated fats and trans fat.
  - Choose fat-free or 1 percent fat dairy products.
  - Avoid consumption of trans fatty acids, found in foods containing partially hydrogenated vegetable oils, such as fried foods, margarines, and commercial baked goods.
  - Aim to limit dietary cholesterol to no more than 300 mg per day.
  - Cut back on drinks and foods with added sugar.
  - Aim to eat less than 2,300 mg of salt per day.
  - If you drink alcohol, drink in moderation—for women, no more than one drink per day, and for men, no more than two drinks per day.

It's Not Just Personal...

People in Mediterranean countries have lower rates of heart disease than people in the United States and other parts of the developed world. It's not clear whether the Mediterranean diet—rich in fruits, vegetables, olive oil, and fish—is responsible for this difference (see Chapter 7), or whether other lifestyle factors, such as physical activity and social support systems, also play an important role. More research is needed to make these relationships clearer.

Source: Data from the American Heart Association, www.americanheart.org.

You Make the Call

Screening for Cardiovascular Disease in Athletes: How Much Is Enough?

Sudden cardiac arrest is the most common cause of death in young athletes (those younger than age 35). Vigorous exercise is a trigger for lethal arrhythmias in athletes with unrecognized heart disease, typically congenital disease. On average, only 11 percent of athletes will survive a sudden cardiac arrest—a worse outcome than might be expected, given their age, fitness level, and the fact that many of these events are witnessed. The low survival rates may be due to the underlying congenital disease, the exertion at the time of arrest, or slow recognition by bystanders of what has happened. These low survival rates highlight the critical importance of early recognition of underlying disease.

Currently, there are no nationally mandated screening standards for high school athletes in the United States. Many states do require preparticipation sports physicals for middle or high school students participating in organized sports, and the National College Athletic Association (NCAA) has recently mandated a preparticipation evaluation for all Division I, II, and III athletes. The traditional evaluation involves a visit to a health care provider for review of an athlete's personal and family history and a physical exam, with findings suggestive of heart disease prompting further evaluation. This screening has limitations, however, because 60–80 percent of athletes have no symptoms, many have no family history of CVD or don't know their family history, and results of physical exams are normal in many people with congenital heart problems.

In 1979 a national program that added electrocardiogram (ECG) screening to the traditional screening was started in Italy. The addition of ECG identified many asymptomatic athletes whose conditions would have gone unrecognized by traditional screening. Since adding ECG screening, the incidence of sudden cardiac death among athletes in Italy has been reduced by 90 percent. The European Society of Cardiology (ESC) and the International Olympic Committee (IOC) recently adopted similar recommendations.

Some health experts think the United States should add ECG screening as a national preparticipation requirement for high school and college athletes, pointing to the healthy young people whose lives would be saved. The prohibiting factor is cost: If national screening were adopted, an estimated 10 million athletes would require screening at a theoretical cost of $2 billion dollars a year or approximately $330,000 for each athlete detected with cardiac disease. Another problem is the number of false-positive results that would occur—abnormal ECG findings in athletes who do not have underlying cardiac disease. An estimated 10 percent of results could be false positives. With further evaluation, only 2 percent of these athletes would be found to have cardiac disease, and 8 percent would have had to go through the stress of an additional workup and temporary disqualification from their sport unnecessarily.

In a 2007 review the American Heart Association did not recommend the addition of ECG screening for American athletes. Although they found the ESC and IOC recommendations an "admirable proposal deserving serious consideration," they concluded that such a program was unrealistic in the United States due to the financial resources, staffing, and logistics required for a national screening program.

Proponents of the additional ECG screening argue that any measures that save the lives of otherwise healthy young adults are worth the time and money invested. Opponents respond that such measures are unrealistic and impractical at this time. What do you think?

PROS

- Because survival rates from sudden cardiac arrest are very low, prevention is critical.

- Although it may be expensive and result in some false positives, the ECG is a straightforward, noninvasive test, and further evaluation is done with another noninvasive test, the echocardiogram.

- Italy demonstrated the will to save lives by adding ECG screening to its other athletic screening requirements. If a small country like Italy can institute such screening, a large, wealthy country like the Untied States should be able to do so, too.

- Cost should not be a factor when the lives of otherwise healthy young adults are at stake.

CONS

- The high rate of false positives from ECGs means that many athletes would be unnecessarily sidelined from their sports while awaiting further evaluation.

- Because of its larger population and geographical size, the United States cannot do ECG screening with the same ease as Italy or other European countries. The United States does not have the infrastructure (staffing, finances) to support a national program adding ECG screening.

- There isn't even a national requirement for the traditional screening (personal history, family history, and physical exam) in the United States right now. Thus, it is unrealistic to talk about adding an ECG requirement.

Source: "Recommendations and Considerations Related to Preparticipation Screening for Cardiovascular Abnormalities in Competitive Athletes: 2007 Update: A Scientific Statement from the American Heart Association Council on Nutrition, Physical Activity, and Metabolism," by B.J. Maron, P.D. Thompson, M.J. Ackerman, et al., 2007, Circulation, 115, pp. 1643–1655.

In Review

1. **What is the cardiovascular system, and how does it work?** The heart, a four-chambered, fist-sized muscle, pumps blood throughout the body (systemic circulation) and to and from the lungs (pulmonary circulation) via the blood vessels—arteries, veins, and capillaries. Arteries carry oxygen-rich blood to the body's cells, and veins carry deoxygenated blood back to the heart and from there to the lungs, where oxygen is replenished.

2. **What is cardiovascular disease?** The disease process underlying most forms of CVD is atherosclerosis, a condition in which the arteries become clogged and blood flow is restricted, causing heart attack, stroke, or peripheral vascular disease. A disturbance in the electrical signals controlling the heartbeat can cause an arrhythmia (disorganized beating) and sudden cardiac arrest. Other forms of CVD are hypertension (high blood pressure), congestive heart failure, heart valve disorders, rheumatic heart disease, congenital heart disease, and cardiomyopathy (disease of the heart muscle). A stroke occurs either when a blood vessel serving the brain is blocked or when a blood vessel in the brain ruptures.

3. **What are the risk factors for CVD?** The six major controllable risk factors are tobacco use, hypertension, unhealthy blood cholesterol levels, physical inactivity, obesity, and diabetes. The five major noncontrollable risk factors are older age, male gender, a genetic predisposition, Black or other minority racial/ethnic status, and postmenopausal status. Numerous other contributing and possible risk factors have been identified, including psychosocial factors such as a hostility-prone personality and chronic stress.

4. **How is CVD diagnosed and treated?** If warranted by family history or symptoms, diagnostic tests can be performed to determine if CVD is present; tests include electrocardiogram, echocardiogram, exercise stress test, blood tests, and a variety of procedures that produce images of the heart and blood vessels. CVD can be managed medically (with drugs) and surgically. Stroke is diagnosed by procedures that produce images of the brain. Some strokes can be treated with drugs, but many cause brain damage requiring rehabilitation.

5. **What are the best ways to avoid CVD?** Eating a heart-healthy diet from a young age is important, as are getting regular exercise, avoiding tobacco use, knowing and managing blood pressure and cholesterol levels, controlling diabetes, and managing stress.

 For a detailed summary of this chapter and a comprehensive set of review questions, visit the Online Learning Center at **www.mhhe.com/teague2e**.

Web Resources

American Heart Association: This organization offers information on diseases and conditions that affect the heart, including a heart and stroke encyclopedia. The site also includes dietary and fitness advice for planning a healthier lifestyle.
www.americanheart.org

Centers for Disease Control and Prevention: A good resource for information on heart-related diseases and conditions, this site features health promotion activities for teens to older adults.
www.cdc.gov

National Heart, Lung, and Blood Institute: Besides information about many heart and vascular diseases and conditions, this site features health assessment tools and recipes for healthy eating.
www.nhlbi.nih.gov

National Institutes of Health: This site is a resource for wide-ranging information on health, including the heart and circulation. NIH's MEDLINEPlus covers more than 700 health topics and offers drug information, a medical encyclopedia, directories, and other resources.
www.nih.gov

National Stroke Association: This organization offers comprehensive information about stroke, including risks, symptoms, treatment approaches, and recovery and rehabilitation.
www.stroke.org

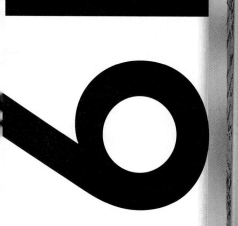

Chapter

19

Cancer
Understanding a Complex Condition

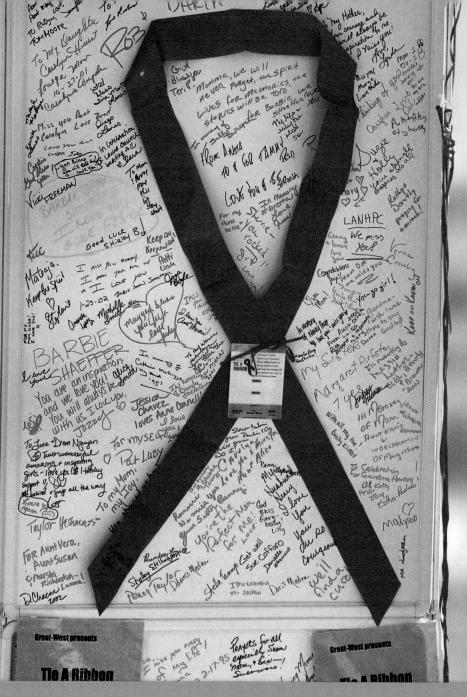

WWW

Your Health Today

www.mhhe.com/teague2e

Go to the Online Learning Center for *Your Health Today* for interactive activities, quizzes, flashcards, Web links, and more resources related to this chapter.

Ever Wonder...

- if it's safer to tan at a tanning salon than in the sun?

- why some people who smoke get lung cancer and others don't?

- if someone who gets cancer can ever be fully cured?

Cancer, the second leading cause of death in the United States, has probably always been part of life. Human remains from thousands of years ago show evidence of cancer; the disease is found in all mammalian species and in many other organisms. Despite its ubiquity, cancer has long been shrouded in mystery, fear, and even shame. In the past, people with cancer often hid their diagnosis; the word *cancer* was not used even in obituaries. Today, with greater understanding of this complex condition, cancer patients have higher survival rates, better prospects for a cure, and more social support. Although there is still much to learn, there is cause for optimism.

The American Cancer society projects an estimated 1.44 million new cancer cases in 2008 and more than 565,000 deaths from cancer, about 1,500 per day. Cancer causes about 23 percent of all deaths in the United States, with lung cancer the leading killer among both men and women. The four most common cancers—lung, colon, breast, and prostate—combined account for nearly half of all cancer deaths[1] (Figure 19.1). In this chapter we provide an overview of the many forms cancer takes and the steps you can follow to reduce your risk of developing this disease.

What Is Cancer?

Cancer is a condition characterized by the uncontrolled growth of cells. It develops from a single cell that goes awry, but a combination of events must occur before the cell turns into a **tumor**. The process by which this occurs is called *clonal growth,* the replication of a single cell such that it produces thousands of copies of itself in an uncontrolled manner. With 30 billion cells in a healthy person, the fact that one out of three people develops cancer is not surprising; what is surprising is that two out of three people do not.

cancer
Condition characterized by the uncontrolled growth of cells.

tumor
Mass of extra tissue.

HEALTHY CELL GROWTH

Healthy cells have a complicated system of checks and balances that control cell growth and division. From the start, beginning with the single-celled fertilized egg, cells develop in contact with other cells, sending and receiving messages about how much space is available for growth. Healthy cells in solid tissues (all tissues except the blood) require the presence of neighboring cells. This tendency to stick together serves as a safety mechanism, discouraging cells from drifting off and starting to grow independently.

Healthy cells divide when needed to replace cells that have died or been sloughed off. Each time a cell divides, there is a possibility that a mutation, an error in DNA replication, will occur. Mutations are always occurring randomly,

Estimated New Cases*		Estimated Deaths	
Male	**Female**	**Male**	**Female**
Prostate 186,320 (25%)	Breast 182,460 (26%)	Lung and bronchus 90,810 (31%)	Lung and bronchus 71,030 (26%)
Lung and bronchus 114,690 (15%)	Lung and bronchus 100,330 (14%)	Prostate 28,660 (10%)	Breast 40,480 (15%)
Colon and rectum 77,250 (10%)	Colon and rectum 71,560 (10%)	Colon and rectum 24,260 (8%)	Colon and rectum 25,700 (9%)
Urinary bladder 51,230 (7%)	Uterine corpus 40,100 (6%)	Pancreas 17,500 (6%)	Pancreas 16,790 (6%)
Non-Hodgkin's lymphoma 35,450 (5%)	Non-Hodgkin's lymphoma 30,670 (4%)	Liver and intrahepatic bile duct 12,570 (4%)	Ovary 15,520 (6%)
Melanoma of the skin 34,950 (5%)	Thyroid 28,410 (4%)	Leukemia 12,460 (4%)	Non-Hodgkin's lymphoma 9,370 (3%)
Kidney and renal pelvis 33,130 (4%)	Melanoma of the skin 27,530 (4%)	Esophagus 11,250 (4%)	Leukemia 9,250 (3%)
Oral cavity and pharynx 25,310 (3%)	Ovary 21,650 (3%)	Urinary bladder 9,950 (3%)	Uterine corpus 7,470 (3%)
Leukemia 25,180 (3%)	Kidney and renal pelvis 21,260 (3%)	Non-Hodgkin's lymphoma 9,790 (3%)	Liver and intrahepatic bile duct 5,840 (2%)
Pancreas 18,770 (3%)	Leukemia 19,090 (3%)	Kidney and renal pelvis 8,100 (3%)	Brain and other nervous system 5,650 (2%)
All sites 745,180 (100%)	All sites 692,000 (100%)	All sites 294,120 (100%)	All sites 271,530 (100%)

*Excludes basal and squamous cell skin cancers and in situ carcinoma except urinary bladder.

figure **19.1** **Leading sites of new cancer cases and deaths, 2008 estimates.**
Source: American Cancer Society Cancer Facts and Figures 2008. *Atlanta: American Cancer Society, Inc. Reprinted with permission.*

but the risk of mutations is increased by exposure to certain substances, such as tobacco smoke, radiation, and toxic chemicals. Certain mutations may start the cell on a path toward cancer. Specific mechanisms are designed to correct genetic mutations and destroy cells with mutations.

As one mechanism, enzymes within the nucleus of each cell scan the DNA as it replicates, looking for errors. If an error is detected, the enzyme backtracks and repairs it. If too much DNA damage is detected and cannot be repaired, cells have a program for self-destruction, or cellular suicide. As another safety mechanism, cells are programmed to divide a certain number of times, and then they become incapable of further division. At this point, the cells die and the particular *cell line* (all the cells that originated from an initial cell) is lost, along with any mutations that might have occurred within it.

The immune system also helps watch for cells that are not growing normally. Cancer cells often display an antigen, like a flag, on their cell surface; when the antigen is detected by the immune cells, the cell is labeled for destruction. If a cell has been infected by a cancer-causing virus, it also displays viral antigens on its surface, and again, the immune system labels and destroys it.

A special protective mechanism exists for certain cells called **stem cells.** These are cells that did not differentiate into specific cell types (for example, nerve cells, skin cells, bone cells) during prenatal development. Instead, they retain the ability to become different cell types, and they are capable of unlimited division. A small number of stem cells are present within most tissue types, where they are needed to replace lost or damaged cell lines. They are found in highest numbers within the skin, blood, lung lining, intestines, endocrine cells, and liver—all tissues with a high rate of turnover and replacement.

stem cells
Undifferentiated cells capable of unlimited division that can give rise to specialized cells.

Because stem cells do not have a predetermined number of cell divisions, they pose a risk for cancer. As a safety mechanism, they are located deep within tissues, where they are protected from factors that increase the risk of genetic mutations, such as exposure to the sun, chemicals, and irritation. Stem cells do have a system of self-destruction if they experience DNA damage or exposure to a toxin.

CANCER CELL GROWTH

Cancer starts from a single cell that undergoes a critical mutation, either as a result of an error in duplication or in response to a **carcinogen** or radiation. This *initiating event* allows a cell to evade one of the restraints placed upon healthy cells. To become a cancer, however, it must escape all the control mechanisms. Usually this process requires a series of 5 to 10 critical mutations within the cell's genetic material. It may take many years for these changes to progress to cancer, or they may never do so.

carcinogen
Cancer-causing substance or agent in the environment.

In time, perhaps a period of years, another mutation, such as one in an **oncogene** (a gene that drives cell growth regardless of signals from surrounding cells), may allow the cell line to divide forever rather than follow its preprogrammed number of divisions. A condition of cell overgrowth, called *hyperplasia*, develops at the site, and some cells may become abnormal, a condition called *dysplasia*. Eventually, a mass of extra tissue—a tumor—may develop.

oncogene
Gene that drives a cell to grow and divide regardless of signals from surrounding cells.

A **benign tumor** grows slowly and is unlikely to spread. Benign tumors are dangerous if they grow in locations where they interfere with normal functioning and cannot be completely removed without destroying healthy tissue, as in the brain. A **malignant tumor** is capable of invading surrounding tissue and spreading. Malignant cells do not stick together as much as normal cells, and as the tumor grows, some cancer cells may break off, enter the lymphatic system or the bloodstream, and travel to nearby lymph nodes or to distant sites in the body. At a new site, the cancerous cell can grow and become a secondary tumor, or **metastasis.** When a cancer spreads from one part of the body to another, it is said to have *metastasized.* The terms *malignant cancer* and *neoplasia* are frequently used interchangeably with *cancer.*

benign tumor
Tumor that grows slowly and is unlikely to spread.

malignant tumor
Tumor that is capable of invading surrounding tissue and spreading.

metastasis
Secondary tumor that appears when cancerous cells spread to other parts of the body.

CLASSIFYING CANCERS

Cancers are classified according to the tissue in which they originate, called the *primary site.* If a cancer originates in the cells lining the colon, for example, it is considered colon cancer, even when it metastasizes to other, secondary sites. The most common sites of metastases are the brain, liver, and bone marrow. Occasionally, the primary site of a cancer cannot be determined. When a cancer is still at its primary site, it is said to be *localized.* When it has metastasized, it is referred to as *invasive.* The greater the extent of metastasis, the poorer the *prognosis* (likely outcome).

Tumors are *graded* on the basis of the degree to which the tumor cells resemble healthy cells of the same tissue type under the microscope. If they are very similar, they are considered well differentiated and low grade (grade I); if they are very different, they are considered poorly differentiated and high grade (grade IV). A poorly differentiated, higher grade cancer grows more quickly, is more aggressive, and is more likely to metastasize.[1]

The *stage* of the disease is a description of how far the cancer has spread. Two systems of staging are used. In the first, there are five categories (stage 0, stage I, stage II, stage III, and stage IV). Stage 0 is also called *cancer in situ,* an early cancer that is present only in the layer of cells where it began. Stage I cancers are generally small and localized to the original site. Stage IV cancers have metastasized to distant sites. Stages II and III are locally advanced and may or may not involve local lymph nodes. Prognosis is related to the stage of a tumor but also depends on the kind of cancer.

In the other staging system, called *TNM*, tumors, nodes, and metastasis are rated based on size and extent of spread. Tumor size is rated from 0 to 4. A T1 tumor is a small local tumor that has not begun to invade local tissue, and a T4 tumor is a large tumor that has invaded surrounding structures. Nodes are rated in a similar way from 0 to 3. N0 means there is no lymph node spread, and N3 means extensive lymph node spread. Metastasis is either M0 (no metastases) or M1 (metastasis). So a cancer might be described as a T1, N2, M0 stage cancer.

TYPES OF CANCER

Different tissues of the body have different risks for cancer, due in part to their different rates of cell division. Four broad types of cancer are distinguished, based on the type of tissue in which they originate. **Carcinomas** arise from epithelial tissue, which includes the skin, the lining of the intestines and body cavities, the surface of body organs, and the outer portions of the glands. Epithelial tissue is frequently shed and replaced. From 80 to 90 percent of all cancers originate in epithelial tissues. **Sarcomas** originate in connective tissue, such as bone, tendon, cartilage, muscle, or fat tissues. **Leukemias** are cancers of the blood and originate in the bone marrow or the lymphatic system. **Lymphomas** originate in the lymph nodes or glands.

carcinomas
Cancers that arise from epithelial tissue.

sarcomas
Cancers that originate in connective tissue.

leukemias
Cancers of the blood, originating in the bone marrow or the lymphatic system.

lymphomas
Cancers that originate in the lymph nodes or glands.

Risk Factors for Cancer

Can cancer be prevented? Because some cancers occur as a result of random genetic mutations, there is an element of chance in the development of the disease. Other cancers are associated with inherited genetic mutations. Still others occur as a result of exposure to carcinogens. Some such exposures can be limited by lifestyle behaviors, such as using sunscreen, but others are beyond individual control and require the involvement of local authorities, the larger society, or even the international community, as in the case of air pollution (see the box "Cancer Incidence and Mortality by Race and Ethnicity").

In this section we consider several risk factors for cancer, as well as ways to reduce them or limit their effect. Risk factors are associated with a higher incidence of a disease but do not determine that the disease will occur. Some people without known risk factors develop cancer, and other people

with multiple risk factors do not. The most significant risk factor for most cancers is age. Advancing age increases the risk for cancer; 78 percent of cancers occur in people aged 55 or older.[1]

FAMILY HISTORY

A family history of cancer increases an individual's risk. As described in Chapter 2, the risk is higher if the cancer occurred in a first-degree relative (parent or sibling) than in a second-degree relative (grandparent, aunt, uncle, or cousin). Risk also varies by the age of the family member at the time of diagnosis and the number of family members with a cancer diagnosis.

Certain cancers, such as breast cancer and colon cancer, appear to have a stronger familial link than other cancers do. Approximately 5–10 percent of women diagnosed with breast cancer have a hereditary form of the disease. Inherited alterations in the genes BRCA1 and BRCA2 (Breast Cancer 1 and Breast Cancer 2) are involved in many of these cases.[2]

Approximately 25 percent of men and women diagnosed with colon cancer have a family history of colon cancer. Mutations have been identified to explain the increased risk for colon cancer in some families, but these account for only 5–6 percent of all colon cancer cases. If a family has two or more members with colon cancer, the possibility of an inherited genetic susceptibility is substantially higher.[3]

Examining your family health tree can help you understand whether you have an increased risk for any cancers. However, genes are not the entire story. Genes interact with environmental exposures and lifestyle behaviors to alter risk. Also influential are socioeconomic and cultural factors, the social determinants of health (see the box "Addressing Cancer Disparities"). If you find you are at increased risk due to family history or other factors, making lifestyle adjustments that can reduce your risk and overcoming barriers to get the recommended screening tests are especially important for you.

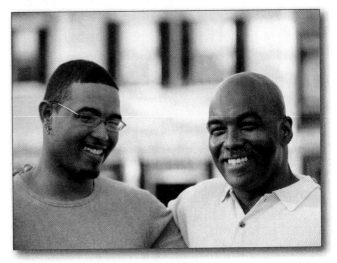

■ A family history of cancer can indicate that a person may have a genetic predisposition to the disease, especially if the cancer occurred in a first-degree relative (like a parent) at an early age. A healthy lifestyle is especially important when this is the case.

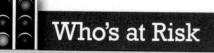

Who's at Risk

Cancer Incidence and Mortality by Race and Ethnicity

Cancer affects people of all races and ethnicities, but disparities in incidence (number of new cases) and mortality (number of deaths) between population groups are striking. For example, Black men have the highest incidence of prostate cancer and are more than twice as likely as White men to die from it. White women have the highest incidence of breast cancer, but Black women are more likely to die from it. Hispanic/Latina women have the highest incidence of cervical cancer, followed by Black women and then White women. Black women are more than twice as likely as White women and Asian American women to die from cervical cancer and somewhat more likely than Hispanic women.

What role is played by genetics in these disparities, and what role is played by the social determinants of health? Genetic differences are believed to play a minimal role. Most of the disparities are believed to be attributable to such factors as socioeconomic barriers to early cancer detection and treatment. These barriers are discussed further in the Public Health in Action box later in this chapter.

Cancer Incidence and Mortality by Race and Ethnicity, per 100,000 population

	White	African American	Asian American/ Pacific Islander	American Indian/ Alaska Native	Hispanic/Latino
Incidence					
All sites					
Male	556.7	663.7	359.9	321.2	421.3
Female	423.9	396.9	285.8	282.4	314.2
Prostate	161.4	255.5	96.5	68.2	140.8
Breast	132.5	118.3	89.0	69.8	89.3
Lung/bronchus					
Male	81.0	110.6	55.1	53.7	44.7
Female	54.6	53.7	27.7	36.7	25.2
Colon/rectum					
Male	60.4	72.6	49.7	42.1	47.5
Female	44.0	55.0	35.3	39.6	32.9
Uterine cervix	8.5	11.4	8.0	6.6	13.8
Mortality					
All sites					
Male	234.7	321.8	141.7	187.9	162.2
Female	161.4	189.3	96.7	141.2	106.7
Prostate	25.6	62.3	11.3	21.5	21.2
Breast	25.0	33.8	12.6	16.1	16.1
Lung/bronchus					
Male	72.6	95.8	38.3	49.6	36.0
Female	42.1	39.8	18.5	32.7	14.6
Colon/rectum					
Male	22.9	32.7	15.0	20.6	17.0
Female	15.9	22.9	10.3	14.3	11.1
Uterine cervix	2.3	4.9	2.4	4.0	3.3

Sources: Adapted from American Cancer Society, Surveillance Research, 2008; "Cancer Facts and Figures 2008," American Cancer Society. Original data: "SEER Cancer Statistics Review, 1975–2004," by L.A.G. Ries, D. Melbert, M. Krapcho, et al., National Cancer Institute, retrieved from www.seer.cancer.gov/csr/1975_2004/.

LIFESTYLE FACTORS

Most of the genetic mutations that eventually become cancer occur during an individual's lifetime, either as a mistake during cell division or in response to environmental factors, as noted earlier. Some environmental agents (carcinogens) have a direct impact on a cell, causing an initial genetic alteration that can lead to cancer. Other agents, called *cancer promoters*, have a less direct effect, enhancing the possibility that a cancer will develop if an initiating event has already occurred in a cell.

Tobacco Use and Cancer Risk   Tobacco use is the leading preventable cause of cancer in the United States. It is responsi-

Public Health in Action

Addressing Cancer Disparities

Do you live in rural America? Do you earn less money than the average American? Have you attended college? Your answers to these questions are indicators of whether or not you are likely to develop cancer someday and how likely you are to die from it.

Although the number of new cases of cancer and the number of deaths from cancer are reported by race and ethnicity, factors such as income, education, geographical location, housing, and cultural beliefs are believed to be stronger indicators of risk. These factors influence risk behaviors (such as tobacco use), access to health care, and quality of health care.

As an example, let's consider cancer screening tests. Getting the recommended tests in a timely way increases the likelihood that a cancer will be detected or diagnosed at an earlier, more treatable stage. Rural Americans are less likely than urban Americans to receive cancer screening, in part because fewer physicians practice in rural communities. Rural residents are also less likely than urban residents to have health insurance. Rural jobs are lower paying than urban jobs, and lower paying jobs are less likely to offer health insurance than higher paying jobs. The cost of individual health insurance is prohibitive for most poor people, so they go without insurance. Uninsured people are significantly less likely to receive cancer screening tests. As a result, if they do develop cancer, it is diagnosed at a later, less treatable stage, and their chances of survival are reduced. Like other disparities, higher cancer mortality in rural populations is influenced by a complex array of factors and conditions.

In an attempt to reduce barriers to screening for breast and cervical cancer, the Centers for Disease Control and Prevention (CDC) implemented the National Breast and Cervical Cancer Early Detection Program in 1990. The program provides low-income, uninsured, and underserved women access to breast and cervical cancer screening, including clinical breast exams, Pap tests, mammograms, and further diagnostic testing or treatment as necessary. Since 1991 the program has served 3.1 million women throughout all 50 states, the District of Columbia, 5 U.S. territories, and 12 American Indian/Alaskan Native tribes or tribal organizations.

Legislation is pending to authorize a National Colorectal Cancer Screening Program that would operate in a similar way. At present, an estimated 40 percent of individuals who should be screened for colorectal cancer have not been screened. The lowest screening rates are among racial and ethnic minorities and the uninsured. Addressing the economic factors influencing access to cancer screening is just one way to reduce cancer disparities.

Sources: "Use of Colorectal Cancer Tests—United States, 2002, 2004, and 2006," Centers for Disease Control and Prevention, 2008, Morbidity and Mortality Weekly Report, 57 *(10), pp. 253–258; National Healthcare Disparities Report, 2006,* Centers for Disease Control and Prevention, Agency for Healthcare Research and Quality, U.S. Department of Health and Human Services.

ble for 30 percent of all cancer deaths and 87 percent of all lung cancer deaths. Lung cancer occurs in smokers 20 times more often than in nonsmokers. Smokers are more likely than non-smokers to die from their lung cancer—23 times more likely if they are men and 13 times more likely if they are women.[1]

Tobacco use increases the risk of cancers of the mouth, throat, lung, and esophagus by direct exposure to the chemicals (over 50 known carcinogens) in tobacco smoke. It increases the risk of other cancers, including bladder, pancreas, stomach, liver, kidney, and bone-marrow cancers, because other chemicals from tobacco are absorbed into the bloodstream and travel to distant sites. Individual risk from tobacco use depends on the age at which the person starts smoking, the number of years the person smokes, the number of cigarettes smoked per day, and the type of cigarettes smoked, with higher tar content being more dangerous.[1, 4]

Dietary Patterns and Cancer Risk   For people who do not use tobacco products, nutrition and physical activity are the most significant contributors to cancer risk. Dietary patterns can be protective or harmful, depending on the choice of foods. Diets rich in fruits, vegetables, and whole grains appear to decrease the risk for many cancers, including lung, colon, rectal, breast, stomach, and ovarian cancers. Diets high in fiber appear to decrease the risk of colon cancer and possibly the risk of breast, rectal, pharyngeal, and stomach cancers.

Among the fruits and vegetables, those rich in carotenoids appear to confer additional benefits; these include dark yellow or orange vegetables and fruits (melon, carrots, sweet potatoes) and dark green leafy vegetables (broccoli, spinach, collard greens). Researchers have tried to determine exactly which components of the fruits and vegetables are beneficial, but studies have had mixed results. The National Cancer Institute recommends eating from 5 to 9 servings a day of fruits and vegetables in their National 5-a-Day for Better Health program.

Diets high in fat have been associated with several types of cancer, including breast, colon, and prostate cancers. Eating red meat and processed meats has been associated with an increased risk of cancer; the American Institute for Cancer Research recommends limiting consumption of red meat to 18 ounces per week and avoiding processed meats.[1, 4–6] Grilling meat, poultry, and fish produces cancer-causing compounds, especially if fat drips onto hot coals, causing smoke and flare-ups. Measures that reduce this risk include trimming fat from meat, marinating or microwaving meat before grilling, and keeping meat portions small so they require a shorter time on the grill.

Additionally, some foods contain toxins from the environment that may cause or promote cancer. Levels of toxins in food that are deemed safe are determined by government policies and regulations, so consumers have little or no control over this source of risk, except to follow the recommendations for food intake, such as limiting intake of fish caught in certain locations and buying organic foods.

Overweight and Obesity and Cancer Risk Overweight and obesity increase the risk of developing many types of cancer as well as the risk of dying from cancer once it occurs. Overweight and obesity not only make it harder to detect cancers at an early stage but also delay diagnosis and may make treatment more difficult.

Although it is not clear how fat cells contribute to an increased risk of cancer, several pathways are possible. Fat cells produce hormones, some of which (such as estrogen) are linked to cancer. Fat cells may trigger an inflammatory reaction, alter insulin production, or release proteins that trigger cell growth, all of which may contribute to the development of cancer. Fat cells may also accumulate more environmental toxins.[1, 4, 7]

Physical Activity and Cancer Risk Physical activity is associated with a reduced risk for colon cancer and probably a reduced risk for breast, prostate, and uterine cancers. Physical activity can help you maintain a healthy body weight and thus further reduce risk. It also alters body functions in a positive way; for example, by increasing the rate that food travels through the intestines, it reduces the exposure of the bowel lining to potential carcinogens. Appropriate exercise after a cancer diagnosis and during treatment can help people eat better, feel less tired, and recover faster.[1]

Alcohol Consumption and Cancer Risk Alcohol consumption of more than one serving a day for women and two servings a day for men increases the risk for cancers of the mouth, throat, esophagus, liver, and breast. Regular intake of a few drinks per week may increase risk of breast cancer. Alcohol and tobacco used together amplify the risk for cancer and are associated with a greater risk than either one alone. Red wine does not appear to offer a protective effect against cancer; wine, beer, and hard liquor all increase risk.[1, 8]

ENVIRONMENTAL FACTORS

Some cancers are caused by exposure to carcinogens in the environment, but some exposures are more controllable than others.

Ultraviolet Radiation Ultraviolet radiation, the rays of energy that come from the sun (or sun lamps and tanning beds), can damage DNA and cause skin cancer. The sun's

ultraviolet radiation has two types of rays: ultraviolet B (UVB) and ultraviolet A (UVA). UVB rays are more likely to cause sunburns and have long been associated with skin cancers. UVA rays tend to pass deeper into the skin and are now believed to cause skin cancer and premature aging of the skin.

The risk for the two milder forms of skin cancer, basal cell and squamous cell carcinomas, is cumulative; the more sun exposure over the years, the higher the risk. The risk for melanoma, the most dangerous form of skin cancer, appears to be related more to the timing and number of sunburns. Sunburns that occur during childhood seem to be the most dangerous, and the more sunburns, the greater the risk.

People who live in certain regions of the world have a higher risk of developing skin cancers because of their location close to the equator or in areas affected by the hole in the ozone layer of the atmosphere. As discussed in Chapter 23, the ozone layer, which protects the earth from the sun's damaging UV rays, is being disrupted by chemical pollution and is thinning over Antarctica and southern portions of the globe.

Australia has one of the highest rates of skin cancer in the world, presumably because of this environmental condition. In 1981 a national campaign was initiated to slow rapidly rising skin cancer rates. The "Slip, Slop, Slap" campaign focused on three preventive measures: slip into the shade, slop on some sunscreen, and slap on a hat. Since then, the program has evolved into the SunSmart campaign, with two additional steps—seek shade and slide on some sunglasses. The campaign has produced positive changes in sun-protective behaviors.[9]

The Australian population supports this campaign, particularly its focus on children. Schools can be registered as "SunSmart," meaning they have a sun protection

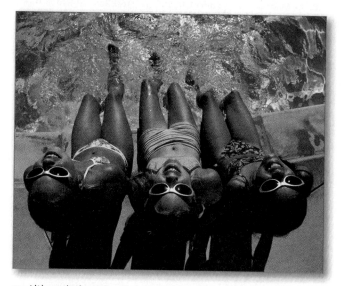

■ Although the risks of sun exposure are well known and include not only skin cancer but premature aging of the skin, tanning is still popular in the United States.

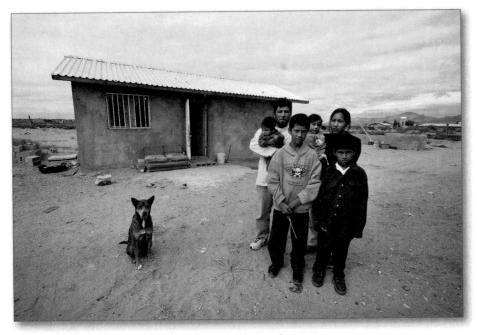

■ Being poor and living in a rural locale are risk factors for cancer. This low-income family living in the desert has less access to well-paying jobs, health insurance, health information, and health care services, including cancer screening tests, than a more affluent family living in an urban environment.

policy that meets minimum requirements, they schedule outdoor activities at low-UV times, they have increased shade areas, and they educate children about skin cancer protective behaviors.[9] In the United States, there has been limited progress in reducing sunburns and increasing sun-protective practices among children and adolescents.[10]

Other Forms of Radiation   Ionizing radiation, radiation with enough energy to displace electrons from atoms, can also cause cancer. The free electrons can enter human cells and cause damage. An estimated 82 percent of ionizing radiation comes from natural sources, such as radon (a naturally occurring radioactive gas in the ground in certain regions of the world) and cosmic rays (particles from the universe). The other 18 percent is from human-made sources, such as medical X-rays, nuclear medicine, and consumer products (such as tobacco, building materials, and television and computer screens).[11]

Residents in many parts of North America are exposed to low levels of radon in their homes, particularly homes with basements. In regions known to have high levels of radon in the ground, testing of homes is recommended, followed by the installation of a ventilation system if levels are found to be elevated.

Nuclear fallout is an environmental source of radiation. Survivors of atom bomb explosions and tests have high levels of cancer, particularly cancers of the bone marrow and thyroid. The nuclear reactors used in power plants have not been shown to emit enough ionizing radiation to place surrounding communities at risk. However, accidental releases of radioactive gases have occurred, and

accidents at power plants, such as the one at Chernobyl in 1986, have contaminated land for miles around and caused an untold number of cancers in those exposed to radiation and radioactive debris.

Radiation in medical settings is used in treatment of cancers or diagnostic imaging. High-dose radiation for cancer treatment has been shown to increase risk for leukemia and thyroid and breast cancer years later. Lower levels of radiation are used in diagnostic X-rays and CT scans. The amount of radiation per procedure is low, but exposures can accumulate if someone needs many tests. To reduce risk, the number of medical procedures should be minimized as much as possible, especially in children.[11]

Chemical and Physical Carcinogens   Many other substances in the environment have been associated with different forms of cancer. Environmental carcinogens include metals (such as arsenic, mercury, and lead), natural fibers (such as asbestos and silica), combustion by-products (including motor vehicle exhaust, diesel exhaust, soot, and polycyclic aromatic hydrocarbons), solvents (benzene, toluene), polychlorinated biphenyls, and pesticides. Your exposure to environmental carcinogens varies depending on where you live, where you work, what your hobbies and recreational activities are, and what you eat, among other factors. Exposures are higher and rates of cancer are higher in cities, farming states, and industrial areas and near hazardous waste sites.[12]

Infectious Agents   One risk from infectious disease occurs when a virus infects a cell and activates gene replication in order to produce copies of itself. Any time gene replication is activated, there is a chance of mutation. Another risk occurs when an infection causes a chronic irritation, prompting cell division and again increasing the chance of mutation.

Some viruses are known to cause cancer. Human papillomavirus (HPV) is linked to cancers of the cervix, anus, vagina, penis, and mouth. The hepatitis B and C viruses are associated with liver cancer. Certain strains of Epstein-Barr virus, which causes mononucleosis, are associated with Hodgkin's lymphoma, non-Hodgkin's lymphoma, and some stomach cancers. Human immunodeficiency virus (HIV) suppresses the immune system and allows several types of cancer to develop. The only bacterium linked to cancer thus far is *Helicobacter pylori,* which causes a chronic irritation of the stomach lining and is associated with stomach ulcers and an increased risk of stomach cancer.[4, 13]

Common Cancers

Since 1930 changes have occurred in the rates of different cancers in the United States (Figure 19.2). The most dramatic changes in overall rates can be seen for stomach, lung, and uterine cancers. A drop in mortality for stomach cancer occurred in both sexes early in the 20th century and is believed to be the result of changes in food processing. The dramatic increase in lung cancer for both sexes is believed to be the result of higher rates of smoking. Rates of smoking increased among women about 20 to 30 years after they increased in men, and there has been a corresponding increase in lung cancer among women; rates have just

recently started to level off. The reduction in mortality from uterine cancer among women corresponds to the introduction of the Pap test to screen for cervical cancer (considered a form of uterine cancer).

In this section we consider some of the most common cancers. For each, we describe risk factors, signs and symptoms of the disease, screening tests and detection, and treatments.

LUNG CANCER

The leading cause of cancer death for both men and women in the United States and the second most commonly diagnosed cancer is lung cancer. In 1987 lung cancer overtook breast cancer as the leading cause of cancer death for American women. The incidence rates are declining for men and have reached a plateau for women.[1]

The leading risk factor for lung cancer is the use of tobacco products in any form. A genetic link has been identified that makes people more likely to become addicted to tobacco, makes it harder to quit, and increases the risk of lung cancer.[14, 15] Other risk factors are exposures to carcinogenic chemicals, arsenic, radon, asbestos, radiation, air pollution, and environmental tobacco smoke. Recently, experts determined that dietary supplements containing beta-carotene, a form of vitamin A, further increases the risk for lung cancer in people who smoke. Reducing risk factors, especially exposure to tobacco smoke and environmental tobacco smoke, is the first line of defense against this disease.

Signs and symptoms of lung cancer include coughing, blood-streaked sputum, chest pain, difficulty breathing, and recurrent lung infections. Unfortunately, symptoms do not appear in most people until the disease is advanced, a factor that frequently delays detection of the disease. There is currently no routine screening test for lung cancer. Chest X-rays, examination of sputum, and a form of computerized tomography called *spiral CT* can detect early-stage lung cancer, but there is no evidence that utilizing these tests increases survival from lung cancer. A large study called the National Lung Screening Trial is under way to determine whether screening high-risk, heavy smokers by these methods can improve survival.[16]

If symptoms suggest lung cancer and an abnormality is found on an X-ray or CT scan, the diagnosis is confirmed by a biopsy, performed either by surgery or by **bronchoscopy.** People with small tumors that can be removed surgically have the best prognosis. For more advanced cancers or for people who are unable to tolerate surgery, radiation or a combination of radiation and chemotherapy is used. If the cancer has spread to distant sites, radiation and

bronchoscopy
Procedure in which a fiber-optic device is inserted into the lungs to allow the health care provider to examine lung tissue for signs of cancer.

chemotherapy can be used for *palliative care* (care provided to give temporary relief of symptoms but not to cure the cancer). The 1-year survival rate for lung cancer is 41 percent, and the 5-year survival rate is 15 percent.[1]

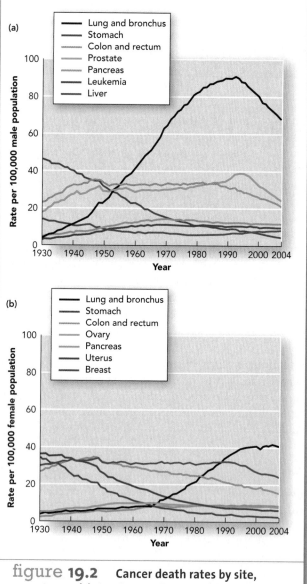

figure **19.2** **Cancer death rates by site, 1930–2004; (a) death rates for men; (b) death rates for women.**
Source: American Cancer Society, Inc. www.cancer.org. Reprinted with permission.

Colon and Rectal Cancer The third leading cause of cancer death and the third most commonly diagnosed cancer is colon and rectal cancer (also called colorectal cancer). During the 1990s, the incidence of colon and rectal cancer declined in the United States in both men and women, along with the number of deaths from the disease. The decrease is thought to be due to improved screening and treatment and the early detection and removal of **colon polyps.**[1]

colon polyps
Growths in the colon that may progress to colon cancer.

The most important risk factor for colorectal cancer is age. More than 90 percent of colorectal cancers are diagnosed in people over age 50. A personal or family history of colon polyps or inflammatory bowel disease also increases risk, as does a family history of colorectal cancer, especially in a first-degree relative. Other factors associated with an increased risk for colon and rectal cancer include smoking, alcohol use, obesity, physical inactivity, a diet high in fat or red or processed meat, and inadequate amounts of fruits and vegetables. Aspirin and hormone replacement therapy may reduce the risk for colon and rectal cancer.[1]

Warning signs of colorectal cancer include a change in bowel movements, change in stool size or shape, pain in the abdomen, or blood in the stool. The signs do not usually occur until the disease is fairly advanced. Screening tests are available that can enhance early detection of polyps or cancer.

flexible sigmoidoscopy
Procedure in which a fiber-optic device is inserted in the colon to allow the health care provider to examine the lower third of the colon for polyps or cancer.

colonoscopy
Procedure in which a fiber-optic device is inserted in the colon to allow the health care provider to examine the entire colon for polyps or cancer.

double-contrast barium enema
Test for colon polyps or cancer in which contrast material is inserted into the colon and X-rays are taken of the abdomen, revealing alterations in the lining of the colon if polyps or cancer is present.

CT colonography
Screen for colon polyps or cancer using a CT scanner.

Four techniques can be used to "visualize" the colon. In a **flexible sigmoidoscopy**, a thin, flexible fiber-optic tube is inserted into the rectum and moved through the lower third of the colon. In a **colonoscopy**, a longer scope is used and the entire colon is viewed (Figure 19.3). If a polyp is found, it can be biopsied during the procedure. In a **double-contrast barium enema** the colon is partially filled with a contrast material and then X-rays are taken. A colon cancer or polyp will alter the lining of the colon and can be seen. In **CT colonography** (or virtual colonoscopy), a CT scanner is used to take multiple pictures of the colon and can detect polyps or cancer.

Several other tests can be used that primarily screen for colon cancer but are not as good at detecting polyps. These include the fecal occult blood test, the stool immunochemical test, and the stool DNA test. The first two screen for trace

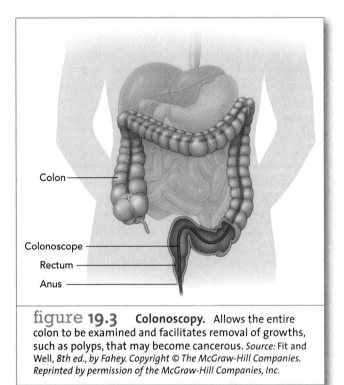

figure 19.3 **Colonoscopy.** Allows the entire colon to be examined and facilitates removal of growths, such as polyps, that may become cancerous. *Source:* Fit and Well, *8th ed., by Fahey. Copyright © The McGraw-Hill Companies. Reprinted by permission of the McGraw-Hill Companies, Inc.*

amounts of blood, which can signal a cancer or a bleeding polyp. The DNA test looks for changes in DNA known to be related to colon cancer.[17]

The American Cancer Society recommends that people of average risk start colorectal cancer screening at age 50. For people with higher than average risk (for example, someone who has a close family member with colon cancer or polyps), earlier and more frequent screening may be recommended.

Surgery is the most common treatment for colon and rectal cancer; it can cure the cancer if it has not spread. Chemotherapy and/or radiation are added if the cancer is large or has spread to other areas. The 1-year survival rate for all stages of colorectal cancer is 82 percent; the 5-year survival rate is 64 percent.

BREAST CANCER

The second leading cause of cancer death in women and the most commonly diagnosed non-skin cancer in women is breast cancer. It was the leading cause of cancer death in women for many years, but it has been surpassed by lung cancer. Breast cancer occurs in men as well as women, but it is less common. There were an estimated 1,990 cases of breast cancer in men in the United States in 2008.[1]

There are both controllable and noncontrollable risk factors for breast cancer. Among the noncontrollable factors are early onset of menarche (first menstruation), late onset of menopause, family history of breast cancer in a first-degree relative, older age, and higher socioeconomic class. As mentioned earlier in this chapter and discussed in Chapter 2, two genes have been identified that are associated with an increased risk of breast cancer, called BRCA1 and BRCA2. Although inherited susceptibility accounts for only 5 percent of all breast cancer cases, having these genes confers a lifetime risk of developing the disease ranging from 35 to 85 percent. Some women with these genes choose to have their breasts and/or ovaries removed to lower their risk of developing breast or ovarian cancer. The estrogen-blocking drugs tamoxifen and raloxifene can also reduce risk.

Controllable risk factors for breast cancer that increase risk include never having children or having a first child after age 30, being obese after menopause, taking hormone replacement therapy, and drinking more than two alcoholic beverages a day. Breastfeeding, engaging in moderate or vigorous exercise, and maintaining a healthy body weight are all associated with decreased risk.

Early stages of breast cancer have either no symptoms or symptoms that may be detected only by a mammogram. Symptoms of later stages include a persistent lump; swelling, redness, or bumpiness of the skin; and nipple discharge. Breast pain or tenderness is common in women without cancer and is usually not a cause for concern; more likely explanations are hormonal changes, infection, or breast cysts, which are rarely cancerous.

Breast cancer can be detected at an early stage by a mammogram, a low-dose X-ray of the breast. The effectiveness of mammography in detecting cancer depends on several factors, including the size of the cancer, the density of the breasts, and the skills of the radiologist. Although mammograms cannot detect all cancers, they have been shown to decrease the number of women who die from breast cancer.

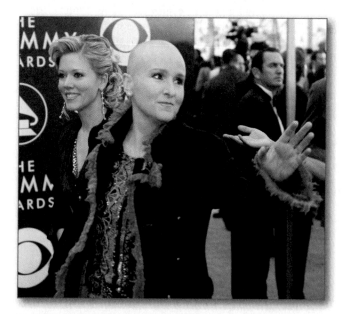

■ When Melissa Etheridge found a lump in her breast, she acted quickly, having lost an aunt and a grandmother to breast cancer. She underwent surgery, radiation, and chemotherapy in 2004 but was able to attend the Grammys 5 months later. Etheridge decided to attend bald to support those who watching who were also undergoing chemo.

The American Cancer Society recommends annual mammograms for all women aged 40 and older.

Another screening technique for breast cancer is breast exam. The American Cancer Society recommends that women in their 20s and 30s have a clinical breast exam (CBE) performed by a health care provider every 2 to 3 years and that women over 40 have a breast exam performed by their health care provider annually near the time of their mammogram. The ACS also suggests that beginning in their 20s, women should be told about the benefits and limitations of performing a breast self-exam (BSE) every month (see the box "Breast Self-Exam"). The ACS considers it acceptable for women to choose not to do self-exams or to do them only occasionally.

Any suspicious lumps, changes, or mammogram findings that are suggestive of cancer are typically followed by a biopsy so that cells or tissues can be evaluated under the microscope, the only way to make a definitive diagnosis. There are several noncancerous causes of lumps in the breast; in younger women, a lump is much more likely to be caused by a cyst or a benign tumor called a fibroadenoma. Other screening tools, including ultrasound and magnetic resonance imaging (MRI), are sometimes used to help determine whether a lump or abnormality is cancerous.

Surgery is usually the first line of treatment for breast cancer, either a lumpectomy (removal of a section of the breast around the cancer) or a mastectomy (removal of the entire breast). Lymph nodes under the arm on the affected side are often tested to determine whether the cancer has spread from the breast. Radiation, chemotherapy, and hormonal therapy are frequently used in the treatment of breast cancer.

The 5-year survival rate for all stages of breast cancer is 86.6 percent. For cancer that is localized (no lymph node involvement), it is 98 percent; for cancer that has spread regionally (only local lymph node involvement), it is 84 percent; and for cancer that has distant metastases, it is 27 percent.[1]

PROSTATE CANCER

The second most common cause of cancer death in men and the most commonly diagnosed cancer in men is prostate cancer. The incidence of prostate cancer is significantly higher among Black men than White men, as is the death rate. The number of diagnosed cases of prostate cancer increased in the early 1990s, probably as a result of better screening, and has leveled off since 1995. Death rates declined during the same period, although death rates for Black men remain twice as high as those for White men.[1]

The most important risk factor for prostate cancer is age. More than 70 percent of prostate cancer cases are diagnosed in men aged 65 and older. Other risk factors include a family history of prostate cancer, being Black, and possibly having a high-fat diet. The risk of dying from prostate cancer appears to increase with increasing body weight.

Highlight on Health

Breast Self-Exam

Performing a monthly breast self-exam (BSE) can help you learn how your breasts normally feel so you can identify any changes that occur. Almost all women have some lumps and bumps in their breast tissue that change throughout the month. The best time to do your exam is a few days after your period when the breast tissue is least tender. If you no longer menstruate or have very irregular periods, do the exam on the same day every month.

If you choose to do a BSE, follow these steps:

- Lie down and put a pillow under your right shoulder. Place your right arm behind your head.

- Use the finger pads of your three middle fingers on your left hand to feel for lumps or thickening in your right breast. Use overlapping dime-sized circular motions of the finger pads to feel the breast tissue.

- Use three different levels of pressure—light, medium, and firm—to feel all the breast tissue. Use each pressure level to feel the breast tissue before moving on to the next spot. If you're not sure how hard to press, talk with your health care provider. A firm ridge in the lower curve of each breast is normal.

- Move around the breast in an up-and-down pattern starting at an imaginary line drawn straight down your side from the underarm and move across the breast to the middle of the chest (breast bone).

- Repeat the exam on your left breast, using the finger pads of the right hand and moving the pillow under your left shoulder.

- While standing in front of a mirror with your hands pressing firmly down on your hips, look at your breasts for any changes of size, shape, contour, or dimpling. (Pressing down on your hips contracts the chest wall muscles and enhances any breast changes.)

- Examine each underarm while sitting up or standing and with your arm only slightly raised so you can easily feel in the area.

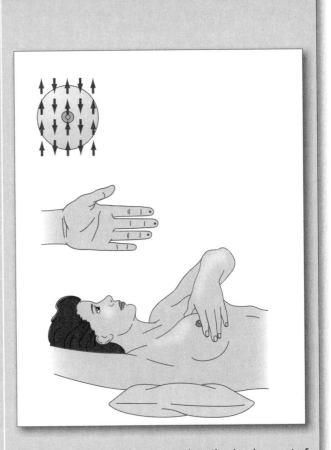

If you notice any change—such as the development of a lump or swelling, skin irritation or dimpling, nipple pain or retraction, redness or scaliness of the nipple or skin, or a discharge other than breast milk—see your health care provider right away for an evaluation. Most of the time, these changes are not cancer.

These BSE guidelines represent a change in previous recommendations, based on an extensive review of the medical literature and input from an expert advisory group.

In its early stages, prostate cancer usually has no signs or symptoms. Advanced prostate cancer can be associated with difficulty urinating, pain in the pelvic region, pain with urination, or blood in the urine. These symptoms can also be caused by more common, noncancerous conditions, such as benign enlargement of the prostate gland and bladder infections.

Two tests are available to detect prostate cancer at an early, asymptomatic stage. One is a *digital rectal exam,* in which a health care provider inserts a gloved finger into the rectum and palpates the prostate gland. The other is the *prostate-specific antigen (PSA) test,* a blood test that detects levels of a substance made by the prostate (prostate-specific antigen) that are elevated when certain conditions are present, including benign prostate enlargement, infection, and prostate cancer. If PSA levels are elevated, a rectal ultrasound and prostate biopsy can be performed to assess and diagnose the cause.

The American Cancer Society recommends that all men discuss with their health care providers whether they should have a digital rectal exam and PSA screening annually starting at age 50; the ACS also recommends that Black men and men with a family history of prostate cancer begin having screening done at age 45.[1]

The routine use of PSA testing is controversial, because many prostate cancers progress slowly and would not cause symptoms before a man died of other causes. The difficulty of determining which prostate cancers are slow growing and which may progress more quickly complicates treatment decisions once a cancer has been detected. Treatments for prostate cancer can themselves cause problems, including erectile dysfunction and incontinence (inability to control the flow of urine). These side effects have to be balanced against the risk that the cancer will progress and spread.

Treatment for prostate cancer depends on the stage of the cancer and the man's age and other health conditions. In its early stages and in a younger man, prostate cancer is usually treated with surgery (removal of the prostate gland) and radiation, sometimes in combination with chemotherapy, radiation, and hormonal medication, which blocks the effects of testosterone and can cause tumors to shrink. Later stages are treated with chemotherapy, radiation, and hormonal medication. Radiation is sometimes administered by the implantation of radioactive seeds, which destroy cancer tissue and leave normal prostate tissue intact.

The 5-year survival rate for all stages of prostate cancer is 98 percent. For cancers detected at local or regional stages, the 5-year survival rate is 100 percent. In studies that follow prostate cancer for more than 5 years, the survival rate decreases to 91 percent at 10 years and to 76 percent at 15 years.[1]

CANCERS OF THE FEMALE REPRODUCTIVE SYSTEM

Cancer can develop throughout the female reproductive system but occurs more frequently in the cervix, uterus, and ovaries.

Cervical Cancer The ACS projected an estimated 11,070 new cases of cervical cancer in 2008 and an estimated 3,870 deaths. The incidence of this cancer and the number of related deaths have declined sharply in the past few decades as a result of improved detection and treatment of precursor lesions, primarily by means of the Pap test.

As described in Chapter 17, cervical cancer is closely related to infection with certain strains of the human papillomavirus (HPV). However, HPV infection is common in women, and the majority of women never develop cervical cancer. Persistent infection and progression to cancer is influenced by other factors, such as tobacco use, immunosuppression, multiple births, early sexual activity, multiple sex partners, socioeconomic status, and nutritional status. Currently two vaccines are available and reduce the risk of HPV infection, as described in Chapter 17.

Cervical cancer develops at a specific site on the cervix, at the opening of the cervix into the vagina. In its early stages, it usually does not cause any symptoms. Warning signs of more advanced cancer include abnormal vaginal discharge or abnormal vaginal bleeding. Pain in the pelvic region can be a late sign of cervical cancer.

Early detection through the Pap test has significantly reduced the rates of cervical cancer and mortality. The Pap test, recommended for all women, is performed as part of a pelvic exam. A small sample of cells is collected from the cervix with a swab or brush, placed on a slide or into a liquid suspension, processed, and then examined under the microscope to detect cells that may be abnormal. Pap tests are good but not perfect, occasionally giving either a **false negative** or a **false positive**. DNA tests can be used with liquid Pap suspensions to identify DNA strains and are particularly helpful if the Pap results are unclear.

false negative
A negative test result when a disease is actually present.

false positive
A positive test result when no disease is actually present.

Treatment for cervical cancer involves removing or destroying precursor cells. Several methods are available, including electrocoagulation (the destruction of tissue locally by intense heat), cryotherapy (the destruction of tissue locally by intense cold), and surgery. Invasive cervical cancer is treated with a combination of surgery, local radiation, and chemotherapy.

Uterine Cancer Also called *endometrial cancer,* uterine cancer usually develops in the endometrium, the lining of the uterus. Uterine cancer is diagnosed more often in White women than in Black women, but the death rate among Black women is nearly twice the rate among White women. Black women tend to have more advanced cancer when they are diagnosed, perhaps as a result of having less access to health care.

The risk for uterine cancer is related to a woman's exposure to estrogen, so factors that increase estrogen—such as obesity and estrogen replacement therapy without progesterone—increase risk. Other factors associated with increased risk include young age at menarche, late-onset menopause, irregular ovulation, and infrequent periods. Pregnancy and oral contraceptive pills reduce the risk of uterine cancer. Warning signs of uterine cancer include abnormal uterine bleeding (spotting between periods or spotting after menopause), pelvic pain, and low back pain. Pain is usually a late sign of uterine cancer.

Uterine cancer is frequently detected at an early stage in postmenopausal women because of vaginal bleeding. An endometrial biopsy is performed to collect cells and tissue from the uterus to determine whether the bleeding is due to cancer or a less serious condition. If uterine cancer is diagnosed, a hysterectomy—surgical removal of the uterus—is usually performed. Depending on the stage of cancer, other treatment methods may also be used, including radiation, chemotherapy, and hormonal therapy.

Ovarian Cancer The leading gynecological cause of cancer death and the fifth overall cause of cancer death in women is ovarian cancer. Ovarian cancer has a low rate of survival because most cases are not diagnosed until they have spread beyond the ovaries. If ovarian cancer is diagnosed early, survival is as high as 95 percent. Between 90 and 95 percent of women with ovarian cancer have no risk factors.

The strongest risk factor is a family history of ovarian cancer in a first-degree relative, especially if the BRCA1 or BRCA2 gene is involved. Women with either of these genetic mutations have a 20–60 percent chance of developing ovarian cancer. Risk is also increased in women with a personal history of breast, colon, or endometrial cancer. Factors that reduce risk include use of oral contraceptive pills, pregnancy, and breastfeeding. Avoidance of postmenopausal hormone replacement therapy may also reduce risk. Women with the BRCA1 or BRCA2 gene mutations may consider more aggressive measures to reduce risk, including removal of the ovaries and fallopian tubes.

The early stages of ovarian cancer have few signs or symptoms. At later stages, a woman may notice swelling of the abdomen, bloating, or a vague pain in the lower abdomen. A screen to increase early detection would be beneficial, given the improved survival with early diagnosis. However, to date, no such screen has proven successful.[18, 19] Most women, as part of their annual checkup with a Pap test, undergo a "bimanual exam," in which a health care provider feels the uterus and ovaries with two gloved fingers in the vagina and a hand on the lower abdomen. The exam occasionally detects ovarian cancer but usually only when the disease is advanced.

Several blood tests have been evaluated for use as a screening tool. Testing for the protein marker CA 125 is the most likely to date. Blood levels of this protein are elevated in 50 percent of women with stage I ovarian cancer and in 90 percent of women with stage II cancer. The marker is currently used to monitor progression and treatment in women with confirmed ovarian cancer. However, because CA 125 can be elevated for other reasons, many women will have false-positive results.

Another potential screening tool is a pelvic ultrasound, in which sound waves are used to visualize the ovaries and show whether they are enlarged or contain a mass. This test also has a high false-positive rate. It may be that the combination of CA 125 and ultrasound will become an effective screen for early detection of ovarian cancer. At present, there is no generally recommended screen. The combination of pelvic exam, ultrasound, and CA 125 level may be offered to women at high risk.[1, 18, 19]

Treatment for ovarian cancer depends on the stage at diagnosis. Typically, all or part of the ovaries, uterus, and fallopian tubes are surgically removed and the lymph nodes are biopsied to determine whether the cancer has spread. Chemotherapy and radiation may then be recommended. Treatment options currently under investigation include vaccinations, targeted drugs, and immunotherapy.[20]

SKIN CANCER

The three forms of skin cancer are basal cell cancer, squamous cell cancer, and melanoma. More than 1 million cases of basal cell and squamous cell cancers occur each year in the United States. Most of these are curable, although both can be disfiguring and, if ignored, fatal. Melanoma is a less common but more serious form of skin cancer. Skin cancers occur in all racial and ethnic groups, but they are more common in people with lighter skin colors.

All forms of skin cancers are linked directly to ultraviolet light exposure—both UVA and UVB.[21] The most effective way to reduce risk for skin cancer is to limit UV exposure, whether from the sun or from the UV lights in tanning salons. Recommended ways of achieving this goal, in order of importance, are staying out of the sun during midday (10:00 a.m. to 4:00 p.m.), wearing protective clothing (including a hat to shade the face and neck, long sleeves, and long pants), using a broad-spectrum sunscreen with a **sun protective factor (SPF)** of 15 or higher, and wearing sunglasses that offer UV protection (see the box "Sunscreen and Other Sun Protection Products"). Parents should be particularly vigilant about protecting their children.

> **sun protective factor (SPF)** Measure of the degree to which a sunscreen protects the skin from damaging UV radiation from the sun.

Melanoma   Because it is capable of spreading quickly to almost any part of the body, melanoma is a particularly dangerous form of cancer. Rates of melanoma increased from 1970 to 2000 but have been stable since 2000, and mortality from this cancer has decreased for people under age 50, probably due to earlier detection.

The risk of melanoma is greatest for people with a personal history of melanoma, a large number of moles (especially those that are large or unusual in shape or color), or a family member with melanoma. The risk is greater in people

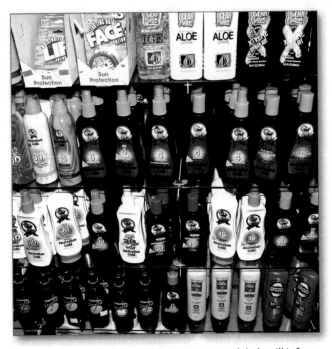

■ Under proposed FDA regulations, sunscreen labels will inform consumers about both UVB and UVA protection.

Consumer Clipboard

Sunscreen and Other Sun Protection Products

Sun exposure is the most preventable risk factor for skin cancers. Sunscreens, if used properly, can offer protection against the damaging effects of UV radiation. Historically, sunscreen products protected primarily against UVB exposure, which has long been known to cause sunburns and skin damage and is associated with skin cancer. Increasing data now indicate that UVA exposure also causes skin cancer, in addition to aging (wrinkling and sagging) and other skin damage. UVA penetrates the skin more deeply than UVB and is responsible for tanning. The FDA has proposed new sunscreen labeling regulations designed to provide consumers with the information they need about UVA and UVB radiation so that they can make wise purchasing decisions.

Currently, sunscreen labels display the SPF (sun protective factor) of the product. (SPF may stand for *sunburn protective factor* on the new labels.) SPF indicates the amount of time you can stay in the sun without burning compared to how long you could stay if you weren't wearing the sunscreen. An SPF of 15 means that a person can stay out in the sun 15 times longer than he or she could without sunscreen before a sunburn would occur. SPF refers to UVB protection only. Currently the highest SPF recognized by the FDA is 30+, but the new label will allow SPFs up to 50+.

Some FDA-approved sunscreens protect against both UVB and UVA by including ingredients that block UVA radiation, such as titanium dioxide and zinc oxide. A sunscreen containing the ingredient Mexoryl also blocks UVA. The new FDA proposals call for products to indicate the amount of UVA protection they provide using the following star system:

- 1 star * = low UVA protection
- 2 stars ** = medium UVA protection
- 3 stars *** = high UVA protection
- 4 stars **** = very high UVA protection

Labels will also have to state clearly if the product provides no UVA protection. In addition, labels will have to carry the following message:

Warning: UV exposure from the sun increases the risk of skin cancer, premature skin aging, and other skin damage. It is important to decrease UV exposure by limiting time in the sun, wearing protective clothing, and using a sunscreen.

The FDA recommends that consumers use a water-resistant sunscreen with an SPF of at least 15 that provides UVA and UVB protection to all exposed skin. Sunscreen should be applied liberally to all sun-exposed areas. Most people do not apply enough. An average-sized adult in a swimsuit needs about 4 ounces of sunscreen for one application. It should be applied at least 20 to 30 minutes before going outside—it takes that long for sunscreen to be absorbed. It should also be reapplied frequently, at least every 2 hours and/or after swimming or sweating.

Combination products, such as sunscreen and insect repellant, result in a reduction in the effect of SPF by up to one-third. When using a combination product, use one with a higher SPF and reapply it more frequently. The protectiveness of clothing can vary. Hats typically offer an SPF between 3 and 6; summer-weight clothing has an SPF of about 6.5; newer sun-protective clothing can have an SPF up to 30+.

The UV index is a rating system developed by the National Weather Service and the Environmental Protection Agency to predict UV levels in the next few days on a scale of 1 to 10+. If UV levels are going to be unusually high, a UV alert may be issued. You can check the UV index at www.epa.gov/sunwise/uvindex.html.

Sources: "American Academy of Dermatology Association Issues Statement in Response to the Food and Drug Administration's 2007 Proposed Sunscreen Rule," American Academy of Dermatology, retrieved from www.aad.org/media/background/press/FDASunscreen.html; "2007 Sunscreen Proposed Rule," U.S. Food and Drug Administration, retrieved from www.fda.gov/cder/drug/infopage/sunscreen/default.htm; "EPA Sunwise," U.S. Environmental Protection Agency, retrieved from www.epa.gov/sunwise/uvindex.html.

with fair skin and sun sensitivity (burning easily). Rates in Whites are 10 times greater than rates in Blacks, but the disease does occur in Blacks. Melanoma can occur on any part of the body, but it is directly related to sun exposure, especially intermittent, acute UV light exposure, as from exposure to sunlight (sunburns) or to UV light in tanning salons. Exposure during childhood or adolescence may be particularly dangerous.

Melanomas usually develop in pigmented, or dark, areas on the skin. Signs suggestive of melanoma are changes in a mole: a sudden darkening or change in color, spread of color outward into previously normal skin, an irregular border,

pain, itchiness, bleeding, or crusting. You can monitor your skin for these signs by using the "ABCD" test for melanoma (Figure 19.4).

Early detection of skin cancer usually occurs as a result of individuals' monitoring their own skin and visiting a health care provider for evaluation of any changes or progressive growth. The ACS recommends that people have a skin exam (visual inspection of the skin all over the body) as part of a regular physical examination every 3 years between ages 20 and 40 and annually after age 40.

Treatment for melanoma begins with surgically excising (cutting out) and doing a biopsy of any suspicious lesions. If

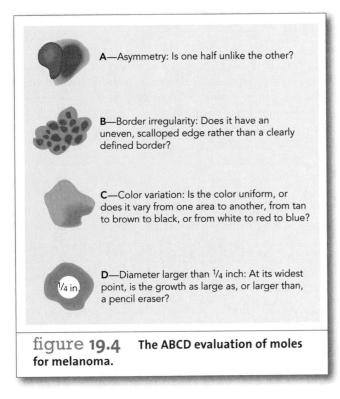

A—Asymmetry: Is one half unlike the other?

B—Border irregularity: Does it have an uneven, scalloped edge rather than a clearly defined border?

C—Color variation: Is the color uniform, or does it vary from one area to another, from tan to brown to black, or from white to red to blue?

D—Diameter larger than ¼ inch: At its widest point, is the growth as large as, or larger than, a pencil eraser?

¼ in.

figure **19.4** The ABCD evaluation of moles for melanoma.

melanoma is confirmed, a larger area of surrounding skin is removed, which improves the chance of survival. The prognosis is based on the size and depth of the melanoma. Chemotherapy and immunotherapy can be added for advanced stages. The overall 5-year survival rate for melanoma is 91 percent; if the melanoma is diagnosed at an early stage, the 5-year survival rate is 99 percent.[1]

Basal Cell and Squamous Cell Carcinomas Sun-exposed areas of the body are susceptible to basal cell and squamous cell cancers. People at high risk include those with fair skin; blonde, red, or light brown hair; blue, green, or hazel eyes; and freckles and moles. Other risk factors are cumulative sun exposure and age, with rates increasing after age 50. However, both types are increasing among younger people.

The signs of a basal cell cancer include new skin growth; a raised, domelike lesion with a pearl-like edge or border; or a sore that bleeds and scabs but never completely heals. The signs of a squamous cell cancer include a red, scaly area that does not go away; a sore that bleeds and does not heal; or a raised, crusty sore. Squamous cell cancers often develop from a precancerous spot called an actinic keratosis, a red, rough spot that develops in a sun-exposed area.

Early detection of basal and squamous cell cancers involves monitoring the skin and having any persistent changes evaluated. The ACS recommends the same skin exams for these cancers as for melanoma. Treatment usually involves local removal and destruction of the cancer by surgery, heat, or freezing, with radiation therapy sometimes an option.[1]

TESTICULAR CANCER

Although testicular cancer accounts for only 1 percent of all cancers in men, it is the most common malignancy in men 20 to 35 years of age. The ACS projected an estimated 8,090 new cases of testicular cancer in 2008 and an estimated 380 deaths. The incidence of testicular cancer has nearly doubled worldwide over the past 40 years. It is not clear why this increase is occurring, but some researchers speculate that it could be due to fetal exposure to higher levels of estrogen during prenatal development as a result of environmental toxins. Because of improved treatment methods, however, the survival rate has increased. In the United States, testicular cancer occurs nearly 4.5 times more often in White men than in Black men. Rates for men of Hispanic, Asian, and Native American backgrounds fall between those for White and Black men.[22, 23]

The risk for testicular cancer is 3 to 17 times higher in men with a history of an undescended testicle (one of the testes fails to descend into the scrotum and is retained in the abdomen or inguinal canal). However, only 7–10 percent of men diagnosed with testicular cancer have a history of this condition. Other risk factors include a family history of testicular cancer, a personal history of testicular cancer in the other testicle, abnormal development of the testes, and infertility or abnormal sperm.[23]

Warning signs of testicular cancer include a painless lump on the testicle and swelling or discomfort in the scrotum. Most testicular cancer is detected by an individual, either unintentionally or during a testicular self-exam. Back pain and difficulty breathing can develop in the later stages after the cancer metastasizes.

For men who have a testicle that is undescended, a surgical procedure early in life can move the testicle into the scrotum. Whether this actually reduces the risk of cancer developing in the testis is unclear, but the repositioning allows for earlier detection of cancer if it does develop. The ACS recommends a testicular exam by a health care provider every 3 years for men over age 20 and annually after age 40.

Men can also perform a self-exam, although there are no specific recommendations for how often it should be performed (see the box "Testicle Self-Exam"). If a lump is detected, an ultrasound is performed, and if the ultrasound suggests cancer, a biopsy is performed to confirm the diagnosis.

Testicular cancer is treated with surgery to remove the testicle; depending on the stage of disease, radiation or chemotherapy may be needed as well. Testicular cancer is highly treatable, with more than 90 percent of cases at all stages being cured. The cure rate is 99 percent if the cancer is diagnosed at an early stage. Even in a man with a late-stage diagnosis and extensive metastases, testicular cancer can be cured. International cycling champion Lance Armstrong, after being diagnosed at age 25 with advanced-stage testicular cancer with metastases to the brain and lungs, was successfully treated and went on to win the world's most prestigious cycling events.

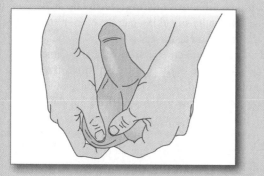

Highlight on Health

Testicle Self-Exam

The testicle self-exam has not been studied enough to show whether it reduces the death rate from testicular cancer. For this reason, the ACS has not set a recommendation for this self-exam for the general population. Testicular cancer is often first detected by a man noticing a change in his own testicles, so some health providers do teach and recommend it.

Follow these steps to perform a self-exam:

- Stand in front of a mirror. Look for any changes or swelling on the skin of the scrotum.

- Examine each testicle with both hands. Place your index and middle fingers under the testicle with the thumbs placed on top. Roll the testicle gently between the thumbs and fingers. It's normal for one testicle to be slightly larger than the other.

- Find the epididymis, the soft, tubelike structure behind the testicle that collects and carries sperm. If you are familiar with this structure, you won't mistake it for a suspicious lump. Cancerous lumps usually are found on the sides of the testicle but also can appear on the front.

If you find a lump, see your doctor right away. Testicular cancer is highly curable, especially when it's detected and treated early. In almost all cases, testicular cancer occurs in only one testicle, and men can maintain full sexual and reproductive function with the other testicle.

ORAL CANCER

Cancers that develop in the mouth or the pharynx (the back of the throat), which can involve the lips, tongue, gums, or throat, are classified as oral cancers. The ACS projected an estimated 35,310 new cases of cancers of the oral cavity and pharynx in 2008 and an estimated 7,590 deaths. The rate of new cases has been declining since the 1980s, and death rates have remained stable since 2000. Oral cancers are more common in men than in women.[1]

The major risk factor for oral cancers is tobacco use (smoking cigarettes, cigars, or a pipe or using smokeless tobacco); high levels of alcohol consumption also increase the risk. Early signs of oral cancer include a sore in the mouth that does not heal or bleeds easily; a lump or bump that does not go away or that increases in size; or a patch of redness or whiteness along the gums or skin lining the inside of the cheeks. Late signs of oral cancer can include pain or difficulty swallowing or chewing.

Oral cancers are usually detected by a doctor or dentist, or the individual may report a sore that does not heal. A biopsy is necessary to confirm the diagnosis. Treatment usually starts with surgery to remove as much as possible of the cancer, along with local radiation. If the cancer is advanced, chemotherapy can be added. The 5-year survival rate for all stages of oral cancer is 59 percent.

LEUKEMIA

Leukemia is a group of cancers that originate in the bone marrow or other parts of the body where white blood cells form. Leukemia is the overproduction of one type of white blood cell, which prevents the normal growth and function of other blood cells and can lead to increased risk of infection, anemia, and bleeding. The ACS projected an estimated 44,270 new cases of leukemia in 2008 and an estimated 21,710 deaths.

Risk factors include cigarette smoking and exposure to certain chemicals, particularly benzene, a chemical found in gasoline products and in cigarette smoke. Ionizing radiation can increase the risk for several types of leukemia; people who survive other cancers are at risk for developing leukemia as a result of radiation treatment. Infection with a virus, human T-cell leukemia/lymphoma virus (HTLV-1), can increase the risk of leukemia and lymphoma, another cancer of the white blood cells.

Symptoms of leukemia often occur because healthy white blood cells, red blood cells, and platelets are unable to perform their functions. These symptoms include fatigue, increased incidence of infection, and easy bleeding and bruising. Symptoms can appear suddenly in acute leukemia, but in chronic leukemia, they may appear gradually.

Because the symptoms are fairly nonspecific, early detection of leukemia can be challenging. There is no recommended screening test, but a health care provider can diagnose leukemia with a blood test or bone marrow biopsy if symptoms are present. The most effective treatment is chemotherapy. Therapy can also include blood transfusion, antibiotics, drugs to boost the function of healthy blood cells, and drugs to reduce the side effects of chemotherapy. Bone marrow transplantation can be effective for certain types of leukemia.

LYMPHOMA

Cancers that originate in the lymph system, part of the body's immune system, are called lymphomas. There are two main types: Hodgkin's lymphoma and non-Hodgkin's lymphoma. Lymphomas can start almost anywhere, since the lymph system exists throughout the body (Figure 19.5). Of the estimated 74,340 cases of lymphoma in 2008, 66,120 will be non-Hodgkin's lymphoma (89 percent). In the past 30 years, rates of lymphoma have nearly doubled. About 95 percent of lymphomas occur in adults, with an average age at diagnosis in the 60s. However, a childhood form of lymphoma exists.[1]

Factors that increase risk for lymphoma include infections, medications, or genetic changes that weaken the immune system. HIV infection explains some of the increase in lymphoma rates. Radiation, herbicides, insecticides, and some chemical exposures also increase risk. However, the majority of people with lymphoma do not have clearly identified risk factors.

Symptoms of lymphoma depend on where it originates. A swollen lymph node is a common presentation, but the majority of swollen lymph nodes are not due to lymphoma. If the lymphoma originates in the thymus, it can cause a cough or shortness of breath; in the abdomen, it can cause swelling or pain. Other general symptoms associated with lymphoma include weight loss, fever, drenching night sweats, and severe itchiness.

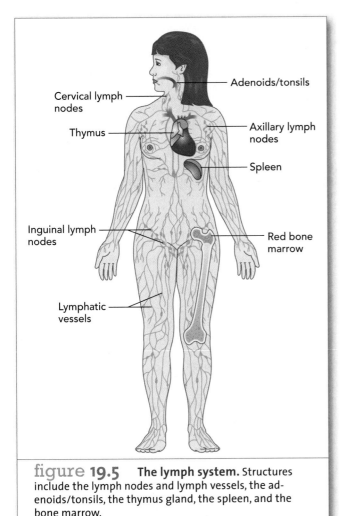

figure 19.5 **The lymph system.** Structures include the lymph nodes and lymph vessels, the adenoids/tonsils, the thymus gland, the spleen, and the bone marrow.

Diagnosis is made by a biopsy of the swollen lymph node or other tissue. Imaging studies, such as chest X-ray, CT scans, and MRIs, are important to determine if and how far the lymphoma has spread. Treatment often includes a combination of surgery, chemotherapy, and radiation. Treatment can sometimes involve immunotherapy or bone marrow transplant. The 5-year survival rate for non-Hodgkin's lymphoma is 63 percent.[1]

Cancer Screening

Early detection is the key to successful treatment of cancer, and **screening tests** are the key to early detection. Cancer screening involves trying to identify risk factors, precancerous lesions, or undetected cancers in an asymptomatic person. An ideal screening test would always detect precursors or cancer at an early, treatable stage and never produce a false negative or false positive result. A false negative means that a cancer is missed and remains undetected and untreated. A false positive creates trauma for the person diagnosed and sometimes leads to unnecessary surgery.

screening test
Test given to a large group of people to identify a smaller group of people who are at higher risk for a specific disease or condition.

Unfortunately, no screening test meets the ideal. The ACS screening recommendations for breast, colon, prostate, uterine, and cervical cancers are summarized in the box "ACS Cancer Detection Guidelines." No screening recommendations exist for some cancers, including lung and ovarian cancers, because to date, no test has been shown to improve detection without increasing harm.

Genetic screening can also be done to assess cancer risk. At this time, it is being reserved for members of high-risk families, that is, families with multiple members with cancer.

Cancer Treatments

Surgery is the oldest treatment for cancer; newer options include chemotherapy, radiation, biological therapies, bone marrow transplantation, and gene therapy.

SURGERY

Surgery remains a mainstay in diagnosis and treatment of cancer. When a cancer is detected early and is small and localized, surgery can cure it, as when an *in situ* cancer of the breast is removed via a lumpectomy. Sometimes an organ affected by cancer can be removed surgically without threatening life, as in the case of prostate or testicular cancer. Certain cancers are unlikely to spread widely, such as a basal cell carcinoma, and surgery often cures these cancers as well. If a cancer has spread, surgery may still be performed as part of the treatment.

Highlight on Health

ACS Cancer Detection Guidelines

Regular physical exams should include examinations for cancers of the thyroid, oral cavity, skin, lymph nodes, testes, and ovaries. Special tests for certain cancer sites are recommended as outlined below.

Breast Cancer

- Yearly mammograms starting at age 40 and continuing for as long as a woman is in good health.

- Clinical breast exam should be part of a periodic health exam, about every 3 years for women in their 20s and 30s and every year for women 40 and over.

- Women should know how their breasts normally feel and report any breast change promptly to their health care providers. Breast self-exam is an option for women starting in their 20s.

- Women at high risk (greater than 20 percent lifetime risk) should get an MRI and a mammogram every year. Women at moderately increased risk (15–20 percent lifetime risk) should talk with their doctors about the benefits and limitations of adding MRI screening to their yearly mammogram. Yearly MRI screening is not recommended for women whose lifetime risk of breast cancer is less than 15 percent.

Colon and Rectal Cancer

Beginning at age 50, both men and women at *average risk* should use one of the screening tests below. The tests that are designed to find both early cancer and polyps are preferred if these tests are available to you and you are willing to have one of these more invasive tests.

Tests that find polyps and cancer

- Flexible sigmoidoscopy every 5 years*
- Colonoscopy every 10 years
- Double-contrast barium enema every 5 years*
- CT colonography (virtual colonoscopy) every 5 years*

Tests that mainly find cancer

- Fecal occult blood test (FOBT) every year*,**
- Fecal immunochemical test (FIT) every year*,**
- Stool DNA test, interval uncertain*

All positive tests should be followed up with colonoscopy.

People should begin colorectal cancer screening earlier and/or undergo screening more often if they have any of the risk factors described in the chapter, such as a personal or family history of colon polyps or colon cancer; a personal history of chronic inflammatory bowel disease; or a family history of a hereditary colorectal cancer syndrome.

---

*Colonoscopy should be done if test results are positive.

**For FOBT or FIT used as a screening test, the take-home multiple sample method should be used. A FOBT or FIT done during a digital rectal exam in the doctor's office is not adequate for screening.

CHEMOTHERAPY

Chemotherapy is a drug treatment administered to the entire body to kill any cancer cells that may have escaped from the local site to the blood, lymph system, or another part of the body. More than 50 chemotherapy medicines have been developed; different combinations are used for different cancers. All chemotherapeutic drugs operate by a similar mechanism—they interfere with rapid cell division. Because cancer cells divide more rapidly than normal cells, they are more vulnerable than healthy cells to destruction by chemotherapy.

Other normal tissues that divide rapidly are also harmed by chemotherapy, including the hair, stomach lining, and white blood cells. The timing and dosage must be carefully adjusted so the drugs kill cancer cells but do not damage normal cells beyond repair. Scientists are developing new chemotherapy techniques that focus on the features that make cancer cells unique. For instance, targeted chemotherapy drugs can distinguish antigen markers on the surface of cancer cells, so they can kill those cells with less harm to normal cells.

RADIATION

Radiation causes damage to cells by altering their DNA; it can be used to destroy cancer cells with minimal damage to surrounding tissues. Radiation is a local treatment that can be used before or after surgery or in conjunction with chemotherapy. It can also be used to control pain in patients with cancer that cannot be cured.

BIOLOGICAL THERAPIES

Biological therapies enhance the immune system's ability to fight cancer (an approach called **immunotherapy**) or reduce the side effects of chemotherapy. One kind of immunotherapy is a vaccine that can be developed after a person has been diagnosed with a cancer. Administering the vaccine can boost the immune response to the cancer and may help prevent a recurrence. Vaccines for several types of cancers, including melanoma and cancers of the breast,

immunotherapy
Administration of drugs or other substances that enhance the ability of the immune system to fight cancer.

Cervical cancer

- Women should begin cervical cancer screening about 3 years after they begin having vaginal intercourse, but no later than when they are 21 years old. Screening should be done every year with the regular Pap test or every 2 years with the liquid-based Pap test.

- Beginning at age 30, women who have had three normal Pap test results in a row may get screened every 2 to 3 years. Another option is to get screened every 3 years (but not more frequently) with either the conventional or liquid-based Pap test, plus the HPV DNA test. Women who have certain risk factors such as diethylstilbestrol (DES) exposure before birth, HIV infection, or a weakened immune system due to organ transplant, chemotherapy, or chronic steroid use should continue to be screened annually.

- Women 70 years of age or older who have had three or more normal Pap tests in a row and no abnormal Pap tests results in the last 10 years may choose to stop having cervical cancer screening. Women with a history of cervical cancer, DES exposure before birth, HIV infection, or a weakened immune system should continue to have screening as long as they are in good health.

- Women who have had a total hysterectomy (removal of the uterus and cervix) may also choose to stop having cervical cancer screening, unless the surgery was done as a treatment for cervical cancer or precancer. Women who have had a hysterectomy without removal of the cervix should continue to follow the guidelines above.

Endometrial (Uterine) Cancer

At the time of menopause, all women should be informed about the risks and symptoms of endometrial cancer and strongly encouraged to report any unexpected bleeding or spotting to their doctors. For women with or at high risk for hereditary non-polyposis colon cancer, annual screening should be offered for endometrial cancer with endometrial biopsy beginning at age 35.

Prostate Cancer

Both the prostate-specific antigen (PSA) blood test and digital rectal examination (DRE) should be *offered* annually, beginning at age 50, to men who have at least a 10-year life expectancy. Men at high risk (Black men and men with a strong family history of one or more first-degree relatives [father, brothers] diagnosed before age 65) should begin testing at age 45. Men at even higher risk, due to multiple first-degree relatives affected at an early age, could begin testing at age 40. Depending on the results of this initial test, no further testing might be needed until age 45.

Information should be provided to all men about what is known and what is uncertain about the benefits, limitations, and harms of early detection and treatment of prostate cancer so that they can make an informed decision about testing.

Men who ask their doctor to make the decision on their behalf should be tested. Discouraging testing is not appropriate. Also, not offering testing is not appropriate.

Source: American Cancer Society Guidelines for the Early Detection of Cancer. Reprinted by permission of the American Cancer Society, Inc., from www.cancer.org. All rights reserved.

colon, ovary, and prostate, are under investigation. Vaccines can also be used to prevent cancer, as in the case of the HPV vaccine for cervical cancer.

Medications can also be used to boost the immune response. Such drugs as interleukin-2, herceptin, and interferon-alpha are used to treat some cancers. Other medications improve the health of damaged immune system components by increasing the numbers of white blood cells, red blood cells, or platelets.[24]

Immunotherapy also includes boosting the immune system with social support, whether in the form of friends, family, or cancer support groups. Prolonged cancer survival is associated with good support systems and a positive outlook.

BONE MARROW TRANSPLANTATION

Bone marrow transplantation was initially used for cancer of the white blood cells (leukemia, lymphoma). Now it is sometimes used for other cancers when healthy bone marrow cells are killed by high doses of chemotherapy. This treatment approach is controversial for some types of cancer because of complications from high-dose chemotherapy and the high risk of infection. Additionally, data have not conclusively shown a significantly improved survival rate for some cancers.

GENE THERAPY AND GENETIC TESTING

Gene therapy could be used in several different ways to improve cancer treatment. In theory, mutated genes could be replaced with functional genes, decreasing the risk that cancer will occur or stopping a cancer that has started to develop. Genes could be inserted into immune cells to increase their ability to fight cancer cells, or they could be inserted into the cancer cells themselves, causing them to self-destruct or making the cancer more susceptible to chemotherapy. The use of gene therapy for cancer treatment is still in the clinical trials stage at this time.[24]

Genetic testing may also become important in cancer treatment. It could allow physicians to predict more accurately how a cancer will behave, which chemotherapy drugs will work best against it, which patients will benefit from chemotherapy, and which patients can skip this treatment.

COMPLEMENTARY AND ALTERNATIVE MEDICINE

The role of complementary and alternative medicine (CAM) in cancer treatment is currently a hot topic for research. Cancer patients and survivors frequently use CAM practices as an adjunct to standard treatment options, often with the goal of reducing the side effects of cancer or cancer treatment, speeding recovery, improving pain control, and increasing chances of survival. Dietary and nutritional supplements are the most commonly used practices, with 60–80 percent of cancer survivors reporting use (compared to 50 percent of the general population). However, there is concern that supplements may interfere with traditional treatments, so they are not generally recommended. Instead, experts recommend a healthy, balanced diet.

Some CAM practices have been shown to be of benefit and include acupuncture (to reduce chemo-induced nausea and vomiting and to reduce cancer pain or surgical pain), massage (to reduce cancer-related fatigue), hypnosis (to reduce pain, nausea, and vomiting), Qigong (to reduce pain and increase activity), and meditation or mindfulness practices (to reduce stress, improve mood, possibly boost immune function).[25–27] For more on this topic, see Chapter 20.

TREATMENTS ON THE HORIZON: CLINICAL TRIALS

Studies designed by researchers and physicians to test different drugs and treatment regimens are known as **clinical trials.** Participants in clinical trials are patients with cancer who enroll both in the hopes of finding a better treatment for their own cancer and in the interest of furthering cancer research in general.

clinical trials
Studies designed by researchers and physicians to test different drugs and treatment regimens.

Once enrolled in the study, participants are usually randomly assigned to either a group receiving a new drug or a group receiving the standard treatment. In rare situations, usually when there is no effective treatment, one group of patients may receive a placebo (a "sugar pill" that has no effect). If cancer is advancing in a patient who is receiving the placebo, he or she may be switched to the group receiving the drug. For more information about new and ongoing clinical trials, visit the Web site of the National Cancer Institute.

Living With Cancer

As a result of improved screening and treatment, cancer is no longer seen as a death sentence; rather, it is seen, in many cases, as a chronic disease that can be managed. In the United States the survival rate for all stages and types of cancer combined is 63 percent. Many cancers are now curable or controllable, and cancer survivors often return to a healthy life. An estimated 10 million people living in the United States have a history of cancer. Some are cancer free, others are undergoing treatment, and others are in remission.

As a chronic disease, however, cancer does change the way a person lives his or her life. Many issues and questions arise for people when they are living with a cancer diagnosis, undergoing treatment, or becoming cancer survivors. For suggestions on dealing with some of these issues, see the box "Living With Cancer."

Important discoveries in the areas of cancer biology, genetics, screening, and treatment have transformed the face of cancer. Greater knowledge of risk factors has led to more effective prevention strategies. Mortality is declining, survival rates are rising, and the quality of life for those with cancer is improving. The future holds great promise for continuing progress.

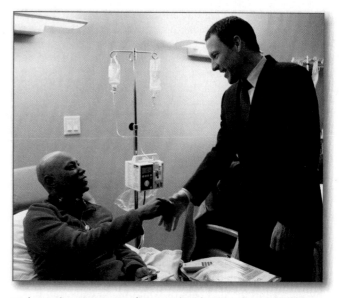

■ Lance Armstrong was diagnosed with testicular cancer that had metastasized to his brain and lungs when he was 25. He founded the Lance Armstrong Foundation, with the goal of supporting quality of life for people affected by cancer, before he knew whether he would survive. Here, he greets a patient during a hospital tour in Texas.

Challenges & Choices

Living With Cancer

If you or a friend or family member receives a diagnosis of cancer, many issues will arise that you probably have never had to deal with before. Here are some suggestions that may help in this difficult time:

- Participate in decisions about your treatment and care to the greatest extent possible, or ask the person with cancer how much he or she wants to be involved in treatment decisions. Maintaining a sense of control is associated with better health outcomes.

- Be an informed consumer. Gather information about your cancer (or your family member's cancer). If you have questions, write them down and ask your health care provider at the next appointment. Make sure you are comfortable with the health team's technical expertise and emotional support.

- Consider how you will interact with family members, friends, and acquaintances. With whom will you share the diagnosis and when? Who will provide you with emotional support? If you need assistance, who might help with tasks, such as driving to appointments, cooking meals, or shopping? If you have a friend or family member with cancer, consider your strengths and what you can offer—perhaps a day spent helping in the garden or taking a child on an outing.

- Consider school or work obligations. You may have to take time off for treatment, and you may experience job discrimination. The Rehabilitation Act and the Americans with Disabilities Act are two federal laws that protect cancer patients. Your health insurance cannot drop you even if you leave your job (although your rates may go up and you may have to pay for it yourself).

- Enlist support. A cancer support group can offer information, teach coping skills, and give you a place to voice your concerns and share your experiences. You can find support groups through your health care team, church, or community or on the Internet.

- Know what physical changes are likely to occur. For example, some cancer treatments have side effects that change how you feel on a daily basis; others change your appearance, as when chemotherapy causes hair loss. Your sense of identity may be affected, as you adapt to the changes in your health. As a support person, remembering the "whole" person and not just focusing on the cancer-related changes can be helpful.

- If you or your partner is about to start a treatment that affects your future fertility and you want to have children, consider the possibility of sperm or egg donation and freezing.

- If you have spiritual beliefs or practices, they can be an important part of life now. Research suggests that people with a sense of spirituality have a better quality of life while living with cancer than those who are not spiritual.

- Understand and follow recommendations for ongoing monitoring. People with cancer have an increased risk of developing a second cancer, as a result of either a genetic predisposition or the cancer treatment itself. Know what is recommended to help reduce your risk of future disease or complications.

- Coping with a cancer diagnosis and treatment can be exhausting. Supporting someone with cancer can also lead to burnout. In either situation, it is important not to think about the cancer all the time. Caregivers should try not to feel guilty about enjoying life and activities. They also need to be able to ask for help so that they can remain supportive in the long run.

It's Not Just Personal . . .

Throughout the world, cancer support groups range from a dozen people who meet monthly in a cancer center to large online groups whose members log on at any time to share their ups and downs. These groups may be organized in different ways—according to the type of cancer, the stage of cancer experience, or the coping skills needed. What they offer in common is a sense of togetherness and hope.

You Make the Call

What Do You Do With Conflicting Health Recommendations?

In the late 1990s the CDC began to report a rise in cases of rickets, a vitamin D deficiency disease not seen for decades. Rickets causes bone softening and deformities in children and bone loss and fractures in adults. The reason for the resurgence of the crippling disease was, in part, avoidance of sun exposure by parents who were protecting their children from the risks of sunburn and future skin cancer, as recommended by health experts. The story of vitamin D deficiency versus risk of skin cancer points to the complexity of current health advisories.

Vitamin D is an essential micronutrient for humans. It is needed for the development and maintenance of bones and teeth and a healthy immune system. Higher levels are associated with lower rates of colon, prostate, breast, esophageal, and pancreatic cancers and improved survival among melanoma patients. Lower levels are associated with multiple health problems, including reduced calcium absorption, osteoporosis (thinning of the bones), autoimmune disorders, and an increased risk of heart disease. Extreme vitamin D deficiency causes rickets.

The body's major source of vitamin D is sunlight. Exposure to sunlight, specifically UVB, triggers synthesis of vitamin D in skin cells. An estimated 20–30 percent of people in some areas of the United States have moderate to severe vitamin D deficiency, mostly because of lack of sun exposure. Risk is greatest in northern latitudes, in individuals who are homebound, and in people with dark skin. Anything that diminishes sun exposure increases the chance of vitamin D deficiency.

At the same time that sun exposure is needed for vitamin D synthesis, it is also the most dangerous risk factor for skin cancer. To reduce the risk of skin cancer, including melanoma, people are advised to avoid being in the sun during peak hours (10 a.m. to 4 p.m.), to stay in the shade, to wear protective hats and clothing, and to use sunscreen. A sunscreen with an SPF of 15 absorbs 99 percent of the UVB radiation in sunlight, reducing the risk for sunburn and skin cancer—but it also decreases the synthesis of vitamin D by 99 percent.

How do we balance these conflicting health recommendations? The Recommended Daily Allowance for vitamin D is 400 international units (IUs). How long do you have to be in the sun to get that amount? Recommendations vary from 10 to 15 minutes of sun exposure without sunscreen twice a week to 30 minutes outside per day.

Vitamin D can also be obtained from a few foods, including salmon, mackerel, sardines, cod liver oil, and some fortified milks, yogurts, and cereals. Vitamin and mineral supplements are not generally recommended as a substitute for a balanced diet, but the Institute of Medicine does recommend 200 IUs of vitamin D a day for people under age 50 and 400–600 IUs for people over age 50. The National Osteoporosis Foundation recommends that postmenopausal women take 800–1,000 IUs per day. Some data suggest that these recommendations may be too low—it may be that all people need up to 1,000 IUs per day.

At present, there is no routine recommendation to check vitamin D levels in the general public. Thus, according to some experts, it makes sense to get sun exposure to ensure that adequate amounts of this micronutrient are being obtained. Others disagree. What do you think?

Pros

- Sunlight is a natural way to get the vitamin D we need.
- The benefits of a moderate amount of sun exposure outweigh the risk of skin cancer.
- Even if sun exposure increases the risk of skin cancer, adequate levels of vitamin D reduce the risk of other kinds of cancer and improve survival among people with melanoma—the worst kind of skin cancer.

Cons

- Sun exposure is linked directly to skin cancer—the most common form of cancer—and avoiding time in the sun is recommended by the CDC, the American Cancer Society, and other leading health organizations.
- You can get vitamin D from other, safer sources, including some fish and vitamin supplements.
- Sun exposure causes skin damage and premature aging. It's an irresponsible health behavior choice to spend time in the sun without sunscreen.

Source: "Vitamin D Deficiency: A Worldwide Problem With Health Consequences," by M.F. Holick and T.C. Chen, 2008, American Journal of Clinical Nutrition, 87 (4), pp. 1080–1086.

In Review

1. **What is cancer?** Cancer, the second leading cause of death in the United States, is a condition characterized by an uncontrolled growth of cells, which develop into a tumor and have the potential to spread to other parts of the body.

2. **What causes cancer?** Cancer can be caused by random genetic mutations, a genetic predisposition, or exposure to carcinogens. Usually a combination of innate and environmental factors is involved. Risk factors include a family history of cancer; lifestyle factors like tobacco use, poor nutrition, overweight and obesity, physical inactivity, and alcohol consumption; and environmental factors like exposure to UV radiation, infectious agents, and chemical and physical carcinogens.

3. **What are the most common cancers?** The leading cause of cancer death for both men and women is lung cancer, and the third leading cause for both men and women is colorectal cancer. The second leading cause of cancer death for women is breast cancer and for men, prostate cancer. Cancers of the female reproductive system include cervical, uterine, and ovarian cancer. Testicular cancer, though rare, is the most common cancer among young men. Two types of skin cancer, basal cell and squamous cell carcinomas, are highly curable, but melanoma is an aggressive and dangerous form of skin cancer. Oral cancer is associated with tobacco and alcohol use. Leukemia is a cancer of the blood cells, and lymphoma is a cancer that arises in the lymph system.

4. **How is cancer detected and treated?** Many cancers can be detected by screening tests like mammograms; for other cancers, there are no reliable screening tests, and symptoms appear only when the cancer is advanced. The traditional treatment is surgery to remove the cancer; other treatments include chemotherapy, radiation, and, most recently, gene therapy. Millions of people have survived cancer and live with it as a chronic condition.

www For a detailed summary of this chapter and a comprehensive set of review questions, visit the Online Learning Center at **www.mhhe.com/teague2e**.

Web Resources

American Cancer Society: The ACS site features topics such as learning about cancer, treatment options, treatment decision tools, clinical trials, and coping strategies. Its Statistics and Facts and Figures are valuable resources for health care consumers.
www.cancer.org

American Institute for Cancer Research: This organization offers resources for cancer prevention, a free information program for cancer patients about living with cancer, and news about the latest advances in cancer research.
www.aicr.org

Centers for Disease Control and Prevention: The cancer section of this site provides facts on all types of cancers. Its links lead to information on risk factors, prevention, survivorship, and statistics.
www.cdc.gov

National Cancer Institute: This site offers a wide range of cancer information, including types, treatments, terminology, support and resources, screening and testing, statistics, and research.
www.cancer.gov

National Coalition for Cancer Survivorship: This organization focuses on survivorship issues, such as palliative care and management of symptoms. It offers a cancer survival toolbox and a resource guide with links to other helpful sites.
www.canceradvocacy.org

Chapter

20

Complementary and Alternative Medicine
Health Choices in a Changing Society

Ever Wonder...

- how acupuncture is supposed to work?

- how to evaluate alternative medical practices?

- if you should tell your doctor about vitamins or herbal remedies you are taking?

WWW

Your Health Today

www.mhhe.com/teague2e

Go to the Online Learning Center for *Your Health Today* for interactive activities, quizzes, flashcards, Web links, and more resources related to this chapter.

If you catch a cold, do you eat chicken soup, take vitamin C and echinacea, or get an acupuncture treatment? If you develop lower back pain, do you start a regimen of stretching exercises, take pain medication, or see a chiropractor? Many health care options are available in our society, and most people are aware of the different conventional health care providers they can consult, including physicians, psychologists, pharmacists, and so on.

In the last 20 years, however, the use of **complementary and alternative medicine (CAM)** has grown dramatically in the United States and Canada. Some CAM practices have a degree of acceptance in conventional health care, such as chiropractic care and massage therapy; others, such as magnetic-field therapies and other forms of energy medicine, remain well outside the mainstream. In this chapter we explore some of these practices and provide guidelines to help you choose among CAM, conventional medicine, and self-care when you have a health problem.

> **complementary and alternative medicine (CAM)**
> As defined by the NCCAM, "a group of diverse medical and health care systems, practices, and products that are not presently considered to be part of conventional medicine."

Approaches to Health Care

As discussed in Chapter 1, health-related beliefs and practices are largely defined by a person's cultural background. In most industrialized countries, ideas about medicine are conditioned by Western tradition; in other countries, different systems and sets of ideas have developed, in many cases over hundreds if not thousands of years. Recently, ideas and practices from other traditions have gained acceptance in Western medicine, as noted throughout this book. They include ideas about mind-body connections, the role of spirituality in wellness, and the importance of relationships and social support, among others (see the box "What Is Holistic Health Care").

In recognition of such ideas, Congress established the Office of Alternative Medicine in 1991 and expanded it into the National Center for Complementary and Alternative Medicine (NCCAM) in 1998. The NCCAM is an institute of the National Institutes of Health, which is an agency of the U.S. Department of Health and Human Services.

The goals of the NCCAM are to support scientific investigation of complementary and alternative healing practices, to train research-ers to explore these practices, and to disseminate authoritative information. The NCCAM funds and conducts rigorous laboratory-based and clinical research projects and supports the integration of proven CAM practices into conventional medicine. In this way, the center acts as a clearinghouse for information about CAM and a bridge between the two traditions.

In this section we consider features that have traditionally been part of Western medicine, and we contrast them with the features that characterize CAM practices. Remember that medical practices considered complementary or alternative in the United States may be, and are likely to be, part of the mainstream medical system in other cultures.

CONVENTIONAL MEDICINE

The term **conventional medicine** refers to the dominant health care system in the United States, Canada, and much of Europe and other parts of the developed world. Other terms for this system include *Western medicine, biomedicine,* and *allopathic medicine.*

Characteristics of Conventional Medicine As discussed in Chapter 1, Western medicine has traditionally considered illness to be the result of pathogens like bacteria and viruses or organic changes in the body. Health is restored, according to this model, when a medical practitioner treats the illness with drugs, vaccines, or surgery. Along with public health measures that improved safety of

> **conventional medicine**
> The dominant health care system in the United States, Canada, and much of Europe and the rest of the developed world; also referred to as *Western medicine, biomedicine,* and *allopathic medicine.*

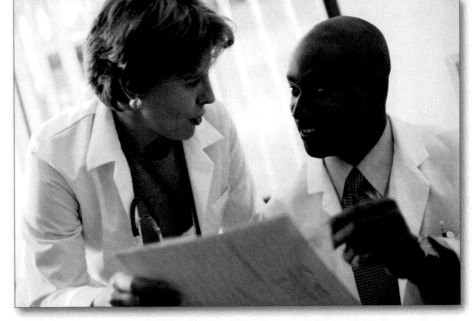

■ In conventional Western medicine, treatment is often provided by a team of licensed or certified health care professionals who share a set of ideas and beliefs about the causes of illness and how it should be treated.

the food and water supply, this medical intervention model has been highly successful in reducing the incidence of infectious diseases, enhancing quality of life, and lengthening life expectancy for people living in developed countries of the world.

Other characteristic ideas underlying conventional medicine include the following:

- The body is somewhat like a machine; it can be broken down into parts that, in the case of illness, need to be fixed. The idea that the whole can be reduced to its parts—that the whole is not greater than the sum of its parts—is a way of thinking known as *reductionist*. The discovery of bacteria supported the search for isolated, external causes of disease and the tendency to treat diseases by destroying pathogens or limiting the damage they do.

- An illness is defined by a set of symptoms that are similar in everyone who has the illness. Thus, large populations can be given the same treatments for a particular disease, as in an antibiotic for an infection.

- Investigations into the causes of disease and treatments for them are conducted using the scientific method, which is based on empirical, observable evidence and controlled studies that can be verified and replicated by other researchers.

Conventional Health Care Providers　The practitioners of conventional medicine include an array of providers who often work side by side. Physicians in conventional medicine hold an M.D. (medical doctor) or D.O. (doctor of osteopathy) degree. Physicians often specialize in a specific part of the body: Cardiologists focus on the heart and blood vessels, neurosurgeons focus on brain surgery, orthopedists focus on bones and joints, and so on. Family physicians, pediatricians, and internists are considered generalists within conventional medicine.

Other conventional providers include dentists, optometrists, podiatrists, and allied health care providers. This last category of trained professionals includes registered nurses, nurse practitioners, licensed vocational nurses, physician

Highlight on Health

What Is Holistic Health Care?

We often hear about the holistic approach to health and health care. What is meant by holistic health care, and how does it differ from conventional health care?

The core idea of holism is that all things are interconnected and that the interacting parts make up an organized whole, or *system*. Smaller systems are embedded in an ever-widening succession of increasingly complex systems. The whole is seen as something unique created from the relationships among the parts, and studying the entire system as well as the relationships within the system reveals more than can be understood from studying the parts alone. In other words, the whole is greater than the sum of its parts.

When applied to health and health care, holism means that the person is considered as a whole—mind, body, and spirit. In conventional Western practice, these aspects of human experience have been treated as separate entities, with the body assigned to the realm of medicine, the mind to the realm of psychology, and the spirit to the realm of religion or spirituality. The holistic model brings the wisdom of these disciplines together, attending to the whole person. A holistic health practitioner might ask questions about physical symptoms, family relationships, life circumstances, and recent events. For example, persistent stomach aches may be part of a grief experience over the loss of a loved one, and a holistic health practitioner might not only treat the stomach ailment but also refer a patient to a grief counselor or a spiritual advisor.

Recent research in neuroscience has offered some explanations for the connections between mind and body. Scientists have found that receptors for certain kinds of brain chemicals (neuropeptides) are located throughout the body, including the digestive system, the cardiovascular system, the muscles, and the skin. This biochemical network connects every part of the body, providing the basis for a body-wide communication system on a cellular level. In holistic health, the terms *mind-body* and *mind-body-spirit* are used to describe this unity. Examples of the interconnections among thoughts, emotions, and physiological reactions include the fight-or-flight response, the effect of anger and hostility on cardiovascular health, and the placebo effect; even blushing and crying are evidence of these interrelationships.

On a larger scale, the principles of holism can be applied to environmental health. We are part of a network of people living in and using the resources of nature on a relatively small planet. We interact in social circles composed of family and friends; we are part of a community; and we share the planet with a wide variety of people from different ethnic groups and cultures. We also live in the natural world of plants and animals. We breathe the air, drink the water, and use the natural resources provided by the planet. All of these things are interconnected and work together to form what we have come to see as the web of life. We need to see ourselves as an integral part of this larger system of life, not just as users of it. Our individual wellness is interconnected with the wellness of the planet and with all the living things that depend on it for life. This is the essence of the holistic world view, of which holistic health care is one expression.

Special thanks go to Kathi Fuller, Charlene Brown, and Jennifer Mills of Western Michigan University for their contribution to this box.

assistants, physical therapists, registered dietitians, nurse midwives, and medical assistants. Standards of practice and credentialing policies for providers are established by states and by professional medical associations.

COMPLEMENTARY AND ALTERNATIVE MEDICINE

As defined by the NCCAM, complementary and alternative medicine is "a group of diverse medical and health care systems, practices, and products that are not presently considered to be part of conventional medicine."[1] Note that practices considered complementary or alternative are "not presently" considered part of conventional medicine, but as they are studied and evaluated, they may be adopted into conventional medicine in the future.

Complementary medicine is a group of practices used together with conventional medicine. The use of acupuncture to reduce pain after surgery would be considered a complement to conventional medicine. **Alternative medicine** is a group of practices used as an alternative to conventional medicine. The use of a special diet instead of chemotherapy as a treatment for cancer would be considered an alternative to conventional medicine.

Integrative medicine combines conventional medicine and CAM practices.[1] Sometimes a conventional health care provider and a CAM provider will work together to provide integrative medicine. At other times, a conventional provider will have training in certain CAM practices and integrate both forms of medicine. For example, some physicians and dentists obtain training in acupuncture and incorporate it into their medical or dental practices.[2] (For a different approach to health care, see the box "What Is Holistic Health Care?")

complementary medicine
Group of practices used together with conventional medicine.

alternative medicine
Group of practices used as an alternative to conventional medicine.

integrative medicine
Use of conventional medicine in combination with CAM practices that have been proven safe and effective.

Characteristics of Complementary and Alternative Medicine CAM approaches encompass a vast array of practices that have developed in different cultures all over the world. Although they are extremely diverse, many have certain characteristics in common, including the following:

- The body is believed to have an inherent balance or ability to heal itself; treatments are aimed at restoring the balance or enhancing the body's self-healing capabilities.

- The whole person is treated, taking into account the physical, mental, emotional, and spiritual dimensions, rather than focusing on a particular part of the body or a specific pathogenic process.

- Each person is unique, so diagnosis and treatment are individualized. Symptoms of a cold in one person might require a different treatment than would similar symptoms in another person. The focus tends to be on the imbalance

Highlight on Health

Domains of CAM and Representative Practices

Provider-based practices are indicated with an asterisk (*). Those without an asterisk can be performed without a provider.

Mind-Body Practices
Biofeedback*
Deep breathing
Guided imagery or visualization
Hypnosis*
Meditation
Prayer for health purposes
Progressive relaxation
T'ai chi
Yoga

Biologically Based Practices
Dietary supplements
Herbal medicines
Megavitamins

Manipulative and Body-Based Practices
Chiropractic care*
Massage therapy*
Rolfing*
Feldenkrais*

Energy Therapies
Magnetic-field therapies
Qigong
Reiki*

Whole Medical Systems
Homeopathy*
Naturopathy*
Ayurvedic medicine*
Traditional Chinese Medicine*

Source: National Center for Complementary and Alternative Medicine, www.nccam.nih.gov.

in a person that allows him or her to be susceptible to illness rather than on the pathogen causing illness in many people.

- Many practices use a combination of interventions, often involving of many medications or medicinal substances at the same time, in addition to recommended behaviors, rather than a single intervention or pill.

CAM Providers Some CAM practices have well-established training programs with licensing and credentialing procedures similar to those in place for conventional pro-

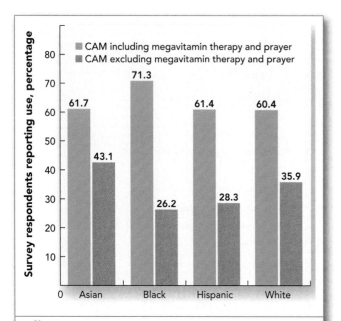

figure **20.1** **Use of CAM therapies, by ethnicity and race.**
Source: "The Use of Complementary and Alternative Medicine in the United States," National Center for Complementary and Alternative Medicine, 2007, retrieved May 18, 2008, from http://nccam.nih.gov/news/camsurvey_fs1.htm#use.

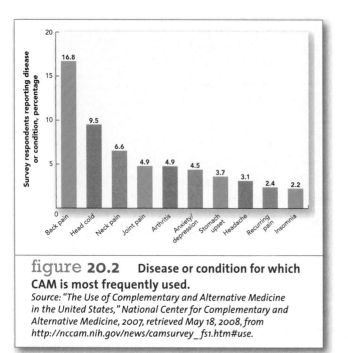

figure **20.2** **Disease or condition for which CAM is most frequently used.**
Source: "The Use of Complementary and Alternative Medicine in the United States," National Center for Complementary and Alternative Medicine, 2007, retrieved May 18, 2008, from http://nccam.nih.gov/news/camsurvey_fs1.htm#use.

viders. To become a chiropractor or acupuncturist in many states requires a formal training program and passage of state licensing exams. Most states have minimum requirements for training and licensure for massage therapists. Other practices, such as homeopathy, hypnosis, or Reiki, are not regulated consistently from state to state. Training programs vary, and licensure, when required, is by the state, making it difficult for the consumer to evaluate a provider's background and competence.[3]

Classification and Use of CAM Practices In an attempt to organize the diverse range of practices included in CAM, the NCCAM has identified four domains—mind-body interventions, biologically based therapies, manipulative and body-based therapies, and energy therapies—in addition to whole medical systems, which cut across the four domains and employ practices from some or all of them (see the box "Domains of CAM and Representative Practices").

The most recent national survey on the use of CAM remains the 2004 National Health Interview Survey, in which more than 30,000 Americans reported on their health-related behaviors, including their use of CAM. According to this survey, 62 percent of Americans use some form of CAM, when megavitamin therapy and prayer for health purposes are included. When these two interventions are excluded, 36 percent report using some form of CAM. The most commonly used domain of CAM is mind-body medicine, when prayer for health reasons in included.[4]

More recent survey data from subsets of the U.S. population suggest that the trend continues toward ongoing integration of CAM practices into mainstream medicine. According to the American Hospital Association, the use of CAM services by patients as reported by hospitals increased from 6 percent in 1998 to 26.5 percent in 2005. Many hospitals are incorporating different CAM modalities for outpatients, including massage, t'ai chi, yoga, Qigong, and relaxation techniques.

Insurance and health maintenance organization coverage for CAM practices continues to increase, with the majority covering chiropractic care, approximately 40 percent covering acupuncture, and 37 percent covering massage. Many states have mandates for insurance to cover CAM practices, although such mandates do not help those too poor to have health insurance (see the box "Poverty and Health Inequities").[5, 6]

CAM practices are more commonly used by women than by men, by people with higher educational levels and higher income, by people who have been hospitalized in the past year, by smokers, and by Asians more than other ethnic groups (when megavitamin therapy and prayer are excluded) (Figure 20.1). However, some of the surveys may underestimate CAM practices among minority populations, because home remedies that may be considered CAM by Western health care practitioners may be seen as everyday practices in these groups. CAM use also appears to increase with age.

People report using CAM for a variety of reasons, including that they believe it will improve health when combined with conventional medicine, they think it would

Public Health in Action

Poverty and Health Inequities

Although the United States spends more money per person on health care than any other nation, it ranks 30th in life expectancy, behind countries such as Japan, Canada, Germany, United Arab Emirates, Chile, and South Korea. Even within the United States, there are inequities in life expectancy. Certain parts of the country, such as the Deep South, areas along the Mississippi River, and areas in Appalachia, have had worsening life expectancy rates since the early 1980s. The increases in mortality appear to be due to cancer, diabetes, chronic lung disease, HIV/AIDS, and homicide. Clearly, the American health care system is not serving the health needs of all the people.

The biggest factor in health inequality in the United States appears to be income. Poverty and lower socioeconomic status predict poorer health, and the larger the economic gap between different segments of the population, the worse the national health picture. Some experts argue that the greatest health hazard faced by the United States as a nation is the gap between rich and poor. If the top health tip from a lifestyle perspective is "Don't smoke," the top health tip from a social determinants of health perspective might be "Don't be poor."

Why is poverty associated with poorer health? The keys are the cost of health care and lack of health insurance. In 2006, 8.7 million children—11.7 percent of all American children—were uninsured. Insurance rates vary by racial and ethnic group, with 34.1 percent of Hispanic Americans uninsured, compared with 31.4 percent of American Indians/Alaska Natives, 20.5 percent of African Americans, 15.5 percent of Asian Americans, and 10.8 percent of non-Hispanic Whites.

People who don't have insurance use health care services less frequently than do people with insurance. When they do become ill or injured, they have to spend a larger portion of their income on treatment, leaving less money for other necessities for good health, such as food and housing. Uninsured children have fewer checkups, vaccinations, and screening tests, are less likely to receive care for chronic conditions like asthma, and are less likely to receive needed items like eyeglasses. Improving overall health care in the United States depends less on developing new treatments and advanced technologies than it does on improving access to basic care and services that already exist.

How does the use of complementary and alternative medicine play into the complex health care scene in the United States? Although some insurance plans cover selected complementary and alternative practices, most people who use CAM options pay for them out of pocket. Thus those with greater financial means have more access to these forms of medicine as well. Poorer people may be more likely to rely on folk and home remedies, which can be less effective than more standardized CAM products.

Some experts believe that if more CAM practices are included in insurance plans, it may drive up the cost of insurance, leading to the unintended consequence of further limiting access to health care for a subset of the population. Others argue that the inclusion of CAM practices may prove to be more cost effective and in turn reduce health care costs. Including CAM practices may also make it more likely that all aspects of health—physical, mental, social, spiritual—will be addressed. From a public health perspective, the critical issue for our society is deciding where we stand on the basic right of all to have access to health care resources. Once that has been decided, the issue of what to include in basic health care can be addressed.

Sources: "The Reversal of Fortunes: Trends in County Mortality and Cross-Country Mortality Disparities in the United States," by M. Ezzati, A.B. Friedman, S.C. Kulkarni, and C.J. Murray, (2008). PLoS Medicine 5(4): p. e66; "Social Determinants of Health Inequalities," by M. Marmot, 2005, Lancet, 365: pp. 1099–1104; "United States of America: Richest Nation 'Big Gap' Society, Sickest Population," Population Health Forum, http://depts.washington.edu/eqhlth; "Household Income Rises, Poverty Rate Declines, Number Uninsured Up," August 28, 2007, U.S. Census Bureau News, U.S. Department of Commerce, http://www.census.gov/Press-Release/www/releases/archives/income_wealth/010583.html.

be interesting to try, they think conventional medicine will not help, they think conventional medicine is too expensive, and their conventional medical professional recommended it. The most frequently reported reason for using CAM practices is to treat some form of chronic pain (Figure 20.2).[6, 7]

Whole Medical Systems

A whole medical system is a comprehensive group of practices based on a common philosophy. Traditional medicine systems flourish in all cultures; they represent a collection of health practices and approaches incorporating knowledge and beliefs; animal-, mineral-, and plant-based materials;

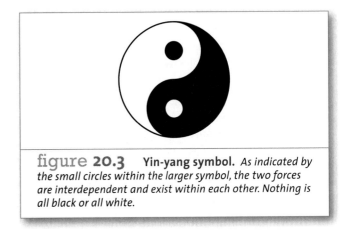

figure 20.3   **Yin-yang symbol.** *As indicated by the small circles within the larger symbol, the two forces are interdependent and exist within each other. Nothing is all black or all white.*

spiritual therapy; and manual therapy. In Africa, Asia, and Latin America, traditional medicines are used by the majority of the population for health care.

Some of the more widely known whole medical systems in the United States and Canada are Traditional Chinese Medicine; Ayurveda, a medical system developed in India; and two Western medical systems, homeopathy and naturopathy. Native American medicine is another example of a traditional system that developed in North America.[8]

TRADITIONAL CHINESE MEDICINE

A well-developed medical system that has been in use in China for nearly 3,000 years, **Traditional Chinese Medicine (TCM)** focuses on maintaining or restoring the physical, mental, and spiritual well-being of the individual. A basic concept is that good health stems from the free flow of **qi (chi)**, vital energy or life force, through the body. Qi moves through the body along several *meridians,* or pathways, each of which is linked with an internal organ or organ system. Illness occurs when the flow of qi is blocked, usually as a result of an imbalance between yin and yang, two opposing but inseparable principles. *Yin* represents the inactive, internal, cold, and dark; *yang* represents the active, external, hot, and bright. Yin and yang are interdependent; each exists within the other, as can be seen in the yin-yang symbol (Figure 20.3.). Good health requires balance and harmony between yin and yang; a deficiency or an excess of one or the other causes a disruption in the flow of qi, resulting in illness.

Diagnosis in TCM involves evaluating an individual for signs of imbalance. Complexion, posture, body fluids, appearance of the tongue, and the quality of pulse in various locations of the body can all be used in diagnosis. The primary treatment methods are herbal medicines, acupuncture, and dietary modification. Preventing illness in TCM involves maintaining a proper lifestyle, which includes eating a balanced diet, getting regular sleep, avoiding excessive stress, and getting adequate exercise. T'ai chi and Qigong are specific mind-body forms of exercise that developed within TCM (both are described later in the chapter).[9, 10]

Herbal Medicine   Specific herbal remedies are believed to strengthen the blood, body, or organs that are imbalanced or weak. Different herbs have different actions and functions, but each one contains dozens of active compounds. Usually, several herbs are combined in a formula, and the proportions and dosage are adjusted to suit the characteristics of the particular patient. Chinese herbal remedies are difficult to evaluate or even analyze because of this variation. Herbal medicine is discussed more fully later in the chapter.

Traditional Chinese Medicine (TCM)
Well-developed medical system originating in China; focus is on maintaining or restoring the physical, mental, and spiritual well-being of the individual.

qi (chi)
Vital energy or life force, believed to flow through the body; a concept in TCM and other forms of CAM.

Acupuncture and Acupressure   Long, thin needles are inserted at certain points in the skin to stimulate the flow of qi in **acupuncture**. Pressure applied with the fingers or hands at these same locations is referred to as **acupressure**. The acupuncturist assesses the individual by questioning, observing, and performing a physical exam that focuses on the tongue, pulse, and any painful trigger points, which correlate with pathways and organs that need rebalancing. Needles are inserted in a pattern that opens blockages and restores energy flow. Treatment usually takes about 30 minutes and may be repeated weekly for 5 to 10 sessions. Practitioners may also use **moxibustion,** a treatment in which heat is applied to acupuncture points by burning an herb called moxa.

In the United States, acupuncture is used primarily to treat muscular problems. Limited studies indicate that acupuncture can help relieve both acute and chronic pain. It is also used to decrease nausea and vomiting during pregnancy and cancer treatment, and studies suggest it may be helpful in substance withdrawal and drug treatment programs. Millions of Americans use acupuncture each year, with relatively few complications reported.

The FDA requires that acupuncturists use sterile, disposable needles to reduce the risk of spreading infection from person to person. Some mild side effects sometimes occur, including sleepiness, fatigue, and pain at the needle site. Very rarely, life-threatening complications have occurred, including serious infection, shortness of breath, organ punctures, and spinal cord injuries.[9, 10]

acupuncture
Treatment method in TCM involving the insertion of long, thin needles at certain points in the skin to stimulate the flow of qi.

acupressure
A treatment involving the use of pressure at certain points of the body to stimulate the flow of qi.

moxibustion
Treatment in which heat is applied to acupuncture points by burning an herb called moxa.

Dietary Modification   Modifying the diet is a key part of TCM. Certain foods are believed to have specific properties— for example, some foods are yin foods and others are yang foods—and they are prescribed to help restore balance between yin and yang properties in the individual seeking treatment. Ginger, a yang food, is believed to promote good digestion by increasing circulation and the secretion of stomach fluids. Garlic, another yang food, improves energy. Chinese yams, sweet potatoes, and whole grains are yin foods; they calm and slow the body, promoting rest.[9]

AYURVEDA

One of the oldest healing systems in the world, **Ayurvedic medicine** has been practiced in India for 5,000 years. It emphasizes balance among the body, mind, and spirit and sets a goal of restoring harmony to the individual. Three energy sources,

Ayurvedic medicine
Traditional medical system of India; focus is on restoring balance among the body, mind, and spirit.

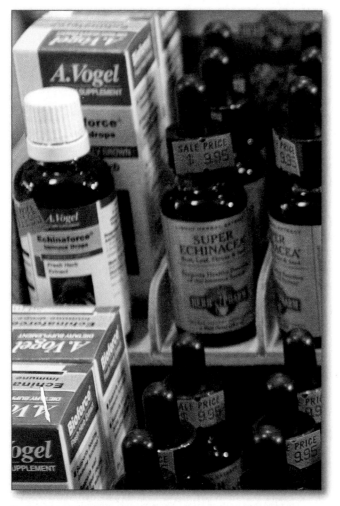

■ Homeopathic remedies include several types of Echinacea, used for conditions associated with the immune system. These include infections, inflammation, colds, flu, allergies, and skin conditions.

called *doshas,* are believed to be present within everyone and everything. *Vatta* is the energy of movement and consists of space and air. *Pitta* is the energy of metabolism and digestion and consists of fire and water. *Kapha* is the energy that forms body structure and holds cells together; it consists of earth and water.

Each person has a unique combination of the three doshas at birth. One or more can be dominant, and seven different combinations are possible. When your three doshas are in balance, you are in good health. When there is an imbalance in your doshas, your body is susceptible to disease. Even if you have a bacterial or viral infection, an Ayurvedic health provider will try to determine why you are susceptible to infection at this particular time.[11]

Ayurvedic practitioners work by helping you align your individual lifestyle with your particular constitution and health history. Assessment involves questioning and observation, especially of the pulse, tongue, eyes, and body fluids. Treatment options include dietary modification, exercises, yoga, meditation, massage, herbal tonics, and controlled breathing.[11]

There is no formalized Ayurvedic training or licensing system in the United States. Some U.S.-trained health care providers complete short courses in India or the United States and incorporate elements of Ayurvedic medicine in their practices.

HOMEOPATHY

A set of principles developed by German chemist and physician Samuel Hahnemann in the 19th century is the basis for **homeopathy.** One principle of homeopathy is the law of similars, or "like cures like." According to this principle, a substance that causes disease in a healthy person can cure the same symptoms in a sick person. For instance, large doses of a plant bark called cinchona will cause a healthy person to develop a fever; homeopaths believe that if a person has a fever, taking a remedy made from diluted cinchona will help the person recover faster.

homeopathy
Medical system based on a set of principles developed by Samuel Hahnemann in the 19th century; principles include the law of similars and the principle of minimal dose.

A second principle of homeopathy is the principle of minimal dose. According to this principle, using the smallest possible dose will have the greatest effect. Homeopathic remedies are intended to encourage the body to heal itself; thus a single small dose is often enough. Remedies are derived from many natural sources, including plants, animals, chemicals, metals, and minerals, and are made through a process called *succession,* a series of shaking and diluting. Solutions are often so diluted that no chemical evidence of the original substance remains.

The third principle of homeopathy is prescribing for the individual. According to this principle, every patient is unique. Treatment in homeopathy is prescribed based not only on the medical diagnosis but also on the specific patient's personality characteristics and emotional and physical responses.

Studying the effectiveness of this system in large groups of people is difficult because of the uniqueness of each individual treatment plan. The studies that have been conducted have had mixed results, with some showing no improvements and others showing benefits. Homeopathy may be beneficial in treating allergies, acute diarrhea in children, and arthritis and in reducing the duration of influenza.[12, 13]

There does not appear to be significant risk associated with homeopathy except the possible risk of delaying diagnosis or the use of other treatments that have been proven to be efficacious. Some studies have shown minor, limited side effects, such as headaches, tiredness, and symptom aggravation, and some problems have arisen due to mislabeling of homeopathic products. The cost of homeopathic medications is typically less than that of pharmaceutical medications, but people in the United States spend more than $200 million on homeopathic treatments each year.

In Europe, homeopathy is practiced as a separate health profession, but in the United States, it is practiced as a subset of another profession. It is a standard component of naturopathy training; medical doctors, osteopaths, chiropractors, and acupuncturists sometimes take courses in homeopathy and integrate it into their practice.

NATUROPATHY

naturopathy
Health system based on the principle that the body can heal itself if stimulated to do so, especially through nutrition.

The main principle of **naturopathy** is that the body has the ability to heal itself, and its goal is to stimulate the body to do so, especially through nutrition. Health is believed to be the natural order if one lives wisely and simply. The focus of naturopathy is on cleansing and strengthening the body rather than on treating the symptoms of a specific illness.

Assessment may include interviewing, observation, evaluation of body fluids, hair analysis, and iridology (a detailed microscopic evaluation of the iris of the eye to aid in diagnosis of disease and illness). Treatments include a variety of noninvasive therapeutic practices, including dietary modification, nutritional supplements, herbal remedies, hydrotherapy, massage and joint manipulation, homeopathy, acupuncture, biofeedback, stress reduction techniques, and lifestyle counseling.

Several colleges of naturopathy now exist in the United States. Naturopaths complete a 4-year training program and then take a licensing exam, although only some states currently license or regulate naturopaths. Only scant data for evaluating naturopathy as a complete system of medicine are available.[14]

NATIVE AMERICAN MEDICINE

Native American tribes throughout North America developed a system of medicine that varied from tribe to tribe but shared certain features. A common thread is the integral relationship of humans with one another, the natural environment, and the spiritual world. Healing and spirituality merge; physical well-being is associated with spiritual balance and illness with imbalance.

Native American healers, sometimes called shamans or medicine men or women, are considered to have spiritual powers or ties to the supernatural. The ability to heal is seen as a gift, often passed down through several generations of the same family. In addition, through a process of observation or apprenticeship, the healer usually learns the medicinal uses of roots, herbs, and other plants.

Illness can have internal or external causes. Internal causes are primarily negative thoughts about oneself or others or the breaking of taboos. External causes might be poisons, traumas, ghosts, witchcraft, or negative thoughts sent from another person. Although a causal agent may be external, individuals are more susceptible if there is an imbalance in their spirit. Techniques that aid in diagnosis and treatment include vision quests, dream interpretation, purification ceremonies, and the use of sweat lodges. Specific remedies may include prayer, healing touch, herbal teas, tinctures, charms, and healing rituals.[15]

Domains of Complementary and Alternative Medicine

The four categories of CAM identified by the NCCAM, as noted earlier, are mind-body practices, biologically based practices, manipulative and body-based practices, and energy therapies.

MIND-BODY PRACTICES

Mind-body practices are based on the premise that the mind influences the body in ways that can promote or detract from well-being. Perceptions, beliefs, and patterns of thinking can have a powerful effect on the immune system, endocrine system, cardiovascular system, digestive system, and other parts of the body. For example, as discussed in Chapters 5 and 18, chronic anger and hostility can cause the release of stress hormones, which can damage the lining of arteries and contribute to cardiovascular disease. Conversely, techniques that enhance stress management, relaxation, and coping skills are beneficial adjuncts to treatment for people with coronary heart disease and pain-related conditions such as arthritis.

Several mind-body practices have been described in this book in the context of mental health, spirituality, and stress management. They include deep breathing, prayer, meditation, progressive relaxation, visualization, yoga, and biofeedback. Many of these practices have health benefits. For example, mindfulness meditation has been shown to decrease chronic pain and anxiety and improve general psychological health when practiced as part of a stress reduction program. Progressive relaxation has been found useful in reducing stress, tension, headaches, and sleep difficulties. Yoga may be beneficial for low back pain, hypertension, arthritis, and sleep difficulties and can improve coordination and flexibility. Biofeedback has proved useful in treating headaches, low back pain, seizures, and incontinence.[1]

The risk associated with mind-body therapies as an adjunct to conventional care is minimal. Most are inexpensive and relatively easy to learn, and they can be integrated into regular self-care. Many people have a daily mind-body practice. In this section we briefly consider two forms of mind-body medicine, hypnosis and t'ai chi.

Hypnosis   **Hypnosis** (or *hypnotherapy*) is the use of intentional relaxation and focusing exercises to produce an altered state of consciousness (a trancelike state) in which a person is more responsive to suggestions or more in control of pain. About 10–15 percent of the adult population is highly susceptible to hypnosis, and 70–80 percent is moderately susceptible. Children are more susceptible to hypnosis than adults. Hypnosis can be performed by a trained professional, or people can be taught to do self-hypnosis.

hypnosis
Use of intentional relaxation and focusing exercises to produce an altered state of consciousness in which a person is more responsive to suggestion.

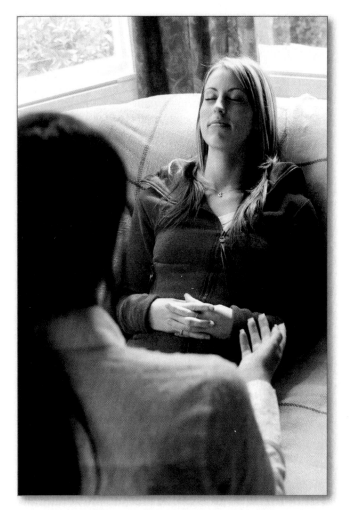

■ Studies suggest that hypnosis, when administered by a trained hypnotherapist, can be used to help people change negative behaviors such as smoking and overeating, reduce fears and anxieties, manage pain, and ease the symptoms of asthma.

When hypnosis is used for health purposes, the hypnotist may make suggestions that may help with behavior change, such as quitting smoking. The person may find it easier to follow suggestions made during hypnosis but is not compelled to do so. Self-hypnosis, which can include visualization and relaxation techniques, can be used to reduce pain in acute and chronic health conditions.

Many different kinds of practitioners may use hypnosis, including family physicians, anesthesiologists, naturopaths, and psychologists. It has been shown to be effective in reducing the acute pain associated with surgery, certain medical procedures, and childbirth. It has also been effective in reducing the chronic pain associated with cancer treatment, migraine headaches, and irritable bowel syndrome.[16]

T'ai Chi As noted in Chapter 5, **t'ai chi,** or **t'ai chi ch'uan,** originated in China as a martial art and has developed into a system of slow, fluid movements through a series of meditative poses. It incorporates breathing, stretching, and stimulation of various organs and organ systems as identified in TCM. In the United States, t'ai chi has evolved into a popular form of exercise that facilitates body awareness and the flow of energy. It is used to reduce stress; promote relaxation; and improve aerobic fitness, strength, flexibility, and coordination.

Preliminary studies suggest that practicing t'ai chi may improve physical functioning for older adults, improve blood circulation, reduce anxiety and depression, and increase bone density in women after menopause. There appear to be some minimal risks, particularly for people with balance problems, especially if the practice is initiated without proper training. Overall, however, these are mild exercises that can be performed daily for 15 minutes to several hours and should be considered safe for most people. If you are interested in learning t'ai chi, the best approach is to look for a class with a qualified teacher.

BIOLOGICALLY BASED PRACTICES

Biologically based practices include the use of vitamins, minerals, dietary supplements, herbal remedies, functional foods, and dietary regimens. CAM practitioners frequently incorporate diet into their treatments, but recommendations are usually based on the individual patient's makeup. Therapeutic diets often involve limiting or excluding certain foods, such as processed foods, refined sugars, or wheat products, for a set period of time. Dietary regimens are usually used as an adjunct or complement to other therapy.

Dietary Supplements Dietary supplements include vitamins, minerals, herbs, enzymes, and metabolites. Both conventional and CAM practitioners recommend that adequate micronutrients be obtained from a balanced diet, but they occasionally recommend supplements in order to reach certain Recommended Daily Allowances (RDAs). CAM practitioners sometimes recommend high-dose supplementation or the use of megavitamins—taking vitamins well in excess of the RDAs.

For example, megadoses of vitamin C (4 grams a day) are sometimes recommended to ward off the common cold. A large review of studies to date showed no effect if taken to prevent colds but did show a possible effect, at megadoses of 8 grams a day, in reducing the length and severity of a cold when taken at the onset of symptoms.[17] High doses of water-soluble vitamins, such as vitamins C, B_3, and B_6, do not pose a significant risk if taken for short periods, but it is possible to overdose on the fat-soluble vitamins (vitamins A, D, E, and K), even with a short course of treatment.

Supplementation of minerals and trace elements can also be part of CAM. For many minerals, there are no clearly established RDAs, and high-dose supplementation for short periods is sometimes recommended by CAM practitioners. For example, zinc is believed to boost the immune system. Studies remain inconclusive about whether zinc lozenges and nasal sprays shorten the course and severity

t'ai chi (t'ai chi ch'uan)
System of slow, fluid movements through a series of meditative poses, incorporating breathing, stretching, and stimulation of various organs and organ systems.

Highlight on Health

Regulation of Drugs Vs. Regulation of Herbs

Pharmaceutical drugs and herbal medicines follow very different routes to the pharmacy or the health food store, and if problems arise after they are on the market, different processes and outcomes can be expected. Consider the case of Vioxx, a nonsteroidal anti-inflammatory medication widely prescribed for chronic pain, especially the pain of arthritis. Although Vioxx was known to have some potential health risks, its benefits were thought to outweigh the risks.

In September 2004, however, the FDA ordered the removal of Vioxx from the market after studies revealed that it caused a significantly increased risk of heart disease and stroke. Despite rigorous clinical trials, this risk had not become apparent until the drug was used for several years by the general population. The manufacturer pulled the drug from the market, and drugs from the same family were subjected to close scrutiny for similar problems.

A different path was followed with ephedra, a stimulant used in Chinese medicine to treat asthma and other respiratory and lung conditions. Derived from the plant called Ma Huang in Chinese herbology, ephedra was included in many dietary supplements and herbal medicines, mainly for the purposes of losing weight and boosting athletic performance. It was known to increase blood pressure, cause heart arrhythmias, and have other effects on the cardiovascular system.

After it was on the market for years, ephedra was associated with cases of heart attack, seizure, and stroke as well as numerous deaths. In April 2004 the FDA banned the sale of products containing ephedra, stating that its use posed "a significant and unreasonable risk to human health" and that the risks far outweighed the benefits of the drug.

The ban was promptly challenged by a Utah-based company that manufactured ephedra products. The company claimed that the FDA had not proven that ephedra actually caused the health problems or that adverse events occurred when the drug was taken at the doses recommended by the manufacturer. A Utah judge agreed with the manufacturer and ruled that the FDA did not have the power to ban a dietary supplement based on weighing risks against benefits (a standard used for pharmaceutical drugs).

The judge pointed out that the Dietary Supplement and Health Education Act (DSHEA) of 1994, under which the FDA is empowered to regulate herbs, was meant to protect the public's access to dietary supplements and herbal products. The DSHEA does not require a manufacturer to show that a dietary supplement confers a benefit or to prove its safety, the judge pointed out; rather, the onus is on the FDA to show that it is unsafe. In 2006, however, a U.S. Court of Appeals upheld the ban on ephedra. Thus, at this time, no dose of ephedra is considered safe, and the sale of products containing ephedra is illegal in the United States. The FDA is seeking an amendment to the DSHEA to make manufacturers of dietary supplements and herbal remedies demonstrate the safety of their products once a safety issue has been raised.

Source: "FDA's Statement on Tenth Circuit's Ruling to Uphold FDA Decision Banning Dietary Supplements Containing Ephedrine Alkaloids," U.S. Food and Drug Administration, 2006, retrieved May 15, 2008, from www.fda.gov/bbd/topics/NEWS/2006/NEW01434.html.

of the common cold. Some studies have shown a positive effect if zinc is started within 24 hours of onset of symptoms. Of concern, however, are recent reports showing a risk of potentially permanent loss of the sense of smell with intranasal zinc.[18]

High-dose dietary supplementation should not exceed the upper limits of safety (ULs) established for some vitamins and minerals (see Chapter 7). When upper limits have not been established, harm may still result from high doses; thus the best course is caution.

_____

herbal remedies or **botanicals**
Products derived from plants and other natural substances, used to treat illness and promote health.

Herbal Remedies **Herbal remedies,** or **botanicals,** include a vast array of products derived from plants and other natural substances. They are a major part of all systems of traditional medicine and the original source of more than 25 percent of pharmaceutical drugs used today.

For example, wild yams were previously a source of the progesterone used in birth control pills and hormone replacement therapy, and the heart medication digitalis comes from the foxglove plant. Pharmaceutical companies are engaged in an ongoing search for new sources of drugs in the natural world and in research aimed at identifying the active ingredients in known plant remedies.

The list of potential medicinal herbs is lengthy, and for most, use dates back hundreds, if not thousands, of years. Only a few herbal medicines have been investigated in controlled clinical studies. Ginkgo biloba has long been believed to have anti-inflammatory and anti-aging effects. Clinical trials show that it does appear to slow the deterioration of brain function in people with Alzheimer's disease and ease the leg pain associated with peripheral vascular disease (narrowing of the blood vessels in the legs).[19]

St. John's wort appears to be beneficial for people with mild depression, and kava kava appears to be useful in treating anxiety, though both herbs have side effects and interact with prescription drugs.[20, 21] Various forms of echinacea stimulate the immune system and are believed to help people with colds recover faster. Valerian may help with insomnia. Besides these, other popular herbal products in the United States include ginseng, garlic supplements, peppermint, ginger, and soy supplements.

Many people assume that herbs are safe because they are "natural," but herbs can have powerful effects, sometimes adverse ones, and safety is a major concern in the use of herbal remedies. Under the Dietary Supplement and Health Education Act (DSHEA) of 1994, herbal medicines and dietary supplements are subject to less stringent regulations than pharmaceutical drugs (see the box "Regulation of Drugs Vs. Regulation of Herbs"). When new pharmaceutical medications are produced, they must undergo rigorous tests for safety, efficacy, and side effects before the FDA will approve their release. The burden is on the manufacturer to prove the safety and efficacy of the product; drugs are considered "guilty until proven innocent."

Dietary and herbal supplements, on the other hand, are released to the market and then removed or banned only if they prove to be unsafe. The burden is on the public and the FDA to demonstrate that the product is not safe; these products are considered "innocent until proven guilty." Herbs listed by the FDA as harmful include belladonna, scotchbroom, comfrey, lobelia, and pennyroyal. Golden seal has potentially serious side effects, and kava kava has been associated with liver damage.

An important safety issue is contamination. Herbal products have been found to contain lead, mercury, arsenic, bacteria, pesticides, and herbicides. Other problems can be caused if manufacturers accidentally or deliberately substitute one plant species for another. If you take any herbal products, purchase those made by reputable manufacturers.[22]

Another issue is the lack of standardization in herbal remedies and associated variation in the quantity of active ingredient in a dose. For many herbs, the "correct" dose is unknown. There is also individual variation in response to herbs; in other words, two people might have different responses to the same herb.

When herbs are homegrown or eaten as medicinal foods, standardization may not be an issue. However, when herbs are processed and sold, lack of standardization makes it difficult for consumers to know if they are getting a product with active ingredients. Lack of standardization also makes it difficult to compare the effects of herbal treatments because it is unclear exactly what dose each person is taking.

Another issue is interaction of herbs with other drugs. This is especially worrisome because many users of herbal supplements do not tell their health care providers they are taking them. Examples of drug-herb interactions are extensive. St. John's wort can trigger serotonin syndrome (a cluster of symptoms including confusion, fever, hallucinations, nausea, and sweating) when combined with the class of antidepressants known as SSRIs. St. John's wort can also cause irregular menstrual bleeding, and it can decrease the effectiveness of birth control pills. Echinacea can increase risk for liver damage when combined with acetaminophen or statin-type drugs (cholesterol-lowering medications). Licorice, an herb used for stomach problems, can cause extremely low levels of potassium in people taking some blood pressure medications.

To reduce risk of drug-herb interaction, inform your physician of any herbal medications you are taking, especially if you are also taking prescription drugs. Pregnant and breastfeeding women are generally advised not to take herbal medicines, given the lack of knowledge about them and the high potential risk to the unborn or nursing child.[22, 23]

In the past, an advantage of herbal medicines was that they were locally grown and lower in cost than prescription medications. This is no longer the case; herbal remedies are now a multibillion-dollar industry. Sales of herbal remedies are doubling every 4 years, and herbs are moving into mainstream supermarkets and drugstores. The cost of drugs, including prescription, over-the-counter, and herbal medicines, is rising faster than any other health care cost. Because money spent in one area takes away from money spent in another, research needs to be continued on the efficacy and safety of herbal medicines, and consumers need to make informed decisions about where to spend their medical dollars.[24]

MANIPULATIVE AND BODY-BASED PRACTICES

Manipulative and body-based practices focus on the body's structures and systems—the bones, joints, muscles, soft tissues, and circulatory system. Practitioners use touch, pressure, manipulation, and other techniques to help the body overcome illness and heal itself.[1]

Osteopathic Medicine Osteopathic medicine has been so well integrated into mainstream practice that it is usually considered a form of conventional medicine rather than a form of CAM. **Osteopathy** is a health system developed in the United States at the end of the 19th century by physician Andrew Taylor Still. Through personal experience, Still came to believe that healing could be achieved through manipulation of the musculoskeletal system without the use of drugs. He believed that manipulation of the bones and muscles could improve blood circulation and balance the functioning of the nerves, thereby allowing the body to heal.

osteopathy
Health system developed by Andrew Taylor Still that focuses on healing through manipulation of the musculoskeletal system; now considered a form of conventional medicine.

Osteopathic physicians receive a medical education comparable to that of conventional physicians and are subject to the same licensing regulations, but their training includes osteopathic manipulation techniques and their focus is on treating the whole person. Since the introduction of antibiotics in the 1940s, most osteopaths have included the use of drugs in their practice. In some settings, it can be difficult to distinguish osteopaths (D.O.s) from conventional physicians (M.D.s).[25]

Chiropractic Medicine **Chiropractic medicine** was developed by American physician Daniel David Palmer in the 1890s. Palmer believed that most illnesses were the result of **subluxation** of the spine—a misalignment, displacement, or dislocation of vertebrae in the spinal column. Such a misalignment interrupts the flow of energy and signals from the brain to the rest of the body, causing illness. Relocating the misaligned joints restores the balance of energy and health.

chiropractic medicine
Health system developed by Daniel David Palmer that focuses on realigning dislocated vertebrae to restore the flow of energy from the brain to the rest of the body.

subluxation
In chiropractic medicine, a misalignment, displacement, or dislocation of vertebrae in the spinal column.

Chiropractors receive their training in a 4-year post-college program at an accredited chiropractic college; upon completion of the program, they receive a Doctor of Chiropractic (D.C.) degree. Chiropractic medicine is licensed in all 50 states and the District of Columbia. It is widely accepted as a form of manual healing; many health insurance plans cover chiropractic treatments.

Studies of the effectiveness of chiropractic have focused on its use in treating low back pain and neck pain. Some studies have shown it to be as effective as standard treatment for low back pain, and others have shown it to be more effective. Other studies suggest a possible benefit in other painful conditions, such as fibromyalgia (a chronic pain condition), carpal tunnel syndrome, and osteoarthritis. Like all treatments, chiropractic has some risks associated with it. Patients can experience mild discomfort, headache, and tiredness after treatment. Serious side effects are rare but can include paralysis and stroke.[26, 27]

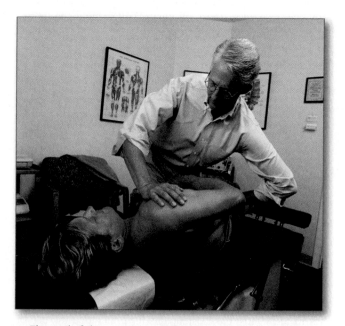

■ The goal of chiropractic medicine is to support the body's ability to heal itself by correcting spinal alignment problems. The chiropractor performs adjustments or manipulations by applying sudden force to joints.

Massage Therapy and Bodywork Massage therapy involves the application of pressure to the skin and muscles. It can be used for a range of purposes, including increasing blood flow and inducing relaxation; relieving pressure, pain, and restricted movement (clinical massage); and improving posture, movement, and body awareness (movement reeducation). Massage is believed to promote healing by boosting the immune system and stimulating the release of natural painkillers. It is part of many treatment modalities and has been shown to be beneficial for reducing anxiety, depression, and pain and improving immune function.

There are more than 75 different types of massage. Swedish massage involves long smooth strokes and kneading motions along the skin, working all parts of the body. Deep tissue massage uses heavier strokes to reach muscles lying at a deeper level in the body. Shiatsu massage, or acupressure, involves pressure applied at acupuncture points to improve the flow of qi. Some limited studies of acupressure have shown it to be effective in reducing nausea, headaches, and some pain. It has been used in palliative care and may produce an improvement in energy level.

Bodywork encompasses a number of physical healing methods. One form of bodywork, Rolfing, was developed in the 1950s by Ida Rolf. She believed that adhesions and scarring in the fascia (the soft tissue covering muscles) can restrict the body's ability to move smoothly, which in turn impairs emotional well-being. She developed a technique of applying deep pressure to the fascia with the thumbs, fingers, and elbows to release these adhesions. Typically, the client undergoes a series of sessions, and with each session, deeper pressure is applied, at times to the point of pain. Although there have been few studies of Rolfing, proponents claim that it can reduce chronic pain, improve posture and movement, and provide an improved sense of well-being.[28]

ENERGY THERAPIES

Energy therapies are among the most controversial CAM practices. Their underlying idea is that humans are infused with energy and that this energy can be modified to influence health. Many CAM practices include the idea that a disruption or imbalance of energy, whether called life force, vital energy, qi, dosha, or something else, is at the root of illness and that the restoration of balance promotes health.

Some forms of energy can be measured, and their use in treating illness is well incorporated into conventional medicine. Light therapy is used to treat seasonal affective disorder, a form of depression associated with low exposure to sunlight, and psoriasis, a skin condition. Electromagnets (magnets that pulsate in response to an intermittent electrical current) are used to treat nonhealing bone fractures (although magnetic-field therapies are not part of standard medical treatment). Other forms of energy cannot be measured by means currently available, and their use in treating illness is considered complementary or alternative. We consider here magnetic-field therapies, Qigong, Reiki, and therapeutic touch.[29]

Magnetic-Field Therapies   Magnets produce a measurable energy called a magnetic field. They have long been used in attempts to treat pain, especially chronic pain, such as occurs in arthritis. It is estimated that Americans currently spend $500 million per year on magnets for pain. There is no proven mechanism by which magnets might work, but some hypotheses are that they may affect cell function, alter blood flow to an area, affect how nerve cells respond to pain, or affect the production of immune cells.[30]

Limited studies have been conducted on magnets, and their results have been mixed. If magnets are going to reduce pain, they usually do so in a week or two. Except for cost, there do not appear to be any significant risks associated with magnets, although they are not recommended for women who are pregnant or for people with an implanted medical device, such as a defibrillator or pacemaker.

Qigong
Chinese energy therapy that combines physical movement and breathing to enhance the flow of qi and boost immune functioning.

Qigong   A Chinese energy therapy, **Qigong** (pronounced "chi-kung") combines physical movement and breathing to enhance the flow of qi and boost immune functioning. Therapy can be administered by a practitioner, who redirects the patient's energy through light touch or massage, or the individual can practice self-healing Qigong by performing a series of movements and exercises. The exercises can be movement oriented, involving very slow, dancelike movements that are believed to promote energy balance and maintain suppleness, or they can be oriented more toward meditation and internal energy flow with minimal external movement. In China, Qigong is widely used in hospitals and clinics to treat asthma, arthritis, stress, allergies, hypertension, and chronic pain. Qigong providers are rare in the United States and Canada.

Therapeutic Touch and Reiki   Like many other CAM therapies, **therapeutic touch** is based on the idea that illness results from a disturbance in the flow of a person's life energy. Related to the ancient practice of "laying-on of hands," therapeutic touch involves a practitioner passing his or her hands over a patient's body to detect imbalances and redirect energy, thus promoting healing. Some studies have suggested that therapeutic touch can be effective in wound healing, osteoarthritis, migraine headaches, and anxiety.[29]

therapeutic touch
Therapy in which a practitioner passes his or her hands over a patient's body to detect imbalances and redirect energy, thus promoting healing.

Reiki (pronounced "ray-kee") is a Japanese energy therapy in which the practitioner uses a number of different hand positions over the patient's body to channel and direct healing energy. Although Reiki has been used for thousands of

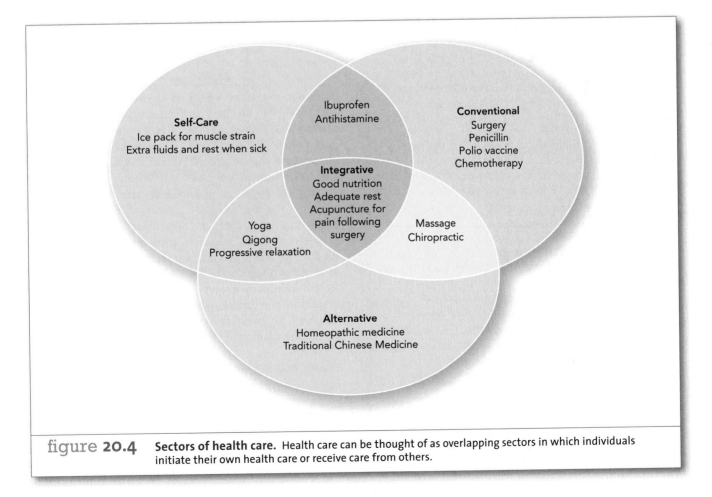

figure **20.4**   **Sectors of health care.** Health care can be thought of as overlapping sectors in which individuals initiate their own health care or receive care from others.

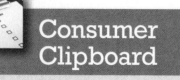

Consumer Clipboard

Questions to Ask When Considering Health Care Choices

When making health care decisions, you need to think about your options in terms of several different dimensions.

- **Safety** All activities have some risk associated with them. For example, the pain reliever acetaminophen (Tylenol) is sold over the counter and is safe for most people, but it can aggravate problems in people who have liver disease and can cause liver failure if taken in too high a dose. For any health care choice you are considering, ask whether the benefits outweigh the risks. What possible side effects are reported with the proposed diagnostic or treatment plan? How does this plan compare with other options? What risk is associated with not choosing another treatment option or with delaying another treatment?

- **Efficacy** How likely are you to get a benefit from the treatment option? Are there studies or data confirming benefits? Have other options been shown to be beneficial? Evidence is available for some complementary and alternative treatments, but for others, you may have to base your decisions on other people's experience. The problem is that people respond differently to illness and to treatments. You might recover from a cold in 3 days after taking vitamin C and echinacea, and your friend might take the same remedies but still have the cold for 10 days. You would not really know whether the vitamins and herbs shortened the course of the illness or not. It could be that you would have recovered in 3 days without any treatment and your friend would have been sick for 3 weeks if she had not taken the vitamins and herbs.

- **Cost** How expensive is each option? Cost includes not just the dollar amount you pay but also the cost of any side effects that choice may cause, any cost associated with not making another choice, and time that you may gain or lose. For example, a person who delays surgery and chemotherapy for melanoma in order to try a less drastic alternative approach may have to pay a heavy cost in lost treatment time.

- **Qualifications of the provider** How qualified is the health care provider? Find out about licensing requirements and other regulations in the field, and check your provider's background. Also find out whether your provider has a financial stake in the option he or she is recommending. If so, is that a source of bias in the advice you are receiving?

years, there are few studies confirming its beneficial effects. It is being studied as an adjunct to treatment of fibromyalgia, heart disease, and cancer and in patients with AIDS.

Reiki
Japanese energy therapy in which the practitioner uses a number of different hand positions over the patient's body to channel and direct healing energy.

Making Informed Health Care Choices

When you are sick, how do you know whether to see your regular health care provider, to seek out a complementary or alternative treatment, or to treat the illness yourself? In general, conventional medicine is highly effective in treating a wide range of illnesses, including infectious diseases and acute and chronic conditions like heart disease, diabetes, and cancer. CAM can be effective in such areas as boosting your immune system, improving energy levels, relieving pain, managing stress, and addressing other symptoms as described in this chapter. Self-care is probably the most commonly used health option. A view of these intersecting areas of health care is shown in Figure 20.4.

EVALUATING CAM CHOICES

As the NCCAM advances in its mission of investigating CAM therapies in rigorous scientific studies, more information will emerge about the safety and efficacy of these practices. For now, if you are interested in using a CAM approach, you will need to educate yourself and make informed choices (see the box "Questions to Ask When Considering Health Care Choices").

The NCCAM recommends that you begin your investigation by consulting with your regular physician or health care provider to find out if there are conventional treatments that address your condition. It is especially important to discuss any CAM treatments you are considering with your physician if you take prescription medications, since drug interactions can be dangerous.

If your physician is knowledgeable about the CAM approach you are considering, he or she may be able to help you make a decision about using it. Otherwise, you may have to investigate it by yourself at the library or on the Internet. Remember to use reliable Web sites, like those of major universities, the NCCAM, and the FDA, and look for government-sponsored clinical trials. Be wary of commercial Web sites that want to sell you a product. Refer to Chapter 1 for guidelines on being an informed consumer of health care information.[31]

CHOOSING SELF-CARE

Self-care involves actions you take on behalf of your own health. It includes observing your own symptoms (physical, mental, or emotional), evaluating your external environment (such as cultural practices, housing, or opportunities for physical activity), gathering information and advice, making informed decisions about a course of action, and then either treating yourself or seeking professional care. Self-care is practiced every day, whether it means putting ice on a strained muscle, eating chicken soup for a cold, taking an antihistamine for allergies, doing relaxation exercises for stress, or seeking support from a clergyperson for a personal problem.

Medical self-care—treating a physical problem, like a headache—is sometimes distinguished from health promotion self-care—taking action to maintain and improve health with activities related to high-level wellness. Medical symptoms are experienced quite frequently—on average, individuals are faced with some symptoms of medical problems 1 out of every 3 days. Symptoms suggesting that high-level wellness has not been achieved may be more subtle—for example, a person may have a low energy level or feel bored and discontented.

Both conventional medicine and CAM include recommendations for self-care practices, such as balanced nutrition, exercise, adequate sleep, deep breathing, and relaxation. If you have symptoms that are severe, unusual, persistent, or recurrent, it is generally recommended that you see a health care provider.

INFLUENCES ON HEALTH CARE CHOICES

Ideas and beliefs about health and health care choices are influenced by multiple factors. Your family of origin shapes your initial patterns of health behaviors and decisions. As you move into adulthood, other factors become important, such as where you live, how much money you have, the health insurance plans available to you, the health information you have access to, any medical conditions you develop, your friends, peers, and coworkers, and other aspects of the social environment. These influences continue to change as you grow older, move to different parts of the country, change jobs, and so on.

The media have been an important influence on health at least since the middle of the 20th century. They disseminate health information, and they also popularize different diets, products, treatments, and attitudes, influencing consumers to follow trends and fads. Most newspapers have health sections, and more than 50 different health-related consumer magazines appear monthly. Internet resources allow individuals to research symptoms, diseases, and treatment options, and Internet advertisers bombard viewers with their messages.

A relatively new influence on how people define health and illness is **direct-to-consumer advertising.** In the past, pharmaceutical companies marketed their products primarily to health care providers, but in 1997, changes made by the FDA in advertising regulations allowed manufacturers to take their campaigns directly to the public. Between 1996 and 2005, spending on direct-to-consumer advertising skyrocketed from approximately $985 million to $ 4.2 billion. The most heavily mar-

direct-to-consumer advertising
Marketing of products directly to consumers instead of to health care providers.

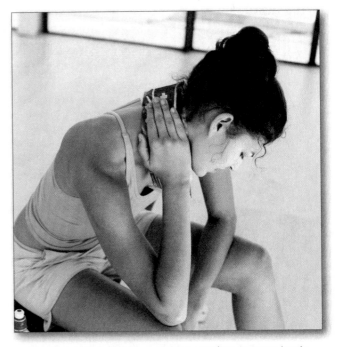

■ People practice self-care every day, as when a person treats a stiff or strained neck with ice. However, symptoms that are severe, unusual, persistent, or recurrent should prompt a visit to a health care provider.

keted drugs are for allergies, high cholesterol, depression, insomnia, and pain. Drugs for hair loss, acne, erectile dysfunction, and sexual desire disorder in women are also commonly advertised. Drugs that are advertised in the media are usually the most recently developed and the most expensive.

Direct-to-consumer ads may educate consumers about new medications for health conditions, or they may motivate people to seek treatment for an untreated illness. Physicians report that they are prescribing drugs for patients who ask for them by name after seeing ads on television or in magazines.

However, these ads are designed primarily to create feelings of inadequacy about having certain conditions and a sense of need for the advertised product. Ad campaigns not only sell products but also help shape a society's views of health and illness, especially by medicalizing physical differences and personality traits. Most ads show people losing control of some aspect of their lives and regaining control by using the advertised drug. As in all decisions, it pays to use your critical thinking skills and to be an informed consumer of messages about health and illness (see the box "Medical Fraud and Quackery").

SUPPORTING INTEGRATIVE MEDICINE

Many people believe that the future of health care lies in a convergence of conventional medicine and CAM practices that have been shown to be safe and effective, known as integrative medicine. Proponents of integrative medicine suggest that it might provide more effective and comprehensive medical treatment for all.

Who's at Risk

Medical Fraud and Quackery

There have always been people who searched for miracle cures, whether for aches and pains, chronic diseases, or normal aging, and there have always been others willing to exploit those hopes. Centuries ago, peddlers traveled from town to town selling creams, tonics, and elixirs to treat a wide range of ailments, real and contrived. In the Old West, the "snake oil salesman" sold remedies from the back of a wagon and hoped to get out of town before his customers realized they had been duped. Nowadays, exotic potions, pills, and medical devices are promoted on TV, on the Internet, and in magazines—as in the past, targeting people at risk for exploitation.

What makes people vulnerable to medical fraud and quackery? One factor is naïveté: Some people believe that anything that appears in print or on the news has to be true or it would not be allowed by law. They may also assume that people would not lie about their experiences, so they take anecdotes and personal testimonials at face value. Others are mistrustful of the medical profession, the health care system, or the government and are ready to believe in any alternative approach to a problem. The people at greatest risk for medical fraud, however, are those with chronic, incurable diseases. When conventional medicine fails or has nothing more to offer, des-peration makes some people vulnerable to deception and exploitation.

Complicating the issue is the fact that an ineffective or bogus treatment may sometimes appear to be helpful. A number of factors may be at work when this occurs. The illness may have run its natural course, be in remission, or have been misdiagnosed in the first place. The individual may be experiencing the placebo effect, in which a person who has received a "sugar pill" gets relief from symptoms or just feels better. Or the person may be experiencing any number of cognitive distortions, such as selective memory, under the influence of a strong desire to believe. The scientific method was developed to help overcome many such factors.

How can you protect yourself against medical fraud and quackery? Consumer advocates recommend that you be wary of anyone who claims to have the cure for a previously incurable disease and of devices or medicines that are said to be miraculous, secret, or foolproof. Other warning signs of fraud include the exclusive use of anecdotes and testimonials to support claims, the assertion that a conspiracy exists to suppress existing cures, the claim that positive thinking can cure disease, and the sale of vitamins or supplements by a health care practitioner. If you or a family member has a chronic health problem, discuss treatment options with multiple sources to ensure that you are not being taken advantage of while in a vulnerable state.

Sources: "CDRH Promises Crackdown on Risky Devices," by J.G. Dickinson, February 2008, Washington Wrap Up, www.devicelink.com/mddi/archive/08/02/006 .html; "Vulnerability to Quackery," S. Barrett, 2005, retrieved July 8, 2008, from www.quackwatch.org/01QuackeryRelatedTopics/quackvul.html.

Another benefit of integrative medicine might be a reduction in health care spending, which currently is spiraling out of control in the United States. In 2007, 16 percent of the U.S. gross domestic product (GDP) was spent on health care, compared to an average of 10 percent in other industrialized countries. The cost of health care as a percentage of GDP is increasing faster than any other part of the economy. Recent tallies show that the total health care expenditure in the United States in 2007 was $2.3 trillion.[32]

At the same time, consumers are spending out-of-pocket money for CAM therapies. In 1997 (the most recent national cost estimates) the U.S. public spent $36–$47 billion on CAM. Of this amount, $12–$20 billion was paid to professional CAM health care providers and $5 billion was spent on herbal medicines. These expenditures rival the out-of-pocket payments made for conventional treatments. Combining conventional medicine and CAM might be a way of consolidating some of this spending.[7]

A key component in the future of integrative medicine is the work of the NCCAM in funding and conducting rigorous scientific studies of CAM therapies and in identifying the most cost-effective ways of maximizing health. Another key component of integrative medicine is the conventional medical system's primary care provider. Such providers are sometimes described as gatekeepers, meaning that they make decisions about who can see specialists and CAM providers, when they can see them, and for what conditions.

A new role for the primary care provider might be that of pathfinder. In this role, providers might be expected to be knowledgeable about various CAM therapies, or they might be trained in certain CAM techniques. With this added knowledge and training, they would be better equipped to guide people through the increasingly complex medical systems that await the next generation of health care consumers.

You Make the Call

Should CAM Be Covered by Health Insurance?

If your primary care physician refers you to a specialist, such as an endocrinologist, a cardiologist, or an oncologist, your health insurance will very likely pay for your care. If your primary care physician were to refer you to a chiropractor, an acupuncturist, or a massage therapist, or if you decided to seek such treatment on your own, your visits might or might not be covered by your insurance. Should all health care options be equally accessible to consumers? Should insurance plans cover CAM practices the same way they cover conventional treatments? And who should decide what kind of practitioners people can see?

Proponents of health insurance coverage for CAM therapies point out that many of these practices have been in existence far longer than Western medicine. They have been developed to meet the health needs of people all over the world and have been proven safe and effective through time. Proponents note that CAM practices tend to be less invasive, less costly, and safer than conventional medicine; they also comment that conventional care tends to be directed toward the very sick and the elderly rather than toward the general population and that not enough attention is paid to disease prevention and health promotion. CAM systems incorporate prevention into their underlying belief systems; by focusing on health promotion, they arguably decrease the cost and burden of chronic disease to individuals and society. Finally, proponents argue that by providing access to only one type of health care, insurance plans are not speaking to the needs of a diverse population.

Opponents point out that many health practices deemed useful in the past have been shown to have limited value; in time, they have been replaced by safer, more effective options. The fact that a practice is old and traditional does not necessarily mean that it has been proven by time. Opponents agree that prevention is important, but they point out that even well-supported, proven prevention practices that are recommended by conventional providers are not well used by the general population. Giving people additional choices will just increase confusion and create resistance to prevention practices that have clearly been proven beneficial, such as vaccinations and Pap tests.

Opponents also point out that although many alternative treatments appear to be relatively safe, they are not without risk. Due to the current lack of organization, licensing, and regulation of some CAM practitioners in the United States, some health care providers are inadequately trained and may cause harm to patients. Finally, although preventive practices may decrease the cost and burden of chronic disease, there is little evidence that patients receiving CAM care have lower health care costs. In fact, most patients receiving CAM care continue to receive conventional care; expanding insurance coverage may simply further increase health care spending in the United States.

Should health insurance cover CAM treatments? What do you think?

Pros

- CAM practices have been proven by time; they are less invasive, less costly, and safer than conventional medicine.

- CAM practices tend to focus on health promotion and prevention of illness for the whole population, whereas conventional medicine directs most of its attention to the very ill and elderly.

- Providing insurance coverage for both conventional and CAM practices promotes access to health care for a diverse population.

Cons

- Many CAM practices have not been proven safe or effective. Providing insurance coverage for unproven treatments may mislead consumers into thinking these treatments have more legitimacy than they do.

- Training and licensing are not regulated for many CAM providers, making it difficult or impossible to evaluate their qualifications and competence. Insurance coverage should not be extended to practitioners who may cause more harm than good.

- Adding CAM practices to insurance plans would complicate health services and may reduce the use of proven tests and treatments, such as Pap tests.

- The health care system is already financially overburdened; adding coverage for unproven practices just adds to the burden.

In Review

1. **What is complementary and alternative medicine?** CAM is defined as a group of practices and products that are not presently considered part of conventional medicine. CAM and conventional medicine operate according to different beliefs and principles concerning the nature of the body, of health, and of illness and disease. Whereas conventional medicine dominates the health care scene in the developed world, CAM is more common in developing societies.

2. **What are the different types of CAM?** CAM practices are classified as whole medical systems (for example, Traditional Chinese Medicine, Ayurvedic medicine) and practices falling into four domains—mind-body interventions (for example, yoga, meditation, prayer, hypnosis), biologically based therapies (dietary supplements, herbal remedies), body-based therapies (chiropractic medicine, massage), and energy therapies (magnets, Qigong, Reiki).

3. **How can a consumer make reasonable decisions about using CAM?** It's important to use critical thinking skills when evaluating a CAM practice or practitioner; it's also important to inform your physician about any CAM treatments you are using. For many ailments, self-care is the best option. The future may lie in integrative medicine, the convergence of conventional medicine and CAM practices that have been shown to be safe and effective.

For a detailed summary of this chapter and a comprehensive set of review questions, visit the Online Learning Center at **www.mhhe.com/teague2e**.

Web Resources

American Academy of Medical Acupuncture: This site provides information about acupuncture, including conditions appropriate for this method, FAQs, articles by physicians, and research.
www.medicalacupuncture.org

American Chiropractic Association: This organization's site offers information on back pain, chiropractic medicine, news, and current research on chiropractic.
www.amerchiro.org

American Medical Association: The AMA site provides online news about health issues and offers many articles about complementary and alternative medicine.
www.ama-assn.org

American Osteopathic Association: This site addresses various health issues in terms of the osteopathic approach.
www.osteopathic.org

MayoClinic.com: The Mayo Clinic site offers interactive health tools, and features information on complementary and alternative medicine, including drugs and dietary supplements.
www.mayoclinic.com

National Center for Complementary and Alternative Medicine: This site features background information on understanding CAM, major areas of this approach, alerts and advisories, treatment information, dietary and herbal supplements, and clinical trials.
http://nccam.nih.gov

National Center for Homeopathy: Offering information on what homeopathy is, this site provides research supporting the effectiveness of homeopathy and guides you in finding a homeopathic practitioner.
www.homeopathic.org

National Council Against Health Fraud: This organization's consumer information sheets address a wide variety of topics, including complementary and alternative medicine.
www.ncahf.org

Office of Dietary Supplements, National Institutes of Health: This site offers information on specific dietary supplements, nutrient recommendations, and consumer safety.
http://dietary-supplements.info.nih.gov

PART SIX

Challenges to Your Health

Certain problems, such as violent crime, natural disasters, and environmental issues, seem beyond the scope of individual action, and in fact, they are problems that must be addressed at the national and global levels. Still, there are actions every person can take to avoid or prepare for these challenges, reduce their impact, and contribute to a healthier world. The chapters in Part 6 offer steps toward solutions.

Think It Over

- If your neighborhood or community isn't safe, are there actions you can take to make it safer?

- Are you prepared for the kinds of extreme weather conditions or natural disasters that may occur in your area, such as floods, earthquakes, or tornadoes? If not, what's keeping you from preparing?

- What are you doing today to reduce your impact on the environment?

Chapter 2

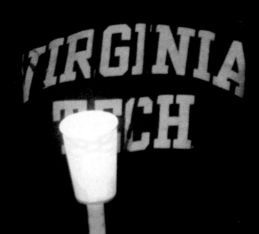

Violence Prevention and Protection

Your Health Today

www.mhhe.com/teague2e

Go to the Online Learning Center for *Your Health Today* for interactive activities, quizzes, flashcards, Web links, and more resources related to this chapter.

Ever Wonder...

- how safe your campus is?
- if campus communication systems have been improved since the shootings at Virginia Tech?
- if airport security is better than it was before September 11, 2001?

More than many of the other health topics discussed in this text, violence is a societal issue. Although violent acts are committed by individuals, the causes of violence are rooted in social and cultural conditions. This does not mean that people who commit violent crimes are not held accountable for their actions—they are. In fact, the United States incarcerates a larger proportion of its population than does any other nation.[1] It does mean that taking action individually to reduce violence is difficult for people, unlike deciding to improve their diet or get more exercise. What you as an individual can do about violence falls into two categories: knowing how to reduce your own risk of encountering violence and working to create safer communities and to prevent violence in society. This chapter gives an overall picture of violence in the United States and provides guidelines on how you can keep yourself safe.

Violence in the United States

Violence is defined as the use of force or the threat of force to inflict intentional injury, physical or psychological, on oneself or another person. Murder, robbery, and **assault** are all violent crimes, but violence also occurs in association with child abuse, sexual harassment, suicide, and several other kinds of conduct.

CRIME RATES AND VIOLENCE FACTS

The United States is commonly believed to be one of the most violent nations in the industrialized world. Actually, rates of violent crime in the United States are lower than those in many other developed countries, except in one area—homicide, especially homicide committed with a firearm. The number of firearm homicides is higher in the United States than in any other country; it is almost 15 times higher than in Canada.[2, 3] Most experts attribute this difference to the ready availability of firearms in the United States.[4]

The U.S. Federal Bureau of Investigation (FBI) and the Department of Justice count cases of homicide, assault, robbery, and rape as violent crimes. *Aggravated assault* accounts for about two-thirds of violent crime and robbery for less than one-third; rape accounts for about 7 percent and homicide about 1 percent. Firearms are involved in about a third of all violent crimes and in about 70 percent of homicides. Among women killed in the United States, about a third are killed by their husbands or boyfriends. About one in five child homicide victims is killed by a family member.[2]

violence
Use of force or the threat of force to inflict intentional injury, physical or psychological, on oneself or another person.

assault
Attack by one person on another using force or the threat of force to intentionally inflict injury. *Aggravated assault* is an attack that causes bodily injury, usually with a weapon or other means capable of producing grave bodily harm or death. *Simple assault* is an attack without a weapon that causes less serious physical harm.

WHAT ACCOUNTS FOR VIOLENCE?

Although the causes of violent crime are complex, some risk factors can be identified. Risk factors are not causes; rather, they are factors that increase the likelihood that a person will engage in a behavior or suffer harm. Age and sex are among the most reliable risk factors for violence.[5] The typical offender is a young male between the ages of 14 to 24. Forty-four percent of those arrested for violent crimes are under 25 years of age. Men are much more likely to commit a violent act than women are; 82 percent of those arrested for violent crimes are men.[6] Women do commit violent acts, but it is often in self-defense.

Being a member of a minority group is a significant risk factor for violence. Although Blacks make up 12 percent of the population, they make up nearly half (47 percent) of all homicide victims (Figure 21.1).[7] The probability of being murdered before the age of 45 is 2.21 percent for Black men, compared with 0.29 percent for white men.[8] Similarly, Blacks account for 52 percent of homicide offenders. Thirty-seven percent of those arrested for violent crimes are Black, 60.5 percent are White, and the remainder are Native American, Asian, or Pacific Islander. (People of Hispanic ethnic origin are included in the racial categories "Black" and "White" in these statistics.)

Like risk factors for mental illness, risk factors for violence occur at many levels. Risk factors at the societal and cultural levels—social determinants of health—include poverty, poor schools, disorganized neighborhoods, use of alcohol and drugs, availability of guns, exposure to media violence, and lack of economic, educational, and employment opportunities. Violence is also more common on college campuses than in the general population, perhaps because of the transient nature of the community.

Risk factors at the family level include child abuse, substance abuse or criminal activity by family members, lack of positive role models, and chaotic family organization. There

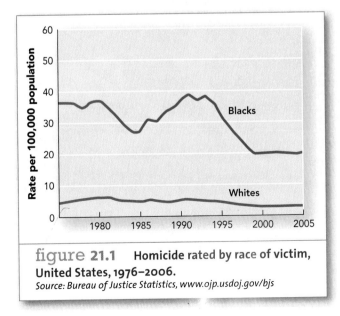

figure 21.1 Homicide rated by race of victim, United States, 1976–2006.
Source: Bureau of Justice Statistics, www.ojp.usdoj.gov/bjs

is a higher risk of violence when parents are not involved in children's lives, do not supervise their activities, and use harsh, lax, or inconsistent discipline.

Risk factors at the individual level include such biological factors as genetics, brain structure, brain chemistry, and medical disorders; low intelligence; certain personality traits, such as aggressiveness and poor impulse control; and a history of previous criminal or antisocial behavior.[5] Other individual risk factors include attention deficit disorder and hyperactivity in children; deficits in cognitive and social cognitive functioning; poor impulse and behavior control; and early antisocial and aggressive behaviors.

Problems are exacerbated for children who do poorly in school, are rejected by classmates, associate with deviant peers, and become involved with gangs. Conversely, protective factors, which buffer young people from the effects of risk factors, include high IQ, a positive social orientation, and involvement in school activities.[9] No single factor is sufficient to explain why violence occurs or why levels of violent crime rise or decline in different time periods.

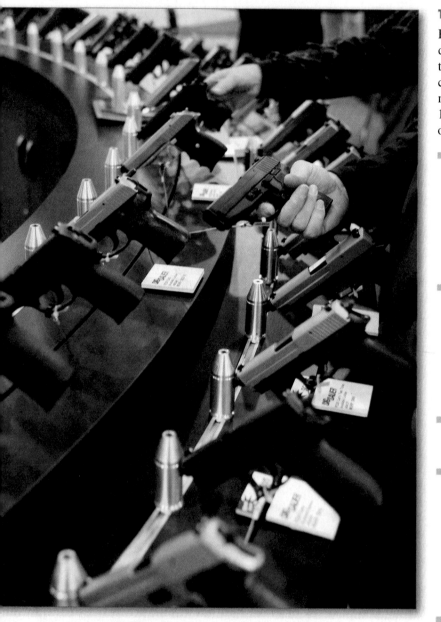

■ The availability of firearms in the Untied States is linked with higher rates of firearm-related homicide than in other developed countries, and states with the highest rates of gun ownership have higher rates of suicide than states with lower rates of gun ownership. Firearms safety training is essential for anyone who owns a gun.

TRENDS IN VIOLENT CRIME

Rates of violent crime in the United States declined precipitously from the early 1990s to 2004. In 2005 and 2006, rates of all violent crimes except forcible rape increased. The estimated rate of violent crime in 2006 was 473.5 per 100,000 inhabitants.[7] Experts proposed a variety of explanations for violent crime trends:[1]

- *Demographics.* Rates of violence fall when the segment of the population responsible for most occurrences of violent crime—young men aged 14 to 24—decreases in size. This commonly offered argument is inadequate to explain the decline in crime in the 1990s, however, because the size of this group changed very little between 1994 and 2003.

- *Crack cocaine.* The boom in crack cocaine in the 1980s, accompanied by drug wars and gun violence, was followed by a steep decline in demand for crack in the early 1990s. Marijuana replaced crack as the drug of choice among younger drug users; the marijuana trade is associated with less violence than is the trade in crack.

- *Economic expansion.* The economy improved in the 1990s, creating more opportunities for people to earn a living in legitimate ways.

- *Law enforcement and incarceration.* Mandatory sentencing policies, as exemplified by "three strikes" laws (automatic maximum sentences for people convicted of a third felony, even a nonviolent one), and the sharp increase in incarceration rates in the 1980s and 1990s removed many criminals from the streets. The prison population in the United States quadrupled between 1980 and 2000.

- *Expansion of resources for victims.* Resources for those affected by domestic violence increased in the 1980s and 1990s, including hotlines, shelters, legal advocates, and increased availability of judicial protections (such as restraining orders).

None of these explanations is sufficient by itself to explain the drop in crime from the 1990s to 2004 or the increase in 2005 and 2006. Some combination of these factors and others is probably responsible for the overall trend. More research is needed to determine what policies and programs are effective and actually result in a reduction in violent crime. Areas for study include, among others, responses to drug offenses other than imprisonment, effective interventions in domestic violence, and approaches to gangs and gun use by young people.

Youth Violence

Among people aged 10 to 24, homicide is the second leading cause of death in the United States (unintentional injuries, or accidents, are the first).[10, 11]

SCHOOL VIOLENCE

Mass shootings in schools are shocking but rare occurrences. The rate of school violence in 2005 (6 deaths per 1,000 students) was less than half the rate in 1994. Homicide rates in 2005 were 13 deaths per 100,000 students, compared to 42 per 100,000 students in 1991–1992. Despite the decline in the prevalence of students reporting being victims of crime at school in the past few years, nearly 7 in 10 teachers and students still feel school violence is a major problem.[12]

zero-tolerance policy
Policy stating that any student who brings weapons or drugs to school will be expelled.

Schools have responded to violence primarily by tightening security and strengthening punitive measures.[13] Two federal laws, the Gun-Free Schools Act and the Safe and Drug-Free Schools Act, both passed by Congress in 1994, created a **zero-tolerance policy** that calls for expelling any student who brings weapons or drugs to school. The teachers' union, the American Federation of Teachers, strongly supports zero-tolerance policies, claiming that principals need to be able to respond quickly, decisively, and fairly to acts or threats of violence and drug abuse.[13]

However, some child advocates, educators, parents, and citizens consider zero-tolerance initiatives too inflexible. Children have been expelled from school for wearing Halloween costumes with paper swords and bringing plastic knives in lunch bags. Experts recommend

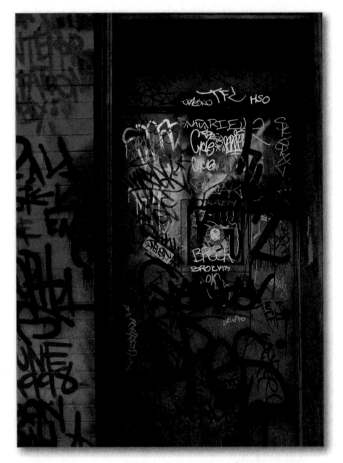

■ Although some graffiti rises to the status of art, most is simple vandalism. When graffiti is not promptly removed, it sends a message of neglect, hurting neighborhoods and communities and lowering quality of life.

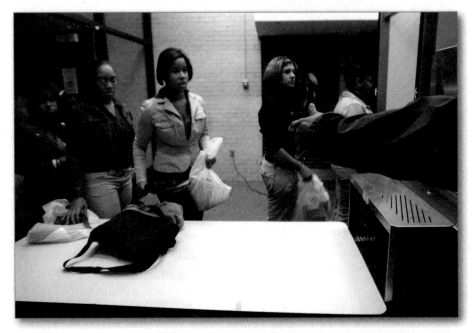

■ Metal detectors were installed at Success Tech Academy in Cleveland after a student shot four people and then killed himself in October 2007. Following the incident, the school system set up an anonymous hotline where students could report threats and suspicious behavior by their fellow students.

such measures as providing mental health services for students, social support for families, classes in anger management, and more extracurricular activities that will get students involved in school and positive peer relationships. They also endorse measures that would reduce access to guns by children and adolescents.

YOUTH GANGS

Youth gangs are associations of adolescents and young adults aged 12 to 24 organized to control a territory, usually in an inner city, and to conduct illegal activities like drug trafficking. Gangs are associated with violence not just because of their illegal activities but because violence is part of members' lives, in their families and communities, before they ever join a gang. Many gang members derive a sense of belonging, purpose, and self-esteem not otherwise available in their lives, as well as security, protection, and a source of income, from gang membership.[14]

youth gangs
Associations of adolescents and young adults aged 12 to 24 organized to control a territory and conduct illegal activities.

Efforts to reduce gang violence focus on preventing adolescents from joining gangs by keeping them in school and providing opportunities for legitimate success, such as meaningful employment opportunities. Community social controls can be increased by strengthening social institutions, such as schools and churches, and encouraging parents and community leaders to play a role in supervising adolescents' activities. Programs are needed in prisons, such as job training and drug treatment programs, that prevent the recycling of adult gang members back into the community crime scene. Finally, efforts to remove guns from the streets need to be enhanced.[15] Several cities have model programs in place, aimed at reducing gang violence through these strategies and others.

Violence on the College Campus

Would you think a community was safe that, in the past year, had 1 murder, 2 rapes, 13 robberies, 20 aggravated assaults, 190 burglaries, 66 car thefts, 160 arrests for alcohol violations, 158 arrests for drug violations, and 32 arrests for weapon violations? Would it surprise you to learn that this community is a university campus, a place traditionally viewed as a tranquil environment for intellectual pursuits (see the box "Violence and College Students")?[16]

Most colleges have responded to campus violence by raising the visibility of campus security officers, tightening security controls, and implementing stringent discipline programs.[17] Two federal laws regulate how campus crime is treated. The Jeanne Clery Disclosure of Campus Security Policy and Campus Crime Statistics Act (originally known

Who's at Risk

Violence and College Students

A 2005 survey revealed the following facts about violence on college campuses.

- For every 1,000 women on a college campus, there are about 35 incidents of rape. Approximately 15–20 percent of college students experienced forced intercourse during their college years. About 15–20 percent of college men acknowledged forced intercourse. Only 5 percent of attempted and completed rapes were reported to law enforcement.

- Non-Hispanic Whites are more likely than students of other races to be victims of overall violence. Black students are somewhat more likely than White students to experience a simple assault.

- Male students are twice as likely as female students to be victims of overall violence. Out of every 14 college men, 1 had been physically assaulted or raped by an intimate partner.

- More than one-third of lesbian, gay, bisexual, and transgender undergraduate students experienced harassment. Some 20 percent of faculty, staff, and students feared for their physical safety because of their sexual orientation or gender identity.

- Between 25 and 30 percent of college women and between 11 and 17 percent of college men were stalked. Most of the victims knew their stalker. Stalking is more prevalent among college students than in the general population. About 10 percent of stalking incidents resulted in forced or attempted sexual contact.

- Some 15 percent of college women and 9.2 percent of college men were in emotionally abusive relationships; 2.4 percent of women and 1.3 percent of men were in a physically abusive relationship; and 1.7 percent of women and 1.0 percent of men were in a sexually abusive relationship.

- Alcohol and other drugs were implicated in 55–74 percent of sexual assaults on college campuses.

- About 93 percent of crimes against students occurred off campus. Strangers committed 58 percent of all violent crimes against students. Only 35 percent of violent crimes against students were reported to law enforcement.

Source: Campus Violence White Paper, *by J. Carr, February 5, 2005, Baltimore, MD: American College Health Association.*

as the Campus Security Act) requires colleges and universities receiving federal funding to disclose information about crime on and around their campuses. Clery was a 19-year-old student at Lehigh University who was raped and murdered in her residence hall in 1986. The law was amended in 2000 to require colleges to inform the community about where they can obtain information about convicted, registered sex offenders enrolled as students or working or volunteering on campus.

The Campus Sexual Assault Victims' Bill of Rights Act requires college administrators to provide justice, medical treatment, and psychological counseling for crime victims and survivors. Amendments to this law require colleges to promote educational awareness programs on sexual assault, facilitate the reporting of sexual assault, and help survivors who want to change their academic and living situations, among other requirements. Schools that fail to comply may lose federal funds, including student loan funding.

The deadliest incident of campus violence in U.S. history, in which 32 people died, occurred at Virginia Polytechnic Institute and State University (Virginia Tech) in 2007. A nonprofit victims' rights organization called Security on Campus (SOC) requested a federal investigation of the school's response to the shootings, which consisted of two attacks separated by about 2 hours. SOC claimed that the school violated the Jeanne Clery Act by failing to issue warnings in a timely way.

In response to the Virginia Tech incident, colleges and universities across the country have revamped their security plans. Multiple means of contact by e-mail, phone messages, text messaging, and siren and/or verbal warnings from communication towers on campus have been implemented. Some creative plans include the use of Web-capable cell phones so that students, faculty, and staff can view live feeds from campuswide security cameras, and the use of special cell phones carried by students that can signal campus police in the event of safety problems and locate students via Global Positioning System (GPS) trackers. The U.S. Department of Education provides data on the safety of college campuses. To find out about your campus, visit www.ope.ed.gov/security/search.asp.

HAZING

A controversial practice on many campuses, hazing is associated especially with fraternities, sororities, and athletic teams. According to the Fraternities Executive Association, **hazing** is "any action taken or situation created intentionally, whether on or off fraternity premises, to produce mental or physical discomfort, embarrassment, or ridicule."[18] Hazing is typically imposed as an initiation rite or a requirement for joining an organization.

Hazing activities have included kidnapping, alcohol chugging, forced swallowing of food and non-

hazing
Actions taken to cause mental or physical discomfort, embarrassment, or ridicule in individuals seeking to join an organization.

food items, sleep deprivation, beatings, and calisthenics to the point of exhaustion. Deaths have occurred as a result of hazing, most often fraternity hazing. A common cause is alcohol poisoning, but death can also occur from such practices as forcing pledges to drink huge quantities of water, which causes "water intoxication" and death from swelling of the brain stem. The number of deaths is difficult to determine accurately, because causes of death may be listed as accidents, alcohol overdoses, suicides, stabbings, shootings, and fires without indicating that the deaths occurred during a hazing acitivity.[19]

Although sorority hazing has caused fewer injuries and deaths than fraternity hazing, a significant number of sorority women have died of alcohol poisoning and alcohol-related falls and car crashes. Campus hazing is also practiced by clubs, bands, and athletic teams. At one university, 80 percent of responding college athletes reported that they had faced questionable or unacceptable initiation activities, including kidnapping and beating.

Hazing is illegal in many states and may be either a misdemeanor or a felony, depending on the state and the severity of the offense. Parents whose children have died in these senseless incidents have filed wrongful death suits against both colleges and fraternities. Hazing has also been reported as an initiation rite among firefighters, police officers, and employee groups.

FREE SPEECH VS. HATE SPEECH

College and university campuses are places where debate and free expression are encouraged in the service of learning and intellectual freedom. Because of this commitment, institutions of higher education often find themselves at the center of free speech controversies. Maintaining an atmosphere of civility that allows respect for different opinions while

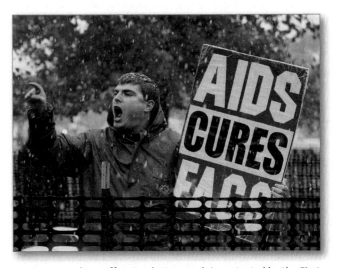

■ No matter how offensive, hate speech is protected by the First Amendment. Some experts recommend increasing conversation, debate, and diversity on campus as a way to expose and combat bigotry.

protecting people from the violence that may be incited by offensive speech has become a major challenge.[20]

hate speech
Verbal, written, or symbolic acts that convey a grossly negative view of particular persons or groups based on their gender, ethnicity, race, religion, sexual orientation, or disability.

Hate speech—defined as verbal, written, or symbolic acts that convey a grossly negative view of particular persons or groups based on their gender, ethnicity, race, religion, sexual orientation, or disability[20]—is particularly troublesome. Its intent is to humiliate or harm rather than to convey ideas or information, and it has the potential to incite violence. Epithets, slurs, taunts, insults, and intimidation are common modes of hate speech; posters, flyers, letters, phone calls, e-mail, Web sites, and even T-shirts are media by which the message is distributed.

Some schools have adopted speech codes that require civility in discourse for all campus community members.[20] Some of these codes have been struck down by the courts as a violation of First Amendment rights. According to the rulings, hate speech must be proven to inflict real, not trivial, harm before it can be regulated. The U.S. Supreme Court has made it clear that colleges and universities cannot suppress speech simply because it is offensive. For this reason, many colleges and universities have adopted conduct codes that regulate certain actions associated with hate speech but not the speech itself.[20]

Sexual Violence

Sexual violence includes not just rape but also sexual harassment, stalking, and other forms of forcible or coercive sexual activity.

SEXUAL ASSAULT

In most states, the term *rape* has been replaced by the more comprehensive term *sexual assault,* which includes different kinds of attacks and varying degrees of severity. **Sexual assault** is any sexual behavior that is forced on someone without his or her consent. At the least, the victim is made to feel uncomfortable and intimidated; at the worst, he or she is physically and emotionally harmed.[21] Sexual assault includes forced sexual intercourse (rape), forced sodomy (oral or anal sexual acts), child molestation, incest, fondling, and attempts to commit any of these acts. Sexual assaults may be classified as misdemeanors or felonies. Another category of victimization is called **sexual coercion,** defined as imposing sexual activity on someone through the threat of nonphysical punishment, promise of reward, or verbal pressure rather than through force or threat of force.

sexual assault
Any sexual behavior that is forced on someone without his or her consent.

sexual coercion
The imposition of sexual activity on someone through the threat of nonphysical punishment, promise of reward, or verbal pressure rather than through force or threat of force.

According to different studies, 25–60 percent of men (15–25 percent of college men) have engaged in sexual assault and coercive sexual behavior.[22] The causes of this behavior are complex. Perpetrators may have been socialized in a way that promotes male power and encourages controlling behavior by males; they may not have the same understanding of sexual situations that women and other men do. They may accept stereotypes about gender roles and relationships. They may have had early sexual experiences, or they may have predisposing personality traits, such as irresponsibility or lack of social conscience.

Also involved are situational factors, including time and place of assault, use of alcohol and other drugs, and the relationship between victim and perpetrator. No matter what their characteristics, only about 2 percent of men who rape ever go to prison.[23] Rape prevention efforts need to focus on changing the environment that promotes violence against women.

Rape   A study called the Sexual Victimization of College Women Survey found that about 35 women per 1,000 female students were victims of completed or attempted rape in any given academic year (fall and spring semesters). Rape was defined as unwanted vaginal, anal, or oral penetration by penis, finger, or object by force or threat of force.[22] Thus, a college with 10,000 female students could experience more than 350 rapes a year. These researchers estimated that 20–25 percent of college women experience completed or attempted rape during their college years. In 2005 the rate of forcible rape in the general population was 31.7 per 100,000 women.[23]

More than half of rape and sexual assault victims are under the age of 18, and one in five are under the age of 12.[24] When a victim is younger than the "age of consent," usually 18, the perpetrator can be charged with **statutory rape** whether there was consent or not. Only 25–50 percent of all rapes are reported to the police, for a variety of reasons.[22] Victims may be embarrassed or traumatized, may not be sure that what happened to them qualifies as rape, may think they won't be believed, may blame themselves or feel guilty, or may not want to identify someone they know as a rapist.

statutory rape
Sexual intercourse with someone under the "age of consent," usually 18, whether consent is given or not.

Relatively few rapes are **stranger rapes,** that is, rapes committed by someone unknown to the victim. In about 60 percent of rapes and sexual assaults, the victim knows the perpetrator.[23] In 40 percent of cases, the perpetrator is a friend or an acquaintance; **acquaintance rape** can be committed by a classmate, coworker, or someone else casually known to the victim. Unfortunately, only about 16 percent of acquaintance rapes are reported to the police.[25] **Date rape,** sexual assault by a boyfriend or

stranger rape
Rape committed by someone unknown to the victim.

acquaintance rape
Rape committed by someone known to the victim.

date rape
Rape committed by someone with whom the victim has a dating relationship.

someone with whom the victim has a dating relationship, is a type of acquaintance rape. In about 18 percent of rapes and sexual assaults, the perpetrator is the victim's intimate partner or husband.[23] Many states now allow rape charges to be brought by a woman against her husband.

Acquaintance rape survivors are more likely to have consumed alcohol or drugs before the assault, possibly reducing their awareness of signs of aggression in the rapist or their ability to respond to violence. (For more reasons to monitor alcohol consumption, see the box "Alcohol, Rape, and Responsibility: Tips for Women and Men.") One study found that 75 percent of men and 50 percent of women involved in campus acquaintance rapes had been drinking before the sexual assault.[26]

Sexual predators also use so-called date rape drugs, including rohypnol, gamma hydroxybutyrate (GHB), ketamine, and Ecstasy, to incapacitate their victims. To avoid this risk, drink bottled beverages, watch bartenders mix your drink, and do not ever leave drinks unattended. For more on date rape drugs, see Chapter 12.

Male Rape In about 5 percent of completed and attempted rapes in the United States, the victim is male. About 1 in 33 men reports being a victim of a completed or attempted rape in his lifetime.[27] Like women, men are reluctant to report that they have been raped. They may feel embarrassed or ashamed, or they may not want to believe they have been raped. Law enforcement personnel, medical personnel, and social service agencies may be less supportive of male rape victims than of female rape victims because of similar misperceptions and misinformation.[27] The law is clear, however, on defining forced penetration as rape or sodomy. Male rape victims require the same level of medical treatment, counseling, and support as female victims.

Effects of Rape Rape is a crime about dominance, power, and control, not about sex. Victims are intimidated and made to feel helpless. For many victims, the effects of rape can be profoundly traumatic and long lasting. Physical injuries usually heal quickly, but psychological pain can endure.

Victims often experience fear, anxiety, phobias, guilt, nightmares, depression, substance abuse, sleep disorders, sexual dysfunctions, and social withdrawal. They may develop rape-related post-traumatic stress disorder, experiencing flashbacks and impaired functioning. Between 4 and 30 percent of victims contract an STD from the rape, and many worry that they may have been infected with HIV.[28] Some state laws now mandate HIV testing of an alleged rapist if the victim requests it.

Many victims blame themselves for the rape, and our society tends to foster self-blame. Myths about rape include the false beliefs that women or men who are raped did something to provoke it, put themselves in dangerous situations and so deserved it, or could have fought off their attacker. The fact is that no matter what a person does, nobody ever has the right to rape.

Highlight on Health

Alcohol, Rape, and Responsibility: Tips for Women and Men

Alcohol can increase your risk of being involved in rape, whether as a victim or as a perpetrator. Keep the following points in mind when deciding whether and how much to drink:

- Being intoxicated impairs your ability to communicate clearly, making it harder for you to state your expectations and limits regarding sexual activity.

- Being intoxicated impairs your ability to assess a situation that makes you vulnerable to assault and reduces your ability to defend yourself.

- Being intoxicated impairs your ability to make responsible decisions. Alcohol can diminish normal inhibitions against behaving aggressively.

- Being intoxicated makes it harder for you to listen carefully to your companion. A person who is drunk is not necessarily willing to have sexual intercourse. Having sex with someone who is too intoxicated to give informed consent is legally considered rape.

- Criminal law does not distinguish between acquaintance rape and stranger rape. Forced sexual intercourse of any kind is rape.

- Even if someone uses poor judgment by engaging in unwise behavior, such as drinking to excess or walking alone in an isolated area, the responsibility for sexual assault lies entirely with the person who uses force.

- Being drunk is not an excuse for using threats, intimidation, or physical force to coerce another person, and it does not reduce your responsibility for such behavior in either a criminal court or a college disciplinary hearing.

- If you do not pay attention to a refusal of sexual advances, you may commit an act punishable by permanent expulsion from school or imprisonment.

Source: Judith Scott, University Sexual Harassment Officer, University of North Carolina at Chapel Hill, 104 Vance Hall, CB 1040, Chapel Hill, NC 27599; 919-962-3026, 1991, rev. 8/97.

What to Do if You Are Raped If you are raped, you may or may not be able to fight back. There is not a way to respond that works in all cases, and authorities recommend that you do whatever you need to do and can do to survive. It may be yelling, screaming, kicking, and fighting; it may be threatening to call the police; or it may be appeasing the perpetrator by going along. No matter how you respond, remember

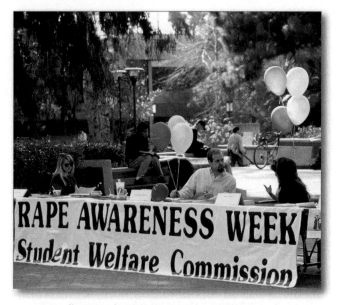

■ Many colleges and universities sponsor a Rape Awareness Week during the school year, often in conjunction with a Take Back the Night march and rally. A growing number of male rape survivors are participating in these events.

that your attacker is violating your rights and committing a crime; rape is not your fault.

After the rape, seek help as soon as you can. If you choose to call the police, there is a better chance that the perpetrator will be brought to justice and will be prevented from raping others. To preserve evidence, do not shower, change your clothes, or clean or straighten the crime scene. You may want to write down everything you can remember about the attack, because memory is diminished during and after traumatic events. Include what the assailant looked like, what he said, his language and use of slang, the kind of sexual activities he wanted, and any threats or weapons he used. Writing this down can help you regain your sense of control, in addition to helping the police find and arrest the attacker.

When the police arrive, tell them exactly what happened, being straightforward and truthful. Most likely they will take you to the hospital, where you will be given a rape exam. A physician may prescribe antibiotics and antiviral medications to decrease your chance of contracting an STD and hormonal medications to prevent pregnancy. In some communities, police departments have sexual assault response teams consisting of law enforcement officers, legal advocates, and medical personnel to help you.

Rape counseling is critical to your recovery from the attack. Talking about the rape, either one-on-one with a rape counselor or in a rape survivors' support group, can help you come to terms with your reactions and feelings. Rape crisis hotlines are available when you need immediate help, although research suggests an increasing reluctance among young people to use the phone to discuss sexual assault. One such hotline is the Rape, Abuse, Incest National Network (RAINN) hotline at (800) 656-HOPE. It takes time to recover from rape, so be patient and take care of yourself.

CHILD SEXUAL ABUSE

Any interaction between a child and an adult or an older child for the sexual gratification of the perpetrator is defined as **child sexual abuse.** This definition includes intercourse, fondling, and viewing or taking pornographic pictures. Rates of child sexual abuse are difficult to verify because many cases go unreported.

The most frequently abused children are age 9 to 11.[29] Girls are sexually abused three times as often as boys.[6] The abuse is usually committed by a family member or other person known to the family. **Incest,** sexual activity between family members, is a particularly traumatic form of child sexual abuse because of the profound betrayal of trust involved.

Victims of sexual abuse usually suffer long-term effects, including anxiety, depression, post-traumatic stress disorder, and sexual dysfunctions. The seriousness of these problems is influenced by the frequency of abuse, the kind of sexual abuse, the child's age when the abuse began, the child's relationship with the abuser, the number of perpetrators, the victim's sex, and the perpetrator's sex. The most common form of child sexual abuse is abuse of a girl by her father, stepfather, brother, or uncle. Abuse of a boy by his mother is rare.[29]

Sex Offenders   Child sexual abusers may or may not be pedophiles. A pedophile is a person who is sexually attracted to and aroused by children. Pedophiles often claim to "love" children and seek opportunities to be around them.

Individuals who are not pedophiles and abuse or molest children are more likely to be opportunists with psychological problems and poor impulse control. Many such individuals spend little time around children, interact with them only sexually, and often dislike them. They are commonly described as predatory, antisocial, and exploitative.

Convicted sex offenders are required to register with the Division of Criminal Justice Services in the state in which they reside. These agencies are authorized to disclose the location of sex offenders if it is considered necessary to protect the public. Sex offenders receive different classifications depending on the risk they are believed to pose to the community. If the risk is believed to be high, they may be required to register for life; if the risk is considered less, they may be allowed to register for shorter periods.

There are more than 500,000 registered offenders in the United States. The location of one in five of these offenders is not known because they have evaded state laws or exploited loopholes in registration laws. The Adam Walsh Child Safety and Protection Act of 2007 enhanced penalties for child sexual abuse, tightened registration requirements for sex offenders, and contained measures to combat Internet predators.

child sexual abuse
Any interaction between a child and an adult or an older child for the sexual gratification of the perpetrator.

incest
Sexual activity between family members.

A biometric database that stores images of sex offenders' irises is a new high-tech weapon used to track sex offenders. Law enforcement agents photograph the offender's iris (a unique identifier) and enter it into a national database, called the Sex Offender Registry and Identification System (SORES). Enforcement agencies can scan the irises of people suspected of committing crimes to see if they are registered in SORES. The American Civil Liberties Union objects to this practice as a violation of privacy rights under the Fourth Amendment.

Internet Predators Pedophiles and other sex offenders have found a community on the Internet, where they exchange stories and buy and sell child pornography. Sexual predators have also accessed social networking sites like Facebook and MySpace. State justice department officials are pushing for state and federal laws that will require these sites to protect users under age 18 through age identity verification and parental consent.[30] Some opponents to these controls argue that there is no simple way to screen for sexual predators, identify underage users masquerading as adults, or ensure that underage users have parental permission.

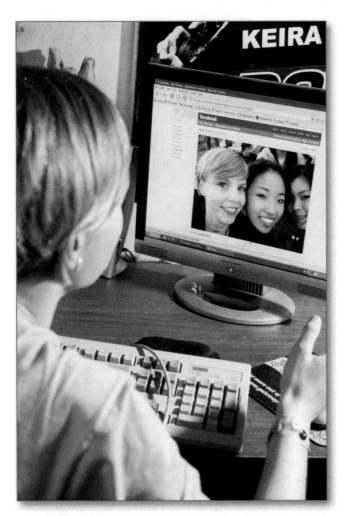

■ Many teens interact safely with strangers online every day. What puts them at risk is giving out their names and other personal information and meeting strangers in person.

The sites themselves, however, are pursuing technologies that can effectively protect users from potential abuses. MySpace, for example, contracted with a national database of convicted sex offenders to detect offenders who were using their site. In one week, MySpace deleted 29,000 convicted sex offenders from its site. In the future, social networking sites will likely face fraud charges if they misrepresent the security of their sites and, possibly, lawsuits if users fall prey to sex offenders and other abusers.

SEXUAL HARASSMENT

Sexual harassment includes two broad types of behavior or situations:

■ A person in a position of authority, such as an employer or a teacher, offers benefits for sexual favors or threatens retaliation for the withholding of sex.

■ Suggestive language or intimidating conduct creates a hostile atmosphere that interferes with a person's work or academic performance.

For example, a manager may seek sexual favors from an employee under the threat of job loss or demotion, or a professor may give a lower grade to a student who rejects his advances. A hostile environment can be created by visual images (for example, sexually explicit photos), language (for example, jokes, derogatory comments, obscene e-mails), or behavior (for example, inappropriate touching). Of all sexual harassment claims, 95 percent result from actions that create a hostile environment.[31]

> **sexual harassment**
> Behavior in which a person in authority offers benefits for sexual favors or threatens retaliation if sexual favors are withheld, or sexually oriented behavior that creates an intimidating or hostile environment that interferes with a person's work or academic performance.

Educational institutions that receive federal money are required to establish policies and grievance procedures for sexual harassment to ensure that complaints are properly investigated and corrective measures taken. If they fail to comply, they can lose their federal funds and be sued by the harassed person. Under federal regulations, colleges and universities are liable for sexual harassment perpetrated by their faculty or staff, regardless of whether the advance is accepted or rejected. About 60 percent of college women and men report being sexually harassed. Only about 10 percent report this harassment to university officials.

If you have experienced sexual harassment, keep a written record of all incidents of harassment, including the date, time, place, people involved, words or actions, and any witnesses. If you can, speak up and tell your harasser that the behavior is unacceptable to you. If you do not feel comfortable confronting the harasser in person, consider doing so by letter.

If confrontation does not change the harasser's behavior, complain to a manager or supervisor. If that person does not respond properly to your complaint, consider using your organization's internal grievance procedures. Legal remedies are also available to you through your state Human Rights Commission and the federal Equal Employment Opportunity

Commission. The threat of a lawsuit may end the harassment, but if it doesn't, don't give up. People who sexually harass others are sexual predators who will continue their unacceptable behavior until stopped.

STALKING AND CYBERSTALKING

Another form of potentially dangerous conduct is **stalking,** in which a person repeatedly and maliciously follows, harasses, or threatens another person. Women are four times as likely as men to be victims of stalking; it is estimated that 1 in 12 women and 1 in 8 college women have been stalked. Four out of five victims know their stalker, who is often a former partner or boyfriend who wants to control or intimidate the victim.[32] In some cases, however, the stalker is a stranger or an acquaintance who has become obsessed with the victim and may have delusional beliefs about their relationship.[33]

stalking
Malicious following, harassing, or threatening of one person by another.

The harassment typically includes surveillance at work, school, or home; frequent disturbing telephone calls; vandalism of the target's property; physical encounters; and attempts to get the victim's family and friends to aid the stalker. Targets of stalkers live in constant fear. They may be forced to change their lives significantly to avoid the stalker. If someone is stalking you, tell your family, friends, and coworkers so that they do not unwittingly divulge information about you.

Many states have passed laws to protect individuals who are being stalked, but in some cases it is difficult to arrest and prosecute stalkers without violating their rights, such as the right to be present in a public place. If you plan to report a stalker to the police, keep a written record of all stalking incidents. Include dates, times, locations, witnesses, and types of incidents (personal encounters, telephone calls, e-mails). Some law enforcement departments and social service agencies provide forms for recording this information.

A variation on stalking is **cyberstalking,** the use of electronic media to pursue, harass, or contact another person who has not solicited the contact.[34] Online stalkers may send threatening, harassing, sexually provocative, or other unwanted e-mails to the target, or attack or impersonate the person on bulletin boards or in chat rooms. Laws against cyberstalking are in place in some states, but prosecution is hampered by Internet protocols that preserve anonymity as well as by constitutional protection of free speech rights. For guidelines on protecting yourself from stalking and cyberstalking, see the box "Tips on Handling a Stalker."

cyberstalking
Use of electronic media to pursue, harass, or contact another person who has not solicited the contact.

Family and Intimate Partner Violence

Violence in families can be directed at any family member, but women, children, and older adults are the most vulnerable. A *family* is defined by the U.S. Census Bureau as a group consisting of two or more persons related by marriage, birth, or adoption and living together in a household.[6] Because this usage excludes dating or cohabiting partners, gay and lesbian partners, and divorced partners, the Census Bureau also uses the term *intimate partners,* which includes all these relationships as well as married partners. Violence between intimate partners is called **intimate partner violence** or **domestic violence.** The rate of assaults among intimate partners is about 47 per 1,000 women and 32 per 1,000 men. Intimate partner violence results in about 2 million injuries and 1,300 deaths each year.[29]

intimate partner violence or **domestic violence**
Violence between two partners in an intimate relationship.

FAMILY VIOLENCE

Family violence is a broad term that includes several forms of violence and abuse. In this section we consider child abuse, elder abuse, and abuse of persons with disabilities.

Child Abuse   Maltreatment of a child, or **child abuse,** includes physical abuse, sexual abuse, emotional abuse, and neglect. It occurs in all cultural, ethnic, and socioeconomic groups, with the highest rates of abuse occurring among the poorest children and among those who are disabled.[35] The highest number of victims are among newborns and infants, who are the most fragile, followed by teenagers.

child abuse
Maltreatment of a child; can be physical, sexual, or emotional abuse or neglect.

Abusive parents often lack the emotional resources to cope with the stress of childrearing; they may not be knowledgeable about normal child development and have unrealistic expectations of their children. Some may have been abused themselves as children. Social determinants like unemployment, poverty, and isolation can be contributing factors, as well as alcohol or drug abuse. When a case of child abuse comes to light, the abusive parent or guardian is usually removed from the home to keep the child safe. Therapy typically focuses on the abuser but includes all family members.[36]

Elder Abuse   Maltreatment of an older adult, or **elder abuse,** can include physical abuse (slapping, bruising); sexual abuse; emotional abuse (humiliating, threatening, intimidating); financial abuse (illegal or improper exploitation of funds); and neglect (abandonment, denial of food or health-related services). The legal determination of whether these actions constitute abuse varies from state to state and depends on their frequency, duration, and intensity. Inconsistent definitions have made it difficult to obtain accurate incidence data,[29] but estimates are that 4–10 percent of people age 65 and older are abused in the United States.[6]

elder abuse
Maltreatment of an older adult; can be physical, sexual, emotional, or financial abuse or neglect.

The abuser is usually a family member, often an adult child, who is taking care of an aging parent or other elderly

Challenges & Choices

Tips on Handling a Stalker

The National Center for Victims of Crime provides the following practical tips for dealing with a stalker:

- If you feel you are in imminent danger, go immediately to a safe place such as a police station, the home of a friend, or a domestic violence shelter; at a minimum, go to a public place where you will be near other people.
- If you know your stalker, consider getting a restraining order.
- Notify police if the stalker commits illegal acts such as entering your residence without permission or destroying your property.
- Document all evidence of stalking. Take photos of any injuries or vandalized property, save answering machine tapes with stalking messages, and keep a detailed written log.
- Consider getting assistance from domestic violence shelters, rape crisis counselors or programs, and victim-assistance coordinators in the prosecutor's office.

To protect yourself from cyberstalking, follow these guidelines:

- Create a gender-neutral, nonprovocative e-mail address. This address should not reveal your general geographic area or your whole name.
- Do not include personal information in your profile.

- Avoid attaching an e-mail signature to your outgoing mail; you may be providing information you do not want revealed to some people.
- When posting information to newsgroups, use a third-party e-mail site such as Yahoo or Hotmail or an anonymous e-mail service that strips out the identity information of the original sender.
- If you are being stalked online and know the stalker, experts recommend that you send the person a clear written warning that the communication is unwanted and must stop immediately. This message should be delivered only once. No matter what response you receive, do not contact the stalker again.
- If the harassment continues, contact the stalker's Internet Service Provider (ISP) and complain about its client; contact your own ISP as well to inform it about what is going on.
- Keep evidence, including e-mails, postings, or other communications, in both electronic and print form.
- Under no circumstances should you agree to meet face-to-face with the stalker. Face-to-face meetings can be very dangerous.

It's Not Just Personal . . .

Australia, India, the United Kingdom, and at least 45 states in the United States have laws against cyberstalking. In many other countries, cyberstalking can be prosecuted under laws against stalking and criminal harassment.

Sources: National Center for Victims of Crime, www.ncvc.org; Cyberstalking: Risk Management, www.crimelibrary.com.

---

relative. Abuse is more likely when the older person is frail, disabled, or impaired, such as by Alzheimer's disease or a physical ailment. It is also more likely when the abuser has substance abuse problems, has a mental illness, or is financially dependent on the older person.[6] Social isolation of the family and lack of community resources also contribute. Research suggests that daughters are more likely to be abusive through neglect than through physical abuse; they are also more likely than sons to be caring for parents who have severe health problems.[29]

Interventions for elder abuse include counseling and support groups for caregivers; battered women's services tailored to the needs of older women; family counseling that attempts to improve relationships within the family; and community services such as Meals on Wheels, home health programs, and elder day care.

Violence Against Persons With Disabilities Children and adults with disabilities are especially vulnerable to abuse by family members; research indicates that they are abused five times more often than those who are not dis-

abled.[29] Because disabled persons often depend on others to report abuse, their abusers are less likely than others to be prosecuted and convicted. One intervention strategy to prevent this form of abuse is to include personal safety training in programs for disabled individuals. When this approach is not feasible, strategies focus on making reporting laws more stringent, improving services to families with a disabled family member, and, where abuse occurs in institutional settings, improving the screening and hiring of staff.[29]

Intimate Partner Violence Intimate partner violence, or domestic violence, is defined as abuse by a person against his or her partner in an intimate relationship. This definition includes the intentional use of fear and humiliation to control another person. The vast majority of domestic violence victims—95–98 percent—are women.[36] The American Medical Association has stated that the home is more dangerous for women than city streets.[37]

Cycle of Abuse Domestic violence is usually characterized by a cycle of abuse, a recurring pattern of escalating

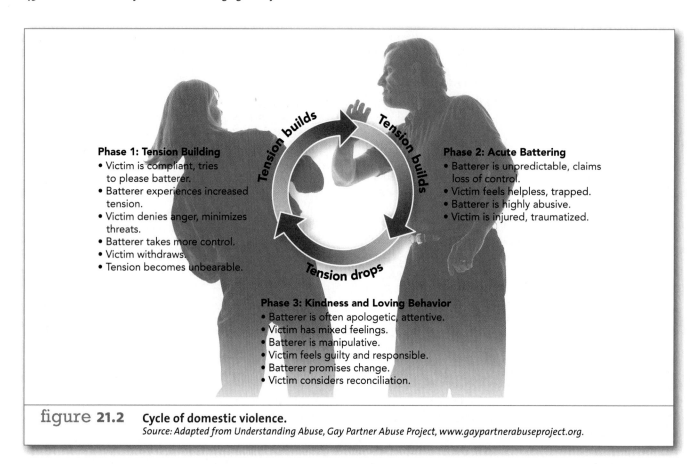

Phase 1: Tension Building
- Victim is compliant, tries to please batterer.
- Batterer experiences increased tension.
- Victim denies anger, minimizes threats.
- Batterer takes more control.
- Victim withdraws.
- Tension becomes unbearable.

Phase 2: Acute Battering
- Batterer is unpredictable, claims loss of control.
- Victim feels helpless, trapped.
- Batterer is highly abusive.
- Victim is injured, traumatized.

Phase 3: Kindness and Loving Behavior
- Batterer is often apologetic, attentive.
- Victim has mixed feelings.
- Batterer is manipulative.
- Victim feels guilty and responsible.
- Batterer promises change.
- Victim considers reconciliation.

figure **21.2**   **Cycle of domestic violence.**
Source: Adapted from Understanding Abuse, Gay Partner Abuse Project, www.gaypartnerabuseproject.org.

violence. If the couple is heterosexual, the pattern is sometimes referred to as **battered woman syndrome**, but it can occur in any relationship, including gay male and lesbian partnerships.

Typically, tension builds up in the relationship until there is a violent outburst, followed by a "honeymoon" period in which the abuser is contrite, ashamed, apologetic, and nonviolent.[29] Often he begs his partner to forgive him and promises it will never happen again. Unless the abuser gets help, however, the violence does recur and the cycle repeats itself, almost always becoming more severe (Figure 21.2).

battered woman syndrome
Cycle of abuse in an intimate relationship, characterized by escalating tension, a violent episode, and a period of lowered tension and nonviolence.

Research indicates that men who batter are more likely to abuse drugs and alcohol, suffer from mental illness, and have financial problems. They need help in dealing with the problems that cause them to act violently.

Most women who are battered eventually leave their abusive relationships, but they may make several attempts before they succeed. Battered women's shelters provide a safe haven where the woman and her children cannot be found by the abuser. They provide housing, food, and resources to help the woman start a new life. When shelters aren't available, private homes are sometimes available as safe houses, and churches, community centers, and YWCAs may also offer temporary facilities.[29]

A variety of social determinants can make it more difficult for some women to receive protection from domestic violence. In rural areas, women often have little or no access to shelters, safe homes, or social service agencies. Older women may be less able to access help, either because of physical impairment or generational attitudes; they may also be subjected to both partner battering and elder abuse. Cultural factors, ethnic traditions, and racism may hinder a woman's ability to obtain help. Women who are not citizens may fear being turned over to the U.S. Citizenship and Naturalization Services and deported. Men in abusive relationships may also have difficulty finding support, because fewer services are available for men. Lesbians and gay men, similarly, may have limited access to appropriate support.[29]

Dating Violence   Dating violence is widespread. Researchers estimate that one in nine high school students and one in five college students have been physically abused in dating relationships.[38] The Centers for Disease Control and Prevention (CDC) reports that about 25 percent of adolescents are victims of verbal, physical, emotional, or sexual abuse each year. Dating abuse occurs more frequently among Black students (13.9 percent) than among Hispanic students (9.3 percent) or White students (7.0 percent).[39]

Some studies suggest that males and females inflict and receive dating violence in equal proportion, but women inflicting violence are usually defending themselves. Other studies find that twice as many women as men are victims of dating violence and that women are more likely to be physically injured. Studies show that individuals at risk for dating violence are more likely than others to have been sexually assaulted, to have peers who have been sexually victimized, and to accept dating violence. Perpetrators are more likely than others to abuse alcohol or drugs, to have adversarial attitudes toward others, to have sexually aggressive peers, and to accept dating violence.[40]

The FBI reports that 20 percent of female homicide victims are 14 to 18 years old.[23] Most killings occur in dating relationships characterized by control and physical abuse. Despite the seriousness of dating violence, young girls face more barriers in finding help than adult women do. Many states require a parent's or guardian's permission before granting a protective order to a minor, and community shelters and counseling programs often require an adult's permission before admitting a minor. Families, schools, and communities need to work together to educate young people about what behavior is acceptable and unacceptable in a relationship.

Unhealthy relationships with the potential for abuse often involve power and control issues. One partner may make all the significant decisions, set numerous rules, restrict his or her partner's visits to friends and family, monitor phone calls and e-mails, control the couple's money, and be obsessed with what the partner is doing at all times. The abusive person may embarrass his or her partner in front of others and use derogatory names for the partner. Other signs of an unhealthy relationship are excessive jealousy, intimidation, and explosive anger. If you recognize any of these signs in your relationships, you may want to consider getting help to deal with these issues or ending the relationship.[29]

Resources for Survivors of Intimate Partner Violence If you are concerned that someone you know may be in an abusive relationship, try talking to the person about the nature of the relationship and giving him or her information about resources available in your community. Encourage the person to maintain contact with friends and family members while getting support to leave the relationship and begin building a new life.[29]

Women who decide to leave abusive relationships may be overwhelmed by the prospect of finding another place to live, supporting themselves and their children, and changing their lifestyle. They need to assess their options for financial support, employment, health care, housing, and education. Help is available from social service agencies, educational programs, hotlines, shelters, advocacy organizations, and informational books and packets provided by national, state, and local organizations.

Workplace Violence, Hate Crime, and Terrorism

Violence can occur where there are high levels of stress, where there is bias, and where there is perceived injustice. In most cases, however, multiple risk factors are present; very often, the perpetrator of violence is psychologically disturbed.

VIOLENCE IN THE WORKPLACE

Workplace violence is defined as violent acts, including physical assault and threats of assault, directed toward persons at work or on duty. It can include threatening or aggressive behavior, verbal abuse, intimidation, or harassment. It can be committed by strangers, customers or clients, coworkers, or people with personal relationships with workers. People in some occupations are at higher risk of experiencing workplace violence. Workers with the most dangerous jobs are police officers, followed by security guards, taxi drivers, prison guards, bartenders, mental health professionals, convenience and liquor store clerks, and schoolteachers.[23]

The National Institute for Occupational Safety and Health estimates that about 20 workers are murdered and 18,000 are assaulted each week while at work.[23] Employers can take measures to lower the risk of workplace violence, such as careful pre-employment screening, appropriate security measures in the workplace, the establishment of procedures for resolving disputes, awareness training for employees and management, and employee assistance programs that provide counseling for employees experiencing psychological problems or high levels of stress. Individuals can also be alert to warning signs of possible violence by others in the workplace, such as extreme changes in behavior, outbursts, conflicts with others, or bringing a weapon to work.

HATE CRIME

A **hate crime** is defined as a crime motivated by bias against the victim's ethnicity, race, religion, sexual orientation, or disability. Hate crimes tend to be excessively brutal, are frequently inflicted at random on people the perpetrators do not know, and are often committed by multiple perpetrators.[41]

hate crime
Crime motivated by bias against the victim's ethnicity, race, religion, sexual orientation, or disability.

In 2006 9,080 hate crime offenses were reported in the United States, involving 9,642 victims and 7,324 offenders. More than half of these crimes were committed because of the offender's racial bias (primarily anti-Black); 18 percent were committed because of the offender's religious bias (primarily anti-Jewish); 16 percent because of the offender's sexual orientation bias (primarily anti–gay men); 14 percent because of the offender's ethnic or national origin bias (primarily anti-Hispanic); and less than 0.5 percent because of the offender's bias against persons with physical or mental disabilities.[41]

Most states have hate crime laws in place, as does the federal government. Many colleges and universities have policies prohibiting hate crimes and harassment of individuals in targeted groups, as well as programs that promote cultural knowledge and diversity.[42] Because hate crimes against lesbian, gay, bisexual, and transgender (LGBT) persons have increased on campuses in recent years,[43] many colleges and universities have specific policies forbidding violence directed toward LGBT students.[43] Many colleges have hotlines for reporting hate crimes; there are also local, state, and federal hotlines for getting information about and reporting hate crimes.

TERRORISM

Terrorism is a form of violence directed against persons or property, including civilian populations, for the purpose of instilling fear and engendering a sense of helplessness. Often, terrorist acts are committed in supposed furtherance of political or social aims. Internationally, terrorist acts include kidnappings, murders, and bombings of churches, mosques, nightclubs, buses, and city streets. In the United States, such acts have included the 1993 bombing of the World Trade Center in New York City, the 1995 bombing of the Federal Building in Oklahoma City, and the September 11, 2001, attacks on the World Trade Center in New York City and the Pentagon in Washington, D.C.

terrorism
Violence directed against persons or property, including civilian populations, for the purpose of instilling fear and engendering a sense of helplessness.

Since the September 11 attacks, psychologists have established that people's deepest fears involve uncontrollable catastrophic events that are likely to affect future generations. Americans most fear the use of weapons of mass destruction—nuclear, chemical, and biological weapons—that could cause massive casualties.[44]

In response to the September 11 attacks, the U.S. government created the Department of Homeland Security to prevent and guard against future attacks and the Homeland Security Advisory System, a color-coded warning system, to alert citizens of the likelihood of attack. In 2005 Congress passed a counterterrorism measure called the Real ID Act

(see the box "The Real ID"). In 2007 Congress passed the John Doe provision as part of the renewal of the Homeland Security bill. This provision protects people who report suspicious activity from being sued by those they report.

In addition, the Federal Emergency Management Agency (FEMA) publishes a booklet, *Are You Ready? An In-Depth Guide to Citizen Preparedness,* that provides guidelines on being ready for any kind of disaster, including terrorist attack. Instructions for obtaining free copies of the booklet are available at the FEMA Web site (www.fema.gov).

Public Health in Action

The Real ID

The Real ID Act, passed by Congress in 2005, establishes minimum standards for driver's licenses and state-issued identification cards. When the law goes into effect, applicants will have to provide the following documentation in order to obtain a license or ID card: a photo or a nonphoto ID that includes full legal name and birth date, documentation of birth date, documentation of legal status and Social Security number, and documentation showing name and principal residence address. The license or ID card, in turn, will include the person's full legal name, date of birth, sex, driver's license or identification number, photograph, residence address, and signature. The card will have physical security features designed to prevent tampering, counterfeiting, or duplication and be machine-readable by a technology common to all the states. States will be required to share their vehicle databases with other states.

The Real ID Act has created considerable controversy. Criticisms are that (1) it will be costly to implement for individuals ($20 more for a standardized, tamper-proof license) and states ($10.7–$14.6 billion), (2) it is a violation of privacy rights, since it creates large federal and state databases containing sensitive private information, (3) it will increase the likelihood that illegal immigrants will drive without driver's licenses or insurance (however, states can still issue driving privilege certificates/cards in lieu of regular driver's licenses, allowing people to obtain liability insurance), and (4) it is not a true national ID system, since the states are still responsible for issuing cards and maintaining databases.

All states must have programs in place to comply with the Real ID Act by 2010, and all driver's licenses and identification cards must be in compliance by 2013. If a state does not comply with this act, residents of that state will not be able to use their driver's licenses to get on a plane or enter a federal building.

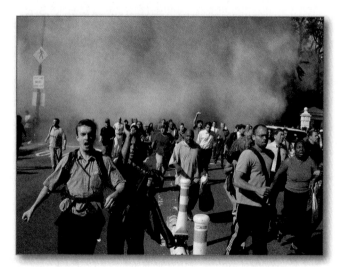

■ Some people still suffer from symptoms of posttraumatic stress disorder as a result of the terrorist attacks of September 11, 2001, including individuals who weren't there but viewed the events on television.

Challenges & Choices

Protecting Yourself From Violence

In Your House or Apartment

- Keep doors and windows locked, even when you are at home.
- Before you open your door, make sure the caller is legitimate. If you are expecting a repairperson, insist on proper identification. If the person wants to use your phone, offer to make the call for him or her but do not let the person inside.
- If you have children, tell them not to open the door to strangers.
- If you are a woman living alone, use only your initials on your mailbox and in telephone directories.
- If you live in an apartment building, avoid being alone in the laundry room or garage, especially late at night.

On Campus and in Public Places

- Be aware of your surroundings; avoid walking through secluded areas and high-crime neighborhoods.
- Avoid listening to music on headphones; it reduces your attention to warning signs that may be occurring around you.
- Stay with others when possible; groups of three or more are rarely attacked.
- Act and walk in a confident manner. Most assaults occur because the assailant perceives an opportunity to attack someone who appears vulnerable.

- Walk close to the curb, facing oncoming traffic. You will be less vulnerable to attacks from people in cars or hiding in doorways, alleys, or bushes.
- When carrying packages or luggage, try to keep one arm free.
- Hold your purse firmly under your arm with the strap over your opposite shoulder. Avoid carrying a wallet in a hip pocket, or transfer money and credit cards to a front pocket.
- When you are in any public place, do not display large amounts of cash. Be alert when using an ATM.
- Rely on your instincts. If you think you are being followed, walk quickly to a lighted area. If you feel that you are in immediate danger, scream and run.
- Encourage older and disabled persons to use community transportation services.
- If you jog, do so with a partner. Vary your route and the time you run, and if you run at night, be sure the area is well lit. Don't wear headphones while jogging.
- Consider taking a class in self-defense.

It's Not Just Personal ...

Whereas young people are most likely to be victims of violent crime, people over 65 are most likely to be victims of property crime (burglary, auto theft, property theft). Ninety percent of crimes committed against older adults are property crimes, compared with 40 percent of crimes committed against people aged 12 to 24.

Source: Adapted from Safety: A Personal Focus *(pp. 178–180), by D.L. Bever, 1996, New York: McGraw-Hill.*

Preventing Violence

Although protecting yourself from terrorism is difficult, there are ways you can limit your risks in life; for strategies and tips, see the boxes "Protecting Yourself From Violence" and "Preventing Identity Theft." At the same time, self-protection measures must be part of a more comprehensive approach that addresses violence at the societal level. Current efforts to curb violence focus primarily on arresting and imprisoning offenders. Strategies are also needed that prevent violence before it occurs—that is, interventions that change the social conditions underlying violence.

THE ROLE OF GUNS: FACILITATING VIOLENCE

As noted earlier, firearms, especially handguns, play a large role in the high death rate associated with crime in the United States. Guns contribute to the lethality of any incident involving violence.

Gun control is a controversial issue in the United States. The Second Amendment to the U.S. Constitution protects the right of citizens to "keep and bear arms," a right that was important in colonial times but that may not be as important today. The gun industry, along with its powerful lobby and many clubs, organizations, and individual enthusiasts, defends the right of Americans to own guns with minimal restrictions. Some laws are in place regulating gun sales, such as computerized background checks on persons seeking to buy guns, aimed at screening out convicted felons and certain other groups.

Proponents of gun control support these and other measures, including waiting periods for gun purchases, licensing of guns, and restrictions on access to guns by young people.[45] Proponents of gun control also support the design of safer guns, such as guns with trigger locks, but gun manufacturers point out that gun owners frequently do not use the locks, and the U.S. Congress has concluded that locks are effective only with children younger than age 6.[46]

Consumer Clipboard

Preventing Identity Theft

If anyone has ever used your name, address, Social Security number (SSN), bank or credit card account number, or other identifying information without your knowledge with the intent to commit fraud or other crimes, you have been the victim of identity theft.

Identity thieves obtain information from businesses or institutions by stealing records, conning or bribing employees, or hacking into computers. They can use "skimming" devices to steal credit and debit account numbers as your card is being processed. Low-tech approaches include rummaging through your trash, stealing wallets and purses, stealing mail, or stealing personal information from your home. In some cases, identity thieves obtain the information directly from you—by luring you into a scam or by posing as a legitimate businessperson or government official.

Someone who steals your account numbers can buy big-ticket items, such as computers, and quickly resell them. They can take out an auto loan or establish phone or wireless service in your name. They can drain your current bank account or open a new one in your name. They can file for bankruptcy under your name or give your name to the police during an arrest.

Here are some tips to minimize your chance of being a victim of identity theft:

- Don't give out personal information on the phone, via mail, or over the Internet unless you've initiated the contact or know for sure whom you're dealing with.

- Don't carry your SSN with you; instead, keep it in a secure place. Give your SSN only when absolutely necessary.

- Protect all personal information in your home and at work.

- Deposit all mail in mailboxes or at your local post office.

- Guard your trash by shredding all billing, medical, and business documents.

- Carry only the ID information and credit and debit cards that you really need.

- Choose passwords for your credit card, bank, and phone accounts with care. Don't use your mother's maiden name, your birth date, the last four digits of your SSN, your phone number, or a series of consecutive numbers.

- Pay attention to your billing cycles. A missing bill could mean that someone has taken over your account.

- Watch out for promotional scams in the form of phony offers.

- Keep your computer secure with a firewall, virus-protection software, and password protection for key files. Before disposing of a computer, remove all data with a "wipe" utility program.

If you are the victim of identity theft, take these steps:

- For financial account information, such as credit card or bank accounts, close those accounts immediately.

- For SSNs, call the toll-free fraud number of any of the three major credit bureaus and place an initial fraud alert on your credit reports. Review those credit reports.

- For driver's license or other ID documents, contact the issuing agency about placing fraud flags.

- File a report with your local police. Get a copy of the police report.

- File a complaint with the Federal Trade Commission so that this information can be added to its database.

Source: Data from Federal Trade Commission, www.consumer.gov/idtheft.

The gun industry has come under fire in recent years for its marketing practices, which include targeting women, children, and minorities. The marketing campaign aimed at women focuses on three themes—empowerment, protection, and participation in shooting sports.[47] Playing on women's fears of rape, gun-wielding assailants, and terrorist acts, these campaigns encourage women to buy guns despite statistics showing that guns in the home are much more likely to kill a family member than a stranger.[47]

The gun industry has also used a variety of strategies to cultivate children as gun enthusiasts, including advertising in youth magazines, financing shooting ranges, providing gun training programs for schools, and manufacturing smaller firearms for children. The huge number of video games that involve shooting also stimulate children's interest in guns.

The gun industry can be expected to increase its marketing to ethnic minorities as well. Rates of gun ownership by Blacks and Hispanics are considerably lower than that for Whites, even though death rates from firearms are higher.[48] The complex issues surrounding the manufacture, sale, and ownership of guns are likely to be part of our national debate for some time to come.

THE ROLE OF MEDIA AND ENTERTAINMENT: GLORIFYING VIOLENCE

Killing, maiming, torture, and rape are all part of the fare served up by the media and entertainment industries in our culture. Violent acts occur much more frequently in movies and television shows than they do in real life.[49] Exposure to such images may lead to increased fearfulness, depression, and pessimism, particularly in children.[49] Repeated exposure to violence may also lead to habituation and **desensitization,** a raised threshold for reaction to violence and a loss of compassion. Repeated exposure to graphic images of violence also feeds the appetite for more intense violence.[49]

desensitization
Raised threshold of reaction to violence and a loss of compassion.

The American Academy of Pediatrics and five other prominent medical groups concluded in 2000 that there is a connection between violence in mass media and increases in both acceptance of aggressive attitudes and aggressive behavior in children.[50] Reports from the National Academy of Sciences and the CDC have supported these conclusions.[49] The entertainment industry maintains that these studies demonstrate only possible associations between media violence and aggression. Media defenders warn that attempts at regulation would border on censorship.

In response to this information, communities have organized boycotts of products of companies that sponsor violent and sexually explicit programs. Parents are using blocking technologies to keep their children from seeing selected television programs and Internet sites. The entertainment industry has started to regulate itself, primarily to avoid government regulation.[49] The video rental industry, for example, has introduced a "Pledge to Parents," promising that movies rated R (restricted) and video games rated M (mature) will not be rented to children under age 17, and the National Association of Theater Owners has promised to enforce the movie ratings system vigorously.

SUPPORTING FAMILIES AND COMMUNITIES

In a healthy society, families carry out a vital function: teaching children self-control. Individuals with high levels of self-control are less likely to engage in criminal acts than are those with less self-control. Families can also teach children constructive ways to deal with anger, frustration, and destructive impulses. When children show signs of delinquency, schools and communities can provide parental education and support.

Positive family interventions emphasize consistent parenting, clear rules and appropriate consequences, supervision of children's activities, and constructive management of family conflicts. There is no evidence that nontraditional families with young or single parents are any less effective than traditional families at instilling values in children.[51]

The health of individuals and families is supported by healthy communities. Common sense suggests that safe physical environments—those with well-lit streets, for example—are less conducive to criminal activity than are run-down environments. Communities where neighbors look out for one another, as with neighborhood watch programs, are less inviting to criminals. Communities also have to support social changes that enhance economic and social stability.[52] To bring about change, communities have used strategies such as the following:[52, 53]

- Cleaning up trash and graffiti and fixing broken windows.
- Providing organized leisure activities and mentoring programs for youth.
- Encouraging parent involvement in school activities.
- Supporting low-income housing to curb an exodus of middle-income residents of all races.
- Maintaining municipal services.
- Curtailing street-corner loitering, panhandling, prostitution, and public drinking.
- Increasing police presence in high-risk areas.

Individuals who want to take action against violence have a variety of options, from volunteering at women's shelters to supporting public policies that address the root causes of violence in our society. Keeping a sense of perspective about violence is important, however. Some observers have suggested that Americans live in a media-driven "culture of fear," frightened by overblown accounts of crime, drugs, and violence.[54] The key is to take media portrayals of violence with a grain of salt while using your common sense to keep yourself safe.

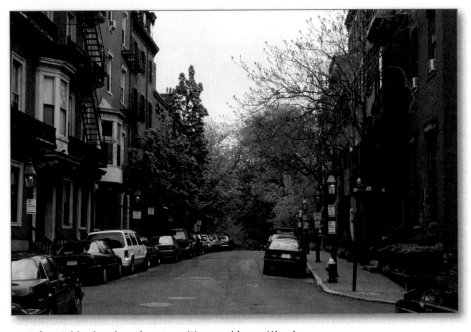

- Safe neighborhoods and communities provide a setting in which individuals have the opportunity to pursue wellness.

You Make the Call

Is Backscatter Body Scanning a Security Improvement or an Invasion of Privacy?

Airport security has undergone many significant changes since the terrorist acts of September 11, 2001. Better training for airport screeners, strengthening of cockpit doors, use of air marshals on flights, and pat-down searches of random passengers are a few of the safety measures now in place. New technology is also being developed for safer airline travel, and the Transportation Safety Administration (TSA) is field-testing a variety of new systems. For example, passenger screening portals may use a gadget to shoot puffs of air at passengers to loosen particles that may reveal the presence of explosive residue. Fingerprint and iris checkers are being used to prevent unauthorized people from accessing secure areas.

The system creating particular controversy, however, is backscatter body scanning—the use of low-energy X-rays that scatter rather than penetrate materials. Backscatter scanners can easily detect weapons, dangerous substances, or bombs being carried on a person's body. The rays, considered harmless, can "see" though clothing and provide a detailed image of a person's naked body. Backscatter portals are currently being used at airports to search travelers suspected by U.S. Customs of carrying illegal drugs, and they have been tested in selected airports. They are also being used in prisons, at foreign embassies in the United States, and at London's Heathrow Airport.

Advocates of backscatter body scanning say that it is needed to enhance airport security and is less invasive than pat-downs. Opponents believe backscatter body scanning is an invasion of privacy and constitutes a "virtual strip search." They argue that routine screening, physical inspection, and observation of behavior provide the safety needed for air travel. What do you think?

PROS

- Backscatter body scanning can significantly reduce the "hassle" factor in passenger screening in secure areas. It can cover crowded security entrances without the need for screening of individual travelers with hand wands.

- Backscatter portals can be used throughout the airport. They can be linked to closed-circuit television cameras that automatically pick out and follow suspicious subjects. They can send an instant alert message to nearby security personnel to stop suspicious passengers for questioning.

- The seminude image problem can be solved by overlaying the body with graphics that shield nipples and genitalia.

- Although backscatter portals are expensive, costing between $100,000 and $200,000 each, overall cost can be reduced by using dummy as well as live devices. Passengers will not be aware of which devices are live.

- Software can be used with backscatter portals that will identify unusual behavior, providing another layer of protection against terrorist acts.

CONS

- Backscatter scanning provides images of the body that violate individual privacy rights. Many people may object to being scanned for religious or ethical reasons.

- This technology cannot detect weapons hidden in body folds and is not as effective as a body cavity search.

- The images from backscatter portals are capable of being permanently stored and viewed at later times, creating an ongoing potential for privacy violations. Many women subjected to backscatter screening have complained to the Federal Aviation Administration that it is a form of sexual abuse.

- Backscatter scanning may produce a high level of false alarms, increasing the likelihood of delays, passenger complaints, and reduced vigilance by screeners.

- Vigilance by passengers is more effective in identifying potential terrorist activity than costly gadgets and technology.

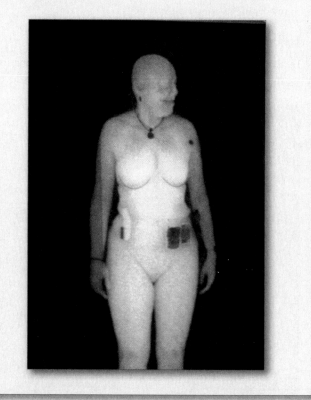

Sources: "Spotlight on Surveillance: Transportation Agency's Plan to X-Ray Travelers Should Be Stripped of Funding," *Electronic Privacy Information Center,* retrieved June 16, 2008, from http://epic.org/privacy/surveillance/spotlight/0605/; "New Screening Technology Is Nigh," *Wired News,* retrieved June 16, 2008, from www.wired.com/news/privacy/0,65366-1.html?tw=wn_story_page_next1.

In Review

1. **How does violence affect personal health?** Many people are the victims of violence and of violent crimes, which include homicide, assault, robbery, and rape. Compared with other developed countries, the United States has higher rates of homicide, especially homicide committed with a firearm.

2. **What risk factors are associated with being the victim or perpetrator of violence?** Sex (male) and age (teen, young adult) are the most reliable risk factors for violence; being a member of a minority group is another significant risk factor. Other risk factors occur at the individual, family, societal, and cultural levels.

3. **What forms does violence take in our society?** Teens and young adults commit violent acts in schools and as members of youth gangs. Crimes on college campuses include assaults, rapes, and very rare but high-profile mass shootings. Sexual violence includes sexual assault, child sexual abuse, sexual harassment, and stalking and cyberstalking. Family violence includes child and elder abuse, intimate partner violence, and dating violence. Violence can also occur in the workplace or take the form of a hate crime. Terrorism is violence intended to create fear and helplessness.

4. **What can be done about violence?** Individuals can take simple measures to protect themselves, such as being aware of their surroundings, avoiding secluded areas, and keeping doors and windows locked. They can also support measures that change the societal conditions underlying violence. Some of these conditions are the availability of handguns and the depiction of violence in movies, video games, and other forms of entertainment. Strong families and healthy communities make it harder for a culture of violence to take root.

www For a detailed summary of this chapter and a comprehensive set of review questions, visit the Online Learning Center at **www.mhhe.com/teague2e**.

Web Resources

National Center for Victims of Crime: This Web site offers information on the cycle of abuse, child abuse, rape, domestic violence, stalking, dating violence, and violence against women.
www.ncvc.org

National Coalition Against Domestic Violence: This organization offers information packets and guides about violence, including teen dating violence. It features a directory of domestic violence programs throughout the United States.
www.ncadv.org

National Organization for Victim Assistance: Online publications of this organization cover topics such as crisis intervention, the psychological trauma of crime, supportive counseling, victims' rights and services, and the Victims Movement.
www.trynova.org

National Sexual Violence Resource Center: This site operates as a collection and distribution center for information, statistics, and resources on sexual violence. Its

publications include newsletters, a directory of projects working toward the end of sexual violence, and news releases.
www.nsvrc.org

Prevent Child Abuse America: This organization is dedicated to building awareness of child abuse and providing education on the abuse and neglect of children. Its publications include tips for parents, information for kids, newsletters, and fact sheets.
www.preventchildabuse.org

Rape, Abuse, and Incest National Network (RAINN): This site provides information about what to do if you or a friend is sexually assaulted, how to reduce your risk of sexual assault, and how to protect your child from sexual abuse. RAINN also offers "A Parent's Guide to Internet Safety" (FBI publication) and operates the free, confidential National Sexual Assault Hotline (1-800-656-HOPE).
www.rainn.org

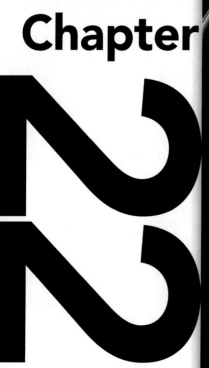

22

Injury
Creating Safe
Environments

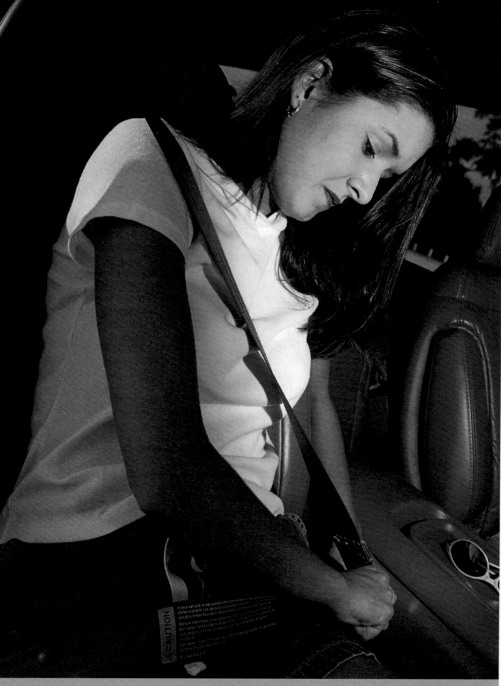

WWW

Your Health Today

www.mhhe.com/teague2e

Go to the Online Learning Center for *Your Health Today* for interactive activities, quizzes, flashcards, Web links, and more resources related to this chapter.

Ever Wonder...

- how your bike and bike helmet should fit?

- if it's safe to talk on your cell phone while you're driving?

- how to do the Heimlich maneuver?

Unintentional injuries are the leading cause of death for children and adults between the ages of 1 and 39 and the fifth leading cause of death for Americans of all ages. Millions of people also suffer nonfatal injuries every year.

Public health experts now avoid the term *accident* in referring to these incidents, because it implies that injury is a chance occurrence or unpreventable mishap over which individuals have no control.[1] These experts emphasize that injuries are preventable if people adopt behaviors that promote safety and if society does its part in reducing environmental hazards. Examples of safety-promoting behaviors are wearing safety belts in cars, keeping medications in locked cabinets out of the reach of children, and having working smoke detectors in the home.

Unintentional injuries are injuries that are not purposefully inflicted,[1] in contrast to intentional injuries like homicides, assaults, or rapes. The leading cause of unintentional injury death for Americans of all ages is motor vehicle crashes, followed by poisoning, falls, choking, and drowning (see the box "Americans and Unintentional Injuries").

unintentional injuries
Injuries that are not purposefully inflicted.

Common causes of injury death are different for different age groups. For example, for infants under 1 year of age, the leading cause of injury death is suffocation; for children aged 1 to 14, the second leading cause (after motor vehicle crashes) is drowning, and the third is fire and flames. For individuals aged 15 to 54, the second leading cause (after motor vehicle crashes) is poisoning, typically from drugs. For those over 75 years of age, the leading cause of injury death is falls.[2]

Leading causes of injury death also vary by ethnicity and race. For Blacks and people of Hispanic background, the second leading cause of death is poisoning, whereas for non-Hispanic Whites and all other groups, it is falls. Blacks and Hispanics are also more likely to die from drownings and fires than from suffocation, while the opposite is true for Whites and other groups.

Across all groups, however, more males than females die from unintentional injuries from birth to age 80, and males have a higher rate of death per 100,000 people than females throughout the life span (Figure 22.1). For males, the greatest number of deaths occurs at age 21, and totals remain high until the early 50s; for females, the greatest number of deaths occurs after age 75.[2] In this chapter we provide an overview of unintentional injuries and include guidelines and tips that will help you keep yourself safe.

Motor Vehicle Safety

Motor vehicle crashes account for 44 percent of all unintentional injury deaths. The highest number of motor vehicle deaths occurs in the young and the old—those aged 16–19 and those aged 75 and older. Men are more likely than women to be killed in car crashes. Women are more likely to be involved in car crashes, fatal and nonfatal combined, than men.[2–4]

Who's at Risk

Americans and Unintentional Injuries

- Someone dies in an alcohol-related motor vehicle crash every 31 minutes, and someone is injured every 2 minutes. Male drivers involved in crashes are twice as likely as female drivers to have a blood alcohol concentration (BAC) of 0.8 percent or higher.

- Drivers aged 65 and older have higher motor-vehicle-related death rates per mile driven than drivers in all other age groups except teen drivers. Rates of motor-vehicle-related injuries are twice as high for older men as they are for older women.

- On average, a pedestrian death occurs every 111 minutes, and a pedestrian injury occurs every 8 minutes. About one-fifth of pedestrians killed or injured are children between the ages of 5 and 9. The pedestrian fatality rate is twice as high for men as it is for women.

- Someone dies in a fire every 134 minutes, and someone is injured every 29 minutes. Those at greatest risk for fire-related death and injury are children aged 4 or younger, adults aged 65 or older, the poorest Americans, Blacks, Native Americans, people living in rural areas, and people living in manufactured homes or substandard housing.

- On average, nine unintentional drownings occur every day. A Centers for Disease Control and Prevention study of self-reported swimming ability found that men are more likely to have greater swimming ability than women. Blacks reported the most limited swimming ability among all races and ethnic groups. Alcohol use is involved in about 25–50 percent of adolescent and adult deaths associated with water recreation.

- Unintentional poisoning is second only to motor vehicle crashes as a cause of injury death for Blacks and Hispanics. Native Americans have the highest death rate from unintentional poisoning. Men are more than twice as likely as women to die from unintentional poisoning.

Source: CDC Injury Fact Book, Centers for Disease Control and Prevention, retrieved September 8, 2008, from www.cdc.gov/ncipc/fact_book/factbook.html.

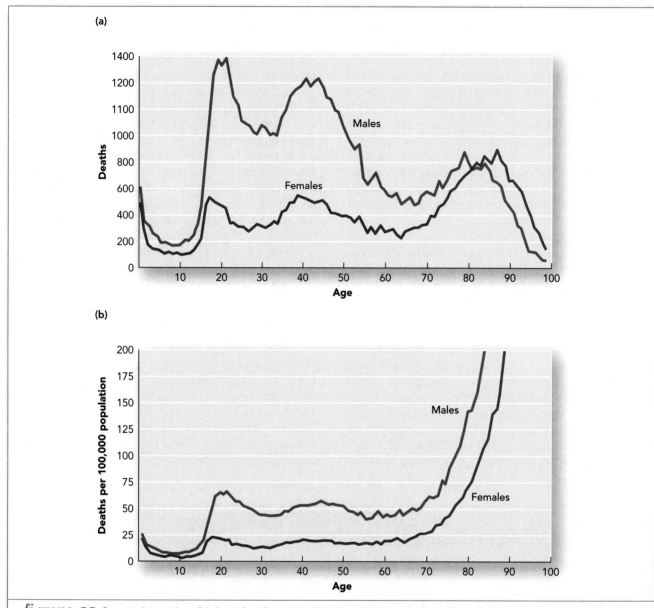

(a)

(b)

figure 22.1   **Unintentional injury deaths, United States, 2001—total number of deaths and rates of death per 100,000 population.** (a) Unintentional injury deaths by sex and age. More males than females die from unintentional injuries at all ages from birth to age 80. (b) Unintentional injury death rates by sex and age. As people become older, their rates of death from unintentional injury soar. *Source: Injury Facts, 2004, National Safety Council.*

FACTORS CONTRIBUTING TO MOTOR VEHICLE CRASHES

improper driving
The cause of most motor vehicle crashes, including speeding, failing to yield right of way, following too closely, and passing on a yellow line.

About 85 percent of motor vehicle crashes are believed to be caused by **improper driving,** defined as speeding, failing to yield the right of way, disregarding signals and stop signs, making improper turns, and following too closely, among other driving behaviors. Speeding is especially dangerous; it is a major factor in most fatal crashes. Speeding-related crashes decrease with

driver age.[5] **Defensive driving** can help you reduce your risk of injury at the hands of people who drive improperly (see the box "Defensive Driving").

In addition to improper driving, factors contributing to motor vehicle crashes include driver inattention, aggressive driving, alcohol-impaired driving, and environmental hazards.

defensive driving
Responsible driving that anticipates potential hazards and monitors changing environmental conditions.

Driver Inattention   The National Highway Traffic Safety Administration (NHTSA) estimates that at least 25 percent of highway crashes involve some form of driver inattention.[6] Drivers under age 20 are the most likely to be involved in distraction-related crashes. Talking on a cell phone is a major source of distraction, and many states and countries have passed laws restricting cell phone use while driving. Some states have banned cell phone use while driving altogether, and others have mandated hands-free devices only.[7] Studies have found that it is not using the phone per se that causes distraction so much as shifting attention to the conversation and away from driving. As the number of distracting devices inside cars increases (navigation systems, computers, televisions, DVD players), more states are passing legislation to limit the use of electronic devices in motor vehicles.

Drowsiness is a major source of driver inattention. As described in Chapter 6, driving while you are drowsy can be as dangerous as driving under the influence of alcohol. Drowsiness reduces awareness of your surroundings, impairs judgment, and slows reaction time. Thirty-three percent of traffic accidents are associated with sleepiness, and fatigue is the leading cause of fatal crashes in people aged 18 to 25.[3, 8]

road rage
Extreme form of aggressive driving in which a driver becomes enraged at another driver's behaviors and one or both drivers take increasingly aggressive actions, such as passing and cutting in or attempting to physically injure the other driver.

Aggressive Driving   The NHTSA estimates that two-thirds of all traffic fatalities are associated with overly aggressive driving behavior.[3] An aggressive driver is someone who tailgates, speeds, runs red lights, changes lanes without signaling, and makes illegal turns.

Aggressive driving can escalate into **road rage**.[9] This extreme form of aggressive driving may occur when a driver becomes enraged at another driver's poor driving behaviors, such as sudden merging or lane changing, or it may occur when one driver provokes another

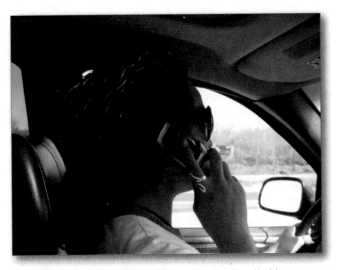

■ Using a cell phone while driving—whether handheld or hands-free—reduces the brain's ability to process information and react quickly. Some states prohibit the use of handheld phones while driving, and some prohibit text messaging. In no state are all types of cell phone use by drivers banned.

Challenges & Choices

Defensive Driving

Defensive driving means anticipating potential hazards by keeping your eyes on other drivers and monitoring changing environmental conditions. The National Safety Council stresses nine defensive driving guidelines:

■ Don't start the engine without securing each passenger in the car, including children and pets. Safety belts save thousands of lives each year. Lock all doors.

■ Remember that driving too fast or too slow can increase the likelihood of collisions.

■ If you plan to drink, designate a driver who won't drink. Alcohol is a factor in almost half of all fatal motor vehicle crashes.

■ Be alert. If you notice that a car is straddling the center line, weaving, making wide turns, stopping abruptly, or responding slowly to traffic signals, the driver may be impaired.

■ Avoid an impaired driver by turning right at the nearest corner or exiting at the nearest exit. If it appears that an oncoming car is crossing into your lane, pull over to the roadside, sound the horn, and flash your lights.

■ Notify the police immediately after seeing a motorist who is driving suspiciously.

■ Follow the rules of the road. Don't contest the "right of way" or try to race another car during a merge. Respect other motorists.

■ Don't follow too closely. You can determine an appropriate following distance by using the "three-second rule." Select a fixed object on the road ahead, such as a sign or an overpass. When the car in front of you passes it, count "one one thousand, two one thousand, three one thousand." If you pass the object before you complete the count, you are following too closely. In poor driving conditions, double or triple your distance (to 6 or 9 seconds).

■ While driving, be cautious, aware, and responsible.

It's Not Just Personal . . .

According to the National Safety Council's *Injury Facts*, 44,700 people died in motor vehicle crashes in the United States in 2008, a decline of 2 percent from 2004. There were also 2.4 million motor vehicle-related disability injuries that year.

Source: Fact Sheet on Driving Defensively, National Safety Council, www.nsc.org. Permission to reprint granted by the National Safety Council, a membership organization dedicated to protecting life and promoting health.

with a curse or gesture and the second driver retaliates. One or both drivers may take more aggressive actions, such as flashing bright lights, passing and cutting in, or attempting to damage the other's vehicle or physically injure the other driver. The irrational thoughts of a driver in the grip of road rage may last for minutes or hours. Road rage has been implicated in numerous fatal car crashes; people who experience this kind of uncontrolled anger need to seek help in managing their anger.

Alcohol-Impaired Driving About 3 in 10 Americans are involved in an alcohol-related crash at some point in their lives. Nearly 40 percent of those killed in these crashes are people other than the drinking driver. Male drivers are twice as likely as female drivers to be intoxicated when involved in fatal vehicle crashes. Rates appear to be higher among White men than among Hispanic and Black men. Among people who binge drink, 14.6 percent say they have driven while impaired, a rate 30 times higher than the rate for non–binge drinkers.[2, 3, 10, 11]

Research has established that the risks of a motor vehicle crash and of a fatal crash increase as blood alcohol concentration increases (Table 22.1). Data also show that the more demanding the driving task, the lower the BAC at which impairment begins.[11, 12] These risks are even greater for drivers under age 21, who are likely to have less driving experience.

Drinking and driving laws and penalties are set by the states, but the federal government uses its leverage to influence state legislation. In 1984 Congress passed the National Minimum Drinking Age Act, which required states to set the legal drinking age at 21 or risk losing federal funding. In 1995 Congress amended the act to encourage the states to pass legislation making it illegal for persons under 21 to drive after drinking alcohol and setting legal BAC limits of 0–0.02 percent for drivers under 21. By 1998 all states had complied with these zero-tolerance limits for minors.[11]

Public health experts estimate that these laws have reduced alcohol-related crashes by 20 percent.[11]

Studies show that more than 90 percent of Americans favor the idea of using a **designated driver**,[12] an individual in a group who abstains from drinking alcohol on a particular occasion and drives for the others, who do not abstain. Whether this practice has reduced alcohol-related crashes is not clear, but it appears that the use of designated drivers is increasing.[12] Community campaigns have not only promoted the use of designated drivers but also encouraged individuals to take a bus or cab or walk when they have been drinking.

designated driver
A person in a group who abstains from drinking alcohol and drives for the others.

Many drugs other than alcohol impair the ability to drive safely. They include illicit drugs such as marijuana and heroin, prescription drugs, and over-the-counter drugs such as sleep aids. Driving safety requires mental alertness, clear vision, physical coordination, and the ability to react quickly. Any drugs that induce dizziness, light-headedness, nausea, drowsiness, fatigue, nervousness, or fuzzy thinking make driving dangerous. If you take any drugs that could impair driving, arrange to be picked up, use public transportation, or stay where you are until the drug effects wear off.

Environmental Hazards Environmental hazards account for less than 5 percent of vehicle crashes, but when combined with human error, they account for 27 percent. Environmental hazards can be natural, such as snow, ice, wind, poor visibility, or glare, or of human origin, such as construction zones, broken-down cars on the side of the road, or drunk drivers. To reduce the number and lethality of injuries that occur as a result of environmental factors, states and local communities use such measures as ice-melting chemicals, crash cushions, breakaway signs and light poles, and median barriers and guard rails.[1]

APPROACHES TO MOTOR VEHICLE SAFETY

Motor vehicle safety is addressed by a variety of measures, including testing cars to make sure they meet NHTSA standards, designing effective restraint systems and increasing the likelihood that people will use them, and developing new safety technology.

NHTSA Standards **Crash worthiness** is a measurement of how well a car performs in a crash in terms of damage to the car and other vehicles and injury to people.[13] All cars sold in the United States must pass a test that measures the effectiveness of the vehicle's structural design in preventing occupants from being ejected, trapped, burned, or crushed in a 30-mph (miles per hour) collision. The test also determines a vehicle's ability to absorb, control, or reduce crash impacts on occupants.[13]

crash worthiness
Measurement of the impact of car crashes on people and property.

Table 22.1	Blood Alcohol Concentrations and Fatal Motor Vehicle Crashes
Compared with drivers who have not consumed alcohol . . .	
If you drive with blood alcohol concentration (BAC) in this range:	**Then your chances of being killed in a single-vehicle crash increase by:**
0.02–0.04 percent	1.4 times
0.05–0.09 percent	11 times
0.10–0.14 percent	48 times
0.14 percent and above	380 times

Sources: "Alcohol and Health," 2000, National Institute on Alcohol Abuse and Alcoholism; "A Review of the Literature on the Effects of Low Doses of Alcohol on Driving-Related Skills," by H. Moskowitz and D. Fiorentino, April 2000, U.S. Department of Transportation.

Restraint Systems During a car crash, there are really two collisions. The first collision happens when one car hits another car or a structure. The **second collision** occurs when unbelted occupants are thrown against the windshield or other structures inside the car, such as the steering wheel, or against other passengers. Most injuries are incurred in the second collision.[1] The hard surfaces inside the car are potential sources of death during any crash, whether front, side, or rear impact.

second collision
Impact of an unbelted occupant with the windshield, steering wheel, doors, dashboard, or other passengers after a collision with another vehicle or object (first collision).

Because many people resisted using safety belts when they were first installed in cars, public information campaigns, incentive programs, and seat belt reminder systems in vehicles were introduced to encourage usage; most of these measures had little effect. Mandatory safety belt laws have proved more effective; today, 49 states and the District of Columbia have such laws in place (New Hampshire requires seat belt use by those under 18 only). In 2005 more than half of the people killed in motor vehicle crashes were not wearing safety belts.

Air bags—fabric cushions that instantly inflate during a collision—are a kind of **passive restraint** that protects front seat passengers from impact with the interior of the vehicle in a crash. Generally, sensing devices in the dashboard inflate air bags at impacts of 12 mph or more. The bags deflate seconds after the impact. Front air bags do not protect occupants against side-impact collisions, which account for 30 percent of crash deaths, and cars are now being equipped with side-impact protection systems.[13]

passive restraint
A safety device that does not require vehicle occupants to engage it.

Infants and children need to be secured in child seats placed in the back seat and anchored by the vehicle's safety belts. Child seats effectively protect small children from injuries that occur when children are thrown from the car or slammed into the car's interior during a crash. Infants should ride in carriers in which they are in a semireclining position facing the rear of the car. Infants and toddlers should not ride in the front seats of cars with air bags, because air bags can deploy with enough force to cause severe head and neck injuries in very young children. For maximum protection, children aged 12 and under should always ride in the back seat. Injuries resulting from motor vehicle crashes are the leading cause of death for children ages 1 to 14.[14, 15]

New Safety Technology Automakers are continually developing new safety technology. New devices will include an intricate network of sensors embedded in bumpers, doors, and seats that anticipate a crash and direct the car's safety devices to work in harmony with one another. For example, to prevent neck injuries and broken ribs, air bags will fire at a precise velocity, or not at all, while safety belts retract to snug occupants into their seats and then, a fraction of a second later, slacken to enable them to "ride down the crash." Airbags that drop from the roof to protect the head will also be available.[13] Computer sensor devices will prevent tipovers and wheel spin by activating brakes together at one time and slowing the engine to prevent vehicle swerving or skidding.[16]

Emergency notification systems are being developed that will automatically call for help when an air bag deploys or allow drivers to call with the push of a button. The goal of these systems is to reduce the number of people who die from their crash injuries before they reach the hospital. Some systems will go even further by sending information that will help rescuers determine the type of assistance needed.[17]

Another invention is a lane-drifting system, which uses a camera linked to a computer that monitors the vehicle's distance to the left and right of lane markings. If the computer senses an unintended lane departure, whether from the driver falling asleep or fiddling with a CD player, it applies torque to the steering wheel to ease the vehicle back into the proper lane.[18]

Other developments include a system that uses forward-facing cameras in the vehicle's side-view mirrors to give drivers a 360-degree view of the road; a system that uses lasers and radar to sense the cars ahead and brakes the car if it gets too close to other vehicles; electronic feelers that detect danger ahead and steer the vehicle out of harm's way; intelligent highways that use global positioning satellites and road sensors to warn drivers of hazards in their path; autopilots that use robotic technology as a navigation system to safely guide vehicles to driver destinations; and electronic stability control (ESC). Ninety-five percent of all vehicles sold in the United States will come with ESC by 2011.[17, 18]

MOTORCYCLE SAFETY

Motorcyclists are about 5 times more likely than passenger car occupants to die in a motor vehicle crash and about 26 times more likely to be injured. Contributing factors in these crashes are lack of proper training, distraction, alcohol, and

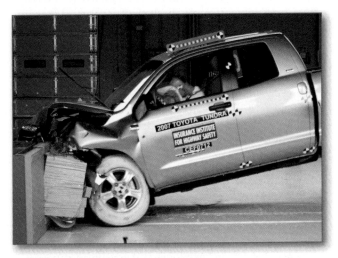

■ A federal program in place since 1979 rates cars for crash safety on a five-star scale. Starting in 2012, a new program will add an overall safety rating that combines scores from front-end, side, and rollover tests.

environmental conditions (weather, roadway surface, equipment malfunction). The Motorcycle Safety Foundation (MSF) has a program called the Rider Education and Training System that promotes lifelong learning for motorcyclists (you can visit their Web site at www.msf-usa.org). However, the MSF reports that about 65 percent of all collisions between motorcycles and other types of vehicles were precipitated by a vehicle operator other than the motorcyclist, usually because the driver failed to see the motorcycle.

Wearing a helmet reduces a motorcyclist's risks of both fatal injury and traumatic brain injury. A study by the NHSTA found that about half of unhelmeted riders suffered a head injury in a crash, compared with about 35 percent of those wearing a helmet.[8] Despite these safety benefits, most motorcyclists choose not to wear helmets, unless state law requires it.[2, 3, 19–21]

PEDESTRIAN SAFETY

Pedestrians account for about 13 percent of traffic-related deaths, second to vehicle occupants. About one out of every six pedestrian deaths occurs in a hit-and-run incident. About 45 percent of pedestrian deaths occur when pedestrians enter or cross streets, and 10 percent occur when pedestrians are walking in the roadway.[2, 3, 22]

The highest number of pedestrian deaths occurs among men aged 35–44, but the highest death rate per 100,000 people occurs among those aged 75 and older. The pedestrian fatality rate for men is about twice that for women, and the rate of nonfatal pedestrian injuries is also higher for men.

The pedestrian fatality rate for Blacks is almost twice that for Whites, and for American Indians and Native Alaskans it is nearly three times as high. Hispanics die from pedestrian incidents at a rate 1.8 times higher than that for non-Hispanics.[23] Safety experts believe this difference can be partly attributed to the fact that members of these groups generally walk more than Whites, because they own fewer cars. Children and older adults are also especially vulnerable to pedestrian deaths and injuries.[1, 2]

Child Safety Young children are often unaware of potential dangers posed by running into a street, do not have accurate perception of vehicle distance and speed, and may not understand traffic signs and signals.[22] Parents can overestimate their children's ability to cross the street on their own. Because children are small, drivers often don't see them. Schools and communities need to work together to provide traffic education programs and safe roads and streets to reduce pedestrian injuries and deaths among children.

Older Adult Safety Although pedestrian deaths make up about one-seventh of all traffic-related fatalities, almost one-third of people aged 70 or older killed in traffic are pedestrians.[23] Inadequate safety islands and traffic lights that do not allow enough time for older people to cross the street contribute to the risk for older adults. Other factors include declining vision and physical impairments in older people. To improve pedestrian safety, communities have introduced traffic-calming measures (speed bumps, lower speed limits), pedestrian crosswalk signs that display the number of seconds left on the green light, cameras that record vehicles that run red lights, and pedestrian safety education programs.[22]

Recreational Safety

Injuries occur in a wide variety of recreational activities and sports, including football, basketball, soccer, swimming, skateboarding, snowboarding, inline skating, and many others. Wearing the right safety equipment and clothing for the activity significantly reduces the risk of injury. For example, inline skaters should wear helmets, wrist pads, elbow and knee pads, and long pants and long-sleeved shirts. Anyone engaging in a sport or recreational activity should refrain from drinking alcohol beforehand.

BICYCLE SAFETY

Collisions between bicycles and motor vehicles result in many deaths and nonfatal disabling injuries.[2] A successful bicycle safety program combines the use of safety equipment with injury-reducing behaviors. Three important considerations are making sure your bicycle fits you properly, wearing a helmet, and employing safe cycling practices.

The Right Fit When your bicycle fits you properly, you are more comfortable and have more control. Several factors

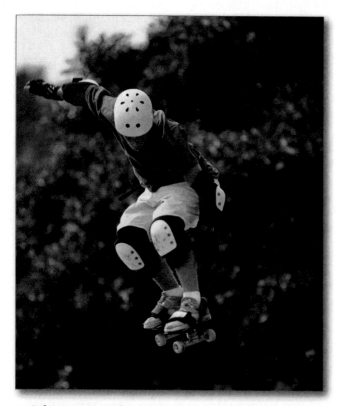

■ Safety equipment for skateboarding includes wrist guards, knee and elbow pads, and a helmet. About 50,000 skateboarding injuries are treated in hospital emergency rooms each year.

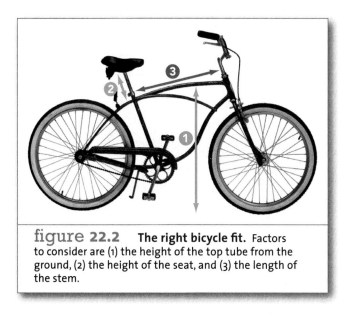

figure 22.2 **The right bicycle fit.** Factors to consider are (1) the height of the top tube from the ground, (2) the height of the seat, and (3) the length of the stem.

determine the appropriate fit (Figure 22.2).[1] One is the size of the bike and the height of the top tube from the ground. On a road bike, you should be able to straddle the bar with both feet flat on the ground and about a one-inch gap between your crotch and the bar. If this is not the case, the bike is too large or too small for you.

Another factor is the height of the seat. When you are cycling, your legs should be fully extended, but not overextended, at the bottom of the cycling stroke. Sit on your bike and completely extend one leg straight down while someone holds the bike for you. Make sure the heel of your foot reaches the pedal in its lowest position. If you have to stretch your toes or shift your weight to reach the pedals, the seat is too high.

A third factor is stem length, the distance from the front of the seat to the handlebars. If this distance is too long or too short, you will put excessive strain on your back or excessive weight on your hands and wrists. Stem length should be equal to the length of your arm from elbow to fingertips. Other factors in the right fit include seat angle (start with the seat level with the ground, then tip it up or down a few degrees if you experience discomfort), seat fore and aft position (your knee should be above the pedal axle), and handlebar height. Different guidelines can apply for mountain bikes and other kinds of bikes. For the best fit, consult with the staff in a bike shop.

Bicycle Helmets Head trauma is involved in most of the bicycle-related injuries and deaths that occur every year. Bicycle helmets are estimated to reduce the risk of head injury by 85 percent and the risk of brain injury by 88 percent. About 39 percent of adults and 69 percent of children under age 16 wear bike helmets on a regular basis. Among those who don't wear helmets, reasons include cost, discomfort, and lack of knowledge about their effectiveness. Bicycle safety programs in elementary schools provide information for young cyclists and encourage helmet use, and 19 states, the District of Columbia, and many local communities have

Highlight on Health

Choosing the Right Helmet

Whether you are bicycling, skating, or skateboarding, you need to wear the right helmet to prevent head injury in case you fall or crash. The Snell Memorial Foundation, a nonprofit organization that tests and develops helmet safety standards, advises trying on several different helmets before purchasing one. Here are some tips for selecting the right one:

- Remember these four s's: size, strap, straight, and sticker.
  - **Size:** The helmet should sit comfortably on your head, fitting snugly but not squeezing your head. When the straps are fastened, you should not be able to pull it off or move it in any direction. Most helmets come with pads you can fasten inside the helmet to adjust the fit.
  - **Strap:** Make sure the chin strap fits snugly and that the V in the straps meets under the ear.
  - **Straight:** Wear a helmet low on the forehead, about two finger widths above your eyebrows, and not tilted in any direction.
  - **Sticker:** Look for a manufacturer's sticker citing the U.S. Consumer Product Safety Commission standard. You can also look for independent certification by the Snell Foundation or the Safety Equipment Institute.
- Replace your helmet according to the helmet's instruction manual. Some helmets need to be replaced after a certain number of years or after you have been in a crash. Skateboarding helmets are designed for multiple knocks.
- Establish a "helmet habit." Children are more likely to wear helmets if their parents do and if they're introduced to them early. Always wear a helmet when participating in an activity that can cause head injury.

Source: Choose the Right Helmet for Your Favorite Summer Sport, National Safety Council, www.nsc.org. Reprinted by permission.

laws requiring the use of helmets.[2] For tips on buying a bicycle helmet, see the box "Choosing the Right Helmet."

Safe Cycling Practices The biggest safety problem for bicyclists is making themselves visible to other vehicle operators. If you are a cyclist, your safety in traffic depends on your being visible, riding in a predictable manner, and knowing the rules of the road.[1] Reflective tape, brightly colored cycling clothes and safety vests, portable leg or arm lights, and headlights are effective for making riders visible. Air-powered horns can add another dimension to safety.

Bicycles are considered vehicles and must follow all traffic laws that apply to cars, including stopping at traffic lights and stop signs and signaling before turning. Obeying traffic laws also helps drivers of other vehicles anticipate your actions. Use bike lanes where they are available; otherwise, ride in the right lane of traffic along the line made by the right wheel of a vehicle. Watch for parked cars and people opening car doors. Know the local laws and regulations governing bicycle traffic.

ALL-TERRAIN VEHICLE SAFETY

Deaths related to all-terrain vehicles (ATVs) have increased significantly in recent years. One million new ATVs are sold every year, and more than 7 million are now in use. The Consumer Product Safety Commission estimates that there are nearly 600 ATV-related deaths and 100,000 injuries every year, caused by rollovers, excessive speed, falls, and collision with stationary objects. One-third of these deaths and injuries are accounted for by children under the age of 16. Often a child is riding an adult-sized ATV, which can reach speeds as high as 75 mph. About one-third of ATV accidents occur on public roads. The ATV's slightly deflated balloon-style tires, limited suspension, and high center of gravity create too much tire traction while turning on asphalt, resulting in rollovers.

To confront the problem, states are passing laws to mandate helmet use and restrict ATV use by age. The American Academy of Pediatrics and the Consumer Federation of America have called for legislation to prohibit use of four-wheel off-road vehicles by children under 16 years of age. States are also opening ATV parks that provide groomed trails for a fee.[24]

WATER SAFETY

Overall, about nine people drown every day in the United States; 80 percent of them are male.[25] More than one-third of adults are unable to swim the length of a pool 24 yards long.[26] Women report less swimming ability than men, although fewer women drown. More than half of all drowning victims are White non-Hispanic males, although this group has the lowest drowning rate per 100,000 persons. Black males have the highest drowning rate per 100,000 persons, followed by non-Hispanic males of other races (for example, Asian, Pacific Islander, American Indian), Hispanic males, and non-Hispanic White males. The lowest drowning rate occurs among Hispanic females.[1–3]

Boating Safety Nearly 70 percent of boating-related deaths are due to drowning. About 9 out of every 10 victims were not wearing life jackets, or **personal flotation devices (PFDs).** Most swimming-associated deaths occur in the late spring and summer months, when the weather is usually warm.

personal flotation device (PFD)
Life jacket worn while participating in water sports.

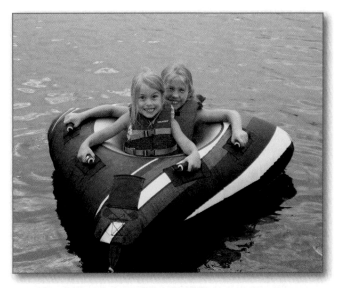

■ Water safety means always wearing a personal flotation device, or life jacket, when in or on the water. For children, parental supervision is also essential.

Boating deaths, however, occur as early as March and as late as October, when water may be cold. Water temperature of less than 70° F can numb your arms and legs and make it difficult to hold on to objects. In cold water, people who are older or not physically fit are more susceptible to cardiac arrest. Cold water cools the body 25 times faster than air of the same temperature does, and hypothermia (loss of body temperature) can cause respiratory failure even if the person does not drown.[1, 2]

If you are on a boat that turns over, stay with the boat, where you are more likely to be spotted and rescued, rather than trying to swim to shore. Good swimmers can usually swim up to 0.8 mile in 50° F water before hypothermia occurs. Poor swimmers may be able to swim only about 100 yards. A swimmer may not accurately estimate the distance to the shore, and wind and currents may make it difficult to reach land. If you are close to shore, however, and immediate rescue is unlikely, attempting to swim to shore may be your best option.[1]

Between 25 and 50 percent of deaths associated with water recreation involve alcohol, as do 60 percent of recreational boating deaths.[25, 26] Many states have laws covering intoxication by people operating boats that are comparable to those covering intoxication by drivers of motor vehicles. Operating any vehicle, including any boat, under the influence of alcohol or drugs is illegal under the criminal code in Canada.

Waterskiing and Personal Watercraft Each year about 50 water-skiers die and about 25,000 are injured.[3] Most of these injuries occur when the skier falls into the water, comes in contact with the boat propeller, collides with an obstacle, or becomes entangled with the tow rope.[1] If you water-ski, make sure you receive training, ski within your ability, learn water survival techniques, use a personal flotation device, and know how to swim.

Jet-skis, or wave runners—boats less than 12 feet long that are powered by an inboard engine and a jet pump mechanism—are popular personal watercraft. Deaths and injuries associated with these boats have more than doubled since their introduction in the mid-1980s.[25] Most injuries involve blunt trauma to the legs, torso, or head. In some states, people under the age of 16 cannot legally operate a motorboat with more than 15 horsepower, including personal watercraft, unless supervised by a person on board who is 18 or older.

Personal flotation devices are essential protection for anyone participating in boating, waterskiing, or personal watercraft recreation. PFDs are made of buoyant material; various types have been designed for different watercraft. Check with your local jurisdiction for rules and regulations governing PFDs for your recreational activity.

HUNTING SAFETY

Hunters who use firearms need to know the rules of gun use and storage to prevent unintentional injuries. If you hunt, never point a gun at anything but a hunting target, and never put your finger on the trigger until you are ready to fire. When you are walking, place your fingers on the outside of the trigger guard and point the barrel downward in front of you. Remove cartridges or shells from guns when crossing a fence, ditch, or stream. If you hunt in a group, walk or stand side by side with other hunters and designate a zone of fire for each hunter. Make sure you see your target clearly before firing, and unload your gun before getting into a vehicle.[1]

Nearly two-thirds of unintentional injuries caused by firearms occur in the home.[3] Children in a home where guns are kept should be taught about their potential dangers and their proper use. Guns should be stored unloaded in a locked rack, cabinet, closet, or drawer well out of children's reach. Safety experts also recommend using a trigger lock, which prevents the trigger from being moved backward and discharging the gun. Some communities provide firearm storage, which is the safest option of all.

Home Safety

Although more deaths occur each year in motor vehicle crashes than in any other category of unintentional injury, the highest number of injuries occurs in the home. In fact, nearly 40 percent of all disabling injuries occur in the home.[1] Home injuries and deaths occur primarily as a result of falls, fires, poisonings, and choking and suffocation.

FALLS

Falls are the most common cause of injury in the home. They are responsible for more open wounds, fractures, and brain injuries than any other cause of injury.[3] Falls are the most common cause of injury visits to the emergency room for two groups: young children and older adults.

Young Children and Falls About 70 deaths occur each year when children fall out of windows; 25 percent of the children are 11 years of age or younger.[1] Other injuries occur when babies roll off beds or young children fall down stairs. Parents can lower the risk of fall-related injuries by supervising children, buying products that promote safety (such as nonslip rugs), and modifying the home (for example, installing gates at the tops of stairs and guards on windows).

Older Adults and Falls Older adults have the highest rate of injury and death from falls of any age group. One of every three persons over age 65 falls each year, and two-thirds of those who fall do so again within 6 months. Falls account for one-third of the deaths from unintentional injuries among older adults.[2, 27, 28] Older adults often suffer hip fractures when they fall and, because of poor healing, end up being confined to convalescent hospitals and nursing homes.

Older adults are more susceptible to falls than are younger people because of medical problems, changes in skeletal composition, poor balance, limited vision, muscular weakness, and medications.[28] Environmental factors like slippery floors, loose rugs, and poor lighting also play a role.[29]

As the American population grows older, fall-related injuries are expected to increase. To make the home safer, older adults or their caregivers should make sure surfaces are clear of objects or conditions that could lead to a fall (for example, electrical cords inside, snow and ice outside); install hand rails and nonslip applications in bathtubs; and make sure rooms and stairways are well lit.

FIRES

Of all fire-related deaths and injuries, 65–85 percent occur in homes. About 50 percent of the homes in which a fire fatality occurred did not have smoke detectors. Older adults are particularly at risk for injury and death in home fires; although they make up about 12 percent of the population, adults over age 65 account for about 30 percent of all fire fatalities.[30, 31]

Fires in the home are associated with smoking (especially smoking in bed), cooking, fireplaces and chimneys, electrical wiring and cords, and appliances, particularly electric heaters. You can reduce your risk of fire injury by changing careless behaviors, correcting faulty equipment, and having smoke detectors and fire extinguishers in your home. You can also improve your chances by having an emergency plan in place and knowing what to do in case of fire.

Lithium Batteries A new source of fire danger is lithium batteries, which power portable electronic equipment (laptop computers, cell phones, CD players). Any electronic device purchased since 2002 operates with a rechargeable lithium ion battery. These batteries contain a separator that prevents positive and negative electrodes from touching each other. Most also contain a flammable liquid. If the separator fails, a spark may be ignited or the battery may explode, causing a liquid fire. Low-cost and counterfeit batteries have a higher risk of separator failure.

Between 2000 and 2006, there were 15 documented cases of airplane fires caused by lithium batteries.[32] Although passengers want to be able to carry their electronic equipment with them onto planes, safety regulators are studying the fire risks posed by lithium batteries and are considering banning them in both carry-on and checked luggage. Battery manufacturers say that proper maintenance of lithium batteries significantly reduces the risk of failure. Safe handling tips include keeping batteries in their original packaging, insulating batteries against impact, not storing lithium batteries in checked luggage, and never carrying cracked, damaged, or recalled batteries onto a plane.[32]

Smoke Detectors and Fire Extinguishers   Experts estimate that deaths from home fires could be reduced by 40–55 percent if smoke-sensing devices were installed in every home.[31] Your home should have at least one smoke detector on every level, placed on a ceiling or a wall 6–12 inches from the ceiling. Building codes in some local jurisdictions require a smoke alarm in every bedroom.

You can purchase battery-operated smoke detectors or models powered by household current, which are available with battery backup systems. If you have battery-powered detectors, replace the batteries every 6–12 months. Because many people fail to replace old batteries, the more costly household-wired detectors are recommended.[1]

Research indicates that young children are not easily roused from deep sleep by the sound of a smoke alarm, but they are roused by the sound of their mother's voice calling their names. Smoke alarms are available that can be programmed for this purpose.

Home fire extinguishers are intended to knock down a fire long enough to allow the occupants to escape; most discharge their extinguishing agent for only about 30 seconds.[31] Use an extinguisher only on the type of fire for which it is designed; the wrong agent may intensify or spread a fire. A Class A fire consists of burning trash, wood, paper, or textile materials. Class B fires involve flammable products such as oil, gasoline, grease, paint, or alcohol. Class C fires involve electrical equipment. Many extinguishers contain a multipurpose dry chemical and are labeled ABC, meaning they can be used on any type of fire. They can be purchased in hardware stores.

Sprinkler systems are used in many commercial buildings, and most states have laws requiring sprinkler systems in newly constructed apartments, condominiums, and other multifamily dwellings.[31] Located in the ceiling of each room, the sprinklers activate at 160° F to 165° F. Sprinklers are now affordable for private homes. College and university students are experiencing a growing number of fire-related injuries in both on-campus and off-campus housing (see the box "Campus Fire Safety").

In Case of Fire   Having an emergency plan will help you react quickly in case of fire. Make sure every room in your

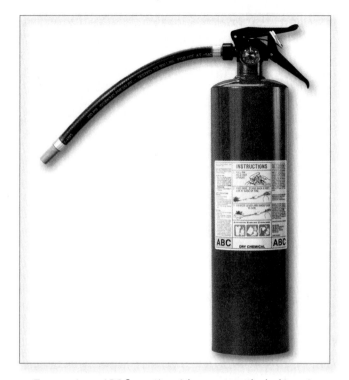

■ To operate an ABC fire extinguisher, remove the locking pin, point the nozzle at the base of the fire, squeeze the handle, and use a sweeping motion as the extinguisher discharges. Although they discharge for less than a minute, even small fire extinguishers can give people time to escape a fire.

house has two escape routes, and designate a place away from the house where occupants or family members will meet once they are outside. The National Fire Protection Association recommends that families practice fire drills to make sure everyone, especially children, knows what to do in case of fire.

If a fire does occur in your home, leave the house as quickly as possible. Make sure that everyone gets out, and don't go back into the house once you are outside. If someone is missing when you get outside, tell the firefighters. If you are in a burning structure, avoid smoke inhalation by crawling along the floor toward a door or window, covering your mouth and nose with a wet cloth. If your clothes catch fire, drop to the ground and roll to extinguish the flames; do not run.

POISONINGS

A poison is any substance harmful to the body that is ingested, inhaled, injected, or absorbed through the skin.[33] Poisoning can be intentional or unintentional. Intentional poisonings (to commit suicide) account for about 20 percent of poisoning incidents. About half of all unintentional poisoning deaths are from drug overdoses, primarily illicit drugs like cocaine and heroin. Alcohol poisoning accounts for a small percentage of poisoning deaths, but alcohol may be involved in poisoning deaths from other drugs. The death rate from poisoning is more than twice as high in males as in females.

Children are especially vulnerable to accidental poisoning in the home. The most common cause of poisoning in

Public Health in Action

Campus Fire Safety

In one week in May 2008, fires on three different college campuses in New York, Texas, and Ohio forced the evacuation of students from their housing. Although no one was killed or seriously injured in these incidents, fires do claim the lives of college students every year. In a one-year period from 2006 to 2007, 113 college students died in house fires. Ninety percent of these fires were in off-campus housing, and 76 percent were within 2 miles of the college campus. Off-campus housing is often old and densely packed with students living in multiple small rooms. Simple, easy-to-follow escape routes may be lacking. Often there are no sprinkler systems or smoke alarms (or students disconnect alarms). The use of alcohol—the most common factor associated with off-campus fires—can make it hard for students to save themselves and rescue others in a fire.

The Center for Campus Fire Safety (CCFS) is a group of fire safety experts that provides a variety of educational programs for college administrators, faculty, staff, students, and parents. The *Princeton Review* has worked in conjunction with the CCFS to provide a fire safety rating for U.S. colleges and universities (www.princetonreview.com/college/research/articles/firesafety/). The CCFS will also contact the college of your choice to obtain information about its fire safety record and prevention programs.

Many college campuses have implemented a training program, "The Great Escape on Campus," developed by the CCFS. It is designed to teach students the importance of escape planning and early evacuation in residence halls, fraternity and sorority houses, and off-campus housing. The program also includes free smoke machines that assist colleges in conducting fire safety simulation exercises.

When looking for a place to live on campus, consider whether the residence is equipped with smoke alarms, automatic sprinkler systems, and fire extinguishers; whether the staff and students are trained in fire prevention and the use of fire extinguishers; whether smoking, candles, and halogen lamps are prohibited; whether electrical appliances and power strips have to be certified; and whether the fire department is notified when fire alarm systems are activated. For off-campus housing, adaptations of these considerations should be applied.

The CCFS reminds everyone of a few simple fire survival tips that should be exercised no matter what the housing situation:

- Always know two ways out. Have an exit strategy!
- Install, maintain, and regularly test smoke alarms and portable fire extinguishers.
- Live in housing protected by a fire sprinkler system.
- Inspect exit doors and windows and make sure they are working properly.
- Conduct fire drills and practice escape routes.
- Take each and every alarm seriously.
- Treat all intentional fire-setting behavior as the crime it is.

Source: "Questions to Ask," Center for Campus Fire Safety, retrieved May 20, 2008, from www.campusfiresafety.org; "Three University Related Fires in One Week," Center for Campus Fire Safety, retrieved May 20, 2008, www.campusfiresafety.org/press/ThreeCloseCalls.pdf.

children is ingestion of household products, including cleaning products, furniture polishes, insecticides and herbicides, products containing lye or acids, and petroleum-based substances like kerosene, lighter fluid, turpentine, and solvents. All such products should be kept well out of the reach of children and stored in a locked cupboard or one with childproof safety latches. Federal law requires that many of these products be sold in containers with child-resistant caps.[34]

Prescription and over-the-counter (OTC) drugs can be poisonous if taken in excess quantities or in improper combinations.[34] To help patients avoid medication errors, drug manufacturers now include patient package inserts with prescription drugs that provide information for the consumer, such

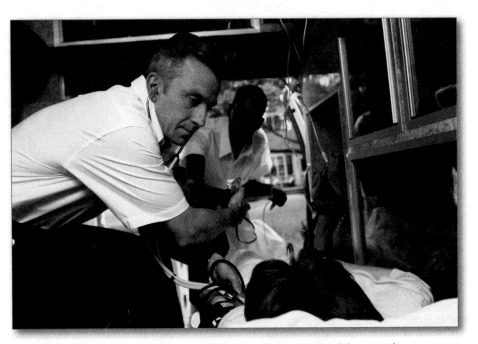

According to the CDC, more than 50 people die from unintentional drug overdoses every day in the U.S. The rate of lethal overdoses has increased dramatically in the last 10 years, making poisoning the second leading cause of unintentional death.

Highlight on Health

The Heimlich Maneuver

The Heimlich maneuver is used to dislodge an object blocking the airway of a person who is choking. To perform this maneuver (also referred to as abdominal thrusts), follow these four steps:

1. Stand behind the person and put your arms around his or her waist.

2. Make a fist with one hand and place the thumb side of your fist against the victim's upper abdomen, just below the rib cage and above the navel.

3. Grasp your fist with your other hand and thrust upward. Do not squeeze the rib cage. Confine the force of your thrust to your hands.

4. Repeat the upward thrusts until the object is expelled.

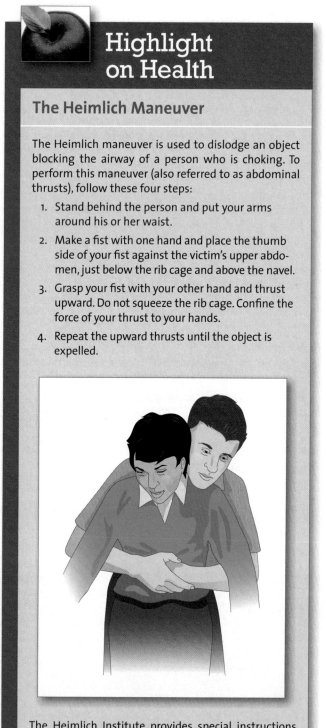

The Heimlich Institute provides special instructions for rescuing infants and children, people the rescuer cannot reach around, people with asthma, and people who are unconscious. For details, visit its Web site at www.heimlichinstitute.org.

To protect consumers against malicious tampering with products, the U.S. Food and Drug Administration requires tamper-resistant or tamper-evident packaging for all OTC drug products, along with a label informing consumers about this safety feature. Federal law requires that many OTC drugs be sold in containers with child-resistant closures, although a patient may request an easy-open container.

Another poisoning hazard in the home is gases and vapors, such as carbon monoxide or natural gas. Carbon monoxide is a major component of motor vehicle exhaust; to avoid poisoning by this lethal gas, never leave your car engine running in a closed garage. Natural gas is used to operate many home appliances, such as furnaces, stoves, and clothes dryers. Although natural gas is odorless, producers add a gas with an odor so that leaks can be detected. If you smell gas, check to see if the gas is turned on but not lit on a stove burner or other appliance; if you cannot find the source of the leak, leave the area and call your utility company.

If you or someone you are with has been poisoned, seek medical advice and treatment immediately.[34] If the skin has been exposed to a toxic substance, wash the area with soap and warm water. If the product contacted the eyes, flush them with warm water. If a poison has been ingested, do not induce vomiting unless instructed to do so. Some poisons cause more damage when vomited than they do in the stomach. Signs that a person has ingested or inhaled a poisonous substance include difficulty breathing or speaking, dizziness, unconsciousness, foaming or burning of the mouth, cramps, nausea, and vomiting.

In all cases of toxic contamination or poisoning, call 911, your local poison control center, or the national poison control hotline (1-800-222-1222). Be prepared to report the person's condition, age, and weight; the product consumed; and when the product was consumed. You may be instructed to administer first aid immediately. After administering first aid, you may need to take the person to the emergency room; if you do, take the poisonous substance with you.

CHOKING AND SUFFOCATION

Death rates for choking are highest in children under 4 years of age and adults over 65 years of age. Rates soar in adults over 75 years of age. Most choking emergencies occur when a piece of food or a swallowed object becomes lodged in the throat, blocking the tracheal opening and cutting the oxygen supply to the lungs. Muscles in the trachea may spasm and wrap tightly around the object.[1]

Children are at risk for choking on small objects they put in their mouths or accidentally ingest, such as part of a toy or a balloon. Children under age 3 should not play with toys with small parts; most toys sold in the United States have warning labels if they have small parts. Children can also choke on hard candies, raw carrots, popcorn, and other small, hard foods.

Older adults with poorly fitting dentures or missing teeth are at risk for choking because they may not adequately chew their food. Alcohol is a contributing factor in choking deaths, since it slows reflexes, desensitizes the back of the

as the purpose of the medication, possible side effects, drug interactions, and contraindications (conditions under which individuals should not take the drug). Pill boxes with a space for each day of the week are available to help patients take medications correctly. Pharmacists have begun taking a more active role in patient education as well.

mouth, and may cause a person to pay less attention to eating. The risk of choking can be reduced by cutting food into reasonably small pieces, chewing well, not rushing, and not talking or laughing while eating.

A person whose airway is obstructed may gasp for breath, make choking sounds, clutch the throat, or look flushed and strained. If a person's airway is only partially blocked, he or she may cough forcefully. Do not slap

Heimlich maneuver
Technique used to help a person who is choking.

someone on the back if he or she is coughing; usually the coughing will clear the obstruction. If the person continues to have difficulty breathing, coughing is shallow, the person is not coughing, or the person cannot talk or breathe, a rescue technique like the **Heimlich maneuver** is needed (see the box "The Heimlich Maneuver").

Suffocation occurs when a person's air supply is cut off. The death rate for suffocation is highest in infants and small children. Infants sometimes suffocate when they become entangled in their crib bedding or when plastic materials cover their mouths and noses. Balloons and plastic bags may pose a suffocation risk.

TEMPERATURE-RELATED INJURIES

Each year scores of people die from excessive heat, particularly older adults and people with weak hearts. The danger is highest for people 75 years of age and older. High temperatures can be exacerbated by high humidity, which prevents the evaporation of perspiration from the skin and makes it difficult for the body to control its core temperature. A temperature of 95° F combined with 75 percent humidity produces a heat index (the temperature the body feels) of 130°F, which can cause heatstroke, a life-threatening condition.[35] See Chapter 8 for more information on heatstroke and guidelines on how to treat it.

Temperatures inside vehicles can quickly reach dangerous levels. On average, 36 children die of hyperthermia in vehicles each year. These children may be forgotten or unintentionally left in the vehicle by an adult, or they may have been playing in an unattended vehicle. There has been a 10-fold increase in child vehicle hyperthermia fatalities since the early 1990s, perhaps because children are being placed in back seats to protect them from air bag deployment injuries. Children riding in the back seat are more likely to be forgotten by an adult.[35]

Vehicle child hyperthermia deaths can occur when the ambient temperature outside is as low as 70° F. Children's thermoregulatory systems are not as efficient as those of adults, so their core body temperature can rise three to five times faster than an adult's. Children should never be left in a vehicle, even if the windows are down, or allowed to play in an unattended vehicle, and adults should establish a "look before you leave" policy any time they vacate a vehicle.

Excessive cold is dangerous as well and can lead to hypothermia, a condition in which body temperature drops to dangerously low levels. See Chapter 8 for more informa-

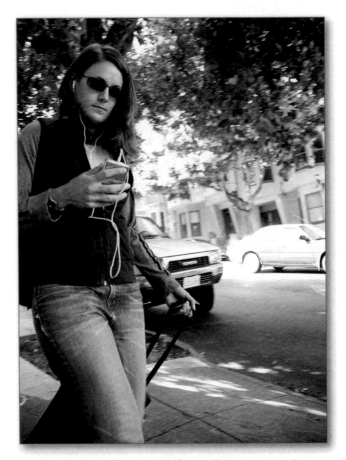

■ Many audio devices now include a package insert warning about the dangers of hearing loss from listening at high volumes.

tion on hypothermia and guidelines on how to avoid it. If you are with someone who is experiencing hypothermia, seek medical treatment immediately. If you cannot get to an emergency room, take measures to prevent further heat loss, such as removing wet clothing. Warm the body by giving warm liquids and immersing the person in a warm bath. Do not give the person alcohol, because it makes blood vessels dilate, resulting in further loss of body heat.

EXCESSIVE NOISE

Exposure to loud noise can damage hearing and lead to permanent hearing loss. Some **noise-induced hearing loss (NIHL)** is inevitable and irreversible as we age, so people should protect their hearing from additional, avoidable damage. The loudness of sound is measured in decibels (dB). Normal conversation occurs at 50 dB to 60 dB, a subway train and a chainsaw are approximately 100 dB, and loud music is approximately 120 dB. Hearing damage begins after 8 hours of continuous exposure to 90 dB, 4 hours of exposure to 95 dB, 2 hours of exposure to 100 dB, and 1 hour of exposure to 105 dB. Noise levels above 125 dB cause pain.[36]

noise-induced hearing loss (NIHL)
Damage to the inner ear, causing gradual hearing loss, as a result of exposure to noise over a period of years.

Consumer Clipboard

MP3 Players and Hearing Loss

Some MP3 and iPod users who listen to music at high volumes have been found to have hearing loss comparable to that found in aging adults. Noise levels from these portable media players can reach 115 to 125 decibels. Exposure to 125 decibels for an hour can cause permanent hearing loss, as can exposure to 115 decibels for half a minute per day. If you have listened to music at the highest volume for even a few seconds, or if you have felt pain in your ears from loud music, you may already have experienced some hearing damage.

Loud noise destroys hair cells at the nerve endings in the inner ear. These tiny hair cells translate sound vibrations into electrical currents that go to the brain. Noise-induced hearing loss is usually a gradual process that can take 10 to 20 years. Early symptoms of hearing loss include ringing or buzzing in the ears; difficulty understanding speech, especially in noisy settings; and a slight muffling of sounds. More serious symptoms include dizziness, discomfort, and pain in the ears. People who listen to loud music should have their hearing tested periodically, because hearing loss can be unnoticeable until damage is extensive.

Consumer complaints have led iPod and MP3 manufacturers to develop solutions to noise-induced hearing problems. In 2006, in response to a lawsuit charging that iPod use caused hearing damage, Apple announced a free download of software for the iPod Nano that allows listeners to set a volume limit. Manufacturers have also developed different kinds of headphones to address hearing loss issues. "Isolator" earphones sit deeper in the ear canal and block out external sound, so that volume does not have to be cranked up so high. "Supra-aural" headphones sit on top of the ears and deliver sound at lower decibel levels.

However, researchers have found that it is not so much the type of earphone that makes a difference in hearing loss as it is the volume level. Listeners are advised to protect their hearing by avoiding prolonged exposure to sounds above 85 decibels. Another recommendation is the 60 percent/60 minute rule—using MP3 players at volume levels no more than 60 percent of maximum and no more than 1 hour a day. Sound is too loud if it prevents normal conversation, if you have to shout to be heard, if it causes ringing in your ears, if you have trouble hearing for a few hours after exposure, or if the person next to you can hear the music from your headphones. Since most people experience a gradual loss of hearing as they grow older, it is important to use safe listening strategies to protect your hearing while you are young.

Sources: "Researchers Recommend Safe Listening Levels for iPod," Hearing Loss Web, 2006, retrieved May 26, 2008, from www.hearinglossweb.com/Medical/Causes/nihl/mus/safe.htm; "Prevent Tech-Related Hearing Loss," by G. Hughes, 2006, retrieved May 26, 2008, from http://tech.yahoo.com/blog/hughes/35.

Common sources of environmental noise include machinery, power tools, traffic, airplanes, and construction. Loud music is also a hazard. When you listen to loud music for a prolonged period, you experience a "temporary threshold shift" that makes you less sensitive to high volumes. In effect, the ears adapt to the environment by anesthetizing themselves. Music at concerts and clubs can be dangerously loud and can damage hearing (see the box "MP3 Players and Hearing Loss"). To protect your hearing, limit your exposure to excessively loud music, and keep the volume down if you listen to music on headphones.

PROVIDING EMERGENCY AID

You can help provide care to other people who have been injured or are in life-threatening situations if you learn first aid and emergency rescue techniques. The Heimlich maneuver, as noted earlier, is used to help someone who is choking. **Pulmonary resuscitation** is used to rescue someone who is not breathing; it is also known as mouth-to-mouth resuscitation or artificial respiration. **Cardiopulmonary resuscitation (CPR)** is used when someone is not breathing and a pulse cannot be found. It consists of mouth-to-mouth resuscitation to restore breathing, accompanied by chest compressions to restore heartbeat. In 2008 the American Heart Association announced that hands-only CPR—with chest compressions only—is just as effective for sudden cardiac arrest as standard CPR with mouth-to-mouth breathing.

Training is required to perform CPR; many organizations offer classes, including the American Heart Association and the American Red Cross. Check the yellow pages or your community or campus resource center for information on where to take a class in first aid or rescue techniques.

pulmonary resuscitation
Technique used to rescue a person who is not breathing; also known as mouth-to-mouth resuscitation or artificial respiration.

cardiopulmonary resuscitation (CPR)
Technique used when a person is not breathing and a pulse cannot be found; differs from pulmonary resuscitation by including chest compressions to restore heartbeat.

Work Safety

Safety in the workplace improved steadily throughout the 20th century as a result of occupational laws and advances in safety technology. Male workers over the age of 65 are at the highest risk of fatal injury on the job, and male workers aged 25–35 are at the highest risk of nonfatal injury. Nearly twice as many men are injured as women.[2] The part of the body most frequently injured is the back, accounting for 24 percent of total injuries.

BACK INJURY

Nearly two in three people have at least one episode of back pain in their lifetime. Acute back pain usually clears up in a few days with or without medical treatment; chronic pain lasts longer than a month. A common cause of chronic back pain is an inflamed or herniated disc, which occurs when one of the cartilaginous discs between the vertebrae in the spine bulges or ruptures, compressing a spinal nerve. The pressure causes back pain, and it may also cause a painful muscle spasm or pain or weakness in the leg.[37]

Improper lifting of heavy objects is a major cause of back injury. When you are lifting an object, do not bend at the waist. Instead, bend your knees and hips and lower your body toward the ground, keeping your back as upright as you can. Keep your feet about shoulder-width apart. Grasp the object and lift it gradually with straight arms, using your leg muscles

to stand up. If you have to turn while holding the object, move your feet to new positions; do not twist your torso. Put the object down by reversing these steps (Figure 22.3).

Although not necessarily related to work, another common source of back pain is carrying a heavy backpack. Backpacks should weigh no more than 10–20 percent of a person's body weight. If you use a backpack, buy one with wide, padded shoulder straps, a waist strap, and a padded back to distribute weight and enhance comfort. Tighten both shoulder straps so that the backpack is held close to your back with the bottom about 2 inches above your waist. Carry heavier items in the center of your backpack. Follow proper lifting techniques when picking something up while wearing a backpack.

Other factors contributing to back pain and injury are obesity, stress, poor posture, and poor physical fitness. To reduce your risk of injury and back pain, do exercises that strengthen your back and abdominal muscles. Try to maintain good posture when you are standing and sitting. Diet

---

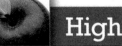

Highlight on Health

Your Computer Workstation

Ergonomics is the study of workplace design for the purpose of fitting environments to the physical and mental characteristics of the people who use them. Ergonomic principles can be used to create a workstation that minimizes your risk of strain or injury.

The main elements to consider are your chair, your desk, and the components of your computer. Adjust your chair so that your hips are slightly higher than your knees; this position pitches your pelvis slightly forward, allowing your back to maintain its natural curvature. A downward lip at the forward edge of the chair takes pressure off the back of your knees. If you don't have an adjustable chair, try putting some extra cushioning at the back of your chair to raise your hips slightly. Place your feet flat on the floor or on a footrest slightly in front of your knees.

Place your monitor on your desk directly in front of you. If you place it to the side, you risk injuring your neck by continually turning your head to see the screen. (You should also protect your neck when talking on the phone by using a headset rather than cradling the phone between your ear and your shoulder.) When you are sitting, you should be an arm's length from the monitor, about 2 to 2 ¹/₂ feet. Set the height of the monitor so that your eyes are level with the top of the screen; you should be looking downward at the middle of the screen. If you wear reading glasses or bifocals, don't tip your head upward to read the screen.

Place the keyboard so that the angle of your elbows is 90 degrees or greater and your wrists are in a neutral position, tilted neither up nor down. Your wrists, hands, and forearms should be parallel to the floor. If you have

a keyboard tray, you may find it comfortable to tilt the back of the tray slightly down. You may also want to use a wrist support on the tray at the front of the keyboard, but resting your wrists on the support while you are typing is not recommended. Keyboards with separated sections for the right and left hands may also be helpful. The computer mouse should be at the same level as the keyboard.

When using the computer for long periods of time, take frequent breaks, getting up to stretch and move around. If you have a laptop computer, try to use it with separate components (monitor, keyboard, mouse) so that you can adjust them to the right position. If you don't have separate components, it's even more important to take frequent breaks.

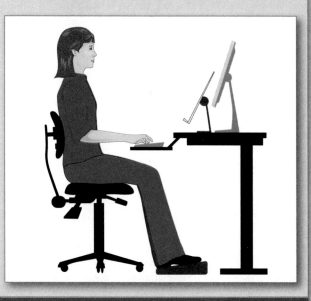

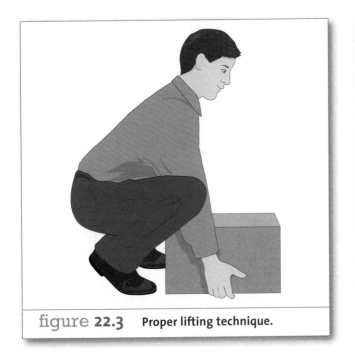

figure **22.3** **Proper lifting technique.**

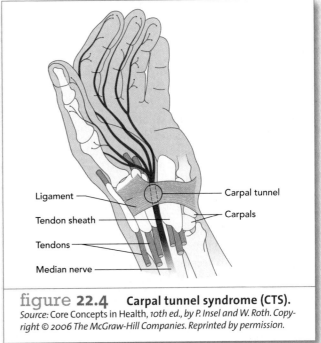

figure **22.4** **Carpal tunnel syndrome (CTS).**
Source: Core Concepts in Health, 10th ed., by P. Insel and W. Roth. Copyright © 2006 The McGraw-Hill Companies. Reprinted by permission.

and exercise can help you reduce excess abdominal weight, which places stress on the lower back.

COMPUTER USE

Extensive computer use can cause strain on the neck, back, arms, hands, and eyes. If your body is not properly aligned while you are using your computer, you may end up with irritated or pinched nerves, inflamed tendons, or headaches. Research on computer workstations has provided information on how to minimize this strain on the body (see the box "Your Computer Workstation").

Excessive computer use can also affect your vision, causing eyestrain, irritated eyes, blurred vision, and headaches. Rest your eyes by refocusing them periodically, such as by looking at something in the distance. To relieve dry, irritated eyes, use lubricating eye drops and make sure air vents in the room are not directing air toward your eyes. Adjust window blinds and lighting to reduce excessive brightness in the room and glare, the reflection of light on a viewing surface. An antireflective shield attached to your monitor can also reduce glare. To facilitate ease of reading, use black type on a white background whenever possible, and avoid extreme contrast on your screen.

REPETITIVE STRAIN INJURIES

repetitive strain injuries
Injuries to soft tissues that can occur when motions and tasks are repeatedly performed in ergonomically incorrect ways.

When motions and tasks are repeatedly performed in ergonomically incorrect ways, injuries to the soft tissues can occur that are known as **repetitive strain injuries.** A common repetitive strain injury is **carpal tunnel syndrome (CTS),** the compression of the median nerve in the wrist caused by certain repetitive

uses of the hands, including computer work, video game playing, and text messaging. The median nerve is located inside a "tunnel" created by the carpals (wrist bones) and tendons in the hand (Figure 22.4). When the tendons become inflamed through overuse or incorrect use, they compress the median nerve. The symptoms of CTS are numbness, tingling, pain, and weakness in the hand, especially in the thumb and first three fingers. Symptoms are often worse at night.

carpal tunnel syndrome (CTS)
Compression of the median nerve in the wrist caused by repetitive use of the hands.

If untreated, CTS can damage the median nerve and the muscles at the base of the thumb. The first steps in addressing this condition are correcting ergonomic problems in the workstation, taking frequent breaks from repetitive tasks, and doing exercises that stretch and flex the wrists and hands. If symptoms persist, a physician may recommend a night splint that keeps the hand and wrist immobile during sleep to reduce inflammation of the tendons. Other treatments include injections of steroids to reduce inflammation and, in severe cases, surgery to reduce pressure on the nerve.[38, 39]

Natural Disasters

A sudden event resulting in loss of life, severe injury, or property damage is typically defined as a *disaster*.[3] Disasters can be caused by humans, as in the case of terrorist attacks, or by natural forces. Tornadoes, hurricanes, floods, wildfires, and earthquakes are among the most devastating natural disasters that occur in the United States and around the world. In 2004 an earthquake under the Indian Ocean caused a tidal wave, or *tsunami*, that swept onto the islands and coastal areas of Indonesia, India, and other countries bordering the ocean, killing an estimated 250,000 people. In 2005 Hurricane Katrina devastated New Orleans and the U.S. Gulf Coast, causing loss of life and billions of dollars of damage.

In May 2008 a cyclone (the name for a hurricane in the Indian Ocean) hit Myanmar (Burma), flooding the low-lying coastal delta that was home to millions of people. The death toll reached into the tens or even hundreds of thousands and an estimated 2 million people lost their homes. In the same month in 2008, a magnitude 7.8 earthquake struck southwestern China, killing an estimated 60,000 people.

When natural disasters occur on this scale, governments and international aid organizations have to provide the assistance and relief that people need to recover. Individuals can help themselves by preparing as much as they can for the types of disasters that are likely to occur where they live (for example, tornadoes in the Midwest, hurricanes on the East Coast). The National Center for Environmental Health (part of the CDC)

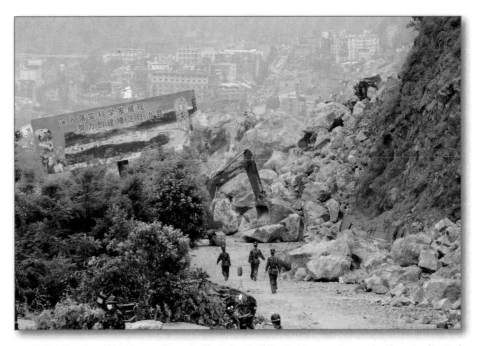

■ Major disasters, like the earthquake that struck China in May 2008, require the coordinated responses of governments and international organizations. The Red Cross and Red Crescent were among the aid agencies that contributed money to support relief and recovery efforts after the China earthquake.

provides detailed information on preparedness for all types of events, including natural disasters and severe weather emergencies. Visit their Web site at www.cdc.gov/nceh.

You Make the Call

Should Vehicles Be Equipped With Event Data Recorders?

In this hypothetical scenario, a motorist driving on an interstate collides with a highway patrol car parked on the shoulder, killing the officer in the car. The motorist is charged with reckless driving. Unbeknownst to the motorist, however, his car is equipped with an event data recorder, commonly referred to as an electronic control module (ECM), or black box. This device reveals that the motorist's driving speed was 30 miles per hour above the posted legal limit. The charge against the driver is upgraded from reckless driving to vehicular homicide.

The ECM is a palm-sized microcomputer embedded in a vehicle's air bag. This device collects and stores data from sensors in the event of incidents severe enough to deploy the air bag as well as incidents that are not severe enough to deploy the air bag. Information is collected up to 5 seconds before impact and includes engine/vehicle

speed, brake status, throttle position, and whether the seat belt switch is on or off. Computer software information translates the recorded data into plain language for analysis. About 300 hours worth of information can be stored in an ECM.

Most people are not aware that their vehicles may be equipped with an ECM. As of 2006 almost one-third of vehicles on American roads had an ECM, and 64 percent of new vehicles manufactured in 2006 were equipped with an ECM. The National Highway Traffic Safety Administration recommended that all vehicles manufactured in 2008 have an ECM installed.

Equipping vehicles with an ECM as a "snitch" device, however, has become controversial. Proponents argue that ECMs offer benefits to motorists, insurance companies, car rental agencies, law enforcement agencies, and parents. Opponents argue that ECMs violate privacy rights, unfairly stack the deck against motorists, and may provide inaccurate information. What do you think?

Continued...

Continued...

PROS

- Consumers can use the information collected by ECMs to support liability cases against car manufacturers that design or make unsafe vehicles. This information can also be used to help settle disputes between motorists as well as to exonerate motorists who have wrongfully been issued a traffic citation.

- When combined with global positioning systems, ECMs can serve as a surveillance device that insurance companies can use to create driver risk profiles. These profiles can be used to adjust premium rates or discontinue policies. Rental car companies can also use the information from ECMs to fine renters who exceed certain speed limits. Such measures are good business practices because they protect companies from damage and loss.

- Parents can use ECMs to collect information about the driving habits of their teenagers. This information can be downloaded onto personal computers. Computer software may be developed to trigger alarms when teenage drivers exceed certain speed limits.

- The ECM is not used as a stand-alone device by law enforcement to investigate car crashes. It is used in conjunction with physical evidence, such as impact data, skid marks, and position of vehicles.

CONS

- The use of information from ECMs is a violation of privacy rights under the Fourth Amendment. Insurance companies do not have a right to the information gathered by ECMs, nor do rental car agencies.

- If the federal government starts to require that all vehicles be equipped with ECMs, motorists will be forced to have a self-surveillance device in their cars, something that many people would object to. In effect, your car would be spying on you.

- Combined with global positioning systems, ECMs could be used by law enforcement officers to issue speeding tickets for infractions that are not witnessed in person, and insurance companies could cancel policies based solely on electronic data. These actions are violations of the right of due process.

- No industry or government standards ensure the reliability of ECMs. If motorists tried to use the information collected by ECMs to settle liability cases or disputes, such information would likely be inadmissible.

- At the very least, auto manuals should inform owners that their vehicles are equipped with ECMs.

Sources: "Psst, Your Car Is Watching You," by M. Roosevelt, August 14, 2006, Time, pp. 58, 59; "Automobile Black Boxes," by P. Zucker, retrieved June 17, 2008, from www.expertlaw.com/library/accidents/auto_black_boxes.html; "Car Black Boxes: Safety or Spy Feature?" by J. Harper, retrieved June 17, 2008, from www.foxnews.com/story/0,2933,141048,00.html.

In Review

1. **How does injury affect personal health?** Unintentional injuries are the fifth leading cause of death in the United States and the leading cause of death for children and adults aged 1 to 39. Public health experts believe that injuries are preventable if people adopt behaviors that promote safety and if society takes steps to reduce environmental hazards.

2. **What are the leading causes of injury-related death?** The top cause for all age groups is motor vehicle crashes, followed by falls, poisoning, choking, and drowning. Common causes vary by age and race/ethnicity, but males are more likely than females to die from unintentional injuries across all groups until age 80.

3. **How are unintentional injuries categorized?** Motor vehicle crashes are a major category, as are recreational injuries (for example, bicycling, boating, and hunting injuries), home injuries (falls, fires, poisonings, choking), and work injuries (back injuries, computer workstation injuries, repetitive strain injuries). Natural disasters such as floods, hurricanes, and tornadoes also account for a significant number of injuries each year.

4. **How can injuries be prevented?** For each type of injury, appropriate safety measures are recommended. They include wearing appropriate safety equipment; avoiding the use of alcohol; having training; knowing the laws, regulations, and one's own physical limits; reducing environmental hazards; knowing how to provide aid; and being prepared. Society and the government play a role in endeavors such as developing safety technology, enacting laws to protect workers, and providing assistance in the event of a natural disaster.

 For a detailed summary of this chapter and a comprehensive set of review questions, visit the Online Learning Center at **www.mhhe.com/teague2e**.

Web Resources

American Automobile Association Foundation for Traffic Safety: This organization offers educational materials for drivers, pedestrians, bicyclists, and others. Its Web site features FAQs, online quizzes on driving safety, and links to other resources.
www.aaafts.org

American Red Cross: Highlighting news, safety tips, and disaster updates, this Web site features information on various emergencies, including blackouts, earthquakes, tornadoes, fires, floods, mudslides, and hurricanes.
www.redcross.org

National Center for Injury Prevention and Control: This organization's Web site includes information on various injury-related topics, including falls, fires, and motor vehicles. Injury care information is also featured.
www.cdc.gov/ncipc

National Highway Traffic Safety Administration: For information about traffic safety, news, vehicles and equipment, research, and laws and regulations, this organization is an authoritative resource.
www.nhtsa.dot.gov

National Safety Council: This council publishes *Injury Facts,* an annual compilation of statistics on injuries. Its Web site features information on driving, ergonomics, first aid, and preparedness, among other topics.
www.nsc.org

U.S. Consumer Product Safety Commission: This government organization oversees the testing of products for safety and issues product recalls as necessary. Its publications include safety information for all-terrain vehicles, bicycle safety, child safety, poison prevention, and household products.
www.cpsc.go

Chapter 23

Environmental Issues
Making a Difference

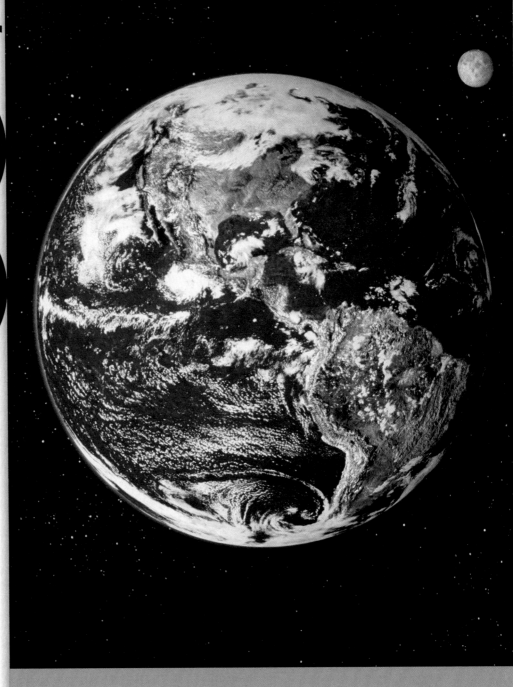

WWW

Your Health Today

www.mhhe.com/teague2e

Go to the Online Learning Center for *Your Health Today* for interactive activities, quizzes, flashcards, Web links, and more resources related to this chapter.

Ever Wonder...

- about the environmental cost of a fast-food burger?

- what the effects of climate change will be?

- what you as an individual can do for the environment?

When we look at **environmental health** issues, we become aware that our lives are part of the intricate web of living organisms and nonliving natural resources that make Earth a single, vital ecosystem. Only recently have people come to realize that the planet's resources are not infinite. We have also realized that many human activities have damaged the integrity of our ecosystem and threatened our own health. The possible enormity of this damage leaves many of us overwhelmed.

environmental health
The area of health concerns that focuses on the interactions of humans with all aspects of their environment.

There are actions that can be taken, however, if individuals and societies recognize that resources are limited and if they take responsibility for protecting and preserving these resources. For example, colleges and universities are "going green," and students are becoming proactive in driving their schools to adopt environment-friendly policies and programs.

The field of environmental health has traditionally been concerned with infectious diseases associated with contaminated water, food, waste, and other pollutants. Recently, the field has expanded to encompass pollutants that result from human and industrial activities and that cause chronic diseases and global environmental damage. Major issues today include climate change, the depletion of resources, especially energy resources, and world overpopulation—the issue that underlies and amplifies all our environmental concerns (see the box "Global Climate Change and Health").

Water and Water Quality

Although water is an abundant resource on earth, much of it is not suitable for drinking or other use by humans. Scientists estimate that only about 14 one-thousandths (0.014 percent) of the earth's water is readily available for human use.[1] Usable water supplies are further diminished by human activities that destroy or pollute natural ecological systems.

WATER SUPPLIES AND SHORTAGES

The earth's supply of water is continuously collected, purified, and distributed in a natural process called the *water cycle*. The water we use has two sources: surface water and groundwater. *Surface water* is precipitation that is stored in lakes, reservoirs, and wetlands (swamps, marshes, bogs) on the surface of the earth. It is renewed fairly rapidly in areas where precipitation occurs 12 to 20 days a year.

Groundwater is precipitation that sinks into the ground. This water is stored in giant underground reservoirs called *aquifers* and slowly moves to areas where it is discharged, such as a stream, a river, a lake, or an ocean, as part of the water cycle. Groundwater makes up 95 percent of the world's supply of freshwater.[2] In North America, about half of the drinking water comes from groundwater supplies.

Since 1900 the world use of water has increased nearly ninefold, and per person use has quadrupled. Withdrawal rates of surface water are projected to double in the next 20 years and exceed reliable sources in a growing number of areas. In the United States and Canada, water supplies are abundant, but much of our water is contaminated by industrial and agricultural wastes or is in the wrong place at the wrong time.[1, 2] Conflicts between regions and states over water supplies have existed throughout U.S. history and are likely to intensify in the future, especially as people migrate and industries relocate to the West and Southwest.[3]

Individuals can play an important role in water conservation. Most of our "drinking water" in the United States is used for toilet flushing, bathing, cooking, lawn watering, clothes and dish washing, and cleaning. For tips on reducing your personal use of water, see the box "You Can Help Conserve Water."

Communities can also support water conservation measures, such as by promoting xeriscaping—replacement of lawns in dry climates with vegetation adapted to arid conditions—and by passing building codes that require water-efficient fixtures and appliances.

WATER POLLUTION

Water pollution refers to any chemical, biological, or physical change in water quality that has a harmful impact on living organisms or makes water unsuitable for desired use.[4] The U.S. Environmental Protection Agency (EPA) claims that all but a few of the surface-water reservoirs in the United States are contaminated by discharge pollutants at specific

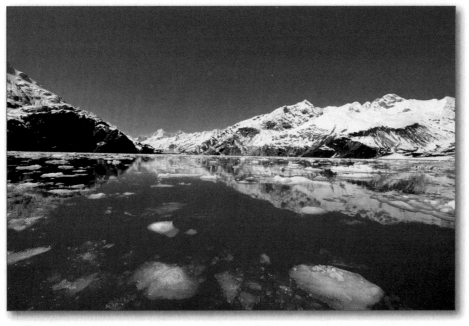

■ Melting ice and shrinking glaciers are just some of the signs of global warming and climate change.

Who's at Risk

Global Climate Change and Health

- Scientists project that global temperatures could rise by 1.0–4.5° F by 2050 and by 2.2–10.0° F by the close of the 21st century. This rise in temperatures would significantly increase heat-related deaths. Older adults, obese individuals, and children are at highest risk for heat-related deaths.

- As a result of global warming, pollen blooms will occur 10 days earlier in 2017 than they did in 2007 and be more severe. Tropical diseases like West Nile virus, malaria, yellow fever, and dengue fever may become more prevalent and expand to new areas in the United States.

- The Environmental Protection Agency projects that seawater in the United States will rise by 39 inches by the end of the 21st century. The rise in seawater would place 22,000 square miles of the United States under water. The most vulnerable areas are southern Florida, the Chesapeake Bay region, New Orleans, and San Francisco.

- One-sixth of the world's population does not have access to safe water. Half of the world's population suffers from a waterborne disease at any given moment. Problems with safe water are especially prevalent in developing nations.

- According to the United Nations Environment Program, a 10 percent thinning of the ozone layer of the atmosphere would cause an additional 300,000 cases of non-melanoma skin cancer worldwide, 4,500 cases of malignant melanoma, and 1.5 million cases of cataracts each year.

- Analysts project that global carrying capacity—the number of people the earth can support at subsistence level—is 50 billion people. However, cultural carrying capacity—the number of people the earth can support at an optimum standard of living—is about 9 billion people. World population is expected to hit this number by about 2050. Because there are not enough energy resources to meet the optimal standard of living needs for everyone, we can expect to see continuing conflict over world resources, especially between developed and developing nations.

Sources: Climate Change 2007: The Physical Science Basis, Intergovernmental Panel on Climate Change, 2007, Geneva, Switzerland; "Global Warming: Early Signs," Intergovernmental Panel on Climate Change, 1999, retrieved June 18, 2008, from www.climatehotmap.org; "Get Out Your Handkerchief," by S. Begley, June 4, 2007, Newsweek, p. 62; "Future Sea Level Changes," U.S. Environmental Protection Agency, retrieved June 18, 2008, from www.epa.gov/climatechange/science/futureslc.html.

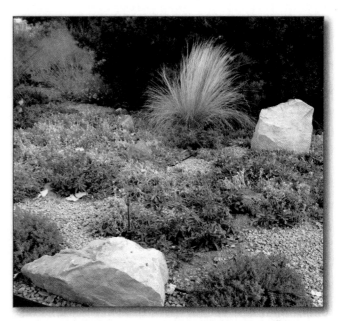

■ Xeriscaping saves water by using native plants, avoiding supplemental irrigation, and preventing the loss of water to evaporation and run-off—without sacrificing the aesthetic appeal of a beautiful garden.

locations through sewers, pipes, or ditches. Sources for these pollutants include factories, sewage treatment plants that remove some but not all pollutants, active and abandoned mines, oil spills, and agricultural feedlots. Runoff from large land areas such as croplands, golf courses, lawns, and parking lots also pollutes surface water.[1]

water pollution
Any chemical, biological, or physical change in water quality that has a harmful impact on living organisms or makes water unsuitable for desired use.

Cleaning up pollutants that reach aquifers lying deep in the ground is very difficult. The main sources of groundwater contamination are storage lagoons, septic tanks, landfills, hazardous waste dumps, and underground storage tanks filled with gasoline, oil, solvents, and hazardous waste. Such tanks can corrode and leak after 25 to 40 years. Groundwater is also contaminated when individuals dump or spill oil, gasoline, paint thinners, or other organic solvents onto the ground.[1,2]

SAFE DRINKING WATER

In the United States, the Safe Drinking Water Act of 1974 established many health standards for drinking water. About 8 percent of people in the United States, primarily farmers and rural residents, rely on their own private drinking water supplies. Owners of private wells are not required to comply with EPA health standards, but people using private water supplies must take special precautions to ensure water safety.[1]

About 1 in 15 households in the United States uses bottled water as the main source of drinking water.[2] Bottled

Challenges & Choices

You Can Help Conserve Water

Americans use about 100 gallons of water per person a day for domestic purposes. This rate is three times the per capita average for the world as a whole. Here are some tips to help you conserve water:

Bathroom   About 65 percent of residential water is used in the bathroom. The toilet accounts for 40 percent of all water used in the home.

- Install a low-flow toilet, which saves about 30 gallons of water per day.
- Install water-saving showerheads and flow restrictors on all faucets. If you can fill a 1-gallon bucket in 15 seconds, you need a more efficient fixture.
- Turn off sink faucets when brushing your teeth, shaving, or washing. An open faucet sends about 7 gallons of water down the drain every minute.
- Repair leaks promptly. A faucet that leaks one drop a second can waste 200 gallons of water in a month. You can test for toilet leaks by adding a few drops of food coloring to the water in the toilet tank. If you have a leak, some color will show up in the toilet bowl within minutes.
- Take shorter showers. Cutting your shower time by 1 minute saves about 500 gallons of water a year.

Laundry   About 15 percent of residential water is used in the laundry room.

- When buying a new washing machine, purchase a front-loading machine that fills at different levels for loads of different sizes.
- Wash your clothes only when you have a full load. If you must wash small loads, select the lowest possible water-level setting.

- Buy appliances with an "Energy Star" label. An Energy Star washing machine can save up to 7,000 gallons of water a year.

Kitchen   About 10 percent of residential water is used for drinking and cooking.

- Run your dishwasher only when you have a full load. Use the short cycle and let your dishes air-dry.
- If you wash your dishes by hand, do not let the water run continuously.
- Start a compost pile instead of using a garbage disposal. Garbage disposals and water softener systems use large amounts of water.

Outdoors   About 10 percent of residential water is used outdoors.

- Water your lawn and plants early in the morning and in the evening, minimizing loss of water through evaporation in the midday heat.
- Install drip irrigation systems for gardens and flower beds.
- Landscape with native plants, which adapt to local annual precipitation.
- Wash your car using a bucket for soapy water; use the hose only for rinsing. If you use a commercial car wash, choose one that recycles water.

It's Not Just Personal . . .

The U.S. Geological Survey (www.usgs.gov) estimates that approximately 408 billion gallons of water per day were withdrawn for all uses in the United States in the year 2000. The largest uses were for thermoelectric power and irrigation, with California, Texas, and Florida accounting for about one-fourth of all water withdrawals in that year.

Sources: One Makes the Difference, by J.B. Hill, 2002, New York: HarperCollins; Living in the Environment, by G.T. Miller, 2002, Belmont, CA: Wadsworth/ Thomson Learning; Water on Tap: A Consumer's Guide to the Nation's Drinking Water, U.S. Environmental Protection Agency, Washington, DC: Office of Water, 1997.

water is just as vulnerable to contamination as tap water, however. If you use bottled water, look for the trademark International Bottled Water Association for assurance of contaminant-free water.[2]

In some older homes, contamination from lead water pipes or lead solder on pipes is a concern. Exposure to lead can cause serious health problems, especially in children. To minimize lead exposure, let the water run for a minute or so after turning on the tap; this can flush away lead that may have leached into the water.[2] Cold water is less likely to contain lead that has been leached from supply pipes, so use only cold water for cooking and preparing infant formula.

Both lead water pipes and lead solder on pipes have been banned in the United States.

Ensuring a sustainable water supply for ourselves and future generations will require several strategies. Consumers and businesses need to use water-saving technologies; farmers and the agriculture industry need to develop ways to irrigate crops more efficiently; and government and policy makers must manage water basins and groundwater fairly and effectively. Such strategies are likely to be controversial and difficult to implement, but failure to address our water-related problems will lead to economic and health problems, increased environmental degradation, and loss of biodiversity.

Air and Air Quality

Like water, air is an essential resource that many of us take for granted until it becomes polluted and hazardous to our health.

EARTH'S ATMOSPHERE

The atmosphere is the whole mass of air surrounding the earth. The innermost layer of atmosphere is called the *troposphere*, or lower atmosphere. This layer contains about 80 percent of the earth's air and extends 11 miles above sea level at the equator and about 5 miles above the poles. The second layer is the *stratosphere*, or upper atmosphere. It extends from 11 to 30 miles above Earth's surface.

Ninety-nine percent of the air in the lower atmosphere consists of nitrogen (78 percent) and oxygen (21 percent). The remaining 1 percent consists of carbon dioxide, argon, and trace amounts of several other gases. Composition of gases in the upper atmosphere is similar except there is much less water vapor and much more ozone.[5]

The presence of certain gases in the lower atmosphere helps regulate the earth's temperature by trapping heat from the sun and preventing it from radiating back into space, a process called the **greenhouse effect.** Without the greenhouse effect, the surface of the earth would be much colder and less hospitable to life.[5, 6] The two most important **greenhouse gases** are carbon dioxide and water vapor.

An important component of the upper atmosphere is **ozone,** an odorless, colorless gas composed of three atoms of oxygen. Ozone forms naturally in the upper atmosphere and provides a protective layer that shields us from the sun's harmful ultraviolet (UV) radiation waves. This shield prevents about 95 percent of the sun's UV rays from reaching the earth's surface.[1] Although it is protective in the upper atmosphere, ozone in the lower atmosphere is hazardous to health; ground-level ozone is discussed in the next section.

AIR POLLUTION

Air pollution is the presence of one or more chemicals in the atmosphere of sufficient quality and in sufficient quantity to cause harm to life.[1] A few hundred years ago, most air pollution occurred as a result of natural events, such as dust storms and sandstorms, forest fires, and volcanic eruptions. These natural pollutants still exist today, but since the Industrial Revolution in the 18th century, human activities have become the primary source of air pollutants.

The EPA designates the six air pollutants of the greatest concern as "criteria pollutants"; they are carbon monoxide, sulfur dioxide, nitrogen dioxide, suspended particulate matter, ground-level ozone, and metal and metal compounds. All of these pollutants cause respiratory problems; some of them also cause cancer, heart disease, and birth defects.[1, 7]

The EPA uses a measure of air pollution called the **Air Quality Index (AQI)** to provide the public with a daily report on air conditions and any associated health warnings. The AQI measures five individual pollutants in local communities on a scale of 0 to 500 and provides an overall air quality value and recommendations for outdoor activity levels. The higher the number, the less healthy the air. For example, at 30, air quality is considered good; at 100 or higher, air is considered unhealthy for sensitive groups, such as people with asthma; at 200, air is considered very unhealthy; and at 300 or higher,

greenhouse effect
Warming of the earth's surface by heat trapped by gases in the lower atmosphere.

greenhouse gases
Gases that help trap heat in the lower atmosphere and radiate it back to the earth; they include carbon dioxide, water vapor, and others.

ozone
Odorless, colorless gas composed of three atoms of oxygen; in the upper atmosphere, ozone forms a protective shield blocking UV radiation from the sun; at ground level, ozone is a dangerous pollutant.

air pollution
Presence of one or more chemicals in the atmosphere of sufficient quality and in sufficient quantity to cause harm to life.

Air Quality Index (AQI)
Measure of air pollution issued daily by the EPA.

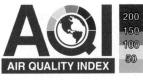

Pollutant: Particles
Today's Forecast: 130
Quality: Unhealthy for Sensitive Groups
People with heart or lung disease, older adults, and children are at risk.

(a)

Air Quality Index (AQI): Carbon Monoxide (CO)

Index Values	Levels of Health Concern	Cautionary Statements
0 - 50	Good	None
51 - 100*	Moderate	None
101 - 150	Unhealthy for Sensitive Groups	People with heart disease, such as angina, should reduce heavy exertion and avoid sources of CO, such as heavy traffic.
151 - 200	Unhealthy	People with heart disease, such as angina, should reduce moderate exertion and avoid sources of CO, such as heavy traffic.
201 - 300	Very Unhealthy	People with heart disease, such as angina, should reduce exertion and avoid sources of CO, such as heavy traffic.
301 - 500	Hazardous	People with heart disease, such as angina, should reduce exertion and avoid sources of CO, such as heavy traffic. Everyone else should reduce heavy exertion.

*An AQI of 100 for carbon monoxide corresponds to a CO level of 9 parts per million (averaged over 8 hours)

(b)

figure **23.1** **The EPA's Air Quality Index.**
(a) A sample AQI report in a newspaper. (b) An AQI chart for carbon monoxide. *Source:* Air Quality Index: A Guide to Air Quality and Your Health, *U.S. EPA, 2004, www.epa.gov.*

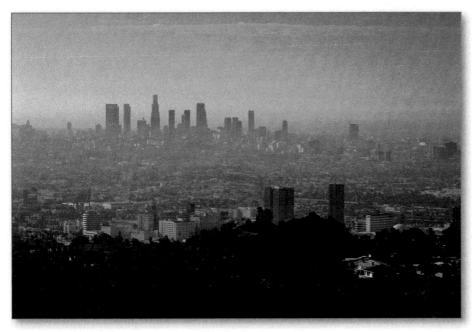

■ Photochemical smog and poor air quality plague Los Angeles not only because of motor vehicle exhaust but also because of the city's climate, shifting wind and weather conditions, and topographical features.

it is considered hazardous. (Levels above 300 almost never occur in U.S. communities.)

The EPA provides charts for four pollutants: ozone, particle pollution, carbon monoxide, and sulfur dioxide. (Levels of nitrogen dioxide are usually so low that they pose little direct threat to health, so a chart is not provided for this pollutant.) The AQI chart for carbon monoxide is shown in Figure 23.1. Levels of health concern are associated with different colors so that the public can quickly understand air quality warnings.[1] The AQI is available in newspapers, on television broadcasts, and on state or local pollution agency Web sites. The EPA also provides maps on its Web site that track and forecast ozone levels in cities and regions.

Ozone Ground-level ozone is a hazard. Ozone is a highly reactive gas that is poisonous to most living organisms. It causes respiratory irritation, aggravates respiratory and heart disease, and damages the lungs. Physical activity or outdoor work requiring exertion and deep breathing results in deeper penetration of ozone in the lungs. For unknown reasons, about one in three people has an unusual susceptibility to ozone. Also at greater risk are active children with respiratory disorders (such as asthma), adults with respiratory diseases (such as emphysema), and older adults (because respiratory function declines with age).[1, 8]

Particulate Matter Another hazardous component of air pollution is **particulate matter,** particles or droplets of dust, soot, oil, metals, or other compounds suspended in the air. The measurement unit for these particles is the micron (a human hair is about 70 microns in

diameter), and the smaller the particle, the more likely it is to cause health damage. Scientists believe that small particles that remain in the lungs for a long time irritate and damage alveoli, the tiny air sacs in the lungs.[1] Ultrafine particles may also trigger an immune system response that alters blood chemistry and blood pressure, contributing to heart disease and lung disease.[7]

Smog One of the primary sources of outdoor air pollutants is **smog,** a mixture of pollutants in the lower atmosphere that makes the air hazy. There are two types of smog: industrial smog and photochemical smog. **Industrial smog** is caused primarily by the burning of large amounts of coal and oil for heating, manufacturing, and the production of electrical power.[9] This type of smog occurs mostly in cold weather and produces a low-lying layer of pollution close to the earth's surface. Industrial smog is no longer a major problem in most developed countries. Coal and heavy oil are burned only in large furnaces or boiler systems that maintain strict pollution control, and waste gases are removed via tall smokestacks that transfer pollutants to downwind areas. This type of smog is still very much a problem in developing countries, however.

Photochemical smog is the type of smog that sits as a thick haze over many cities in the summer. It forms when pollutants from motor vehicle exhaust, industry, and other sources combine in the presence of sunlight and heat, producing large amounts of ozone and more than 100 other chemicals. All modern cities have photochemical smog, but it is much more prevalent in sunny, warm, dry climates with high population density and high use of **fossil fuels** (oil, coal, and natural gas) in transportation and industry.

Photochemical smog problems can be amplified by a temperature inversion.[1] Under normal conditions, the air at the earth's surface is heated by the sun and rises to mix with cool air above it. Surface air is

particulate matter
Particles or droplets of dust, soot, oil, metals, or other compounds suspended in the air.

smog
Mixture of pollutants in the lower atmosphere that makes the air hazy.

industrial smog
Type of air pollution that forms mostly in cold weather and is caused primarily by burning large amounts of coal and oil.

photochemical smog
Type of air pollution that forms when pollutants from motor vehicle exhaust, industry, and other sources combine in the presence of sunlight and heat, producing ozone and more than 100 other chemicals.

fossil fuels
Oil, coal, and natural gas—fuels that were produced over the course of millions of years by the pressure and heat of the earth acting on the buried remains of plants and animals containing carbon; they are typically extracted from the earth by drilling.

Challenges & Choices

You Can Help Improve Outdoor Air Quality

Small changes in individual behaviors and lifestyles can add up to big changes in greenhouse gas emissions.

- Walk, bike, skate, carpool, or use public transportation instead of driving your car. Each gallon of gas used by a car contributes about 20 pounds of carbon dioxide to the atmosphere. If all Americans between the ages of 10 and 74 replaced 30 minutes of driving with walking or biking, they would cut carbon dioxide emissions by 64 million tons a year.

- Get regular tune-ups for your car. A well-running car produces about 475 fewer pounds of carbon dioxide than a poorly tuned car.

- Check your tires to make sure they are inflated to the right pressure. When tires are properly inflated, your car uses less gas.

- Make sure your car's air conditioner isn't leaking chemicals, and limit your use of it to only the hottest days.

- If you are buying a car, consider an electric or a hybrid car that does not rely heavily on gasoline. If you don't get a hybrid, look for a car that gets good gas mileage.

- Turn down your home heating thermostat by at least 1 degree. You can cut energy consumption by as much as 10 percent for each degree.

- Buy the most energy-efficient homes, lights, and appliances available. Use compact fluorescent bulbs in lamps. Lighting accounts for about 20 percent of the total electricity used in the United States; refrigerators consume about 7 percent of total electricity.

- Turn down the thermostat on your water heater to between 110° and 120° F. Insulate hot water pipes. Hot water heaters consume about 20 percent of all energy used in a home.

- Keep houseplants to help clean the air in your home, and plant shade trees outside.

It's Not Just Personal . . .
The EPA notes that significant air pollution is transported between nations via weather changes. In the summer months, upper air winds allow for the transport of airborne pollutants to the United States from Mexico and Central America.

Sources: Living in the Environment, by G.T. Miller, 2002, Belmont, CA: Wadsworth/Thomson Learning; Clear Skies Initiative, U.S. EPA, www.epa.gov; "Driving Up the Cost of Clean Air," by D.C. Holzman, 2005, Health Perspectives, 113 (4), pp. A246–A249.

replaced by cooler air that in turn is heated and rises, creating a natural circulation process. In a **temperature inversion,** a warm layer of air moves in over a cooler layer, trapping it so that the air cannot circulate. Pollutants at ground level can build up to dangerous levels if the inversion lasts more than a few days.

Some types of topography are particularly favorable to temperature inversions and photochemical smog. A town or city located in a valley surrounded by mountains is susceptible during cold and cloudy seasons because surrounding mountains block out the winter sun. Very large cities with mountains on three sides and the ocean on the other side, extensive automobile use, and a sunny climate with light winds have ideal conditions for temperature inversions and smog. These are the conditions that account for the very high level of photochemical smog in Los Angeles.

The Clean Air Act of 1990 required the EPA to set national emission standards for more than 100 different air pollutants. These standards have led to continued improvements in air quality by encouraging use of public transporta-

temperature inversion
Weather condition in which a warm layer of air moves in over a cooler layer, trapping pollutants in the air near the earth's surface.

tion, non-gas-burning automobiles, the use of scrubbers to clean polluted air from smoke stacks, reduced use of fossil fuels, and increased use of renewable energy.[1]

In addition, the 2002 Clear Skies Initiative amendment to the 1990 Clean Air Act set mandatory caps that substantially reduce emissions of sulfur dioxide, nitrogen oxide, and mercury from coal-fired electric power generation.[9] Individuals can also take steps to improve outdoor air quality (see the box "You Can Help Improve Outdoor Air Quality).

Acid Deposition and Precipitation Another major source of outdoor air pollutants is **acid deposition,** which occurs when acidic pollutants drop out of the atmosphere onto the earth's surface. The two major pollutants involved in acid deposition are sulfur dioxide from coal-burning power plants and nitrogen dioxide from motor vehicle emissions.

Acid deposition can be dry or wet. Dry deposition occurs when acidic gases and particulate matter are blown by winds onto buildings, homes, cars, and trees or washed from surface areas by rainstorms. Dry deposition causes damage to stone, metal, and paint and necessitates repair to public monuments and build-

acid deposition
Depositing of acidic pollutants from the atmosphere on the earth's surface, in either dry or wet form.

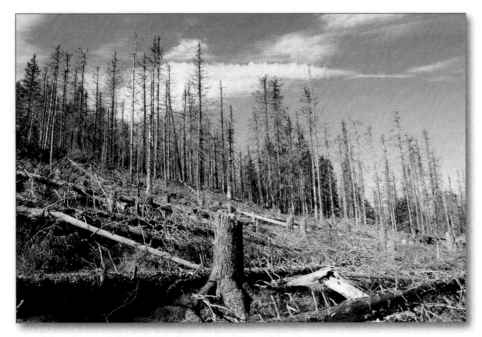

■ Acid rain damages trees by stripping nutrients from leaves, dissolving and washing away nutrients in the soil, and causing the release of toxic substances in the soil. Weakened trees are more susceptible to harm from environmental factors, especially cold weather.

ings totaling millions of dollars every year. Dry deposition accounts for nearly half of the acid deposition falling from the atmosphere.[10]

Wet deposition, or **acid precipitation,** occurs when acidic pollutants mix with moisture in the atmosphere and fall to earth as acid rain, snow, sleet, hail, or fog. This type of acid deposition has devastated lakes, streams, and forests in certain parts of the world, killing trees, fish, and aquatic wildlife. The pollutants in acid precipitation also cause respiratory problems in vulnerable individuals.

acid precipitation
Mixing of acidic pollutants in the atmosphere with moisture and their precipitation in the form of rain, snow, sleet, hail, or fog.

The degree of environmental damage from acid deposition depends on the ability of the soil to neutralize acid. Where soils are alkaline, such as in parts of the U.S. Midwest, there is less damage. Where soils are neutral or acidic, as in the northwestern United States, northeastern North America, and many parts of Canada and Europe, damage is extensive.

chlorofluorocarbons (CFCs)
Chemicals used as coolants, propellants, solvents, and foaming agents that destroy ozone in the upper atmosphere.

THINNING OF THE OZONE LAYER OF THE ATMOSPHERE

Every spring and early summer, a massive "hole" appears in the ozone layer of the atmosphere over Antarctica. This thinning of the ozone layer is caused by **chlorofluorocarbons (CFCs),** chemicals used as coolants in refrigeration and air-conditioning units, as propellants in aerosol sprays, as solvents in cleaning products, and as foaming agents in some rigid foam products.[11] When these chemicals are released or leak into the air, they slowly rise into the upper atmosphere, where chlorine atoms destroy ozone.

Without the protection of the ozone layer, humans are at risk for more severe sunburns, more skin cancers, more cataracts (clouding of the lens in the eye, causing blindness), and suppression of the immune system, which increases the risk for infectious diseases.[1, 11]

International agreements under the 1989 Montreal Protocol and subsequent treaties called for the reduction and eventual elimination of CFC production by 2000. This protocol is currently supported by 160 nations. However, because it takes CFCs 11–20 years to reach the upper atmosphere, it will be at least 50 years before the ozone layer begins to recover.[1] In the meantime, the hole continues to grow. During certain times of the year, it extends into populated areas of South America and Australia, and people living there are advised to stay indoors during critical periods and wear sunscreen and hats when they go outdoors.

GLOBAL WARMING AND CLIMATE CHANGE

For the past few hundred years, human activities have increased the amount of greenhouse gases in the lower atmosphere. These activities—burning fossil fuels, burning forests, cultivating cropland, raising cattle and other livestock on a mass basis, producing fertilizers, creating landfills—have significantly increased levels of carbon dioxide, methane, nitrous oxide, ozone, and other greenhouse gases. The intensification of the greenhouse effect has led to **global warming,** a gradual rise in the average temperature of the earth's surface (Figure 23.2).

global warming
Gradual rise in the average temperature of the earth's surface, caused by an increase in greenhouse gases in the lower atmosphere.

According to the National Academy of Sciences, the surface temperature of the earth has risen 1.1–1.3° F in the past century, but research suggests that most global warming has taken place in the last 50 years. Signs of global warming include melting of the ice caps and of glaciers, northward migration of some warm-climate fish, the bleaching of coral found in tropical areas, and the rise of sea levels by 4 to 8 inches over the past century.[1, 11–14]

Predicted Effects of Climate Change Agriculture, water resources, forests, wildlife, and coastal areas are all vulnerable to the effects of global warming and climate change. Melting glaciers and polar ice sheets may cause sea

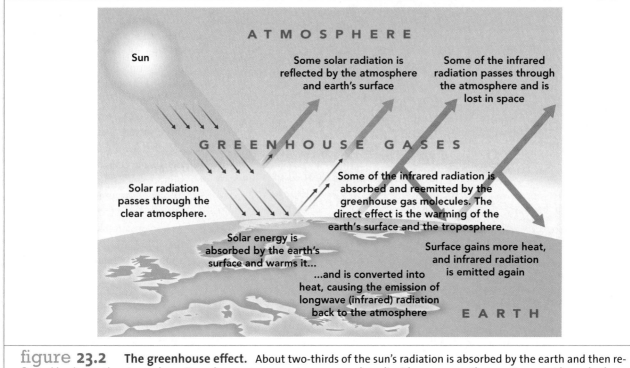

figure **23.2** **The greenhouse effect.** About two-thirds of the sun's radiation is absorbed by the earth and then re-flected back into the atmosphere. Greenhouse gases—water vapor, carbon dioxide, ozone, methane, nitrous oxide, and others—trap infrared radiation from the earth, warming the atmosphere. Human activities are causing greenhouse gas levels in the atmosphere to increase, which in turn increases the temperature of the earth. *Source: Reprinted with permission from* Information on Climate Change, *United Nations Environment Programme (UNEP).*

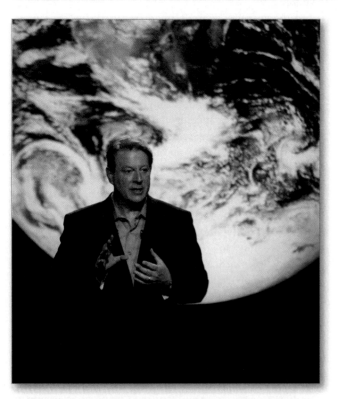

■ Al Gore spoke out for the environment in his 2006 documen-tary film about global warming, *An Inconvenient Truth*. The former Vice President won the 2007 Nobel Peace Prize for his role in increasing public awareness about climate change.

levels to rise by 39 inches by the end of the 21st century. Seawater would encroach on Wall Street in New York City and many of the major airports and interstates in Louisiana, Florida, North Carolina, Texas, and New Jersey.

As climate changes, storms are expected to become more frequent and intense; some areas are likely to receive more rain while others become drier. These changes will affect the kinds of food that can be grown and shift the nature of agri-culture throughout the world. Crop damage may increase because agricultural pests and diseases flourish in warmer weather.[1, 15, 16, 17]

Climate change is likely to have many adverse impacts on health, with significant loss of life. More frequent and severe heat waves would cause more heat-related deaths and illnesses. Heat causes more deaths in the United States than hurricanes, lightning, tornadoes, and floods combined. Mos-quito-borne illnesses would increase, especially in the south-ern parts of the United States. Air quality would decline, because pollution is worse in warmer weather. Older adults and people with cardiovascular and respiratory disorders would be particularly vulnerable to adverse health effects of global warming.[17]

What Can Be Done? To address global climate change, 38 nations signed the Kyoto Protocol, a United Nations–sponsored international agreement, in 1997. The protocol called for nations to cut their emissions of greenhouse gases, particularly carbon dioxide, by about 5.2 percent below 1990 levels by 2012. This market-based treaty allows countries and private companies to trade and sell their greenhouse gas emission allowances to other countries and businesses. It also encourages private companies to develop new technologies that reduce greenhouse gas emissions.

The Kyoto Protocol was to take effect when ratified by 55 countries responsible for 55 percent of global greenhouse gas emissions. The United States signed the treaty in 1998 but withdrew in 2001, citing insufficiently conclusive evidence of global warming and potential strain on the economy, including probable job losses.

Although 120 nations had signed the protocol by 2007, the nonparticipation of the United States, by far the greatest producer of greenhouse gases in the world, was a serious obstacle to its success. The United States has introduced its own emissions reduction plan for the nation, which calls for voluntary participation by all sectors of the economy. This plan was signed into law by the U.S. Senate in 2002.

Substantial reduction in carbon dioxide emissions will require massive changes in industrial processes, transportation, energy sources, and personal lifestyles.[3] Cost estimates to meet standards run into the billions of dollars, to be shouldered not just by businesses but also by consumers through higher car prices, higher gas prices, and costlier car maintenance to meet federal emission controls.

One promising approach to the problem is the promotion of hybrid gas-electric cars and cars with high fuel economy and low emissions. It has been estimated that hybrid gas-electric cars could reduce the pollution that causes global warming by at least one-third.[18, 19] Institutions, communities, and individuals can also take steps to prevent climate change (see the box "The Greening of College Campuses").

INDOOR AIR POLLUTION

Levels of air pollution indoors can be higher and more hazardous than levels of air pollution outside. On average, Americans spend between 80 and 90 percent of their time indoors.[20] Spending extensive time indoors magnifies health risks from indoor air pollutants, possibly to 50 times the health risks experienced outdoors. Eleven of the most common air pollutants are usually two to five times higher inside the home than outside.[1] The EPA estimates that exposure to indoor air pollutants causes 6,000 cases of cancer every year in the United States.[20]

Pollutants inside the home include allergens, such as dust mites and animal dander; mold and mildew; and chemicals, usually as fumes or vapors. You can reduce many of the biological pollutants (allergens, mold, bacteria) by keeping the house clean, keeping pets clean, washing bedding weekly, and maintaining the relative humidity between 30 and 50 percent. According to the EPA, the most dangerous indoor air pollutants are environmental tobacco smoke (dis-

Public Health in Action

The Greening of College Campuses

The presidents of many of the leading higher education institutions in the United States met in 2007 to pledge their schools to the "green college campus" movement. By reducing the "carbon footprint" of their campuses and promoting energy conservation, colleges and universities can have a significant impact on climate change. According to the EPA, schools that use more energy-efficient equipment, lighting, and mechanical systems in residences, classrooms, offices, and laboratories can reduce their carbon footprint as well as lower their operating costs.

Some of the actions and initiatives that are part of the green college movement are living in green buildings, developing sustainable food programs (using organic and locally grown food), sponsoring daily conservation messages, turning off lights and computers, using compact fluorescent bulbs, and encouraging students to buy energy-efficient appliances for dorm rooms. Many schools have undertaken environmental projects and educational campaigns. Middlebury College, Lewis and Clark College, the University of Colorado, and the University of Buffalo have been identified as having model sustainable energy programs on their campuses. Brown University and Harvard University have developed extensive educational campaigns that can provide useful information to other colleges and universities. Harvard also pays undergraduate students to deliver conservation messages to their peers.

Many colleges and universities use Earth Day to hold events that promote environmental stewardship. The next generation of campus buildings, including sports stadiums, will most likely be built with reusable materials, be designed to conserve water, and be powered by alternative energy. More important, the next generation of students will understand the significance of climate change and be ready to take the green movement with them when they leave campus.

cussed in Chapter 12), formaldehyde, radon, carbon monoxide, mold, and polybrominated diphenyl ethers.[20, 21]

Formaldehyde Formaldehyde is a colorless gas that is commonly used in the construction of household materials, such as those used in furniture, drapes, and fiberboard. Vapors can seep out of these materials into the home. Daily exposures to this irritating gas can cause chronic breathing problems, dizziness, skin rash, headaches, sore throat, sinus infections, and eye irritation.[22]

Radon Colorless, odorless, and tasteless, **radon** is a radioactive gas that occurs naturally in some soils, rocks, and building materials. It can seep into homes through dirt floors and cracks in foundations. When it becomes attached to dust particles, radon can be inhaled. It has been definitively linked to lung cancer but not other respiratory diseases, such as asthma.[23] Your chances of getting lung cancer from radon exposure depend on the level of radon in your home, the amount of time you spend in your home, and whether you are a smoker or an ex-smoker. Smokers and ex-smokers already have lung tissue damage that makes them more susceptible to radon-related lung cancer.[1] If you are interested in finding a qualified radon professional to test levels in your home, contact your state radon office or the National Environmental Health Association.

radon
Radioactive gas that occurs naturally in some soils, rocks, and building materials and is hazardous to human health.

Carbon Monoxide Carbon monoxide is produced by the incomplete burning of fuels containing carbon. This gas impairs the transport of oxygen in the blood. Symptoms of carbon monoxide poisoning include mental confusion, irregular heartbeat, dizziness, blurred vision, mild nausea, and headache. Severe poisoning can cause seizures, coma, and death. Fetuses and very young children are especially vulnerable to the toxic effects of carbon monoxide.

High concentrations of carbon monoxide indoors are very dangerous. Gas stoves, space heaters, furnaces, fireplaces, wood-burning stoves, and cigarette smoke are common sources. If you or family members experience symptoms of carbon monoxide poisoning, turn off combustion appliances and leave the contaminated area immediately. If the symptoms are serious, go to a hospital emergency center.[24]

Mold Basements with relative humidity above 60 percent often have walls and floors blackened by mold colonies. Some people have an allergic reaction to airborne mold spores; symptoms include coughing, sneezing, wheezing, eye irritation, and headaches. Mold can also bother people without allergies; mold spores inflame lung tissues and produce chemicals called mycotoxins that are hazardous when inhaled. If you regularly sneeze, cough, or have trouble breathing when you are in certain parts of your home, mold may be the problem. You may need to consult an expert to identify and remove sources of mold.[21]

Polybrominated Diphenyl Ethers (PBDEs) PBDEs are flame retardant chemicals used in plastic and foam products, such as furniture cushions and carpet pads; hard casings for televisions, telephones, computers, and other electronic equipment; and insulation for cables and wires.[22] PBDEs seep or leach out of these products and enter the environment, showing up in house dust, soil, and plants and animals. They have been found in human breast milk, tissue, and blood.

The major health concern is that PBDEs can accumulate in human tissue and may cause chromosome abnormalities.

Children who spend a lot of time at floor level are at greater risk for exposure by ingestion and inhalation.[23] PBDEs are under study by government-sponsored scientific endeavors, and some manufacturers of computers and office equipment have voluntarily stopped using them in their products.

Waste Management

Waste products are a natural outcome of the process of living on earth, but humans tend to generate large quantities of waste that must be managed in safe and satisfactory ways. Industrial processes and a "throwaway" attitude among consumers both contribute to the problem of excessive waste in our society.

SOLID WASTE

Solid waste is any unwanted or discarded material that is not a liquid or gas. The United States generates nearly 12 billion tons of solid waste each year. Ninety-nine percent of this waste is produced by mining, oil and natural gas production, agriculture, and industrial activities. The remaining 1 percent is municipal solid waste, commonly called garbage and refuse, from businesses and homes.

solid waste
Any unwanted or discarded material that is not a liquid or gas; garbage.

The United States leads the world in garbage production, generating about 1,600 pounds per person per year. Canada ranks third.[1, 25] The main components of garbage are paper products (including packaging and junk mail), yard waste, plastics, metals, glass, and wood. Food waste is not a major contributor to garbage because most is processed in garbage disposals and directed into sewage systems.

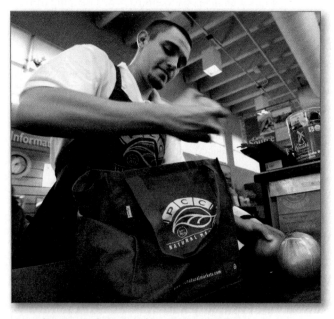

■ Both paper and plastic take energy to produce and burden landfills when discarded. The best choice for shopping is a reusable cloth bag.

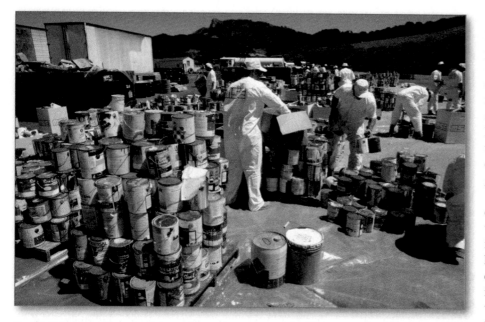

■ There is no good way to dispose of some hazardous materials. Experts recommend buying fewer products containing toxic contaminants.

Methods of managing solid waste have traditionally included burning, burying, and shipping wastes to other states or countries. Most of these methods were problematic and are now subject to numerous regulations. The principal method of dealing with solid waste today is burying it in sanitary landfills; this method is used to dispose of 54 percent of municipal solid waste in the United States and 80 percent in Canada.[1] **Sanitary landfills** are carefully selected sites where waste is buried, sometimes in plastic-lined containers or pits; they are designed to prevent leaching into water supplies and soil for at least 10 to 40 years.

A second method of dealing with solid waste is burning it in large city incinerators. Temperatures inside these incinerators exceed 1800° F, which prevents air pollution. In some cases, energy generated by the burning of refuse is sold as electricity to offset the cost of the incinerators, a waste management technique called waste-to-energy recovery.[1]

HAZARDOUS WASTE

Hazardous waste is any discarded solid or liquid material that meets one or more of four criteria: (1) the material contains a toxic, carcinogenic, or mutagenic compound at levels that exceed EPA safety standards (for example, solvents, pesticides); (2) it catches fire easily (for example, gasoline, oil-based paints); (3) it is reactive or unstable enough to explode or release toxic fumes (for example, chlorine, chlorine bleach); or (4) it corrodes metal containers (for example, drain cleaners, industrial cleaners).[1]

sanitary landfills
Carefully selected sites where waste is buried, sometimes in plastic-lined containers or pits; they are designed to prevent leaching into water supplies and soil for at least 10 to 40 years.

The EPA estimates that 12 trillion tons of hazardous material are produced each year in the United States.[25] The top five chemical compounds of concern are arsenic, lead, mercury, vinyl chloride, and polychlorinated biphenyls, or PCBs (used to insulate electrical transformers). Nearly 75 percent of the world's hazardous wastes is generated by the United States.[1]

Direct exposure to hazardous waste poses health hazards, whether it is touched, inhaled, or ingested. Safe handling measures have significantly reduced direct exposure to hazardous waste, but indirect exposure occurs when wastes leak from sanitary landfills and contaminate water supplies. Such leaks are suspected of causing cancer, respiratory diseases, neurological damage, developmental deficits, and other health problems in people in neighboring communities.

Today, federal laws drastically restrict the storage of hazardous waste in sanitary landfills.[25] Much of it is stored in ponds, pits, buildings, and specialized hazardous landfills or disposed of by injection into deep underground wells.

Household Hazardous Waste Hazardous waste is also generated in the home. It is estimated that the average home accumulates about 100 pounds of household hazardous waste (HHW) annually.[25] This waste includes batteries, paints, cleaners, oils, and pesticides, often stored in closets, basements, and garages. These products pose serious health threats. Farmworkers suffer the most from pesticide poisoning. About 25 farmworkers die each year in the United States, and nearly 300,000 suffer pesticide-related illness.[26]

Disposal of HHW is also a problem. Hazardous waste should not be poured down the drain, onto the ground, or into storm drains, nor should it be disposed of in the trash. Many communities have special collection days or permanent collection facilities for such waste. The best strategy is to limit your purchase of these items.

hazardous waste
Any discarded solid or liquid material that contains a toxic, carcinogenic, or mutagenic compound at levels that exceed EPA safety standards; catches fire easily; is reactive or unstable enough to explode or release toxic fumes; or corrodes metal containers.

Emergent Contaminants A growing concern today is *emergent contaminants,* products that are showing up in local rivers and other water sources. They include pharmaceuticals, cosmetics, antibacterial soap, shampoo, shaving lotion, skin cream, dishwashing liquids, plastic, flame retardants, and many other chemical compounds. It is not clear whether these contaminants have health effects. Alone, they occur in minute quantities—you would have to drink 17,000 gallons of contaminated water to ingest the equivalent of one 200-mg ibuprofen tablet—but collectively they can form a "cocktail" of chemicals. Some experts believe these compounds can disrupt the endocrine system and play havoc with hormones, including estrogen, androgen, and thyroid hormones.

Medical Waste The EPA has specific regulations pertaining to **medical waste,** any solid or liquid waste that is generated in the medical diagnosis, treatment, or immunization of human beings or animals. It includes used needles and syringes, used culture dishes and other glassware, discarded

medical waste
Any solid or liquid waste generated in the medical diagnosis, treatment, or immunization of human beings or animals.

surgical gloves, blood and blood products, tissue samples, and any materials contaminated by contact with such products. Medical waste disposal is strictly regulated by the states to prevent the spread of bloodborne pathogens and infectious disease. Public exposure to medical waste is very rare due to these regulations.

Radiation and Radioactive Waste Low-level radiation is used in medical and dental procedures, such as chest X-rays, dental X-rays, nuclear medicine diagnosis, and radiation therapy. Although these uses have contributed to improvements in health in some areas, exposure to X-rays should be limited. Recently, concern has grown about other sources of low-level radiation, such as televisions, computer monitors, microwave ovens, and cell phones. These devices do emit low levels of radiation, but research has so far been inconclusive on their health effects, if any.[1]

Disposal of radioactive waste is problematic. Waste with low levels of radioactivity, such as radioactive isotopes used in medicine, is often disposed of in landfills and near-surface burials, an approach that may lead to contamination of groundwater. High-level radioactive waste, generated by the production of nuclear weapons and the operation of nuclear power plants, is dangerous for tens of thousands of years; developing deposit sites that can offer this kind of protection is a challenge that has to be faced by the United States and other world powers.

APPROACHES TO WASTE MANAGEMENT: RECYCLING AND MORE

Most citizens do not want landfills, incinerators, and hazardous waste repositories located in their communities. This understandable "not in my backyard" attitude frustrates waste management operators and government officials. Many citizens argue that the real problem is not where to dispose of waste but how to stop producing so much of it.[1]

Many communities have established recycling programs to help address the problem of excessive waste. **Recycling** is a circle, or loop, program in which materials that would otherwise be discarded are collected, sorted, cleaned, and processed into raw materials to make new products. Today, the United States has the highest recycling rate of any industrialized country. Americans recycle 28 percent of their waste.[1]

recycling
Circle, or loop, program in which materials that would otherwise be discarded are collected, sorted, cleaned, and processed into raw materials to make new products.

Many communities provide curbside pickup of paper, glass, metals, certain types of plastics, and yard material, and many states have deposit/refund programs to encourage recycling of beverage containers made of glass or aluminum. Communities with these laws report that 90 percent of glass and can beverage containers are returned.[27]

Besides recycling household items, individuals can take many other actions to help control and prevent waste. These include buying recyclable, reusable, or compostable products; composting yard trimmings; using rechargeable batteries; using reusable cloth bags for grocery shopping; reducing use of paper towels and other paper products; buying products with as little Styrofoam, cardboard, or paper packaging as possible; and stopping junk mail by contacting the Direct Marketing Association (www.thedma.org).

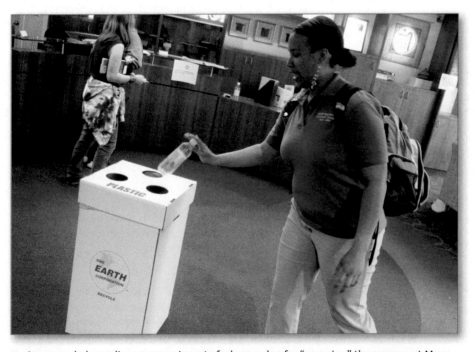

■ An expanded recycling program is part of a larger plan for "greening" the campus at Mary Baldwin College in Staunton, Virginia. College students across the country are driving the movement for sustainable living solutions on campus and in their communities.

Ecosystems and Biodiversity

An **ecosystem** is an interconnected community of organisms living together in a physical environment as a balanced, mutually supportive system. A frog pond in a meadow is an ecosystem; so is our planet. **Biodiversity,** or biological diversity, is the variety of different animal and plant species on earth, numbering in the millions, and the genetic variation in their gene pools—the material used in the process of evolution when changing environmental conditions require that species adapt or die out.[3]

ecosystem
Interconnected community of organisms living together in a physical environment as a balanced, mutually supportive system.

biodiversity
Variety of different animal and plant species on earth and the genetic variation in their gene pools.

An ecologically and biologically diverse planet offers innumerable benefits to humans. Twenty-five percent of medicines used in North America are derived from natural substances contained in plants and animals.[28] Choices in food, fuel, and lumber are enhanced by the variety of life-forms on the planet. Wild areas provide abundant opportunities for recreation, retreat, and refreshment. Most important, natural ecosystems promote the health of the planet, playing a role in climate maintenance, water cycling, soil production, waste disposal, and pest control.

Unfortunately, human activities have significantly disrupted these ecosystems and caused a decline in biodiversity. Nearly 50 percent of the earth's land surface has been disturbed or degraded by human activities.[1] Forests, grasslands, and wetlands have been converted for urban expansion and agricultural, industrial, and recreational use. Every year, hundreds of plant and animal species become extinct, and thousands more are at risk of extinction. The processes involved in this pattern of disruption include deforestation, desertification, and loss of freshwater resources.

DEFORESTATION

Deforestation is the removal of trees from a forested area without adequate replanting. When trees are cut down faster than they are replaced, forests become a nonrenewable resource. In the past 8,000 years, human activity has reduced the world's forests by about 46 percent, mostly in the past 3 decades.[1]

deforestation
Removal of trees from a forested area without adequate replanting.

In North America, the size and health of forests have been slightly improved since 1920 by reforestation. Some ecologists believe, however, that replacing *old-growth forests* (those that have flourished for several hundred years without interference from human activities or natural disasters) with *second-growth forests* (those that have been replanted following human activities or natural disasters) causes an overall reduction in biodiversity. Others claim that national parks and forests, tree farms, and lumber companies' reforestation programs are sufficient to preserve forest biodiversity. Year-round recreational use of national forests, including use of snowmobiles and all-terrain vehicles, hiking, mountain biking, cross-country skiing, camping, swimming, and hunting, also threatens the natural habitats of animals and plants. Heavy use of national forests results in noise, litter, pollution, and vandalism.[1]

In tropical areas of the world—in Africa, Asia, and Central and South America—deforestation has resulted in significant declines in tropical forests (see the box "Palm Oil: Harmful to Health, Rainforest, and Biodiversity"). About 90 percent of forest loss is occurring in tropical forests. Although tropical forests make up only 6 percent of the world's land, they are home to between 50 and 90 percent of all terrestrial species. At present deforestation rates, 50 percent of tropical species could be extinct by 2042.[1, 3, 28] Such an extinction could carry a heavy price, because tropical plants play an important role in removing some of the excess carbon dioxide that human activity puts into the atmosphere.

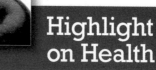

Highlight on Health

Palm Oil: Harmful to Health, Rain Forests, and Biodiversity

Palm oil is used worldwide as a cooking oil and as an ingredient in processed and packaged foods. It is commonly found in margarine, soups, sauces, crackers, and other baked goods. It is attractive to consumers because of its taste, cooking properties, and low price compared with similar oils. However, unlike other vegetable oils, palm oil contains primarily saturated fatty acids (as do other tropical oils, including coconut oil) and thus, when consumed, can increase cholesterol levels in the blood and contribute to heart disease.

Aside from the effect of palm oil on health, the production of palm oil contributes to environmental degradation. Most of the palm trees in the world grow on plantations in Southeast Asia, where tropical forests have been destroyed to make room for them. An estimated 70 percent of all the species of plants and animals in the world are believed to live in tropical forests. The destruction of 15,000 square miles of tropical forest causes loss of habitat for about 75 rhinos, 40 Asian elephant families, and 50 to 75 tigers.

What can you do? Stop buying palm oil. Better choices are safflower, canola, sunflower, corn, and soy oils. Check the ingredients on baked goods and make a different choice when you find products that contain palm oil. Consumers can make a difference in demand for a product, even on the other side of the world.

Source: From "Why Is Palm Oil Replacing Tropic Rain Forests? Why Are Biofuels Fueling Deforestation?" by R.A. Bultler, 2006, http:news.mongabay.com/2006/0425-oil_palm.html.

DESERTIFICATION

Another process of environmental degradation is **desertification,** the conversion of once fruitful land into infertile wasteland, or desert. A desert is a terrestrial region in which evaporation exceeds precipitation and the average annual precipitation is less than 10 inches.[29] Every day, on average, 40 square miles of land are turned into desert by droughts in combination with human activities, such as livestock grazing, poor irrigation techniques, and overplanting of crops.[30] Unlike natural deserts, human-created deserts are associated with worldwide famines. Some scientists believe that global warming contributes to desertification, because climate change produces droughts in areas that once had adequate rainfall.[1]

desertification
Conversion of once fruitful land into desert.

LOSS OF FRESHWATER RESOURCES

Rivers, lakes, and wetlands occupy only about 1 percent of the earth's surface, but they provide trillions of dollars worth of ecological and economic services. The causes of freshwater degradation and loss of biodiversity are the same as those for terrestrial ecosystems.[3] Freshwater species are actually more at risk of extinction than land-based species. Nearly half of all freshwater species are now threatened with extinction.[1]

Many rivers in North America are threatened by industrial, agricultural, and city wastes as well as disruption of water flow by dams, channelization, and diversion of water for agricultural irrigation. The National Wild and Scenic Rivers Act (NWSRA) of 1968 protects rivers with outstanding scenic, recreational, geological, wildlife, historical, or cultural values from development, but only 0.2 percent of the 3.5 million miles of waterways in the United States are protected by the NWSRA. Environmentalists have lobbied Congress to increase designated waterway lengths to 2 percent, a proposal opposed by many developers and some local communities.[1]

Lakes are threatened by acid precipitation and pollution, which kill plant and animal life. Sewage and agricultural runoff also pollute lakes and deplete oxygen in the water. Some lakes shrank or dried up when humans withdrew more water from them than could be replaced by rainfall. Another threat is the intentional or unintentional introduction of non-native species of fish and other organisms into lakes, which disrupts the balance of the ecosystem and usually results in the extinction of native species.

Wetlands are vulnerable as well. Swamps, marshes, and bogs are vital ecological resources for wildlife and the environment. They provide breeding areas and habitats for wildlife, store enormous amounts of water, keep the water table high during droughts, and help prevent flooding.[31] Despite their vital ecological roles, wetlands are often viewed as wasteland and considered fair game for draining, building, and agriculture. They are also vulnerable to industrial and agricultural runoff and human sewage, all of which destroy animal and plant life. The U.S. Fish and Wildlife Service estimates that more than 50 percent of wetlands in the United States have been destroyed in the past two centuries.[1]

PROTECTING ECOSYSTEMS

Stringent federal and state protection of animal and plant habitats in forests, deserts, and wetlands is a component of sustainable land management programs. The United States has several laws in place protecting endangered species, and many species are protected by international agreements. Genetically improved trees and tree farms can be part of a successful forest management program. Business and industry can help preserve forests by recycling paper, using fiber that does not come from trees to make paper, and using wood efficiently.

Individuals can help preserve forests by reusing and recycling paper products, refusing to buy products or materials made from endangered or threatened species, purchasing wood products with the Good Wood Seal, and stopping junk mail. Individuals can also let their elected representatives know that they are in favor of environmental protections, and they can support groups taking action to preserve natural habitats.[32]

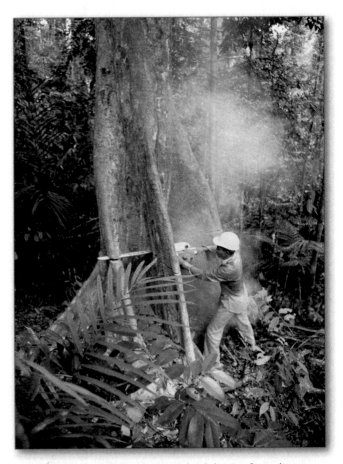

■ Logging, industrial development, land clearing for cash crops and cattle grazing, and even tourism are factors behind rainforest destruction. Rainforests are home to thousands of species of plants and animals and absorb huge quantities of carbon dioxide, the primary greenhouse gas in our atmosphere.

Energy Resources

Although the United States contains 4.5 percent of the world's population, it uses 24 percent of the world's commercial energy. Energy use per person in North America is nearly 50 percent higher than in Germany, France, Japan, or the United Kingdom and 100 times higher than in India or China. Nonrenewable energy resources provide 91 percent of the commercial energy used in the United States, 84 percent from fossil fuels and 7 percent from nuclear power.[1] Dependence on oil, coal, and natural gas is the primary cause of air pollution, water pollution, and global warming.[28]

The United States has only 2 percent of world oil reserves and thus is heavily dependent on foreign oil to meet its energy needs.[19] Environmentalists believe the solution lies not in the relentless pursuit of fossil fuels but in energy conservation. They argue that our efforts should focus on reducing the ecological effects of current energy practices, diminishing energy waste, and shifting toward renewable, nonpolluting energy sources such as water, wind, geothermal, and solar power.[1] When we conserve energy, they point out, we lower the demand on commercial energy sources, which in turn reduces the emission of air pollutants and greenhouse gases (see the box "Eating Green").

World Population Growth

Overpopulation increases the severity of every environmental problem on our planet. The world's population grew slowly until about 1750, when living conditions began to improve as a result of the Industrial Revolution. Since then, it has grown exponentially (Figure 23.3). World population reached 1 billion in about 1800, 1.6 billion in 1900, 2 billion in 1930, and 3 billion in 1960. A billion people were added between 1960 and 1975 and another billion between 1975 and 1987.[33] By the year 2000, world population stood at 6.1 billion, and by 2005, it reached 6.5 billion. The United Nations predicts that world population will reach 9.1 billion by 2050 and stabilize at about 10 billion in 2200.[34] Much of the population growth will take place in the less developed countries of Africa, Asia, and Latin America.

HOW MANY PEOPLE CAN THE PLANET SUPPORT?

The projected growth in the world's population has raised a vital question: How many people can the planet support? The answer depends on whether we are talking about the number of people the earth can support at subsistence levels—referred to as *global carrying capacity*—or the number the earth can support at an optimum standard of living—

Challenges & Choices

Eating Green

The United Nations Food and Agriculture Organization reports that the meat sector of agriculture is responsible for 18 percent of the world's greenhouse gas emissions. The production of large amounts of red meat also takes a significant toll on the environment by requiring large amounts of land, the diversion of huge quantities of water for irrigation, and the use of toxic chemicals as pesticides and fertilizers. Much of the land in the Midwest is now used to grow grain for animal feed to meet Americans' demand for beef. Here are some of the costs:

- It takes 1,600 calories from oil, gas, and other fossil fuels to produce 100 calories worth of grain-fed beef. In comparison, it takes only 500 calories of fossil fuels to produce 100 calories worth of chicken.

- 14 trillion gallons of irrigation water are used each year to produce feed for livestock.

- A large feedlot of 50,000 cattle produces as much manure as a city of several million people. Methane (a greenhouse gas) from this manure is 23 times more potent than equal amounts of carbon dioxide.

- Pesticides used in the Midwest to raise beef have washed into the Mississippi River, creating a large,

oxygen-depleted "dead zone" where bottom-dwelling water life cannot survive.

In contrast, greater reliance on a plant-based diet— a "green" diet—can help preserve the integrity of the environment:

- It takes only 50 calories from fossil fuels to produce 100 calories worth of plant foods.

- A low-meat diet uses 41 percent less energy and generates 37 percent less greenhouse gas emissions than a high-meat diet.

- If the typical American switched to an all-plant diet, the estimated reduction in carbon dioxide emitted each year would be 430 million tons, or 6 percent of the nation's greenhouse gas emissions.

It's Not Just Personal . . .

The CDC is considering a public health promotion campaign that would address issues related to global warming and the obesity epidemic at the same time. The campaign would encourage Americans to shift away from heavy meat consumption toward a plant-based diet and to walk or ride a bike rather than drive a car.

Source: "Eating Green," by J. Jacobson, September 2007, Nutrition Action Newsletter, pp. 3–7.

referred to as *cultural carrying capacity.* Subsistence living includes enough food, water, land, and energy to survive. An optimum standard of living includes the luxuries that are part of life in the developed world, such as plentiful food, indoor plumbing, cars, and air conditioning.

As noted earlier, analysts estimate that the global carrying capacity of the earth is 50 billion people,[35] but the cultural carrying capacity is much less. If luxuries are minimized, the cultural carrying capacity could be well above the population of 9 billion projected for 2050. If luxuries are maximized, it is probably lower than the current population of 6 billion. In other words, there are probably not enough resources, especially energy resources, to extend an optimum standard of living to everyone alive on the planet right now.

These global inequities may only be magnified in the future, with the world's 200-some nations coexisting in a finite global environment with very different standards of living. Currently, at least 2 billion people in the world are poorer than the 34 million people living below the official poverty line in the United States. This discrepancy increases by a million people every year.[1]

APPROACHES TO POPULATION CONTROL

If standards of living are to be improved for all the people on the planet, population growth has to be slowed. Approaches to population control include extending **family planning** resources, which help people make informed decisions about the number and spacing of their children, to women and couples around the world; empower-

family planning
Informed decisions that individuals and couples make about the number and spacing of their children; most family planning programs provide information on birth control, birth spacing, breastfeeding, and prenatal care.

ing women and increasing their access to educational and employment opportunities; reducing poverty and infant mortality and improving access to health care, all of which encourage parents to have fewer, healthier children; and offering incentives (such as salary bonuses, free education) and disincentives (such as higher taxes) to promote smaller families.

Family planning programs alone could have a significant effect if implemented in developing countries, according to the United Nations. The success of family planning

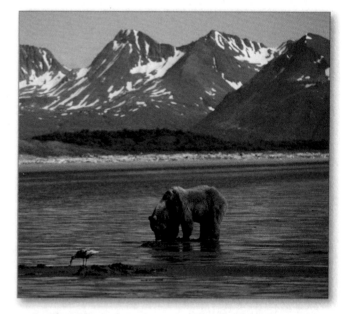

■ People are becoming more aware that the planet is a single, intricate, and sometimes fragile ecosystem that includes plants, animals, water, air, and all the interdependent patterns of life on earth.

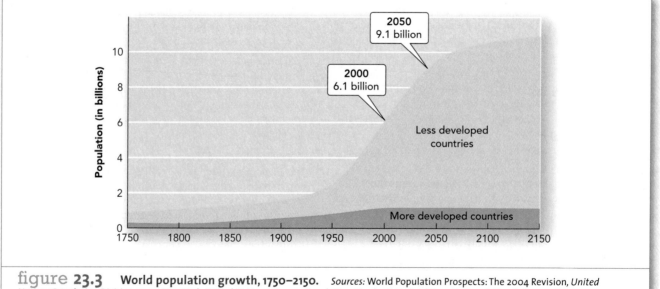

figure **23.3** **World population growth, 1750–2150.** *Sources:* World Population Prospects: The 2004 Revision, *United Nations Population Division, 2005, New York: United Nations; Human Population: Fundamentals of Growth, Population Reference Bureau, www.prb.org/; Historical Estimates of World Population, U.S. Census Bureau, 2005, www.census.gov.*

Consumer Clipboard

What College Students Can Do

College students can do their part for planetary health by living an environmentally conscious lifestyle. Here are a few examples:

- Recycle computers, cell phones, CDs, iPods, MP3 players, and other electronic equipment to help solve the electronic waste problem. You can find electronics recycling programs in your state through the National Recycling Coalition. CDs and DVDs can be recycled through eRecycle (www.erecycle.org) and GreenDisc (www .greendisc.com). You can also be an advocate for computer recycling through the Electronics Take Back Campaign (www.computertakeback.com).

- Use fewer personal care items (cosmetics, toothpaste, deodorant) that spill down the drain. Cosmetics that contain fewer solvents are less harmful to the environment. To find out more about the ingredients in cosmetics that you use, visit the Campaign for Safe Cosmetics (www.safecosmetics.org).

- Plug your electronic devices into a power strip and turn off the power strip when not in use. Turned-off electronic devices still use energy, called phantom electricity. Phantom electricity is responsible for more than 75 million tons of carbon dioxide emissions each year in the United States.

- Buy an energy-efficient car or truck. Vehicles are responsible for about 25 percent of the world's greenhouse gas emissions. One gallon of gas produces 20 pounds of carbon dioxide. The American Council for an Energy-Efficient Economy's *Green Book* will help you evaluate the carbon dioxide impact of your current vehicle or a vehicle you are planning to buy.

- Paper or plastic? Plastic bag production produces less water pollution, air pollution, and solid waste than paper, but plastic bags take more than 1,000 years to degrade. Paper is biodegradable and is a renewable resource, but paper bags take more energy to produce than plastic bags. Your best choice is reusable cloth bags for grocery shopping.

- Buy more of your food from local markets. A typical meat travels about 22,000 miles to reach the U.S dinner plate. A California lettuce travels 2,973 miles to reach New York City, and a Hawaiian pineapple travels 3,943 miles to reach the Midwest. The energy resources used for food transportation and the pollution generated contribute to many of our environmental problems. Many college campuses are now placing a priority on locally grown food. Learn more at www.localharvest.org and www.foodroutes.org.

Sources: Global Warming Survival Handbook, *by D.E. Rothschild, 2007, United Kingdom: Live Earth;* Wake Up and Smell the Planet, *edited by B. Davis, 2007, Seattle: Skipstone.*

programs in developing nations has been mixed, however. Minimal success has been attained in some very populous countries, including many countries in Africa and Latin America, primarily for cultural and religious reasons.[1]

A SUSTAINABLE PLANET

A resource management tool called the *ecological footprint* can be used to compare human consumption of natural resources with the planet's ecological capacity to regenerate used resources. In other words, it provides a comparison of a lifestyle and pattern of consumption with the earth's ability to provide for this pattern. Ecological footprints can reveal how sustainable a particular lifestyle is and can point out inequities of resource use and consumption.

Currently the ecological footprint of the United States is the largest in the world. Americans consume more resources,

generate more pollution, and discard more waste than any other people on the globe. If China and India were to catch up to the United States in ecological footprint, a second planet Earth would be needed to meet world resource requirements.

Even though environmental health involves human activities all over the globe, each of us can take actions today to reduce the size of the American ecological footprint (see the box "What College Students Can Do"). The Earth Day organization (www.earthday.net/footprint/info.asp) provides an ecological footprint quiz that estimates how much productive land and water you need to support what you use and what you discard. This quiz will enable you to compare your personal ecological footprint to the footprints of other people and what is available on planet Earth. You can use this information to shift your personal lifestyle toward a more sustainable and earth-friendly one.

You Make the Call

Is Recycling Worth the Trouble?

In the 1960s and 1970s, many landfills around the country reached their capacity and closed, prompting a sense of crisis in many communities and an interest in developing long-term waste disposal plans. One of the proposed solutions was recycling, which grew in popularity as environmental awareness increased. In the 1970s and 1980s, recycling became a popular fund-raising activity for community groups, and the slogan "Recycling Pays" was used to encourage consumers to recycle. By the late 1980s, some states were setting up deposit/refund programs for beverage containers and passing other recycling laws; programs were becoming more formalized.

At the same time, recycling was becoming a victim of its own success: Supply exceeded demand for some recyclable materials, and the public was becoming aware that it cost money to recycle—sometimes more money than simply throwing something in the garbage. Costs of recycling included collection and processing of materials, promotion and administration of programs, capital investment in equipment and containers, labor costs, and the fees that are charged to process certain materials. In some cases, consumers objected to recycling practices, such as having to pay refundable deposits on beverages, and some retail merchants complained about having to store returned bottles and cans.

As costs increased and objections surfaced, questions arose about whether recycling was worth the time and money. Some people were concerned about reports that recycling sometimes increases rather than decreases pollution, and others wondered whether there even was a "garbage crisis." One commentator, writing in the *New York Times* in 1996, called recycling the U.S. public's "rite of atonement for the sin of excess."

Supporters of recycling assert that the point is not necessarily to save money but to save the planet. Recycling slows the filling of landfills and conserves natural resources. It is environmentally sound, whereas unlimited consumption and waste production are not. Supporters point to research showing that although recycling of some materials, such as newsprint, actually creates more pollution than processing virgin materials, the overall environmental advantages of recycling are beyond doubt. Even if landfills do not contain hazardous materials, they emit methane, a greenhouse gas, as waste decomposes. One expert states that U.S. landfills are one of the biggest contributors to global methane emissions. Supporters also point out that recycling can save money: Landfill and incineration fees are avoided; recycled products are sold; and recycled products cost less to produce than products made from virgin materials.

Recycling—a worthwhile endeavor or a waste of time and money? What do you think?

PROS

- There is a limit to the amount of land available for landfills, especially since no community wants a landfill in its backyard. Landfills are potentially dangerous (if they contain hazardous wastes) and produce methane, a greenhouse gas. Recycling reduces the amount of waste that has to be disposed of in landfills.

- Recycling reduces water pollution (for example, from paper mills) and air pollution (from methane gas and incinerators).

- Recycling conserves natural resources. Less land has to be allocated for landfills; less fuel is used to run incinerators; trees, forests, and habitats are preserved and biodiversity is protected.

- People throughout the world are interdependent; we need to be aware of our relationships and responsibilities to others. Recycling helps us reduce our impact on the global environment.

- Well-run recycling programs can make money.

CONS

- Recycling is not good business. In a capitalist economy, any program must prove its economic value, and recycling has not done that. It costs more to run recycling programs than to run a landfill.

- Landfills are the logical choice for garbage disposal; they are safe, cheap, and convenient. Most do not contain hazardous waste.

- Some forms of recycling actually cause pollution, as when newsprint is processed.

- Recycling programs allow people to delude themselves into thinking they are doing something for the environment, while actually they are still consuming goods, using energy, and creating waste at the same excessive levels.

In Review

1. **What is environmental health?** Traditionally, environmental health focused on the conditions that contributed to infectious diseases, such as contaminated food and water, insects and rodents, and the disposal of waste. Today the field encompasses a broad range of issues, from global climate change to overpopulation. The key principle underlying environmental health is that we inhabit a small planet with infinite interconnections and finite resources.

2. **What are the key issues in environmental health today?** Key issues include water quality and quantity; air pollution, global warming, and climate change; management of waste, including hazardous and radioactive waste; loss of biodiversity and ecosystems; depletion of energy resources; and world overpopulation.

3. **What can people do to make a difference?** There are innumerable small and large steps individuals can take every day to make a difference in the environment, from recycling to conserving energy to reducing their ecological footprint. Information is widely available about how individuals can move toward a more sustainable and earth-friendly lifestyle.

WWW For a detailed summary of this chapter and a comprehensive set of review questions, visit the Online Learning Center at **www.mhhe.com/teague2e**.

Web Resources

CDC National Center for Environmental Health: This Web site provides information on environmental topics such as the elimination of chemical weapons, earthquakes, lead poisoning, and cancer clusters. The organization offers fact sheets, brochures, and other publications. www.cdc.gov/nceh

Natural Resources Defense Council: This Web site features weekly Web picks and a current legislative watch. Its Guide to Green Living includes ideas for green gifts, how to live green, and buying energy-efficient appliances. www.nrdc.org

U.S. Environmental Protection Agency: The EPA site offers news and information on topics such as acid rain, environmental laws, hazardous waste, oil spills, ozone, radon, and wetlands. Click on "where you live," enter your zip code, and find out environmental information about your community. www.epa.gov

U.S. Geological Survey: Focusing on the study of our landscape, natural resources, and natural hazards, USGS provides information on a variety of science topics, including climate, oceans and coastline, water resources, and plants and animals. www.usgs.gov

World Watch Institute: This independent research organization focuses on critical global issues, looking for practical solutions. It offers a wide range of publications and online features on such topics as global security, population, and climate change. www.worldwatch.org

World Wildlife Fund: This organization is dedicated to protecting endangered wildlife and preserving wild places. Its Global 200 is a scientific ranking of critical terrestrial, freshwater, and marine habitats that must be protected to preserve the "web of life." www.wwfus.org

Add It Up!

Part 1   Scoring Your Lifestyle

For each item, indicate whether you always, some-times, or never engage in the behavior.

	Almost Always	Sometimes	Almost Never
CIGARETTE SMOKING			
If you *never smoke*, enter a score of 10 for this section and go to the next section on *Alcohol and Drugs*.			
1. I avoid smoking cigarettes.	2	1	0
2. I smoke only low-tar and low-nicotine cigarettes *or* I smoke a pipe or cigars.	2	1	0

Smoking Score: _____

Alcohol and Drugs

	Almost Always	Sometimes	Almost Never
1. I avoid drinking alcoholic beverages *or* I drink no more than one or two drinks a day.	4	1	0
2. I avoid using alcohol or other drugs (especially illegal drugs) as a way of handling stressful situations or the problems in my life.	2	1	0
3. I am careful not to drink alcohol when taking certain medicines (for example, medicine for sleeping, pain, colds and allergies) or when pregnant.	2	1	0
4. I read and follow the label directions when using prescribed and over-the-counter drugs.	2	1	0

Alcohol and Drugs Score: _____

Eating Habits

	Almost Always	Sometimes	Almost Never
1. I eat a variety of foods each day, such as fruits and vegetables, whole-grain breads and cereals, lean meats, dairy products, dried peas and beans, and nuts and seeds.	4	1	0
2. I limit the amount of fat, saturated fat, and cholesterol I eat (including fat on meats, eggs, butter, cream, shortenings, and organ meats such as liver).	2	1	0
3. I limit the amount of salt I eat by cooking with only small amounts, not adding salt at the table, and avoiding salty snacks.	2	1	0
4. I avoid eating too much sugar (especially frequent snacks of sticky candy or soft drinks).	2	1	0

Eating Habits Score: _____

Exercise/Fitness

	Almost Always	Sometimes	Almost Never
1. I maintain a desired weight, avoiding overweight and underweight.	3	1	0
2. I do vigorous exercises for 15–30 minutes at least three times a week (examples include running, swimming, brisk walking).	3	1	0

	Almost Always	Sometimes	Almost Never
3. I do exercises that enhance my muscle tone for 15–30 minutes at least three times a week (examples include yoga and calisthenics).	2	1	0
4. I use part of my leisure time participating in individual, family, or team activities that increase my level of fitness (such as gardening, bowling, golf, and baseball).	2	1	0

Exercise/Fitness Score: _____

Stress Control

1. I have a job or do other work that I enjoy.	2	1	0
2. I find it easy to relax and express my feelings freely.	2	1	0
3. I recognize early, and prepare for, events or situations likely to be stressful for me.	2	1	0
4. I have close friends, relatives, or others whom I can talk to about personal matters and call on for help when needed.	2	1	0
5. I participate in group activities (such as church and community organizations) or hobbies that I enjoy.	2	1	0

Stress Control Score: _____

Safety

1. I wear a seat belt while riding in a car.	2	1	0
2. I avoid driving while under the influence of alcohol and other drugs.	2	1	0
3. I obey traffic rules and the speed limit when driving.	2	1	0
4. I am careful when using potentially harmful products or substances (such as household cleaners, poisons, and electrical devices).	2	1	0
5. I avoid smoking in bed.	2	1	0

Safety Score: _____

What Your Scores Mean to YOU

Scores of 9 and 10

Excellent! Your answers show that you are aware of the importance of this area to your health. More important, you are putting your knowledge to work for you by practicing good health habits. As long as you continue to do so, this area should not pose a serious health risk. It's likely that you are setting an example for your family and friends to follow. Because you got a very high test score on this part of the test, you may want to consider other areas where your scores indicate room for improvement.

Scores of 6 to 8

Your health practices in this area are good, but there is room for improvement. Look again at the items you answered with a "Sometimes" or "Almost Never." What changes can you make to improve your score? Even a small change can often help you achieve better health.

Scores of 3 to 5

Your health risks are showing! Would you like more information about the risks you are facing and why it is important for you to change these behaviors? Perhaps you need help in deciding how to successfully make the changes you desire. In either case, help is available.

Scores of 0 to 2

Obviously, you were concerned enough about your health to take the test, but your answers show that you may be taking serious and unnecessary risks with your health. Perhaps you are not aware of the risks and what to do about them. You can easily get the information and help you need to improve, if you wish. The next step is up to you.

SOURCE: U.S. Public Health Service, www.usphs.org.

Part 2   Signing a Behavior Change Contract

Signing a behavior change contract can be an effective strategy for changing a health behavior. Use this contract or adapt it to suit your own program.

I, _____, agree to _____
            (name)   (behavior you want to change)

_____.

I will begin my program on _____, and I expect to reach my goal on _____.
                                    (date)   (date)

I will use the following tools to help me reach my goal: _____.
                                                                    (journals, exercise buddies, social support, etc.)

When I reach my goal, I will reward myself as follows: _____.
                                                                            (reward)

I have recruited _____ to help me reach my goal by _____
                            (name)   (helping strategies)

_____.

In signing this contract, I assert my commitment to reaching my goal.

Signature _____   Date _____

Witness's signature _____   Date _____

SOURCE: Adapted from *Core Concepts in Health* (11th ed.), Wellness Worksheet 5, by P. M. Insel and T. Walton Roth, 2010, New York: McGraw-Hill.

How do we live to our fullest potential and become every-thing that we are capable of becoming? Dr. Abraham Maslow called the person who is in the process of developing his or her full potential "self-actualizing." For Maslow, self-actualized living is the ultimate achievement in the development of the human personality. Listed here are 15 characteristics of self-actualizing people. After carefully reading the descriptions, rate yourself on each characteristic on a scale from 1 to 10.

Score

1. **Reality-based perceptions:** Self-actualizing people have a more efficient perception of reality and a more comfortable relationship with it. They have an ability to detect the phony and the inaccurate in both people and things.

   1　2　3　4　5　6　7　8　9　10　_____

2. **Acceptance:** Self-actualizing people have the ability to accept themselves, other people, and nature as they are. They are not defensive, enjoy living, and are genuine.

   1　2　3　4　5　6　7　8　9　10　_____

3. **Spontaneity:** Self-actualizing people behave with spontaneity, simplicity, and naturalness. They are serene and characterized by lack of worry.

   1　2　3　4　5　6　7　8　9　10　_____

4. **Problem-centered:** Self-actualizing people focus on problems and people outside themselves. They are not self-centered and often choose to help others. This involvement is sometimes seen as a mission in life.

   1　2　3　4　5　6　7　8　9　10　_____

5. **Need for privacy and downtime:** Self-actualizing people enjoy solitude and aloneness.

   1　2　3　4　5　6　7　8　9　10　_____

6. **Autonomy and independence:** Self-actualizing people act independently of culture and environment. They are capable of doing things for themselves and making decisions on their own. They believe in who and what they are.

   1　2　3　4　5　6　7　8　9　10　_____

7. **Sense of wonder and appreciation:** Self-actualizing people experience a continuing freshness of appreciation about the world. They tend to have rich emotional reactions, are intensely alert and alive to things around them, and live the present moment to the fullest.

   1　2　3　4　5　6　7　8　9　10　_____

8. **Periodic peak experiences:** Most self-actualizing people have had profound spiritual experiences, although not necessarily religious in character. These are referred to as peak experiences.

   1　2　3　4　5　6　7　8　9　10　_____

9. **Identification with all of humankind:** Self-actualizing people have deep empathy and compassion for others.

   1　2　3　4　5　6　7　8　9　10　_____

10. **Deep relationships:** Self-actualizing people have profound and meaningful interpersonal relationships with a few people. They tend to select friends who exhibit self-actualizing characteristics.

    1　2　3　4　5　6　7　8　9　10　_____

11. **Democratic values:** A self-actualizing person does not discriminate against others, being virtually unaware of

differences in social class, race, or color. He or she respects everyone as potential contributors to his or her knowledge, merely because they are human beings.

1   2   3   4   5   6   7   8   9   10   _____

12. Strong ethical sense: Self-actualizing persons are highly ethical. They clearly distinguish between means and ends and subordinate means to ends. They follow their own set of internal moral values.

1   2   3   4   5   6   7   8   9   10   _____

13. Sense of humor: The self-actualizing person has a philosophical, unhostile sense of humor. He can laugh at himself but does not make jokes that will hurt others.

1   2   3   4   5   6   7   8   9   10   _____

14. Creativeness: The self-actualizing person has greatly increased, original creativeness that carries over into everything he or she does.

1   2   3   4   5   6   7   8   9   10   _____

15. Independence from culture and environment: Self-actualizing people are autonomous and have an ability to transcend the environment rather than just cope. They are capable of making decisions on their own.

1   2   3   4   5   6   7   8   9   10   _____

16. Aware of imperfections: Self-actualizing people are aware of the fact that they are not perfect, that they are as human as the next person, and that there are constantly new things to learn and new ways to grow.

1   2   3   4   5   6   7   8   9   10   _____

TOTAL _____

What are your strengths in moving toward being a self-actualizing person? What are your weaker characteristics? Why? What might you do to make your score higher on any given characteristic? The highest possible total is 160 points. How close are you?

SOURCE: From "Characteristics of a Self-Actualizing Person: An Evaluation Instrument," by R. Boyum, Ed.D., University of Wisconsin Counseling Services. www.uwec.edu/counsel/pubs/chars.htm.

Add It Up!

How would you rate your satisfaction with life? Below are five statements that you may agree with or disagree with. Read each one and then select the response that best describes how strongly you agree or disagree.

7 Strongly agree

6 Agree

5 Slightly agree

4 Neither agree nor disagree

3 Slightly disagree

2 Disagree

1 Strongly disagree

1 In most ways, my life is close to my ideal.

2 The conditions of my life are excellent.

3 I am completely satisfied with my life.

4 So far I've gotten the most important things I want in life.

5 If I could live my life over, I would change nothing.

Scoring

Add up the total number of points you scored. Your total should be between 5 and 35.

Understanding Your Score

30–35 Highly satisfied. People who score in this range love their lives and feel that the major domains of life—school, family, friends, leisure, personal development—are going very well.

Life is not perfect, but this is as good as life gets. Being satisfied does not mean being complacent, however. In fact, growth and change may be sources of satisfaction.

25–29 Satisfied. People who score in this range like their lives and feel that the major domains of life are going well. Life is not perfect, but it's mostly good.

20–24 Slightly satisfied. Most people score in this range. Some are mostly satisfied with most domains of their lives but see the need for improvement in each area. Others are satisfied with most domains but have one or two areas in which they would like to see large improvements.

15–19 Slightly below average. People who score in this range usually have small but significant problems in several areas of their lives or one area that represents a substantial prob-

lem. For those who score in this range because of a recent event, things will usually improve over time and satisfaction will generally move back up. For those who are continually dissatisfied with many areas of life, some changes or reflection might be in order. Sometimes a certain amount of dissatisfaction can provide motivation for change.

10–14 Dissatisfied. People who score in this range are substantially dissatisfied with their lives and have a number of areas that are not going very well or one or two areas that are going very badly. If life dissatisfaction is a response to a recent event such as the death of a loved one or a significant problem at work, there may be a return to a former level of higher satisfaction over time. If life dissatisfaction has been persistent for some time, then changes are in order, both in attitudes and in life activities. A person with life satisfaction in this range is often not functioning very well, and the help of a friend or a professional may be appropriate.

5–9 Extremely dissatisfied. People who score in this range are extremely unhappy with their current lives. The dissatisfaction may be due to a recent event, or it may be due to an ongoing problem like alcoholism or addiction. Whatever the reason, the help of a friend or a professional is strongly recommended.

Components of Life Satisfaction

As noted in Chapter 4, one of the most important influences on happiness and life satisfaction is social relationships. People with high life satisfaction tend to have supportive family and friends, whereas those who do not have close friends and family members are more likely to be dissatisfied.

Another factor that influences life satisfaction is work, school, or performance in an important role such as homemaker or grandparent. When a person enjoys his or her work and feels it is meaningful, the person is likely to have higher life satisfaction. Having important goals that derive from one's values also increases life satisfaction.

A third factor is personal—satisfaction with the self, one's religious or spiritual life, learning and growth, or leisure. For most people, these are sources of satisfaction.

Add It Up!

This adaptation of the Holmes-Rahe Social Readjustment Scale has been modified to apply to young adults. If you have experienced any of the events listed here in the last 12 months, check that item.

1.	Death of a close family member	_____ 100
2.	Death of a close friend	_____ 73
3.	Divorce of parents	_____ 65
4.	Jail term	_____ 63
5.	Major personal injury or illness	_____ 63
6.	Marriage	_____ 58
7.	Firing from a job	_____ 50
8.	Failure in an important course	_____ 47
9.	Change in health of a family member	_____ 45
10.	Pregnancy	_____ 45
11.	Sex problems	_____ 44
12.	Serious argument with close friend	_____ 40
13.	Change in financial status	_____ 39
14.	Change of major	_____ 39
15.	Trouble with parents	_____ 39
16.	New girlfriend or boyfriend	_____ 37
17.	Increase in workload at school	_____ 37
18.	Outstanding personal achievement	_____ 36
19.	First quarter/semester in college	_____ 36
20.	Change in living conditions	_____ 31

21.	Serious argument with an instructor	_____ 30
22.	Lower grades than expected	_____ 29
23.	Change in sleeping habits	_____ 29
24.	Change in social activities	_____ 29
25.	Change in eating habits	_____ 28
26.	Chronic car trouble	_____ 26
27.	Change in the number of family get-togethers	_____ 26
28.	Too many missed classes	_____ 25
29.	Change of college	_____ 24
30.	Dropping of more than one class	_____ 23
31.	Minor traffic violations	_____ 20

TOTAL _____

Scoring

Now total your points. A score of 300 or more is considered high and puts you at risk for developing a serious stress-related health problem. A score between 150 and 300 is considered moderately high, giving you about a 50–50 chance of developing a stress-related health problem. Even a score below 150 puts you at some risk for stress-related illness. If you do have an accumulation of stressful life events, you can improve your chances of staying well by practicing stress management and relaxation techniques, as described in this chapter.

SOURCES: Adapted from "The Social Readjustment Rating Scale," by Thomas H. Holmes and Richard H. Rahe, *Journal of Psychosomatic Research, 11*, issue 2, August, 1967. Copyright © Elsevier Science, Inc. Used with permission. All rights reserved; *Core Concepts in Health,* 4th ed., by P. M. Insel and W. T. Roth, 1985, Palo Alto, CA: Mayfield.

Add It Up!

Part 1　How sleepy are you?

The Epworth Sleepiness Scale is an informal sleep latency test that can help you evaluate how sleepy you are during the day, a key symptom of many sleep disorders. To evaluate your daytime sleepiness, use the scale from 0 to 3 to rate how likely you would be to doze off in the situations listed here.

```
0 = Would never doze
1 = Slight chance of dozing
2 = Moderate chance of dozing
3 = High chance of dozing
```

Situation	Chance of Dozing
Sitting and reading	_____
Watching television	_____
Sitting inactive in a public place (for example, a theater or a meeting)	_____
Riding in a car for an hour without a break	_____
Lying down in the afternoon	_____
Sitting and talking to someone	_____
Sitting quietly after lunch (when you have had no alcohol)	_____
Sitting in a car stopped in traffic	_____
	TOTAL _____

INTERPRETATION

0–8　You are probably not suffering from excessive daytime sleepiness.

9–14　You need to think seriously about getting more sleep.

15+　You should probably consult your physician, describing all your sleep-related symptoms.

Part 2　Do you have symptoms of a sleep disorder?

Ask yourself the following questions:

- Do you have trouble falling asleep three nights a week or more?

- Do you wake frequently during the night?

- Do you wake up too early and find it difficult to get back to sleep?

- Do you wake up unrefreshed?

- Do you snore loudly?

- Are you aware of gasping for breath or not breathing while you are sleeping, or has anyone ever told you that you do this?

- Do you feel sleepy during the day or doze off watching TV, reading, driving, or engaged in daily activities, even though you get 8 hours of sleep a night?

- Do you have nightmares?

- Do you feel unpleasant, tingling, creeping sensations in your legs while trying to sleep?

If you answer yes to any of these questions, it is possible that you are suffering from a sleep disorder. The first step to take is to make sure you have good sleep habits and practices, as described in Chapter 6. If you are doing everything you can to ensure a good night's sleep, consult your physician. He or she may refer you to a sleep disorder specialist.

SOURCE: Part 1: Adapted from National Sleep Foundation, 2002, www.sleepfoundation.org. Epworth Sleepiness Scale developed by Dr. Murray Jones; used by permission of Dr. Murray Jones. Part 2: Adapted from National Sleep Foundation, 2004, www.sleepfoundation.org.

Add It Up!

On average, Americans eat out more than four times a week. How does your restaurant diet measure up? Answer each question, then total your points.

Breakfast

1. **Which are you most likely to get on your bagel or English muffin?**

   a) nothing or hummus   (+5)

   b) jam or jelly   (+2)

   c) light cream cheese   (−1)

   d) margarine   (−1)

   e) butter   (−2)

   f) regular cream cheese   (−3)

2. **Which breakfast pastry do you order most often?**

   a) low-fat muffin   (+1)

   b) regular muffin   (o)

   c) doughnut   (−1)

   d) cake doughnut   (−2)

   e) chocolate-coated doughnut (−3)

   f) croissant or scone   (−4)

   g) pecan roll or Danish   (−5)

3. **Which is closest to the breakfast you typically order?**

   a) hot or cold cereal   (+3)

   b) eggs and toast   (−1)

   c) pancakes or French toast   (−3)

   d) Belgian waffle   (−5)

   e) ham-and-cheese omelette   (−5)

4. **Which beverage are you most likely to order at Starbucks?**

   a) coffee, regular   (o)

   b) Frappuccino coffee   (−1)

   c) cappuccino   (−2)

   d) caffè latte   (−3)

   e) caffè mocha   (−4)

Lunch

5. **Which sandwich do you most often order?**

   a) turkey   (+4)

   b) roast beef   (+3)

   c) chicken salad   (+1)

   d) tuna salad   (o)

   e) corned beef   (−1)

   f) ham or egg salad   (−2)

   g) bacon-lettuce-and-tomato sandwich (−3)

   h) grilled cheese   (−4)

6. **What do you usually order on your sandwiches?**

   a) lettuce, tomato, or onion (+3)

   b) mustard   (o)

   c) mayonnaise   (−1)

   d) cheese   (−3)

7. **What do you get to go with your sandwich?**

   a) fruit or garden salad   (+5)

   b) cole slaw   (+1)

   c) potato salad   (o)

   d) potato chips   (−1)

   e) french fries   (−3)

8. **Which are you most likely to order at McDonald's?**

   a) Grilled chicken sandwich   (+4)

   b) hamburger   (+2)

   c) Chicken McNuggets (6)   (−1)

   d) Quarter Pounder   (−2)

   e) Big Mac   (−3)

   f) Quarter Pounder with Cheese (−3)

9. **What do you get with—or instead of—a burger, order of nuggets, etc., at McDonald's?**

   a) side salad   (+5)

   b) Fruit 'n Yogurt Parfait   (+4)

   c) baked apple pie   (−2)

   d) french fries (large)   (−3)

e) shake (medium)   (−4)

f) shake (large)   (−5)

g) McFlurry (16 oz.)   (−6)

10. Which kind of pizza comes closest to what you usually order?

a) cheeseless with grilled vegetables, chicken, or shrimp   (+5)

b) half the cheese   (+1)

c) cheese   (−2)

d) pepperoni   (−3)

e) beef or sausage   (−4)

Snacks

11. Which are you most likely to snack on at the mall?

a) fruit shake   (+3)

b) soft pretzel, no butter or cheese   (+1)

c) soft pretzel with butter or cheese   (−1)

d) Mrs. Fields or other gourmet cookie   (−3)

e) Cinnabon or similar roll   (−4)

f) Mrs. Fields Double Fudge Brownie   (−4)

12. Which snack do you typically get at a movie theater?

a) nothing   (+5)

b) Twizzlers   (−1)

c) Junior Mints (1/2 box)   (−2)

d) Raisinets or Milk Duds (1/2)   (−2)

e) Whoppers (1/2)   (−2)

f) M&M's (1/2)   (−3)

g) Reese's Pieces (1/2)   (−4)

h) small popcorn   (−4)

i) medium popcorn (1/2)   (−5)

j) large popcorn (1/2)   (−6)

13. Which is closest to what you typically order at an ice cream shop?

a) low-fat frozen yogurt   (+3)

b) low-fat ice cream   (+3)

c) sorbet, sherbet, or ices   (+2)

d) regular ice cream   (−2)

e) gourmet ice cream   (−3)

f) hot fudge sundae   (−5)

g) milk shake   (−5)

14. What do you typically get on your ice cream?

a) nothing   (+5)

b) fruit   (+4)

c) nuts   (+2)

d) chocolate chips or candy   (−1)

e) crumbled cookies   (−1)

f) syrup or sprinkles   (−1)

g) hot fudge   (−2)

h) chocolate dip or coating   (−3)

Dinner

15. Which is closest to what you typically order as an appetizer?

a) salad   (+5)

b) unbuttered bread   (+2)

c) garlic bread   (−1)

d) Buffalo wings   (−2)

e) fried calamari (1/2 portion)   (−2)

f) cheese nachos (1/2)   (−3)

g) fried mozzarella sticks (1/2)   (−3)

h) deep-fried onion (1/2)   (−5)

i) stuffed potato skins (1/2)   (−5)

j) cheese fries (1/2)   (−7)

16. Which is closest to what you typically order at a Chinese restaurant?

a) Hunan tofu   (+5)

b) shrimp with garlic sauce   (+5)

c) stir-fried vegetables   (+5)

d) Szechuan shrimp   (+5)

e) chicken chow mein   (+3)

f) beef with broccoli   (+2)

g) moo shu pork   (0)

h) house lo mein   (−1)

i) house fried rice   (−3)

j) kung pao chicken   (−3)

k) General Tso's chicken   (−4)

l) orange or crispy beef   (−4)

m) sweet and sour pork   (−4)

17. **Which is closest to what you typically order at an Italian restaurant?**

    a) linguine with red clam sauce (+5)

    b) spaghetti with marinara sauce (+5)

    c) linguine with white clam sauce (+4)

    d) spaghetti with meat sauce (+2)

    e) cheese ravioli (−1)

    f) spaghetti and meatballs (−1)

    g) spaghetti and sausage (−1)

    h) cheese manicotti (−4)

    i) veal or eggplant Parmigiana (−4)

    j) lasagna (−5)

    k) fettuccine Alfredo (−8)

18. **Which is closest to what you typically order at a Mexican restaurant?**

    a) chicken, vegetable, or shrimp fajitas (+5)

    b) 2 chicken tacos (crispy or soft) (+2)

    c) 1 chicken burrito (+1)

    d) 2 beef or chicken enchiladas (−1)

    e) 1 beef burrito (−3)

    f) beef chimichanga (−5)

    g) taco salad or 2 chile rellenos (−6)

19. **Which is closest to what you order at a seafood restaurant?**

    a) grilled fish or shellfish (+5)

    b) fried fish or shrimp (−1)

    c) fried clams (−5)

    d) fried seafood combo (−5)

20. **Which is closest to what you typically order at a steak house?**

    a) grilled chicken or fish (+5)

    b) sirloin or filet mignon (+1)

    c) pork chops (−1)

    d) New York strip steak (−4)

    e) rib eye steak (−4)

    f) T-bone steak (−5)

    g) porterhouse steak (−6)

    h) prime rib (16 oz.) (−7)

21. **Which kind of potato do you most often order as a side dish?**

    a) baked potato with sour cream (1 tablespoon or less) (+5)

    b) mashed potatoes with gravy (+3)

    c) baked potato with sour cream (3 tablespoons) (+1)

    d) baked potato with butter (−1)

    e) baked potato with sour cream and butter (−3)

    f) french fries (−3)

    g) "loaded" baked potato (with bacon, butter, cheese, and sour cream) (−5)

22. **Which is closest to what you typically order at a family-style restaurant?**

    a) chicken stir-fry or pot roast (+3)

    b) grilled or roasted chicken (+3)

    c) turkey and stuffing (+1)

    d) chicken Caesar salad (0)

    e) chicken fingers or nuggets (−2)

    f) hamburger (−3)

    g) chef salad or chicken pot pie (−4)

    h) meat loaf (−5)

23. **Which side dish is closest to what you typically order?**

    a) salad or vegetable of the day (+5)

    b) rice pilaf or mashed potatoes (+3)

    c) macaroni and cheese (−1)

    d) french fries or creamed spinach (−3)

    e) onion rings (−5)

24. **Which is closest to what you typically order at a Greek restaurant?**

    a) chicken souvlaki (+5)

    b) lamb or pork souvlaki (+4)

    c) Greek salad (−1)

    d) spanakopita (spinach pie) (−1)

    e) dolmades (meat-stuffed grape leaves) (−3)

    f) gyro sandwich (−5)

    g) moussaka (−5)

25. **Which is closest to the dessert you typically order?**

     a) sorbet   (+2)

     b) pumpkin pie   (+1)

     c) baklava or chocolate cake   (−1)

     d) apple pie or chocolate mousse   (−3)

     e) cheesecake   (−6)

     f) fudge brownie sundae   (−6)

Scoring

75 or more Lookin' good. You know your way around a menu.

54–74 Could be worse. A few changes and you're set.

25–49 Could be better. Think about brown-bagging it.

24 or less Stay home. Don't leave home without a guide to healthy restaurant eating!

Add It Up!

People give many different reasons when asked why they don't get more exercise. To find out what the major barriers to exercise and physical activity are in your life, complete the following quiz. Indicate how likely you are to consider the following statements a barrier by using this key: Very likely = 3, Somewhat likely = 2, Somewhat unlikely = 1, Very unlikely = 0.

_____ 1. My day is so busy now, I just don't think I can make the time to include physical activity in my regular schedule.

_____ 2. None of my family members or friends likes to do anything active, so I don't have a chance to exercise.

_____ 3. I'm just too tired after work to get any exercise.

_____ 4. I've been thinking about getting more exercise, but I just can't seem to get started.

_____ 5. I'm getting older, so exercise can be risky.

_____ 6. I don't get enough exercise because I have never learned the skills for any sport.

_____ 7. I don't have access to jogging trails, swimming pools, or bike paths.

_____ 8. Physical activity takes too much time away from other commitments like home, work, and family.

_____ 9. I'm embarrassed about how I will look when I exercise with others.

_____ 10. I don't get enough sleep as it is. I just couldn't get up early or stay up late to get some exercise.

_____ 11. It's easier for me to find excuses not to exercise than to go out and do something.

_____ 12. I know of too many people who have hurt themselves by overdoing it with exercise.

_____ 13. I really can't see learning a new sport at my age.

_____ 14. It's just too expensive. You have to take a class or join a club or buy the right equipment.

_____ 15. My free times during the day are too short to include exercise.

_____ 16. My usual social activities with family or friends do not include physical activity.

_____ 17. I'm too tired during the week and need the weekend to catch up on my rest.

_____ 18. I want to get more exercise, but I just can't seem to make myself stick to anything.

_____ 19. I'm afraid I might injure myself or have a heart attack.

_____ 20. I'm not good enough at any physical activity to make it fun.

_____ 21. If we had exercise facilities and showers at work, I would be more likely to exercise.

Scoring

Enter your individual scores for each statement on the following lines. For example, enter your scores for statements 1, 8, and 15 on the first three lines, and add each group of three scores. Barriers to exercise and physical activity fall into the seven categories shown. A score of 5 or above in any category indicates that this is a significant barrier for you. For ideas on how to overcome these and other barriers, see the box "Strategies for Overcoming Barriers to Physical Activity" on p. 000.

____ + ____ + ____ = _____
 1   8   15   Lack of time

____ + ____ + ____ = _____
 2   9   16   Social influence

____ + ____ + ____ = _____
 3   10   17   Lack of energy

____ + ____ + ____ = _____
 4   11   18   Lack of willpower

____ + ____ + ____ = _____
 5   12   19   Fear of injury

____ + ____ + ____ = _____
 6   13   20   Lack of skill

____ + ____ + ____ = _____
 7   14   21   Lack of resources

SOURCE: Barriers to Being Active Quiz, 2003, Centers for Disease Control and Prevention, www.cdc.gov.

Add It Up!

Chapter 9
What Are Your Daily Energy Needs?

You can *estimate* your daily energy needs by (1) determining your BMR and (2) determining your energy expenditure above BMR from physical activity. Combining the two numbers gives you an estimate of your total energy requirement. This will require fine-tuning based on your body composition, metabolism, and activity and is intended as a start.

1. First, estimate your BMR, the minimum energy required to maintain your body's functions at rest. Begin by converting your weight in pounds to weight in kilograms. Then multiply by the BMR factor, which is estimated at 1.0 calories/kg/hour for men and 0.9 for women. Then multiply by 24 hours to get your daily energy needs from BMR.

   - Let's look at Gary, a 30-year-old, 180-pound man.

$$\frac{180 \text{ lb}}{2.2 \text{ lb/kg}} = 82 \text{ kg}$$

$$82 \text{ kg} \times 1 \text{ calories/kg/hour} = 82 \text{ calories/hour}$$

$$82 \text{ calories/hour} \times 24 \text{ hours/day} = 1{,}968 \text{ calories/day}$$

Gary's BMR—the energy he uses every day just to stay alive—is 1,968 calories.

   - Now let's look at Lisa, a 24-year-old, 115-pound woman.

$$\frac{115 \text{ lb}}{2.2 \text{ lb/kg}} = 52 \text{ kg}$$

$$52 \text{ kg} \times 0.9 \text{ calories/kg/hour} = 47 \text{ calories/hour}$$

$$47 \text{ calories/hour} \times 24 \text{ hours/day} = 1{,}128 \text{ calories/day}$$

Lisa's BMR is 1,128 calories per day.

   - Now calculate your own BMR.

Your weight in lbs _____ /2.2 lb/kg = _____ kg

_____ kg × 1 (men) = _____ calories/hour

_____ kg × 0.9 (women) = _____ calories/hour

_____ calories/hour × 24 hours/day = _____ calories/day

2. Next, estimate your voluntary muscle activity level. The following table gives approximations according to the amount of muscular work you typically perform in a day. To select the category appropriate for you, think in terms of muscle use, not just activity.

Lifestyle	BMR Factor
Sedentary (mostly sitting)	0.4–0.5
Lightly active lifestyles (such as a student)	0.55–0.65
Moderately active (such as a nurse)	0.65–0.7
Highly active (such as a bicycle messenger or an athlete)	0.75–1

A certain amount of honest guesswork is necessary. If you have a sedentary job but walk or bicycle to work every day, you could change your classification to lightly active (or even higher, depending on distance). If you have a moderately active job but spend all your leisure time on the couch, consider downgrading your classification to lightly active. Competitive athletes in training may actually need to increase the factor above 1.

   - Let's assume that Gary works in an office. He does walk around to talk to coworkers, go to the cafeteria for lunch, make photocopies, and do other everyday activities. We'll assess his lifestyle as sedentary but on the high side of activity for that category, say 0.5. To estimate Gary's energy expenditure above BMR, we multiply his BMR by this factor:

$$1{,}968 \text{ calories/day} \times 0.50 = 984 \text{ calories/day}$$

   - Let's assume that Lisa works as a stock clerk in a computer store. She spends a lot of time walking around and sometimes lifts fairly heavy merchandise. She doesn't own a car and rides her bike several miles to and from work each day and also for many errands, so she's at the high end of moderately active, say 0.7. To estimate Lisa's energy expenditure above BMR, we multiply her BMR by this factor:

$$1{,}128 \text{ calories/day} \times 0.70 = 790 \text{ calories/day}$$

Note that although Lisa is much more active than Gary, she uses less energy because of her lower body weight.

   - Now calculate your own estimated energy expenditure from physical activity.

_____ calories/day × BMR factor _____ = _____ calories/day

3. To find your total daily energy needs, add your BMR and your estimated energy expenditure.

   - For Gary, this is

$$1{,}968 \text{ calories/day} + 984 \text{ calories/day}$$

$$= 2{,}952 \text{ calories/day}$$

- For Lisa, it is

  1,128 calories/day + 790 calories/day

  = 1,918 calories/day

Because several estimates are used in this method, total daily energy needs should be expressed as a 100-calorie range roughly centered on the final calculated value, which would be about 2,900–3,000 calories/day for Gary and about 1,870–1,970 calories/day for Lisa.

- Now calculate your total daily energy needs.

  BMR calories/day _____ + physical activity

  calories/day _____ = _____ total calories/day

Finally, compare your daily energy needs with your daily calorie intake.

Your daily energy needs: _____

Your daily calorie intake: _____

Remember, if you want to lose weight, you need to take in less energy than you use up. You can shift the balance by increasing your activity level or decreasing your food intake. Moderate changes in both intake and activity level are the safest way to lose weight.

Add It Up!

This exercise is designed to help you think about your body image and eating patterns. It is not intended to diagnose an eating disorder. If you answer yes to any of the questions, you may benefit from talking to a counselor or health care provider. If you mark yes for several questions, you may have serious body image concerns and may have disordered eating. A professional consultation is recommended.

Check if any of the following statements are true or mostly true for you:

☐ 1. I feel more in control when I restrict the amount of food that I eat.

☐ 2. I consistently compare the way I look to others and perceive myself to be too heavy.

☐ 3. I would do almost anything to look more muscular and ripped.

☐ 4. I make sure to exercise whenever I feel as though I have eaten too much.

☐ 5. I would agree to cosmetic surgery if it were free.

☐ 6. I am dissatisfied with my body size and shape.

☐ 7. I am anxious about how people perceive or judge me.

☐ 8. I have patterns or rituals around food and eating, and I follow them in order to improve my appearance.

☐ 9. I feel anxious about gaining weight.

☐ 10. I feel as though I am constantly on a diet.

☐ 11. I eat to make myself feel better when I am sad, upset, or lonely.

☐ 12. I feel good about myself only when I weigh a certain amount or look a certain way.

☐ 13. I believe that people would think less of me if I gained weight.

☐ 14. I often skip meals to lose weight.

☐ 15. If I work hard enough, I can look like a professional athlete.

☐ 16. I frequently feel anxious or depressed because of concerns about my appearance.

☐ 17. My preoccupation with food makes it hard to concentrate on my work or school.

☐ 18. I get excluded from social groups because of how I look.

☐ 19. I sometimes feel obsessed about food.

☐ 20. I often talk negatively about my body in a serious way to myself or others.

Add It Up!

Compared with non-binge drinkers, binge drinkers are more likely to experience negative consequences from drinking. Primary consequences are alcohol-related problems experienced by the drinker. Secondary consequences are alcohol-related problems experienced by those around the drinker. For each of the items listed here, indicate on a scale of 1 to 5 whether this event would be very important to you (5), somewhat important (4), neither important nor unimportant (3), somewhat unimportant (2), or very unimportant (1).

Primary Consequences

	Important				Unimportant
Did something regrettable	5	4	3	2	1
Missed a class	5	4	3	2	1
Got behind in schoolwork	5	4	3	2	1
Argued with friends	5	4	3	2	1
Drove after drinking alcohol	5	4	3	2	1
Engaged in unplanned sex	5	4	3	2	1
Had unprotected sex	5	4	3	2	1
Got hurt or injured	5	4	3	2	1
Got into trouble with police or college authorities	5	4	3	2	1
Damaged property	5	4	3	2	1
Had a poor performance on an exam	5	4	3	2	1
Engaged in pranks	5	4	3	2	1
Made unwanted sexual advances	5	4	3	2	1

Secondary Consequences

Experienced unwanted sexual advances	5	4	3	2	1
Had studying disrupted	5	4	3	2	1
Had sleep disrupted	5	4	3	2	1
Had to take care of a drunk fellow student	5	4	3	2	1
Been insulted or humiliated	5	4	3	2	1
Had my property damaged	5	4	3	2	1
Was physically assaulted	5	4	3	2	1

Scoring

Add up your points for Primary Consequences: _____

Add up your points for Secondary Consequences: _____

Interpreting Your Scores

PRIMARY CONSEQUENCES

59–65 Consequences of binge drinking are very important to you.

46–58 Consequences of binge drinking are somewhat important to you.

33–45 Consequences of binge drinking are neither important nor unimportant to you; you are neutral toward them.

13–32 Consequences of binge drinking are of little or no importance to you.

SECONDARY CONSEQUENCES

32–35 The secondhand effects of binge drinking are very important to you.

25–31 The secondhand effects of binge drinking are somewhat important to you.

18–24 The secondhand effects of binge drinking are neither important nor unimportant to you; you are neutral toward them.

7–17 The secondhand effects of binge drinking are of little or no importance to you.

If the consequences of binge drinking are important to you, now is the time to take action to change your behavior or to influence those around you to change their behavior.

SOURCE: Adapted from "Trends in College Binge Drinking During a Period of Increased Prevention Efforts: Findings from the Harvard School of Public Health College Study Surveys: 1993–2001," by H. Wechsler et al., 2002, *Journal of American College Health, 50*, p. 207.

Add It Up!

If you wonder whether you are becoming dependent on a drug, ask yourself the following questions. Answer yes (Y) or no (N).

_____ 1. Do you take the drug regularly?

_____ 2. Have you been taking the drug for a long time?

_____ 3. Do you always take the drug in certain situations or when you're with certain people?

_____ 4. Do you find it difficult to stop using the drug? Do you feel powerless to quit?

_____ 5. Have you tried repeatedly to cut down or control your use of the drug?

_____ 6. Do you need to take a larger dose of the drug in order to get the same high you're used to?

_____ 7. Do you feel specific symptoms if you cut back or stop using the drug?

_____ 8. Do you frequently take another psychoactive substance to relieve withdrawal symptoms?

_____ 9. Do you take the drug to feel "normal"?

_____10. Do you go to extreme lengths or put yourself in dangerous situations to get the drug?

_____11. Do you hide your drug use from others? Have you ever lied about what you're using or how much you use?

_____12. Do people close to you ask you about your drug use?

_____13. Are you spending more and more time with people who use the same drug as you?

_____14. Do you think about the drug when you're not high, figuring out ways to get it?

_____15. If you stop taking the drug, do you feel bad until you can take it again?

_____16. Does the drug interfere with your ability to study, work, or socialize?

_____17. Do you skip important school, work, social, or recreational activities in order to obtain or use the drug?

_____18. Do you continue to use the drug despite a physical or mental disorder or despite a significant problem that you know is worsened by drug use?

_____19. Have you developed a mental or physical condition or disorder because of prolonged drug use?

_____20. Have you done something dangerous or that you regret while under the influence of the drug?

The more questions you answered yes, the more likely it is that you are becoming dependent on a drug. If the problem is still in its early stages, try the behavior change strategies suggested for alcohol-related behaviors at the end of Chapter 11 (p. 000). If the problem is more serious, talk to your physician or to a health care provider at your student health center before it gets worse.

If you think a friend or family member is developing a drug problem, you may want to talk to the person about your concerns. Be prepared for the person to deny that there is a problem or to get angry at you. Provide the person with information about treatment resources in the community or on your campus. The less judgmental and more supportive you can be, the more likely it is that you will be able to help.

SOURCE: _Core Concepts in Health_ (11th ed.), Wellness Worksheet #47, by P. M. Insel and W. T. Roth. Copyright © 2009 The McGraw-Hill Companies. Reprinted by permission of The McGraw-Hill Companies.

Add It Up!

People smoke for different reasons—for example, to enhance mood, to relieve tension, or to have something in their hands. If you are a smoker, knowing why you smoke will give you tools to help you quit. For each of the following statements, circle one number indicating how often the statement is true for you.

	Never	Seldom	Sometimes	Often	Always
A. I smoke cigarettes in order to keep from slowing down.	1	2	3	4	5
B. Handling a cigarette is part of my enjoyment in smoking.	1	2	3	4	5
C. Smoking cigarettes is pleasant and relaxing.	1	2	3	4	5
D. I light up a cigarette when I feel angry about something.	1	2	3	4	5
E. When I run out of cigarettes, I find it unbearable until I can get them.	1	2	3	4	5
F. I smoke cigarettes automatically, without even being aware of it.	1	2	3	4	5
G. I smoke cigarettes to stimulate myself, to perk myself up.	1	2	3	4	5
H. Part of my enjoyment in smoking a cigarette comes from the steps I take to light up.	1	2	3	4	5
I. I find cigarettes pleasurable.	1	2	3	4	5
J. When I feel uncomfortable or upset about something, I light up a cigarette.	1	2	3	4	5
K. When I am not smoking a cigarette, I am very much aware of it.	1	2	3	4	5
L. I light up a cigarette without realizing I still have one burning in the ashtray.	1	2	3	4	5
M. I smoke cigarettes to give me a lift.	1	2	3	4	5
N. When I smoke a cigarette, part of my enjoyment is watching the smoke as I exhale it.	1	2	3	4	5
O. I want a cigarette most when I am comfortable and relaxed.	1	2	3	4	5
P. When I feel blue or want to take my mind off cares and worries, I smoke a cigarette.	1	2	3	4	5
Q. I get a real gnawing hunger for a cigarette when I haven't smoked for a while.	1	2	3	4	5
R. I've found a cigarette in my mouth and not remembered putting it there.	1	2	3	4	5

Scoring

Enter the number you have circled for each question in the spaces on the next page. Add the three scores on each line to get your totals. Most people smoke for one or more of six broad reasons: (1) stimulation, a sense of increased energy; (2) handling, the satisfaction of manipulating things; (3) pleasurable feelings, a state of enhanced well-being; (4) a decrease in negative feelings and tension; (5) psychological addiction, a complex pattern of craving for tobacco; (6) habit, an automatic response to environmental stimuli or internal craving.

			Totals
___ +	___ +	___ =	_____
A	G	M	Stimulation
___ +	___ +	___ =	_____
B	H	N	Handling
___ +	___ +	___ =	_____
C	I	O	Pleasurable feelings
___ +	___ +	___ =	_____
D	J	P	Crutch: tension reduction
___ +	___ +	___ =	_____
E	K	Q	Craving: psychological addiction
___ +	___ +	___ =	_____
F	L	R	Habit

Interpreting Your Score

The highest score possible in a category is 15. A score of 11 or above on any factor suggests that this factor is an important source of satisfaction for you. The higher your score, the more important a particular factor is in your smoking. Your smoking cessation efforts should include strategies that help you address each of the dimensions that strongly influence your smoking. Here are some suggestions:

Stimulation: Try substituting a brisk walk or some other form of exercise.

Handling: Try playing with a pen or pencil, a smooth stone, or a coin. If you want to have something in your mouth, try sugarless gum.

Pleasurable feelings: Try exercising, socializing, or eating or drinking low-calorie foods or drinks.

Tension reduction: Same as pleasurable feelings.

Craving: Quitting may be especially hard for you. However, many smokers with this primary motivation have a low risk of relapse because once they quit, they never want to have to go through it again. Nicotine replacement therapy can help.

Habit: Quitting may be relatively easy for you. Ask yourself, Do I really want this cigarette?

SOURCE: "Why Do You Smoke?" NIH Publication No. 93-1822. Reprinted October 1992, U.S. Department of Health and Human Services.

Add It Up!

How does Sternberg's triangular love model relate to your relationships? Consider an important love relationship you have had with someone in the last few years. Read the following statements and rate your agreement with each one, on a scale of 1 to 9, with 1 indicating you don't agree at all, 5 indicating you agree moderately, and 9 indicating you agree strongly. After rating all the items, consult the scoring key at the end of the scale.

1	2	3		4	5	6		7	8	9
Not at all				**Moderately**				**Strongly**		

Intimacy Component

_____ 1.   I actively support my partner's well-being.

_____ 2.   I have a warm relationship with my partner.

_____ 3.   I can count on my partner in times of need.

_____ 4.   My partner can count on me in times of need.

_____ 5.   I am willing to share my possessions and myself with my partner.

_____ 6.   I receive considerable emotional support from my partner.

_____ 7.   I give considerable emotional support to my partner.

_____ 8.   I communicate well with my partner.

_____ 9.   I value my partner greatly in my life.

_____ 10.   I feel close to my partner.

_____ 11.   I have a comfortable relationship with my partner.

_____ 12.   I feel that I really understand my partner.

_____ 13.   I feel that my partner really understands me.

_____ 14.   I feel that I can really trust my partner.

_____ 15.   I share deeply personal information about myself with my partner.

Passion Component

_____ 16.   Just seeing my partner excites me.

_____ 17.   I find myself thinking about my partner frequently during the day.

_____ 18.   My relationship with my partner is very romantic.

_____ 19.   I find my partner very attractive.

_____ 20.   I idealize my partner.

_____ 21.   I cannot imagine another person making me as happy as my partner does.

_____ 22.   I would rather be with my partner than with anyone else.

_____ 23.   Nothing is more important to me than my relationship with my partner.

_____ 24.   I especially like physical contact with my partner.

_____ 25.   There is something almost "magical" about my relationship with my partner.

_____ 26.   I adore my partner.

_____ 27.   I cannot imagine life without my partner.

_____ 28.   My relationship with my partner is passionate.

_____ 29.   When I see romantic movies and read romantic books, I think of my partner.

_____ 30.   I fantasize about my partner.

Decision/Commitment Component

_____ 31.   I know that I care about my partner.

_____ 32.   I am committed to maintaining my relationship with my partner.

_____ 33.   Because of my commitment to my partner, I would not let other people come between us.

_____ 34.   I have confidence in the stability of my relationship with my partner.

_____ 35.   I could not let anything get in the way of my commitment to my partner.

_____ 36.   I expect my love for my partner to last for the rest of my life.

_____ 37.   I will always feel a strong responsibility for my partner.

_____ 38.   I view my commitment to my partner as a solid one.

_____ 39.   I cannot imagine ending my relationship with my partner.

_____ 40.   I am certain of my love for my partner.

_____ 41.   I view my relationship with my partner as permanent.

_____ **42.**   I view my relationship with my partner as a good decision.

_____ **43.**   I feel a sense of responsibility toward my partner.

_____ **44.**   I plan to continue my relationship with my partner.

_____ **45.**   Even when my partner is hard to deal with, I remain committed to our relationship.

Scoring Key

Add your ratings for each of the three sections—intimacy, passion, and decision/commitment—and write the totals in the blanks below. Divide the score from each section by 15 to get an average score for each section.

_____ $\div 15 =$ _____

Intimacy score   Intimacy average

_____ $\div 15 =$ _____

Passion score   Passion average

_____ $\div 15 =$ _____

Decision/   Decision/
commitment score   commitment
                                     average

Each average score can range from 1 (low agreement) to 9 (strong agreement). If your average score on any component is 7–9, that component is a very strong part of your relationship. If your average score on any component is 1–3, that component is not a very strong part of your relationship. If your average score on any component is 4–6, that component is a moderately strong part of your relationship. Refer to the chapter discussion for an overall characterization of your relationship based on your scores. Remember, though, that relationships change over time—intimacy can deepen, commitment can grow, and even passion can be renewed. Remember, too, that a relationship does not have to fit a model to be a satisfying and important part of your life.

SOURCE: Sternberg's Triangular Love Scale, adapted from _The Triangle of Love,_ by Robert J. Sternberg. Reprinted by permission of Robert J. Sternberg.

Add It Up!

Sexual problems in a relationship can often be traced to the emotional dimension of the relationship, to general sexual misinformation, or to inadequate communication between partners. Many people prefer not to think about sexual problems, but self-reflection is the vital first step in addressing them. If you think you might be experiencing a sexual problem in your relationship, consider the following five questions and answer them as honestly as you can. Use a scale of 1 to 5, with 1 representing "not at all," 3 representing "somewhat," and 5 representing "very much." Then read the discussion that follows the questions.

1. Do you think about the problem often?   1   2   3   4   5

2. Has the problem affected your self-image?   1   2   3   4   5

3. Do you fear discussing the problem with your partner?   1   2   3   4   5

4. Does the problem affect your daily life?   1   2   3   4   5

5. Have you sought advice or thought about seeking advice about the problem from a friend?   1   2   3   4   5

Scoring

1. Determining whether there is a sexual problem in your relationship is the critical first step. The amount of time you spend worrying or thinking about the problem is an indicator of its seriousness. A high score here indicates greater seriousness and a greater need to address the problem. For example, if you feel anxious much of the day as you visualize what may happen later that evening, you need to address the problem.

2. Does the problem affect how you feel about your body? Does it damage your ability to develop relationships? For example, do you avoid intimate relationships out of fear that a sexual encounter will embarrass you? A high score on this question indicates that this problem may be damaging your self-esteem and your ability to develop healthy relationships.

3. People often complain that their partner does not understand the depth of their frustration or anxiety about a sexual problem. A high score here indicates fear or reluctance to discuss the issue with your partner. Sexual problems affect both partners and have to be addressed by both. Fear and withdrawal isolate you and increase the distance in the relationship.

4. A high score on this question is a warning that the problem is affecting areas of your life other than your sexual relationship. For example, a preoccupation with feelings of sexual inadequacy may interfere with your ability to concentrate at work or make you feel depressed or short-tempered at home. These feelings can snowball into overall dissatisfaction with the relationship and eventually destroy it. Sexual dissatisfaction is a primary cause of divorce in the United States and Canada.

5. Seeking advice about a sexual problem from a friend is probably not a good idea. Many partners would consider it a betrayal of trust. Discussion of sexual problems is best kept within the relationship. If you cannot resolve the problem by yourselves, first rule out physical or medical causes and then seek help from a counselor or sex therapist. A valuable source for referrals is the American Association of Sex Educators, Counselors, and Therapists.

SOURCE: Adapted from *The Sexual Male: Problems and Solutions,* by R. Milstein and J. Slowinski, 1999, New York: W. W. Norton & Company.

Add It Up!

If you are sexually active, are you and your partner at risk for an unintended pregnancy? If you or your partner does become pregnant, are there likely to be difficulties during pregnancy or health problems in your child? And have you thought about your options if you or your partner should become pregnant? Answer the following questions to assess your risks.

1. Have you ever felt pressured in a relationship to have sex when you did not want to do so?   Yes   No

2. In your relationships, do you feel you can express your views with a partner and have him or her respect your opinion?   Yes   No

3. Do you always avoid having sex while under the influence of drugs or alcohol?   Yes   No

4. Do you discuss your partner's and your own history of sexually transmitted diseases before initiating sexual contact?   Yes   No

5. If you have had an STD in the past, has it been completely treated?   Yes   No

6. Do you discuss your partner's and your own thoughts and feelings about unintended pregnancy before initiating sexual contact?   Yes   No

7. Do you know your partner's thoughts about having children in the future?   Yes   No

8. Do you use an effective method of contraception every time you have sexual intercourse?   Yes   No

9. Do you use a method of contraception that protects you against STDs?   Yes   No

10. If you are a woman, do you get the recommended amount of folic acid in your diet or with supplements?   Yes   No

11. If you are a woman, do you avoid smoking, drinking, and using recreational drugs?   Yes   No

12. Are you between the ages of 18 and 35?   Yes   No

13. Do you know if you are at risk for sickle cell disease, Tay-Sachs disease, or cystic fibrosis?   Yes   No

14. Do you know your family health history for congenital birth defects, including Down syndrome?   Yes   No

15. If you become pregnant, do you know what your three choices are?   Yes   No

16. If you are considering parenthood, do you feel ready—in terms of your financial resources, educational goals, relationship status, and emotional maturity—to have a baby at this point in your life?   Yes   No

17. Is either abortion or adoption an acceptable choice for you?   Yes   No

If you answered yes to 12 or more questions, you are well educated about communicating with your partners and knowing your risks for unintended pregnancy and the possible outcomes. If you answered yes to 9–11 questions, you are probably taking some risks; it would be a good idea to learn more about your own health and communication with partners. If you answered yes to fewer than 9 questions, you are taking significant risks and may be on your way to an unintended pregnancy.

Add It Up!

Many people think they can judge the likelihood that someone is infected with HIV by how the person looks or whether the person is in a high-risk group. In fact, risk is determined by behaviors, not appearance or membership in a group. Answer the following questions to find out whether your behaviors, past or present, have put you at risk for contracting HIV infection.

Your past behaviors

1. Did you receive a blood transfusion or other blood product before 1985?

2. Have you ever had sex?

3. Have you ever had sex with someone whose HIV status you didn't know?

4. Have you ever had sex while under the influence of drugs or alcohol?

5. Have you ever exchanged sex for drugs or money?

6. Have you ever had sex with a prostitute?

7. Have you had sex with more than one person during your lifetime?

8. Have you ever had unprotected sex (sex without a condom)?

9. Have you ever been the recipient in anal sex?

10. Have you ever had a sexual partner who has been the recipient in anal sex?

11. Have you ever had a sexually transmitted disease?

12. Have you ever had a genital injury (such as a tear or scrape) occur during sex?

13. Have you ever had an injection drug user as a sexual partner?

14. Have you ever used injection drugs?

15. Have you ever used the same needle that someone else used to inject drugs?

16. Have you ever worked in a health care setting?

17. Have you ever been exposed to someone else's blood or body fluids (such as vaginal secretions or semen)?

18. If so, did the fluid make contact with a break in your skin, with your eyes, or with mucous membranes (such as the mouth)?

19. Have you ever accidentally been stuck with a needle contaminated with someone else's blood?

Your current behaviors

1. Are you sexually active?

2. Do you have sex with partners whose HIV status you don't know?

3. Do you sometimes have sex while under the influence of alcohol or drugs?

4. Do you have sex with prostitutes?

5. Do you exchange sex for drugs or money?

6. Do you have sex with multiple partners (even if you tend to have only one partner at any given time)?

7. Do you ever have unprotected sex (sex without a condom)?

8. Are you the recipient in anal sex?

9. Do you have a sexual partner who has been the recipient in anal sex?

10. Do you have rough sex or sex without lubrication, so that genital injury could occur?

11. Do you have an injection drug user as a sexual partner?

12. Do you use injection drugs?

13. Do you share needles for injection drug use?

14. Do you work in a health care setting?

If you answered yes to more than three questions about your past behaviors, there is a possibility that you have been infected with HIV, and you should consider getting tested. If you answered yes to three or more questions about your current behaviors, you are putting yourself at risk for HIV infection. Although you can't eliminate all risk in life, you can improve your chances by practicing safer sex (using a condom), avoiding injection drug use, and using universal precautions if you work in a health care setting.

Add It Up!

The National Heart, Lung, and Blood Institute, a division of the National Institutes of Health, used data from the Framingham Heart Study to create an assessment that can be used to determine your risk of developing coronary heart disease in the next 10 years. Evaluate yourself on each of the risk factors (Steps 1–6), enter and add your points (Step 7), and find out your risk (Step 8). You can compare your risk to that of a man or woman the same age as you with average and low risk (Step 9). If your risk is higher than you would like it to be, make sure you are practicing the healthy lifestyle habits described in the chapter.

Step 1

Age	
Years	Points
30-34	–9
35-39	–4
40-44	0
45-49	3
50-54	6
55-59	7
60-64	8
65-69	8
70-74	8

Step 2

Total Cholesterol		
(mg/dl)	(mmol/L)	Points
<160	≤4.14	–2
160-199	4.15-5.17	0
200-239	5.18-6.21	1
240-279	6.22-7.24	1
≥280	≥7.25	3

Key	
Color	Risk
Green	Very low
White	Low
Yellow	Moderate
Rose	High
Red	Very high

Step 3

HDL - Cholesterol		
(mg/dl)	(mmol/L)	Points
<35	≤0.90	5
35-44	0.91-1.16	2
45-49	1.17-1.29	1
50-59	1.30-1.55	0
≥60	≥1.56	–3

Step 4

Blood Pressure					
Systolic (mmHg)	Diastolic (mmHg)				
	<80	<80	<80	<80	<80
<120	–3 pts				
120–129		0 pts			
130–139			0 pts		
140–159				2 pts	
≥160					3 pts

Note: When systolic and diastolic pressures provide different estimates for point scores, use the higher number.

Step 5

Diabetes	
	Points
No	0
Yes	4

Step 6

Smoker	
	Points
No	0
Yes	2

Risk estimates were derived from the experience of NHLBI's Framingham Heart Study, a predominantly Caucasian population in Massachusetts, USA.

Step 7 Sum from steps 1–6.

Adding Up the Points	
Age	_____
Total Cholesterol	_____
HDL Cholesterol	_____
Blood Pressure	_____
Diabetes	_____
Smoker	_____
Point Total	_____

Step 8 Determine CHD risk from point total.

CHD Risk	
Point Total	10-Yr CHD Risk
≤–2	1%
–1	2%
0	2%
1	2%
2	3%
3	3%
4	4%
5	4%
6	5%
7	6%
8	7%
9	8%
10	10%
11	11%
12	13%
13	15%
14	18%
15	20%
16	24%
≥17	≥27%

Step 9 Compare to women of the same age.

Comparative Risk		
Age (years)	Average 10-Yr CHD Risk	Low* 10-Yr CHD Risk
30-34	<1%	<1%
35-39	1%	<1%
40-44	2%	2%
45-49	5%	3%
50-54	8%	5%
55-59	12%	7%
60-64	12%	8%
65-69	13%	8%
70-74	14%	8%

*Low risk was calculated for a woman the same age, normal blood pressure, total cholesterol 160–199 mg/dL, HDL cholesterol 55 mg/dL, nonsmoker, no diabetes.

Add It Up!

The more risk factors you have for a particular cancer, the greater the likelihood that you will develop that cancer. In the lists below for six common cancers—lung, colon, breast, prostate, cervical, and melanoma—check any risk factors that apply to you. The more items you check, the more important it is that you adopt healthy lifestyle behaviors and have regular screening tests. There is no score.

Lung cancer risk factors

_____ Age greater than 40

_____ Family history of lung cancer

_____ Smoking cigarettes

_____ Smoking cigars

_____ Exposure to environmental tobacco smoke

_____ Exposure to air pollution

_____ Exposure to workplace chemicals

_____ Fewer than three servings of vegetables per day

_____ Fewer than three servings of fruit per day

Colon cancer risk factors

_____ Age greater than 50 (average age at diagnosis: 73)

_____ Family history of colon cancer

_____ Overweight

_____ More than one serving of red meat per day

_____ Fewer than three servings of vegetables per day

_____ More than one alcoholic drink per day

_____ Less than 30 minutes of physical activity per day

_____ Having inflammatory bowel disease for 10 years or more

Lower risk associated with:

- Taking a multivitamin with folate every day
- Taking birth control pills for at least 5 years
- Taking postmenopausal hormones for at least 5 years
- Taking aspirin regularly for more than 15 years
- Having regular screening tests

Breast cancer risk factors

_____ Age greater than 40 (average age at diagnosis: 62)

_____ Female sex

_____ Family history of breast cancer

_____ Jewish ethnicity, especially Ashkenazi descent

_____ Overweight

_____ Fewer than three servings of vegetables per day

_____ More than two alcoholic drinks per day

_____ Having had hyperplasia (benign breast disease)

Longer exposure to estrogen:

_____ Early age at menarche

_____ Older age at birth of first child

_____ Older age at menopause

_____ Fewer than two children

_____ Breastfeeding for less than one year combined for all pregnancies

_____ Currently taking birth control pills

_____ Taking postmenopausal hormones for 5 years or more

Prostate cancer risk factors

_____ Age greater than 55

_____ Family history of prostate cancer

_____ Five or more servings per day of foods containing animal fat

_____ Having had a vasectomy

_____ African American ethnicity

Lower risk associated with:

- Asian ethnicity
- At least one serving per day of tomato-based food

Cervical cancer risk factors

_____ Older age (average age at diagnosis: 47)

_____ Smoking cigarettes

_____ Having had sex at an early age

_____ Having had many sexual partners

_____ Having had an STD, especially HPV

_____ Having given birth to two or more children

Lower risk associated with:

- Using a condom or diaphragm on every occasion of sexual intercourse
- Having regular Pap tests

Melanoma risk factors

_____ Older age (average age at diagnosis: 57)

_____ Family history of melanoma

_____ Light-colored hair and eyes

_____ Having had severe, repeated sunburns in childhood

_____ Exposure to ultraviolet radiation

_____ Taking immunosuppressive drugs (for example, after organ transplant)

Lower risk associated with:

- Protecting the skin from the sun
- Regular self-examination of the skin

SOURCE: Adapted from "Your Disease Risk," Harvard Center for Cancer Prevention, www.yourdiseaserisk.harvard.edu.

Informed consumers share important information with their health care providers and don't hesitate to ask questions. Use the following checklists to make sure you are working effectively with your health care provider, whether a conventional provider or a CAM practitioner.

When seeing a health care provider, do you share the following information?

_____ I have allergies; I am allergic to _____.

_____ I am pregnant or trying to get pregnant.

_____ I am breastfeeding.

_____ I have other medical problems.

_____ I have other symptoms.

_____ I am taking other medications (prescription, over-the-counter, dietary supplements, herbal remedies).

_____ I am being treated, or plan to seek treatment, by another health care provider.

When seeing a CAM practitioner, do you ask the following questions?

_____ How does this treatment work?

_____ Will it be effective for my condition?

_____ Are there any scientific studies supporting the use of this treatment for my condition? Where can I read about them?

_____ What improvements can I expect to see and when?

_____ What risks are associated with the treatment?

_____ Does the treatment have side effects?

_____ How long will treatment last, and how many treatments will I need?

_____ How much do treatments cost?

_____ Is this treatment covered by health insurance?

_____ What is your background in this type of therapy?

_____ Are providers in your field licensed or certified by the state or a professional organization?

_____ Is there a Web site I can visit for more information on this therapy?

When being given a prescription for a medication or an herbal remedy, do you ask the following questions?

_____ For what condition of mine are you prescribing this medicine?

_____ What is this medicine supposed to do?

_____ How do I take this medicine?

- What is the administration route?
- How much do I take?
- How often do I take it?
- At what time of the day?
- With meals or without food?
- How long should I take it?

_____ What should I do if I miss a dose?

_____ When will the medicine begin to work?

_____ How will I know if the medicine is working?

_____ What should I do if it doesn't seem to work?

_____ What side effects should I watch for?

- What should I do if they occur?
- How long will they last?
- How can I reduce the side effects?

_____ While using this medicine, should I avoid:

- Driving or operating machines?
- Drinking alcohol?
- Eating certain foods?
- Taking certain medications (prescription, over-the-counter, dietary supplements, herbal remedies)?

_____ Are there any other precautions?

_____ How should I store the medicine?

- At room temperature?
- In the refrigerator?
- Away from heat, sunlight, or humidity?

_____ Can I get refills? How many?

_____ Are there any special instructions about how to use this medicine?

When taking medication, do you follow these precautions?

_____ I take the medication exactly as directed.

_____ I do not share medications with anyone else, even if they have a similar condition.

_____ I do not leave my medications where children or pets can get them.

_____ I discard unused or expired medications.

_____ I know what to do in case of an overdose by myself or a child.

_____ I keep the telephone numbers of my health care provider and pharmacy handy.

_____ I keep the telephone number of the poison control center handy (800-222-1212).

SOURCE: Data from "Just Ask! A Dozen Questions to Help You Understand Your Medicines," U.S. Pharmacopeia, www.usp.org.

Add It Up!

Violence does not have to be part of your everyday life. To see how well you are protecting yourself from unsafe situations, consider the following statements and decide whether each one is always, sometimes, or never true for you.

General Safety Considerations	Always	Sometimes	Never
I am aware of my surroundings.			
I tell someone where I'm going whenever I leave home.			
I'm careful about giving personal information or my daily schedule to people I don't know.			
I vary my daily routine and walking patterns.			
If I walk at night, I walk with others.			
Auto Safety	**Always**	**Sometimes**	**Never**
I look in the backseat before I get in my car.			
I look around before parking, stopping, or getting into or out of my car.			
I keep my car doors locked at all times.			
I have a plan of action in case my car breaks down.			
I scan ahead of me and behind me, with my mirrors, for potential dangers.			
I avoid dangerous, high-risk places whenever possible.			
If hit from behind, I drive to the nearest police station or well-lit, populated area, motioning for the person who hit me to follow.			
If I notice anyone loitering near my car, I go straight to a safe place and call the police.			
I never hitchhike.			
ATM Safety	**Always**	**Sometimes**	**Never**
I avoid using ATMs at night.			
I try to take someone with me when I use an ATM.			
I look for suspicious people or activity before entering or driving into an ATM area.			
I do not write my personal identification number on any paper I carry with me.			
I take all my ATM and credit card receipts with me to avoid leaving behind personal information.			
Violence, Rape, and Homicide	**Always**	**Sometimes**	**Never**
I carefully limit my alcohol intake at parties.			
I do not drink alcohol on a first date.			

	Always	Sometimes	Never
I refuse to be with anyone who seems violent.			
I do not allow anyone to strike me.			
I don't stay around anyone who has a gun and is drinking alcohol or using other drugs.			
I break off any relationship that is verbally or physically abusive.			
Ramps and Parking Lots	**Always**	**Sometimes**	**Never**
I park in well-lit areas.			
I avoid walking down ramps in parking lots if there are other options.			
I keep my arms as free as possible when walking to my car.			
I check the backseat of my car before getting in.			
Public Transportation	**Always**	**Sometimes**	**Never**
While waiting for transportation, I am aware of my immediate surroundings.			
While waiting for transportation, I place myself so that I am protected from behind.			
I hold items under my arm so that they will be difficult to grab.			
While riding on buses or trains, I look aware and alert.			

Scoring

Give yourself 3 points for each "Always" answer, 2 points for each "Sometimes," and 0 points for each "Never."

Your Score	Your Risk
90–99	You are probably safe as long as you continue to follow these precautions.
80–89	You may need to reexamine some of your habits and make changes to improve your safety.
79 or less	You may need to make significant changes in your habits to improve your safety.

SOURCE: Adapted from *Wellness: Concepts and Applications,* 5th ed., by D. J. Anspaugh, M. H. Hamrick, and F. D. Rosato. Copyright © 2005 The McGraw-Hill Companies. Reprinted by permission of The McGraw-Hill Companies.

Add It Up!

The National Highway Traffic Safety Administration describes an aggressive driver as someone who "commits a combination of moving traffic offenses so as to endanger other persons or property." The NHTSA recommends avoiding the challenges and confrontations of such risk drivers. Do you ever exhibit any of the behaviors of an aggressive driver? To find out, answer yes or no to the following questions:

		Yes	No
1.	Overtake other vehicles only on the left?	___	___
2.	Avoid blocking passing lanes?	___	___
3.	Yield to faster traffic by moving to the right?	___	___
4.	Keep to the right as much as possible on narrow streets and at intersections?	___	___
5.	Maintain appropriate distance when following other motorists, bicyclists, and motorcyclists?	___	___
6.	Leave an appropriate distance between your vehicle and the one you have passed when cutting in after passing?	___	___
7.	Yield to pedestrians?	___	___
8.	Come to a complete stop at stop signs and before making a right turn on red?	___	___
9.	Stop for red traffic lights?	___	___
10.	Approach intersections and pedestrians slowly to show your intention and ability to stop?	___	___
11.	Follow right-of-way rules at four-way stops?	___	___
12.	Drive below posted speed limits when conditions warrant?	___	___
13.	Drive at slower speeds in construction zones?	___	___
14.	Maintain speeds appropriate for conditions?	___	___
15.	Use vehicle turn signals for all turns and lane changes?	___	___
16.	Make eye contact and signal intentions when necessary?	___	___
17.	Acknowledge intentions of others?	___	___

		Yes	No
18.	Use your horn sparingly around pedestrians, at night, and near hospitals?	___	___
19.	Avoid unnecessary use of high-beam headlights?	___	___
20.	Yield and move to the right for emergency vehicles?	___	___
21.	Refrain from flashing headlights to signal a desire to pass?	___	___
22.	Drive trucks at posted speeds and in the correct lanes, changing lanes at proper speeds?	___	___
23.	Make slow U-turns?	___	___
24.	Maintain proper speeds around roadway crashes?	___	___
25.	Avoid returning inappropriate gestures?	___	___
26.	Avoid challenging other drivers?	___	___
27.	Try to get out of the way of aggressive drivers?	___	___
28.	Refrain from using high-occupancy-vehicle or carpool lanes to pass vehicles?	___	___
29.	Focus on driving and avoid distracting activities such as smoking, using a cell phone, reading, or shaving?	___	___
30.	Avoid driving when drowsy?	___	___
31.	Avoid blocking the right-hand turn lane?	___	___
32.	Avoid taking more than one parking space?	___	___
33.	Avoid parking in a disabled space if you are not disabled?	___	___
34.	Avoid letting your door hit the car parked next to you?	___	___
35.	Avoid stopping in the road to talk with a pedestrian or other driver?	___	___
36.	Avoid playing loud music that can be heard in neighboring cars?	___	___

Scoring

Count the number of "no" answers and use the following ranges to determine your level of hostility on the road.

1–3 Excellent. You are a responsible driver who behaves like an adult on the road.

4–7 Good. Pay attention to improving in your "no" areas.

8–11 Fair. You need to reevaluate your dangerous behaviors.

12+ Poor. You need to change your aggressive driving habits; you are endangering yourself and others.

SOURCE: National Highway Traffic Safety Administration, www.nhtsa.dot.gov.

Add It Up!

Do you have a lifestyle that promotes the health of the environment, or are you contributing to pollution and waste? Answer the following statements by indicating whether each one is true for you regularly, sometimes, or never.

	Regularly	Sometimes	Never
1. I keep my car in good operating condition and get oil or fluid leaks fixed immediately.	___	___	___
2. I use mass transit, walk, or bike instead of using my car.	___	___	___
3. I don't allow people to smoke in my home, and I make sure my home is well ventilated.	___	___	___
4. I store and dispose of household cleaners, solvents, and pesticides properly.	___	___	___
5. I recycle plastic, glass, aluminum cans, newspapers, and paper products.	___	___	___
6. I turn off lights when leaving a room.	___	___	___
7. I buy products with the least amount of packaging.	___	___	___
8. I take my own cloth shopping bag to the grocery store instead of using the store's paper or plastic bags.	___	___	___
9. I use rechargeable batteries and recycle them batteries after their useful life period is over.	___	___	___
10. I use cloth dish towels and washable sponges rather than paper products.	___	___	___
11. I avoid turning on my car air conditioner.	___	___	___
12. I water my lawn and/or outdoor plants early in the morning or in the evening.	___	___	___
13. I wear a sweater at home when it's cold rather than raise the thermostat.	___	___	___
14. I do not let tap water run continuously when I shave and/or brush my teeth.	___	___	___
15. I use compact fluorescent bulbs in lamps and lighting fixtures.	___	___	___
16. I try to produce as little garbage as possible.	___	___	___
17. I participate in community cleanup days.	___	___	___
18. I read labels on household products and buy the least toxic ones available.	___	___	___
19. I run the washing machine and the dishwasher only with full loads.	___	___	___
20. I write to my local and state elected officials to support environmentally friendly legislation.	___	___	___

Scoring

Give yourself 2 points for each activity you do regularly, 1 point for each activity you do sometimes, and 0 points for each activity you never do.

Interpretation

35–40   Very environmentally friendly. You are helping to heal the planet. Keep up the great work.

30–34   Above average. Your lifestyle contributes to a healthy environment.

25–29   Average. You are on the right track, but you can do more.

20–24   Below average. Look for ways to improve your record.

Under 20   Environmentally unfriendly. There are many changes you can make to develop a more environmentally friendly lifestyle.

44. Kübler-Ross, E. (1997). *On death and dying.* New York: Simon & Schuster Adult Publishing Group.

45. Moss, E., & Dobson, K. (2006). Psychology, spirituality and end of life care: An ethical integration. *Canadian Psychology, 47* (4), 284–299.

46. Can you die of a broken heart? (2002, January). *Harvard Mental Health Letter.*

47. Zamora, D. (2003). Death from a broken heart. www.WebMd.com.

48. Gesensway, D. (1998, May). Talking about end-of-life issues. *ACP Observer.*

49. Oliver, S. L. (1998). *What the dying teach us: Lessons on living.* Binghamton, NY: The Haworth Press.

50. Braude, S. (2003). *Immortal remains: The evidence for life after death.* Lanham, MD: Rowman & Littlefield.

51. Evidence of "life after death" (2000, October 23). BBC News. http://news.bbc.co.uk.

Chapter 5

1. American Psychological Association. (2007). *Stress in America.* Washington, DC: American Psychological Association.

2. Blonna, R. (2005). *Coping with stress in a changing world* (3rd ed.). New York: McGraw-Hill.

3. Benson, H. (1993). The relaxation response. In D. P. Goleman & J. Gurin (Eds.), *Mind-body medicine: How to use your mind for better health* (pp. 233–257). Yonkers, NY: Consumer Reports Books.

4. Selye, H. (1956). *The stress of life.* New York: McGraw-Hill.

5. Hafen, B. Q., Karren, K. J., Frandsen, K. J., & Smith, N. L. (1996). *Mind/body health: The effects of attitudes, emotions, and relationships.* Boston: Allyn & Bacon.

6. Stress: It is deadly. (2005). www.holisticonline.com.

7. Benson, H. (2006). *Stress Management: Techniques for preventing and easing stress.* Cambridge, MA: Harvard Medical School Press.

8. Kiecolt-Glaser, J. K., et al. (2002). Psychoneuroimmunology: Psychological influences on immune function and health. *Journal of Consulting and Clinical Psychology, 70,* 537–547.

9. Wittstein, I. S., et al. (2005). Neurohumoral features of myocardial stunning due to sudden emotional stress. *New England Journal of Medicine, 352* (6), 539–548.

10. Girdano, D. A., Dusek, D. E., & Everly, G. S., Jr. (2005). *Controlling stress and tension* (7th ed.). San Francisco: Benjamin Cummings.

11. Whitehead, W. E. (1993). Gut feelings: Stress and the GI tract. In D. P. Goleman & J. Gurin (Eds.), *Mind-body medicine: How to use your mind for better health* (pp. 161–176). Yonkers, NY: Consumer Reports Books.

12. National Institute of Diabetic and Digestive and Kidney Diseases. (2006). *Irritable bowel syndrome.* Rockville, MD: Author.

13. American Psychiatric Association. (2000). *Diagnostic and statistical manual of mental disorders* (4th ed., Text Revision [*DSM-IV-TR*]). Washington, DC: American Psychiatric Association Press.

14. Friedman, M., & Rosenman, R. H. (1982). *Type A behavior and your heart.* New York: Fawcett Books.

15. Williams, R. (1989). *The trusting heart: Great news about type A behavior.* New York: Random House.

16. Seligman, M. (1998). *Learned optimism: How to change your mind and your life.* New York: Pocket Books.

17. Kobasa, S. O. (1984, September). How much stress can you survive? *American Health,* 71–72.

18. Maddi, S. (2002). The story of hardiness: Twenty years of theorizing, research and practice. *Consulting Psychology: Practice & Research, 54* (3), 175–185.

19. Holmes, T., & Rahe, R. (1967). The social readjustment rating scale. *Journal of Psychosomatic Research, 11,* 213–218.

20. Segerstrom, S. C., & Miller, G. E. (2004). Psychological stress and the human immune system: A meta-analytic study of 30 years of inquiry. *Psychological Bulletin, 130* (4), 610–630.

21. Greenberg, J. (1984). A study of the effects of stress on the health of college students: Implications for school health education. *Health Education, 15,* 11–15.

22. Greenberg, J. (1981). A study of stressors in the college student population. *Health Education, 12,* 8–12.

23. American College Health Association. (2007). American College Health Association national college health assessment spring 2006 reference group data report (abridged). *Journal of American College Health, 55* (4), 198.

24. Reisberg, L. (2000, January 18). Students' stress is rising, especially among young women. *Chronicle of Higher Education,* A49–A52.

25. Gleick, J. (2000). *Faster: The acceleration of just about everything.* New York: Vintage Books.

26. Kraft, U. (2006, June–July). Burned out. *Scientific American,* pp. 29–33.

27. Pines, A. M. (1993). Burnout, an existential perspective. In W. B. Schaufeli, C. Maslach, & T. Marek (Eds.), *Professional burnout: Recent developments in theory and research.* Philadelphia: Taylor & Francis.

28. Lyons, A. (2003). Economic downturns impact health. http://web.aces.uiuc.edu.

29. Shay, J. (1996, July/August). Shattered lives. *Family Therapy Networker,* pp. 46–54.

30. Meyer, I. H. (2003). Prejudice, social stress, and mental health in lesbian, gay and bisexual populations: Conceptual issues and research evidence. *Psychological Bulletin, 129* (5), 674–697.

31. Vaccaro, P. (2000, September). The 80/20 principle of time management. *Family Practice Management.*

32. Ornish, D. (1998). *Love and survival: 8 pathways to intimacy and health.* New York: Harper Perennial.

33. Sacks, M. H. (1993). Exercise for stress control. In D. P. Goleman & J. Gurin (Eds.), *Mind-body medicine: How to use your mind for better health* (pp. 315–327). Yonkers, NY: Consumer Reports Books.

34. Davis, M., McKay, M., & Eshelman, E. R. (2000). *The relaxation and stress reduction workbook* (5th ed.). Oakland, CA: New Harbinger Publications.

35. Schwartz, M., & Andrasik, F. (Eds.). (2003). *Biofeedback: A practitioner's guide* (3rd ed.). New York: Guilford Publications.

Chapter 6

1. National Sleep Foundation. (2006). 2005 Sleep in America poll, executive report. www.sleepfoundation.org.

2. National Sleep Foundation. (2005). Facts and stats. www.sleepfoundation.org.

3. Institute of Medicine. (2006). *Sleep disorders and sleep deprivation.* Washington, DC: National Academies Press.

4. Gangwisch, J. E., Heymsfield, S. B., Boden-Albala, B., et al. (2006). Short sleep deprivation as a risk factor for hypertension: Analyses of the First National Health and Nutrition Examination Survey. *Hypertension, 47,* 833–839.

5. Schenck, C. H. (2007). *Sleep: The mysteries, the problems and the solutions.* New York: Penguin Books.

6. Chokrovefy, T., Thomas, R. J., & Bhatt, M. (2005). *Atlas of sleep medicine.* San Diego, CA: Butterworth-Heinemann.

7. Zee, P. C., & Turek, F. W. (2006). Sleep and health. *Archives of Internal Medicine, 166* (16), 1686–1688.

8. Nilsson, J. P., Soderstrom, M., Karlson, S. U., et al. (2005). Less effective executive functioning after one night's sleep deprivation. *Journal of Sleep Research, 14* (1), 1–6.

9. Klauer, S. G., Dingus, T. A., Neale, V. L., Sudweeks, J. D., & Ramsey, D. J. (2006). *The impact of driver inattention on near-crash/crash risk: An analysis using the 100-car naturalistic driving study data* (DOT HS810594). Washington, DC: U.S. Department of Transportation.

10. Maruff, P., Falleti, M. G., Collie, A., et al. (2005). Fatigue-related impairment in the speed, accuracy and variability of psychomotor performance: Comparison with blood alcohol levels. *Journal of Sleep Research, 14* (1), 21–27.

11. Shen, J., Bolty, L. C. P., Chung, S. A., et al. (2005). Fatigue and shift work. *Journal of Sleep Research, 15* (1), 1–5.

12. Epstein, L. J. (2007). *A good night's sleep.* New York: McGraw-Hill.

13. Moore, R. Y. The neurobiology of sleep-wake regulation. www.medscape.com/viewarticle/491041.

14. Roehrs, T., Kapke, A., Roth, T., et al. (2006). Sex differences in the polysomnographic sleep of young adults: A community based study. *Sleep Medicine, 7* (1), 49–53.

15. State of the Science Panel. (2005). National Institutes of Health State of the Science Conference: Manifestations and management of chronic insomnia in adults, June 13–15. *Sleep, 28,* 1049–1057.

16. Kantrowitz, B. (2006, April 24). The quest for rest. *Newsweek,* pp. 51–56.

17. Dement, W. C., & Vaughn, C. (2000). *The promise of sleep.* New York: Delacorte Press/Random House.

18. Rosenthal, L. (2005). Excessive daytime sleepiness: From an unknown medical condition to a known public health risk. *Sleep Medicine, 6* (6), 485–486.

19. Rauchs, G., Desgranges, B., Foret, J., et al. (2005). The relationships between memory systems and sleep stages. *Journal of Sleep Research, 14* (2), 123–140.

20. Ferreni, A. F., & Ferreni, R. L. (2006). *Health in the later years.* New York: McGraw-Hill.

References

21. Ancoli-Israel, S. (2005). Normal sleep at different ages: Sleep in older adults. In *SRS Basics of Sleep Guide*. Westchester, IL: American Academy of Sleep Medicine.

22. National Sleep Foundation. (2007). Stressed-out American women have no time for sleep [press release]. www.sleepfoundation.org.

23. Chokroverty, S. (1999). *Sleep disorders medicine: Basic science, technical considerations, and clinical aspects* (2nd ed.). Boston: Butterworth-Heinemann.

24. Guilleninault, C., & Robinson, A. (2006). Central sleep apnea, upper airway resistance and sleep. *Sleep Medicine, 7* (2), 189–191.

25. Hiestand, D. M., Britz, P., Goldman, M., & Phillips, B. (2006). Prevalence of symptoms and risk of sleep apnea in the US population: Results from the National Sleep Foundation Sleep in America poll. *Chest, 130* (3), 780–786.

26. Wang, H., Newton, G. E., Floras, J. S., et al. (2007). Influence of obstructive sleep apnea on mortality in patients with heart failure. *Journal of American Cardiology, 49,* 1625–1631.

27. Artz, M. A., Young, T., Finn, L., et al. (2006). Sleepiness and sleep in patients with both systolic heart failure and obstructive sleep apnea. *Archives of Internal Medicine, 166,* 1716–1722.

28. American Academy of Sleep Medicine. (2005). *The international classification of sleep disorders*. Westchester, IL: American Academy of Sleep Medicine.

29. Practice parameters for the use of laser-assisted uvulopalatoplasty: An update for 2000. (2001). Position paper. *Sleep, 24* (5), 603–619.

30. Practice parameters for the treatment of narcolepsy: An update for 2000. (2001). Position paper. *Sleep, 24* (4), 451–456.

31. Wesenten, N. J., William, D., Kilgore, S., & Balkin, T. J. (2005). Performance and alertness effects of caffeine, dextroamphetamine, and modafinil during sleep deprivation. *Journal of Sleep Research, 14* (3), 255–266.

32. Boggan, B. Alcohol, chemistry and you: Ethanol and sleep. www.chemcases.com/alcohol/alc-09.htm.

33. Wetter, D. W., & Young, T. B. (1994). The relation between cigarette smoking and sleep disturbance. *Preventive Medicine, 23,* 328–334.

34. National Sleep Foundation. (2006). Sleep aids. www.sleepfoundation.org.

35. Maas, J. B. (1998). *Power sleep*. New York: Villard Books/Random House.

36. O'Hanlon, B. (2000). *Overcoming sleep disorders: A natural approach*. Freedom, CA: Crossing Press.

Chapter 7

1. Wardlaw, G. M., & Smith, A. M. (2006). *Contemporary nutrition*. New York: McGraw-Hill.

2. Wardlaw, G. M., Hampl, J. S., & DiSilvestro, R. A. (2008). *Perspectives in nutrition*. New York: McGraw-Hill.

3. Sizer, F., & Whitney, E. (2006). *Nutrition: Concepts and controversies*. Belmont, CA: Wadsworth/Thomson Learning.

4. Willet, D. C. (2005). Diet and cancer. *Journal of the American Medical Association, 293* (12), 233–234.

5. *Dietary reference intakes for energy, carbohydrate, fiber, fat, fatty acids, cholesterol, protein, and amino acids (macronutrients)*. (2002). Washington, DC: National Academies Press.

6. Park, Y., Hunter, D. J., Spielgelman, D., et al. (2005). Dietary fiber intake and risk of colorectal cancer. *Journal of the American Medical Association, 294* (2), 2849–2857.

7. Baron, J. A. (2005). Dietary fiber and colorectal cancer: An on-going saga. *Journal of the American Medical Association, 293* (22), 86–89.

8. U.S. Department of Agriculture. (2005). *2005 Dietary guidelines for Americans*. www.health.gov/dietaryguidelines.

9. Tholstrup, T., Raff, M., Basu, S., et al. (2006). Effects of butter high in ruminant trans and monounsaturated fatty acids on lipoproteins, incorporation of fatty acids into lipid classes, plasma c-reactive protein, oxidative stress, hemostatic variables, and insulin in healthy young men. *American Journal of Clinical Nutrition, 83* (2), 237–243.

10. Rasmussen, B. M., Vessey, B., Lusitupa, M., et al. (2006). Effects of dietary saturated, monounsaturated, and n-3fatty acids on blood pressure in healthy subjects. *American Journal of Clinical Nutrition, 83* (2), 221–226.

11. Mozafarrian, D., Katan, M. B., Scherio, A., et al. (2006). Trans fatty acids and cardiovascular disease. *New England Journal of Medicine, 354* (15), 1601–1613.

12. Harvard Medical School. (2007, February 13). The dish on fish. *Health Newsletter*. www.health.harvard.edu.

13. Schumann, K., Borch-Johnsen, B., Hentze, M. W., & Marx, J. M. (2002). Tolerable upper intakes for dietary iron set by the U.S. Food and Nutrition Board. *American Journal of Clinical Nutrition, 76* (3), 499–500.

14. Morris, C. D., & Carson, S. (2003). Routine vitamin supplementation to prevent cardiovascular disease: A summary of the evidence for the U.S. Preventive Services Task Force. *Annals of Internal Medicine, 139* (1), 56–70.

15. The antioxidant responsive element (ARE) may explain the protective effects of cruciferous vegetables on cancer. (2003). *Nutrition Reviews, 61* (7), 250–254.

16. Willett, C. W. (2001). *Eat, drink and be healthy*. New York: Simon & Schuster.

17. Munro, I. C., et al. (2003). Soy isoflavones: A safety review. *Nutrition Reviews, 61* (1), 1–33.

18. Giovannucci, E. (1999). Tomatoes, tomato-based products, lycopene and cancer: Review of the epidemiogic literature. *Journal of the National Cancer Institute, 91,* 317–331.

19. Nuovo, J. (1999). AHA statement on antioxidants and coronary disease. *American Family Physician, 59* (10).

20. USDA. (2004). Q&As, revision of the Food Guidance System. www.usda.gov.

21. U.S. Food and Drug Administration. (2007). Final rule promotes safe use of dietary supplements. www.fda.gov/consumer/updates/dietarysupps062207.html.

22. Sabate, J. (2003). The contribution of vegetarian diets to health and disease: A paradigm shift. *American Journal of Clinical Nutrition, 78* (3), 502–507.

23. Borta, S. (2006). Consumer perspectives on food labels. *American Journal of Clinical Nutrition, 83* (5), 1235S.

24. Jacobson, M. F. (2006). *Liquid candy: How soft drinks are harming Americans' health*. Washington, DC: Center for Science in the Public Interest.

25. Popkin, B. M., Armstrong, L. E., Brat, G. M., et al. (2006). A new proposed guidance system for beverage consumption in the United States. *American Journal of Clinical Nutrition, 83* (3), 529–542.

26. Popkin, B. M. (2006). Pour better or pour worse. Center for Science in the Public Interest *Nutrition Action Healthletter, 33* (5), 1–5.

27. High blood pressure: The end of an epidemic. (2000, December 3–9). *Nutrition Action Healthletter*.

28. Dahl, R. (2006). Food safety: Allergen labels take effect. *Environmental Health Perspectives, 114* (1), A24.

29. Bostwick, H. (2006). McDonald's french fry lawsuit: More than meets the fry. www.lawsuitsearch.com/product-liability/.

30. Liebman, B., & Schardt, D. (2006). Bar exam: Engergy bars flunk. Center for Science in the Public Interest *Nutrition Action Healthletter, 27* (6), 10–12.

31. Severson, K. (2006). Energy drinks are fueling concerns. *New York Times*, June 19, p. 9.

32. Barston, S. (2008). *Healthy fast food: Guide to healthy fast food restaurants*. www.helpguide.org/life/fast_food_nutrition.htm.

33. Use of nutritive and nonnutritive sweeteners. (1998). Position of the American Dietetic Association. *Journal of the American Dietetic Association, 98,* 581–687.

34. Schardt, D. (2007). Organic food: Worth the price. Center for Science in the Public Interest *Nutrition Action Healthletter, 34* (6), 1, 2–8.

35. Barrett, J., Jarvis, W. T., Kroger, M., & London, W. M. (2007). *Consumer health: A guide to intelligent decisions*. Dubuque, IA: Brown & Benchmark.

36. Castro, I. A., Barroso, L. P., & Sinnecker, P. (2005). Functional foods for coronary heart disease risk reduction: A meta-analysis using a multivariate approach. *American Journal of Clinical Nutrition, 82* (1), 32–40.

37. Taylor, C. L. (2004). Regulator's framework for functional foods and dietary supplements. *Nutrition Reviews, 62* (2), 55–59.

38. Centers for Disease Control and Prevention: Incidence of foodborne illnesses. (1999). Preliminary data from the foodborne disease active surveillance network (food net). *Morbidity and Mortality Weekly Report, 48* (9), 189–194.

39. Centers for Disease Control and Prevention, Division of Bacterial and Mycotic Diseases. *Escherichia coli O157:H7*. www.cdc.gov/nczved/dfbmd/disease_listing/stec_gi.html.

40. Centers for Disease Control and Prevention, Division of Bacterial and Mycotic Diseases. *Campylobacter infections*. www.cdc.gov/ncidod/dbmd/diseaseinfo/campylobacter_g.htm.

41. Fox, N. (1999). *It was probably something you ate*. New York: Penguin Books.

42. Greene, L. W., & Ottoson, J. M. (2001). *Community and population health*. Dubuque, IA: WCB/McGraw-Hill.

43. Food irradiation. (2000). *Journal of the American Dietetic Association, 100,* 246–253.

44. Brown, K. (2001). Seeds of concern. *Scientific American, 284* (4), 60–61.

Chapter 8

1. U.S. Department of Health and Human Services. (2005). Fact sheet: Physical activity and health. http://fitness.gov.

2. Corbin, C. B., & Pangrazi, R. (2000). *Definitions: Health fitness and physical activity.* President's Council on Physical Fitness and Sports, 3 (9), 1–8.

3. Warburton, D., Nicol, C. W., & Bredin, S. D. (2006). Health benefits of physical activity: The evidence. *Canadian Medical Association Journal, 174,* 801–809.

4. Holmes, M. D., Chen, W. Y., Feskanich, D., et al. (2005). Physical activity and survival after breast cancer diagnosis. *Journal of the American Medical Association, 173* (20), 2479–2486.

5. Irwin, M. L., McTiernan, A., Bernstein, L., et al. (2005). Relationships of obesity and physical activity with c-peptide, leptin and insulin-like growth factors in breast cancer survivors. *Cancer Epidemiology, Biomarkers, and Prevention, 14,* 2881–2888.

6. Simon, H. B. (2006). *The no sweat exercise plan.* New York: McGraw-Hill.

7. Finauls, J., Gerard, L., & Filaire, E. (2006). Oxidative stress: Relationships with exercise and training. *Journal of the American Medical Association, 36* (4), 327–358.

8. Katarina, B. (2005). Physical activity in the prevention and amelioration of osteoporosis in women: Interaction of mechanical, hormonal and dietary factors. *Sports Medicine, 35* (9), 779–830.

9. Bruunsgard, H. (2005). Physical activity modulation of systemic low-level inflammation. *Journal of the American Medical Association, 78,* 819–835.

10. Frontier, W. R. (2006). *Exercise in rehabilitation medicine.* Champaign, IL: Human Kinetics.

11. Jakicic, J. M., Marcus, B. H., Gallagher, K. I., Napolitano, M., & Lang, W. (2003). Effect of exercise duration and intensity on weight loss in overweight, sedentary women: A randomized trial. *Journal of the American Medical Association, 290* (1), 1377–1379.

12. Poon, L. W. (2006). *Active living, cognitive function and aging.* Champaign, IL: Human Kinetics.

13. U.S. Preventive Services Task Force. (2005). *Guide to clinical prevention services* (3rd ed.). Alexandria, VA: International Medical Publishing.

14. Center for Science in the Public Interest. (2005). While you wait: The cost of inactivity. *Nutrition Action Healthletter, 32* (10), 3–6.

15. Trine, M. R. (1999). Physical activity and quality of life. In J. Rippe (Ed.), *Lifestyle medicine.* Malden, MA: Blackwell Science.

16. American College of Sports Medicine. (2003). *ACSM Fitness Book* (3rd ed.). Champaign, IL: Human Kinetics.

17. Pate, R. R. (2007). Physical activity and public health. Updated recommendation for adults from the American College of Sports Medicine and the American Heart Association. *Circulation, 116,* 1081–1093. http://circ.ahajournals.org/cgi/reprint/circulationaha.107.185649.

18. Lee, I.-M., Sesso, H. D., Oguma, Y., et al. (2004). The "weekend warrior" and risk of mortality. *American Journal of Epidemiology, 160* (7), 636–641.

19. Larew, K., Hunter, G. R., Larson-Meyer, D. E., Newcomer, B. R., McCarthy, J. P., & Weinsier, R. L. (2003). Muscle metabolic function, exercise performance, and weight gain. *Medicine and Science in Sports and Exercise, 35* (2), 230–236.

20. American College of Sports Medicine. (1998). Position stand: Exercise and physical activity for older adults. *Medicine and Science in Sports and Exercise, 30,* 992–1008.

21. President's Council on Physical Fitness and Sports. (2005). *Progression and resistance training* (series 6, no. 3). Rockville, MD: U.S. Department of Health and Human Services.

22. American College of Sports Medicine. (2002). Position stand: Progression models in resistance training for healthy adults. *Medicine and Science in Sports and Exercise, 34* (3), 64–380.

23. Stoppani, J. (2006). *Encyclopedia of muscle and strength.* Champaign, IL: Human Kinetics.

24. Hunter, J. P., & Marshall, R. N. (2002). Effects of power and flexibility training on vertical jump technique. *Medicine and Science in Sports and Exercise, 34* (3), 478–486.

25. Kibler, W. B., Press, J., & Sciascia, A. (2006). The role of core stability in athletic function. *Sports Medicine, 36* (3), 189–198.

26. Benardot, D. (2006). *Advanced sports nutrition.* Champaign, IL: Human Kinetics.

27. Williams, M. H. (2005). *Nutrition for health, fitness and sport* (7th ed.). New York: McGraw-Hill.

28. Cardwell, G. (2006). *Gold medal nutrition.* Champaign, IL: Human Kinetics.

29. Schrier, I. (2005). When and how to stretch. *Physician and Sports Medicine, 33* (3), 22–26.

30. Sports Fitness Advisor. (2008, July). PNF stretching. www.sport-fitness-advisor.com/pnfstretching.html.

31. Centers for Disease Control and Prevention. (2006). Adult participation in recommended levels of physical activity—United States 2001–2003. *Journal of the American Medical Association, 295* (9), 25–27.

32. Iknoian, T. (2005). *Fitness walking.* Champaign, IL: Human Kinetics.

33. Oguma, Y., & Shinoda-Tagawa, T. (2004). Physical activity decreases cardiovascular disease risk in women: Review and meta-analysis. *American Journal of Preventive Medicine, 26* (5), 407–418.

34. 10,000 Steps Program. (2003). Shape Up America. www.shapeup.org.

35. Tudor-Locke, C. E., & Myers, A. M. (2001). Methodological considerations for researchers and practitioners using pedometers to measure physical ambulatory patients. *Research Quarterly for Exercise and Sport, 72* (1), 1–12.

36. Harvard Medical School. (2006). A little bit at a time: Eating and exercising in bits and pieces. www.health.harvard.edu/fhg/updates/A-little-at-a-time-Eating-and-exercising-in-bits-and-pieces.shtml.

37. Eberle, S. G. (2000). *Endurance sports nutrition.* Champaign, IL: Human Kinetics.

38. Antol, J. D. (1999). High-altitude acclimatization and illness. In J. Rippe (Ed.), *Lifestyle medicine.* Malden, MA: Blackwell Science.

39. Schneider, M., Bernacsch, D., Weymann, J., Holle, R., & Bartsch, P. (2002). Acute mountain sickness: Influence of susceptibility, pre-exposure, and ascent rate. *Medicine and Science in Sports and Exercise, 34* (12), 1863–1867.

40. Schnirring, L. (2003). New hydration recommendations: Risk of hyponatremia plays a big role. *Physician and Sports Medicine, 31* (7), 15–18.

41. American College of Sports Medicine. (1996). Position stand: Heat and cold illness during distance running. *Medicine and Science in Sports and Exercise, 28,* i–x.

42. Schnirring, L. (2005). Experts issue hyponatremia consensus. *Physician and Sports Medicine, 33* (8), 18–19.

43. Linn, S. W., & Gong, H. (1999). Air pollution exercise, nutrition, and health. In J. Rippe (Ed.), *Lifestyle medicine.* Malden, MA: Blackwell Science.

44. Trost, S. G., & Pate, R. R. (1999). Physical activity in children and youth. In J. Rippe (Ed.), *Lifestyle medicine.* Malden, MA: Blackwell Science.

45. Schnirring, L. (2005). Groups endorse ECG screening for athletes. *Physician and Sports Medicine, 33* (3), 12–15.

46. Nieman, D. C. (1998). *The exercise-health connection.* Champaign, IL: Human Kinetics.

47. Nelson, M. E., et al. (2007). Physical activity and public health in older adults: Recommendation from the American College of Sports Medicine and the American Heart Association. *Circulation.* www.circ.ahajournals.org/cgi/reprint/circulationaha.107.185650v1.

48. Jones, J. C. (2005). *Physical activity instruction for older adults.* Champaign, IL: Human Kinetics.

49. Armitage, C. J. (2005). Can the theory of planned behavior predict the maintenance of physical activity? *Health Psychology, 24* (3), 235–245.

50. Blair, S. N., Dunn, A. L., Marcus, B. H., Carpenter, R. A., & Jaret, P. (2001). *Active living every day.* Champaign, IL: Human Kinetics.

51. Rafferty, A. P., Reeves, M. J., McGee, H. B., & Pirarnik, J. M. (2002). Physical activity patterns among walkers and compliance with public health recommendations. *Medicine and Science in Sports and Exercise, 34* (81), 1255–1261.

52. Centers for Disease Control and Prevention. (2005). Creating or improving access to places for physical activity is recommended to increase physical activity. www.thecommunityguide.org/pa/pa-int-create-access.pdf.

53. Duany, A. (n.d.). Smartcode: A comprehensive form-based planning ordinance. www.smartcodecentral.com.

54. Erving, R., et al. (2003). Relationship between urban sprawl and physical activity, obesity, mortality. *American Journal of Health Promotion, 8* (1), 47–52.

55. Mansnerus, L. (2003). New Jersey is running out of open land it can build on. *New York Times,* May 24. www.nytimes.com.

56. Centers for Disease Control and Prevention. (n.d.). Physical activity resources for health professionals: Active environments. www.cdc.gov/nccdphp/dnpa/physical/health_professionals/active_environments/index.htm.

Chapter 9

1. Ogden, C. L., Carroll, M. D., MacDowell, M. A., et al. (2007). Obesity among adults in the United States, no change since 2003–2004. *National Center for Health Statistics Data Brief, 1.* Hyattsville, MD: National Center for Health Statistics.

2. Centers for Disease Control and Prevention. (2008). U.S. obesity trends, 1985–2007. www.cdc.gov.

3. World Health Organization. (n.d.) Global strategy on diet, physical activity and health: Obesity and overweight. www.who.int/dietphysicalactivity/publications/facts/obesity/en/.

4. Ogden, C. L., Carroll, M. D., & Flegal, K. M. (2008). High body mass index for age among U.S. children and adolescents, 2003–2006. *Journal of the American Medical Association, 299*(20), 2401–2405.

5. Nader, P. R., O'Brien, M., Houts, R., et al. (2006). Identifying risk for obesity in early childhood. *Pediatrics, 118* (3), e594–e601.

6. National Heart, Lung, and Blood Institute, Obesity Education Initiative. (2007). Aim for a healthy weight: Information for patients and the public. www.nhlbi.nih.gov/health/public/heart/obesity/lose_wt/risk.htm.

7. National Center for Health Statistics. (n.d.) National Health and Nutrition Survey. 2000 CDC growth charts: United States. www.cdc.gov/growthcharts/.

8. Gallagher, D., Heymsfield, S. B., Heo, M., et al. (2000). Healthy percentage body fat ranges: An approach for developing guidelines based on body mass index. *American Journal of Clinical Nutrition, 72* (3), 694–701.

9. Bray, G. A. (2003). *An atlas of obesity and weight control.* New York: Parthenon Publishing Group.

10. Waller, D. K., Shaw, G. M., Rasmussen, S. A., et al. (2007). Prepregnancy obesity as a risk factor for structural birth defects. *Archives of Pediatrics and Adolescent Medicine, 161* (8), 725–814.

11. Manson, J. E., Bassuk, S. S., Hu, F. B., et al. (2007). Estimating the number of deaths due to obesity: Can the divergent findings be reconciled? *Journal of Women's Health, 16* (2), 168–176.

12. Field, B., Wren, A., Cooke, D., & Bloom, S. (2008). Gut hormones as potential new targets for appetite regulation and the treatment of obesity. *Drugs, 68* (2), 147–163.

13. Schulz, L. O., Bennett, P. H., Ravussin, E., et al. (2006). Effects of traditional and western environments on prevalence of type 2 diabetes in Pima Indians in Mexico and the U.S. *Diabetes Care, 29*, 1866–1871.

14. Nelsen, M. C., Neumark-Stzainer, D., Hannan, P. J., et al. (2006). Longitudinal and secular trends in physical activity and sedentary behavior during adolescence. *Pediatrics, 118* (6), e1627–e1634.

15. Gunderson, E., & Abrams, B. (2000). Epidemiology of gestational weight gain and body weight changes after pregnancy. *Epidemiology Reviews, 22* (2), 261–274.

16. Wang, Y., & Beydom, M. A. (2007). The obesity epidemic in the United States—Gender, age, socioeconomic, racial/ethnic, and geographic characteristics: A systematic review and meta-regression analysis. *Epidemiologic Review, 29* (1), 6–28.

17. Darmon, N. and Drewnowski, A. (2008). Does social class predict diet quality? *American Journal of Clinical Nutrition, 87*(5), 1107–1117.

18. French, S. A., Strory, M., & Jeffery, T. W. (2001). Environmental influences on eating and physical activity. *Annual Review of Public Health, 22*, 309–335.

19. Neilsen, S. J., & Popkin, B. M. (2003). Patterns and trends in food portion sizes 1977–1998. *Journal of the American Medical Association, 289*, 450–453.

20. National Center for Chronic Disease Prevention and Health Promotion, Division of Nutrition and Physical Activity. (2006). Do increased portion sizes affect how much we eat? (Research to Practice Series, No. 2.) Centers for Disease Control and Prevention. www.cdc.gov/nccdphp/dnpa/nutrition/pdf/portion_size_research.pdf.

21. Dietz, W. H., & Gortmaker, S. L. (2001). Preventing obesity in children and adolescents. *Annual Review of Public Health, 22*, 337–353.

22. Frank, L. D., Andresen, M. A., & Schmid, T. L. (2004). Obesity relationship with community design, physical activity and time spent in cars. *American Journal of Preventive Medicine, 27* (2), 87–96.

23. Papas, M. A., Alberg, A. J., Ewing, R., et al. (2007). The built environment and obesity. *Epidemiological Reviews, 29*, 129–143.

24. Holmes, G. (2006). Nielsen Media Research reports television's popularity is still growing. www.nielsenmedia.com/nc/portal/site/Public/menuitem.55dc65b4a7d5adff3f65936147a062a0/?vgnextoid=4156527aacccd010VgnVCM100000ac0a260aRCRD.

25. Marshall, S. J., Biddle, S. H., Gorely, T., et al. (2004). Relationship between media use, body fatness and physical activity in children and youth: A meta analysis. *International Journal of Obesity and Related Metabolic Disorders, 28* (10), 1238–1246.

26. Bowman, S. A. (2006). Television-viewing characteristics of adults: Correlations to eating practices and overweight and health status. *Preventing Chronic Disease* [serial online], April. www.cdc.gov/pcd/issues/2006/apr/05_0139.htm.

27. Christakis, N. A., & Fowler, J. H. (2007). The spread of obesity in a large social network over 32 years. *The New England Journal of Medicine, 357* (4), 370–379.

28. U.S. weight loss market to reach $58 billion in 2007. PRWeb Press Release. www.prwebdirect.com/releases/2007/4/prweb520127.php.

29. Tsai, A. G., & Wadden, T. A. (2005). Systematic review: An evaluation of major commercial weight loss programs in the United States. *Annals of Internal Medicine, 142* (1), 56–67.

30. Moyers, S. B. (2005). Medications as adjunct therapy for weight loss: Approved and off-label agents in use. *Journal of the American Dietetic Association, 105* (6), 948–959.

31. Rumsfeld, J. S., & Nallamothu, B. K. (2008). The hope and fear of rimonabant. *Journal of the American Medical Association, 299*, 1601–1602.

32. DeMaria, E. J. (2007). Bariatric surgery for morbid obesity. *The New England Journal of Medicine, 356* (21), 2176–2183.

33. National Association to Advance Fat Acceptance. www.naafa.org.

34. Spark, A. (2001). Health at any size: The self-acceptance non-diet movement. *Journal of the American Medical Association, 56* (2), 69–72.

35. Position of the American Dietetic Association: Total diet approach to communicating food and nutrition information. (2007). *Journal of the American Dietetic Association, 107*, 1224–1232.

36. Wansink, B., & Van Ittersum, K. (2007). Portion size me: Downsizing our consumption norms. *Journal of the American Dietetic Association, 107* (7), 1103–1106.

37. Hu, F. B., et al. (2003). Television watching and other sedentary behaviors in relation to risk of obesity and type 2 diabetes mellitus in women. *Journal of the American Medical Association, 289* (14), 1729–1880.

Chapter 10

1. National Eating Disorders Association. (2006). Statistics: Eating disorders and their precursors. www.nationaleatingdisorders.org.

2. Morris, A. M., & Katzman, D. K. (2003). The impact of the media on eating disorders in children and adolescents. *Adolescent Medicine, 14* (1), 109–118.

3. Derenne, J. L., & Beresin, E. V. (2006). Body image, media, and eating disorders. *Academic Psychiatry, 30* (3), 257–261.

4. Striegel-Moore, R. H., & Bulik, C. M. (2007). Risk factors for eating disorders. *American Psychologist, 62* (3), 181–198.

5. Agliata, D., & Tantleff-Dunn, S. (2004). The impact of media exposure on males' body image. *Journal of Social and Clinical Psychology, 23* (1), 7–22.

6. Grieve, F. G. (2007). A conceptual model of factors contributing to the development of muscle dysmorphia. *Eating Disorders, 15*, 63–80.

7. Cafri, G., Thompson, J. K., Ricciardell, L., & McCabe, M. (2005). Pursuit of the muscular ideal: Physical and psychological consequences and putative risk factors. *Clinical Psychology Review, 25* (2), 215–239.

8. Hoek, H. W., & van Hoeken, D. (2003). Review of the prevalence and incidence of eating disorders. *International Journal of Eating Disorders, 34*, 383–396.

9. Hudson, J. I., Hiripi, E., Pope, H. G., & Kessler, R. C. (2007). The prevalence and correlates of eating disorders in the National Comorbidity Survey Replication. *Biological Psychiatry, 61*, 348–358.

10. Shaw, H., Ramirez, L., Trost, A., Randall, P., Stice, E. (2004). Body image and eating disturbances across ethnic groups: More similarities than differences. *Psychology of Addictive Behaviors, 18* (1), 12–18.

11. Ricciardelli, L. A., McCabe, M. P., Williams, R. J., & Thompson, J. K. (2007). The role of ethnicity and culture in body image and disordered eating among males. *Clinical Psychology Review, 27*, 582–606.

12. Becker, A. E. (2007). Culture and eating disorders classification. *International Journal of Eating Disorders, 40* (Suppl. 3), S111–S116.

13. Toro, J., Galilea, B., Martinez-Mallen, E., et al. (2005). Eating disorders in Spanish female athletes. *International Journal of Sports Medicine, 26*, 693–700.

14. Bonci, C. M., Bonci, L. J., et al. (2008). National Athletic Trainers' Association position statement on preventing, detecting, and managing disordered eating. *Journal of Athletic Training, 43* (1), 80–108.

15. Fairburn, C. G., & Harrison, P. J. (2003). Eating disorders. *Lancet, 361*, 407–416.

16. Feldman, M. B., & Meyer, I. H. (2007). Eating disorders in diverse lesbian, gay and bisexual populations. *International Journal of Eating Disorders, 40* (3), 218–226.

17. Costin, C. (1999). *The eating disorder sourcebook: A comprehensive guide to causes, treatments and prevention of eating disorders.* Lincolnwood, IL: Lowell House.

18. American Psychiatric Association. (2000). *Diagnostic and statistical manual of mental disorders* (4th ed., text revision). Washington, DC: American Psychiatric Association.

19. Yager, Y. (2008). Binge eating disorder: The search for better treatments. *American Journal of Psychiatry, 165,* 4–6.

20. Wilfley, D. E., Bishop, M. E., Wilson, G. T., & Agras, A. S. (2007). Classification of eating disorders: Toward DSM-V. *International Journal of Eating Disorders, 40* (Suppl. 3), S123–S129.

21. Zipfel, S., Lowe, B., Reas, D. L., Deter, H. C., & Herzog, W. (2000). Long-term prognosis in anorexia nervosa: Lessons from a 21-year follow up study. *Lancet, 355,* 721.

22. Chavez, M., & Insel, T. R. (2007). Eating disorders; National Institute of Mental Health's perspective. *American Psychologist, 62* (3), 159–166.

23. American Society of Plastic Surgeons. (2007). 2000/2005/2006 National plastic surgery statistics. Cosmetic and reconstructive procedure trends. www.plasticsurgery.org/media/statistics/loader.cfm?url=/commonspot/security/getfile.cfm?&PageID=23628.

24. Mariwalla, K., & Dover, J. S. (2006). The use of lasers for decorative tattoo removal. *Skin Therapy Letter, 11* (5), 8–11.

Chapter 11

1. Wechsler, H., & Wuethrich, B. (2002). *Dying to drink: Confronting binge drinking on college campuses.* New York: Rodale Books.

2. National Campus Safety Awareness Month. (2006). High risk drinking. www.campussafetymonth.org/high_risk_drinking.

3. Weitzman, E., & Chen, Y. (2005). Risk modifying effect of social capital on heavy alcohol consumption, alcohol abuse, harms, and secondhand effects: National survey findings. *Journal of Epidemiology, 59* (4), 303–309.

4. American Pyschiatric Association. (2000). *Diagnostic and statistical manual of mental disorders* (4th ed., Text Revision [*DSM-IV-TR*]). Washington, DC: American Psychiatric Association Press.

5. National Institute on Alcohol Abuse and Alcoholism; National Institutes of Health. (2000). *Alcohol and health.* Washington, DC: U.S. Department of Health and Human Services.

6. U.S. Department of Health and Human Services. (1998). *Substance abuse among older adults* (Treatment Improvement Protocol, Vol. 26, Ch. 2). http://ncadistore.samhsa.gov/catalog/productDetails.aspx?ProductID=13287.

7. Ferrini, A. F., & Ferreni, R. L. (2008). *Health in the later years* (3rd ed.) New York: McGraw-Hill.

8. Ksir, C., Hart, C. L., & Ray, O. (2006). *Drugs, society, and human behavior* (11th ed.). New York: McGraw-Hill.

9. Office of Applied Studies. (2006). Alcohol and drug use: 2004–2005. *National Survey on Drug Use and Health* (DHHS Publication No. SMA 05-4061). Rockville, MD: U.S. Department of Health and Human Services.

10. Huff, R. M., & Kline, M. V. (1999). Health promotion in the context of culture. In R. M. Huff & M. V. Kline (Eds.), *Promoting health in multicultural populations.* Thousand Oaks, CA: Sage Publications.

11. Hodge, F. S., & Fredericks, L. (1999). American Indian and Alaska native populations in the United States: An overview. In R. M. Huff & M. V. Kline (Eds.), *Promoting health in multicultural populations.* Thousand Oaks, CA: Sage Publications.

12. Wild, T. C. (2002). Personal drinking and sociocultural drinking norms: A representative population study. *Journal of Studies on Alcohol, 63* (4), 469–475.

13. Morse, R. M., & Flavin, D. K. (1992). The definition of alcoholism: The Joint Committee of the National Council on Alcoholism and Drug Dependence, and the American Society of Addiction Medicine to Study the Definition and Criteria for the Diagnoses of Alcoholism. *Journal of the American Medical Association, 263,* 1012–1014.

14. Springer, K., & Kantrowitz, B. (2004, May 16). Alcohol's deadly triple threat. *Newsweek,* 90–102.

15. National Center on Addiction and Substance Abuse. (2007). *Wasting the best and the brightest: Substance abuse at America's colleges and universities.* New York: Columbia University.

16. Wechsler, H., Lee, J. E., Kuo, M., & Lee, H. (2000). College binge drinking in the 1990s: A continuing problem. Results of the Harvard School of Public Health 1999 College Alcohol Study. www.hsph.harvard.edu.

17. Wechsler, H. (2000). College binge drinking in the 1990s: A continuing problem. Results of the Harvard School of Public Health 1999 College Alcohol Study. *Journal of American College Health, 48,* 199–210.

18. Wechsler, H., Lee, J. E., Nelson, T. F., and Kuo, M. (2002). Underage college students: Drinking behavior, access to alcohol, and the influence of deterrence policies. Findings from the Harvard School of Public Health College Study. *Journal of American College Health, 50* (5), 223–236.

19. Costello, B. J., Anderson, B. J., & Stein, M. D. (2006). Heavy episodic drinking among adolescents: A test of hypotheses derived from control theory. *Journal of Drug and Alcohol Education, 50* (1), 35–55.

20. Okoro, C. A., Brewer, R. D., Darmi, T. S., Moriarity, D. G., Giles, W. H., & Mokdad, A. H. (2004). Binge drinking and health-related quality of life: Do popular perceptions match reality? *American Journal of Preventative Medicine, 26* (3), 230–233.

21. Nelson, T. F., Naimi, T. S., Brewer, R. D., et al. (2005). The state sets the rate: The relationship among state-specific college binge drinking rates, and selected state alcohol control policies. *American Journal of Public Health, 95* (3), 441–446.

22. Mohler-Kuo, M., Dowdall, G. W., Koss, M., et al. (2004). Correlates of rape while intoxicated in a national sample of college women. *Journal of Studies on Alcohol, 65* (1), 37–45.

23. Wechsler, H., Lee, J. E., Nelson, T. F., & Lee, H. (2001). Drinking levels, alcohol problems, and second-hand effects in substance-free college residences: Results of a national study. *Journal of Studies on Alcohol, 62* (1), 23–31.

24. Alcohol: Problems and Solutions Web site. (2007). Binge drinking. www2.potsdam.edu/hansondj/BingeDrinking.html.

25. Higher Education Center. (2000). Note to the field: On "binge drinking." www.higheredcenter.org/press-releases/001020.html.

26. Martins, M. P., Page, J. C., Mowry, S., et al. (2006). Differences between actual and perceived standard norms: An examination of alcohol use, drug use, and sexual behavior. *Journal of American College Health, 54* (5), 295–300.

27. Neighbors, C., Dillard, A. J., Lewis, M. L., et al. (2006). Normative misperceptions and temporal precedence of perceived norms and drinking. *Journal of Studies on Alcohol, 67* (2), 290–300.

28. Clapp, J., Lange, J. E., & Perkins, H. W. (2006). Success and failure in social norms interventions. *Journal of Studies on Alcohol, 67* (3), 482–485.

29. National Institute on Alcohol Abuse and Alcoholism. (2002). *A call to action: Changing the culture of drinking at U.S. colleges.* Washington, DC: U.S. Department of Health and Human Services.

30. Green, T. C., Lord, S., Thum, C., et al. (2005). My student body: A high-risk drinking prevention Web site for college students. *Journal of American College Health, 53* (6), 263–274.

31. Barry, K. L., & Blow, F. C. (2006). Substance safety. In S. Goring and J. Arnold (Eds.), *Health promotion in practice.* San Francisco: Jossey-Bass.

32. White, A. M. (2006). How does alcohol impair memory? www.duke.edu/~amwhite/Blackouts/blackouts14.html.

33. White, A. M. (2006). Alcohol-induced blackouts. www.duke.edu/~amwhite/Blackouts/blackouts4.html.

34. American Medical Association. (n.d.). Brain damage risks. www.ama-assn.org.

35. Sheffield, F. D., Dorkes, J., Del Boca, F., et al. (2005). Binge drinking and alcohol-related problems for prevention policy. *Journal of American College Health, 54* (3), 137–141.

36. U.S. Department of Agriculture (2005). *2005 Dietary guidelines for Americans.* www.health.gov/dietaryguidelines.

37. Chesson, H. W., Harrison, P., & Stall, R. (2003). Changes in alcohol consumption and in sexually transmitted disease incidence rates in the United States: 1983–1998. *Journal of Studies on Alcohol, 64* (5), 623–630.

38. Giancola, P. R. (2002). Alcohol-related aggression during the college years: Theories, risk factors, and policy implications. In National Institute on Alcohol Abuse and Alcoholism, *A call to action: Changing the culture of drinking at U.S. colleges.* Washington, DC: U.S. Department of Health and Human Services.

39. Simon, H. B. (2002). *The Harvard Medical School guide to men's health.* New York: The Free Press.

40. National Institute on Alcohol Abuse and Alcoholism. (2000). *10th special report to the U.S. Congress on alcohol and health.* Washington, DC: U.S. Department of Health and Human Services.

41. Vasilaki, E. I., Hosier, S., & Cox, W. M. (2006). The efficacy of motivational interviewing as in brief intervention for excessive drinking. *Alcohol and Alcoholism, 41* (3), 328–335.

42. Brink, S. (2001, May 7). Your brain on alcohol. *U.S. News & World Report,* 50–57.

43. Helmkamp, J. C., Hungerford, D. W., Williams, J. M., et al. (2003). Screening and brief intervention for alcohol problems among college students in a university hospital emergency department. *Journal of American College Health, 52* (1), 7–10.

44. Weitzman, E. L., & Nelson, T. F. (2004). College student drinking and the prevention paradox: Implications for prevention and harm reduction. *Journal of Drug Education, 34* (3), 247–266.

45. Peele, S. (2004, March/April). The new prohibitionists: Our attitudes toward alcoholism and doing more harm than good. *The Science News*, 14–19.

46. Oglivie, H. (2001). *Alternatives to abstinence: Controlled drinking and other approaches to managing alcoholism.* New York: Hatherleigh Press.

47. Wagenarr, A. C., & Toomey, T. L. (2000, March). Effects of minimum drinking age laws: Review and analyses of the literature from 1960 to 2000. *Journal of Studies of Alcohol.*

48. Williams, J., Chaloupka, F. J., & Wechsler, H. (2002). Are there differential effects of price and policy on college students' drinking intensity? *National Bureau of Economic Research I*, Working paper 8702.

49. Harwood, E. M., Erickson, D. J., Fabian L. E. A., et al. (2003). Effects of communities, neighborhoods and stores on retail pricing and promotion of beer. *Journal of Studies on Alcohol, 64* (5), 720–726.

Chapter 12

1. Substance Abuse and Mental Health Services Administration. (2007). *Results from the 2006 National Survey on Drug Use and Health: National Findings* (Office of Applied Studies, NSDUH Series H-32, DHHS Publication No. SMA 07-4293). Rockville, MD: Author.

2. National Center on Addiction and Substance Abuse. (2007). *Wasting the best and the brightest: Substance abuse at America's colleges and universities.* New York: Columbia University.

3. American Psychiatric Association. (2000). *Diagnostic and statistical manual of mental disorders* (4th ed., Text Revision [*DSM-IV-TR*]). Washington, DC: American Psychiatric Association Press.

4. Saal, D., Dong, Y., Bonci, A., & Malenka, R. C. (2003). Drugs of abuse and stress trigger a common synaptic adaptation in dopamine neurons. *Neuron, 37* (4), 577–582.

5. National Institute on Drug Abuse. (2007). Info-Facts: Crack and cocaine. www.nida.nih.gov/Infofacts/cocaine.html.

6. National Institute on Drug Abuse. (2006). Info-Facts: Methamphetamine. www.nida.nih.gov/InfoFacts/methamphetamine.html.

7. National Institute on Drug Abuse. (2006). InfoFacts: MDMA (Ecstasy). www.nida.nih.gov/Infofacts/ecstasy.html.

8. Ksir, C., Hart, C. L., & Ray, O. (2006). *Drugs, society, and human behavior* (11th ed.). New York: McGraw-Hill.

9. National Institute on Drug Abuse. (2006). InfoFacts: Heroin. www.nida.nih.gov/Infofacts/heroin.html.

10. NIDA Research Report. (2001, March). Hallucinogens and dissociative drugs. www.nida.nih.gov.

11. Substance Abuse and Mental Health Services Administration. (2003). *Emergency department trends from the drug abuse warning network, final estimates 1995–2002.* Rockville, MD: Office of Applied Studies.

12. National Institute on Drug Abuse. (2006). Info-Facts: Inhalants. www.drugabuse.gov/Infofacts/Inhalants.html.

13. National Institute on Drug Abuse. (2006). Info-Facts: Marijuana. www.nida.nih.gov/Infofacts/marijuana.html.

14. National Institute on Drug Abuse. (2004). *Marijuana: Facts for teens* (NIH Publication No. 04-4037). www.nida.nih.gov/MarijBroch/Marijteens.html.

15. National Drug Intelligence Center. (2006). The impact of drugs on society. In *National drug threat assessment 2006.* www.usdoj.gov/ndic/pubs11/18862/impact.htm.

16. Substance Abuse and Mental Health Services Administration. (2007). Emergency room visits climb for misuse of prescription and over-the-counter drugs. www.samhsa.gov/newsroom/advisories/0703135521.aspx.

17. Glaze, S. (1995). Treating addiction. *Congressional Quarterly Researcher, 5* (1), 1–24.

18. Califano, J. (1998). Crime and punishment—and treatment too. National Center on Addiction and Substance Abuse at Columbia University. www.casacolumbia.org.

19. Marlatt, G. A. (Ed.). (1998). *Harm reduction: Pragmatic strategies for managing high-risk behaviors.* New York: Guilford Press.

20. Drug Policy Alliance. (2004). Reducing harm: Treatment and beyond. www.drugpolicy.org.

21. National Institute on Drug Abuse. (2006). Info-Facts: Drug addiction and treatment methods. www.nida.nih.gov/Infofacts/treatmeth.html.

Chapter 13

1. National Center on Addiction and Substance Abuse. (2007). *Wasting the best and the brightest: Substance abuse at America's colleges and universities.* New York: Columbia University.

2. American Lung Association. (2007). Smoking and teens fact sheet. www.lungusa.org/site/pp.asp?c=dvLUK9O0E&b=39871.

3. National Center for Health Statistics. (2007). *Health, United States,* 2007. Hyattsville, MD: Author.

4. U.S. Department of Health and Human Services. (2000). *Tobacco use among U.S. racial/ethnic minority groups—African Americans, American Indians and Alaska Natives, Asian Americans and Pacific Islanders, and Hispanics: A report of the surgeon general.* Atlanta, GA: Author.

5. American Lung Association. (2007). Smoking and American Indians/Alaska Natives fact sheet. www.lungusa.org/site/pp.asp?c=dvLUK9O0E&b=35999.

6. Das, S. K. (2003). Harmful health effects of cigarette smoking. *Molecular and Cellular Biochemistry, 253* (1–2), 159–165.

7. Krogh, D. (1999). *Smoking: The artificial passion.* New York: W. H. Freeman and Company.

8. Centers for Disease Control and Prevention. (2007). Fact sheet: Hookahs. www.cdc.gov/tobacco/data_statistics/Factsheets/hookahs.htm.

9. The Bacchus Network. (n.d.). Top facts: Beedies and clove cigarettes. www.tobaccofreeu.org/pdf/bedi_kreteks_web_2.pdf.

10. Hoffman, D., Hoffman, I., & El-Bayoumy, K. (2001). The less harmful cigarette: A controversial issue. *Chemical Research in Toxicology, 14* (7), 767–790.

11. Watson, C. H., Polzin, G. M., Calafat, A. M., & Ashley, D. L. (2003). Determination of tar, nicotine, and carbon monoxide yields in the smoke of bidi cigarettes. *Nicotine & Tobacco Research, 5* (5), 747–753.

12. Rahman, M., & Fukij, T. (2000). Bidi smoking and health. *Public Health, 114* (2), 123–127.

13. Soldz, S., & Dorsey, E. (2005). Youth attitudes and beliefs toward alternative tobacco products: Cigars, bidis and kreteks. *Health Education and Behavior, 32* (4), 549–566.

14. U.S. Department of Health and Human Services. (2005). *2004 National Survey on Drug Use and Health* (DHHS Publication No. SMA 05-4061). Rockville, MD: Author.

15. National Cancer Institute. (n.d.). Fact sheet: Questions and answers about cigar smoking and cancer. www.cancer.gov/cancertopics/factsheet/tobacco/cigars.

16. Shaper, A. G., Wannamethee, S. G., & Walker, M. (2003). Pipe and cigar smoking and major cardiovascular events, cancer incidence and all-cause mortality in middle-aged British men. *International Journal of Epidemiology, 32* (5), 802–808.

17. McNeil, A., Bedi, R., Islam, S., et al. (2006). Levels of toxins in oral tobacco products in the UK. *Tobacco Control, 15* (1), 64–67.

18. National Cancer Institute. (n.d.). Fact sheet: Smokeless tobacco and cancer: Questions and answers. www.cancer.gov/cancertopics/factsheet/Tobacco/smokeless.

19. Swedish tobacco product may cut cancer risk. (2007). www.msnbc.msn.com/id/18594133.

20. Hatsukami, D. K., & Severson, H. H. (1999). Oral spit tobacco: Addiction, prevention, and treatment. *Journal of Nicotine and Tobacco Research, 1,* 21–44.

21. U.S. Department of Health and Human Services. (2004). *The health consequences of smoking: A report of the surgeon general.* Atlanta, GA: Author.

22. Ulrich, J., Meyer, C., Jurgen, H., et al. (2006). Predictors of increased body mass index following cessation of smoking. *American Journal of Addiction, 15* (2), 192–197.

23. Goren, S. S., & Schnoll, R. A. (2006). Smoking cessation. In S. S. Goren and J. Arnold (Eds.), *Health promotion in practice.* San Francisco: Jossey-Bass.

24. Glantz, S. A. (1996). *The cigarette papers.* Berkeley, CA: University of California Press.

25. Levington, S. (2003). The importance of cholesterol, blood pressure, and smoking for coronary heart disease. *European Heart Journal, 24* (19), 1703–1704.

26. National Cancer Institute. (n.d.). Fact sheet: Cigarette smoking and cancer: Questions and answers. www.cancer.gov/cancertopics/factsheet/tobacco/cancer.

27. Kozlowski, L. T., Henningfield, J. E., & Brigham, J. (2001). *Cigarettes, nicotine, and health: A biobehavioral approach.* Thousand Oaks, CA: Sage Publications.

28. Harris, J. E. (2005). Cigarette smoke components and disease: Cigarette smoke is far more than a triad of "tar," nicotine, and carbon monoxide. *Smoking and Tobacco Control Monograph No. 7.* Bethesda, MD: National Cancer Institute, 59–70.

29. National Center on Addiction and Substance Abuse. (2006). *Women under the influence.* New York: Columbia University.

30. Patel, J. D., Bach, P. B., & Kris, M. G. (2004). Lung cancer in US women: A contemporary epidemic. *Journal of the American Medical Association, 291,* 1763–1768.

31. DeMarini, D. M., & Preston, J. (2005). Smoking while pregnant: Transplacental mutagenesis of the fetus by tobacco smoke. *Journal of the American Medical Association, 293* (10), 1264–1265.

32. Chapman, S. (2006). Erectile dysfunction and smoking: Subverting tobacco industry images and masculine potency. *Tobacco Control, 15* (2), 73–74.

33. U.S. Department of Health and Human Services. (2006). *The health consequences of involuntary exposure to tobacco smoke: A report of the U.S. surgeon general.* Rockville, MD: Author.

34. Henningfield, J. E. (2000). Tobacco dependence treatment: Scientific challenges, public health opportunities. *Tobacco Control, 9* (suppl. 1), 13–110.

35. Davies, G. M., Willner, P., James, D. L., & Morgan, M. J. (2004). Influence of nicotine gum on acute cravings for cigarettes. *Journal of Psychopharmacology, 18* (1), 83–87.

36. Glantz, S. A. (2003). *Tobacco biology and politics.* Waco, TX: Health Edco.

37. Fiore, M. C., Bailey, W. C., Cohen, S. S., et al. (2000). *Treating tobacco use and dependence: Clinical practice guideline.* Rockville, MD: U.S. Department of Health and Human Services, Public Health Service.

38. Schuurmans, M. M., Diacon, A. H., Van Biljon, X., & Bolliger, C. T. (2004). Effect of pretreatment with nicotine patch on withdrawal symptoms and abstinence rates in smokers subsequently quitting with the nicotine patch: A randomized controlled trial. *Addiction, 99* (5), 634–640.

39. Larabee, L. C. (2005). To what extent do smokers plan quit attempts? *Tobacco Control, 14* (6), 425–428.

40. Bonnie, R. J., Stratton, K., & Wallace, R. B. (Eds.). (2007). *Ending the tobacco problem: A blueprint for the nation.* Washington, DC: National Academies Press.

41. Americans for Nonsmokers' Rights. (2003). Recipe for a smoke free society. www.no-smoke.org.

42. Kessler, D. (2001). *A question of intent: The great American battle with a deadly industry.* New York: Public Affairs.

43. Gallus, S., Schiaffino, A., LaVecchia, C., et al. (2006). Price and cigarette consumption in Europe. *Tobacco Control, 15* (2), 120–124.

44. Novak, S. P., Reardon, S. F., Raudenbush, S. W., et al. (2006). Retail tobacco outlet density and youth cigarette smoking: A propensity-modeling approach. *American Journal of Public Health, 96* (4), 670–676.

45. Givel, M., & Glanz, S. A. (2004). The global settlement with the tobacco industry 6 years later. *American Journal of Public Health, 94* (2), 218–224.

46. National Cancer Institute. The truth about "light" cigarettes: Questions and answers. U.S. National Institute of Health. www.cancer.gov/cancertopics/factsheet/tobacco/lightcigarettes.

47. Burns, D., Shanks, T., Major, J., & Thun, M. (2002). Evidence on disease risk in public health consequences of low-yield cigarettes. *Smoking and Tobacco Control Monograph, 13.* Washington, DC: National Cancer Institute.

48. Mecklenburg, R. E. (2003). Public health issues in treating tobacco use. *American Journal of the Medical Sciences, 326* (4), 255–261.

Chapter 14

1. Social support: A buffer against life's ills. (2005). www.mayoclinic.com.

2. Mental Health America. (2008). Social connectedness and health survey. www.nmha.org.

3. Smith-Lovin, L. (2006). Social isolation in America: Changes in core discussion networks over two decades. *American Sociological Review, 71,* 353–375.

4. Gottman, J., Gottman, J. S., & DeClaire, J. (2006). *10 Lessons to Transform Your Marriage.* New York: Three Rivers Press.

5. Pines, A. M. (2005). *Falling in love: Why we choose the lovers we choose.* New York: Routledge Press.

6. Fisher, H. (2004). *Why we love: The nature and chemistry of romantic love.* New York: Henry Holt.

7. Moreland, R. L., & Beach, S. (1992). Exposure effects in the classroom: The development of affinity among students. *Journal of Experimental Social Psychology, 28,* 255–276.

8. Glenn, N., & Marquardt, E. (2001). Hanging out, hooking up, and hoping for Mr. Right. Institute for American Values. www.americanvalues.org.

9. Sternberg, R. J. (2006). *The new psychology of love.* New Haven, CT: Yale University Press.

10. Jungsik, K., & Hatfield, E. (2004). Love types and subjective well-being: A cross-cultural study. *Social Behavior and Personality: An International Journal, 32,* 173–182.

11. Tannen, D. (2002). *I only say this because I love you.* New York: Random House.

12. Gallup Organization. (2000, December). Gallup poll: Traits of males and females.

13. Kinsey, A. C., Pomeroy, W. B., & Martin, C. E. (1948). *Sexual behavior in the human male.* Reprint edition, 1998. Bloomington, IN: Indiana University Press.

14. Kinsey, A. C., Pomeroy, W. B., Martin, C. E., & Gebhard, P. H. (1953). *Sexual behavior in the human female.* Reprint edition, 1998. Bloomington, IN: Indiana University Press.

15. Hill, D., Rozanski, C., & Willoughby, B. (2007). Gender identity disorders in childhood and adolescence: A critical inquiry. *International Journal of Sexual Health, 19,* 57–74.

16. Whitehead, B. D., & Popenoe, D. (2006). The state of our unions: The social health of marriage in America. http://marriage.rutgers.edu/publications/soou/textsoou2006.htm.

17. Olson, D. H., & Olson, A. K. (2000). *Empowering couples: Building on your strengths.* Minneapolis, MN: Life Innovations.

18. Weaver, J. (2007). Cheating hearts: Who's doing it and why. www.msnbc.msn.com/id/17951664.

19. Bepko, C., & Johnson, T. (2000). Gay and lesbian couples in therapy: Perspectives for the contemporary family therapist. *Journal of Marital and Family Therapy, 26* (4), 409–419.

20. van Wormer, K., Wells, U., & Boes, M. (2000). *Social work with lesbians, gays, and bisexuals: A strengths perspective.* Boston: Allyn & Bacon.

21. Gottman, J., & Levenson, R. L. (2004). 12-year study of gay and lesbian couples. Gottman Institute. www.gottman.com.

22. Brumbaugh, S. M., Sanchez, L. A., Nock, S. L., & Wright, J. D. (2008). Attitudes toward gay marriage in states undergoing marriage law transformation. *Journal of Marriage and the Family, 70,* 345–359.

23. Cohan, C., & Kleinbaum, S. (2000). Toward a greater understanding of the cohabitation effect: Premarital cohabitation and marital communication. *Journal of Marriage and Family, 64,*180–192.

24. Fields, J. (2004, November). America's families and living arrangements, 2003. *Current Population Reports,* 1–25. Washington, D.C.: U.S. Census Bureau.

25. Olson, D. H., & Defrain, J. (2003). *Marriage and families: Intimacy, diversity, and strength* (4th ed.). New York: McGraw-Hill.

Chapter 15

1. Hutcherson, H. (2002). *What your mother never told you about sex.* New York: G. P. Putnam's Sons.

2. Abramson, P. R., & Pinkerton, S. D. (1995). *With pleasure: Thoughts on the nature of human sexuality.* New York: Oxford University Press.

3. Levin, R. J. (2006). The breast/nipple areola complex and human sexuality. *Sexual and Relationship Therapy, 21* (2), 237–249.

4. Sanders, S. A. (2006). Issue 3: Is Masters and Johnson's model an accurate description of sexual response? In T. Williams (Ed.), *Taking sides: Clashing views and controversial issues in human sexuality.* New York: McGraw-Hill.

5. Basson, R. (2000). The female sexual response: A different model. *Journal of Sex and Marital Therapy, 26,* 51–65.

6. Godson, S. (2002). *The sex book.* London: Cassell Illustrated.

7. Wingert, P., & Kantrowitz, B. (2007, January 15). The new prime time. *Newsweek,* 39–50, 53–54.

8. Prentice, R. L., Langer, R. D., Stafanick, M., et al. (2006). Combined analysis of Women's Health Initiative observational and clinical data on postmenopausal hormone treatment and cardiovascular disease. *American Journal of Epidemiology, 163* (7), 600–607.

9. Wald, M. (2005). Male infertility: Causal cures. *Sexuality, Reproduction and Menopause, 3* (2), 83–87.

10. Federman, D. D., & Walford, G. A. (2007, January 15). Is male menopause real? *Newsweek,* 58–60.

11. Youn, G. (2006). Subjective sexual arousal in response to erotica: Effects of gender, guided fantasy, erotic stimulation and duration of exposure. *Archives of Sexual Behavior, 35* (1), 87–97.

12. Bullough, V. L. (2005). Masturbation: 100 years ago and now. *Journal of Sex Research, 42* (2), 175–176.

13. American Psychiatric Association. (2005). *Diagnostic and statistical manual of mental disorders* (4th ed., Text Revision [*DSM-IV-TR*]). Washington, DC: Author.

14. Milsten, R., & Slowinski, J. (1999). *The sexual male: Problems and solutions.* New York: W. W. Norton and Company.

15. U.S. Department of Health and Human Services. (2004). The surgeon general's call to action to promote sexual health and responsible sexual behavior. www.ejhs.org/volume4/calltoaction.htm.

16. King, S. R., & Lamb, D. J. (2006). Why we lose interest in sex: Do neurosteroids play a role? *Sexuality, Reproduction and Menopause, 4* (1), 20–23.

17. Heiman, J. R. (2000). Orgasmic disorders in women. In S. R. Leiblum & R. C. Rosen (Eds.), *Principles and practice of sex therapy.* New York: Guilford Press.

18. Orgasmic dysfunction. (n.d.). MedlinePlus Medical Encyclopedia. www.nlm.nih.gov/medlineplus/ency/article/001953.htm.

19. Crawford, M., and Popp, D. (2003). Sexual double standards: A review and methodological critique of two decades of research. *The Journal of Sex Research, 40* (1), 13–26.

20. Silverhorn, D. U. (2006). *Human physiology: An integrated approach* (4th ed.). San Francisco: Benjamin Cummings.

21. Levin, R. J. (2005). The mechanisms of human ejaculation: A critical analysis. *Sexual and Relationship Therapy, 20* (1), 123–131.

22. Peterson, K. S. (2001, March 21). Young men add Viagra to their drug arsenal. *USA Today.* www.usatoday.com/news/health/ 2001-03-21-viagra-abuse.htm.

23. Cramer, E., & Strossen, N. (2006). Is pornography harmful to women? In T. Williams (Ed.), *Taking sides: Clashing views in human sexuality.* New York: McGraw-Hill.

24. Maticka-Tyndale, E., Lewis, J., & Street, M. (2005). Making a place for escort work: A case study. *Journal of Sex Research, 42* (1), 46–53.

25. Bovard, J., & Volkonsky, A. (2006). Should prostitution be legal? In T. Williams (Ed.), *Taking sides: Clashing views in human sexuality.* New York: McGraw-Hill.

Chapter 16

1. National Center for Health Statistics. (2007). *Health United States with chartbook on trends in the health of Americans.* Hyattsville, MD: Author.

2. Hatcher, R. A., Trussell, J., Nelson, A.L., Cates, W., et al. (2004). *Contraceptive technology* (19th rev. ed.). New York: Ardent Media.

3. Santelli, J. S., Lindberg, L. D., Finer, L. B., & Singh, S. (2007). Explaining recent declines in adolescent pregnancy in the United States: The contribution of abstinence and improved contraceptive use. *American Journal of Public Health, 91* (1), 150–156.

4. Cole, J. A., Norman, H., Doherty, M., & Walker, A. M. (2007). Venous thromboembolism, myocardial infarction and stroke among transdermal contraceptive system users. *Obstetrics and Gynecology, 109* (2), 339–346.

5. FemCap—A new non-hormonal, latex-free birth control method. www.femcap.com/index .htm.

6. U.S. Department of Agriculture. (2007). *Expenditures on children by families, 2006* (Center for Nutrition and Policy Promotion Publication No. 1528-2006). www.cnpp.usda.gov/Publications/ CRC/crc2006.pdf.

7. Schlangen, R. (2006). Global illegal abortion: Where there is no "Roe": An examination of the impact of illegal abortion around the world (Issue brief). www.plannedparenthood.org/ issues-action/international/global-abortion-6480 .htm.

8. Shulman, L. P., & Ling, F. W. (2007). Overview of pregnancy termination. www.uptodate.com.

9. Chandra, A., Martinez, G. M., Mosher, W. D., & Abma, J. C. (2005). Fertility, family planning and reproductive health of U.S. women: Data from the 2002 National Survey of Family Growth. National Center for Health Statistics. *Vital Health Statistics, 23* (25).

10. Lewis, B. H., Legato, M., & Fisch, H. (2006). Medical implications of the male biological clock. *Journal of the American Medical Association, 296* (19), 2369–2371.

11. Institute of Medicine. (2007). *Weight gain: Influence of pregnancy weight on maternal and child health: Workshop report.* www.iom.edu/ CMS/12552/31379/41424.aspx.

12. U.S. Department of Agriculture. (2005). 2005 *Dietary guidelines for Americans.* www.health .gov/dietaryguidelines.

13. U.S. Environmental Protection Agency. (2004). What you need to know about mercury in fish and shellfish. EPA and FDA advice for: Women who might become pregnant, women who are pregnant, nursing mothers and young children. Updated July 19, 2007. www.epa.gov/ waterscience/fishadvice/advice.html.

14. Chasnoff, I. J., et al. (2005). The 4P's Plus screen for substance use in pregnancy: Clinical application and outcomes. *Journal of Perinatology, 25,* 368–374.

15. Cunningham, R. G., et al. (2005). *Williams obstetrics* (22nd ed.). New York: McGraw-Hill.

Chapter 17

1. Playfair, J., & Bancroft, G. (2008). *Infection and immunity* (3rd ed.). New York: Oxford University Press.

2. Centers for Disease Control and Prevention. (n.d.). Parasitic diseases. www.cdc.gov/ncidod/ dpd/index.htm.

3. Centers for Disease Control and Prevention. (1999). Achievements in public health, 1900–1999: Impact of vaccines universally recommended for children—United States, 1990–1998. *Morbidity and Mortality Weekly Report, 48* (12), 243–248.

4. Roush, S. W., Murphy, T. V., et al. (2007). Historical comparisons of morbidity and mortality for vaccine-preventable diseases in the United States. *Journal of the American Medical Association, 298* (18), 2155–2163.

5. Segerstrom, S. C., & Miller, G. E. (2004). Psychological stress and the human immune system: A meta-analytic study of 30 years of inquiry. *Psychological Bulletin, 130* (4), 601–630.

6. The Organ Procurement and Trasnplantation Network. (2006). SRTR annual report: Transplant data 1996–2005. http://optn.org/AR2006/ default.htm.

7. Kleinman, S. (2007). Laboratory testing of donated blood. www.uptodateonline.com/ patients/content/topic.do?topicKey= ~4eeeQG5TGIXHOa.

8. Dodd, R. Y., Notari, E. P., & Stramer, S. L. (2006). Current prevalence and incidence of infectious disease markers and estimated window period risk in the American Red Cross blood donor population. *Transfusion, 42,* 975.

9. Centers for Disease Control and Prevention. (2004). Investigation of rabies infections in organ donor and transplant recipients—Alabama, Arkansas, Oklahoma, Texas. *Morbidity and Mortality Weekly Report, 53* (26), 586–589.

10. Centers for Disease Control and Prevention. (2007). Blood donor screening for Chagas disease, United States 2006–2007. *Morbidity and Mortality Weekly Report, 56* (7), 141–143.

11. Centers for Disease Control and Prevention. (2007). Multistate outbreak of salmonella serotype Tennessee infections associated with peanut butter—United States, 2006–2007. *Morbidity and Mortality Weekly Report, 56* (21), 521–524.

12. World Health Organization. (2007). Five keys to safer food. www.who.int/foodsafety/ publications/consumer/5keys/en/index.html.

13. World Health Organization–Western Pacific Region. (2004). SARS. www.wpro.who.

14. Centers for Disease Control and Prevention. (n.d.). Sexually transmitted diseases treatment guidelines 2006. www.cdc.gov/STD/treatment/ default.htm.

15. Holmes, K. K., Levine, R., & Weaver, M. (2004). Effectiveness of condoms in preventing sexually transmitted infections. *Bulletin of the World Health Organization, 82* (6), 454–461.

16. Centers for Disease Control and Prevention. (n.d.). Frequently asked questions about hepatitis C. www.cdc.gov/ncidod/diseases/hepatitis/c/faq .htm#1b.

17. Centers for Disease Control and Prevention. (2006). Methicillin-resistant *Staphylococcus aureus* skin infections among tattoo recipients— Ohio, Kentucky, and Vermont, 2004–2005. *Mortality and Morbidity Weekly Report, 55* (24), 677–679.

18. Centers for Disease Control and Prevention. (2007). Antimicrobial Resistance Interagency Task Force. 2006 annual report. www.cdc.gov/ drugresistance/actionplan/2006report/index.htm.

19. Klevens, R. M., Morrison, M. A., Nadle, J., et al. (2007). Invasive methicillin-resistant *Staphylococcus aureus* infections in the United States. *Journal of the American Medical Association, 298* (15), 1763–1771.

20. Atkinson, W., Hamborsky, J., McIntyre, L., & Wolfe, S. (Eds.) (2007). *Epidemiology and prevention of vaccine-preventable diseases* (10th ed.). Washington, DC: Public Health Foundation.

21. National Institute of Child Health and Human Development. (2006). Autism and the MMR vaccine. www.nichd.nih.gov/publications/pubs/ autism/mmr/.

22. World Health Organization. (2007). Rotavirus position paper. *Weekly Epidemiological Record, 32* (82), 285–296. www.rotavirus.org/ documents/WHO_position_paper_rotavirus _2007.pdf.

23. Gerberding, J. L. (2007, June 6). Statement before the Committee on Homeland Security, United States House of Representatives. www .hhs.gov/asl/testify/2007/06/t20070606a.html.

24. World Health Organization. (2006). *The stop TB strategy.* http://whqlibdoc.who.int/hq/2006/ WHO_HTM_STB_2006.368_eng.pdf.

25. World Health Organization. (n.d.). *Tuberculosis: XDR-TB; the facts.* www.who.int/tb/challenges/ xdr/facts_nov2007en.pdf.

26. Centers for Disease Control and Prevention. (n.d.). Malaria. www.cdc.gov/malaria.

27. Centers for Disease Control and Prevention. (2003). Local transmission of *Plasmodium vivax* malaria—Palm Beach County, Florida, 2003. *Morbidity and Mortality Weekly Report, 52* (38), 908–911.

28. American College Health Association. (2007). National College Health Assessment data highlights. www.acha-ncha.org/data_highlights.html.

29. Craig, A. S., Wright, S. W., Edwards, K. M., et al. (2007). Outbreak of pertussis on a college campus. *American Journal of Medicine, 120* (4), 364–368.

30. Hutchins, S. S., & Harris, M. L. (2006, June 2). *The mumps outbreak in the Midwest: Implications for college health.* Presented at the American College Health Association annual meeting.

31. Sharp, D. (2007, December 5). USM to ban some students without mumps vaccination from campus. *Boston Globe.*

32. Dellit, T. H., & Duchin, J. (2007). *Guidelines for evaluation and management of community-associated methicillin-resistant* Staphylococcus aureus *skin and soft tissue infections in outpatient settings.* www.metrokc.gov/health/providers/epidemiology/MRSA-guidelines.pdf.

33. Foxman, B. (2002). Epidemiology of urinary tract infections: Incidence, morbidity and economic costs. *American Journal of Medicine, 113* (S1), 5–13.

34. World Health Organization. (2007). *AIDS epidemic update.* Joint United Nations Programme on HIV/AIDS. http://data.unaids.org/pub/EPISlides/2007/2007_epiupdate_en.pdf.

35. Hall, H. I., Song, R., Rhodes, P., et al. (2008). Estimation of HIV incidence in the United States. *Journal of the American Medical Association, 300*(5), 520–529.

36. Keele, B. F., Heuverswyn, F. V., Li, Y., et al. (2006). Chimpanzee reservoirs of pandemic and nonpandemic HIV-1. *Science, 313* (5786), 523–526.

37. Kassutto, S., & Rosenberg, E. S. (2004). Primary HIV type 1 infection. HIV/AIDS. *Clinical Infectious Disease, 38* (10), 1447–1453.

38. Branson, B. M., Handsfield, H. H., Lampe, M. A., et al. (2006). Revised recommendations for HIV testing of adults, adolescents, and pregnant women in health-care settings. *Morbidity and Mortality Recommendations and Reports, 55* (RR14), 1–17.

39. Centers for Disease Control and Prevention. (2003). *Exposure to blood: What healthcare personnel need to know.* www.cdc.gov/ncidod/dhqp/pdf/bbp/Exp_to_Blood.pdf.

40. Greenwald, J. L., Burstein, G. R., Pincus, J., & Branson, B. (2006). A rapid review of rapid HIV antibody tests. *Current Infectious Disease Reports, 8*, 125–131.

41. U.S. Department of Health and Human Services. (2007). HIV testing. www.fda.gov/oashi/aids/test.html.

42. World Health Organization. (2007). *Towards universal access: Scaling up priority HIV/AIDS interventions in the health sector.* www.who.int/hiv/mediacentre/univeral_access_progress_report_en.pdf.

43. Stephenson, J. (2007). HIV vaccine concerns? *Journal of the American Medical Association, 298* (23), 2733.

44. Garber, D. A., Silvestri, G., & Feinberg, M. B. (2004). Prospects for an AIDS vaccine: Three big questions, no easy answers. *The Lancet Infectious Diseases, 4*, 397–413.

45. World Health Organization. (2008). Microbicides. www.who.int/hiv/topics/microbicides/microbicides/en/.

46. Centers for Disease Control and Prevention. (2007). Trends in reportable sexually transmitted diseases in the United States, 2006. National surveillance data for chlamydia, gonorrhea and syphilis. www.cdc.gov/STD/STATS/trends2006.htm.

47. Centers for Disease Control and Prevention. (2008). Sexually transmitted disease surveillance, 2006 supplement. Chlamydia Prevalence Monitoring Project *Annual Report 2006—revised 2008*.

48. Miller, W. C., et al. (2004). Prevalence of chlamydia and gonorrhea infection among 18-26 year old young adults in the U.S. *Journal of the American Medical Association, 291* (18), 2229–2236.

49. Beigi, R. H., & Wiesenfeld, H. C. (2003). Pelvic inflammatory disease: New diagnostic criteria and treatment. *Obstetrics and Gynecology Clinics of North America, 30* (4), 777–793.

50. U.S. Preventive Services Task Force. (2004). Screening for syphilis infection. www.ahrq.gov/clinic/USpstf/uspssyph.htm.

51. Centers for Disease Control and Prevention. (2007). *Human papillomavirus: HPV information for clinicians.* www.cdc.gov/std/hpv/common-clinicians/ClinicianBro-fp.pdf.

Chapter 18

1. American Heart Association. (2008). Heart disease and stroke statistics—2008 update. www.americanheart.org.

2. Strong, J. P. (1999). Prevalence and extent of atherosclerosis in adolescents and young adults: Implications for prevention from Pathobiological Determination of Atherosclerosis in Youth Study. *Journal of the American Medical Association, 281* (8), 727–735.

3. Canto, J. G., Goldberg, R. J., Hand, M. M., et al. (2007). Symptom presentation in women with acute coronary syndromes: Myth vs reality. *Archives of Internal Medicine, 167* (22): 2405–2413.

4. National Heart, Lung, and Blood Institute. (2003). *Seventh report of the Joint National Committee on Prevention, Detection, Evaluation and Treatment of High Blood Pressure.* www.nhlbi.nih.gov/guidelines/hypertension/.

5. National Heart, Lung, and Blood Institute. (2007). Congenital heart defects. www.nhlbi.nih.gov/health/dci/diseases/chd/chd_what.html.

6. Maron, B. J., Thompson, P. D., Ackerman, M. J., et al. (2007). Recommendations and considerations related to preparticipation screening for cardiovascular abnormalities in competitive athletes: 2007 update: A scientific statement from the American Heart Association Council on Nutrition, Physical Activity, and Metabolism. *Circulation, 115*, 1643–1655.

7. National Heart, Lung, and Blood Institute. (1948). The Framingham Heart Study. www.framingham.com/heart.

8. Yusuf, S., Hawken, S., Ounpuu, S., et al. (2004). Effect of potentially modifiable risk factors associated with myocardial infarction in 52 countries (the INTERHEART study): Case-control study. *Lancet, 364* (9438), 937–952.

9. Ambrose, J. A., & Barva, R. S. (2004). The pathophysiology of cigarette smoking and cardiovascular disease: An update. *Journal of the American College of Cardiology, 43* (10), 1731–1737.

10. Watson, K. E., & Topol, E. J. (2004). Pathobiology of atherosclerosis: Are there racial and ethnic differences? *Reviews of Cardiovascular Medicine, 5* (Suppl. 3), S14–S21.

11. Executive summary of the third report of the National Cholesterol Education Program Expert Panel on Detection, Evaluation, and Treatment of High Blood Cholesterol in Adults (2001). *Journal of the American Medical Association, 285* (19), 2486–2497.

12. Grundy, S. M., et al. (2004). Implications of recent clinical trials for the National Cholesterol Education Program Adult Treatment Panel III guidelines. *Circulation, 110*, 227–239.

13. Centers for Disease Control and Prevention. (2007). Prevalence of regular physical activity among adults—United States, 2001 and 2005. *Morbidity and Mortality Weekly Report, 56*, 1209–1212.

14. Stike, P. C., & Steptoe, A. (2004). Psychosocial factors in the development of coronary artery disease. *Progress in Cardiovascular Diseases, 46* (4), 337–347.

15. Player, M. S., King, D. E., Mainous, A. G., & Geesey, M. E. (2007). Psychosocial factors and progression from prehypertension to hypertension or coronary heart disease. *Annals of Family Medicine, 5*, 403–411.

16. Massing, M. W., et al. (2004). Income, income inequality and cardiovascular disease mortality: Relationship among county populations of the United States, 1985 to 1994. *Southern Medical Journal, 97* (5), 475–484.

17. O'Keefe, J. H., et al. (2004). Psychosocial stress and cardiovascular disease: How to heal a broken heart. *Comprehensive Therapy, 30* (1), 37–43.

18. Wang, T. J., Pencina, M. J., Booth, S. L., et al. (2008). Vitamin D deficiency and risk of cardiovascular disease. *Circulation, 117*, 503–511.

19. Kamstrup, P. R., Benn, M., Tybjaerg-Hansen, A., & Nordestgaard, B. G. (2008). Extreme lipoprotein (a) levels and risk of myocardial infarction in the general population: The Copenhagen City Heart Study. *Circulation, 117*, 176–184.

20. Ridker, P. M., Cushman, M., Stampfer, M. J., et al. (2007). Inflammation, aspirin, and the risk of cardiovascular disease in apparently healthy men. *New England Journal of Medicine, 336* (14), 973–979.

21. Pearson, T. A., et al. (2003). Markers of inflammation and cardiovascular disease. *Circulation, 107*, 499.

22. Clayton, T. C., Thompson, M., & Meade, T. W. (2008). Recent respiratory infection and risk of cardiovascular disease: Case-control study through a general practice database. *European Heart Journal, 29* (1), 96–103.

23. Musher, D. M., Rueda, A. M., Kaka, A. S., & Mapara, S. M. (2007). The association between pneumococcal pneumonia and acute cardiac events. *Clinical Infectious Diseases, 45*, 158–165.

24. Grayston, J. T., Kronmal, R. A., Jackson, L. A., et al. (2005). Azithromycin for the secondary prevention of coronary events. *New England Journal of Medicine, 352* (16), 1637–1645.

25. Cannon, C. P., Braunwald, E., McCabe, C. H., et al. (2005). Antibiotic treatment of *Chlamydia pneumoniae* after acute coronary syndrome. *New England Journal of Medicine, 352* (16), 1646–1654.

26. Khan, O. A., Chau, R., Bertram, C., et al. (2005). Fetal origins of coronary heart disease—Implications for cardiothoracic surgery? *European Journal of Cardio-thoracic Surgery, 27* (6), 1036–1042.

27. Harding, R. (2005). Fetal origins of postnatal health and disease. *Early Human Development, 81* (9), 721–722.

28. Centers for Disease Control and Prevention, National Institutes of Health. (2000). Heart disease and stroke. In *Healthy people 2010.* Bethesda, MD: National Center for Chronic Disease Prevention and Health Promotion. www.healthypeople.gov/Document/HTML/Volume1/12Heart.htm.

29. Office of Minority Health and Health Disparities (OMHD). (n.d.). Eliminate disparities in cardiovascular disease. www.cdc.gov/omhd/AMH/factsheets/cardio.htm.

30. Rossouw, J. E., et al. (2002). Risks and benefits of estrogen plus progestin in healthy postmenopausal women. *Journal of the American Medical Association, 288* (3), 321–333.

31. Kendler, B. S. (2006). Supplemental conditionally essential nutrients in cardiovascular disease therapy. *Journal of Cardiovascular Nursing, 21* (1), 9–16.

32. Grundy, S. M. (2008). Is lowering low density lipoprotein an effective strategy to reduce cardiac risks? *Circulation, 117,* 569–573.

33. Campbell, C. L., Smyth, S., Montalescot, G., & Steinhubl, S. R. (2007). Aspirin dose for the prevention of cardiovascular disease. A systematic review. *Journal of the American Medical Association, 297* (18), 2018–2024.

Chapter 19

1. American Cancer Society. (2008). *Cancer facts and figures 2008.* www.cancer.org.

2. National Cancer Institute. (n.d.). Genetics of breast and ovarian cancer. www.cancer.gov/cancertopics/pdq/genetics/breast-and-ovarian.

3. National Cancer Institute. (n.d.). Genetics of colorectal cancer. www.cancer.gov/cancertopics/pdq/genetics/colorectal/healthprofessional.

4. Irigaray, P., Newby, J. A., Hardell, R. C., et al. (2007). Lifestyle-related factors and environmental agents causing cancer: An overview. *Biomedicine and Pharmacotherapy, 61* (10), 640–658.

5. World Cancer Research Fund/American Institute for Cancer Research. (2007). *Food, nutrition, physical activity and the prevention of cancer: A global perspective.* Washington, DC: Author.

6. Cho, E., Chen, W. Y., Hunter, D. J., et al. (2006). Red meat intake and risk of breast cancer among premenopausal women. *Archives of Internal Medicine, 166* (20), 2253–2259.

7. Renehan, A. G., Tyson, M., Egger, M., et al. (2008). Body-mass index and incidence of cancer: A systematic review and meta-analysis of prospective observational studies. *Lancet, 371* (9612), 569–578.

8. DeNoon, D. J. (2007). Alcohol increases breast cancer risk. WebMD Medical News. www.webmd.com/breast-cancer/news/20070927/alcohol-increases-breast-cancer-risk.

9. The Cancer Council Australia. (n.d.). SunSmart. www.cancer.org.au/cancersmartlifestyle/SunSmart.htm.

10. Cokkinides, V., Weinstock, M., Glanz, K., et al. (2006). Trends in sunburns, sun protection practices, and attitudes toward sun exposure protection and tanning among U.S. adolescents, 1998–2004. *Pediatrics, 118* (3), 853–864.

11. Board on Radiation Effects Research, Committee to Assess Health Risks from Exposure to Low Levels of Ionizing Radiation, National Research Council. (2006). *Health risks from exposure to low levels of ionizing radiation: BEIR VII phase 2.* Washington, DC: National Academies Press.

12. Clapp, R. W., Howe, G. K., & Jacobs, M. M. (2007). Environmental and occupational causes of cancer: A call to act on what we know. *Biomedicine and Pharmacotherapy, 61* (10), 631–639.

13. National Cancer Institute. (n.d.). Human papillomaviruses and cancer: Questions and answers. www.cancer.gov/cancertopics/factsheet/risk/HPV.

14. Hung, R. J., McKay, J. D., Gaborieau, V., et al. (2008). A susceptibility locus for lung cancer maps to nicotinic acetylcholine receptor subunit genes on 15q25. *Nature, 452,* 633–637.

15. Thorgeirsson, T. E., Geller, F., Sulem, P., et al. (2008). A variant associated with nicotine dependence, lung cancer and peripheral arterial disease. *Nature, 452,* 638–642.

16. National Cancer Institute. (2008). Chest X-Ray and Sputum Cytology. Lung cancer screening (PDQ) health professional version. www.cancer.gov/cancertopics/pdq/screening/lung/healthprofessional/allpages/print#Section_16.

17. Levin, B., Lieberman, D. A., McFarland, B., et al. (2008). Screening and surveillance for the early detection of colorectal cancer and adenomatous polyps, 2008: A joint guideline from the American Cancer Society, the US MultiSociety Task Force on Colorectal Cancer and the American College of Radiology. *CA: A Cancer Journal for Clinicians, 58* (3), 130–160.

18. Gagnon, A., & Ye, B. (2008). Discovery and application of protein biomarkers for ovarian cancer. *Current Opinion in Obstetrics and Gynecology, 20* (1), 9–13.

19. Munkarah, A., Chatterjee, M., & Tainsky, M. (2007). Update on ovarian cancer screening. *Current Opinion of Obstetrics and Gynecology, 19* (1), 22–26.

20. National Cancer Institute. (n.d.). Ovarian cancer. www.cancer.gov/cancertopics/types/ovarian/.

21. Runger, T. M., & Kappes, U. P. (2008). Mechanisms of mutation formation with long-wave ultraviolet light (UVA). *Photodermatology, Photoimmunology, and Photomedicine, 24* (1), 2–10.

22. National Cancer Institute. (n.d.). Testicular cancer. www.cancer.gov/cancertopics/types/testicular/.

23. Shaw, J. (2008). Diagnosis and treatment of testicular cancer. *American Family Physician, 77* (4), 469–474.

24. National Cancer Institute. (n.d.). Types of treatment. www.cancer.gov/cancertopics/treatment/types-of-treatment.

25. Velicer, C. M., & Ulrich, C. M. (2008). Vitamin and mineral supplement use among US adults after cancer diagnosis: A systematic review. *Journal of Clinical Oncology, 26* (4), 665–673.

26. Menfee Pujol, L. A., & Monti, D. A. (2007). Managing cancer pain with nonpharmocologic and complementary therapies. *Journal of the American Osteopathic Association, 107* (7), 15–21.

27. National Center for Complementary and Alternative Medicine. (n.d.). Get the facts: Cancer and CAM. http://nccam.nih.gov/health/camcancer/.

Chapter 20

1. National Center for Complementary and Alternative Medicine. (n.d.). What is CAM? www.nccam.nih.gov/health/whatiscam/.

2. Yeh, G. Y., Ryan, M. A., Phillips, R. S., & Baudette, J. F. (2008). Doctor training and practice of acupuncture: Results of a survey. *Journal of Evaluation in Clinical Practice, 14* (3), 439.

3. Eisenberg, D. M., et al. (2002). Credentialing complementary and alternative medical providers. *Annals of Internal Medicine, 137,* 965–973.

4. Barnes, P., Powell-Griner, E., McFann, K., & Nahin, R. (2004). Complementary and alternative medicine use among adults: United States, 2002. *Advance Data from Vital and Health Statistics,* no. 243, 1–20.

5. American Hospital Association. (2008). Hospital statistics. Health forum. Chicago: Author.

6. Institute of Medicine. (2005). *Complementary and alternative medicine in the United States.* Washington, DC: National Academies Press.

7. National Center for Complementary and Alternative Medicine. (2007). The use of complementary and alternative medicine in the United States. http://nccam.nih.gov/news/camsurvey_fs1.htm#use.

8. World Health Organization. (n.d.). Traditional medicine. www.who.int/mediacentre/factsheets/fs134/en/.

9. Lu, H. C. (2007). *Chinese natural cures—Traditional methods for remedy and prevention.* New York: Black Dog and Leventhal Publishers.

10. Ni, M. (2008). *Secrets of self-healing.* New York: Penguin.

11. National Center for Complementary and Alternative Medicine. (2007). What is Ayurvedic medicine? http://nccam.nih.gov/health/ayurveda/.

12. Novella, S., Roy, R., Marcus, D., et al. (2008). A debate: Homeopathy—Quackery or a key to the future of medicine? *Journal of Alternative and Complementary Medicine, 14* (1), 9–15.

13. National Center for Complementary and Alternative Medicine. (2007). *Research report: Questions and answers about homeopathy* (Publication No. D183). www.nccam.nih.gov.

14. National Center for Complementary and Alternative Medicine. (2007). *An introduction to naturopathy* (Publication No. D372). www.nccam.nih.gov.

15. Cohen, K. (2003). *Honoring the medicine: The essential guide to Native American healing.* New York: Random House Ballantine Publishing Group.

16. Rogovik, A. L., & Goldman, R. D. (2007). Hypnosis for treatment of pain in children. *Canadian Family Physician, 53* (5), 823–825.

17. Douglas, R. M., et al. (2007). Vitamin C for preventing and treating the common cold. *Cochrane Database of Systematic Reviews, 18* (3), CD 000980.

18. Caruso, T. J., Prober, C. G., & Gwaltney, J. M. (2007). Treatment of naturally acquired common colds with zinc: A structured review. *Clinical Infectious Diseases, 45* (5), 569–574.

19. Chan, P. C., Xia, Q., & Fu, P. P. (2007). Ginkgo biloba leaf extract: Biological, medicinal, and toxicological effects. *Journal of Environmental Science and Health, Part C, 25* (3), 211–244.

20. Kasper, S., Gastpar, M., Muller, W. E., et al. (2008). Efficacy of St. John's wort extract WS 5570 in acute treatment of mild depression: A reanalysis of data from controlled clinical trials. *European Archives of Psychiatry and Clinical Neuroscience, 258* (1), 59–63.

21. Van der Watt, G., Laugharne, J., & Janca, A. (2008). Complementary and alternative medicine in the treatment of anxiety and depression. *Current Opinion in Psychiatry, 21* (1), 37–42.

22. Grossberg, G. T., & Fox, B. (2007). The *essential herb-drug-vitamin interaction guide.* New York: Broadway Books.

23. Bristol, M. N., Sonnad, S. S., & Guerra, C. (2008). Uninformed complementary and alternative supplement use: A risky behavior for cardiovascular patients. *Complementary Health Practice Review, 13*, 100–126.

24. Gruenwald, J., et al. (2007). *PDR for herbal medicines* (4th ed.). Montvale, NJ: Thomson PDR.

25. American Osteopathic Association. (n.d.). Osteopathic medicine. www.osteopathic.org/index.cfm.

26. National Center for Complementary and Alternative Medicine. (2007). *An introduction to chiropractic* (Publication No. D403). http://nccam.nih.gov/health/chiropractic/.

27. Lawrence, D. J., & Meeker, W. C. (2007). Chiropractic and CAM utilization: A descriptive review. *Chiropractic and Osteopathy, 15* (2), 1–27.

28. Sherman, K. J., Dixon, M. W., et al. (2006). Development of a taxonomy to describe massage treatments for musculoskeletal pain. *BMC Complementary and Alternative Medicine, 6*, 24.

29. National Center for Complementary and Alternative Medicine. (2007). *Backgrounder: Energy medicine: An overview* (Publication No. D235). http://nccam.nih.gov/health/backgrounds/energymed.htm.

30. Winemiller, M. H., et al. (2003). Effect of magnetic vs. sham-magnetic insoles on plantar heel pain: A randomized controlled trial. *Journal of the American Medical Association, 290* (11), 1474–1478.

31. Rakel, D. P., Guerrera, M. P., et al. (2008). CAM education: Promoting a salutogenic focus in health care. *Journal of Alternative and Complementary Medicine, 14* (1), 87–93.

32. Poisal, J. A., et al. (2007). Health spending projections through 2016: Modest changes obscure Part D's impact. *Health Affairs, 21*, W242–W253.

Chapter 21

1. Rosenfeld, R. (2004, February). The case of the unsolved crime decline. *Scientific American.*

2. Bureau of Justice Statistics. (2007). Firearms and crime statistics. www.ojp.usdoj.gov/bjs/guns.htm.

3. Lynch, J. (2002). Crime in international perspective. In J. Q. Wilson & J. Petersilia (Eds.), *Crime: Public policies for crime control* (pp. 5–42). San Francisco: ICS Press.

4. Diaz, T. (2000). *Making a killing: The business of guns in America.* New York: The New Press.

5. Potter, L. B. (2006). Violence prevention. In S. S. Gorin & J. Arnold (Eds.), *Health promotion practice.* San Francisco: Jossey-Bass.

6. Barnett, O. W., Miller-Perrin, C. L., & Perrin, R. D. (2004). *Family violence across the lifespan: An introduction* (2nd ed.). Thousand Oaks, CA: Sage Publications.

7. Bureau of Justice Statistics. (2007). Homicide trends in the U.S. www.ojp.usdoj.gov/bjs/homicide/homtrnd.htm.

8. Davis, G. G., & Muhlhausen, D. B. (2000). Young African-American males: Continuing victims of high homicide rates in urban communities. The Heritage Foundation. www.heritage.org/research/crime.

9. Greenwood, P. W. (2002). Juvenile crime and juvenile justice. In J. Q. Wilson & J. Petersilia (Eds.), *Crime: Public policies for crime control* (pp. 75–108). San Francisco: ICS Press.

10. Bureau of Justice Statistics. (2008). Crime and victims statistics. www.ojp.usdoj.gov/bjs/cvict.htm.

11. National Center for Education Statistics. (2003). Indicators of school crime and safety. http://nces.ed.gov/pubs2004/crime03/.

12. Centers for Disease Control and Prevention. (2007). Youth violence: Fact sheet. www.cdc.gov/ncipc/factsheets/yvfacts.htm.

13. Cauchan, D. (1999, July 13). Schools struggling to balance "zero tolerance," common sense. *USA Today,* 1A–2A.

14. Goodson, B., & Muncie, J. (2006). *Youth crime and justice.* Newbury Park, CA: Sage.

15. Howell, J. C., & Decker, S. H. (1999). The youth gangs, drugs, and violence connection. Office of Juvenile Justice and Delinquency Prevention, *Juvenile Justice Bulletin.* www.ncjrs.org.

16. Security on Campus, Inc. (2006). College university campus crime statistics. www.securityoncampus.org/crimestats/.

17. Willis, E. (2005). Colleges should do more to prevent campus violence, report says. *Chronicle of Higher Education,* February 14. http://chronicle.com/free/2005/02/2005021408n.htm.

18. Newer, H. (2003). *The hazing reader: Examining rites gone wrong in fraternities, professional and amateur athletics, high schools, and the military.* Auckland, New Zealand: Reid Publishing.

19. Nuwer, H. (1999). *Wrongs of passage: Fraternities, sororities, hazing, and binge drinking.* Bloomington, IN: Indiana University Press.

20. Hudson, D. L. (2007). Hate speech and campus speech codes. www.firstamendmentcenter.org/speech/pubcollege/topic.aspx?topic=campus_speech_codes.

21. Carr, J. L. (2005). *Campus violence white paper.* Baltimore, MD: American College Health Association.

22. Fisher, B. S., Cullen, F. T., & Turner, M. G. (2000, December). The sexual victimization of college women. *National Institute of Justice Research Report.* Rockville, MD: National Criminal Justice Reference Center.

23. Bureau of Justice Statistics. (2005). National Crime Victimization Survey, 2005. www.ojp.usdoj.gov/bjs.

24. Tjaden, P., & Thoennes, N. (2000). Full report of the prevalence, incidence, and consequences of violence against women: Findings from the National Violence Against Women Survey. Report NCJ 183781. Washington, DC: National Institute of Justice.

25. National Center for Victims of Crime. (n.d.). Acquaintance rape. www.ncvc.org.

26. Macy, R. J. (2006). Responding in their best interests; contexualizing women's coping with acquaintance sexual aggression. *Violence Against Women, 12* (15), 478–500.

27. Male Survivor Organization. (2007). Myths about male sexual victimization. www.malesurvivor.org/myths.html.

28. Gross, M. N., & Graham-Berman, S. A. (2006). Gender, categories, and science-as-usual: A critical review of gender and PTSD. *Violence Against Women, 12* (4), 393–406.

29. Wallace, H. (2005). *Family violence: Legal, medical and social perspectives.* Boston: Allyn and Bacon.

30. McCarty, C. (2007). New Jersey attorney general subpoenas Facebook over sex offender data. http://news.cnet.com/8301-13577_3-9790064-36.html.

31. U.S. Equal Employment Opportunity Commission. (2008). Sexual harassment. www.eeoc.gov/types/sexual_harassment.html.

32. National Center for Victims of Crime. (n.d.). Stalking. www.ncvc.org.

33. Morewitz, S. J. (2003). *Stalking and violence: New patterns of trauma and obsession.* New York: Kluwer Academic.

34. Crime Library. (n.d.). Cyber-stalking: Risk management. www.crimelibrary.com/criminal_mind/psychology/cyberstalking/6.html.

35. Centers for Disease Control and Prevention, National Center for Injury Prevention and Control. (2004). Child maltreatment: Fact sheet. www.cdc.gov.

36. Theo, A. (2006). *Deviant behaviors.* Boston: Allyn and Bacon.

37. Centers for Disease Control and Prevention. (2006). Intimate partner violence: Fact sheet. www.cdc.gov/ncipc/dvp/ipv_factsheet.pdf.

38. Luthra, R., & Gidycz, C. A. (2006). Dating violence among college men and women: Examination of a theoretical model. *Journal of Interpersonal Violence, 21* (6), 717–731.

39. Centers for Disease Control and Prevention. (2006). Dating abuse fact sheet. www.cdc.gov/ncipc/dvp/datingviolence.htm.

40. Murphy, C. M., Winters, J., O'Farrell, T. J., et al. (2005). Alcohol consumption and intimate partner violence by alcoholic men: Comparing violent and non-violent conflicts. *Psychology of Addictive Behaviors, 19*, 35–42.

41. Perry, B. (2001). *In the name of hate: Understanding hate crimes.* New York: Routledge.

42. Fenske, R. H., & Gordon, L. (1998). Reducing race and ethnic hate crimes on campus: The need for community. In A. M. Hoffman, J. H. Schuh, & R. H. Fenske (Eds.), *Violence on campus: Defining the problems, strategies for action.* Gaithersburg, MD: Aspen Publishers.

43. McPhail, B. A., & Dinitto, D. M. (2006). Prosecutorial perspectives on gender bias and hate crimes. *Violence Against Women, 11* (19), 1162–1185.

44. Stern, J. (2002). *The ultimate terrorists.* Cambridge, MA: Harvard University Press.

45. Cole, T. B., & Johnson, R. M. (2005). Storing guns safely in homes with children and adolescents. *Journal of the American Medical Association, 293* (6), 740–744.

46. Teret, S. P., & Culross, P. L. (2000). Product-oriented approaches to reducing youth gun violence. *The Future of Children, 12* (2), 119.

47. Kelly, C. (2004). *Blown away: American women and guns.* New York: Simon & Schuster.

48. Bok, S. (1999). *Mayhem: Violence as public entertainment.* New York: Basic Books.

49. Minnebo, J. (2006). The relation between psychological distress, television exposure, and television-viewing motives in crime victims. *Media Psychology, 8* (2), 61–63.

50. Farrington, D. P. (2002). Families and crime. In J. Q. Wilson & J. Petersilia (Eds.), *Crime: Public policies for crime control* (pp. 129–148). San Francisco: ICS Press.

51. Samson, R. J. (2002). The community. In J. Q. Wilson & J. Petersilia (Eds.), *Crime: Public policies for crime control* (pp. 225–252). San Francisco: ICS Press.

52. Murray, C. (2002). The physical environment. In J. Q. Wilson & J. Petersilia (Eds.), *Crime: Public policies for crime control* (pp. 349–361). San Francisco: ICS Press.

53. Furedi, F. (2005). *The culture of fear: Why Americans are afraid of the wrong things.* New York: Continuum Intermediate Publishing Group.

Chapter 22

1. Bever, D. L. (1998). *Safety: A personal focus.* New York: WCB and McGraw-Hill.

2. National Safety Council. (2007). *Injury facts, 2007 edition.* Itasca, IL: Author.

3. Centers for Disease Control and Prevention. (2006). *Injury surveillance training manual.* www.ihs.gov/medicalprograms/portlandinjury/pdfs/injurysurveillancetrainingmanual.pdf.

4. National Safety Council. (n.d.). What are the odds of dying? www.nsc.org/research/odds.aspx.

5. National Highway Traffic Safety Administration. (2005). *Analysis of speeding-related fatal motor vehicle traffic* (Publication No. DOT HS 809839). Washington, DC: U.S. Department of Transportation.

6. National Highway Traffic Safety Administration. (2006). *The impact of driver inattention on near crash/crash risk: An analysis using the 100-Car Naturalistic Driving Study data* (Publication No. DOT HS 810594). Washington, DC: U.S. Department of Transportation.

7. Mazzae, E. N., Ranney, T. A., Watson, G. S., & Wightman, J. A. (2005). Hand-held or hands-free: The effects of wireless phone interface type on phone task performance and driver preference. www.nhtsa.gov.

8. Ingree, M., Akerstedt, T., Peters, B., et al. (2006). Subjective sleepiness, simulated driving performance and blink duration: Examining individual differences. *Journal of Sleep Research, 15* (1), 47.

9. Larson, J. (1999). *Road rage.* Tom Doherty Associates.

10. Centers for Disease Control and Prevention. *Preventing injuries in America: Public health in action.* www.cdc.gov.

11. National Highway Traffic Safety Administration. (2005). *Alcohol-related fatalities in 2004* (Publication No. DOT HS 809904). Washington, DC: U.S. Department of Transportation.

12. Dittmer, S. M., Elder, R. W., & Shultz, R. A., et al. (2005). Effectiveness of designated driver programs for reducing alcohol-impaired driving: A systematic review. *American Journal of Preventive Medicine, 28* (5, Suppl 1), 280–287.

13. U.S. Department of Transportation. (2004). *U.S. DOT proposes tougher standard to protect occupants in side-impact crashes.* Washington, DC: National Highway Traffic Safety Administration.

14. Cummings, P., & Rivera, F. P. (2004). Car occupant death according to the testimony use of other occupants: A matched cohort study. *Journal of the American Medical Association, 291* (3), 343–349.

15. Zaza, S., Briss, P. A., & Harris, K. W. (Eds.). (2005). *The guide to community preventive services.* New York: Oxford University Press.

16. Heisler, H. (2002). *Advanced vehicle technology* (2nd ed.). Woburn, MA: Butterworth-Heinemann.

17. Norman, D., and the Nielsen Norman Group. (2004). A time for standards. www.jnd.org/dn.mss/a_time_for_standards.html.

18. Rosenberg, J. (2008). Electronic stability control. www.cars.com/go/advice/Story.jsp?section=safe&story=techStability&subject=safe_tech&referer=.

19. National Highway Traffic Safety Administration. (2004). Motorcycle helmet use laws. *Traffic Safety Facts: Laws.* www.nhtsa.dot.gov/people/injury/new-fact-sheet03/MotorcycleHelmet.pdf.

20. Natalier, K. (2001). Motorcyclists' interpretation of risk and hazard. *Journal of Sociology, 37* (1), 65.

21. Insurance Institute for Highway Safety, Highway Loss Data Institute. (2008). Current U.S. motorcycle and bicycle helmet laws. www.iihs.org/laws/helmetusecurrent.aspx.

22. Retting, R. A., Ferguson, S. A., & McCarthy, A. T. (2003). A review of evidence-based traffic engineering measures to reduce pedestrian–motor vehicle crashes. *American Journal of Public Health, 93* (9), 1456–1462.

23. Office of Disease Prevention and Health Promotion. (2000, January). *Healthy people 2010.* Washington, DC: U.S. Department of Health and Human Services.

24. Praderelli, M. (2005). As ATV usage soars, safety needs to take a front seat. *Midwest Injury Prevention Control, 7* (1), 1.

25. Centers for Disease Control and Prevention. (2008). Water-related injury: Fact sheet. www.cdc.gov/ncipc/factsheets/drown.htm.

26. Saluja, G., Brenner, R. A., Trumble, A., et al. (2006). Swimming pool drownings among U.S. residents aged 5–24 years: Understanding racial/ethnic disparities. *American Journal of Public Health, 96* (4), 778–783.

27. Kannus, P., Parkkari, J., Niemi, S., et al. (2005). Induced deaths among elderly people. *American Journal of Public Health, 95* (3), 422–424.

28. Schwartz, A. V., Nevitt, M. C., Brown, B. W., et al. (2005). Increased falling as a risk factor for fracture among older women: The study of osteoporotic factors. *American Journal of Epidemiology, 16* (2), 180–185.

29. Lehtola, C. J., Becker, W. J., & Brown, C. M. (2004). Preventing injuries from slips, trips, and falls. www.cdc.gov/nasd/docs/d000001-d000100/d000006/d000006.html.

30. Centers for Disease Control and Prevention. (2007). Fire deaths and injuries: Fact sheet. www.cdc.gov/ncipc/factsheets/fire.htm.

31. National Fire Protection Agency. (2006). *Fire in your home.* Washington, DC: Author.

32. Eisler, P., & Levin, A. (2007, March 6). Batteries can pose risk to planes. *USA Today,* p. 3A.

33. Centers for Disease Control and Prevention. (2008). Poisoning in the United States: Fact sheet. www.cdc.gov/ncipc/factsheets/poisoning.htm.

34. Centers for Disease Control and Prevention. (2008). Tips to prevent poisoning. www.cdc.gov/ncipc/factsheets/poisonprevention.htm.

35. Null, J., & Quinn, J. (2005). Heat stress from enclosed vehicles: Moderate ambient temperatures cause significant temperature rise in enclosed vehicles. *Pediatrics, 116* (1), e109–e112.

36. Mestel, R. (2000, April 13). Coping with a noisy world. *The Gazette,* Iowa City, IA, 1D.

37. Dunn, K. M., Jordan, K., & Croft, P. R. (2006). Characterizing the course of low back pain: A latent class analysis. *American Journal of Epidemiology, 163* (8), 754–761.

38. Badia, A. (n.d.). Understanding carpal tunnel syndrome. www.ctsplace.com.

39. Carpal tunnel syndrome: Common ailment, many treatments. (2006). *Safety Compliance Letter, 2462,* 12–13.

Chapter 23

1. Miller, G. T. (2006). *Living in the environment.* Belmont, CA: Wadsworth/Thomson Learning.

2. U.S. Environmental Protection Agency. (n.d.). Ground water: Drinking water: Frequently asked questions. www.epa.gov/ogwdw.

3. Gralla, P. (1994). *How the environment works.* Emeryville, CA: Ziff-Davis Press Books.

4. Organization for Economic Cooperation and Development. (2001). Glossary of statistical terms: Water pollution. http://stats.oecd.org/glossary/detail.asp?ID=2906.

5. Meyers, N., & Kent, J. (2005). *The new atlas of planet management.* Los Angeles: University of California Press.

6. Weinhold, B. (2004). Weather warning: Climate change can be hazardous to your health. *Environmental Health Perspectives, 112* (3), A532–533.

7. Logorio, S., Forostieve, F., Pastelli, R., et al. (2006). Air pollution and lung function among susceptible adult subjects: A panel study. *Environmental Health, 5* (11), 5–11.

8. U.S. Environmental Protection Agency. (1999). Smog—Who does it hurt? www.epa.gov/airnow/health/smog.pdf.

9. Bernstein, M., & Whitman, D. (2005). Smog alert: The challenges of battling ozone pollution. *Environment, 47* (8), 28–36.

10. U.S. Environmental Protection Agency. (2002). Acid rain. www.epa.gov/acidrain.

11. Intergovernmental Panel on Climate Change. (2007). *Climate change 2007: The physical science basis.* Geneva, Switzerland: Author.

12. Tennebaum, D. J. (2005). Global warming: Arctic climate: The heat is on. *Environmental Health Perspectives, 113* (2), A91.

13. Intergovernmental Panel on Climate Change. (n.d.). Global warming: Early warning signs. www.climatehotmap.org.

14. Breslin, K. (2004). Hot new report on climate change. *Environmental Health Perspectives, 112* (3), A157.

15. Begley, S. (2007, June 4). Get out your handkerchief. *Newsweek,* 62.

16. National Oceanic and Atmosphere Administration. (n.d.). Global warming: Frequently asked questions. www.ncdc.noaa.gov/oa/climate/globalwarming.html.

17. U.S. Environmental Protection Agency. (2007). Future sea level changes. www.epa.gov/climatechange/science/futureslc.html.

18. Romm, J. J., & Frank, F. A. (2006). Hybrid vehicles gain traction. *Scientific American, 294* (4), 72–79.

19. Natural Resources Defense Council. (2004). Reducing America's energy dependence. www.nrdc.org/air/transportation/gasprices.asp.

20. U.S. Environmental Protection Agency (n.d.). Indoor air facts no. 4 (revised): Sick building syndrome. www.epa.gov/iaq/pubs/sbs.html.

21. U.S. Environmental Protection Agency. (2003). *A brief guide to mold, moisture and your home.* Office of Air and Radiation. Environments Division. EPA publication 402-K-02-003. Washington, DC: Author.

22. Ahrens, A., Braun, A., Gleich, A. V., et al. (2006). *Hazardous chemicals in products and processes: Substitution as an innovative process.* New York: Springer.

23. Phillips, M. L. (2005). Children's centers study kids and chemicals. *Environmental Health Perspectives, 113* (10), A664–A668.

24. U.S. Environmental Protection Agency. (1996). Protect your family and yourself from carbon monoxide poisoning. www.epa.gov/iaq/pubs/coftsht.html.

25. U.S. Environmental Protection Agency. (n.d.). Household hazardous waste. www.epa.gov/garbage/hhw.htm.

26. U.S. Environmental Protection Agency. (n.d.). Pesticides: Frequently asked questions. www.epa.gov/pesticides/about/faq/htm.

27. U.S. Environmental Protection Agency. (n.d.). Recycling. www.epa.gov/garbage/recycle.htm.

28. Davis, B. (Ed). (2007). *Wake up and smell the planet.* Seattle, WA: Skipstone Press.

29. McKenzie J. F., Pinger, R. R., & Kotecki, J. E. (2002). *An introduction to community health.* Boston: Jones & Bartlett.

30. O'Riordan, T. (2005). Ecodiversity and biodiversity. *Environment, 47* (10), 3.

31. Schantz, S. L. (2005). Editorial: Lakes in crisis. *Environmental Health Perspectives, 113,* (3), A148–A149.

32. Stone, M. K., & Barlow, Z. (Eds.). (2005). *Ecological literacy: Educating our children for a sustainable world.* San Francisco: Sierra Club.

33. Population Reference Bureau. (n.d.). World population data sheets. www.prb.org.

34. United Nations Population Division. (2005). *World population prospects: The 2004 revision.* New York: United Nations.

35. Salmony, S. E. (2006). The human population: Accepting species limits. *Environmental Health Perspectives, 114* (1), A17–A18.

Credits

Chapter 1

p.1: © BananaStock / JupiterImages; p.3: © BananaStock / PunchStock; p.4: © Ryan McVay / Getty Images p.5 © Sonda Dawes / The Image Works; p.5 (bottom left, top to bottom): © Comstock Images / PictureQuest; © Mitch Hrdlicka / Getty Images; © Photodisc / Getty Images; p.5 (bottom right): © Squared Studios / Getty Images; p.6: © David Greedy / Getty Images; p.8: © HFPA, 63rd Annual Golden Globe Awards; p.9: © Brooke Slezak / Getty Images; p.10: © Rachel Epstein / The Image Works; p.11: © The McGraw-Hill Companies, Inc./ Gary He, photographer; p.15: © Tony Freeman / PhotoEdit; p.18 (left): © AP Photo / Ng Han Guan; p.18 (right): PR News Foto / Minnesota Partnership for Action Against Tobacco / AP Photos; p.19 © Newscom

Chapter 2

p.23: © BananaStock / PictureQuest; p.24: © Getty Images / Digital Vision; p.26: © Frank Trapper / Corbis; p.28 (left): © Bilder-Lounge/ SuperStock; p.28 (right): © Custom Medical Stock Photo / Alamy; p.29: © Marion Bull / Alamy; p.30: © Tim Defrisco / Getty Images; p.31: © Jeff Greenberg / PhotoEdit; p.32: © Jack Hollingsworth / Getty Images; p.34: Steve Cole / Getty Images; p.35: © Michael Caulfield / WireImage Awards / Newscom; p.36: © Phototake Inc. / Alamy; p.39: Nicole Bengiveno / The New York Times / Redux; p.40: © BananaStock / PictureQuest

Chapter 3

p.43: © Royalty Free / Corbis; p.44: Photo by Lynn Betts, USDA Natural Resources Conservation Service; p.47: © Purestock / PunchStock; p.48 © AP Photo / Karen Tam; p.53: Getty Images / Digital Vision; p.54: ©AP Photo / Stephen J. Boitano; p.55: © vario images GmbH & Co.KG / Alamy; p.56 (top to bottom): The McGraw-Hill Companies, Inc. / Jill Braaten, photographer; C. Sherburne / PhotoLink / Getty Images; Photodisc Collection / Getty Images; © Ingram Publishing / Fotosearch; © Comstock / PunchStock; © Royalty Free / Corbis; © Janis Christie / Getty Images; © Royalty Free / Corbis; © Royalty Free / Corbis; p.58: National Suicide Prevention Lifeline, U.S. Department of Health and Human Services; p.60: © Bubbles Photolibrary / Alamy; p.61: © Tim Sloan / AFP / Getty Images

Chapter 4

p.64: © Royalty Free / Corbis; p.65: © Jeff Greenberg / PhotoEdit; p. 66: © BananaStock / PictureQuest; p.67: © James Marshall / The Image Works; p.68: © Royalty Free / Corbis; p.69: © Blend Images / Alamy; p.70: D. Falconer / PhotoLink / Getty Images; p. 71: © Anna Pena / Getty Images; p.72: © James Marshall / The Image Works; p.74: © Bob Daemmrich / The Image Works; p.75: © Royalty Free / Corbis; p.77: © Spencer Grant / PhotoEdit

Chapter 5

p.80: © Getty Images; p.83: © Galen Rowell / CORBIS; p. 86: Photo Courtesy of U.S. Army; p. 88 (top): © Peter Hvizdak / The Image Works; p.88 (bottom): © Newscom; p.90: Kent Knudson / PhotoLink / Getty Images; p.91: © AP Photo / Nancy Palmieri; p.92: Eric Audras / Photoalto / PictureQuest; p.93: © Mike Segar / Reuters / Landov; p.94 © Royalty Free / Corbis; p. 95: © Michael Newman / PhotoEdit; p.97: Mike Powell / Digital Vision / Getty Images

Chapter 6

p.100: © Veer; p.103: © PhotoAlto / PunchStock; p.105: Photodisc Collection / Getty Images; p.106: © Photodisc / Getty Images; p.109: Plush Studios / Digital Vision / Getty Images; p.111: Corbis Images / Jupiter Images; p.112 (left): Photo by Eric Erbe / United States Department of Agriculture; p.112 (middle and right): Department of Health and Human Services, Centers for Disease Control and Prevention; p.113: © Tim Boyle / Getty Images; p.115: Courtesy of Carole McDonnell

Chapter 7

p.119: © Ingram Publishing / SuperStock; p.120: © Pixtal / Age footstock; p.121: Janis Christie / Digital Vision / Getty Images; p.123: © Comstock / PunchStock; p.126: Getty Images / Jonelle Weaver; p.131: Source: MyPyramid, 2005, U.S. Department of Agriculture, Center for Nutrition Policy and Promotion; p.137: © David Young-Wolff / PhotoEdit; p.139: © BananaStock / JupiterImages; p.140: Martin Bond / Peter Arnold Inc., p.142: (clockwise): © iStockphoto.com / Romas Bercic; © iStockphoto.com / webking; © iStockphoto.com / Roberto Adrian; © iStockphoto.com / Rebecca Ellis; © iStockphoto.com / Pam R; © iStockphoto.com / Graça Victoria; © PhotoAlto / Punchstock; © iStockphoto.com / Vaska Miokovic; © iStockphoto.com / orix3

Chapter 8

p.146: Rubberball Productions / Getty Images; p.148: Getty Images / Photodisc; p.149: © iStockphoto.com / James Phelps; p.151: Ryan McVay / Getty Images; p.153: © Corbis; p.156: © Stockbyte / PunchStock; p.158: Mark Hamel / Getty Images; p.159: AP Photo / Eckehard Schulz; p.161 (top): Pete Saloutos / Getty Images; p.161 (bottom): Ryan McVay / Getty Images; p.163: © McGraw-Hill Companies, Inc./ Lars. A. Niki, photographer; p.164: © Barry Lewis / Corbis

Chapter 9

p.169: © Digital Vision / Alamy; p.171: © AP Photo / Sue Ogrocki; p.174: © 2007 Getty Images, Inc.; p.175: Scott Olson / Getty Images; p.176: (top to bottom): © iStockphoto.com / Andrew Howe; iStockphoto.com / Feng Yu; © iStockphoto.com / Andrzej Burak; © iStockphoto.com / Victor Burnside; p.177: Image Source / SuperStock; p.179: © Newscom; p.183: © Mario Anzuoni / Reuters / Corbis; p.184: © Doug Menuez / Getty Images; p.185: Paul Burns / Photodisc / Getty Images

Chapter 10

p.188: © BananaStock / PunchStock; p.189 © David J. Green–Lifystyle / Alamy; p.190 (left): © Sunset Boulevard / Sygma / Corbis; p.190 (right): Laura Cavanaugh / Landov; p.192 (top): © Sony Pictures / Photofest; p.192 (bottom): © Royalty Free / Corbis; p. 198: Image Source Black / Jupiter Images; p.199: © BananaStock / PunchStock; p.201: © Digital Vision / Alamy; p.203: © Corbis-All Rights Reserved

Chapter 11

p.208: Digital Vision / Getty Images; p.209 (left to right): © iStockphoto.com / Bjorn Heller; iStockphoto.com / Plainview; iStockphoto.com / Chris Hutchinson; iStockphoto.com / Rebecca Ellis; p.212: © Rudi Von Briel / PhotoEdit; p.213: Jim Arbogast /

Credits

Index

body, routes of administration for, 238f, 239t
caffeine, **244–245**
causing disease, 357
classification of psychoactive, 241f
college and, 252
combating teen abuse of, 250
commonly abused, 242t
demand reduction strategies, 249–252
dependence on, 240
ED, misuse of, 310
effect on body, 238–241
factors influencing effects of, 239–240
fat blocking, 182
harm reduction strategies, 252
for HIV/AIDS, 368
HIV/AIDS caused by injection, 367
illicit, **237**
illicit, and pregnancy, 334–335
illicit use causing disease, 357
illicit, use in lifetime, 234t
incarceration for, -related crimes, 249–250
law enforcement and, 253
misuse, **237**
mucous membrane application, 238–239
for muscle development, 154
for obesity, 181–182
patterns of use, 234–235
performance enhancing, and their effects, 155t
pharmaceutical, **236–237**
during pregnancy, 334–335
prescription, for dieting, 181–182
prevention strategies, 250–251
rates of use, 235
rebound effect from, **245**
regulation of herbs vs. regulation of, 434
skin application, 239
supply reduction strategies, 249
treatment programs, 251–252
trends in illicit use of, 234t
what are, **235–238**
DTs. *See* delirium tremens
Durable Power of Attorney for Health Care
    (DPOAHC), **77**
dysmorphic disorder, body, **200–201**
dyssomnias, **106**, 108–109
dysthymic disorder, **53**

E

E. coli, 141
EAR. *See* Estimated Average Requirement
earthquakes, 480–481
eating. *See also* diet; eating disorders; nutrition
    out, 175–176
    too close to bedtime, 113
eating disorders, **193**, 193–200. *See also* binge-
        eating disorder; nocturnal eating disorder
    components of treatment, 197, 200
    diagnosing, 194–195
    factors contributing to, 194f
    health consequences of, 196–197
    media and, 203
    in men, 191
    night eating syndrome, **109**
    nocturnal, **109**
    recognizing problems, 197

treating, 197–200
echocardiograms, **394**
eclampsia, **336**
ECMs. *See* electronic control modules
ecological footprint, **501**
ecosystems, **497**–498
Ecstasy, 244
    signs of use, 243
ectoparasites, 349
ED. *See* erectile dysfunction
egg donation, pregnancy, 341
Eisenhower, Dwight D., 167
ejaculation, **302**
    dysfunction, 308–309
EKG. *See* electrocardiogram
elective abortion, **330**
electrocardiogram (EKG), **394**
electrolytes, **121–122**
electronic control modules (ECMs), 481–482
embolism, **382**
emergency
    aid, providing, 478
    contraception, **325**
    fires, 474
emotional intelligence, **46–47**
emphysema, **263**
endorphins, **240–241**
energy
    adaptive thermogenesis, 178
    balance, **177–178**
    balance as key to weight control, 177–178
    bars, 137–138
    estimating daily, requirements, 178–179
    resources, 499
    therapies, 427, 436–438
    thermic effect of food, **178**
environment (earth), 485–503
    air quality, 488–494
    biodiversity, **497**–498
    college students and, 501
    colleges and, 493
    creating safe, 465–483
    deforestation, **497**
    ecological footprint on, **501**
    ecosystems, **497**–498
    energy resources, 499
    global warming, **491–493**
    greenhouse effect, 492f
    impact on exercise/physical activity, 161–162
    nature and, 74–75
    palm oil and, 497
    waste management, 494–496
    water quality, 485–487
environmental health, **485**
environmental tobacco smoke, **265–266**
epidemic, **347**
epinephrine, **82**
erectile dysfunction (ED), **308**
    drug misuse and, 310
ergonomics, **479**
Erikson, Erik, 50–51
Erikson's Stages of Development, 51t
erogenous zones, **299**
essential amino acids, **125**
essential nutrients, **121**
Estimated Average Requirement (EAR), **120**
estrogens, **302**

Etheridge, Melissa, 410
ethics, 18–19, 78
ethnicity, **7**
    cardiovascular disease risk and, 394
    disorders, 31–33
    identifying, 20
ethnocentrism, **8**
ethnosensitivity, **8**
eugenics, 40
eustress, 82
exercise, **147**, 152
    activity, 152
    for adolescents, 162–163
    altitude impact on, 161
    American Council on, 168
    benefits of, 148–149
    for better sleep, 112
    cancer risk reduced with, 406
    for children, 162–163
    climbing stairs for, 159
    cognitive benefits of, 148
    disorders, 201–202
    environment impacting, 161–162
    fatigue from, 160
    frequency of, 151
    gaming, 159
    guidelines for, 149–150
    impact of environmental conditions, 161–162
    importance of regular, 396
    intensity of, 151
    Kegel, **307**
    for managing stress, 95
    for older adults, 163
    overexertion during, 160
    for persons with disabilities, 163
    physical benefits of, 148
    during pregnancy, 333
    psychological and emotional benefits of,
        148–149
    shoe selection for, 160
    special considerations, 159–163
    spiritual benefits of, 149
    spirituality and, 149
    strain from extreme temperatures, 161–162
    stress to help with, 148–149
    time and, 151–152
extramarital affairs, 299
extreme drinking, **214**

F

faith, 77
falls, 473
false negatives, **412**
false positives, **412**
family. *See also* relationships
    health tree, **24–25**, 25f
    history of, 24–25
    history of cancer, 403
    history relating to cardiovascular disease, 392,
        394
    planning, **500–501**
    Pride Coalition, 293
    resemblance, 26f
    stress and, 92
FAS. *See* fetal alcohol syndrome

Index

Index